W9-BZQ-299

REVIEW OF MEDICAL PHARMACOLOGY

3
Edition

review of
MEDICAL
PHARMACOLOGY

FREDERICK H. MEYERS, MD

Professor of Pharmacology
School of Medicine
University of California
San Francisco

ERNEST JAWETZ, PhD, MD

Professor of Microbiology
Chairman, Department of Microbiology
Professor of Medicine
Lecturer in Pediatrics
School of Medicine
University of California
San Francisco

ALAN GOLDFIEN, MD

Professor of Medicine
Departments of Medicine and
Obstetrics & Gynecology
and Cardiovascular Research Institute
School of Medicine
University of California
San Francisco

Illustrated by **LAUREL V. SCHAUBERT**

Lange Medical Publications

LOS ALTOS, CALIFORNIA

1972

Copyright © 1968, 1970, 1972

All Rights Reserved By

Lange Medical Publications

Copyright in Canada

Portuguese Edition: *Editora Guanabara Koogan S.A., Rio de Janeiro, Brazil*

International Standard Book Number: *0–87041–152–7*
Library of Congress Catalogue Card Number: *73–182391*

A Concise Medical Library for Practitioner and Student

Review of Medical Pharmacology, 3rd ed. $8.50

Lithographed in USA

RM
360
.M48
1972

Table of Contents

PART VII. CHEMOTHERAPEUTIC AGENTS

PART VIII. TOXICOLOGY

Preface

In preparing the Third Edition of this book, the authors have again attempted to emphasize those aspects of pharmacology that serve the clinical needs of the student and practitioner in medicine, dentistry, nursing, and pharmacy. As in previous editions, the discussion of certain theoretical and research aspects of pharmacology has been drastically limited in order to keep the size and cost of the book within reasonable limits.

Learning how to think clearly about drugs is one of the medical student's most obvious and most difficult duties. Even clinicians with years of experience in prescribing for their patients are often at a loss to know what to accept and what to reject among the annual crop of claims for new drugs or drug modifications. The primary objective of this book is to foster a skeptical attitude toward all new drug claims and even to suggest to the practicing physician that he should occasionally reexamine his prescribing habits and critically reevaluate drugs he may have been using for years.

The voluntary or directed withdrawal from the market of a number of useless drugs validates both the general attitude and the specific negative judgments expressed in previous editions. The present edition, however, also reflects the now established importance of drugs such as levodopa and propranolol previously listed as investigational.

New editions of this book will reappear every 2 years. Any comments the reader may wish to make about any aspect of our presentation—including our deliberate or inadvertent omissions—will be gratefully received.

We wish to express our thanks to everyone who helped with the preparation of this *Review*. Particular thanks go to the following for substantial contributions: Dr. Ilsa P. Caswell, Dr. Milton J. Chatton, Dr. Joseph G. Chusid, Dr. William F. Ganong, Dr. Mervin J. Goldman, Miss Shirley Gullixson, Dr. Harold A. Harper, and Mr. Elliot Poston.

Frederick H. Meyers
Ernest Jawetz
Alan Goldfien

San Francisco, California
June, 1972

Notice

Drugs are commodities regulated by law and administrative orders. If the physician deviates from standards approved by the regulating agency, responsibility for any mishap—even if it is only tenuously related to administration of the drug—is apt to devolve upon the physician alone.

The dosages included in this text are in most instances those that are generally accepted or those suggested by the manufacturer. In some cases, dosages suggested by a more conservative position have been included. When drugs are known to cause frequent or dangerous toxic reactions; when establishment of a maintenance dose is difficult; when parenteral administration requires special precautions; or when the drug is unfamiliar to the prescriber, the manufacturer's package insert or other current FDA-monitored sources of information should be consulted before the drug is administered.

Part I. General Information

1...

Introduction

Pharmacology, for the purpose of this book, is considered to be the body of information that underlies the effective and safe use of drugs in the diagnosis, prevention, or treatment of disease. However, pharmacology includes many controversial areas, and the divergence of opinion begins with the very definition of the field. From the point of view of the practicing physician and medical student rather than the research specialist, pharmacology is a derived or applied science. Understanding how drugs are used and progress in drug therapy require the application and development of special information from many areas, especially organic and analytical chemistry, biochemistry, physiology, and the various clinical specialties.

Many research and laboratory oriented pharmacologists, however, insist that pharmacology is a basic science, and view it as a valid field of investigation independent of its immediate applications. Their approach would emphasize some of the headings in the outline below and minimize others. The emphasis of this book reflects the teaching responsibility of pharmacologists toward students in the professions rather than the needs of research pharmacologists. It deliberately blurs any distinction between pharmacology and therapeutics.

The discussion of most of the groups of drugs in the following chapters of this book is organized according to the outline that begins below. However, several chapters on general pharmacologic or therapeutic subjects precede the chapters in which the drug groups are systematically discussed. Whether these general discussions should be read before or after a store of specific pharmacologic information is acquired depends upon the individual student. The following brief review of the conventionalized outline of what a practitioner should consider before using a particular drug should allow study of the general chapters to be deferred if desired.

History

Information about the history of the development or introduction of a drug group to therapy is not essential to its proper use. The history, however, is usually interesting and often important in the formation of attitudes toward current problems. The brief history of pharmacology at the end of this chapter divides the subject somewhat arbitrarily into periods.

The historical sketches that appear in some chapters are usually selected to illustrate one of the generalizations presented in the outline of the history.

Chemistry

Data on the structure and the chemical properties of compounds used as drugs have different significance and interest to different workers. The person interested in the synthesis of new drugs requires information different from that needed by the person whose ultimate interest is biologic and practical.

A. Chemical and Pharmacologic Classification: A key problem or concept that will be repeatedly emphasized is that the many hundreds of drugs that are available can be classified into a reasonable number of drug groups and subgroups rather than regarded as so many individual agents. The most important function of the information on chemical structure given in the tables or figures is to demonstrate the similarity of related drugs within a group and to suggest a basis for establishing subgroups when important differences are present. In a few cases, minor changes in chemical structure may lead to major changes in the nature or specificity of biologic effect. However, the proliferation of drugs within most groups is not necessarily due to the synthesis of significantly different compounds but is related to the marketing of compounds that are merely imitative of the prototype in the group or subgroup.

B. Structure-Action Relationships: Very few drugs have been "designed" in the sense that chemical theory predicted a desired biologic effect. BAL—the first chelating agent applied in therapy—and most of the antimetabolites introduced since the sulfonamides are compounds whose pharmacologic effects and usefulness were predicted. However, by far the largest number of drugs now in use derive from prototypes that were natural products and from later synthetic counterparts whose chemistry was patterned after the natural product. Drugs whose discovery was purely accidental or stemmed from the empiric preparation and screening of a large number of compounds without a justifiable theoretical basis also contribute to currently used drugs. Much structure-action speculation is retrospective and is of limited practical importance. The application of structure-action theory to the problems of the mechanisms of drug action, on the other hand, represents one of the ultimate goals of pharmacologic thought. The primitive and tentative data available are discussed under the relevant drugs.

Absorption, Distribution, Metabolism, & Excretion

These properties—(1) the absorption from the gastrointestinal tract or the injection site, (2) the distribution of the drug intra- or extracellularly throughout the body, (3) the metabolism or biotransformation of the drug, and (4) its excretion—are discussed together because there are several unifying chemical concepts. The lipid barrier model suggests that the barrier to distribution provided by cells or the cell wall will allow the transfer of lipid-soluble, nonpolar molecules preferentially to water-soluble substances. A more lipid-soluble substance would enter parenchymal cells, but its excretion would be slowed because it would also be well reabsorbed at the renal tubules. The metabolism or biotransformation of drugs by conjugation or chemical alteration converts them to more polar, more water-soluble metabolites that can be more rapidly excreted. The metabolites are usually inactive—ie, drug action is terminated by metabolism—in which case the details of the transformation are of limited practical importance except in following the rate of excretion. However, some metabolites are active or toxic. Some of the possible metabolic paths are discussed in Chapter 2.

Pharmacologic Actions

A. Mechanisms of Action: Discussions of the mechanisms of action of a drug usually involve separate discussions at the physiologic level and at the biochemical level. For most drugs it will be possible to make some statement about the mechanism of action at the level of the organ or functional system or tissue. The site of action, for example, may be localized to an organ such as the spinal cord or even to a functional system such as internuncial or polysynaptic pathways. In some cases, drug action can be explained by an action on chemical mediators liberated by the cell.

Below the organ or tissue level, at the biochemical or subcellular site of drug action, information is available in only a few cases. Some drugs are known to be inhibitors of specific enzymes; a few are metabolic antagonists; and several other biochemical mechanisms have been defined. For most drugs, however, the ultimate mechanism of action is unknown.

It is frequently said that an understanding of mechanism of action is a prerequisite to the rational use of drugs. Such understanding is certainly the goal. However, drugs used in the absence of such information will continue to act after the mechanism of action has been defined exactly as they have during the period of their empiric use.

B. Effects: The observed effects on as many organ systems and tissues as are influenced—ie, the descriptive pharmacology—is the crucial part of the discussion of each drug group since it underlies and explains most of the therapeutic and toxic actions of the drug.

Clinical Uses

The possible therapeutic applications of a drug group cannot simply be listed. Not all of the suggested or even commonly accepted indications for the use of a drug are supported by convincing clinical studies. One cannot even assume that all of the marketed drugs are active. The problems of the clinical evaluation of drugs are discussed in a general way in Chapter 3. For the individual drug groups the indications are listed, and some discussion of the methods of establishing usefulness and therapeutic effectiveness is given.

Adverse Reactions

The use of drugs is not without many dangers and discomforts. Before any drug or combination of drugs is used, the possible toxic effects must be considered so that the physician can be prepared to treat toxic reactions and so that some judgment can be made about the possible benefits as compared with the possible toxic effects. A general discussion of the toxicity of therapeutic agents is presented in Chapter 6. In the discussion of each drug, adverse reactions are listed under one or more of the following categories:

A. Side-Effects: Under this category are discussed effects that are often unavoidable if adequate doses of the drug are given.

B. Overdosage Toxicity: Toxic effects of this type are dose-related—ie, their incidence increases as the dose level is increased.

C. Allergic Reactions: These reactions are not dose-related but depend upon the altered reactivity or hypersensitivity of the patient, usually induced by prior contact with the drug which has acted as an antigen.

D. Drug Abuse: A special form of toxicity is the use for nontherapeutic purposes of drugs that act on the CNS. The misuse of the individual drug is discussed in the relevant chapters (eg, alcohol; see Chapter 24), but drug abuse and habituation as a general problem are discussed in Chapter 7.

Contraindications & Cautions

For each drug there are situations in which its use invites disaster. Most of the contraindications to the use of a drug are predictable from its effects and are easily remembered. Some are unexpected or easily overlooked. For each drug, therefore, a list of contraindications and cautions is presented. This check list in a text or in the physician's mind should be reviewed before a drug is ordered for any patient.

Most contraindications are disease entities or altered physiologic states—eg, morphine is contraindicated in head injury. In other situations, the possible interaction of a drug with one previously administered dictates caution. Drug interactions are discussed at this point in each chapter, and a general discussion of the topic is presented in Chapter 6.

Preparations, Choice of Drug, & Dosage

In many chapters all of the drugs in a group will be discussed as if there were no differences between them or as if the newer compounds did not differ from the prototype. In many cases it does not matter which of a large number of similar compounds is selected for use. In most drug groups, however, there will be compounds or subgroups of compounds that are more efficacious for a particular purpose than others, and these will be discussed when such difference does exist. The importance of the general principles of the technic of drug administration discussed in Chapter 4 will be apparent to the practitioner. They should be reviewed by the student when the selection and ordering of drugs for patients becomes one of his responsibilities.

An especially confusing factor is the multiplicity of names involved. Each drug has a generic or public name—eg, penicillin G—but in addition may be given a protected or trade mark name by one or by many different manufacturers or distributors.

References
A. Chapter References: A list of references is placed at the end of each chapter, but these suggested readings will prove adequate for all purposes only if combined with the general references listed below. Those references in each chapter that are reports of research or observation rather than reviews are usually chosen to cover areas that are judged to be controversial, rapidly changing, or unfamiliar. The emphasis is on clinical aspects of the drug group, and many of the references are from a few of the most readily available journals. Additional comprehensive reviews and summaries of the most recent work should be sought in the sources below.

B. General References: The following publications contain comprehensive discussions of specific drug groups and of the general problems of pharmacology. Their citation will not be repeated in each chapter.

DiPalma, J.R. (editor): *Pharmacology in Medicine,* 4th ed. McGraw-Hill, 1971. Comprehensive text.

Elliott, H.W. (editor): *Annual Review of Pharmacology.* Vols 1–11. Annual Reviews, 1961–1971. Provides references to most recent work.

Ellis, G.P., & G.B. West (editors): *Progress in Medicinal Chemistry.* Vols 1–7. Butterworth, 1961–1970.

Garattini, S., & P.A. Shore (editors): *Advances in Pharmacology and Chemotherapy.* Vols 1–8. Academic Press, 1962–1970.

Goldstein, A., Aranow, L., & S.M. Kalman: *Principles of Drug Action.* Hoeber, 1968. Highly recommended when rigorous, theoretical approach is needed.

Goodman, L.S., & A. Gilman (editors): *The Pharmacological Basis of Therapeutics,* 4th ed. Macmillan, 1970. Comprehensive text.

Jucker, E. (editor): *Progress in Drug Research.* Vols 1–14. Interscience, 1960–1970. Comprehensive, largely nonclinical reviews; many in German or French. Strong emphasis on pharmaceutical chemistry.

Pharmacological Reviews. Williams & Wilkins. (Quarterly.) Comprehensive reviews of areas of current research interest.

Root, W.S., & F.G. Hofmann (editors): *Physiological Pharmacology.* Eleven volumes projected; 4 in print. Academic Press, 1963–1967.

Sollman, T.: *A Manual of Pharmacology,* 8th ed. Saunders, 1957. Useful for data on old and obscure drugs.

The clinical application and evaluation of drugs requires the use of a literature distinct from the above. In addition to the journals of the several specialties and the better general medical journals, *Clinical Pharmacology and Therapeutics* is especially useful. Of the general references listed at the end of Chapter 3, one deserving special emphasis is *The Medical Letter on Drugs and Therapeutics* (Drug and Therapeutic Information, Inc). This valuable fortnightly periodical presents brief, current clinical evaluation of drugs by experts in all of the medical specialties.

HISTORY OF PHARMACOLOGY

The discussion of some of the specific drug groups in the following chapters will begin with the history of their use or discovery. A survey of the history of drug therapy at this point provides one way of outlining or organizing the entire subject. The data presented in subsequent chapters will illustrate the ideas outlined in this section.

Prescientific Period
The prototypes of many modern drug classes derive from natural products that have a long history of folk use. Scholars enjoy searching the records of the oldest cultures for references that can be interpreted as establishing the first use of a drug still used today. It is often assumed that our present more or less rational use of drugs and their natural progenitors in therapy grew out of the primitive experience. Actually, however, only a few folk remedies or contributions of the medicine of earlier cultures have been taken over directly. Most of the active natural products were used originally not as medicines but as magic tools, arrow poisons, cosmetics, or even homicidal agents. The properties of opium have certainly been exploited for 3 millennia, but the specific use of most natural products is based on the intervention of a relatively recent worker. In many cases, modern use could occur only when a sufficient nosologic basis had been developed—eg, only after fevers and dropsy were classified could cinchona bark and digitalis be used properly. Most of the drugs used in therapy prior to the modern period were abandoned along with bleeding and purging.

Therapy to 1800
The development of medicine and biology lagged far behind that of the other sciences. For medieval authoritative systems, the physical sciences substituted observation, quantitative analysis, and the experimental method. Medicine actually regressed from Hippocratic empiricism, and late in the 18th century was scholastic and dependent on pure logic rather than observation. Many systems of medicine were developed, usually with a single pathologic process to explain all disease. These attempts to reach a system of Newtonian unity and comprehensiveness actually inhibited observation and, therefore, progress.

There are more than a few exceptions to the above generalization, and medicine did have its great men. Vesalius, Paré, and Paracelsus were physicians of the Renaissance who trusted their own observations and experience.

More important to the history of therapy are the 17th century Englishmen—eg, Harvey and especially Sydenham—whose empiricism presaged the British clinical school.

First Applications of Experimental Method

At the time of the French Revolution, then, medicine was barely into its descriptive period, only anatomy having reached any maturity. Even general biology was still structural and taxonomic. François Magendie (1783–1855), an instructor of anatomy in Paris, then introduced the experimental method to medicine and biology. He studied the absorption of strychnine in order to challenge some of the vitalistic teaching of the period. A Javanese arrow poison (nux vomica) was administered by various routes and the resulting convulsions and asphyxia described. After studying the action in animals with the cord sectioned or destroyed, Magendie and his collaborating medical student accurately concluded that the spinal cord was the site of action of the active component, which was subsequently isolated and named strychnine. They presented their work in 1809 to the Paris Academy.

Magendie studied many other drugs and physiologic problems. His students isolated a number of alkaloids, and he published a formulary based on only pure, single compounds. His demonstration of the value of the experimental approach was influential.

Not the least of Magendie's contribution was to hire and encourage Claude Bernard (1813–1878). Unlike Magendie, who resisted all generalizations and compared his function as data collector to that of a junkman, Bernard not only contributed to every area of physiology but reflected on the methods of "experimental medicine," as the undifferentiated field of physiology-pharmacology-biochemistry was then called.

Clinical Research

For the development of modern medicine, a revolution in clinical medicine to restore the primacy of observation was as necessary as the application of the experimental method, and it too took place in France. After the Revolution, when all sciences broke with tradition and a new intellectual life was encouraged, the medical schools of the old regime (together with all universities) were simply abolished and new schools established within a few large hospitals. Clinical observations, especially those arising from the new technics of physical diagnosis, were correlated with autopsy data. Progress in the study and classification of disease entities was extremely great during the period 1825–1850. Cabanis, Pinel, and Bichat were the philosophic progenitors of the medical revolution, and Broussais should perhaps be called the founder of the Paris clinical school.

Progress in therapy was not equally rapid. Ineffective remedies had first to be eliminated. The resulting nihilistic attitude toward drugs and the emphasis on diagnosis have persisted. P. Ch. A. Louis (1787–1872), a successor to Broussais and Laennec, introduced his "numerical" or statistical method of describing the natural history of disease and of evaluating therapy. His recognition of observer bias and other still current problems were especially influential in the USA through Oliver Wendell Holmes and others.

Germany & the Rise of the University

Not only were the French ideas immediately very influential in neighboring Germany, but, in response to the imperialism of Napoleon, the unification of Germany began during the period just described. Soon thereafter, the influence of the German university appeared, and by 1850 the Germans led the world in research. The German universities were provincial rather than national, and governmental support was increased by a feeling of competitiveness. Students and faculty moved freely between schools, and the faculties were large enough that time for research as well as teaching was available.

Experimental medicine differentiated into the separate basic sciences. In 1846 Rudolph Buchheim established the first laboratory for experimental pharmacology in Dorpat (Tartu), Estonia. His student, Oswald Schmiedeberg (1838–1921), together with the great physiologist Ludwig, became preeminent and trained many of the pioneers of modern pharmacology whether German, American, British, or other.

American Pharmacology

It has not been many years since it was almost true that syphilis and general anesthesia were the only contributions of the New World to medicine. American medical education initially followed the British provincial pattern, which meant that most practitioners were trained by apprenticeship. However, as British medical training improved during the 19th century with the dominance of hospital schools, American training deteriorated as proprietary and sectarian (eg, homeopathic, chiropractic) undergraduate schools proliferated. Each state controlled licensing of its practitioners, and degrees of doubtful validity were accepted as licenses. A few superior or privileged men were trained at Edinburgh, Paris, and, later, in Germany, but little investigational medicine existed.

In the years just prior to 1890, the State Boards of Medicine began to move against the worst incompetents in medicine, and a few isolated universities began to respond to the social need. The first American pharmacologist, J.J. Abel, returned from his training in Germany to an appointment at the University of Michigan.

An important stimulus to scientific medicine in the USA was provided by Johns Hopkins University. A graduate school more or less patterned after the German university was opened in 1876, and soon thereafter the hospital (1889) and a medical school (1893) were established. J.J. Abel moved from Michigan to Hopkins, and trained most of the academic leaders in pharmacology for the next generation.

The reorganization of the American Medical Association in 1901 and the dramatization of the situation by the Flexner Report (1910) led to the disappearance of the proprietary schools and the emergence of the university-associated medical school. Clinical and laboratory research finally appeared in respectable amounts in the USA.

American pharmacology continued to lag in its development until after World War II, when unprecedented amounts of money were made available for research, first by voluntary agencies and then by the National Institutes of Health. Graduate programs made it possible for a student to enter pharmacology with a research degree rather than an MD, resulting in an increase in the numbers of pharmacologists but also in an alienation from medicine. Finally, the American drug industry expanded to match in size if not in originality its European counterpart.

● ● ●

General References

Ackerknecht, E.H.: Elisha Bartlett and the philosophy of the Paris Clinical School. Bull Hist Med 24:43–60, 1950.

Ackerknecht, E.H.: Medical education in 19th century France. J M Educ 32:148–153, 1957.

Flexner, S., & J.T. Flexner: *William Henry Welch and the Heroic Age of American Medicine*. Viking, 1941.

Olmsted, J.M.D.: *François Magendie*. Schuman, 1944.

Olmsted, J.M.D., & E.H. Olmsted: *Claude Bernard and the Experimental Method in Medicine*. Collier Books, 1961.

Shryock, R.H.: European backgrounds of American medical education. JAMA 194:709–714, 1965.

Silverman, M.: *Magic in a Bottle*. Macmillan, 1941.

2 . . .

Pharmacokinetics & Drug Interactions

The metabolism of each drug or drug group must be studied separately. However, the discussions of this aspect of drug information in subsequent chapters can be greatly shortened by a preliminary general consideration here since the several processes that occur between the time of administration of the drug and the termination of its activity are closely related. The absorption, the distribution within the body, and the excretion of a drug are related processes since they all depend upon the passage of the drug across a series of cellular membranes of similar properties. These plasma membranes or "lipid barriers" are more permeable to uncharged, lipid-soluble drugs than to ionized, water-soluble molecules. The biotransformation or metabolism of drugs is generally a process by which drugs are rendered more water-soluble, less subject to renal tubular reabsorption, and, therefore, more readily excreted.

In the qualitative, descriptive account presented here, it may seem that absorption, distribution, metabolism, and excretion are sequential processes. This is true only in retrospect after the drug has been excreted and its effect finally dissipated. At any given moment, a drug and a variety of metabolic products may be distributed in many compartments—eg, the drug in the lumen of the intestine, the drug and perhaps a conjugate within the cells of the intestinal mucosa, drug and metabolites in the plasma, etc—until excretion occurs in bladder urine, expired air, or feces. Each transfer or metabolic change occurs at its own rate and has its own equilibrium constant. As drugs are ordinarily given—ie, with the exception of a continuous intravenous infusion—a steady state is not achieved. Quantitative or kinetic description of these related processes is ordinarily not possible. It is, however, an important goal of research pharmacology, and the sum of these processes is included under the term pharmacokinetics.

DISTRIBUTION OF DRUGS WITHIN THE BODY

Unit Membrane or Plasma Membrane

The distribution of drugs within the body is hindered by a series of membranes. Some of these membranes, like the skin or a mucosal surface, may be many cells thick; but the barrier to distribution resides in the cell membrane, and some generalities about transport across this membrane apply to many sites.

A. The Lipid-Sieve Model: The unit or plasma membrane surrounds or forms the boundary of all cells and surrounds the nucleus and organelles. Fig 2–1 presents a model of the lipoprotein membrane based on chemical analysis and electronmicroscopic and x-ray diffraction technics. Studies of the permeability of this membrane lead to the conclusion that it is a mosaic with at least 3 functional components. The major component, for drugs if not for physiologically important substances, is the lipid membrane that is permeable to lipid-soluble molecules and impermeable to polar, water-soluble substances. The membrane must in addition contain pores that permit the passage of small water-soluble molecules such as urea, alcohol, and water itself. Finally, the membranes contains channels through which substances can move after they have combined with a specific carrier.

B. Mechanisms of Transfer Across Membrane:

1. Passive transfer—Transfer or transport is said to be passive when the membrane need not generate energy to carry out the process.

a. Filtration, as across the capillary wall, is not an important factor in limiting drug distribution.

b. Simple diffusion—If the rate of transfer across a membrane is proportionate to the concentration gradient, one infers that the process is one of simple

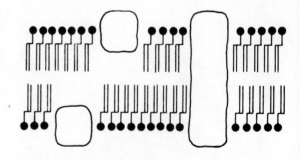

FIG 2–1. Hypothetical model of plasma membrane. The matrix of the membrane is a double layer of phospholipid molecules oriented with the polar heads in contact with intra- and extracellular water. Globular protein masses are embedded in the phospholipid bilayer with charged ionic residues projecting from the surface into water.

diffusion. A water-soluble drug of low molecular weight such as alcohol may diffuse through the aqueous pores of the membrane. Water-soluble drugs of greater molecular weight either do not cross the membrane or are transported by one of the active processes described below. Transfer by simple diffusion is then an important process for the distribution of lipid-soluble drugs. Many drugs—eg, ether or digitoxin—have a lipid solubility or oil-water partition coefficient that favors their transfer regardless of the pH of the medium. However, many drugs are either weak acids or weak bases, and the fraction of molecules present as the lipid-soluble un-ionized form to which the cell is preferentially permeable varies with the pH of the system. The pH within cells or of extracellular fluid cannot, of course, vary greatly. In order for a substance that is not actively transported to act intracellularly, it must either be lipid-soluble at all pH's or, if it is an amine or weak base, it must be largely in the un-ionized form at the pH of the body. It is possible, however, to alter the absorption or excretion of drugs by varying the pH of the gastric contents or the renal tubular urine.

c. Carrier-facilitated diffusion—In this process, the substance to be transported combines with a carrier molecule at one membrane surface and dissociates from it at the other surface. The carrier, a protein, is specific for the transported ion or larger water-soluble molecule that would not otherwise traverse the membrane. The process is still one of diffusion, and a substance cannot be moved against a concentration gradient.

Exchange diffusion is a common variation of carrier-facilitated diffusion in which the carrier combines with one substance at the outer surface to transport it inward and, having dissociated from the first substance, picks up a generally similar molecule at the inner surface and carries it to the outside.

2. Active transport—Active transport is carrier-facilitated but is able to move the substance against a chemical or electrical gradient. Performance of such work or active transport requires energy which is known, in the common examples, to be generated by the action of membrane ATPase. There are a variety of channels or pumps of this type. Each transports a specific chemical type—eg, sodium, organic acids—and related compounds compete for the capacity of the mechanism. Interference with the supply of energy inhibits the system noncompetitively.

Absorption

A. From the Gastrointestinal Tract: This discussion applies to the absorption of drugs after oral administration.

1. Site and rate of absorption—Small, neutral water-soluble molecules—eg, alcohol and water itself—are absorbed from the stomach although the amount absorbed is limited by the rapid emptying time. The absorption of other drugs will vary with the secretory state of the stomach. Aspirin, the most common drug that is a weak acid, exists almost entirely in the un-ionized form at the pH of the secreting stomach, and that lipid-soluble form is well absorbed from the stomach (Fig 2–2). Giving aspirin with a base or with food would increase the fraction present as the salt or water-soluble form and slow its absorption to the rate normally observed in the small intestine. (This may nevertheless be advisable since it reduces gastric irritation.)

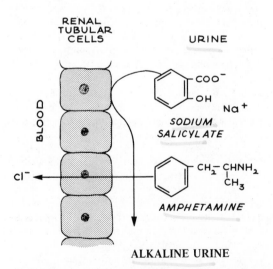

ALKALINE URINE

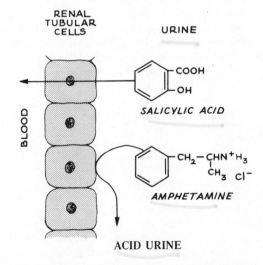

ACID URINE

FIG 2–2. The influence of the pH of the medium on the diffusion of a substance across a cellular barrier illustrated with a diagram of the renal tubule. The excretion of salicylic acid, a metabolite of aspirin, is increased if the renal tubular fluid is alkaline because it then exists as the ionized, less lipid-soluble salt form. The excretion of amphetamine, a weak base, is increased in an acid urine because it then is present as the salt rather than the lipid-soluble free base.

The intracellular and luminal pH influences movement in both directions. Thus, weak bases given by injection can appear in the gastric contents.

2. In the alkaline medium of the small intestine, those drugs that are weak bases exist as the free base and are absorbed from that site.

B. From Injection Sites: The rate of absorption from a subcutaneous or intramuscular injection site is related to the water solubility of the injected substance. The rate of absorption can be slowed and the duration of action of a water-soluble drug prolonged by injecting it as an insoluble complex—eg, procaine penicillin or protamine zinc insulin.

C. From the Skin: The keratinized layer of the skin is a much less permeable barrier than the ordinary cell membrane, and the skin conforms to the lipid barrier model only if the keratinized layer is removed. Absorption of drugs after application to the skin or even penetration for a local effect is difficult to achieve and is discussed separately in Chapter 5. Many drugs are well absorbed from the nonkeratinized epithelium of the mucous membranes of the mouth or pharynx.

Transport Within the Vascular Compartment

Drugs freely and quickly leave the vascular compartment to enter the interstitial fluid. Lipid-soluble drugs pass across the entire membranous surface, but even large, water-soluble molecules are filtered through the large pores of the capillary membrane with the aid of hydrostatic pressure. Thus, distribution of a drug to a particular region of the body will be determined by blood flow to that part rather than by the rate of transfer across the capillary membrane.

Many drugs combine loosely with plasma albumin, and such protein binding could theoretically inactivate a drug and slow its distribution. However, the drug-protein complex dissociates freely and a high concentration of free drugs is maintained. A few clinically important applications are known—eg, the ability of sulfonamides to displace bilirubin from the binding sites on plasma protein and intensify jaundice in the newborn.

Differential Distribution

A. To the CNS: The factors that determine whether or not a drug can reach and act on an intracellular site are similar throughout the body. The CNS is unusual in that drugs can reach even extracellular sites only after passing through glial cells.

Capillaries in the CNS ("within the blood-brain barrier") cannot filter plasma into the interstitial space because interstitial space is very limited in extent and the supporting glial cells are closely opposed to the capillary wall. Drugs that act on peripheral nerve tissue, presumably at an extracellular site, may not reach parenchymal CNS cells if the drugs are in a charged, lipid-insoluble form. Quaternary ammonium derivatives such as curare or acetylcholine, for example, exist entirely in the salt form at body pH and, after intravenous injection, do not act on the CNS however great

their effect on peripheral nerve. They do act on brain and spinal cord if applied directly.

B. To Other Special Sites:

1. To lipid depots and other storage sites—Drugs with high intrinsic lipid solubility and low water solubility may accumulate in high concentration in the adipose tissues of the body—eg, thiopental or the chlorinated hydrocarbon type of insecticide. (The accumulation of thiopental in fat is discussed again below as an example of redistribution as a mechanism of terminating drug action.)

Some other examples of selective accumulation depend upon more than partition coefficient. Colloidal and particulate drugs are taken up by the cells of the reticuloendothelial system; heavy metals concentrate in bone. Physiologically important substances may also accumulate by mechanisms unrelated to solubility—eg, cobalamin (vitamin B_{12}) in the liver or norepinephrine in the specific granules of adrenergic nerve. The concentration of the antimalarial drug quinacrine in parenchymal tissues is several thousand times that in plasma.

2. To sites of metabolism or excretion—The drug and—what is more consistent with the general concepts of distribution across membranes—its more water-soluble metabolites will accumulate at the sites of metabolism and excretion: in the liver if that is the site of biotransformation; in the intestinal contents if secretion is into the bile; or in the kidney if the metabolites are concentrated in tubular urine.

3. To fetal tissues—The distribution of drugs across the placenta is a difficult and incompletely studied problem. The fetal tissues covering the villi are in contact with maternal blood. Some substances move back and forth across this membrane as if it were conforming to the lipid barrier model. The general anesthetic agents, the narcotic analgesics, and the barbiturates reach and depress the fetal CNS as expected, but quaternary ammonium compounds such as succinylcholine do not. However, the fetal barrier is at times permeable to particles as large as red cells.

4. To milk—In animal studies, the appearance of drugs in milk appears to be predictable by reference to the lipid barrier model. Since milk is slightly more acidic than plasma, basic compounds may be concentrated in milk. Small neutral molecules (alcohol) appear in milk in the same concentration as in plasma. Acidic drugs such as penicillin appear in milk (pH 6.6) in concentrations less than in plasma, and bases (erythromycin) are more concentrated in milk.

Verified reports of toxic reactions in nursing infants due to drugs ingested by the mother are few. Drugs that have bad demonstrable effects include the nicotine in cigarettes, bromides, cascara and purified anthroquinones, antithyroid drugs, and phenindione (but not the other anticoagulants). Heroin—but not morphine or codeine—is said to act on the infant. Many drugs—eg, radioactive agents and antimetabolites—are almost certainly dangerous.

TERMINATION OF DRUG ACTION

The processes that terminate drug action determine the duration of action of a drug. If they are altered by disease or concurrent administration of other drugs, the intensity and duration of drug effect may be altered.

ELIMINATION OF UNCHANGED DRUG OR METABOLITE

Elimination by the Lungs

The gases and volatile liquids used as general anesthetics are absorbed and excreted across the pulmonary alveolar membrane. Many other volatile drugs—eg, alcohol or paraldehyde—appear in the expired air but have other more important routes of excretion or metabolism. However, the content of alcohol and certain industrial solvents in alveolar air reflects plasma levels in a consistent way and can be used to quantify the degree of intoxication.

Elimination by the Kidneys

Drugs and their metabolites or conjugates appear in the urine as a result of 2 processes: (1) They appear in the glomerular filtrate; and (2) a greater or lesser fraction is then reabsorbed through the tubular cell to be returned to the plasma. This reabsorptive process is also an example of passive diffusion. The more lipid-soluble the material, the greater the degree of reabsorption. The more water-soluble the material, the greater the fraction that remains in the urine. The excretion of the unmetabolized, lipid-soluble drug can be altered by acidification or alkalinization of the urine. (Fig 2–2.) For example, intoxication with salicylates or barbiturates (both weak acids) is treated by maintaining a high volume of alkaline urine. The weak acids then exist largely in the salt form or the ionized, water-soluble form, and reabsorption is greatly decreased.

The renal tubule is also able to actively transport or secrete organic anions and cations through separate channels.

Other Routes of Elimination

Drug and drug conjugate may appear in the feces subsequent to excretion in the bile or secretion by the colon. Specific drugs may also appear in saliva or sweat in significant amounts.

TERMINATION OF DRUG ACTION BY PROCESSES NOT INVOLVING ELIMINATION OF DRUG

The action of a drug may terminate even though the drug is still present in the body, or, if the change caused by the drug requires a long period for its repair, the effect of a drug may persist long after it has been destroyed or excreted.

Redistribution

The differential distribution of a drug (see above) may be a mechanism for terminating its activity. For example, when the anesthetic thiopental is injected rapidly intravenously, a high plasma level is immediately achieved. The subsequent distribution of thiopental depends upon its high lipid solubility and the blood flow to the various tissues. An effective amount of thiopental is immediately carried to the CNS by the cerebral blood flow. However, over the subsequent 20 minutes the poorly perfused adipose tissue slowly takes up enough thiopental to bring about its withdrawal from the CNS and the termination of the anesthesia. In somewhat the same manner, the action of injected epinephrine or norepinephrine is terminated mostly because the amine enters sympathetic nerve and can no longer act on smooth muscle.

Repair of Drug-Induced Changes

Some drugs that disappear from the body after a few hours cause changes, during their brief residence time, that may take many days for correction. For example, after prothrombin synthesis is inhibited by a coumarin anticoagulant, the effect persists until new protein is synthesized.

Antagonism

The effect of a drug may be terminated by giving its competitive or physiologic antagonist—eg, the effect of morphine can be antagonized by nalorphine or the effect of histamine antagonized by epinephrine.

Physiologic Compensations

Some adaptations or compensations by the organism may decrease or completely abolish the effects of a drug. Other compensations may modify only certain prominent responses such as pulse rate or blood pressure but give the impression of a decreased overall response to the drug.

The familiar compensatory reflexes originating from a change in pressure within carotid and other pressoreceptor areas act whenever a pressor or depressor drug is given. These reflexes cannot modify a drug-induced rise in pressure but may cause a reflex bradycardia that can obscure the primary effect of the drug. Vasoconstrictor drugs (norepinephrine, ephedrine, angiotensin) can reduce cardiac output by increasing the amount of work needed to move the same volume of blood. A long-acting vasoconstrictor such as ephedrine may limit cardiac output enough to limit the rise in blood pressure that it causes. Such a state of reduced response of the blood pressure when the vasoconstricting and other actions are maximal is called tachyphylaxis.

Limited tolerance to the effects of other drugs arises from other compensatory mechanisms. Administration of the potent hypotensive agents—eg, guanethidine or methyldopa—results in an expanded plasma volume and the dose of the drug must be increased a limited amount to maintain the effect.

Tolerance of a qualitatively different kind follows the administration of organic nitrates or the narcotic analgesics. In this case, larger and larger doses must be given to maintain the effect, and tolerance can be made absolute—ie, many previously lethal doses can be given without danger or even much effect.

BIOTRANSFORMATION; ENZYMATIC ALTERATION

Many pharmacologists feel that it is impossible to overemphasize the importance of drug metabolism; others feel that this has already been achieved. In a few cases—eg, the study of cholinesterase or of monoamine metabolism—important information about the mechanism of drug actions and drug interactions has developed. Usually, however, the action of enzymes on drugs, unlike the study of the action of drugs on enzymes, does not often provide information about the mechanism of action of drugs. The process of biotransformation usually reduces or destroys the activity of the drug and hastens its excretion (reduces renal tubular reabsorption) by converting it to a more water-soluble form. More often than not, the process will consist of conjugation or of hydroxylation followed by conjugation. The process of biotransformation of drugs is often called detoxification.

Biotransformation can modify the effects of the drug administered in at least 4 ways:

(1) By forming an inactive metabolite from an active drug: This is the most common mechanism of drug inactivation. The metabolite may itself be further transformed and a mixture of metabolites and conjugates excreted, or the fragments may be lost in the metabolic pool.

(2) By forming an active metabolite from an initially inactive drug: For example, the cholinesterase inhibitor parathion must have a sulfur atom replaced by an oxygen atom before it is active; and the antimalarial chlorguanide and the alpha-adrenergic blocking agent phenoxybenzamine must cyclize before they can become active. (See Fig 11–1 for the reaction that converts phenoxybenzamine to a cyclic compound.)

(3) By forming an active metabolite from an initially active drug: Enzymatic transformation of a drug does not always terminate its action—eg, heroin is converted to morphine, and phenacetin is metabolized to an equally potent analgesic, acetaminophen (Fig 27–2).

(4) By forming a toxic metabolite from an initially less toxic drug: Referring to the same drug (phenacetin) and Fig 27–2, it can be said that the metabolite of phenacetin may be active therapeutically; but the acetaminophen is also responsible for the renal damage that on rare occasions follows the use of phenacetin. The same parent compound, phenacetin, is also transformed into small amounts of an aniline derivative capable of causing methemoglobinemia.

CLASSES & EXAMPLES OF METABOLIC REACTIONS

The metabolism of specific drugs will be discussed in subsequent chapters. In the following paragraphs, the general classes of metabolic reactions will be described briefly and some of the many specific reactions will be cited as examples. Because the conjugation reactions apply to so many drug groups and because the oxidative enzymes of liver microsomes are important in drug interactions, they should be especially noted.

Conjugation Reactions

The conjugation reactions (also often called syntheses or transfer reactions) will be discussed first to emphasize their dual function. They can modify not only the original drug but also common metabolites formed by the reactions listed below. In the latter case, the polarization or increase in water solubility begun by one reaction is intensified by conjugation.

A. Glucuronide Formation: Each of the conjugation or synthetic reactions can be represented by the following reaction:

$$Ab + CD \xrightarrow{\boxed{\text{TRANSFERASE}}} AC + bD$$

where Ab is a drug or drug metabolite with functional group b, and C is the donor molecule activated by combination with D (UDP in the case of glucuronic acid). For example,

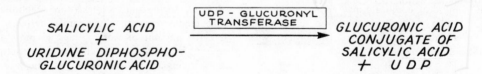

$$\text{SALICYLIC ACID} + \text{URIDINE DIPHOSPHO-GLUCURONIC ACID} \xrightarrow{\boxed{\text{UDP - GLUCURONYL TRANSFERASE}}} \text{GLUCURONIC ACID CONJUGATE OF SALICYLIC ACID} + \text{UDP}$$

If the activated glucuronic acid (UDPGA) reacts with a phenolic or alcoholic hydroxyl group, the resulting conjugate is an ether glucuronide; carboxylic acids react to form ester glucuronides.

**Ether Glucuronide
of Salicylic Acid**

**Ester Glucuronide
of Salicylic Acid**

B. Sulfate Formation: Phenols, alcohols, and aromatic amines can be converted to sulfates or sulfanilic acid derivatives. Active sulfate is provided by adenosine-3-phosphate-5-phosphosulfate (PAPS).

Sulfate of Phenol

C. O-Methylation: A methyl group from S-adenosylmethionine converts a phenolic or alcoholic hydroxyl group to a methoxy group. This reaction is shown in Fig 10–5 since O-methylation is the most important enzymatically governed step in the biotransformation of epinephrine and norepinephrine, the chemical mediators released by the sympatho-adrenal system. The reaction is also important in relation to the pharmacologic actions of corticosteroids.

D. N-Methylation: A methyl group from activated methionine (S-adenosylmethionine) replaces a hydrogen on an amine function or is added to the nitrogen to convert the parent drug to a quaternary amine. The N-methylation of histamine is shown in Fig 19–1.

E. N-Acetylation: The acetyl moiety from acetyl-coenzyme A replaces a hydrogen on an amine or amide group under the influence of various acetyl or acyl transferases. Histamine (Fig 19–1) and the sulfonamides are important examples of drugs that may be acetylated.

F. Other Conjugation Reactions: Glycine and glutamine (and, rarely, serine and lysine) may conjugate with acids. A few toxins may form mercapturic acid derivatives.

Oxidation by Liver Microsomal System

The enzymes in the liver microsomes govern a large number of reactions important in drug metabolism. Furthermore, the activity of the drug-inactivating enzymes is increased during the administration of many long-acting, lipid-soluble drugs. Administration of a drug may therefore increase its own rate of metabolism or decrease the effect of another drug subsequently administered by hastening its oxidation.

The enzymes are contained in the smooth endoplasmic reticulum of liver cells. Rough endoplasmic reticulum—ie, that with ribosomes on its surface—is not involved. Smooth endoplasmic reticulum increases in amount as enzyme activity is induced.

Microsomal enzymes convert lipid-soluble substances to more easily excreted and less active water-soluble metabolites. The first step in the process, prior to conjugation, is usually hydroxylation. Hydroxylation or oxidation of aromatic rings or alkyl side chains occurs at a cytochrome (designated P450 on the basis of its absorption characteristics) where atmospheric oxygen is activated by NADPH and the drug is oxidized by active oxygen. In other words, these enzymes —unlike the dehydrogenases of intermediary metabolism—require NADPH and oxygen. There is little substrate specificity beyond the requirement that the foreign substance be lipid-soluble.

Enzyme induction—or the increase in activity following the administration of, for example, phenobarbital or diphenylhydantoin, or exposure to DDT—depends upon the synthesis of new enzyme.

A variety of reactions are governed by the enzymes, but all can be considered as hydroxylation of the substrate or the direct incorporation of oxygen into the substrate molecule.

The reactions in this group include the following:

(1) Hydroxylation of aromatic rings.

(2) Oxidation (hydroxylation) of alkyl side chains.

(3) N- and O-dealkylation.

(4) Oxidative Deamination: The microsomal enzyme should not be confused with mitochondrial MAO (monoamine oxidase), which is the important enzyme in the transformation of the physiologically important amines—eg, epinephrine, norepinephrine, tyramine, serotonin, and histamine. Microsomal MAO acts on amphetamine, ephedrine, and other phenylisopropylamines if their excretion is slowed (Fig 28–1).

(5) Sulfoxidation: Oxygen may be added to sulfur in a ring structure such as that in chlorpromazine.

In addition to the oxidative reactions, liver microsomes catalyze other reactions—eg, hydrolysis of esters and amides, glucuronide conjugation, and reduction of nitro groups. The activity of these microsomal enzymes can also be modified by the prior or simultaneous administration of other drugs.

Other Oxidations

Other oxidative enzymes are important in the metabolism of relatively few and specific pharmacologic compounds. Detailed reactions are shown in the relevant chapters. These reactions include the following:

(1) Alcohol dehydrogenase of mammalian liver converts ethanol and a few other simple alcohols to the corresponding aldehyde (see Chapter 24).

(2) Aldehyde dehydrogenase converts simple aldehydes, especially acetaldehyde derived from the oxidation of ethanol, to the corresponding acid.

(3) Xanthine oxidase governs the final steps in the synthesis of uric acid. Inhibitors of xanthine oxidase are discussed in Chapter 40.

(4) Monoamine oxidase of mitochondria converts simple monoamines to their corresponding aldehydes, which are then further oxidized to acid or reduced to alcohol (Fig 10–6).

(5) Diamine oxidase is also a mitochondrial flavoprotein but will oxidatively deaminate only compounds with 2 amine functions relatively close together. Histamine is the important diamine (Fig 19–1).

Hydrolysis

Many physiologically important enzymes are hydrolytic—eg, proteases, peptidases, or phosphatases. The acetylcholinesterases which inactivate an important neurohumor have also been well studied (see Chapter 8). There are, in addition, microsomal esterases and others that have been less well characterized. Esters such as procaine and meperidine are examples of drugs that are esters whose activity is destroyed by hydrolysis to an alcohol and acid. Amides—eg, procainamide—are hydrolyzed at a much lower rate. The inactivation of penicillin G depends upon the hydrolytic opening of the lactam ring.

Hydrogenation (Reduction)

This mechanism is not commonly encountered in studies of drug metabolism. Nitrobenzene derivatives—eg, chloramphenicol—may in part be reduced to the amine.

•   •   •

General References

Binns, T.B. (editor): *Absorption and Distribution of Drugs.* Livingstone, 1964.

Conney, A.H.: Pharmacological implications of microsomal enzyme induction. Pharmacol Rev 19:317–366, 1967.

Remmer, H.: The role of the liver in drug metabolism. Am J Med 49:617–629, 1970.

Schanker, L.S.: Passage of drugs across body membranes. Pharmacol Rev 14:501–530, 1962.

Shuster, L.: Metabolism of drugs and toxic substances. Ann Rev Biochem 33:571–596, 1964.

Singer, S.J., & G.L. Nicolson: The fluid mosaic model of the structure of cell membranes. Science 175:720–731, 1972.

Stowe, C.M.: Extrarenal excretion of drugs and chemicals. Ann Rev Pharmacol 8:337–356, 1968.

Williams, R.T.: Detoxication mechanisms in man. Clin Pharmacol Therap 4:234–254, 1963.

3...

The Clinical Evaluation of Drugs

Over the centuries, many ineffective treatments have been confidently prescribed with results that were satisfactory as judged by patient responses. Bleeding and purging were abandoned in spite of predictions of disaster by many physicians, just as present-day efforts to remove ineffective drugs from the market are protested by physicians convinced of the usefulness of even demonstrably inactive substances. The clear lesson is that symptomatic improvement or even cure of disease following the administration of a drug is not evidence that the drug played any role in the clinical result. The evaluation of any therapeutic experience must take into account the variable course of the disease, patient responsiveness even to inactive medication, and possible inadequacies (including bias) of the observer. The principles of clinical drug evaluation apply not only to all areas of medical treatment but to nondrug therapy as well.

The practitioner, responsible for patient care rather than therapeutic research, is rarely able to make adequate measurements and comparisons of drug effects but must depend to a large extent upon the research of other physicians. However, the clinical evaluation of drugs is one activity in medicine that has been dealt with in less than an optimal manner, a fact recognized by recent legislation as well as by current thinking within medicine. In this chapter, the origin of the problems surrounding the evaluation of therapy will be examined; some practical steps in the preliminary evaluation of the large number of available drugs and preparations will be suggested; and, most importantly, the characteristics of an acceptable clinical evaluation of drug efficacy will be outlined.

Origin of the Problems Related to Drug Evaluation

A. Great Progress in Drug Therapy: The remarkable progress in drug therapy during the past 30–40 years has posed a real problem in the evaluation of drugs for both the practitioner and the student. The revolutionary changes in medical practice that have occurred since World War II are largely the result of a revolution in drug therapy. A great many potent and effective therapeutic agents have become available to the modern practitioner during his years of practice—ie, subsequent to his formal medical training. Men who are now the leaders in medical practice and medical education have observed since medical school the development of most of the current antibacterial and antileukemic agents, antihypertensive drugs, antihis-

tamines, oral antidiabetic agents, the anti-inflammatory steroids, the phenothiazine tranquilizers, and other important groups of drugs.

B. Influence of the Diagnostic Orientation of Medicine: The failure to collect and present all of the data needed to evaluate old and new agents is in part due to the traditional diagnostic orientation of medicine carried over from the period of therapeutic nihilism. The elaborate and sophisticated scientific approaches that are applied to diagnostic and physiologic problems in medicine have not been employed in the evaluation of treatment methods. This is a problem not only with drug therapy but with other types of therapy as well. For example, after many years of experience, we are still unable to compare the effectiveness of the several possible treatments for carcinoma of the breast, and the direct relationship between the amount of surgical care provided and the amount available also suggests that some other practices need validation.

C. Economic Factors: The unavoidable problem created by progress in drug therapy is intensified by unnecessary problems which derive from economic factors associated with the use of drugs. The market for American prescription drugs now represents over $4 billion a year at manufacturers' prices. As a result, there has been a great proliferation of drugs and dosage forms as manufacturers compete for a share of the market. There has also been competition between professional sources of drug information and information provided by pharmaceutical industry sources.

D. Governmental Pressure: During the past several years, many episodes of drug toxicity have attracted public attention; the public has concluded that drug costs are in general unreasonably high; and there have been violations of ethics in the course of the clinical evaluation of drugs. For these reasons, the conclusion has been reached both inside and outside the medical profession that the clinical evaluation of drugs poses a special problem. This has resulted in legislative pressure on the pharmaceutical industry, on the profession, and on the government regulatory agencies to provide additional protection against toxic or ineffective drugs and to encourage price competition.

Recognition of the problem and the availability of special funds have led to the emergence of clinical pharmacology as a specialized area of medical research intended to increase the number of acceptable clinical evaluations. Clinical pharmacology so defined will cease to have a function when workers in each clinical specialty undertake the responsibility to carry out acceptable studies on the drugs used by its practitioners. It now appears that clinical pharmacology will come to mean human pharmacology—in contrast to the molecular pharmacology that is developing in the traditional departments.

Evaluation of Drugs by Physicians: Preliminary Steps

A. Maintain a Skeptical Attitude: Physicians vary in their attitudes toward new drugs. A cautious attitude would seem to be justified on a statistical rather than emotional basis by the fact that 100—400 new preparations—new single drugs or new mixtures and dose forms—are introduced each year, whereas only a few are genuinely new or useful. The genuinely new advances quickly find wide recognition within the profession. No one will miss a useful new drug by maintaining a reasonably skeptical attitude, and time will be saved for the study of real problems in drug usage rather than of the unnecessary problem posed by the proliferation of "new" preparations.

B. Acknowledge and Assess the Economic Factors Involved: The drug industry has an essential function to perform and has made outstanding contributions to the health of the world population. However, it is an industry, and one must expect commercial rather than professional attitudes in some representations from its members. The conservative point of view is to regard any commercial source of information as biased whether it is in printed form or presented verbally by detail men.

Subtle as well as obvious forms of advertising should be recognized and in part discounted. These include unsolicited journals and other literature, the distribution of samples that persuade the physician and patient to use trade-marked preparations, and use of the lay press to introduce or publicize a drug.

The volume and easy availability of such information can easily distract the physician from the professionally oriented sources of information listed in the following chapter.

Some apparently technical matters—eg, the use of proprietary mixtures, prescribing by trade name, and the use of special dosage forms—may actually be competitive devices.

These matters of drug economics are further discussed in the section on prescription writing.

C. Drugs Can Be Put in Groups: If each new drug or preparation presented under an attractive but meaningless name were to be regarded as a new problem in evaluation, the burden of drug evaluation would become overwhelming even for the person with a special interest in drugs. Usually the new agent can be related to a familiar drug, and much information and experience already at hand become relevant. For example, many of the drugs said to have new effects and to represent an advance in psychopharmacology are actually closely related to familiar sedative-hypnotics. Even in the genuinely new drug groups—eg, the phenothiazine tranquilizers or the thiazide diuretics—the many compounds available differ only slightly one from another.

D. Laboratory Versus Clinical Results: There is no question but that most current progress in medicine originates in laboratory research. However, laboratory data are directly transferable to the clinic only to the extent that the basic work is complete and accurate and to the extent that the laboratory models imitate the condition of the diseased human. The applicability of a new product of research cannot be assumed but must be determined by a test in the clinical situation. For example, studies of the effect of vasodilator drugs on animals (or even normal human volunteers) are not directly applicable to patients with hypertension or coronary artery disease. This final caution, that the problems of drug evaluation cannot be solely approached in the laboratory, emphasizes our dependence on a well executed clinical trial.

THE CLINICAL TRIAL

The fact that a patient improves after a drug is given does not necessarily mean that the drug was responsible for the change. Before a conclusion about therapeutic usefulness can be reached, the investigator must take into account, measure, or allow for 3 factors other than a pharmacologic effect that can explain an apparent response to medication.

(1) The variable course of the disease process: Colds resolve, ulcers heal and recur, and other diseases run their variable courses whether drugs are used or not. Before an effect can be related to any treatment, a control group must be available and be studied in conjunction with the group receiving the drug. This control group should have received a placebo or a standard drug.

Data for the control group should be collected at the same time as that for the treated group. Control groups selected from the published experience of others ("literature controls") or from earlier experience by the same investigator or at the same hospital are rarely satisfactory. They may be used when a control group is not necessary or justifiable—eg, in the case of a rapidly and uniformly fatal disease.

(2) Patient suggestibility or bias: The reaction of patients or subjects to administered medication does not result entirely from the pharmacologic effect of the active drug contained in the particular dose. The expectation of the patient—generated by the status or the words of the physician; the magic of drugs, especially new drugs in a research setting; and other factors inherent in the personality of the individual—may lead to improvement or deterioration of a symptom or clinical state or to the appearance of side-effects. The nonspecific effects of drugs may be very great on pain, sleep, mood, autonomic functions such as blood pressure, and many other subjective and objective effects.

A physician treating a patient may wish to exploit nonspecific drug effects, but the clinical investigator must measure and evaluate them. A group given no medication will react differently than a group given some medication which might be active or inactive.

The control group in an acceptable clinical trial is, therefore, given a placebo ("I shall please") or dummy medication indistinguishable in every way from the active medication. The patient, of course, is not told whether he is receiving an active or inactive preparation, but he must be told that he is participating in an investigation and that a placebo may be used.

When a symptom or disease state has been well studied and a standard treatment measured and evaluated against a placebo, such standard drug should be used instead of a placebo in further testing of related drugs.

The concept of placebo reactions—and all of the concepts discussed in this section—apply to nondrug therapy as well.

(3) Physician or observer bias: An investigator need not be dishonest to be influenced by his own preconceptions and unconscious bias. In a proper study, he does not know which patient is in the control group and which in the treated group; therefore, he views all patients similarly. When neither the patient nor the observer knows the distribution of subjects into control or treated groups, the study is said to be "double-blind, placebo controlled."

Well controlled clinical evaluations reflecting the above ideas are not the invariable rule in practice today. Indeed, some resistance to the very concept often arises. The traditional authoritative attitudes held by most physicians make it difficult for them to believe that they cannot put complete trust in their individual judgments but must defer to the conclusions of some investigator unknown to them. However, the individual physician combining the responsibilities of evaluation with those of patient care is easily misled by "mere experience." An acceptable evaluation can be done only by executing a carefully prepared experimental design.

The concept of rigidly controlled experimental drug evaluation studies is an important part of current medical philosophy that is now embodied in federal legislation governing the introduction of new drugs.

Characteristics of an Acceptable Clinical Trial

The goal of the double-blind clinical trial is to assay the effectiveness of a drug or other form of treatment against a specific disease or symptom. The trial is carried out after adequate animal toxicity testing has been done and after preliminary experience in humans has established the dosage and provided other pharmacologic data.

Following the sequence outlined by Lasagna and ignoring some of the permissible variations, the characteristics of a good clinical trial would include the following:

A. Careful Planning: The clinical trial must be carefully planned not only to increase the possibility of forming a useful conclusion but also to protect the subject. More than one investigator is usually involved, and the contributions of a clinician, an investigator with a special interest in the clinical pharmacology of the drug involved, and even a statistician are needed. This kind of experiment cannot be modified while the data are being gathered but must be carried out as initially planned in order for the results to be valid.

The planning should be reviewed by a disinterested group whose primary interest is the protection of the subject. They would consider the possible dangers to the subject, the relationship between possible dangers and possible benefits, and the adequacy of the consent form. Review by such a committee is now required by most institutions, granting agencies, and supervisory bodies.

B. Control Groups: A control group of untreated subjects matched to the group receiving therapy is necessary in order to avoid attributing to the treatment effects that are due to variations in the natural course of the disease or symptom. However, the control group is not adequate unless the subjects receive either an inactive or a standard reference medication indistinguishable in its appearance, texture, taste, etc from the active drug. Administration of such a dummy medication or placebo provides control over the nonspecific effects of therapy. The more subjective the response, the more important is the effect of patient expectation and responsiveness.

C. Double-Blind Procedure: The placebo control loses its usefulness unless the patient is unaware of whether he is in the control group (the placebo group), or the treatment group. (However, he must by law be told that he is involved in an experimental study in which an active drug and placebos are included.) In addition, the physician or technician evaluating the results of treatment must also be unaware of which group the subject is in. Any conscious or unconscious bias on the part of the observer is thus controlled.

When the response is completely objective—eg, blood levels of uric acid, creatinine, or similar measurement—control groups would still be necessary but placebo administration would not be required.

D. Random Assignment of Patients to Groups: The control and treated groups must be exactly equivalent. If one group differs from the other in age, severity of disease, willingness to cooperate, or other variables, the effects of treatment will be influenced accordingly. Assignment of patients to groups is best done from a table of random numbers rather than by any device subject to manipulation. If large enough numbers of subjects are used, the groups will be equivalent. In any case, a measure of comparability of the groups is necessary. This is presented by tabulations of age, number of patients with a given symptom in each group, etc.

When a homogeneous group cannot be selected— ie, when the subjects vary widely in some characteristic that will alter their response to the drug being tested— individuals or groups may be paired or matched before the experiment. They are then randomly given the active drug and the placebo or standard. For example, subjects may be matched by placing in subgroups selected for sex, age, or severity of disease.

The technic is varied when it is possible or desirable to test 2 or more medications on the same subject. When this kind of paired comparison is done, the patient becomes his own control. The order of drug administration must then be randomized so that some patients receive the control medication first and others receive it after the "cross-over." The drug or placebo is then randomly assigned to subjects within each subgroup.

E. Statistical Analysis of Data: To establish that a difference between groups is not merely due to variability in response, some statistical measure of variability and significance must be presented. The nature of the analysis is dependent on the design of the experiment and should be established before the drug testing is done. The assistance of a qualified statistician will be necessary for most investigators.

Limitations of the Placebo Controlled Double-Blind Assay

There are data that the type of evaluation described above cannot provide. These limitations must be discussed explicitly since they often are used not as a critique of the double-blind method but as an excuse for not doing a proper trial.

The function of the double-blind study is to establish therapeutic effectiveness and compare the effectiveness of different drugs or other forms of treatment. Such experiments in drug evaluation will not provide information about the general pharmacology of the drug or information about the disease entity being treated. In fact, adequate prior information on dosage and other pharmacologic factors is necessary before a clinical evaluation can be carried out. It is also certainly true that a quantitatively minor drug effect may be missed using the methods just discussed. However, most criticisms of the double-blind studies are actually rationalizations of an unwillingness to perform one of these stereotyped studies. For example, an investigator may state that the conventionalized method is no good because so long as he uses it he cannot establish a drug effect that he knows to exist but which cannot be established by other investigators. Another frequent comment is that a double-blind study cannot be carried out because patient and staff will identify the active compound from the effects on the patient. An example of how such an objection was circumvented is provided by the study discussed in Chapter 25 on the effectiveness of phenothiazine tranquilizers on an institutionalized population in which an "active placebo" was used–ie, the control group received atropine and phenobarbital, a combination that had no therapeutic effect but mimicked the side-effects of the antipsychotic tranquilizer being tested. And, of course, in most studies comparison with a standard drug rather than with an inert placebo is done.

A final objection which must be seriously considered is that it is not proper to deprive a patient of optimal treatment for research purposes. There are very few situations in which the new drug is so dramatically superior to the accepted treatment with which it is being compared that this objection causes real ethical concern. Drug evaluation can be carried out parallel to patient care but must be planned separate from it. One must believe that a definitive evaluation is so valuable that the inconvenience (but never harm) to the patient is justified.

Ethical & Legal Restraints on Human Trials

Important ethical questions arise whenever an investigator uses a human subject. The situation that we are first concerned with relates to the investigative use of chemical substances that are not yet approved for sale as drugs. Because the public health and safety are so clearly involved and because both physicians and manufacturers were sometimes involved in questionable practices, the Federal Food, Drug, & Cosmetic Act was amended in 1962 to establish additional controls. Under the regulations of the Food & Drug Administration (FDA), a new chemical substance may be investigated as a potential drug in the following steps.

A. Preclinical Study: The regulations governing preclinical testing of new drugs are designed to provide as much protection against toxic reactions in humans as possible. (See Chapter 6, Toxicity of Therapeutic Agents.)

B. Clinical Testing of New Drugs: The initial clinical testing of drugs is governed by FDA regulations as well as by the established procedures of clinical pharmacology. Considerable variations are tolerated, but the following stages are defined:

1. Phase I–Following adequate animal studies, the first trials in humans may be undertaken. This stage is not designed to establish or compare usefulness but to establish dosage, duration of action, and other preliminary factors. These tests may in most cases be carried out on normal volunteers, and the investigator may demonstrate his confidence in the preliminary studies and satisfy what some believe to be an ethical obligation by being one of the first subjects. There are perhaps situations where this is not necessary, eg, use of a potential antineoplastic agent may be justified only by the presence of a life-threatening disease.

2. Phase II–When phase I has eliminated the probability of a dangerous and disastrous experience and some preliminary data on dosage are available, the drug is tested for therapeutic effect on a limited number of patients. In this stage, as later, a placebo effect may distort the results, but the use of placebo controls is not required either legally or as a technical consideration until later. Naturally, the data are strengthened if placebo controls are used. The dosages used–a series of dosages must be used–should establish the therapeutic level and the maximum tolerated dose.

3. Phase III–This phase is the controlled clinical bioassay designed to establish the usefulness of a drug under conditions of actual practice. The law requires demonstration of efficacy as well as an evaluation of toxicity, and the FDA requires double-blind, placebo

---

The Nuremberg Code

(1) The voluntary consent of the human subject is absolutely essential.

(2) The experiment should be such as to yield fruitful results for the good of society, unprocurable by other methods or means of study, and not random and unnecessary in nature.

(3) The experiment should be so designed and based on the results of animal experimentation and a knowledge of the natural history of the disease or other problem under study that the anticipated results will justify the performance of the experiment.

(4) The experiment should be so conducted as to avoid all unnecessary physical and mental suffering and injury.

(5) No experiment should be conducted where there is an a priori reason to believe that death or disabling injury will occur; except, perhaps, in those experiments where the experimental physicians also serve as subjects.

(6) The degree of risk to be taken should never exceed that determined by the humanitarian importance of the problem to be solved by the experiment.

(7) Proper preparations should be made and adequate facilities provided to protect the experimental subject against even remote possibilities of injury, disability, or death.

(8) The experiment should be conducted only by scientifically qualified persons. The highest degree of skill and care should be required through all stages of the experiment of those who conduct or engage in the experiment.

(9) During the course of the experiment the human subject should be at liberty to bring the experiment to an end if he has reached the physical or mental state where continuation of the experiment seems to him to be impossible.

(10) During the course of the experiment the scientist in charge must be prepared to terminate the experiment at any stage, if he has probable cause to believe, in the exercise of good faith, superior skill, and careful judgment required of him that a continuation of the experiment is likely to result in injury, disability, or death to the experimental subject.

---

controlled studies. In actual practice, comparison with standard agents already available is almost always more useful than comparison with a placebo.

C. Who Can Carry Out New Drug Investigations: Before a new chemical compound can be tested in humans it must be exempted from the laws forbidding its use as a drug. A sponsor—almost always the company that hopes to market the compound—submits to the FDA a Notice of Claimed Investigational Exemption for a New Drug (IND) summarizing what is known of the compound from prior animal and clinical studies. The sponsor may then proceed with the clinical trials necessary to collect the information required before permission to sell the drug is granted. If an individual investigator wishes to use in research a drug not yet marketed in the USA, or to use a marketed drug in a new therapeutic application, he may act as sponsor by preparing a brief letter.

The sponsor then supplies the drug to physicians for clinical pharmacology investigation (phases I and II) or clinical trial (phase III). The sponsor must collect information from the investigators establishing their competence, and must also secure the researcher's agreement to obtain consent from the subjects receiving the drug.

Principle of Informed Consent

When a patient voluntarily visits a physician he gives implied consent to the performance of usual and expected procedures. Administration of drugs accepted for use does not require special permission from the patient unless the drug is unusually hazardous, in which case the patient or his representative should participate in making the decision to use the drug.

When a new drug is used or when a familiar drug is used as part of an investigation, the patient must give an informed, voluntary consent. By informed consent is meant that he is given all of the information necessary to form a responsible opinion. The information must be provided in understandable (nontechnical) language, and an opportunity for questions and discussion must be offered. Possible adverse effects as well as the possible benefits to others must be described; it must be made clear that the experiment is separate from ordinary treatment.

A consent is voluntary when there is no duress which makes it difficult or impossible for the subject to refuse to participate. The inducement should not be too strong—eg, the fee should be nominal, and the participation of a prisoner (a doubtful practice) should not be made a condition for parole. Both the law (in the case of new drugs) and the consensus of ethical attitudes in the profession make the exceptions necessary for special situations.

• • •

General References*

Barron, B.A., & S.C. Bukantz: The evaluation of new drugs: Current Food and Drug Administration regulations and statistical aspects of clinical trials. Arch Int Med 119:547–556, 1963.

Beecher, H.K.: *Measurement of Subjective Responses: Quantitative Effects of Drugs.* Oxford Univ Press (New York), 1959.

Beecher, H.K.: Ethics and clinical research. New England J Med 274:1354–1360, 1966.

Hill, A.B.: *Principles of Medical Statistics,* 9th ed. Oxford Univ Press, 1971.

Ladimer, I., & R.W. Newman: *Clinical Investigation in Medicine: Legal, Ethical and Moral Aspects. An Anthology and Bibliography.* Boston University Law-Medicine Research Institute, 1963.

Lasagna, L.: The controlled clinical trial: Theory and practice. J Chronic Dis 1:353–367, 1955.

Lasagna, L., & P. Meier: Experimental design and statistical problems. Chap 4, pp 37–60, in: *Clinical Evaluation of New Drugs.* Waife, S.O., & A.P. Shapiro. Harper, 1959.

Lewis, C.E.: Variations in the incidence of surgery. New England J Med 281:880–884, 1969.

Wolf, S.: The pharmacology of placebos. Pharmacol Rev 11:689–704, 1959.

*See also references for Chapters 4 and 6.

4 ...

Technics of Drug Administration

The subject matter covered in this chapter is often called "prescription writing," but much more is involved than the mere form of the order to the pharmacist. Whether the drug is ordered by prescription or by entry in a hospital chart or dispensed directly by the physician, prescribing drugs requires much more than simply a knowledge of drug action. The patient whose doctor is skilled in the practical applications of pharmacy and pharmacology will receive the benefits of drug treatment with greater convenience and effectiveness and at less expense and discomfort.

Prescription writing as such has become less complicated as progress in drug therapy has provided more and more specific remedies. The complex and ineffective mixtures of many crude drugs which were the mainstay of the 19th century pharmacy have been largely replaced by pure agents ordered in a simple prescription written in English.

To the patient, the act of prescribing is of great psychologic import, and nothing should be done to minimize the impact of what is felt to be the climactic part of an office visit.

This chapter deals with the administration and prescribing of drugs used for their systemic effects. The topical application of drugs is discussed in Chapter 5.

REVIEW OF FACTORS MODIFYING DRUG ACTION

Most of the factors modifying drug action are discussed in other chapters. They are summarized here because of their importance at the time that a specific drug is selected and its dose and method of administration prescribed.

Individual Variation

As is true of all biologic responses, the response of any given patient to a drug will be subject to individual variation—ie, the therapeutic dose will be different for different individuals, and toxic effects will also appear at different dosage levels in different patients. With some drugs—eg, penicillin or aspirin—the margin between the therapeutic and the toxic dose is so wide that it is always possible to give a dose greater than would be necessary to achieve a response in the most insensitive patient. With most drugs, however, this is not possible, and each drug administration becomes an exercise in bioassay to establish the dose that will have a therapeutic effect without intolerable or dangerous toxic effects. The average dose is thus a statistical abstraction from which the individual dose varies in a manner described by a normal curve of distribution.

In contrast to this individual variation are unexpected drug responses which depend not upon the dosage of the drug but upon the altered reactivity or allergic sensitization of the patient. (See Chapter 6.)

Absorption

The intensity and duration of the response to a single dose of a drug of a certain size will vary depending upon the rapidity with which blood or tissue levels are achieved. Factors modifying absorption include the following:

A. Solubility: One property of drugs that can be modified to provide a longer duration of effect is their solubility when given by subcutaneous or intramuscular injection. For example, unmodified water-soluble penicillin must be injected as often as 6 times a day to maintain constant therapeutic levels. If the penicillin is combined with procaine and thus rendered less soluble, its absorption from the injection site will continue for more than 12 hours. The solubility of insulin is altered in a similar fashion to increase the duration of effect and, therefore, the convenience to the patient. Drugs administered orally may, however, be well absorbed even though they are insoluble in water.

B. Chemical Properties: A drug may be dispensed in different chemical forms suitable for different routes of administration—eg, neostigmine is dispensed in its quaternary amine form for parenteral use but as the better absorbed salt of a tertiary amine for oral administration. For topical use, local anesthetics or antihistamines may be dispensed as the lipid-soluble free base rather than the water-soluble salt.

Route of Administration

A. Oral: Oral administration is painless, convenient, and economical, and this is therefore the most frequently used route. The onset of action after oral administration is delayed in comparison with the effect after parenteral administration. The major limitations of the oral route are that the drug may not be well absorbed from the gastrointestinal tract; that irritating drugs may cause many local side-effects; that the flavor may be unpleasant; and that some drugs, such as proteins that are digested or steroids that are inactivated by the liver, do not reach the general circulation after oral administration. In an emergency situation, when rapid onset of action is important, or if the patient is unable to swallow, another route must be chosen.

B. Rectal: Certain drugs can be given by suppository or, less commonly, by enema. Drugs that may be irritative when given orally are better tolerated when given by this route, and nausea does not prevent giving the drug.

Those routes of administration listed from this point on are parenteral, by which is meant any route of administration that does not require absorption across an enteric membrane into the portal circulation and immediate transport to drug metabolizing sites in the liver.

C. Subcutaneous: Solutions or suspensions of drugs can be injected into the subcutaneous areolar tissue. When small volumes are injected, the skin overlying the deltoid or triceps muscles is lifted and the needle enters the tent thus formed. When larger volumes are given, the inner surface of the thighs or the back over the thoracic spine (in infants) is preferable. Large volumes of isotonic fluid are absorbed from these sites, and such an injection is often referred to as a hypodermoclysis or clysis. Irritating solutions are more painful if given by this route than if given intramuscularly or intravenously.

D. Intramuscular: Muscle is more vascular and less sensitive than subcutaneous tissue, and irritant solutions or suspensions are better tolerated when given intramuscularly. Absorption from the intramuscular site is somewhat more rapid than from subcutaneous injection sites. Small volumes (2 ml or less) are given into the deltoid. Small or large volumes (up to 10 ml) are given into the gluteal mass underlying the upper, outer quadrant of one buttock or the other. The vastus muscle underlying the lateral surface of the thigh is an alternate area.

E. Intravenous: The intravenous route makes possible accurate control of dosage, rapid dilution of caustic material, and an onset of action that is even more rapid than after intramuscular or subcutaneous administration. The volume of fluid that can be injected intravenously is also greater than is possible by other parenteral routes. Even if the volume and rate of injection are carefully controlled, the intravenous route is far more hazardous than other routes of administration because of the high local concentration of drugs that can result.

F. Intra-arterial: Drugs may be injected into the artery perfusing a specific area of the body in order to achieve a high local concentration in the area before dilution by the entire plasma volume occurs. The injection of x-ray contrast media in arteriography is the most common example of the use of this route. Vasodilators may be given intra-arterially during the vasospastic state following an acute arterial occlusion.

G. Intradermal: A small amount (less than 0.5 ml) of an isotonic material can be injected into the skin. If the injection is properly superficial—ie, into the epidermis only a few cell layers deep—a wheal is formed. Antigens for skin tests are injected in this way. Local anesthetics injected in this manner provide an insensitive area through which a larger needle can be passed without pain for the deeper injection of a local anesthetic.

H. Oral Mucous Membrane: Tablets containing drugs may be placed under the tongue (sublingual) or between the gingival and buccal mucosa. The barrier of the mucous membrane is present, but absorption is much more rapid than after the drug is swallowed. In addition, drugs absorbed from this site enter the systemic rather than the portal circulation. Nitroglycerin, ergot, methyltestosterone, and isoproterenol are examples of drugs conveniently administered in this way.

I. Inhalation: In addition to the volatile anesthetics, microcrystals or aerosols may be rapidly absorbed after inhalation. The effect may be most intense upon the tissues of the lung, but the effect is systemic—ie, absorption is rapid.

J. Intrathecal: X-ray contrast media and spinal anesthetics are frequently given intrathecally. In rare circumstances, a chemotherapeutic agent may be administered in this way.

K. Topical: Drugs may be applied topically, ie, upon the surface of the body. This route is discussed separately in Chapter 5. The important distinction here is between application to the skin and application to a mucosal surface. Drugs are well absorbed across the mucosal surface and a therapeutic effect easily obtained. The intact skin, in contrast, is a barrier to the absorption of most drugs, including many of those suggested for use in this way. Some drugs such as the steroids and some toxins are absorbed after topical application. Important systemic drugs with frequent or dangerous allergic reactions—eg, penicillin—should not be used topically since sensitization frequently occurs.

Interaction With Other Drugs

Two drugs administered simultaneously or sequentially may simply act independently of each other, or they may interact to augment or diminish the expected responses. Obviously, these possible drug interactions should be considered before the drugs are ordered rather than after toxicity or therapeutic failure has occurred.

Examples and details of such drug interactions are discussed in Chapter 2.

Presence of a Disease State

Patients may be unusually sensitive or unusually resistant to a specific drug in the presence of a particular pathologic state. Hypothyroidism, head injury, potassium depletion, respiratory insufficiency, and other states often mentioned as contraindications to drug use alter the sensitivity of the patient.

Drugs that are detoxified by the liver (eg, barbiturates)—or, more importantly, drugs that are excreted by the kidneys—have an extended duration of action or more intense effect if these organs are diseased.

Tolerance

Drug tolerance necessitating an increasing dosage to maintain the initial effect is of several types and is discussed with the individual drugs: narcotic analgesics, sedative-hypnotics, nitrates, the postural hypotensive drugs, and others.

Age & Weight; Pediatric Dosage

When drugs are given to adults, the weight of the subject is only rarely considered in determining the initial dose to be given. Whenever the relative toxicity of the drug permits, a dosage is chosen that is greater than the minimal effective dose for all patients. The dosage of many drugs is that which produces the optimal therapeutic effect or that beyond which intolerable side-effects or toxicity appear. Factors other than body weight are more important sources of variability of response.

In children, however, dosage must be adjusted to body size. The optimal dosage is most dependably determined from the experience of prior investigators or prescribers of the drug. Several general rules are available for calculating pediatric dosage. These are based on age, weight, or body surface area.

A. Age: Young's rule is the most satisfactory of the guides to dosage that are based on age:

$$\frac{Age}{Age + 12} = \text{Fraction of adult dose to be used}$$

Thus, a 12-year-old child would receive half of the adult dose:

$$\frac{12}{12 + 12} = 1/2$$

This child might, however, weigh more or less than the average 12-year-old.

B. Size: Clark's rule approximates the pediatric dosage as 1/150 of the adult dose per pound body weight or 1/70 of the adult dosage per kilogram.

C. Surface Area: Since both of the above rules underestimate the dosage for infants and young children, and since Young's rule also underestimates the dosage for older children, total body surface area provides a better index of the need for drugs and nutrients. Table 4–1 shows the surface area at several ages and the ratio of surface area at these ages to adult surface area—ie, the fraction of the adult dose to be used.

Nomograms from which surface area can be determined are shown on the inside back cover. A rough rule for children is—

$$(0.7 \times \text{weight in lb}) + 10 = \% \text{ of adult dose}$$

or

$$(1.5 \times \text{weight in kg}) + 10 = \% \text{ of adult dose}$$

Doses based on experience are much better than those calculated from any of the above rules. The sen-

TABLE 4–1. Determination of drug dosage from surface area.*

Weight kg	Weight lb	Approximate Age	Surface Area (sq M)	Percentage of Adult Dose
3	6.6	Newborn	0.2	12
6	13.2	3 months	0.3	18
10	22	1 year	0.45	28
20	44	5.5 years	0.8	48
30	66	9 years	1.0	60
40	88	12 years	1.3	78
50	110	14 years	1.5	90
65	143	Adult	1.7	100
70	154	Adult	1.76	103

*Reproduced, with permission, from Silver, Kempe, & Bruyn: *Handbook of Pediatrics,* 9th ed. Lange, 1971.

sitivity or resistance of children to drugs varies with factors other than age or size. In the sections on narcotic analgesics, atropine, amphetamine, and other drugs, pediatric dosage will be discussed further.

PREPARATIONS & DOSAGE FORMS

Most drugs are synthetic in origin. A few are minerals or are extracted from the organs or body fluids of animals, but many are still derived from plants. A **crude drug** is simply that part of the plant containing the drug, untreated except for drying or powdering. Digitalis leaf is an example of a crude drug still in wide use. If an effort is made to partially purify the drug by extraction of the active fraction with water or alcohol, the various extracts and tinctures are known as galenicals—after Galen, who was an influential herbalist in addition to his other activities. The active compound may be purified from the crude drug and used as a **purified preparation**—eg, atropine or digitoxin from belladonna root or digitalis leaf.

Regardless of the source of the drug, it may be available in a variety of forms and containers.

A **tablet** (the most common preparation for oral use) is made by compressing the drug and an inert binder such as starch or lactose into a hard mass which disintegrates in water. A tablet containing a minimum amount of a soluble binder suitable for making a solution for injection is called a tablet triturate or "hypo tablet." These tablets are rarely used today for their original purpose but may be used for sublingual administration. Drugs which are gastric irritants may be "enteric coated" with a substance that will not dissolve until the tablet has entered the intestine. The dependability of these tablets is variable. (Sustained release tablets, designed to release their contents over an extended period, are discussed below.)

A **pill** is an obsolete dosage form made by rolling the drug and a binder into a sphere.

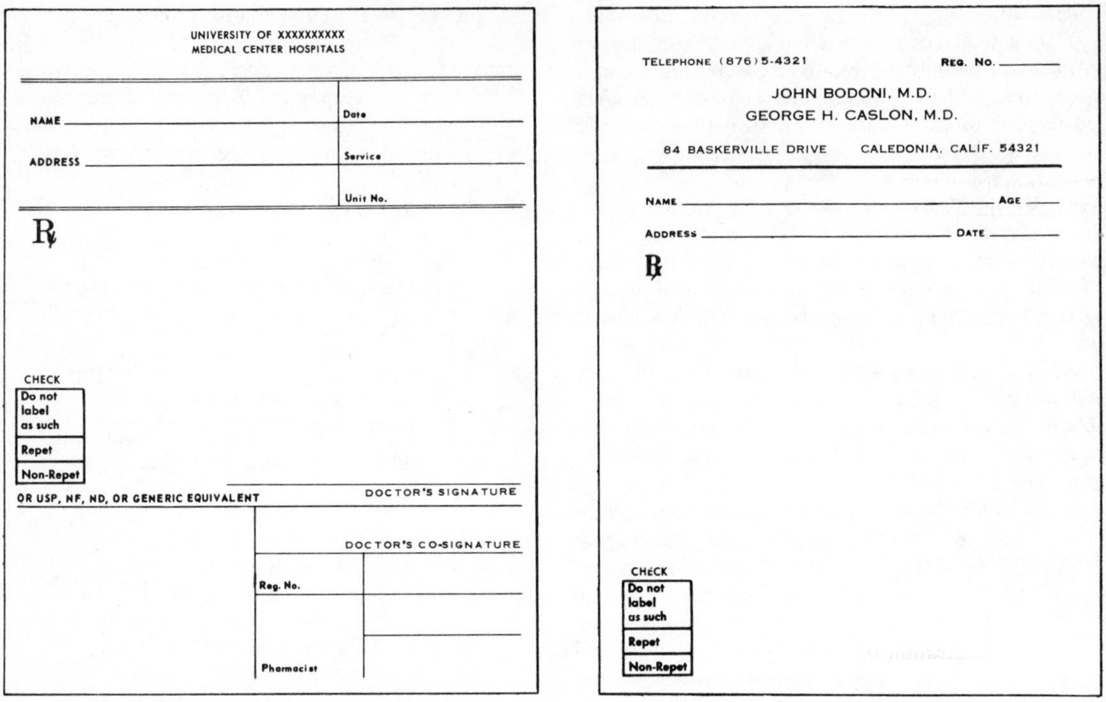
UNIVERSITY OF XXXXXXXXX
MEDICAL CENTER HOSPITALS

NAME ________ Date ________
ADDRESS ________ Service ________
Unit No. ________

℞

CHECK
Do not label as such
Repet
Non-Repet

OR USP, NF, ND, OR GENERIC EQUIVALENT
DOCTOR'S SIGNATURE
DOCTOR'S CO-SIGNATURE
Reg. No.
Pharmacist

TELEPHONE (876) 5-4321 REG. NO. ________
JOHN BODONI, M.D.
GEORGE H. CASLON, M.D.
84 BASKERVILLE DRIVE CALEDONIA, CALIF. 54321

NAME ________ AGE ________
ADDRESS ________ DATE ________

℞

CHECK
Do not label as such
Repet
Non-Repet

FIG 4–1. Examples of 2 prescription forms in use today. Note that the institutional form specifically authorizes generic name dispensing; that each form reminds the physician to record his instructions about refills; and that the name of the drug and dosage will appear on the label unless the physician objects.

Troches and **lozenges** are flavored tablets intended to dissolve slowly when held in the mouth. The released drug acts in the mouth or throat.

Capsules are drug containers made of gelatin that will disintegrate in water.

An **ampule** is a glass container in which solutions of drugs (or dry powder or crystals) can be sterilized and protected until administration. It usually contains a single dose.

Multiple dose vials are rubber stoppered containers from which several doses can be withdrawn, using aseptic technic, without contaminating the solution.

A **solution** is an aqueous preparation of a drug.

An **elixir** is a sweet, aromatic, dilute alcoholic solution of a drug.

A **syrup** contains the drug in a concentrated sugar solution.

A **tincture** is an alcoholic extract of a drug.

Suppositories contain the drug in a waxy or fatty medium that liquefies and liberates the drug after insertion into the rectum or vagina.

A **gel** may be a colloidal suspension of a drug–eg, aluminum hydroxide–or a solution or suspension of a drug in a thickened vehicle. In the latter case, the design may be to keep the drug in contact with the oral or pharyngeal mucosa or to achieve a demulcent effect. In the past, gums were used and the preparation called a mucilage.

Insoluble drugs may be suspended in water for oral administration–eg, milk of magnesia. The thick suspension or the finely divided, amorphous (rather than crystalline) solid may be called a **magma** or mass.

Suspensions of insoluble drugs may also be injected intramuscularly or subcutaneously–eg, procaine penicillin. **Emulsions** are ordinarily only used topically or orally, but one emulsion (vitamin K) is given intravenously.

THE FORM OF A PRESCRIPTION

The form of the practitioner's order to the pharmacist is dictated by tradition, by usage that varies with the locale, and by legal requirements that vary depending upon the drug and the locale.

A prescription may, must, or should include some of the following parts (Fig 4–1):

(1) The date the prescription is written should always be included.

(2) Name of patient.

(3) Address of patient is required only on prescriptions for narcotic and "dangerous" drugs (see below).

(4) Age of young patient may be included to allow pharmacist to intelligently recheck the correctness of the dose.

(5) Superscription: The R (for Latin **recipe**, "take thou of") was modified to ℞ by adding a symbol invoking the aid of Jove.

(6) Inscription: The name of the drug, dose form, and amount per dose. Until recently, the inscription sometimes included multiple ingredients and, theoretically, was adjusted to the individual patient. The pharmacist was then required to "compound" the prescription, ie, to mix the ingredients and manufacture the dose form. Insofar as drugs for systemic administration are concerned, the compounding function has been taken over almost completely by the drug manufacturer.

(7) Subscription: The directions to the pharmacist are now limited to the number of doses to be dispensed.

(8) Signature: This is the instruction to the patient that the pharmacist will transcribe or translate onto the label of the prescription container. This is an important part of the prescription and should be carefully done. To simply state "as directed" is to court misunderstanding or toxicity. Many physicians instruct the pharmacist to "label as such" so that the drug can be identified in case of toxicity or change of doctors, and this practice is generally commended.

(9) Instructions regarding refilling of the prescription: Some indication of the physician's desires about refills should be routinely included in the prescription. These instructions are not only a convenience and courtesy to the patient and pharmacist, but give the physician control over the continued use of a drug. The prescription blank usually offers the prescriber some convenient way of permitting or proscribing refills. Refills may be approved for a certain number of times or through a given date.

Prescriptions for narcotics cannot be refilled. Refills of prescriptions for certain dangerous drugs; most commonly the barbiturates and amphetamines, may be refilled 5 times in the 6 months after the prescription is written if the physician so indicates on the original prescription.

(10) Signature of the licensed practitioner: The prescription must be signed with name and degree. The body of the prescription need not be in the handwriting of the physician, but routine prescriptions that are typed, printed, or stamped are impersonal and usually interpreted as impolite. The address of the prescriber will almost always be printed on the prescription blank, but is required only as noted below. The physician's BNDD* registration number should not be printed on the blank and should be added only on prescriptions for controlled drugs.

WEIGHTS & MEASURES

There are 2 systems of measurement with which the physician must be familiar. The apothecary system is an older system based on arbitrary and unrelated units—eg, grains, ounces. The metric or decimal system

*Bureau of Narcotics & Dangerous Drugs (see p 24).

TABLE 4–2.

Conversion Factors

1 mg	=	1/60 or 1/65 gr
1 gm	=	15 or 15.5 gr
1 kg	=	2.2 lb
1 liter	=	1.06 quarts
1 gr	=	60 or 65 mg
1 fluid ounce	=	30 or 29.57 ml
1 quart	=	1000 or 946.3 ml

Apothecary System (Volume)

1 minim	=	1 drop
60 minims	=	1 fluid dram
8 fluid drams	=	1 fluid ounce
16 fluid ounces	=	1 pint
32 fluid ounces	=	1 quart

Metric System Prefixes

mega (M)	10^6
kilo (k)	10^3
deci (d)	10^{-1}
centi (c)	10^{-2}
milli (m)	10^{-3}
micro (μ)	10^{-6}
millimicro, nano (mμ)	10^{-9}
micromicro, pico ($\mu\mu$)	10^{-12}

is based on related and rationally derived units—eg, centimeters, milliliters or cubic centimeters, grams. Because of the use of the metric system by other sciences, the easier calculations it involves, and its greater accuracy and flexibility, the metric system has been adopted by all official agencies and most teaching hospitals in the USA and British Commonwealth and many other areas.

At present, however, the transition from the apothecary to the metric system in medicine is not complete, and it is still necessary to be familiar with both systems. This duplication is necessary principally because physicians trained to use the apothecary system will assume or expect a familiarity with the obsolescent scale, and some hospitals still retain it as the local standard. In addition, the dosage forms of some older drugs are understood by reference to the older system. Atropine, for example, is available in tablets which contain odd doses in milligrams (0.3, 0.4, 0.6 mg rather than 0.5 and 1 mg) because they derive from the fractional grain doses (1/200, 1/150, 1/100 gr).

Prescriptions for liquids should be written to fit the containers available, and waste is avoided if it is remembered that bottles are still manufactured to contain ounce measurements rather than milliliters (5, 30, 60, 120, 240, and 480 ml are standard bottle sizes).

Newer drugs are dispensed in conformity with the metric system, so that the practitioner who tries to hold to the apothecary system will find himself ordering morphine, gr 1/8, but meperidine, 100 mg (Table 4–2).

For practical purposes, conversion can be accomplished by remembering that—

1 grain (gr) = 0.065 gram (gm) (or 60 mg
 for the usual approximations)
1 gram (gm) = 15 gr
1 ounce (oz) = 30 ml

An ordinary teaspoon will deliver 5 ml, and liquid preparations often contain one dose in 5 ml. In the past, the teaspoon contained 4 ml (1 dram). A tablespoon holds 15 ml (½ oz). A calibrated medicine glass is available in most households to measure 1 oz (30 ml).

When the strength of a solution is expressed in percentage, the meaning is that the solution contains so many parts of solute by weight per 100 parts of solution (W/V). A 5% solution contains 5 gm of solute, with solvent added to make 100 ml.

ABBREVIATIONS

Prescriptions today are no longer written in Latin, but the classical influence persists in a number of abbreviations. The use of these abbreviations is not obligatory nor even recommended, but they are widely used in the signature of the prescription and in orders on hospital charts and are certainly preferable to individual or local coinage.

A few common abbreviations:

āā, of each (ana)
ac, before meals (ante cibum)
ad lib, freely (ad libitum)
bid, twice each day (bis in die)
c̄, with (cum)
gt (plural, gtt), drop(s) (gutta)
gm, gram
gr, grain
h, hour(s)
hs, at bedtime (hora somni, "hour of sleep")
mcg, μg, microgram, 1/1000 mg
mg, milligram, 1/1000 gm
non repet, not to be repeated (refilled) (non repetatur)
pc, after meals (post cibum)
prn, as the need arises (pro re nata)
q, every (quaque); eg, q 4 h, "every 4 hours"
qid, 4 times each day (quater in die)
qs ad, a quantity sufficient to make (quantum sufficiat ad)
repet, to be repeated (repetatur)
s̄, without (sine)
sig, write on label (signa)
s̄s̄, one half (semis)
stat, immediately (statim)
tid, thrice each day (ter in die)

SPECIAL REGULATIONS APPLIED TO THE PRESCRIPTION OF CONTROLLED DRUGS IN THE USA

Drugs with a significant potential for abuse are subject to special regulation not only of their prescription but also of their possession and use in hospital, office, emergency, and research situations. The federal laws were recently modified and codified into the Controlled Substances Act of 1970, and cover narcotics, cocaine, some amphetamines, hallucinogens, marihuana, and the barbiturates and some of the other sedatives.

Responsibility for control and enforcement is assigned to the Department of Justice, Bureau of Narcotic & Dangerous Drugs (BNDD), and many of the rules outlined below can be changed by administrative order.

Annual Registration

After a practitioner (physician, dentist, veterinarian, or other) has received a state license to prescribe and administer drugs, he may apply for federal permission to dispense and prescribe controlled drugs. He is then given a registration or BNDD number which must appear on each prescription for a controlled drug. The registration must be renewed each year.

Schedules of Controlled Drugs

Controlled drugs are placed in different schedules to which different regulations apply. The original listings were established by legislation but are changed by administrative action of the Attorney General as new drugs or new problems appear.

Schedule I consists of drugs whose use is forbidden under all but research conditions—ie, heroin, the hallucinogens, and marihuana (see Table 4–3). These are substances considered to have a high potential for abuse, no currently accepted use in treatment, and whose safety is unestablished even when used under medical supervision.

The usual annual registration and BNDD number applies only to drugs in schedules II–V. A separate registration for research with schedule I substances must be completed before the drugs can be obtained. Since these drugs are investigational, clearance from the Food & Drug Administration must also be provided. Hallucinogens are legally available only from the National Institute of Mental Health.

Schedule II includes substances with high potential for abuse but with currently accepted use in treatment whose use may lead to severe psychologic or physical dependence—ie, the potent analgesics (formerly called class A narcotics), cocaine, and the more widely used amphetamines.

The physician cannot authorize a refill of a prescription for any one of these drugs. A new prescription must be written each time.

TABLE 4–3. Schedules of controlled drugs.

Schedule I: (All use forbidden.)

Narcotics: Heroin and many nonmarketed synthetic narcotics.

Hallucinogens (See Chapter 7 for abbreviations):
LSD
MDA, STP, DMT, DET, mescaline, peyote, bufotenine, ibogaine, psilocybin.

Marihuana, tetrahydrocannabinols.

Schedule II: (No telephoned prescriptions, no refills.)

Narcotics:
Opium
Opium alkaloids and derived phenanthrene alkaloids: Morphine, codeine, hydromorphone (Dilaudid), oxymorphone (Numorphan), oxycodone (dihydrohydroxycodeinone, a component of Percodan)
Designated synthetic drugs: Meperidine (Demerol), alphaprodine (Nisentil), anileridine (Leritine), methadone, levorphanol (Levo-Dromoran), phenazocine (Prinadol)

Stimulants:
Coca leaves and cocaine
Amphetamine
Dextroamphetamine
Methamphetamine
Phenmetrazine (Preludin)
Methylphenidate (Ritalin)
Above in mixtures with other controlled or uncontrolled drugs (Dexamyl, Eskatrol).

Schedule III: (Prescription must be rewritten after 6 months or 5 refills.)

Narcotics: The following opiates in combination with one or more active nonnarcotic ingredients, provided the amount does not exceed that shown:

Codeine and dihydrocodeine: Not to exceed 1800 mg/100 ml or 90 mg/tablet or other dose unit

Dihydrocodeinone (hydrocodone and in Hycodan): Not to exceed 300 mg/100 ml or 15 mg/tablet
Opium: 500 mg/100 ml, or 25 mg/5 ml, or other dosage unit (paregoric).

Narcotic Antagonist: Nalorphine

Depressants:
Barbiturates (except phenobarbital, etc).
Glutethimide (Doriden)
Methyprylon (Noludar)
Phencyclidine (Sernylan, PCP)

Schedule IV: (Prescription must be rewritten after 6 months or 5 refills.)

Depressants:
Chloral hydrate
Chloral betaine (Beta-Chlor)
Ethchlorvynol (Placidyl)
Ethinamate (Valmid)
Meprobamate
Methylphenobarbital (Mebaral)
Paraldehyde
Phenobarbital
Barbital

Schedule V: (As any other [nonnarcotic] prescription drug; may also be dispensed without prescription unless additional state regulations apply.)

Narcotics: The following drugs in combination with other active, nonnarcotic ingredients and provided the amount per 100 ml or 100 gm does not exceed that shown:

Codeine: 200 mg
Dihydrocodeine: 100 mg
Ethylmorphine: 100 mg
Diphenoxylate (not more than 2.5 mg and not less than 0.025 mg of atropine per dosage unit, as in Lomotil)

Telephoned prescriptions for schedule II drugs (Table 4–3) cannot be honored by the pharmacist since he must have a prescription to account for the drugs he dispenses. The order may be phoned to the pharmacist and the actual prescription delivered to the pharmacy or left at the home of the patient where the pharmacist can receive it before delivering the narcotic.

In the case of a bona fide emergency when no other treatment is possible, the pharmacist may (under federal law) allow the physician 72 hours to deliver the written prescription.

Schedule III is defined as a category for drugs with a potential for abuse less than that for substances in schedules I and II. The narcotics included are paregoric and the former "class B narcotics"–notably, mixtures of codeine and aspirin, which are widely used mostly because their prescribing is more convenient.

Short- and intermediate-acting barbiturates and a few other sedatives are also in this schedule. The remainder of the drugs so far recognized as sedatives are placed in schedule IV, where the same prescribing rules apply.

Prescription for drugs in schedule III and IV may be given to the pharmacist by telephone. A new prescription must be provided after 5 refills (if they are authorized by the physician) or after 6 months.

Schedule IV does not differ from schedule III insofar as prescribing practices are concerned but does differ in other matters, eg, penalties for illegal possession.

Schedule V includes those drugs formerly called exempt narcotics. Federal law permits the sale of these mixtures without a prescription, but state laws are more restrictive in some cases. If a doctor dispenses any of these preparations, he must keep a record for 2 years.

Office Supplies

A practitioner is authorized to keep a supply of controlled drugs on hand for emergency use and to dispense to patients.

The drugs listed in schedule II (potent narcotics and amphetamines) cannot be ordered from a pharmacist on a regular prescription nor from a wholesaler on an ordinary order form. A special federal form which is made out in triplicate must be used.

A record must be kept of all controlled drugs received and an inventory made every 2 years. A record must be kept documenting the dispensing of **narcotics** of schedule II and III. At this time it appears that entries on the record of the patient are adequate recordings of the use of other controlled drugs.

Office and emergency supplies of these drugs must be stored in a locked cabinet.

Form of the Prescription

The information required on prescriptions for narcotics or dangerous drugs differs in different states and for different classes of drugs. The prescription should include the date, the address and full name of the patient, and the signature, address, and registry number of the practitioner. It should be written in ink or typewritten. Some states require that, if written, it must be entirely in the handwriting of the doctor. The signature of the prescription should indicate the use intended—eg, "q 4 hours prn cough" or "prn pain, no oftener than q 4 hours" not merely, "q 4 hours" or "as instructed." The doctor must keep a record of each prescription for 2 years. This record is most easily maintained by making a carbon copy of each narcotics prescription. Some states require special prescription blanks which facilitate auditing and prevent forging of prescriptions.

State Regulations

Some states have added regulations more restrictive than the federal law. Several states require that narcotic prescriptions be written on special triplicate forms. At present, the state rules still reflect the old federal law, and many changes can be anticipated as state laws are brought into conformity with the present federal regulations.

LEGAL & ECONOMIC FACTORS IN PRESCRIBING (USA)

Medicine and related professions are subject to licensing and other regulations out of concern for the public health. Similarly, most societies conclude that drugs are different from other commodities and impose special regulations on their manufacture and distribution. Most of these regulations are designed to protect the safety of the patient.

Statutory Regulation of Prescriptions

There are certain common sense obligations associated with prescribing. Regardless of the nature of the drug prescribed, the physician should keep a record of the prescription. This may be in the form of a duplicate of the prescription, but more commonly the prescription is copied into the patient's record. This is essential for the evaluation of therapy and also protects the physician against legal action in the event of a misunderstanding or error in the use of the medication.

The federal regulations on prescribing are contained largely in the Durham-Humphrey Amendment to the Food, Drug, & Cosmetic Act (1952), and the Controlled Substances Act discussed above.

The first statute defined "legend drugs," ie, drugs that must bear the label, "Caution: Federal law prohibits dispensing without prescription." The FDA defines permissible over-the-counter (OTC) drugs, but drugs may be made legend drugs if the manufacturer does not wish the OTC classification.

In the USA, drugs classified as "legend drugs" cannot be refilled unless the refill is authorized by the prescriber. For this reason it is convenient to include on the prescription a statement of the prescriber's desire concerning refills. Lacking this, the pharmacist must obtain permission from the physician for a refill. Such permission is usually obtained by phone.

Telephoned prescriptions are authorized if they are immediately reduced to writing by the pharmacist.

Additional administrative regulations influencing prescribing are issued by the US Food & Drug Administration as the need arises. Drugs may be withdrawn from the market when unexpected toxicity occurs, or special restrictions may be placed on special drugs. For example, 2 antineoplastic agents (methotrexate and triethylenemelamine) may be dispensed by the pharmacist only to a physician, not to a patient.

Drug Prices

The total sales of the US drug industry in 1970 were in excess of $12 billion at manufacturers' selling prices. Over $4 billion, still at manufacturers' prices, represent sales of prescription drugs for humans.

In meeting the need for prescription drugs, the drug industry performs several essential functions. It is, however, an industry rather than a profession, and its competitive efforts have led to several practices that must be regarded as controversial. The interaction between the physician and the drug industry becomes most apparent when the physician chooses a specific preparation and gives the patient no alternative but to buy and pay for that specific product. The following would be regarded by many as an outline of sound practice in selecting and ordering a drug, but attitudes vary widely.

A. Prescribe by Generic Rather Than Brand Names: If an individual (or company) develops a new drug he can, in the USA, secure a patent on the new substance or on the process for producing it. The patent holder is then entitled to exclusive control of the patented substance or process for 17 years. During this period of freedom from competition, developmental costs can be recovered. In anticipation of the expiration of the patent or when the product is not genuinely new, the distributor may attempt to improve his competitive position by advertising a trade name that remains his exclusive property almost indefinitely. The expense of establishing such a protected or registered name invariably increases the cost of a drug. Once the protected name is successfully established, prices can be increased. The wholesale price of an unprotected drug available as a "generic preparation" is usually low, but, when the drug is sold under its trade name, the cost will be higher, sometimes exorbitantly so. At this time, for example, reserpine, 0.25 mg tablets, is offered as a generic preparation at 59 cents per 1000 tablets, but the most familiar brand name preparation costs $39.50 per 1000. Prescribing by generic rather than brand names can, therefore, result in savings on drug costs if the drug is no longer patented, ie, if price competition is possible.

The argument against generic name prescribing is that only by stipulating the manufacturer can the physician be sure that his patient will receive a preparation of the best quality. However, drugs are different from most other commodities in that legal standards of potency, purity, etc are established and only limited variations are permitted. The quality of marketed drugs is monitored by the FDA with expanded facilities; by competing companies; and, during this period of controversy, by individual investigators. All of these efforts now employ blood level studies as well as tablet analysis to establish therapeutic as well as chemical equivalence. Antibiotics are assayed before marketing and each batch individually certified by the FDA. With rare exceptions, there have been no important variations among the products of different suppliers. Generic and brand name drugs may actually come from the same manufacturer.

If the physician prescribes only the products of the largest (ie, most heavily advertising) manufacturers, he will not protect his patient from the rare variations in quality but he will greatly increase the cost of medication not only immediately but in the long run by concentrating the drug industry in a few large companies.

In private practice, the community pharmacist enters the distributive chain, and in some communities he may be reluctant to pass on to the patient the savings inherent in generic name prescribing. However, as medical care becomes more centralized and institutions and governmental agencies contribute more to the cost of medical care, the 5% of the medical care dollar being spent on drugs is subject to more and more control. Many institutions reserve the right to substitute generic for protected names unless the physician offers prior objection. (See the specimen prescription, Fig 4–1.) Generic name prescribing is thus an accomplished fact in a large area of medical practice.

Generic name prescribing can be a burden, since the names are chosen to be as difficult as the registered names are euphonious—eg, chlordiazepoxide or Lib-

rium, prochlorperazine or Compazine. Generic names are proposed by the manufacturer and approved by the United States Adopted Names (USAN) Council, a committee of the American Medical Association, the American Pharmaceutical Association, and the United States Pharmacopeia.

B. Drug Combinations: A patient may often require more than one drug, but rarely should they be given as mixtures of fixed composition. Their varied dosage and duration of action usually require that they be given separately. A few common mixtures are official and used for good medical reasons—eg, trisulfapyrimidines USP, oral contraceptives, dermatologic medications—but more are trade-marked. Many such combinations have their origin in economic rather than scientific considerations since they provide a way of developing a proprietary interest in a combination of drugs that would individually be competitive. Atropine and phenobarbital, for example, offer no way for a distributor to establish a brand name individually, but as combinations they can be marketed with the advantage (higher prices) inherent in a trade-marked or otherwise protected commodity.

In some cases use of the combination can be rejected on the grounds that the mixture is therapeutically irrational—ie, that the 2 drugs are not commonly indicated as part of the same treatment regimen (eg, anti-inflammatory steroid plus a sedative); or that the combination adds a risk without adding a benefit (eg, some antibiotic combinations and antibiotic plus anti-inflammatory steroid ophthalmic topical agents).

However, even when one concedes that each drug in a combination is indicated, it does not follow that they are best given as a combination. The optimal dose of phenobarbital for most patients may vary between 8 and 30 mg/dose. The dosage of anticholinergics must be so individualized that at least a few physicians still prefer to adjust it dropwise, using tincture of belladonna. A combination product with a fixed proportion of phenobarbital and atropine cannot be given with the same precise therapeutic benefit.

Other preparations irrationally combine drugs with slow onset of action and long duration of action (eg, amphetamine) with drugs whose effects are comparatively brief (eg, aspirin, amobarbital).

In most cases, the combinations are more expensive than their separate constituents, a consideration of importance both to the patient and to the agency subsidizing his medical care.

The Food & Drug Administration, acting upon the advice of a NAS-NRL review board, has removed a number of fixed combinations from the market (see Appendix). They propose to require in the future that there be substantial evidence that in fixed combinations of drugs each component contributes to the effect claimed and that the dosage (amount and interval of administration) of each component be appropriate. The evaluation will be gradually extended to include over-the-counter remedies.

C. Prolonged Action Drugs for Oral Administration: Many drugs are available in dosage forms designed to provide sustained action or repeated release of the drug. The idea of reducing the number of doses that have to be taken per day is attractive, and there is no reason why such preparations should not eventually be developed. However, until the technology is improved, these dosage forms must be regarded as nothing more than competitive devices. Most types, notably the coated bead or Spansule type, release the entire dose at almost the same rate as the ordinary tablet. Others allow some of the drug to traverse the gastrointestinal tract unabsorbed and thus reduce the amount of each dose actually available. Specific data on the behavior of some of these preparations are presented in the discussions of the individual drugs, eg, aspirin, iron, antipsychotic tranquilizers.

SOURCES OF CURRENT INFORMATION ON NEW DRUGS

In Chapter 1 are listed the most authoritative sources of general pharmacologic information. In the area of prescribing practices, many physicians feel that they should have some special help in evaluation from the medical literature because of the many new drugs and preparations which continuously appear on the market. Having been told that they should reject industrial sources of information, they look for an authoritative source so that they will be sure to recognize important new drugs and reject the others. As in other areas of medicine, summary authoritative pronouncements should be less influential than a study of the underlying data and experience.

The general and specialty journals publish good drug studies. Several special aids are available for the physician or pharmacist. *Medical Letter* publishes evaluations of current therapy every 2 weeks and has an impressive record for recognizing the significant as well as rejecting the trivial, imitative, or specious. Brief discussions represent the consensus of several physicians with experience with the drug or drug group evaluated. *Clinical Pharmacology and Therapeutics* publishes useful reviews and summaries as well as research papers.

AMA Drug Evaluations (1971) is the latest in a series of volumes sponsored by the AMA Council on Drugs. Most of the space is devoted to discussions of individual agents, including the dosage and available preparations. However, the drugs are grouped according to use, some general discussion is provided, and adverse as well as favorable judgments are expressed. For these reasons, *AMA Drug Evaluations* appears preferable for use to PDR.

Physicians' Desk Reference (PDR) is an annual publication in which manufacturers may buy space to present prescribing information about their products. The material included is similar to the package insert accompanying the product. Toxic reactions and precautions are presented in sufficient detail to shift more responsibility onto the physician than is the case with the usual advertisement. PDR is, however, a convenient source of information about dosage forms.

The *United States Pharmacopeia* (USP) and the *National Formulary* (NF) establish standards of purity, tablet disintegration times, and other criteria of acceptability for a product, and these standards are binding upon the courts. The physician will rarely have occasion to consult these official compendia for prescribing information, but they have some importance to him in an indirect way. Now that the Food & Drug Administration is empowered to require testing of efficacy and is involved in the widespread testing of drugs for biologic availability as well as mere tablet content, the importance of the traditional pharmacopeia is waning.

DRUG INCOMPATIBILITIES

The term "incompatibility" is carried over from the period when individually compounded mixtures could contain ingredients that were chemically, pharmaceutically, or therapeutically incompatible. Therapeutic incompatibilities are now discussed as drug interactions, but an occasional problem of chemical incompatibility arises when drugs for parenteral injection are mixed either in the syringe or in a larger volume of parenteral fluid to be given by continuous intravenous drip.

When acidic and basic solutions of drugs are mixed in the same syringe, one component may be precipitated. For example, the barbiturates are acids and are prepared for injection as very basic sodium salts—ie, as the salt of a weak acid and a strong base. The narcotic analgesics and the atropine alkaloids are bases dispensed as acidic solutions of the hydrochloride or sulfate. If these are mixed in a small volume for intramuscular administration, some of the barbiturate is precipitated. It is true that many injections of such cloudy solutions have been given. In this case, the ultimate solubility being determined by the pH at the injection site, the effects of the members of the mixture are not affected. However, a variable amount of the drug may adhere to the syringe.

When drugs are added to the contents of the infusion bottle for administration over a period of hours, problems of stability as well as solubility may arise. It is actually difficult to conceive of situations in which more than one drug need be added to an infusion fluid. When a continuous intravenous infusion is being given, drugs can usually be injected slowly into the tubing or side arm of the infusion set with few concerns about chemical incompatibility. Examples of a few drugs that do pose problems are:

(1) Tetracycline: Solutions of tetracycline for parenteral use contain large amounts of ascorbic acid. The acid solution hastens the hydrolysis of penicillin and precipitates a number of antibiotics and other drugs. Further examples involving antibiotics are shown in Table 48–3.

(2) Diphenylhydantoin for injection is solubilized with sodium hydroxide.

(3) Heparin is a large, acidic molecule and complexes with many other drugs.

(4) Proteins: Whole blood, protein hydrolysates, and biologicals should not have drugs added because of the theoretical possibility of inactivation by binding.

● ● ●

General References

General

Facts and Comparisons. E.K. Kastrup (editor). Facts and Comparisons, Inc. [Loose-leaf compilation of dosage forms with monthly supplements.]

Cook, E.F., & others: *Remington's Practice of Pharmacy,* 13th ed. Mack Printing Co., 1965.

Pelissier, N.A., & S.L. Burgee, Jr.: Guide to incompatibilities. Hospital Pharm 3:15–32, 1968. [Also package insert for each drug.]

Shirkey, H.C. (editor): *Pediatric Therapy,* 3rd ed. Mosby, 1968.

Wilson, C.O., & T.E. Jones: *American Drug Index.* Lippincott. [Annual. A listing of virtually all drugs and preparations.]

Drug Economics

Feldmann, E.G.: Brand versus generic drugs. J Am Pharm A 9:8–12, 1969.

Harris, R.: *The Real Voice.* Macmillan, 1964. [Summary of Kefauver hearings.]

Hastings, G.E., & R. Kunnes: Predicting prescription prices. New England J Med 277:625–628, 1967.

Leprowski, W.C.: Medicinal chemicals. Economic and social forces bring changes. Chem Eng News, pp 100–104, Sept 1, 1969.

May, C.D.: Selling drugs by "educating" physicians. J M Educ 36:1–23, 1961.

Steele, H.: Monopoly and competition in the ethical drugs market. J Law Econ 5:131–163, 1962.

5...

Dermatologic Application

The discussion of the technics of medication in Chapter 4 emphasizes factors important in ordering drugs used for their general systemic effect. The application of drugs to the skin involves the concepts already mentioned as well as additional matters of technic. For example, the application of drugs to the skin requires consideration not only of the pharmacologic effect of the active agent but also the physical form of the preparation, which may itself have a therapeutic or adjuvant effect. The present chapter, therefore, defines some pharmaceutical preparations used for topical application and lists some of the possible drug actions. The detailed discussion of some topically active drugs and the discussion of drugs used systemically for the treatment of dermatologic manifestations of disease—eg, corticosteroids, antibiotics, antihistamines—will be found in later chapters.

At one time the ability of the physician to order and of the pharmacist to compound individualized prescriptions was very important. With the availability of specific and potent drugs such as the topical and systemic steroids, antibiotics, parasiticides, and fungicides, dermatologic therapy is both simpler and more effective than in the past. As is true also of other areas of medicine, the pharmaceutical industry now prepares most of the standard preparations.

ABSORPTION OF DRUGS THROUGH THE SKIN

A few substances—eg, the cholinesterase inhibitors used as nerve gases and insecticides—are rapidly absorbed after application to the skin. However, such examples are few in number, and it is the impermeability of the skin, which is physiologically essential, that is most impressive in drug studies.

The rate-limiting barrier to percutaneous absorption is the stratum corneum of the epidermis. This dense layer of dead, keratinized cells resists the diffusion of both water-soluble and lipid-soluble substances. In its absence, as when the skin is denuded by some disease process or even after stripping off part of the epithelium by repeated applications of cellophane tape, the skin functions as a lipid barrier similar to other membranes (see Chapter 2).

If drugs are dissolved in solvents that are miscible with both water and lipid solvents, their absorption may be enhanced. The investigative drug DMSO (see p 35) provides the only significant application of this idea.

Hydration of the cornified layer of the epidermis also increases penetration of some drugs, especially the anti-inflammatory steroids. Such a change in the epidermis is accomplished by covering the part with an occlusive dressing such as a polyethylene film. The use of ointments also macerates the underlying skin and is an older technic for improving the absorption of drugs into the skin.

FORMS OF TOPICAL APPLICATION

Topical medication can be applied to the skin dissolved or suspended in a variety of media ranging from simple solutions to greasy ointments. The medium or pharmaceutical form of application has by itself an effect on the skin lesion, and selection of the form in which a topical medication is applied is determined as much by the acuteness or chronicity of the dermatosis as by its specific cause. Acute (recent) lesions are red, burning, blistered, swollen, and weeping. A subacute stage is represented by the subsidence of the above acute changes. In chronic (long-standing) lesions, the skin is thickened by the underlying process or by scratching and is crusted or scaly. A greasy ointment that prevents drainage and drying is unsuitable for application to an acute, weeping lesion; and a powder placed on the surface of a grossly thickened or crusted skin will have little effect. The relation of the preparation selected to the acuteness of the dermatosis is shown in Table 5–1.

Wet Preparations

Baths, soaks, and wet dressings are therapeutically equivalent, the variation selected depending upon the area and extent of involvement. Wet preparations may be used for their inherent cleansing or antipruritic action or may be medicated to achieve additional antipruritic, astringent, or other effects. In either case, continued contact with water is cleansing, maintains drainage from the affected areas, and is a convenient way of heating the skin and causing vasodilatation. Water is keratolytic, leading initially to softening and maceration, but water is ultimately drying in its effect

TABLE 5-1. Types of topical formulations used in acute, subacute, and chronic skin lesions.

	Acute Lesions (weeping, hot, edematous, crusting, recent)	Subacute Lesions (edematous, hot, chapped)	Chronic Lesions (scaling, lichenified, crusting)
Wet preparations (baths, soaks, wet dressings)	X		
Powders, shake lotions	X	X	
Emulsions	X	X	X
Creams	X	X	X
Pastes		X	X
Ointments			X

on the skin. Medicated baths are suitable for application in the most acute lesions.

Some examples of wet preparations are shown in Table 5-2.

Powders

Powders such as zinc oxide, talc (magnesium silicate), and titanium dioxide reduce friction and absorb moisture. In practice, powders are most often applied to the body in the form of shake lotions (see below).

Powders as such are used in intertriginous areas (between the toes, in the groin, beneath the breasts) or as inert carriers of antiparasitic (DDT) or fungistatic agents.

Shake Lotions (Table 5-3.)

Strictly defined, a lotion is a solution or suspension of a medication. It is better to use the term "solution" for the first case and avoid confusion with cosmetic and other uses of the term.

TABLE 5-2. Wet preparations: for baths, soaks, and wet dressings.*

Indications: For acute, red, swollen, itching, infected, weeping, or vesicular lesions.

Technic: (1) Baths: Lukewarm or cool baths for 30 minutes 2-3 times daily as needed. Dry by blotting, not rubbing. The usual home tub contains 20 gal (75 liters) when half-filled. (2) Basin soaks (2-5 quarts of solution) for hands and feet: Soak for 15 minutes twice daily. Solutions must be applied cool (hot for infections). (3) Wet dressings (for localized lesions): Use a Turkish towel; keep saturated with solution. Frequent applications are necessary (eg, 30 minutes 2-4 times a day). Covered dressings should not be used.

Agent	Action†	Range of Concentrations Used	Most Common Strength Used	Preparation of Solution of Most Commonly Employed Strength
Plain tap water		...	...	...
Starch bath	Antipruritic	...	...	2 cups starch or Linit to tub
Proprietary bath oils (Alpha-Keri, Nivea, Lubath, Demol, etc)	Antipruritic	...	...	5-25 ml to tub
Sodium chloride		6:1000-15:1000 (0.6-1.5%)	0.9%	2 tsp/quart water
Sodium bicarbonate	Antipruritic	1:50-1:20 (2-5%)	3%	8 tsp/quart water
Magnesium sulfate (Epsom salts)	Antipruritic	1:50-1:25 (2-4%)	3%	8 tsp/quart water
Aluminum subacetate solution	Astringent	1:200-1:10 (0.5-10%)	5%	Domeboro powder, 2 tsp/quart, or Burow's solution, 50 ml/quart water
Potassium permanganate	Antipruritic, oxidizing, antiseptic, astringent	1:10,000-1:400 (0.01-0.25%)	1:10,000 (0.01%)	One 0.3 gm tablet to 3 quarts water or one 0.1 gm tablet to 1 quart water

*Modified, with permission, from Krupp, M.A., & M.J. Chatton: *Current Diagnosis & Treatment, 1972.* Lange, 1972.

†All of the solutions listed have a drying, soothing, and cleansing action also.

TABLE 5–3. Lotions and emulsions.*

Liquid mixtures containing medicaments in solution or suspension are useful in a wide variety of localized and generalized skin lesions because they are easy to apply and remove. They often have a marked drying effect and must not be used if this effect is undesirable. The following are some useful well known lotions.

Lotion and Action	Prescription		Instructions and Remarks
Calamine lotion (soothing, drying)	Prepared calamine	8	Apply locally 3–4 times daily or as needed. Use for acute dermatitis. Avoid excessive drying by prolonged use of this lotion (as with other nonoily lotions). Add 1% phenol for antipruritic effect.
	Zinc oxide	8	
	Glycerin	2	
	Magma of bentonite	25	
	Lime water, qs ad	100	
Starch lotion (antipruritic, soothing, drying)	Corn starch	24	Apply locally twice daily or as needed for acute dermatitis. This is a useful basic lotion to which other agents may be added.
	Zinc oxide	24	
	Glycerin	12	
	Lime water, qs ad	120	
Coal tar lotion (soothing, drying, keratoplastic)	Coal tar solution	12	Apply locally at night; scrub in morning. Use for subacute dermatitis. A useful mild stimulating lotion. Do not use on hairy or infected areas.
	Zinc oxide	24	
	Starch	24	
	Glycerin	36	
	Water, qs ad	120	
Oily lotion (soothing, drying, lubricating)	Zinc oxide	10	Apply locally 3–4 times daily or as needed for acute dermatitis. Less drying than calamine and starch lotions.
	Olive oil		
	Lime water $\overline{aa}$, qs ad	120	

*Modified, with permission, from Krupp, M.A., & M.J. Chatton: *Current Diagnosis & Treatment, 1972.* Lange, 1972.

Shake lotions, so called because it is essential to shake well before using, are suspensions of fine powders. They provide a convenient way of applying a powder with good contact and adherence to the surface. The benefit of the application is due to the mechanical properties of the powder and to the effect of added agents—eg, 1% phenol for an antipruritic action. The disadvantages of shake lotions are that they may be excessively drying when applied to acute lesions and that they do not penetrate thickened chronic lesions as well as creams or ointments.

Calamine lotion is a familiar example of a shake lotion. Calamine lotion and calamine lotion with phenol are both official (USP) preparations and are available without a prescription. Calamine was originally a zinc carbonate ore colored pink by iron salts present as impurities. Calamine lotion is now prepared from zinc oxide and "prepared calamine," which is actually zinc oxide to which a small amount of ferric oxide has been added for color.

Emulsions

Oil in water emulsions are less drying than lotions, and an oily calamine shake lotion (calamine liniment) may be substituted for calamine lotion.

Creams or Hydrophilic Ointments

Creams should be considered in contrast with the heavier greasy ointments (described below). Their properties are intermediate between those of drying preparations (wet dressings, lotions) and ointments.

Creams contain a high percentage of water but are semisolid in consistency. Hydrophilic ointments are petrolatum in water emulsions stabilized with a detergent such as sodium lauryl sulfate. Polyethylene glycols are more commonly used today than the older hydrophilic ointments. These polymers have the consistency of an oil, cream, or wax, depending upon their molecular weight, but are water-soluble and dissolve most water-soluble drugs.

Creams are water-washable and do not leave the greasy residue that is present after use of an ointment. They are able to absorb fluids from the skin and bring any dissolved medication into good contact with the skin.

Pastes

A paste, in the present context, is a suspension of a powder such as zinc oxide in a greasy ointment base. Pastes are thicker and drier than ointments. They do not penetrate as well as ointments but are less occlusive.

Ointments

Ointments are preparations in which a drug is suspended or dissolved in a grease or oil. Petrolatum, liquid petrolatum (mineral oil), olive oil, lanolin, or other animal fats may be used.

Ointments provide mechanical protection to the underlying skin and penetrate thickened lesions well with their contained medication. They are emollient—ie, they lubricate and soften the surface of the skin and overlying crusts or scales. They do not permit drainage or evaporation from the skin, and continued application (by trapping moisture) causes maceration. They should not be used in hairy areas, where their penetration to the base of the follicle may lead to folliculitis.

Direct Application of Drugs

In some situations the most efficacious means of applying a drug may be as a simple solution, tincture, paint, suspension, or as crystals.

PHARMACOLOGIC ACTIONS OF DRUGS APPLIED TO THE SKIN

The form of the topical medication may itself have important pharmacologic effects—eg, the drying or emollient action of the aqueous or greasy preparations, or the antipruritic effect of baths or soaks. In addition, drugs may be incorporated into the vehicle to exert a variety of local actions.

Antipruritic Actions

The mechanical properties of many of the above vehicles may relieve itching by protecting the skin from the stimulation of scratching, friction, or changes in temperature or by moistening or drying the skin as necessary. In addition, several phenols which may be added to lotions reduce itching by an action on sensory reception. Whether the action is local anesthesia or the substitution of one sensation for another (counterirritation) is not clear.

Lotions, creams, and ointments containing local anesthetics and antihistamines are available, but, unless the skin is badly denuded of epithelium, they are poorly absorbed and have little effect other than that inherent in their mechanical properties. Antihistamines given for their systemic effect are highly useful in treating urticarial lesions, but they have no effect on itching due to other causes. The anti-inflammatory steroids (see below) relieve itching by suppressing the underlying process.

Astringent Actions

Astringents are mild protein precipitants that form a thick coagulum on the surface of an area of acute damage (eg, the alcohol in after-shave lotion) or coagulate and remove overlying debris (eg, the zinc chloride in a mouth wash).

Aluminum subacetate, aluminum acetate (Burow's solution), and potassium permanganate are astringents used in the concentrations shown in Table 5–2.

Keratoplastic Actions

Many chemicals cause an apparent destructive (keratolytic) or stimulant (keratoplastic) action on the epidermis depending upon the concentration used. The process is comparable to the more familiar results of constant rubbing or other trauma to an area of the skin. The trauma may denude an area, or, if it is continued for a longer time, may result in stimulation of the basal layers and produce a much thickened cornified layer which is apparent as a callus. Keratolytic drugs, therefore, are those that remove the

cornified layer by chemical damage. A keratoplastic effect is seen when the drug does not produce rapid destruction and desquamation but a slower or milder process that increases basal layer activity and a thickened cornified layer.

Keratoplastic drugs include the following: (1) salicylic acid, 1–2%; (2) coal tar and other tars; and (3) those substances grouped together as reducing agents—eg, sulfur, chrysarobin, and pyrogallic acid in low concentrations.

Keratolytic Actions

Keratolytic drugs act to damage the cornified layer of the skin which is then sloughed off to whatever depth the agent has acted. The very strong agents such as the caustics used on warts or calluses act by dehydrating the horny tissue. Ointments act by hydrating (macerating) the cornified layer which then separates and is thrown off.

Those drugs listed above as keratoplastic are keratolytic when used in greater concentrations. These and other keratoplastics are salicylic acid, 5–20%; resorcin (resorcinol), 2–30%; chrysarobin, 0.1–10%; and anthralin, 0.1–5%.

Topical agents used in the treatment of **eczema, psoriasis,** and **seborrheic dermatitis** are often discussed as separate groups. The management of these difficult problems has been somewhat simplified by some recently introduced drugs, but definitions of a few old irritants and antiseptics are introduced here.

A. Tar: Crude coal tars are prepared by the destructive distillation of coal, gas, shale, or wood. Their composition is variable.

Tars are keratoplastic and keratolytic. Their effect is intensified by ultraviolet light, which itself alters the epidermis.

Tars have been displaced to a large extent by the corticosteroids but are still used against persistent psoriatic lesions.

Crude coal tar is used in 5–10% concentrations in antiseborrheic shampoos and applied in a thin layer directly to psoriatic lesions. Liquor carbonis detergens is a solution of coal tar with detergent. Ichthammol is tar prepared from fossil fish remains in shale. It is a mild, water-soluble tar. Unless one has a special interest in and experience with these drugs, proprietary preparations of tar should be used.

B. Chrysarobin and Anthralin: These very irritant substances are mentioned for identification and because they suggest the nature of the active component in tar. Chrysarobin is a mixture of hydroxylated polycyclic substances—eg, emodin—from a South American tree. It irritates normal skin, must not be used near the eyes, and stains clothing, hair, and skin.

Anthralin is a pure substance, a trihydroxy anthracene, comparable to chrysarobin but more potent and without its staining properties.

C. Sulfur: Sulfur in fine enough particles (microcrystalline or precipitated and colloidal) is an anti-infective agent and also reduces the activity of the sebaceous glands and dries the skin. Its principal

TABLE 5—4. Some representative dermatologic preparations not detailed in text. For topical antibiotics and corticosteroids, see Index.

Common Name	Prescriptions	Instructions and Remarks
Sulfur-salicylic acid ointment	Sulfur 1–3 Salicylic acid 1–3 Petrolatum, qs ad 100	Apply locally as needed. A potent fungicide. *Note:* Not for acute or subacute lesions.
Ointment of benzoic and salicylic acid (Whitfield's)	Benzoic acid 6 Salicylic acid 3 Polyethylene glycol ointment, qs ad 100	Apply locally at bedtime. Fungicide. Often prescribed in ½–¼ strength. Not for acute or subacute lesions.
Alcoholic Whitfield's solution	Salicylic acid 2 Benzoic acid 4 Alcohol, 40%, qs ad 120	Apply locally. Effective fungicidal combination. May substitute bay rum for alcohol.
Antiseborrheic shampoo	Selsun, Fostex, Sebulex, Capsebon, Alvinine, Sebical	Contain detergents, salicylic acid, sulfur compounds, tar and allantoin, or quinolone. Some may cause excess oiliness.
Ammoniated mercury ointment	Ammoniated mercury 5 Liquid petrolatum 3 Petrolatum, qs ad 100	Apply locally as required for seborrheic dermatitis and psoriasis.
Acne lotion	Sulfur, ppt Zinc sulfate a̅a̅ 3.6 Sodium borate Zinc oxide a̅a̅ 6 Acetone 30 Camphor water Rose water, a̅a̅, qs ad 120	Apply locally at night for acne.
Fungicidal Tolnaftate solution	Tinactin solution, 10 ml	Apply twice daily for dermatophyte (tinea) fungal infections. Ineffective for onychomycosis.
Haloprogin (Halotex)	Solution and cream	
Amphotericin B (Fungizone)	Fungizone lotion, 30 ml	Apply twice daily and as needed for mucocutaneous candidiasis.
Nystatin (Mycostatin)	Nystatin, 100,000 units/gm dusting powder, 15 gm	Dusting powder twice daily for candidiasis.
Gentian violet	1% aqueous solution	Antiseptic (gram-positive organisms) and fungicide (candidiasis).
Acrisorcin cream	Akrinol cream, 50 ml	Apply twice daily for tinea versicolor. Avoid eyes and genitalia.
Sodium thiosulfate	10% aqueous solution	Fungicide (especially for tinea versicolor).
Parasiticidal Gamma-benzene hexachloride (1%) (lindane)	Kwell cream, 60 ml	Apply each night for 3 nights. Useful scabicide.
Chlorophenothane (DDT)	10% in talc (also 2% emulsion)	Apply 15–30 gm twice daily for 2–3 days over the entire surface of underwear, and treat seams on inside of shirt and trousers. Effective against all pediculoses.

remaining use is in the treatment of acne. Many proprietary acne creams, cakes, and lotions contain 4–8% sulfur together with the keratolytic resorcinol.

D. Ammoniated Mercury: This is aminomercuric chloride ($HgNH_2Cl$). It was once used as a 5% ointment as a topical antiseptic and is still occasionally used in psoriasis.

Antibacterial Actions

Antibiotics should be used topically only for the most superficial infections—eg, impetigo or superficial folliculitis or pyoderma. The antibiotic used should have a low sensitizing potential and should preferably not be one of those commonly used systemically.

Systemic antibiotics can profoundly alter dermatologic disease, including some that are not primarily infectious in origin. In acne, for example, tetracycline, 250 mg 1–2 times daily, may reduce pustule formation and possibly alter the general course of the process by modifying the fats elaborated by the skin.

Anti-inflammatory Corticosteroids

The availability of corticosteroids for systemic and topical application has made the treatment of many dermatologic problems much simpler and much more effective. This important drug group is discussed in detail in Chapter 35 where the corticosteroids most commonly used by topical application are listed.

Antifungal Actions

The deep mycoses require treatment with systemically acting drugs such as the antibiotics discussed in Chapter 55. The superficial mycotic infections may also be treated with an orally administered antibiotic, griseofulvin, but the most common fungal infections of the skin are treated with topical agents. The topical antifungal agents may act on the infecting organism to inhibit its growth or they may alter the condition of the cornified layer of the epithelium in which the fungus grows.

A. Dermatophytosis (Athlete's Foot): The prevention and treatment of mild cases of athlete's foot depend upon careful drying of the feet after bathing and the use of dusting powders. Very acute lesions with fissuring and pain may require astringent soaks (see aluminum subacetate in Table 5–2) until the acute process subsides. Thereafter, zincundecate ointment, half-strength Whitfield's ointment, or tolnaftate solution may be used until careful personal hygiene and powders are again adequate.

B. Tinea Capitis (Ringworm of Scalp): Griseofulvin (Grisactin, Grifulvin) is an antibiotic that is deposited in keratinous structures and apparently acts by interfering with reproduction of the fungal elements.

Griseofulvin is employed orally against dermatophyte or "ringworm" fungal infections. It is most effective for ringworm infections of the scalp and quite effective for involvement of the face, neck, and trunk; reasonably effective against ringworm of the groin; and much less effective for involvement of hands and feet. Nail infections are least responsive to griseofulvin therapy.

For ringworm of the scalp, griseofulvin should be given for at least 2 weeks in doses of 0.125 or 0.25 gm 2 times daily. With extensive involvement, the initial daily dose may be 1 gm. The dosage for children is safely predicted on the basis of weight—ie, approximately 10 mg/kg/day. The microcrystalline form of griseofulvin (Grisactin, Grifulvin) is better absorbed than the older preparations.

C. Tinea Corporis (Body Ringworm):

1. Griseofulvin as for tinea capitis.

2. Tolnaftate (Tinactin) is a topical agent that can be used in place of griseofulvin unless the infection involves the nails.

3. Sulfur-salicylic acid ointment. (See Table 5–4.)

Parasiticidal Actions

A. Scabies: Infestation with this mite is easily treated with gamma benzene hexachloride (lindane, Kwell cream). Benzyl benzoate and crotamiton are also effective.

B. Pediculosis: Body, head, and pubic lice are controlled by DDT used on the infected areas and on the clothing. Benzene hexachloride is also useful against crab (pubic) lice.

·   ·   ·

DIMETHYL SULFOXIDE
(DMSO)

DMSO, $(H_3C)_2=S=O$, is a colorless liquid used as a solvent in the paint and other industries. It is highly polar and dissolves a great variety of both water-soluble and lipid-soluble substances. It has had investigational use as a vehicle for drugs and by virtue of its own properties.

DMSO applied topically in concentrations of 70% or greater has an anti-inflammatory action that has been used experimentally for the relief of symptoms associated with arthritis, bursitis, and scleroderma.

Drugs dissolved in DMSO penetrate the keratinized layer of the skin far more rapidly than when they are dissolved in other vehicles. The increased rate of absorption has been shown by measuring both systemic and local effects and is observed with drugs that are water- or lipid-soluble, charged or neutral.

DMSO has a very low acute systemic toxicity and does not alter the toxicity of drugs injected in DMSO rather than in aqueous solutions. Applied topically, especially in greater concentrations (90%), it is a histamine liberator and may cause redness or whealing.

In 3 of the animal species so far studied (dogs, rabbits, and pigs), the chronic administration of large doses of DMSO alters the optical properties of the central area of the lens. The refractive power of the lens becomes more like that of the aqueous than that of the cortical area of the lens, creating the effect of a lens within the lens. Because of this toxic effect (and perhaps also because the clinical investigation of DMSO had become undisciplined in many cases), the drug was briefly deprived of even its investigational status. It is now again available for investigational studies in humans.

Dimethylacetamide and dimethylformamide are solvents with properties similar to DMSO.

•   •   •

General References

Kligman, A.M.: Topical pharmacology and toxicology of dimethyl sulfoxide. JAMA 193:796–804, 923–928, 1965.

Lerner, M.R., & A.B. Lerner: *Dermatologic Medications,* 2nd ed. Year Book, 1960.

Rubin, L.F., & P.A. Mattis: Dimethyl sulfoxide: Lens changes in dogs during oral administration. Science 153:83–84, 1966.

Stoughton, R.B., & W. Fritsch: Influence of dimethyl sulfoxide (DMSO) on human percutaneous absorption. Arch Dermat 90:512–517, 1964.

Sulzberger, M.F., Wolf, J., & V.H. Witten: *Dermatology: Diagnosis and Treatment,* 2nd ed. Year Book, 1961.

6...

Toxicity of Therapeutic Agents

The toxic effects of specific drug groups and individual drugs vary widely as would be predicted from their diverse pharmacologic effects. The adverse reactions that may occur are discussed for individual drugs in the subsequent chapters. There are, however, some aspects of toxicity that are relevant to all drugs, and these will be discussed here. The toxicity of common environmental—ie, nontherapeutic—agents is discussed separately (Chapters 64–66).

The topics to be discussed in this chapter are: (1) the general evaluation of drug toxicity (especially of new drugs) and the problem of identifying and measuring risk; and (2) allergic reactions to drugs.

SIGNIFICANCE OF ANIMAL TOXICITY STUDIES

There are many reasons why toxicity data from experiments on normal animals cannot be directly extended to diseased human beings. Nevertheless, these data do have considerable predictive value, and it is essential that they be collected before a new drug is tried in humans. Dose-related toxicity can usually be predicted in this way, and the potency of a new drug can be compared with older drugs to the extent that the toxic effect is an extension of the desired pharmacologic action.

In most countries, the animal toxicity studies that must precede trials of new drugs in humans are to some extent determined by law or the administrative orders of a regulatory agency. The details mentioned below reflect one suggested set of requirements for preclinical testing.

Acute Toxicity

Acute toxicity is measured by the median lethal dose, or LD_{50}. This is the dose that will kill 50% of a group of animals under stated conditions—ie, it is a statistical expression of the dose which will kill an animal of average sensitivity to the drug. The LD_{50} is an assay, not a measurement. It is not an absolute value but will vary from laboratory to laboratory and even when the assay is repeated in the same laboratory. The experimental conditions of the assay must be standardized. Both the species and the strain of the animals should be recorded, as well as the route of administration, the vehicle in which the drug is dissolved or suspended, and the concentration and volume of the solution injected. Diet, ambient temperature, season, and other variables are not easily controlled; for this reason, a standard related drug should be studied for comparison. In the USA, 4 species must be used, including one nonrodent form. The routes of administration must be those that are to be used in man.

Subacute & Chronic Toxicity

Preliminary to an extended chronic toxicity test, a subacute toxicity experiment is usually the second step in preclinical toxicity testing. It extends for 14–21 days and establishes the minimal toxic and maximal tolerated dose as well as a possible role of cumulation and tolerance. It is essential to the design of an extended toxicity test.

The chronic toxicity experiment is the third step. The drug is given to animals of 2 species for 90 days in at least 3 dosage levels, one of which is the predicted therapeutic level and one the level at which at least minimal toxicity occurs. Growing animals are used for this test, and weight gain during the experiment is compared with that of a control group. Gross and histopathologic examinations are done at the conclusion of the experiment. The chronic toxicity test in dogs must (in the USA) continue for 1 year, but early clinical trials may be initiated after 3 months of testing.

Other Toxicity Tests

Depending upon the anticipated use of the drug, special toxicity tests may be required. If the drug is to be recommended for use in women of childbearing age, possible teratogenicity must be studied. For this purpose the drug is given to both male and female rats prior to the first mating and extending through the production of 2 litters. The results of these animal studies are of questionable validity with respect to the possible effects of the same drug on the human fetus, and for this reason most recently introduced drugs are still considered to be of unestablished safety for use early in pregnancy.

Other drugs may need to be studied in newborn animals or, if they are to be used topically, must be studied for possible irritant effects on the skin. Prospective anesthetic agents are administered for 3 hours a day for at least 5 consecutive days in lieu of the above chronic toxicity tests.

Prediction of Toxicity by Pharmacologic Grouping

While the toxicologic data are being collected, general pharmacologic observations are being made. These usually allow a new drug to be placed in a general chemical or therapeutic drug class and thus frequently permit the prediction of adverse effects by analogy with familiar drugs.

Therapeutic Index

Absolute toxicity is less important than the ratio between the toxic and the therapeutic dose. Reference is often made to a median effective dose or ED_{50}—ie, the dose that is therapeutically effective in 50% of a population similar to that on which the median lethal dose (LD_{50}) was determined. The ratio LD_{50}/ED_{50} is then calculated as a "therapeutic index." However, in very few drug groups is a therapeutic effect measured in animals which is comparable to the desired effect in human beings. Furthermore, because the physician hopes to avoid even an isolated fatality due to direct drug toxicity, the dosage that produces the dose-limiting side-effect or first dangerous toxic sign is of greater importance than the therapeutic index. The concept of a therapeutic index thus has value mainly as an abstraction emphasizing that toxicity is relative rather than absolute.

EVALUATION OF TOXICITY IN THE HUMAN

Investigative Drugs

The first trials on human beings of a potentially useful pharmacologic agent may begin while the chronic animal toxicity tests are still in progress. These earliest human studies are done as part of the phase I testing of a new drug as defined in Chapter 3, and are usually performed on healthy volunteers. This experience serves to uncover any marked toxic effects of the drug which were not apparent during administration to animals and to establish dose, duration of action, and other factors necessary to design further clinical investigations. Further studies on larger groups of patients with the disease or symptom against which the drug is to be used then serve to prove or disprove the usefulness of the preparation. At the same time, they begin to uncover adverse reactions that occur with a low incidence. The number and severity of allergic reactions especially—which cannot be predicted on the basis of animal studies—can be accurately evaluated only after hundreds or thousands of subjects have received the drug.

After this stage in the evaluation of a new drug, a judgment is made by the Food and Drug Administration about whether the possible usefulness of the drug outweighs its possible dangers, and permission to market the drug is given or denied.

Quantitation of Risk of Agents in General Use

When a new drug is released for general use, information about its toxicity may be incomplete. The total number of cases in which the drug has been used, and the number of cases seen by any one investigator, may have been too small to identify dangerous adverse reactions that occur in only one out of hundreds or thousands of patients. A drug remains under "post-marketing surveillance" for an indefinite period and may be withdrawn from the market if unexpected untoward reactions are encountered. However, there are 2 questions about many drugs that remain unanswered even after many years of widespread use: (1) the absolute incidence of adverse reactions, and (2) whether all reactions are recognized or only those that cause obscure rather than familiar signs of diseases.

A. Incidence of Reactions: To make an accurate statement about the frequency with which a particular reaction occurs, it is necessary to know the size and characteristics of the population at risk and the number of reactions. A closed group—eg, those patients on a particular service in one hospital—may be studied, but this group is not necessarily representative of all patients in and out of the hospital who are receiving the drug. Furthermore, the reporting of drug reactions is grossly inadequate. Reactions are often not recognized as drug-induced, or they may not be reported because of the feeling that a professional error is involved or because of the fear of legal action. Monitoring of hospital populations has shown that adverse reactions occur many times oftener than are recognized and recorded.

What is needed is a report of all untoward effects of a drug given to a representative sample of patients of diverse types. Such a system is not now available nor in prospect in spite of the efforts of the FDA to establish one.

Case reports and registries of drug reactions—eg, the now abandoned registry of adverse reactions of the AMA—are not adequate for quantifying the risk with any degree of accuracy. Such registries depend upon volunteered information, and there is no way of knowing what fraction of the total experience is represented. Certainly it is a very small fraction. Adequate epidemiologic studies are available in only a few situations. The example presented in Fig 6—1 has unavoidable limitations but suggests a relation between the amount of a drug used and the incidence of a particular toxic reaction.

In this book, therefore, the attempt to quantitate the frequency of drug reactions will necessarily be expressed in somewhat vague terms—eg, rare, infrequent, common—simply because more precise wording—eg, 9 cases of agranulocytosis per 100,000 administrations—is not forthcoming from the facts at hand.

B. Identification of Reactions: The foregoing suggests that, even in those cases where a causal relation is established between the administration of a drug and the appearance of a toxic effect, information about the absolute incidence of the reaction is often lacking.

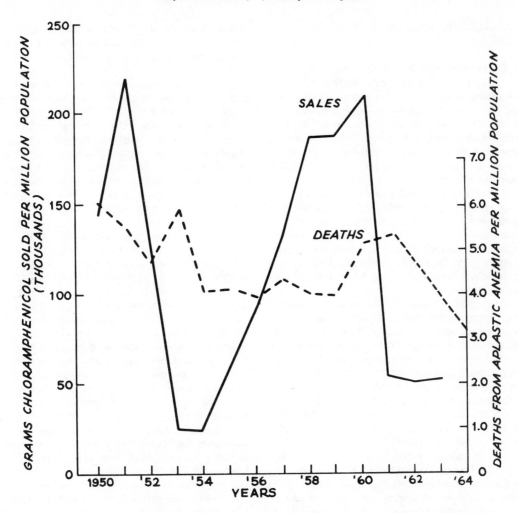

FIG 6-1. The data on the annual sales of chloramphenicol in California illustrate the transient decrease in the prescribing of a drug following public alarm about its toxicity. The increase in the number of cases of aplastic anemia following each sales peak suggests the conclusion (established by more definitive studies) that the use of chloramphenicol is associated with an incidence of aplastic anemia 13 times greater than that seen in the total population. (Redrawn, with additional figures, from California State Department of Health, Report to State Senate: *Chloromycetin—A Study of Antibiotic Drugs.* 1963.)

Another concern is that the causal relation may not be recognized if the reaction occurs infrequently, especially if the toxic reaction resembles a common complaint.

Association of a rare toxic effect of a drug with that drug cannot be accomplished by the study of single cases but only by refined epidemiologic technics. (Consider the similarity with the problem of establishing a causal relationship between cigarette smoking and cancer of the lung.) If the epidemiologic method consists merely of the accumulation of isolated case reports, uncommon toxic effects resembling a common disease would not be recognized and reported as drug-related. If a previously rare disease suddenly occurs more frequently and occurs in clusters in populations or areas of high drug use, the connection is more easily made—eg, phocomelia and thalidomide, renal papillary necrosis and phenacetin, or retroperitoneal fibrosis and methysergide. If thalidomide had merely added to the total of common congenital defects, recognition of its toxicity would have been delayed or its toxicity might not have been recognized at all. The problem of assigning responsibility for a toxic effect is made more difficult by the fact that individuals, whether patients or merely members of the total population, rarely have contact with a single drug. A degree of conservatism in adopting new chemical types of drugs is therefore justified.

Not all therapeutic misadventures are due to factors inherent in the drug itself. Prescribing and nursing errors, usually but not invariably minor, occur in a surprisingly high percentage of administrations.

ALLERGIC REACTIONS TO DRUGS

The occurrence of most adverse reactions to drugs is related to the amount taken or administered, and the exact nature of the toxic effect is determined by the properties of the drug molecule. A given patient may be unusually sensitive or resistant to a particular drug effect, but all patients will respond if the dose is great enough, and the variation in sensitivity or reactivity is normally distributed—ie, if patient response is plotted against the logarithm of the dose, the response values will be symmetrically distributed about the mean.

In contrast, allergic or hypersensitivity reactions depend on reactivity of the patient altered by prior contact with a drug that functions as an allergen or antigen. Signs and symptoms of the allergic reaction are unrelated to the pharmacologic effect of the drug but resemble instead those of other allergic reactions.

Drug molecules (except for those few that are proteins) cannot function as complete antigens but only as haptens—ie, they must chemically react with some homologous protein after administration or contact. The altered body protein is antigenic and the haptenic drug confers specificity. Fortunately, most drugs do not react as readily with protein as the simple molecules used by the immunochemist in his experiments. Penicillin is a well studied example of a drug with a reactive metabolite (penicillenic acid) that is responsible for its antigenicity.

Not all allergic reactions to drugs have been categorized immunochemically. Indeed, there are a few that have not been clearly characterized either as dose-related or allergic. Depending upon the amount of study that a particular reaction has attracted, one or more of the following criteria may be used to establish the allergic nature of an adverse reaction: (1) Circulating or cellular antibodies to the suspect drug can be demonstrated. (2) The process conforms to a known allergic pattern—eg, hives, skin rash, anaphylaxis. (3) After recovery, the process can be precipitated again in its same form by a single test dose. (4) The reaction occurs most frequently after a sensitizing period of administration. (5) The reaction is not related to dosage level (per day) or total amount administered. (The amount of antigen is important in causing sensitization, but thereafter small doses may induce the reaction.) (6) The reaction is relieved by sympathomimetics, antihistamines, or anti-inflammatory steroids.

Some examples of allergic reactions to drugs are discussed in the following section.

Immediate Allergic Reactions

Immediate allergic reactions to drugs depend upon the formation of immunoglobulins of the IgE class. The IgE or reaginic or tissue-fixed antibody specific for the drug hapten is bound to the surface of tissue mast cells or blood basophils. When the drug is subsequently reintroduced, the sensitized cells are degranulated by the reaction of antigen and antibody on their surface, releasing histamine and other substances and causing an anaphylactic or urticarial reaction.

At the same time, antibodies of the IgG and IgM (circulating) class are also formed. These may combine with antigen administered later to keep antigen from reaching tissue-fixed (IgE) antibody and thus block anaphylaxis, or the antigen-antibody complex may be deposited in blood vessels to cause serum sickness or vasculitis. The reaction may appear soon after absorption of the drug or may be delayed for several weeks; the name "immediate" is applied because the reaction to a skin test appears within minutes in those situations in which it is positive.

A. Anaphylaxis: Anaphylaxis is a rare but potentially lethal drug reaction. Anaphylaxis is inherently very dangerous, and delay in recognition, hesitancy in treatment, or lack of preparation for treatment greatly increases the possibility of death.

Anaphylaxis, unlike most other allergic reactions, can be easily studied in animals, and its characteristics are similar in the laboratory and in clinical situations. A sensitizing dose or doses must be given. After a certain minimal period without additional antigen being given, a small challenge dose of antigen causes a reaction due almost entirely to mast cell degranulation. Mast cells of different species contain varying proportions of histamine or serotonin, and the anaphylactic state will vary depending upon which amine is present and upon the reaction of different target organs in different species. Mast cells also contain heparin, kinins, and SRS (slow-reacting substance), which may also contribute to the anaphylactic reaction.

In humans, histamine release leads to bronchiolar constriction; localized edema, often in the laryngeal and glottal region; and vasodilatation with consequent hypotension and shock. Respiratory obstruction due to one or both of the first 2 effects is the cause of death in human anaphylaxis. Urticaria usually appears along with the more dangerous signs.

The treatment of anaphylaxis is outlined in Chapter 19, where the pharmacology of histamine and antihistamines is discussed. In summary, the immediate treatment consists of the injection of epinephrine, 0.5 ml of 1:1000 solution or 0.5 mg IV or IM. This sympathomimetic amine acts as a physiologic antagonist of histamine—ie, it has effects opposite to those of histamine and leads to vasoconstriction, bronchiolar dilatation, and resorption of edema. The antihistamines block further action of histamine but do not reverse changes that have already occurred. The anti-inflammatory steroids inhibit the allergic reaction and suppress allergic inflammation just as they suppress other types of inflammation. Their action is too slow for this situation, however.

Oxygen is of little value since the airway is obstructed. Tracheostomy is often mentioned as advisable, especially when intubation fails. In at least some cases, however, bronchiolar constriction prevents effective respiration even after tracheostomy.

The threat posed by an anaphylactic reaction depends upon the speed with which the reaction occurs after administration of the antigen. Treatment—ie, epinephrine—must be immediately available. If the reaction is delayed as much as 30 minutes after an injection, the situation is less threatening and an antihistamine can be used instead of epinephrine.

Almost all drugs that are injected intravenously and many that are given intramuscularly or subcutaneously have caused anaphylactic reactions. Biologicals containing horse serum and other protein drugs (chymotrypsin, penicillinase, etc) are, of course, most dangerous. Because of its wide use and pronounced allergenicity, intramuscularly administered penicillin was the most common cause of anaphylactic incidents until the adoption of oral penicillin. Anaphylaxis has been reported after oral penicillin and other orally administered drugs, but far less frequently and usually with a slow appearance and progression of signs, permitting effective treatment.

Anaphylaxis is in part mimicked by another process that occurs after rapid intravenous injection and is described as speed shock or nitritoid crisis. Almost any drug, but notably x-ray contrast media today and arsenicals in the past, can, when injected rapidly, alter the blood somehow—presumably by acting on the plasma proteins or other colloids—and cause profound vasodilatation.

B. Other Immediate Reactions: Other immediate allergic reactions are uncommon but not so rare as anaphylaxis. They neither present the same dangers nor require the same instant treatment.

1. Urticaria and angioneurotic edema—Hives and localized edema are caused more often by food allergens than by drugs. Some drugs such as morphine, codeine, and their relatives are able to liberate histamine by a direct action on mast cells. The urticaria thus produced is not allergic in origin.

2. Serum sickness and allied states—Following the administration of a drug or of biologicals containing horse serum or other heterologous serum, antibodies may build up during an incubation period of 5—14 days. There is then a sudden decrease in the amount of antigen circulating and the deposition of antigen-antibody complex in blood vessels. Whether or not the drug is still being administered, there will be the sudden appearance of fever, skin rash, adenopathy, and arthralgia. The state may persist for several days to several weeks and require corticosteroids for its relief.

It appears that the same process can lead to a vasculitis distinguishable from periarteritis by its involvement of smaller vessels and a reversible course.

3. Drug fever—Another variant of serum sickness is the sudden appearance of fever to 104° F or higher 7—21 days after the use of a drug. Drug fever has become less common as antibiotics have replaced the sulfonamides. It is most puzzling when it occurs following treatment of an infection, and a distinction must be made between a possible drug reaction and an apparent relapse. The fever usually lasts 2—3 days after the drug has been discontinued.

4. Asthma and rhinitis—These rare reactions to drugs usually occur in patients with other allergies. Some of the gums—eg, acacia and tragacanth—were frequently involved in this reaction in the past. Aspirin, quinine, sulfonamides, penicillin, and other drugs have also caused isolated cases.

5. Vasculitis—The final manifestation of this general process is a systemic vasculitis resembling polyarteritis nodosa. Penicillin and other drugs have been implicated.

C. Autoimmune Reactions:

1. Thrombocytopenic purpura—The mechanism of this reaction has been established for quinidine. It is not actually autoimmune in that neither platelets nor other homologous proteins function as the antigen. The antigen-antibody complex formed subsequent to the administration of quinidine to a sensitive patient is adsorbed onto the platelets, and they are suddenly agglutinated. Bleeding into the skin may occur, but recovery is rapid since the problem is one of peripheral destruction rather than depression of production.

2. Disseminated lupus erythematosus—The long-continued administration of a number of drugs—especially hydralazine and procainamide but also diphenylhydantoin, trimethadione, isoniazid, and others—may be followed by the appearance of a state indistinguishable clinically and in the laboratory from spontaneously occurring lupus. It is usually mild and usually regresses when the drug is discontinued. A few cases have resulted in permanent damage.

3. Hemolytic anemia—Drugs may cause hemolytic anemias by several mechanisms. They may act directly to cause hemolysis—eg, phenylhydrazine. In patients with an inherited deficiency of glucose-6-phosphate dehydrogenase in the erythrocytes, administration of many drugs—eg, primaquine, nitrofurantoin—will cause an oxidative hemolysis. Finally, at least one drug, methyldopa, can cause hemolytic anemia. In many patients the interaction of methyldopa and some ordinary red cell antigen is apparent as a positive Coombs test—ie, the presence of antibody globulin on the surface of the erythrocyte is established. In a smaller number of patients, actual hemolysis and anemia occur. The process is reversed upon discontinuance of the drug and, if necessary, treatment with corticosteroids.

Delayed Allergic Reactions

In the development of delayed hypersensitivity reactions, the drug-protein combination is identified by small lymphocytes (antigen recognition cells) as foreign. Immune cells differentiate from these AR cells and return to the skin or other antigen-containing tissue to initiate an inflammatory reaction. The inflammatory process precipitated by a delayed reaction reaches a peak only after 24—48 hours.

A. Cutaneous Reactions: Drugs acting as antigens after systemic administration can cause a great variety of cutaneous allergic reactions. Most are of the delayed type and may be a minor morbilliform rash or resemble an atopic or eczematous dermatitis or even progress to an exfoliative dermatitis.

Applied to the skin, drugs may act as primary or direct chemical irritants. However, many drugs function as antigen when applied topically. The occurrence of sensitization depends upon the patient, the drug, and the duration of exposure. For some drugs—eg, penicillin and sulfonamides—the incidence is so high that topical use has had to be abandoned.

B. Agranulocytosis: Some cases of agranulocytosis are associated with an aplastic bone marrow, are not associated with demonstrable antileukocyte antibodies, and are not controlled by corticosteroid administration. Agranulocytosis presumed to be an allergic reaction to the administration of a drug is due to the abrupt peripheral destruction of granulocytes, is associated with a cellular marrow, and usually responds promptly to treatment with corticosteroids and discontinuance of the drug responsible.

The onset of the process is abrupt and immediately severe—ie, it is not a continuation of any dose-related leukopenia and cannot be anticipated even by weekly blood counts.

Treatment other than steroids consists of antibiotics to treat the infections that develop in the absence of granulocytes. Mortality is still estimated to be 20% or higher.

C. Aplastic Anemia: No mechanism for this process has been established. Whether it is allergic or not, an association with the use of certain drugs is quite clear. Of 700 cases of aplastic anemia reported to the AMA Registry in one 7-year period, 45% of the patients had received chloramphenicol and 20% had received no other drug. Phenylbutazone, mephenytoin, gold salts, and chlorinated hydrocarbon insecticides were also implicated.

The condition is one of bone marrow depression, and leukopenia and thrombocytopenia accompany the anemia. Recovery is very slow, and mortality is variously estimated at 50—80%. The reaction may be more easily reversible if detected early. Treatment includes transfusions, antibiotics, and androgens or other anabolic steroids.

Radiation and antimetabolites cause aplastic anemia by a more direct kind of depression. In a fraction (perhaps 1/3) of the cases of aplastic anemia, no association with drugs or environmental toxins can be suggested.

●　●　●

General References

General

Jick, H., & others: Comprehensive drug surveillance. JAMA 213:1455—1460, 1970.

Meyler, L.: *Side Effects of Drugs,* vol 5. Excerpta Medica Foundation, 1966.

Mintz, M: *The Therapeutic Nightmare.* Houghton-Mifflin, 1965.

Moser, R.H.: *Diseases of Medical Progress,* 2nd ed. Thomas, 1964.

Shapiro, S., & others: Fatal drug reactions among medical inpatients. JAMA 216:467—472, 1971.

Smith, J.W., Seidl, L.G., & L.E. Cluff: Studies on the epidemiology of adverse drug reactions. V. Clinical factors influencing susceptibility. Ann Int Med 65:629—640, 1966.

Whipple, H.E. (editor): Evaluation and mechanisms of drug toxicity. Ann New York Acad Sc 123:1—366, 1965.

Drug Allergy

Baer, R., & V.H. Witten: Drug eruptions. Pages 9—37 in: *Year Book of Dermatology.* Year Book, 1960—61.

Carr, E.A., Jr. (chairman): Allergic responses to pharmacologic agents: A symposium. Fed Proc 24:39—54, 1965.

Huguley, C.M., Jr.: Hematological reactions. JAMA 196:408—410, 1966.

James, L.P., Jr., & K.F. Austen: Fatal systemic anaphylaxis in man. New England J Med 270:597—603, 1964.

Lichtenstein, L.M., & P.S. Norman: Human allergic reactions. Am J Med 46:163, 1969.

Wallerstein, R.O., & others: Statewide study of chloramphenicol therapy and fatal aplastic anemia. JAMA 208:2045—2050, 1969.

7...

Drug Abuse

Because the drugs subject to misuse present a variety of hazards, there is no single "drug problem" but a variety of problems. However, a few concepts are applicable to the misuse of drugs of all classes. By reviewing them at this point, overemphasis on drug factors can be avoided and individual and social factors stressed. The pharmacology of marihuana and the hallucinogens is discussed in this chapter also.

It is difficult to rationalize the use of any drug for nontherapeutic purposes. Even drugs that are generally pleasurable and safe and whose use is not only socially approved but in some groups almost mandatory—eg, alcohol—become destructive when used by many individuals. Thus, insofar as personal use of drugs is concerned, the physician should both practice and advise the greatest caution in even experimenting with drug use. However, drug use promises to remain widespread in spite of contrary advice. In fact, the amount of experimentation with drugs—especially among the young—and the variety of agents involved have recently increased greatly, creating both social and pharmacologic problems. The health professional, invested with a presumption of technical expertise and a degree of automatic leadership, must influence the development of attitudes toward users of both old and new drugs so that the damage from both drug effects and the societal reaction can be minimized.

Patterns of Drug Abuse

Drugs are used in different patterns which may vary in their effect on the individual from benign to totally destructive. The terms "addiction" (physical and psychologic dependence) and "habituation" (psychologic dependence) were used in the past to describe some patterns of use, but these inadequate terms have been abandoned even by the expert committees that defined them. The current more or less official terminology (ie, "dependence of the ――― type") obscures the fact that a given drug may be used in a variety of patterns and is even less satisfactory.

In describing and evaluating the hazards of drug use, the following terms allow for the variety of patterns seen, imply a process of progression, and relate drug use to other social and psychologic processes.

A. Experimental Use: Drug use or abuse must begin with experimental or exploratory use, after which the individual may reject the use of the drug or progress to one of the patterns of use described below. This concept is obvious but important. If our goal is abatement rather than treatment of drug problems, our efforts should be aimed at discouraging experimentation with drugs.

B. Social Use: Social drugs are used in groups, and the common examples—alcohol and marihuana—are sedatives that relieve anxiety and facilitate group interaction. When cigarettes, coffee, or soft drinks are used as social drugs, the separation of drug and social factors becomes more complex.

The danger of the social use of drugs, like the danger of experimentation with drugs, is that it exposes those individuals who are vulnerable to a more destructive pattern of use.

C. Episodic Abuse: Excessive amounts of a drug may be used periodically. If the drug is alcohol or other sedative, the user may in his disinhibited state damage himself and others. The abuse is, however, still elective rather than compulsive.

D. Compulsive Abuse: In a number of individuals who have experimented with one drug or another, its use becomes a compulsion—ie, an act based on emotion rather than volition, recognizably irrational even to the user, but senselessly repeated to avoid the anxiety that appears if he does not repeat his compulsive act.

The hazard of developing such a compulsive pattern of use depends in part upon the personality of the individual. However, considering the fraction of the population that at some time adopts a compulsion—eg, cigarette smoking, coffee drinking, nail-picking, or adolescent masturbation—the vulnerability must be so widely distributed as to escape being called abnormal.

The probability of a given act becoming a compulsion also depends upon the sensory or pharmacologic reward that reinforces the behavior. Thus, injected opiates and injected amphetamine carry a great hazard because of the rush or feeling of orgasm that occurs at the time of injection. The mild CNS stimulating properties of nicotine make cigarettes a common vehicle of compulsion; statistically, 85% of adolescents who smoke more than one cigarette become regular smokers and cannot substitute nicotine-free cigarettes. Relief of anxiety by sedatives must also be an important reward or reinforcing factor. The percentage of drinkers of alcohol who become compulsive alcoholics is less than the percentage of heroin users or cigarette smokers who become that dependent, but the wide use of alcohol ensures a huge number of chronic alcoholics.

The compulsive drug user ("addict") has difficulty giving up his habit even when given maximal assistance.

E. Ritual Abuse: Drugs may be used with a philosophic basis or preconception—eg, LSD may be used with the expectation of achieving a religious or psychotherapeutic experience. The ritual pattern of use is not a part of the above sequence—ie, it does not develop from social use nor progress to compulsive abuse. Ritual drugs are not selected to provide some hedonistic reward, and, if the user is protected by other group members during the drug effect, the dangers are minimal. One is not committed by such a judgment to agreement with the philosophic basis for the use of the drug nor to sympathy with any associated life style.

Factors in the Development of Drug Abuse

Drugs are generally misused because they alter mood or behavior, and an understanding of their properties is important to an understanding of their abuse. However, if drug abuse depended entirely on the properties of the drugs, everyone would be using the same drug to the same extent. To understand the geographic, cultural, and temporal variations in the epidemiology of drug use, factors other than the unchanging pharmacologic effects of the drugs must be considered.

A. Individual (Psychologic) Factors in Drug Abuse: Alcohol, the most commonly misused drug, is freely available to all members of our culture, but our patterns of alcohol use vary widely. Some individuals never drink; some drink temperately and intermittently to relieve anxiety or to facilitate participation in social situations; some drink episodically to excess; and a tragically large number develop a compulsive pattern of alcohol misuse that destroys their own and other lives. The same variability occurs in response to contact with other drugs when the personality of the individual is the only variable in the situation. Yet it has not been possible to define a "user personality." Even the compulsive user of "hard" drugs does not differ greatly from the nonusing members of the group from which he comes until he has lived in the drug world for many years. (If he comes from the youthful population of a ghetto, he will probably share some immediately apparent behavioral problem with the population collected there.)

B. Group (Sociologic) Factors: Individuals form attitudes and react as members of groups. The attitudes and problems of their group will condition their use of drugs and their reaction toward people who choose to use drugs.

The social factors that interact with the properties of drugs and the individual personality can be simplified into 2 categories: (1) the attitudes of the dominant group in the culture, and (2) the often conflicting attitudes of members of the several subgroups in our society.

The attitudes of the dominant group are reflected in the laws. In western society, the laws are generally permissive of alcohol and tobacco, which are actually quite harmful, but often impose severe penalties for the mere possession of other drugs.

There are, of course, subgroups of our pluralistic society who feel that the prohibitions against their social drugs are arbitrary and unjustified by the actions of the drug. Conflict between these groups and the dominant group is inevitable.

The youthful subculture, for example, has been adopting marihuana as a social drug comparable to alcohol. The essential similarity of these 2 drugs is discussed below, yet the use of one is treated by the older generation as a serious crime and the use of the other is more than tolerated.

Other groups, at first mature intellectuals but later middle class young whites, experimented with LSD and other "psychedelics" and formed the "hippie" group, many of whom then became nominally "criminal" in their possession and use of illegal drugs but had wide influence on music, art, dress, and the attitudes of the young toward the dominant culture.

In societies such as those in the USA, most of the "drug problem" is actually a conflict between the mores of the dominant culture and the 2 subcultures that have recently gained identity: the blacks and the emerging generation.

Finally, general economic and social factors can act through the individual. Minority groups and the economically distressed contribute disproportionately to the problem of heroin use in the USA, and one opinion holds that they are vulnerable because of their poverty and repression. There have been few paths out of the ghetto, and heroin provides transient escape along with relief of aggressive feelings. The peace in Harlem had been maintained, according to James Baldwin, by Jesus and junk. An alternative opinion holds that the availability of heroin in the central city explains its wider use there; that blacks and other ethnic groups living in large cities at the time of the first epidemic of heroin use (1949–1951) were not more vulnerable, merely more exposed. The recent epidemic (1968–1972) with its involvement of more diverse groups supports the concept. In either case, the groups involved were exposed to the societal reaction mentioned below.

C. Drug Factors: For each drug class and individual drug, the possible patterns of misuse, the effect of abuse on the individual, and the effect on society must be considered. Each of the drug classes used as therapeutic agents is discussed in other chapters. Fuller discussions will be provided here about marihuana and the hallucinogens since these agents have no therapeutic usefulness and are not considered elsewhere.

1. Narcotics or opiates—Heroin, morphine, other alkaloids of opium, and various synthetics are quite dangerous for the individual because of their potential for compulsive misuse. Nevertheless, with society having now expressed its willingness to provide heroin users with huge daily doses of another narcotic, it can no longer be argued that the opiates are inherently and inevitably destructive. The heroin user is either depressed by his drug or shows no effect if he is "maintaining" on a habit of unvarying size. He is driven to antisocial acts not by the drug effect but by a compulsive need to guarantee the availability of the next fix. The dangers and the objections of society must be based on the associated criminal activity resulting from the illegality and expense of heroin—ie, the societal reaction rather than the drug effects.

Tolerance to and physical dependence on the opiates are less important than might be predicted because heroin (owing to its expense) is supplied in diluted form.

Fear of withdrawal is a factor in maintaining the habit and is the first barrier to treatment. However, withdrawal is repeatedly imposed on the average user, either by detention or therapy, without curing him. Heroin users, like alcoholics, often revert to their compulsion after prolonged periods of abstinence (as during incarceration) when physical withdrawal sickness cannot be present.

2. Major sympathomimetic stimulants—The prototype of this class of drugs is cocaine, but methamphetamine is the one most widely used. Methamphetamine (Methedrine, Desoxyn), amphetamine (Benzedrine, Dexedrine), and other diet pills are abused by oral administration, and an occasional case of compulsive oral misuse has followed therapeutic administration. The cause of greatest concern, however, is that, when injected intravenously, methamphetamine ("speed," "crystal"), causes an immediate pleasurable experience that imposes a hazard of compulsive abuse comparable to that of heroin.

An epidemic of intravenous methamphetamine abuse occurred in the young people's ghettos (eg, the Haight-Ashbury neighborhood of San Francisco) during the past few years. Not only was the effectiveness of the drug-dominated individual destroyed, but much violent behavior was generated by the drug effect and by the new, poorly disciplined illegal marketplace. The user found heroin an effective drug to terminate the speed "run," and through this experience progressed to heroin use and probably initiated the present epidemic. Abuse of intravenous amphetamines continues, but comparatively few people are now involved.

3. Minor stimulants—CNS stimulants, such as the nicotine in cigarettes and the caffeine in coffee, are listed here for 2 purposes: first, to point out that there are drugs that have been accepted as social or recreational agents; and second, to suggest that an understanding of the problem and the treatment of compulsive drug misuse is perhaps best developed by studying similar compulsive acts in those who do not regard themselves as "drug users." The compulsive use of cigarettes, for example, is, like heroin use, an act senselessly repeated despite the certainty of damage to the health not so much out of a desire to smoke as because the confirmed smoker cannot face the resulting intense, if transient, anxiety.

4. Sedative-hypnotic drugs—The dangers of misuse—ie, the effect of use on the individual and, through his altered behavior, on his society—are greatest for alcohol or other sedatives. Not only may the altered psychomotor capability and impaired judgment result in irresponsible and criminal acts if the drug acts long enough, but the hazard of developing a compulsive pattern of use is also present. It must be emphasized again that misuse of alcohol is by far the greatest problem in drug abuse.

Sedative-hypnotics that are misused include the following: (1) Alcohol. (2) Barbiturates, meprobamate, glutethimide, diazepam, and other sedatives ordinarily given by prescription. (3) General anesthetics such as ether, nitrous oxide, and phencyclidine (PCP) or the closely related ketamine. Ketamine is used as a general anesthetic and is discussed in Chapter 20, and the chemical structure of PCP is shown at that point. PCP, whether smoked or taken by mouth, is long-acting. (4) Many hydrocarbons other than the familiar general anesthetics. Gasoline and solvents in model airplane glue are the older examples. More recently, the propellants in aerosol spray cans have been used. The fluorinated hydrocarbons or Freons are comparable to halothane or chloroform. (Freon 11 is trichloromonofluoromethane.) The propellants are inhaled from a plastic bag filled from the spray can, and a high initial concentration is inhaled, sometimes causing the cardiac arrest predicted by experience with other halogenated hydrocarbons. Well over 100 fatalities have been documented as a result of this practice. (5) Marihuana (see below).

CANNABIS
(Marihuana, Hashish)

Marihuana is discussed separately from the other sedative-hypnotics because it is not a therapeutic agent and because of the controversy surrounding it. Part of the controversy is generated by the bias of those occupying 2 poles of thought: the dominant feeling that marihuana is a frighteningly dangerous drug in no way comparable to any accepted social drug, and the often equally emotional claim by groups of increasing size that it is a purely beneficent drug in no way comparable to any acceptable social drug.

Additional reluctance to summarize the pharmacology of marihuana stems from the assumption that research on its pharmacology is scant, dated, and of poor quality. Certainly, huge amounts of research remain to be done. However, the clamor for more research is in part a device to defer the changes in the laws that will inevitably come as the emerging generation becomes the majority. Furthermore, the present inability to present a consistent formulation of the pharmacology of marihuana may not be due so much to lack of data as to failure to apply some unifying concept to the fragmentary information available.

The specific data presented below suggest that marihuana is a sedative-hypnotic comparable in its effect to alcohol but that it does not have the same toxicity as alcohol.

Source & Chemistry

The various products that are smoked or ingested derive from one species of easily cultivated hemp, *Cannabis sativa*. The active principle occurs in all leaves but is especially concentrated in the flowering tops of the female plant, where a resin many times as potent as the leaves is exuded. The resin, which may be collected in concentrated form, is known as hashish in the Middle East or charas in India. The term marihuana is used in the western hemisphere to mean the mixed leaves and flowering tops of cannabis. In the USA, the term marihuana (by legal definition) embraces all parts and preparations of cannabis, including the pure resin.

The active constituent of cannabis is probably one of several isomeric tetrahydrocannabinols (THC). The delta^9-THC (Fig 7-1) reproduces the effects of the natural product.

THC is synthesized with difficulty and is not available as an illegal or street drug. The material currently being sold as THC is another sedative, phencyclidine.

Pharmacologic Actions

A. Mechanisms of Action: The effects described below establish that marihuana exerts the same diffuse depression of the CNS as the barbiturates. The ascending reticular activating system is especially sensitive to the action of marihuana; in studies on cats with electrodes implanted in the midbrain reticular formation and some of its rostral connections, the actions of an analogue of THC and thiopental cannot be distinguished.

B. Effects: The effects common to all sedative-hypnotics that provide a basis for classifying a drug as a sedative are discussed in Chapter 23 and summarized in Table 23-1. Marihuana has been shown to exert all of these effects. The actions cannot all be demonstrated after smoking the comparatively weak preparation of the leaves but are demonstrable in experiments using pure THC or synthetic analogues. They are also described in cultures where the more potent hashish is available.

1. Effect of graded doses—Marihuana or other preparations of hemp may cause sedation and can also cause a disinhibited, excited state comparable to intoxication with alcohol or barbiturates or to stage II of anesthesia. The "high" is accompanied by ataxia and impaired performance on tests of psychomotor skills. As with alcohol, one must distinguish between manifest changes in behavior (excitement) and the pharmacologic effect (depression of the CNS). Large enough doses cause a loss of consciousness (general anesthesia), and animals given lethal doses die of respiratory depression.

2. Physical dependence and withdrawal—Clinical observations of hashish smokers suggest that withdrawal symptoms are unusual or mild. Experimentally—ie, for purposes of classification—withdrawal can be shown. After 26-31 days on large doses of a synthetic analogue of THC (synhexyl), abrupt discontinuance of the drug was followed on the third day by a hyper-excitable state relieved by the drug. In another experimental situation, great numbers of marihuana cigarettes were smoked for 39 days, but withdrawal symptoms were not observed after discontinuance.

3. Dreamy state—An additional area of confusion or controversy is introduced when marihuana is characterized as a "mild hallucinogen." The effect referred to is better described as a dreamy state with an increased tendency to fantasize and to accept suggestion. Such a dreamy, hypnagogic state can be induced with alcohol or almost any one of the sedatives or anesthetics under appropriate conditions. The state is most easily produced with nitrous oxide and was a problem during the use of this gas to provide analgesia for dental procedures. Additional examples are the thiopental interview, the street use of phencyclidine, and the transient "hallucinatory" state described during the therapeutic use of chlordiazepoxide (Librium).

If marihuana is classified as a "mild hallucinogen," it will be invested with the mystic values of LSD and rational discussion of its use will become even more difficult.

4. Other effects—Various preparations of cannabis have been shown in animals and humans to be anticonvulsants and to depress polysynaptic spinal cord reflexes—effects that are not important in its use but emphasize the similarity to other sedatives. The drug increases the appetite and has a minor vasodilating effect often apparent as injection of the conjunctivas. Strong preparations may cause vomiting after inhalation. Cross-tolerance with alcohol has been demonstrated in animals.

Absorption, Metabolism, & Excretion

When any cannabis preparation is smoked, the effect quickly reaches a maximum but persists for only a short time—ie, even though the drug remains in the body for a longer period, the effect quickly passes from excitement to a lesser sedative effect. Redistribution of the lipid-soluble THC presumably occurs rapidly, as with thiopental. When larger amounts are ingested by mouth, absorption is slower, the duration of action is longer, and the similarity to alcohol becomes more apparent.

Uses

Cannabis has no therapeutic applications, and the problem of its use as a social drug would not be altered if it did.

Adverse Reactions

A. Disinhibited Behavior: The brief duration of the high achieved by smoking marihuana minimizes the problem of drug-induced criminal activity, but social missteps do occur. Psychomotor performance is impaired if large enough doses are taken. As after the use of alcohol, the manifest behavioral change in any one individual—eg, sedation or excitement—will depend upon the individual and the setting. The assassins, a radical Islamic sect, used hashish and carried out political assassinations, but the assassinations were elaborately planned, not carried out in a drunken state.

B. Potential for Abuse: Marihuana as currently available in the USA ("grass") appears to have a low potential for the development of a compulsive pattern of use. If one looks outside of our culture to the Moslem world, it appears that a compulsive pattern of use of hashish, with results comparable to those of chronic alcoholism, is indeed possible. Alcohol is forbidden in the Moslem world, but hashish is available.

C. Anxiety Reactions: Practically all of the complaints brought to the physician by marihuana smokers are manifestations of anxiety. The experienced user is unconcerned and confident of his ability to minimize overt changes in his behavior. Other individuals may fear the loss of controls or disinhibition, or may feel guilt. The tendency of the youthful subculture to regard grass as "psychedelic" increases anxiety by suggesting toxic effects similar to those popularly ascribed to LSD.

D. Legal: A nonpunitive, understanding attitude will often be interpreted as permissive. Any discussion of marihuana must in fairness, therefore, include a warning about the extreme penalties imposed in most areas for the mere possession of even small amounts of the drug.

E. Progression to Use of Other Drugs: The punitive attitudes toward marihuana users are maintained in part by the excuse that, even if marihuana is not inherently extremely dangerous, its use leads to abuse of heroin and other hard drugs. Virtually all heroin users have had experience with marihuana prior to their use of heroin. They have also had prior contact with alcohol and many other factors for which no causal relationship is suggested. Considering that marihuana use involves millions and is increasing and that heroin abuse involves 100–200 thousand people and has not increased correspondingly, no correlation or progression can be claimed.

Marihuana use can lead to experimentation with other drugs to the extent that criminalization of marihuana use encourages association with neighborhoods, individuals, and subcultures that favor experimentation.

THE HALLUCINOGENS

Drugs from several pharmacologic classes are able to disorganize neural function and produce a toxic psychosis or acute brain syndrome. The toxic state is characterized by alterations in perception that culminate in hallucinations. These agents have been called hallucinogenic, psychotomimetic, or psychedelic drugs. Except for some uncommon ritualistic uses, these drugs were primarily of toxicologic interest until recently, when 2 factors led to an increase in interest concerning them.

The first factor was the assumption that the drug-induced hallucinatory state provided a model of schizophrenia. It was reasoned that, if these chemical agents can cause an altered state that accurately mimics the spontaneously occurring psychosis, they might be useful in the investigation of a postulated biochemical basis for schizophrenia or that descriptions of the experience after experimental induction in volunteers might contribute to our understanding of psychotic behavior. The second reason for renewed interest is that some individuals have attributed great personal value to the "consciousness-expanding" effect of the hallucinogens.

1. LSD ("Acid")

Lysergic acid diethylamide is a chemically modified ergot alkaloid (Table 14–1). Pharmacologically, LSD is unusual in its potency—100 μg causes observable changes in behavior—and in its ability to cause the desired changes in perception with a minimum of sympathomimetic effects. The total duration of its effect is approximately 8 hours. Tolerance develops after a single dose, and the effects cannot be duplicated within 2–3 days.

Pharmacologic Effects

A. Altered Perception: The intensity of behavioral changes depends upon the dose and time since ingestion. Initial effects or the effects of small doses may be limited to variable degrees of euphoria or anxiety and feelings of depersonalization. Subsequently, there is progressive alteration of perception of tactile, visual, and auditory stimuli. Colors and sounds develop unexpected qualities, or objects change appearance. Delusions occur—ie, objects or sounds actually present are falsely perceived. Finally, in a rare person after a large dose, hallucinations may occur—ie, voices or objects are perceived in the absence of any stimuli. At this time, paranoid ideation and panic are common.

When acid or other hallucinogens are knowingly ingested, the subject recognizes that his symptoms are drug-induced—ie, the ability to test reality is retained to a greater or lesser degree, and the drugs do not mimic a true schizophrenic experience.

B. Meaning to the Individual: In the absence of preconditioning or philosophic preparation, the LSD experience is anxiety laden and only an occasional person will use the drug repeatedly for amusement or for the minor euphoria induced. If an individual accepts instruction from an enthusiast or proselytizer, the experience may develop one of 2 meanings, a mystical one or a psychotherapeutic one. Both groups believe that the altered perception extends to abstract ideas as well as to stimuli from physical sources.

The devout hippie uses LSD to achieve mystical understanding. The nature of this psychedelic or "consciousness-expanding" effect of LSD is no more susceptible to description than other mystical or

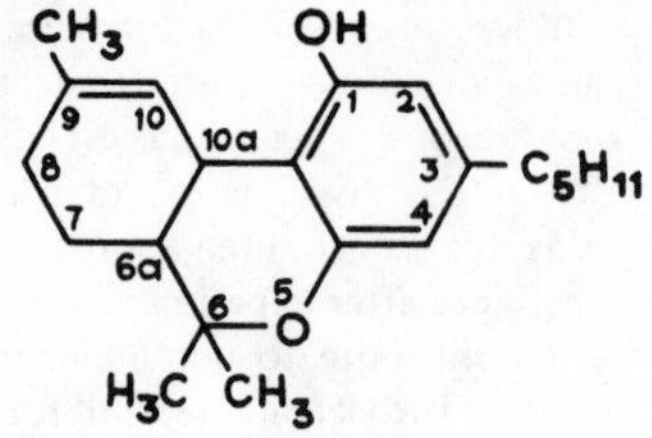

Δ⁹-Trans-tetrahydrocannabinol
(Δ⁹-THC)

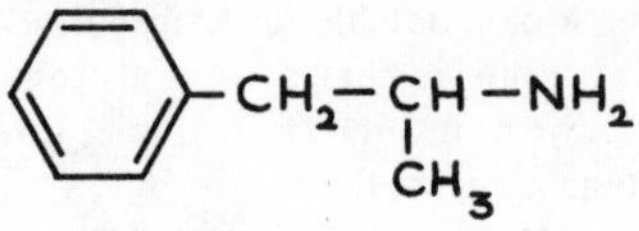

Amphetamine

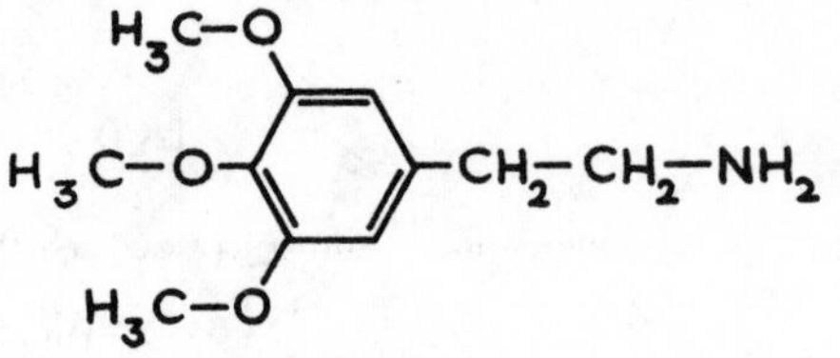

Mescaline

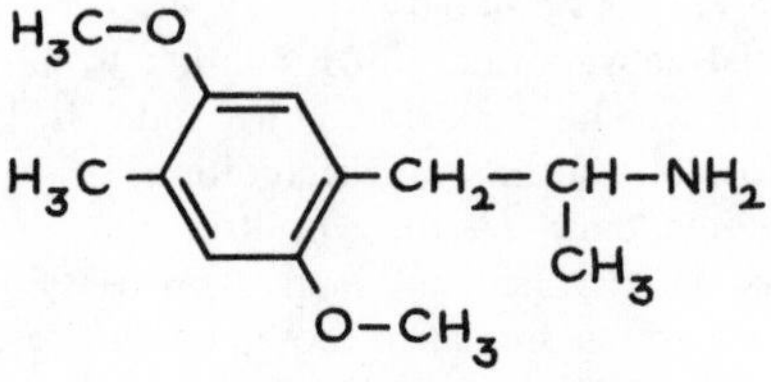

2,5-Dimethoxy-4-methylamphetamine
(STP)

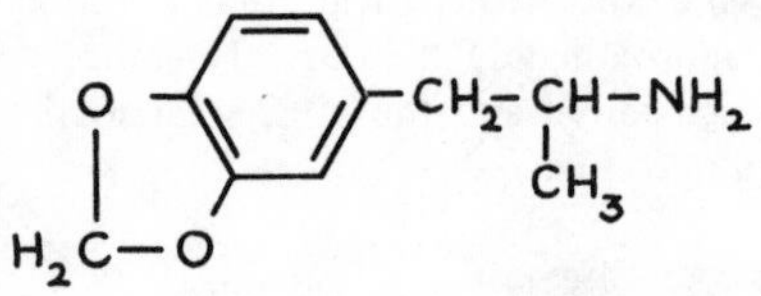

Methylenedioxyamphetamine
(MDA)

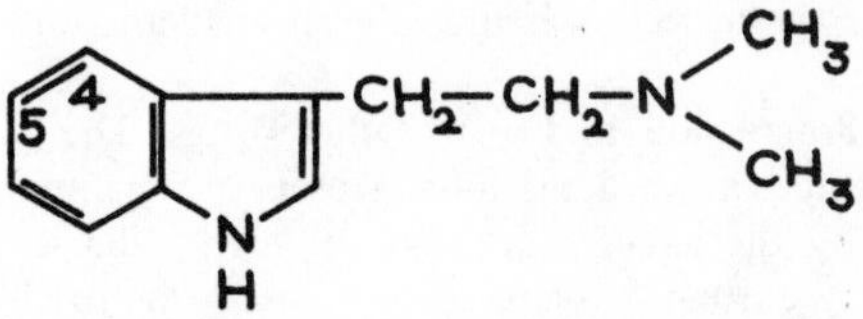

Dimethyltryptamine (DMT)

FIG 7–1. Chemical structures of certain drugs subject to misuse. THC is an active constituent of marihuana. Amphetamine is shown for comparison with 3 ring-substituted sympathomimetic amines used as hallucinogens. DMT is a representative tryptamine derivative (see also Fig 19–3). The structure of LSD is shown in Table 14–1.

religious experiences. Indeed, the analogy to religious conversion first suggested for other drugs by William James is impressive: The requirements are an individual with a need to change; an experience that serves to mark the change; and, afterward, the continued support of a like-minded group.

Another group uses LSD as a substitute or accelerating technic in a process visualized as being close to psychotherapy or psychoanalysis.

Proselytizing for the use of acid has become less effective, and the use of LSD has declined since its peak in 1967.

C. Sympathomimetic Effects: LSD causes a minor elevation in blood pressure, tachycardia, pupillary dilatation, hyperglycemia, tremulousness, awakening, and euphoria.

Clinical Uses

Suggestions that LSD can facilitate psychotherapy or be useful in the treatment of chronic alcoholism are not supported by any controlled studies.

Adverse Reactions

The reaction of an individual to LSD will be strongly conditioned by his predrug personality, his expectations of the drug, his companions, and the setting. The common adverse reactions ("bad trips") are manifestations of anxiety.

A. Anxiety Reactions During the Drug Effect: Somatic feelings of depersonalization, distorted perception, and the content of delusional material may be very alarming and lead to anxiety that may be minor in degree or may lead to panic and uncontrolled excitement at the peak of the drug effect. These reactions are most likely to occur in inexperienced users, in disturbing or threatening environments, or in subjects who have ambivalent attitudes toward the drug experience. Most bad trips are handled within the group of users rather than by a physician.

Treatment usually requires only reassurance that the subject will return to normal when the drug effect dissipates and explanation that the symptoms are drug-related. LSD induces a suggestible or hypnagogic state that makes it easy to inadvertently suggest a bad reaction but also makes it easy to establish the relationship between the drug and the symptom. If the patient cannot be "talked down," drugs may be used. A sedative (anti-anxiety) agent usually is preferable. In a few subjects, the panic may be so intense that it is necessary to terminate the reaction with chlorpromazine (50 mg orally or IM) or similar major antipsychotic tranquilizer.

B. Flashbacks: Flashing (the sudden recurrence of perceptual distortions experienced during a drug experience) is a common occurrence. Flashing is commonly precipitated by the use of other drugs or by some stimulus that reminds the person of the previous experience, but the flashback may be spontaneous. Experienced users recognize them as learned behavior and do not present them as complaints. Patients who are anxious about their drug use, fearing lasting brain damage or other consequences promised by the literature of drug education, may bring the complaint to the physician.

These states do not arise from any pharmacologic effect of LSD but from anxiety and misinterpretation or exaggeration of ordinary perceptions. They can almost always be treated by reassurance and explanation. If drug treatment is necessary, a sedative such as phenobarbital rather than an antipsychotic tranquilizer should be used.

C. Prolonged Psychotic Episodes: There are many reports of prolonged psychotic episodes after LSD use. However, all drug-using communities attract many disturbed people, and it is difficult to separate direct drug effects from episodes precipitated or preordained in the already ill. Acid cannot be exculpated, but it is a mistake to focus on the drug if such interest obscures the underlying problem.

It is similarly difficult to apportion responsibility for suicide among users of "psychedelics." Only a few of the suicide attempts take place while the drug is acting, and the coexistence in the same personality of the tendency toward suicide, drug use, and religious conversion was described long before LSD was used.

D. Chromosomal Damage: LSD has been shown to increase the number of chromosomal breaks in cultured white cells and in cells from skin biopsies. Mutagenic chemicals known to be carcinogenic or teratogenic have the same effect. So, however, do a number of common drugs used without special concern—eg, alcohol, caffeine, menadione, and ergonovine. There are no epidemiologic data that associate LSD with an increased incidence of congenital defects.

The early laboratory studies were probably overinterpreted, but there is no reason to except LSD from the rule that only essential drugs be used during the first trimester of pregnancy. LSD is an ergot derivative capable of contracting the pregnant uterus. Anecdotal evidence suggests that this effect has caused fetal death, so that the caution should actually extend throughout pregnancy.

2. OTHER AGENTS

All of the drugs listed below cause a similar toxic psychosis. The several drugs may also have distinctive side-effects—eg, LSD and the sympathomimetics cause anxiety, pupillary dilatation, and similar sympathomimetic effects; and the parasympatholytic agents add amnesia for the experience. Most of these drugs are discussed in other chapters (see Index).

Sympathomimetic Stimulants

All of these drugs cause side-effects such as anxiety, tremulousness, elevated blood pressure, and pupillary dilatation to a greater extent than does LSD.

A. Methamphetamine, Amphetamine, Cocaine, and Others: Drugs related to amphetamine are misused for their euphoriant effect but not for their hallucinogenic effects. Most individuals who use huge amounts of amphetamine by mouth (up to 2 gm/day) or who use methamphetamine intravenously have experienced the hallucinatory state. Except during a most severe paranoid reaction, they recognize the drug origin of their hallucinatory or euphoric state and avoid hospitalization.

B. Hallucinogenic Amphetamine Congeners: Amphetamine congeners with a lipophilic substituent on the ring may act more rapidly and more intensely on the CNS. Several of these have been used as substitutes for LSD—eg, STP and MDA (Fig 7–1). STP and MDA have properties similar to those of LSD.

C. Peyote and Mescaline: Buttons from a small cactus that grows in the Sonoran Desert have long been chewed to derive the effect of the active principle, mescaline. Use of peyote has been incorporated into the religious rituals of some American Indians. Mescaline (chemically related to epinephrine) was popularized as a hallucinogenic agent in the cities in the early 1950s, and its use paved the way for LSD. Recently, the drug sold as mescaline has been STP.

D. Tryptamine Derivatives: Serotonin or 5-hydroxytryptamine (see Chapter 19) occurs in several areas of the brain. Exogenous serotonin does not reach the cells of the CNS, but a number of other tryptamine derivatives are active as stimulants and hallucinogens and have been used ritually in the past and are now used as LSD equivalents. Psilocybin is the phosphate ester of psilocin (4-hydroxydimethyltryptamine) isolated from a Mexican mushroom and active after oral administration. DMT (dimethyltryptamine) and DET (diethyltryptamine) must be smoked rather than ingested and have a brief duration of action. They were used earlier in the form of ground seeds or cohoba snuff.

Parasympatholytics

Large doses of atropine, scopolamine, and related therapeutic agents cause a toxic psychosis characterized by an unusual degree of excitement, intensely uncomfortable side-effects, and amnesia for the experience. Occasionally, someone intrigued by the publicity given the psychedelic experience but lacking access to the usual drugs will use belladonna or an over-the-counter asthma remedy containing stramonium leaves to achieve an unsatisfactory, uncomfortable effect. Antihistamines and scopolamine (as in nonprescription sleeping tablets) occasionally cause the same excited hallucinatory state.

Sedative-Hypnotics & General Anesthetics

Toxic psychoses resulting from repeated administration of bromides are still seen. However, withdrawal rather than continued administration of hypnotics is the more common cause of delirium. Alcohol is, of course, the most commonly involved drug.

If a protracted stage like that of stage II of anesthesia (disinhibition or excitement) can be induced with one of these drugs—eg, nitrous oxide or phencyclidine—a dream-like state suggestive to some subjects of the hallucinatory experience may occur. Volatile anesthetics have been used in the past to reach such a state, and marihuana is sometimes called a "mild hallucinogen" on the same basis.

Other Drugs & Causes of Hallucinatory States

Drugs such as narcotic antagonists (nalorphine, etc), anti-inflammatory corticosteroids, disulfiram, amantadine, and methysergide, and many disease states such as infections, dehydration, sodium depletion, and any cause of hypoxia may cause a toxic psychosis, with characteristics similar to those deliberately induced. The delusions that appear during a toxic psychosis caused by disease or by a therapeutically administered drug are more varied, are not so easily related to the precipitating cause by the patient, and are typically worse at night or in a strange place such as a hospital.

TREATMENT & ABATEMENT
OF DRUG ABUSE

The treatment and control of drug abuse is a problem that involves public policy and concerns the entire community rather than just the patient and his physician or other therapist. Emotional involvement with this subject is intense, and rational discussion is correspondingly difficult. Present public policy in the USA is based on a punitive attitude toward drug use which conflicts with the attitude of practically all of the professionals in actual contact with the problem.

The Punitive Attitude & Its Influence

This attitude accepts the judgment of the dominant culture about which drugs are acceptable and legislates vigorously against all others. Acts which do no harm to persons or property are defined as criminal, and these "crimes without victims" are punished severely—eg, it is a serious crime to merely possess certain drugs, to possess the equipment to use drugs, or to simply be in a place where drugs are kept or to be with people who possess drugs. There now seems to be a growing public and professional awareness of some of the limitations of this approach.

(1) Most important, the punitive attitude has had limited effectiveness. Prior to the enactment of the Harrison Narcotic Act in 1914, narcotics were easily available even without prescription and were misused by large numbers of people. Opiate use decreased sharply thereafter, and no one advocates a return to the unregulated availability of narcotics. However, the old pattern of oral use of narcotics was comparatively benign when compared with the subsequent patterns of intravenous use in a criminalized scene, and the punitive approach has obviously not prevented the increased use of marihuana, LSD, and other drugs.

(2) The laws are inconsistent. The public has been taught to regard narcotic addiction as the most terrible of crimes. Other drugs, some more dangerous and some less so, are uncritically lumped together as narcotics in the law, and penalties inconsistent with the properties of the drug or the possible social consequences of their use are imposed.

(3) No distinction is made between criminal activity inherent in drug misuse—which, except for alcohol, is quantitatively negligible—and associated criminal activity. By associated criminal activity is meant the provision of illegal drugs and the criminal activity into which the user, to maintain his habit, is forced by restrictive laws.

(4) Enforcement of the drug laws is possible only by the use of informers, entrapment, and search and seizure procedures that are of doubtful constitutional validity and are offensive to some citizens. The laws are not uniformly applied, and the heavy penalties prescribed, together with other defects in the system of criminal justice, make the drug laws vehicles for harassment and repression of certain ethnic groups, neighborhoods, or life styles.

(5) Labeling almost the entire emerging generation as deviant because they are experimenting with grass and acid has intensified the alienation of that group.

Treatment Problems & Technics of Management

A. Individuals Who Acknowledge No Illness: During the foreseeable future, there will continue to be a large number of drug users who regard themselves as neither criminal nor ill. The social drinker sees no reason why he should tell his physician or other advisor about his occasional use of alcohol, and the young users of marihuana view themselves in the same way.

B. Problems Unrelated to Drug Abuse: To the extent that drug use is symptomatic of individual and social ills, expansion of general treatment facilities and social and economic change will have an impact on drug use.

C. Acute Drug Reactions: Acute intoxication with stimulants or depressants, adverse reactions to LSD or other hallucinogens, or withdrawal should be treated as medical problems rather than as police problems. Not only is such care safer and more effective, but, more important, more patients could then be induced to accept aftercare from a medical facility.

D. Compulsive Drug Use: The special treatment procedures applicable to the compulsive use of alcohol and narcotics are discussed in the relevant chapters. The general types of treatment can be summarized as follows:

1. **Psychotherapy**—Conventional psychotherapy is not impressive in this context. Once the compulsive user acknowledges a need to change and himself solicits treatment, a number of different medical or self-help facilities have significant success. The patient learns, usually slowly, to give up his compulsion and is helped by the supervision of his peers and by removal from a threatening environment. The size of the problem is such that community-based facilities rather than the usual medical institutions must be used.

2. **Pharmacologic blockade**—The use of alcohol becomes intolerably sickening after the administration of disulfiram (Alcophobin, Antabuse). Neither the immediate nor the delayed effects of injected heroin appear if a patient is maintained on continuous doses of methadone or a narcotic antagonist.

3. **Regulated access**—Since neither the purely punitive nor the purely medical approach offers a high rate of success in the case of narcotic use, a third alternative embodying the concept of regulated access to the drug is used in some countries. Such a program continues to impose jail sentences for criminal activity but not for mere use or possession. It insists that the addict identify himself and accept treatment and supervision. However, in cases of treatment failure, it offers an alternative to jail by providing maintenance doses of drugs if that is the only way the user can be maintained within the community. This form of treatment removes the user from those associations that initiated or perpetuated his addiction. Such a program is repugnant to many citizens because it tolerates the "stabilized addict."

British law permits dispensing narcotics even for intravenous use, to an addict, and the British experience is usually mentioned in this context. The British population has characteristics different from that of the USA, but the fact remains that in 1970, with a population of 50 million, there were only 1430 known heroin addicts in England (compared with a conservative estimate of 200,000 in the USA). The associated criminal activity in England is negligible when compared to that in the USA.

In the USA, the nearest equivalent is the provision of a daily oral dose of methadone, a narcotic discussed in a later chapter.

Education & Counseling

If the goal of society's effort in this area is control and prevention rather than retribution, only education and counseling offer any real hope. Dissemination of authoritative information would probably reduce experimentation with drugs, but the following cautions must be observed:

(1) The effectiveness of such efforts will be limited by the extent to which drug use is symptomatic of underlying social and individual problems, including frustration due to apparently unalterable economic conditions, ineffective families, and lack of personal goals or resources.

(2) The information presented must be scrupulously accurate and scientifically derived even if it is in conflict with the preconceptions of the teacher. The "student" will have had personal experience with drugs or will be in contact with others who have. If information from a professional source about one drug is known by the experimenter to be inaccurate, he will subsequently reject more accurate data about another drug. Again, marihuana is the drug of central importance because, if our professional proclamations about it to our young people are judged to be palpably inaccurate, our warnings about methamphetamine or heroin will also be rejected. Personal experimentation with drugs is thus encouraged since it is judged to be the individual's only dependable source of drug information. The consequences, already apparent, have been the epidemic of methamphetamine abuse followed now by the occurrence of compulsive heroin use among white middle class youth. It is the professional drug expert's obvious duty to maintain his credibility among those groups who are most apt to need his advice. This must be done even at the risk of disapproval from others in the community who might hope that their proscriptions against all drugs will be uncritically heeded. Unfortunately, the young people who must be dealt with in this context are already partially alienated from the establishment we represent, and they have reserved to themselves the decision about what to believe.

(3) Drugs accepted by the older dominant culture must be examined as objectively as the new drugs. Alcohol and cigarettes must be acknowledged as major problems and condemned as freely as marihuana.

● ● ●

General References

General

Davis, F.: Heads and freaks: Patterns and meanings of drug use among hippies. J Health Social Behavior 9:156–164, 1968.

Flowers, N.C., & L.G. Horan: Nonanoxic aerosol arrhythmias. JAMA 219:33–37, 1972.

Lewin, L.: *Phantastica: Narcotic and Stimulating Drugs.* Dutton, 1964. [Translated from the 2nd German edition (1927).]

Ludwig, A.M., Levine, J., & L.H. Stark: *LSD and Alcoholism: A Clinical Study of Treatment Efficacy.* Thomas, 1970.

New York Academy of Medicine Committee on Public Health: Report on drug addiction. II. Bull New York Acad Med 39:417–473, 1963 **or** Clin Pharmacol Therap 4:425–460, 1963.

Russell, M.A.H.: Cigarette dependence. Brit MJ 2:330–331, 393–395, 1971.

Shick, J.F.E., Smith, D.E., & F.H. Meyers: Patterns of drug use in the Haight-Ashbury neighborhood. Clin Toxicol 2:1, 1970.

Marihuana

Boyd, E.S., & D.A. Meritt: Effects of barbiturates and a tetrahydrocannabinol derivative on recovery cycles of medial lemniscus, thalamus and reticular formation in the cat. J Pharmacol Exper Therap 151:376–384, 1966.

Hollister, L.E., Richards, R.K., & H.K. Gillespie: Comparison of tetrahydrocannabinol and synhexyl in man. Clin Pharmacol Therap 9:783–991, 1968.

Kaplan, J.: *Marijuana: The New Prohibition.* World, 1970.

Lemberger, L., & others: Delta-9-tetrahydrocannabinol: Temporal correlation of the psychologic effects and blood levels after various routes of administration. New England J Med 286:685–688, 1972.

Newman, L.M., & others: Δ^9-Tetrahydrocannabinol and ethyl alcohol: Evidence for cross-tolerance in the rat. Science 175:1022–1023, 1972.

Way, E.L., & H. Isbell (editors): Symposium: Marihuana and its surrogates. Pharmacol Rev 23:263–380, 1971.

Williams, E.G., & others: Studies on marijuana and pyrahexyl compounds. Pub Health Rep 61:1059–1083, 1946.

Hallucinogens

Frosch, W.A., Robbins, E.S., & M. Stern: Untoward reactions to lysergic acid diethylamide (LSD) resulting in hospitalization. New England J Med 273:1235–1239, 1965.

Jacobsen, E.: The clinical pharmacology of the hallucinogens. Clin Pharmacol Therap 4:480–503, 1963.

Ludwig, A.M., & L. Levine: Patterns of hallucinogenic drug abuse. JAMA 191:104–108, 1965.

Part II. Autonomic & Cardiovascular Drugs

8...

Cholinomimetic or Parasympathomimetic Agents

This and the following 3 chapters deal with drugs that either mimic, intensify, or block the effects of the sympathetic and parasympathetic divisions of the autonomic nervous system. The 4 most general types of drug actions are (1) parasympathomimetic, acting like the mediators of parasympathetic nerve activity; (2) parasympatholytic, blocking the effects of the mediators of parasympathetic nerve activity; (3) sympathomimetic, acting like sympathetic nerve or adrenal medullary activity; and (4) sympathoplegic, acting by a variety of mechanisms to decrease sympathetic activity. These drug groups appear first in this survey of classes of drugs because alterations of autonomic nervous system function are also produced by most of the drugs discussed in subsequent chapters even if the drugs do not act primarily on the autonomic nervous system.

FUNCTIONAL ORGANIZATION OF THE AUTONOMIC NERVOUS SYSTEM

The term autonomic nervous system (ANS) is convenient but inaccurate since it is the peripheral organ rather than the nervous system that is autonomic. The "autonomic nervous system" consists of the nervous and humoral mechanisms that modulate and integrate the functions of the autonomous, automatic, or vegetative organs. These organs or functions include heart rate and force of contraction; the caliber of blood vessels; the contraction or relaxation of the smooth muscle of the gut, bladder, and bronchioles; visual accommodation and pupillary size; secretion from exocrine glands; and others.

The widespread interest in drugs modifying these functions is understandable. A significant fraction of all disease entities or altered physiologic states involve the autonomous end organs. Even in those instances where the etiology of the disease is not yet clarified, as in hypertension, the effective treatment may be with drugs acting on the ANS. And the large group of symptoms or disease entities that may be behavioral or psychologic in origin (migraine, asthma, peptic ulcer, neurotic conversion symptoms) must be mediated by the ANS and are usually more amenable to drug therapy than to psychotherapy.

The classification and mechanism of action of drugs that act on autonomic tissues is in large part understandable from the correlation of the anatomy of the ANS with the data on chemical transmission of nerve impulses.

Chemical Transmission

Transmission along a nerve fiber is by the spread or propagation of the wave of depolarization. There is an ultramicroscopic discontinuity or cleft between the terminations of one nerve and the cell body or processes of the next, or between the nerve and the muscle or glandular cells innervated. Transmission across this discontinuity (neuro-effector junction) is not electrical but chemical. A chemical mediator or neurohumor is liberated by the proximal nerve and acts postsynaptically to depolarize the next cell in the series to excite it to conduct, contract, or secrete. Or, if it is an inhibitory agent, it may hyperpolarize the next cell and delay depolarization.

If the ANS is divested of the anatomic complexity that it actually possesses, it can be represented as in Fig 8–1. Such a simplification allows us to correlate chemical transmission and anatomic site. In summary, it will be seen that (1) norepinephrine is the mediator liberated by sympathetic nerve endings and by a few other chromaffin cells; (2) epinephrine and a small fraction of norepinephrine are liberated by the adrenal medulla; and (3) acetylcholine is the mediator at all (both sympathetic and parasympathetic) ganglionic synapses of the ANS, at parasympathetic nerve endings, and at the voluntary nerve-muscle junction.

Sympathetic or Thoracolumbar Division of ANS

A. Sympathetic Nerves: The cell bodies of the preganglionic fibers, comparable to the anterior horn cells of the somatic nervous system, lie in the lateral horn of the spinal cord from T1 through L2 (hence the older designation, thoracolumbar). The myelinated (white) fibers leave the cord over the motor root but run only a short course before synapsing with the postganglionic fiber.

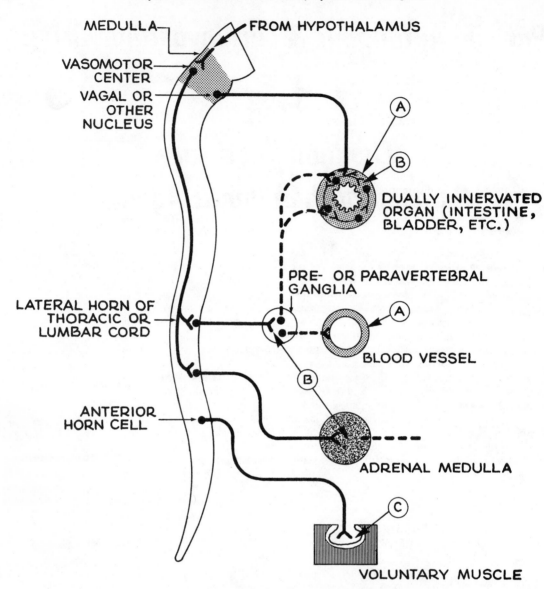

FIG 8–1. Functional organization and chemical transmission in autonomic and somatic efferent nerves. Fibers of cholinergic neurons are shown by solid lines, and the presence of a myelin sheath may be indicated. Fibers of adrenergic neurons are shown by dashed lines. The anatomic basis for the diagram is discussed in the text. The diagram should also be used to visualize the sites of action of the drugs discussed in this and the next 4 chapters. For example, cholinomimetic drugs act at the following sites: *A:* On muscarinic receptors on the effector tissue to contract nonvascular smooth muscle and stimulate exocrine glands but to relax vascular smooth muscle. *B:* On nicotinic receptors at ganglionic synapses where acetylcholine is also the mediator. Postganglionic sympathetic activity is increased, which constricts blood vessels and stimulates the heart. The adrenal medulla is also activated by agents that mimic the effect of preganglionic activity, and epinephrine is released into the circulation. *C:* On receptors on the motor end-plate of voluntary muscle to initiate contraction of single units. Cholinesterase inhibitors act at *A* and *B* by allowing the accumulation of acetylcholine, but not at *C* in blood vessels since no acetylcholine is liberated that can be protected from hydrolysis.

The collection of terminations of the first neuron in the series and the processes and cell bodies of the second neuron is called a sympathetic ganglion. These ganglion cells lie in the ganglia of the paravertebral chain or in the unpaired prevertebral ganglia.

Mediation of the impulse from pre- to postganglionic cell is by the liberation of acetylcholine. The preganglionic fiber is cholinergic, a term applied to nerve fibers that work by liberating acetylcholine.

The properties of the postganglionic fibers explain the diffuse effect of sympathetic nerve activity. There are many more postganglionic than preganglionic fibers, and the distribution of both types of fibers is not segmental, allowing for amplification and a diffuse rather than segmental distribution of postganglionic fibers.

Furthermore, the postganglionic fiber is adrenergic, ie, it exerts its influence on the effector tissue by liberating norepinephrine. This amine, like the epinephrine that enters the circulation from the adrenal medulla, is destroyed comparatively slowly (in minutes) and can exert effects distant from its site of liberation.

A further anatomic fact explains the greater effect of chemical sympathetic block compared with surgical sympathectomy. Not all sympathetic ganglion cells are located in the pre- and paravertebral ganglia. A significant number of ganglion cells lie along an embryologic migratory path between cord and periphery. These intermediate ganglia are accessible to drugs but are not removed by the usual sympathectomy that is based partly on excision of grossly visible ganglia.

The termination of the postganglionic sympathetic fibers involves at least 2 patterns. Adrenergic neurons that are vasomotor in function may terminate in the muscle layers of blood vessels. At least in the case of the intestine and bladder, the postganglionic adrenergic neuron, identified by its content of fluorescent granules of mediator, terminates in close relation to the cholinergic synapses of the parasympathetic division—ie, the effect of norepinephrine on these tissues is probably not due to an action on smooth muscle but to an inhibitory effect on the intrinsic nerves of the organ.

B. The Adrenal Medulla as a Sympathetic Ganglion: The cells of the adrenal medulla have the same embryologic origin, similar staining reactions, and the same innervation by cholinergic sympathetic preganglionic neurons as the sympathetic ganglia. The adrenal medulla can thus be thought of as a sympathetic ganglion made up of cell bodies without axons or postganglionic fibers. As expected, therefore, the secretion of the adrenal medulla (epinephrine) is similar to that of the sympathetic nerves (norepinephrine). It will also be necessary to speak of sympatho-adrenal discharge, since preganglionic discharge will activate both the sympathetic nerves and the adrenal medulla. Epinephrine, since it enters the blood stream and exerts a diffuse, widespread effect, is called a hormone rather than a neurohumor—an unimportant distinction.

C. Other Chromaffin Tissue: Other chromaffin cells that contain stores of norepinephrine that can be liberated by drugs occur in functionally significant numbers in blood vessels and in the atria. The term "intrinsic amine" is sometimes applied to these stores.

Additional data on sympathetic neurons and neuromediators are given in Chapter 10. The suprasegmental control of sympathetic neurons is discussed in Chapter 11.

Parasympathetic or Craniosacral Division

The preganglionic fibers of the parasympathetic nerves arise either from cell bodies in the motor nuclei of the brain stem or of the sacral segments of the cord. They run to or almost to the organ innervated without synapse. Parasympathetic efferent fibers make up part of the oculomotor (III), facial (VII), glossopharyngeal (IX), vagus (X), and pelvic nerves. The first 3 cranial nerves listed (III, VII, and IX) have ganglia close to but outside of the eye and glands innervated from which postganglionic fibers originate. However, all of the autonomic tissues except the uterus have ganglion cells within them. These may be well organized, as in the submucosal and myenteric plexuses of the intestine; or diffuse, as in the bladder, blood vessels, etc. The preganglionic parasympathetic fibers terminate in close relation to the ganglion cells. These ganglionic synapses are acted upon by ganglion stimulant and depressant drugs in the same manner as are the sympathetic ganglia.

It is an oversimplification to say that acetylcholine is the mediator at the parasympathetic postganglionic endings since there may be multiple synapses within the plexus between the preganglionic fiber and the neuro-effector junction.

Concept of Sympathetic-Parasympathetic Antagonism

The development of the concept of chemical mediation and the study of drugs related to the mediators have led to the assumption that drug effects necessarily define the physiologic mechanism. Pharmacologic data have been influential in strengthening the hypothesis that the activity of autonomous organs is controlled by the balance between sympathetic and parasympathetic influences. Sympathomimetic and parasympathomimetic drugs do have generally opposite actions, but the following cautions should be observed in translating that pharmacologic fact into physiologic theory.

Drugs that mimic the effects of mediators act independently of innervation. Acetylcholine acts on tissues that have no parasympathetic innervation. Each of the mediators acts more intensely on denervated effector tissue and will act on noninnervated smooth muscle such as that in umbilical vessels.

Many tissues are not dually innervated. The ciliary body has only parasympathetic innervation. The nictitating membrane, most blood vessels, and uterine muscle have only sympathetic innervation. The salivary glands, which grossly are innervated by both sympathetic and parasympathetic nerves, are made up of 2 cell types, and individuals cells are singly innervated.

The response to drugs said to block one or the other divisions of the ANS is not necessarily the same as the response to extrinsic nerve section. Cutting the parasympathetic "motor" nerves does lead to cardiac acceleration and decreased motility of the fundus of the stomach, but many organs, notably the bladder and pylorus, respond by disastrously heightened activity, and some, such as the small intestine, are not affected at all. Atropine or other drugs that diminish the intensity of all of these functions uniformly must therefore be acting on an intrinsic mechanism distal to the surgically accessible nerves.

The ANS is by definition an efferent system, but the autonomous organs have a rich sensory innervation and many "autonomic" nerves such as the vagus and pelvic nerves are predominantly sensory. Consideration of the reflex regulation of smooth muscle organs is necessary to understand the difference between the effect of blocking drugs and nerve section—eg, bladder contractions are inhibited by atropine but greatly increased by cutting the pelvic nerves, which nerves include sensory fibers from the bladder that are essential to maintain normal, reflexly generated, sympathetic inhibiting tone.

CHOLINOMIMETIC OR PARASYMPATHOMIMETIC DRUGS

Drugs that act like acetylcholine would be expected to simulate or mimic the effects of stimulating the vagus or other parasympathetic nerve. The therapeutic usefulness of drugs of this group does indeed depend upon their **parasympathomimetic** actions. The term "parasympathomimetic" is, therefore, satisfactory at the practical level. However, acetylcholine is the mediator at sites other than parasympathetic neuro-effector junctions, and cholinomimetic drugs have effects other than parasympathomimetic. These additional effects are either sympathomimetic or involve voluntary muscle. Drugs that act like acetylcholine (cholinomimetics) differ in the proportion of parasympathomimetic effects and sympathomimetic and voluntary muscle effects that they exert.

The following 4 groups of cholinomimetic drugs discussed in this chapter differ largely in this manner, although one—the cholinesterase inhibitors—has a different mechanism of action: (1) choline esters, (2) cholinesterase inhibitors, (3) old alkaloids that act like acetylcholine, and (4) nicotine and other facilitants of ganglionic transmission.

CHOLINE ESTERS

These drugs, exemplified by methacholine (Mecholyl) and bethanechol (Urecholine), are comparable to the physiologic mediator, acetylcholine, but are longer acting.

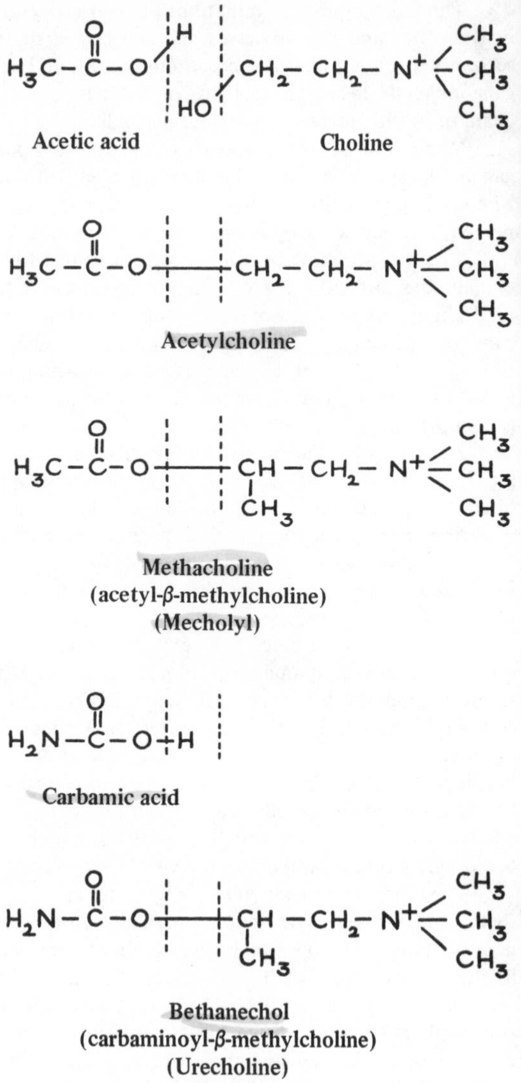

Acetic acid   Choline

Acetylcholine

Methacholine
(acetyl-β-methylcholine)
(Mecholyl)

Carbamic acid

Bethanechol
(carbaminoyl-β-methylcholine)
(Urecholine)

FIG 8–2. Choline esters.

Chemistry: Structure & Resistance to Hydrolysis

However important acetylcholine may be physiologically, its action is too brief for it to be a useful drug. When released from nerve endings, it is hydrolyzed within milliseconds to acetate and virtually inactive choline. If this were not so, it could not mediate the rapidly repetitive movement of a voluntary muscle or even the alteration between accommodation for near and distant vision.

Compounds resistant to hydrolysis by cholinesterase have therefore been prepared. These synthetic drugs have the advantage over some of the older long-acting cholinomimetic alkaloids of being relatively more active as parasympathomimetics and having relatively fewer sympathomimetic actions.

The chemical structure of some of the choline esters in use is shown in Fig 8–2. Addition of a beta-methyl group to acetylcholine slows the rate of destruction. The resulting drug, methacholine (Mecholyl), acts several times as long as acetylcholine but is not long-acting enough to be active when given by mouth. It is occasionally used by injection.

Esterification of choline with carbamic acid rather than acetic acid yields a compound, carbachol, that is no longer hydrolyzed by true cholinesterase and whose longer life in the body permits its oral administration. Addition of the beta-methyl substituent in such a carbamate results in bethanechol (Urecholine), the most widely used member of this group.

Pharmacologic Actions

A. Mechanisms of Action: The choline esters act directly on postganglionic neurons and on effector tissues. The effectors that will be sensitive or responsive to acetylcholine can be predicted in part from knowledge of the sites at which acetylcholine is the chemical mediator. Acetylcholine is released at parasympathetic (postganglionic) neuro-effector junctions, at ganglionic synapses, and at the voluntary nerve-muscle junction. Corresponding to these 3 sites are 3 general effects:

1. Parasympathomimetic (muscarinic)—The choline esters act on the gut, bladder, and other nonvascular smooth muscle and on exocrine glands to increase activity much as would parasympathetic nerve stimulation. Long before the concept of chemical mediation was developed, the effects referred to here as parasympathomimetic were observed to occur after the administration of muscarine, an alkaloid from a mushroom (Fig 8–6); hence the term **muscarinic,** which still persists.

To exert their parasympathomimetic or muscarinic actions, the choline esters act directly on the effector—ie, beyond the nerve ending (postsynaptically) and not through any parasympathetic nerves that may be present. Chronic denervation of parasympathetically innervated organs does not decrease the response to choline esters. On the contrary, sensitivity is increased following degeneration of the extrinsic nerves. (At this point, our interest is in the mechanism of action of acetylcholine. Note, however, that denervation supersensitivity is a more general phenomenon. Whenever a damaged nerve degenerates, the next nerve or tissue [effector] in the chain of cells becomes unusually sensitive to the mediator.)

Tissues lacking parasympathetic innervation may respond to choline esters. For example, blood vessels are dilated by choline esters, and the action is quantitatively far greater than can be explained by the cholinergic dilator mechanism demonstrated for some vascular beds.

2. Sympathomimetic (nicotinic)—Simultaneously with their parasympathomimetic action, all of the cholinomimetic drugs will exert some sympathomimetic effects—eg, vasoconstriction and cardiac stimulation—that are the opposite of the parasympathomimetic action. The sympathomimetic effects were first described for the tobacco alkaloid nicotine. The term **nicotinic** is usually used to encompass also effects on voluntary muscle and the CNS. Since there is some confusion and ambiguity in the use of the term, it is probably better to stipulate whether sympatho-

mimetic, voluntary muscle, or CNS actions are meant. However, the term nicotinic is in use and should be recognized.

The origins of the sympathomimetic effects of the choline esters are as follows:

a. Facilitation of transmission across sympathetic ganglia—Parasympathetic postganglionic fibers are also stimulated, but such action merely reinforces the parasympathomimetic effect.

b. Liberation of adrenal medullary amines—The adrenal medulla is innervated by cholinergic, preganglionic sympathetic neurons, and cholinomimetic drugs cause the liberation of epinephrine and smaller amounts of norepinephrine.

c. Liberation of norepinephrine from chromaffin tissue in the atria and blood vessels.

d. Reflex sympatho-adrenal discharge stimulated by the fall in blood pressure caused by vasodilatation or decreased force of cardiac contraction.

3. Voluntary nerve-muscle junction (nicotinic)—As ordinarily used, the choline esters have negligible effects on voluntary muscle. Their ability to act like acetylcholine at the voluntary nerve-muscle junction can be demonstrated by special technics such as injection into an artery close to the muscle perfused.

The effects of acetylcholine on voluntary muscle are more important in understanding cholinomimetics other than the choline esters. The cholinesterase inhibitors allow the accumulation of high concentrations of acetylcholine, and nicotine acts like a persistent cholinomimetic.

Cholinomimetic drugs act to cause striated muscle contraction in lower concentrations and to cause muscle paralysis when present in greater amounts. Small amounts act to depolarize the motor endplate—a specialized membrane at the site where nerve endings approach the muscle. Depolarization of the motor endplate spreads to the membranes of the muscle cell, and contraction follows. If the acetylcholine effect is intense, depolarization persists, and, if repolarization of the motor endplate does not occur, a flaccid paralysis results.

B. Effects: The parasympathomimetic or muscarinic actions of these drugs are predominantly on nonvascular smooth muscle, on exocrine glands, and on the eye; the effects on the cardiovascular system are the resultant of the parasympathomimetic and sympathomimetic (nicotinic) actions. The consequences of these diametrically opposed effects cannot always be predicted even if specific drugs and dosages are stipulated.

1. Nonvascular smooth muscle is stimulated to contract. Propulsive gastrointestinal activity is increased; the bladder is contracted; the bronchioles are constricted; the pupils are decreased in size by contraction of the sphincter of the pupil; and the ciliary muscle is contracted to accommodate the eye for near vision (Fig 9–1).

2. Exocrine glands—An increase in salivation and perspiration and in the secretions of the mucosa of the respiratory tract occurs. The secretion of gastric acid is not augmented, but increased secretion of gastric enzyme and mucus occurs. The differential effect on gastric secretion is difficult to explain since both the acid-secreting (parietal) cells and chief cells are activated by vagal stimulation.

3. Cardiovascular—The direct effect of choline esters on blood vessels is to dilate them. At the same time, the sympathomimetic mechanisms described above cause vasoconstriction. The net effect is unpredictable; however, even when a net increase in total peripheral resistance occurs, the superficial vessels of the skin usually dilate and a flush and a feeling of warmth is noted. Cardiac rate may also change in either direction. The profound slowing or cardiac arrest so easily demonstrated in animals by the rapid intravenous injection of a choline ester is rare in humans. It has, however, occurred during the treatment of atrial tachycardia with methacholine. The force of cardiac contraction is reduced demonstrably in the laboratory, but clinically the effect is more apt to be the opposite, because of sympatho-adrenal discharge, or to be negligible. The slowing of the rate of AV conduction—ie, prolongation of AV conduction time—is also not prominent under the usual conditions of clinical use.

The mixed vasomotor and cardiac effects lead to a variable response of the blood pressure until the dose is increased, when a fall in blood pressure regularly appears. Of the choline esters in common use, methacholine gives the mixed effect, and bethanechol, in the usual oral doses, has minor cardiovascular effects.

Clinical Uses, Preparations, & Dosages

These are discussed below in the section on cholinesterase inhibitors.

Adverse Reactions

Allergic reactions have not been reported.

A. Side-Effects: Side-effects are cramps (abdominal or epigastric, resembling hunger contractions), uri-nary urgency, a feeling of warmth, nausea, faintness, sweating, or excess salivation.

B. Overdosage Toxicity: Toxicity due to excess doses of choline esters is uncommon, and most cases have followed the injection of methacholine. Syncope (especially with the patient in the upright position), asthma, dyspnea, and AV block have been reported. These drugs are not innocuous, and in one incident 15 deaths occurred as a result of the mistaken injection of an ophthalmic preparation of confusingly labeled carbachol before the labeling was changed.

Treatment of overdosage consists of the prompt injection of atropine, the specific antagonist.

CHOLINESTERASE INHIBITORS

The choline esters just discussed and the alkaloids with an equivalent effect act directly on nerve and effector tissues. The cholinesterase inhibitors act indirectly by inhibiting the enzyme that hydrolyzes acetylcholine, allowing its accumulation at those sites where it is normally liberated.

Source, Chemistry, & Classification

The cholinesterase inhibitors are divided into 3 general groups based upon the reversibility of their combination or chemical reaction with cholinesterase and consequent duration of action.

A. Reversible Inhibitors: These compounds are esters of carbamic acid that react with the enzyme surface to form a carbamylated enzyme that is regenerated by hydrolysis at a slow rate compared to recovery of the enzyme that has reacted with acetylcholine. The duration of their effect (about 4 hours) is brief only by

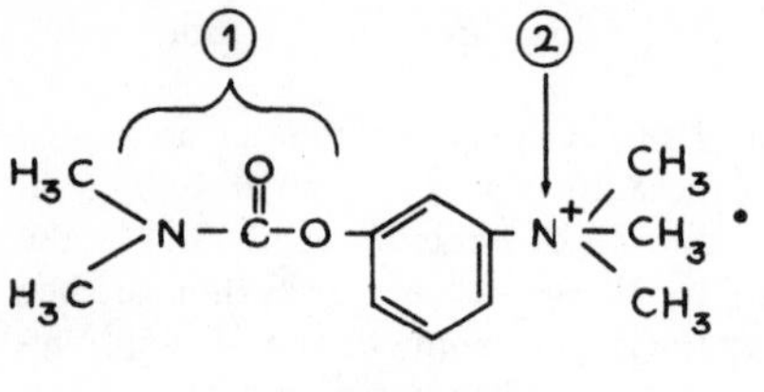

Neostigmine 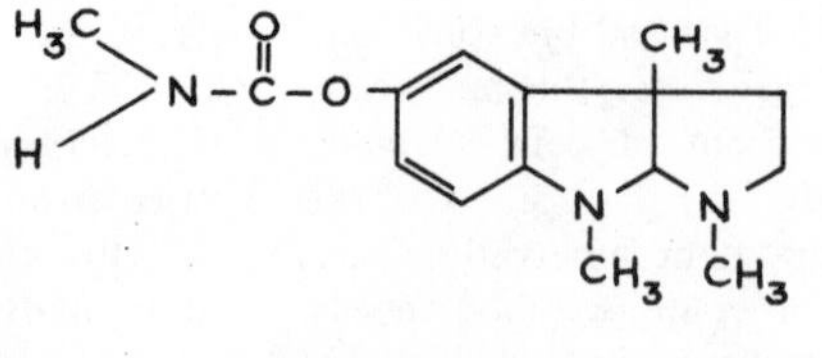   Physostigmine (eserine) 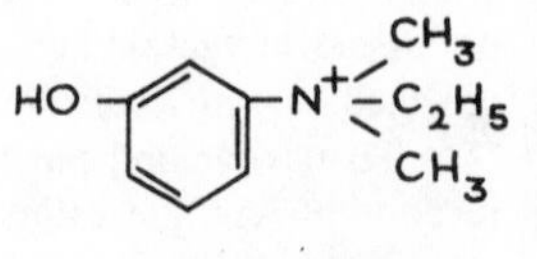   Edrophonium (Tensilon)

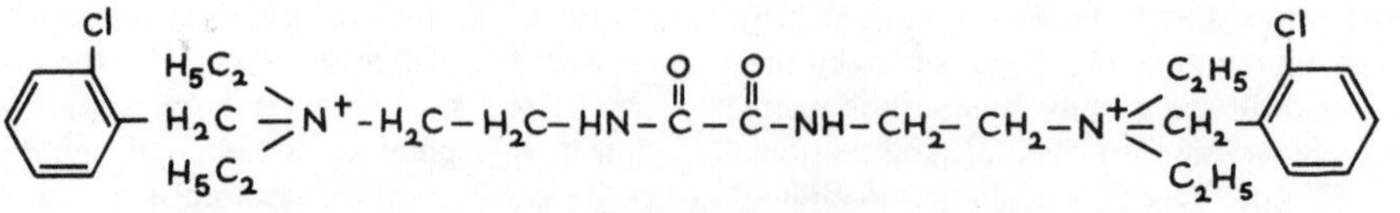

Ambenonium

FIG 8–3. Reversible cholinesterase inhibitors. Neostigmine exemplifies the typical compound that is an ester of a substituted carbamic acid [①] and a phenol bearing a quaternary ammonium group [②]. Physostigmine, the naturally occurring prototype, is a tertiary amine. The remaining 2 compounds are not esters and, for reasons given in the text, have distinctively shorter and longer durations of action.

TABLE 8-1. Representative organophosphorus cholinesterase inhibitors.

$$R_2 - \underset{\underset{O}{\overset{\displaystyle R_1}{|}}}{P} - X$$

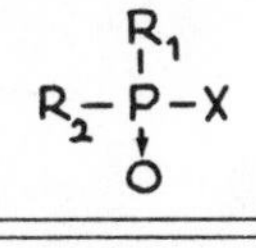

	X	R_1	R_2	Related Compounds
Isofluorophate (Floropryl, DFP)	$-F$	$-O-C_3H_7$	$-O-C_3H_7$	Mipafox, sarin, soman
Tabun	$-CN$	$-N = (CH_3)_2$	$-O-C_2H_5$	
Paraoxon	$-O-\langle\bigcirc\rangle-NO_2$	$-O-C_2H_5$	$-O-C_2H_5$	Parathion,* O-ethyl-O-*p*-nitrophenyl benzenethionophosphonate (EPN)*
Malathion*†	$-S-R_3$	$-O-CH_3$	$-O-CH_3$	Echothiophate (Phospholine)‡
Tetraethylpyrophosphate (TEPP)	$-O-\underset{\underset{O}{\overset{\displaystyle R_1}{|}}}{P}-R_2$	$-O-C_2H_5$	$-O-C_2H_5$	Octamethyl pyrophosphoramide (OMPA)

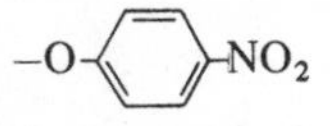

*Sulfur analogues.

†$R_3 = -CH-COO-C_2H_5$
$\quad\quad\quad\quad |$
$\quad\quad\quad CH_2-COO-C_2H_5$

‡$R_3 = -CH_2-CH_2-N^+ \equiv (CH_3)_3$

comparison with the second group, the organophosphates.

1. Physostigmine (eserine)−The prototype of this drug group was introduced into medicine, as is true for many drug classes, following the study of a natural product used in folk practice. Physostigmine was isolated from a Calabar (Nigeria) ordeal bean. (As a test of guilt, a suspect was made to swallow the beans. If he died, he was guilty. Perhaps if he ate the beans rapidly, confident of his innocence, he would promptly vomit them. The test has never been validated.) Physostigmine is a tertiary amine and better absorbed than the quaternary (charged) analogues named below. It is, therefore, still used by instillation into the eye.

2. Neostigmine and analogues−Neostigmine (Prostigmin), pyridostigmine (Mestinon), benzypyrinium (Stigmonene), and demecarium (Humorsol) are synthetic quaternary analogues of physostigmine.

B. Irreversible Inhibitors; Organophosphates: A large number of widely used insecticides, potential war gases, and one therapeutic agent are included in this category. The P−X bond shown in the type structure in Table 8−1 is opened following combination with cholinesterase. The moiety represented by X−eg, fluoride or paranitrophenoxy−is excreted, but the remainder of the molecule reacts with and irreversibly inactivates cholinesterase.

C. Truly Reversible Inhibitors: Edrophonium (Tensilon) consists, in effect, of only the base contained in neostigmine or other substrate for cholinesterase. It combines with cholinesterase only briefly and does not react with it chemically.

Ambenonium (Mytelase) is a biquaternary compound−ie, it is not an ester and is not split by cholinesterase. It attaches persistently to cholinesterase.

Pharmacologic Actions

A. Mechanisms of Action:

1. Cholinesterases−The cholinesterase most importantly related to the chemical mediation of nerve activity is called acetylcholinesterase, or true cholinesterase. It occurs in neurons known to be cholinergic−ie, it is concentrated in nerve terminals and also in the postsynaptic site if it is part of a cholinergic neuron. The neuromuscular junction is also rich in cholinesterase postsynaptically. It is distributed through the CNS in a pattern presumed to identify cholinergic neurons, and is present in red blood cells. The red cell content of cholinesterase can be measured and provides a clinically useful test for intoxication with cholinesterase inhibitors.

True cholinesterase is distinguished from pseudo- or butyrylcholinesterase, which is found in plasma and in glial rather than neuronal cells of the CNS. True cholinesterase hydrolyzes acetylcholine more rapidly, whereas pseudocholinesterase hydrolyzes butyrylcholine more rapidly. True cholinesterase, furthermore, hydrolyzes methacholine but not benzoylcholine; the reverse is true for the pseudo enzyme. The function of pseudocholinesterase is unknown. Both forms are inhibited by the drugs being discussed.

2. Reversible or irreversible inhibition−The action of cholinesterase in hydrolyzing acetylcholine is one of transesterification. The properties of the enzyme surface are conventionally represented as shown in Fig 8−4A, which assumes that the reactive group at the esteratic site is the hydroxyl group of serine.

In the process, the ester (Ach) is first physically attached to the enzyme (E), as diagrammed in Fig 8−4B.

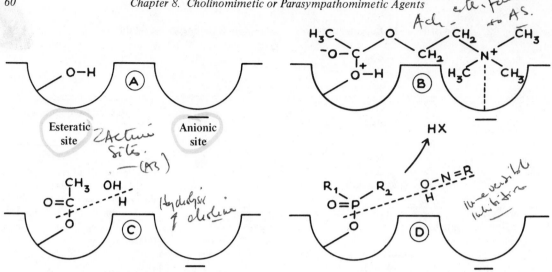

FIG 8–4. Combination of substrate or inhibitor with acetylcholinesterase enzyme. *A:* Representation of the 2 active sites on enzyme. *B:* Acetylcholine is adsorbed to active sites. *C:* Choline is released by hydrolysis and acetylated enzyme formed. Active enzyme is regenerated by hydrolysis of its acetamido derivative. Neostigmine or other reversible inhibitor combines similarly but is more slowly hydrolyzed. *D:* Irreversible inhibitor reacts to form phosphorylated enzyme. Hydrolysis and regeneration of enzyme do not occur in presence of water, but enzyme may be regenerated by reaction with hydroxylamine derivatives.

$$E + Ach \longrightarrow EAch \quad (1)$$

The substrate is hydrolyzed, and the base is released from its attachment to the enzyme surface. The acetyl group, however, reacts at the esteratic site to form an acetamido derivative of the enzyme:

$$EAch \longrightarrow EA + ch \quad (2)$$

The acetylated enzyme is rapidly (1 msec) hydrolyzed to regenerate the enzyme:

$$EA \longrightarrow E + A \quad (3)$$

The comparatively short-acting, reversible inhibitors such as neostigmine are esters that participate in the transesterification sequence, but a carbamylated rather than an acetylated enzyme is formed which is only slowly hydrolyzed to regenerate the enzyme.

The irreversible inhibitors (organic phosphates) react to form a stable, phosphorylated enzyme. There is almost no regeneration of the enzyme by hydrolysis, and the pharmacologic effect persists until new enzyme is synthesized.

The compounds (edrophonium, ambenonium) characterized above as truly reversible inhibitors are not substrates for the enzyme and act by occluding the site of hydrolysis.

3. Role of acetylcholine–The cholinesterase inhibitors, then, act indirectly through acetylcholine liberated in the organism. In therapeutic or mildly toxic doses, their effects will appear only at sites where acetylcholine is being liberated. Only with the most severe intoxications will acetylcholine be blood-borne

and exert a diffuse effect. Thus, blood pressure will be well maintained after cholinesterase inhibition because only a few vessels have cholinergic innervation and most will, therefore, be constricted because of the sympathomimetic effects.

B. Effects: Inhibition of cholinesterase activity will allow the accumulation of acetylcholine at all of the sites where it is liberated. The cholinesterase inhibitors will, therefore, show a mixture of parasympathomimetic (muscarinic) and sympathomimetic and voluntary muscle (nicotinic) effects, as was described above for choline esters. The few differences between the effects of choline esters and esterase inhibitors depend upon the fact that the latter act only where acetylcholine is being liberated.

1. Nonvascular smooth muscle–All nonvascular smooth muscle (of gut, bladder, bronchioles, constrictor of pupil, ciliary muscle) is contracted. The resulting effects are as described above for the choline esters.

2. Exocrine glands–Salivation and sweating are most sensitive to the stimulant effect of cholinomimetic agents. Increased secretions along the respiratory tract (manifest earliest as rhinorrhea) and lacrimation are also seen. Gastric acid secretion is not increased, but mucus and enzyme elaboration is.

3. Cardiovascular–Blood pressure is elevated. A bradycardia is produced at the same time which causes a widened pulse pressure. Thus, systolic pressure rises more than diastolic.

The rise in blood pressure is maintained even in severe intoxications almost until the subject is terminal and acetylcholine actually enters the blood. Facilitation of ganglionic transmission and adrenal medullary stimulation play a part in causing the elevation of blood pressure, but in experimental animals CNS stimulation, by increasing sympathetic outflow, is more important.

Cardiac rate is regularly slowed. The slowing is more regularly seen after administration of cholinesterase inhibitors than after the administration of choline esters because there is no fall in blood pressure to evoke compensatory reflexes.

4. Voluntary muscle—Cholinesterase inhibitors will act on striated muscle as described above for the choline esters, and a few drugs of the neostigmine type will in addition act directly on muscle to increase the force of contraction.

a. Initial stimulation—The common effect of the accumulation of acetylcholine is to mimic or intensify the effects of motor nerve stimulation. Therapeutically, this action is apparent as an amelioration of the weakness or fatigability of voluntary muscle in patients with myasthenia gravis (see below). In toxic doses, the depolarization of the motor endplate by acetylcholine leads to involuntary, incoordinate contraction of small muscle units. These fasciculations are apparent as retraction or undulation of the overlying skin. Only rarely will they be gross enough to briefly lift a limb or turn the head. They are finer and more discrete than preconvulsive jerks but easily apparent compared to fibrillation, the contraction of denervated single fibers which usually requires electromyography for its demonstration.

b. Depolarization block—The accumulation of very large amounts of acetylcholine prevents repolarization of the motor endplate. In the case of organophosphate intoxication, paralysis occurs very late and central respiratory and other muscle paralysis is usually also present. During the therapeutic use of neostigmine and related compounds in the treatment of myasthenia gravis, it is possible to cause depolarization block (cholinergic crisis) by an overdose. Since atropine may already have been given to reduce the muscarinic actions of the drug, the differentiation of cholinergic crisis from inadequately treated disease is difficult.

c. Direct effect—Neostigmine and comparable cholinesterase inhibitors—ie, the reversible inhibitors, excluding physostigmine—act to increase the force of voluntary muscle contraction by a mechanism independent of cholinesterase inhibition. This direct or acetylcholine-like effect of neostigmine is shown by its action on denervated muscle and after complete inhibition of cholinesterase by an organophosphate. The quantitative clinical importance of this effect has not been established.

5. CNS—The CNS effects are demonstrable after administration of reversible inhibitors but are most important in toxic reactions to the organophosphorus type of insecticide. Here again the actions consist of an initial stimulation followed by depression.

The medullary stimulant effects are manifest as increased respiratory volume and elevated blood pressure. The EEG shows a desynchronized or awakening pattern, presumably due to facilitation in the reticular activating system (RAS), which is activated by both cholinomimetic and sympathomimetic drugs. The behavioral correlates of the initial stimulation are anxiety, restlessness, dreaming and nightmares, and insomnia. In animals, sleeping time after a barbiturate is shortened.

With larger doses—ie, with virtually complete inhibition of cholinesterase—the effects include depression, drowsiness, confusion, slurred speech, ataxia, coma, and convulsions. Medullary depression leads to vasodilatation and lowered blood pressure and respiratory paralysis.

Some of the early CNS effects of cholinesterase inhibition are antagonized to some extent by atropine.

Clinical Uses

This section and the subsequent discussions of adverse reactions, contraindications, and preparations and dosages apply to choline esters as well as cholinesterase inhibitors.

A. Postoperative Ileus and Urinary Retention: Following surgical procedures done under general or spinal anesthesia, and especially if intra-abdominal manipulation is necessary, patients may have difficulty in urinating and in restoring gastrointestinal activity. These postoperative changes are due to smooth muscle atony, not to obstruction, and the present discussion does not apply if mechanical obstruction of the gastrointestinal or urinary tract is present.

The decrease in propulsive activity is due to drugs such as morphine and atropine used preoperatively and to an increase in inhibitory sympathetic tone generated by peritoneal irritation and distention by swallowed air. Treatment does not necessarily involve drugs, but measures such as gastric suction designed to reduce distention may be supplemented by cholinomimetic drugs. If parenteral administration is necessary, neostigmine (0.25–0.5 mg subcut) is usually used. If oral medication is possible, as in the case of urinary retention without ileus, bethanechol (Urecholine), 20 mg 3–4 times daily, is used.

B. Glaucoma: Parasympathomimetic drugs constrict the pupil by stimulating the smooth muscle arranged concentrically around the pupil. The miosis so induced pulls the iris away from the anterior chamber angle, facilitates drainage of aqueous humor, and is, therefore, useful in the treatment of glaucoma. At the same time, the ciliary muscle is also contracted and the eye accommodated for near vision. The effect of autonomic drugs on the eye and the treatment of glaucoma are discussed in more detail in association with Fig 9–1.

C. Termination of Curare Action: The use of drugs that weaken or paralyze voluntary muscle as adjuncts to general anesthesia is discussed in Chapter 21. These curariform drugs are of 2 general types. One type acts like a large dose of acetylcholine to cause a depolarization block. The second type, exemplified by the curare alkaloids, acts as a competitive antagonist to acetylcholine at the voluntary nerve-muscle junction. It is often desirable to terminate the action of curare at the conclusion of a surgical procedure and restore the patient's ability to breathe unassisted. For this purpose and in the case of the curare type of blocker, a neostigmine type of cholinesterase inhibitor is used. The mechanisms are to allow the accumulation of acetylcholine and to act directly on muscle as acetylcholine would. Edrophonium (Tensilon) has a brief duration of action and is supposed to have more of the direct action on muscle. It is the most widely used drug in this application.

D. Myasthenia Gravis: Myasthenia gravis attracts an interest disproportionate to its incidence because of its relation to chemical transmission and autoimmune disease. Acetylcholine is released at the voluntary nerve-muscle junction in quanta that reflect the amount held in each presynaptic vesicle. (One or 2 of these units are released each second, resulting in micro-end-plate potentials. When a wave of depolarization arrives, the nerve may liberate several hundred quanta and depolarize the postsynaptic membrane of the motor end-plate.) In myasthenia gravis, the size of each quantum of acetylcholine released is reduced with effects similar to those described for curare. The strength of a repetitive or sustained muscle contraction cannot be maintained. The muscles are affected in the same order as during the development of a curare effect—ie, muscles innervated by cranial nerves (external ocular, facial, palatal, pharyngeal, laryngeal, neck) and small muscles earliest and only later the limbs, intercostals, and diaphragm.

Studies on animals immunized against thymic extract suggest that the defect in acetylcholine synthesis is due to overproduction by the thymus of a hormone (thymin) comparable to the long-acting thyroid stimulator (LATS) demonstrated in thyrotoxicosis.

1. Effect of cholinesterase inhibitors—The accumulation of acetylcholine subsequent to cholinesterase inhibition and, to an undefined extent, the acetylcholine (direct) action of the reversible inhibitors increases strength in most patients with myasthenia. Some patients (and other patients at some time in the course of their disease) have an acetylcholine-insensitive type of block which does not respond to cholinesterase inhibitors.

The several drugs now in use are listed in Table 8–2. The irreversible, organophosphorus type of inhibitors—eg, DFP—have been less satisfactory than the reversible inhibitors listed. The irreversible inhibitors did have the advantage of persisting in their effect overnight and leaving the patient with greater strength in the morning. Should DFP or a similar compound be used, it must not be given when neostigmine is acting since the enzyme will be occupied and the organophosphate metabolized before it can act on the enzyme.

Because atropine does not antagonize the voluntary muscle effects of acetylcholine, parasympathomimetic side-effects can be controlled with atropine. Surprisingly, less than half of the patients treated will require atropine.

2. Other drugs—Ephedrine is said to be of some value in certain patients. This effect was observed before the cholinesterase inhibitors came into use. A typical dosage would be 25 mg morning and noon, and a third dose later in the day if tolerated.

The use of supplementary potassium salts is controversial. No beneficial effect has been quantitatively established by acceptable clinical trials, but some clinicians feel that supplementary potassium is useful even if no deficiency is present.

Germine is a veratrum alkaloid that has given interesting results in the treatment of myasthenia. This investigative drug acts on muscle so that a single stimulus generates not one action potential but a burst of action potentials. This veratrum alkaloid is different in its properties from the alkaloids of veratrum discussed later as a treatment for hypertension.

Some drugs intensify the symptoms of myasthenia gravis: curare and congeners, quinine and quinidine, and parenteral neomycin. Narcotic analgesics and sedatives should be used in smaller doses than usual, especially if the patient is having difficulty in swallowing or breathing.

E. Other Uses: The organophosphorus cholinesterase inhibitors are widely used as insecticides and are potential chemical warfare agents.

Supraventricular tachycardias may be converted to a normal sinus rhythm by drugs and maneuvers that

TABLE 8–2. Cholinesterase inhibitors used in treatment of myasthenia gravis.

	Single Adult Dose	Approximate Duration of Action*	Preparations Available
Neostigmine bromide (Prostigmin)	15 mg orally	3 hours	Tablets, 15 mg
Neostigmine methylsulfate (Prostigmin)	1 mg IM or subcut	2 hours	Injectable (IM or subcut), 0.25 mg/ml, 1 ml; 0.5 mg/ml, 1 and 10 ml; 1 mg/ml, 10 ml
Pyridostigmine (Mestinon)	60 mg orally	4 hours	Tablets, 60 mg Syrup, 60 mg/5 ml
Ambenonium (Mytelase)	10 mg orally	8 hours	Tablets, 25 mg Capsules, 10 mg
Edrophonium (Tensilon)	10 mg IV	†	Injectable (IV), 10 mg/ml, 1 and 10 ml

*Treatment begins with 4 doses each day and is adjusted individually thereafter.
†Used as diagnostic test only.

augment vagal influences on the atria. Neostigmine and methacholine have been used for this purpose, but the application is extremely rare today.

Contraindications & Cautions

Parasympathomimetics should not be used in the presence of obstructive rather than paralytic or hypotonic ileus or urinary retention. Other situations requiring caution are (1) asthma, because of the risk of added bronchiolar constriction; (2) hyperthyroidism, because paroxysmal atrial fibrillation may be precipitated; and (3) peptic ulcer, because the increased motility may cause increased pain.

Adverse Reactions

A. Side-Effects: When cholinesterase inhibitors are used for their parasympathomimetic action, they may cause gastrointestinal cramps or diarrhea, nausea, sweating, or excess salivation. These side-effects cannot be blocked by atropine without at the same time blocking the therapeutic effect, and their uncommon occurrence must be controlled by changing the dosage or using a different preparation.

During the treatment of myasthenia gravis, excessive dosage may cause depolarization block and increased muscle weakness or paralysis. Several methods are available to differentiate "cholinergic crisis" from an exacerbation of the disease. The toxic state may be treated in a number of ways. The dosage of cholinesterase inhibitor can be reduced (with

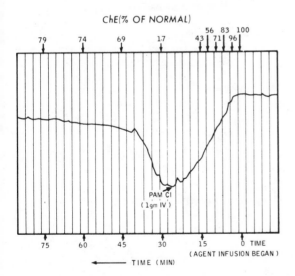

ChE(% OF NORMAL)

FIG 8–5. A continuous record of the circulating cholinesterase of a volunteer subject. At zero time, 4 μg/kg of sarin was given IV. At 27 minutes, blood cholinesterase had fallen to 17% of normal. Pralidoxime given at this time (very soon after administration of the inhibitor) restored the cholinesterase level to 80% of control in 50 minutes. (Reproduced, with permission, from Sim: Diagnosis and therapy for anticholinesterase poisoning. JAMA 192:404, 1965.)

mechanical support for respiration), observing for either improvement or deterioration. An injection of a short-acting inhibitor–eg, edrophonium, 1 mg IV–will result in short-lived intensification of weakness due to overdosage and improvement of weakness if it is due to disease. In theory, pralidoxime, a cholinesterase reactivator described below, could be used to antagonize an excess of neostigmine or other carbamate.

B. Acute Accidental Toxicity: The problem of acute toxicity exists almost entirely because of the use of organophosphate and carbamate inhibitors as insecticides in the agricultural industry. The most widely used insecticides are of 2 general types. The chlorinated hydrocarbons–DDT, chlordane, lindane, aldrin, dieldrin, toxaphene, etc–are chemically stable, water-insoluble but fat-soluble dusts that are persistent contaminants. Their acute toxicity (CNS stimulation) to humans is usually low, but some unresolved concern exists about their chronic toxicity since residues on food are concentrated in body fat.

The second class of insecticides, the cholinesterase inhibitors, are volatile and chemically labile in the presence of moisture, but, under proper weather conditions, the residue on sprayed vegetation may be dangerous for 1–2 weeks. Parathion is water-insoluble and persists for as long as 3 weeks under usual conditions. They are more likely to present immediate treatment problems to the physician than are the chlorinated hydrocarbons.

Examples of the organophosphates involved would include parathion, TEPP, Phosdrin, Thimet, and Systox. Malathion deserves special mention. It is metabolized rapidly by the mammalian and avian body to an inactive derivative, but in insects is converted to the oxy analogue, which is an active metabolite. It is the least toxic of this group and is permitted even in household insecticides. A few insecticides–eg, carbaryl (Sevin) and Prophan–are carbamates comparable to neostigmine in that the carbamylated enzyme is rapidly regenerated. The toxic effects persist for only about 2 hours. The effect of the organophosphates lasts so long that widely spaced exposures have a cumulative effect.

Exposure may be from inhalation, skin contamination, or ingestion. Handlers–eg, aircraft operators, mixers, sprayers–are most likely to be exposed, but drift from an air spray, contamination from work clothes, or unusual and unpredictable circumstances may lead to toxicity in persons not occupationally exposed.

The toxic effects can be anticipated from the parasympathomimetic, sympathomimetic, voluntary muscle, and CNS effects discussed above. The order and occurrence of a given symptom will depend upon the dosage and rate of administration of the toxin. The possible findings may be summarized as follows:

1. Autonomic effects–Nausea, cramps, diarrhea, tenesmus; miosis, ciliary spasm (blurred or painful vision); sweating, salivation, rhinorrhea, lacrimation; bronchial constriction and hypersecretion, with wheezing and dyspnea; urinary frequency and urgency; elevated blood pressure until terminal, and slowed pulse.

2. Voluntary muscle effects—Fasciculations in eyelids, tongue, face, neck, extraocular muscles; generalized fasciculations; and weakness.

3. CNS effects—Dreams and nightmares, giddiness, restlessness, anxiety, tremulousness, fatigability, ataxia, tremors, confusion, paresthesias, convulsions, coma, and central respiratory failure.

The diagnosis can be verified in the clinical laboratory by demonstrating depression of red blood cell cholinesterase. Treatment of an acute intoxication should not await this information, but in chronic, less intense exposures with minimal symptoms it may be useful. Many workers show laboratory evidence of exposure to cholinesterase inhibitors. In the case of parathion, exposure can be quantitatively evaluated by measuring urinary paranitrophenol.

C. Treatment of Acute Toxicity: (See also Chapter 64.) As soon as an airway is assured and respiration assisted and maintained if necessary, remove the patient's clothing and decontaminate the skin as necessary by thorough washing with soap and water.

1. Atropine—The most important part of treatment is atropine, which antagonizes the parasympathomimetic effects, but huge doses may be needed. One effective routine is to give 2–4 mg IV every 5–10 minutes until some sign of atropine effect (eg, pupillary dilatation, tachycardia) appears.

2. Pralidoxime (a reactivator of cholinesterase)—Inhibition of cholinesterase by phosphorylation is theoretically reversible by hydrolysis. The phosphorylated cholinesterase is actually regenerated by hydrolysis but at a rate so slow as to be unimportant. Wilson noted that the rate of regeneration was more rapid when the reaction was with hydroxylamine rather than water. He then developed quaternary ammonium compounds that fitted the anionic site on the enzyme and also contained nucleophilic groups that react with the phosphorus and break the enzyme-phosphorus bond (Fig 8–4D). Pralidoxime (2-PAM; pyridyl-2-aldoxime; Protopam) is the available activator of cholinesterase.

the response, a trial of therapy is advisable in patients with moderate or severe intoxication.

Pralidoxime is most active against the effects of cholinesterase inhibition on voluntary muscle. It is far less effective than atropine against autonomic effects. It is, therefore, a useful supplement to atropine and artificial respiration and often causes dramatic further improvement.

The dosage of pralidoxime is 1 gm IV well diluted and given over at least 5 minutes; this amount may be repeated in 30 minutes. In children, the dose is 25–50 mg/kg.

Pralidoxime (Protopam) is available in vials containing 1 gm/20 ml and as 500 mg tablets.

Preparations Available

Dosages and some preparations available are listed under Clinical Uses (above) or, in the case of pralidoxime (Protopam), under the treatment of adverse reactions to cholinesterase inhibitors.

In addition to those dosage forms listed in Table 8–2, the following are available:

Bethanechol (Urecholine, Myocholine):
   Tablets, 5, 10, and 25 mg
   Injectable (subcut), 5 mg/ml, 1 ml

Demecarium (Humorsol):
   Ophthalmic solution, 0.125 and 0.25%, 5 ml

Neostigmine (Prostigmin):
   Ophthalmic solution, 5%, 7.5 ml

Physostigmine:
   Ophthalmic solution, 0.25 and 0.5%, 15 ml
   Ophthalmic ointment, 0.25%, 1/8 oz

Pilocarpine:
   Hypodermic tablets, 16 mg
   Ophthalmic solution, 1, 2, 3, and 4%, 15 ml
   Ophthalmic ointment, 1 and 2%, 1/8 oz

Pralidoxime

The activity of pralidoxime depends on the nature of the inhibitor—eg, it is quite active after parathion, inactive after OMPA—and on the time elapsed since exposure. As the phosphorylated enzyme "ages," presumably by loss of an alkyl group, it is less readily regenerated. It is most active when used within 24 hours after exposure and is not ordinarily of any value after 36–48 hours. Because of the variables that alter

OLD ALKALOIDS

MUSCARINE

Muscarine occurs in a mushroom, *Amanita muscaria,* and thus has toxicologic significance on rare occasions. Its primary significance is historical. It has the parasympathomimetic properties of acetylcholine but lacks the sympathomimetic and voluntary muscle effects. It was isolated and studied by Schmiedeberg, one of the founders of experimental pharmacology, in 1869. Not until 1914 did the studies of Dale on acetylcholine begin to suggest the importance of that ester.

As a consequence, even today the parasympathomimetic effects of acetylcholine are described as "muscarinic."

It should be briefly emphasized that *Amanita muscaria* contains an atropine-like toxin as often as it contains the cholinomimetic, muscarine. The effects of the very dangerous *A phalloides* are due to a hepatotoxin with a delayed onset of action rather than to any autonomic changes.

PILOCARPINE

Pilocarpine, isolated from a South American shrub, is a tertiary amine with cholinomimetic properties. It has the parasympathomimetic effects described above for acetylcholine but is orally active and especially potent in producing salivation and sweating. Blood pressure and pulse rate changes often show the sympathomimetic or nicotinic effect of pilocarpine. The ganglionic facilitant action is easily blocked by atropine and is therefore often described as nonnicotinic—ie, acting on receptors other than those for acetylcholine.

Pilocarpine has now been almost entirely superseded for systemic use by the drugs mentioned above. It is still the drug most commonly applied topically to the eye in the treatment of glaucoma. In those rare situations in which salivary stimulation is desired, it is also the preferred drug.

ARECOLINE

Arecoline is an alkaloid with predominantly parasympathomimetic effects. It must have some nicotine-like CNS stimulant action, however, to explain its

habitual use in a manner comparable to tobacco. For this purpose, a slice of the nut of a particular palm, *Areca catechu*, is mixed with lime from burned shell and the leaf of a pepper, *Piper betel*. The lime hastens absorption by keeping arecoline in the form of the free base. The pepper contributes the name, betel nut, to the quid.

NICOTINE & OTHER GANGLION STIMULANTS

Nicotine and a few other comparatively unimportant drugs are often discussed as a separate class of drugs, ganglion stimulants. However, their properties are exactly the same as the nicotinic or sympathomimetic properties of cholinomimetic drugs.

NICOTINE

Summary of Pharmacology

Nicotine is an alkaloid isolated from tobacco. The free base is a clear liquid that becomes brown upon exposure to air. It is well absorbed from all body surfaces.

Nicotine exerts a sympathomimetic effect by the same mechanisms as acetylcholine—ie, facilitation of transmission across sympathetic ganglia, adrenal medullary stimulation, and release of norepinephrine from chromaffin tissue in the cardiac atria and arterioles. Muscarinic or parasympathomimetic effects due to stimulation of parasympathetic ganglia occur, especially on the gastrointestinal tract and eye. Acute CNS effects are as described above for cholinesterase

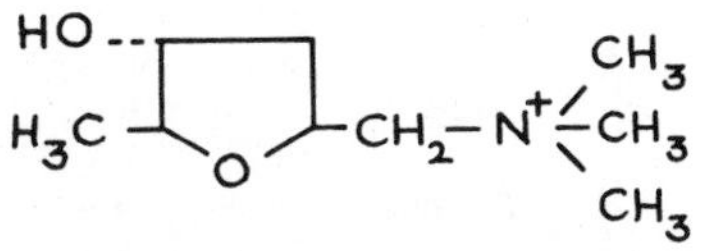

Muscarine

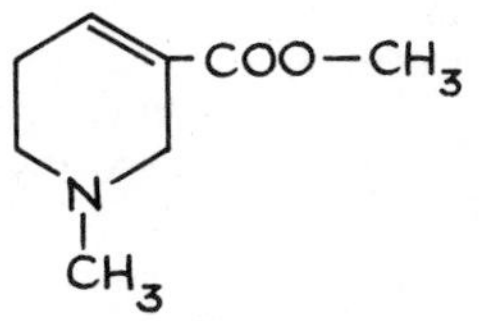

Arecoline

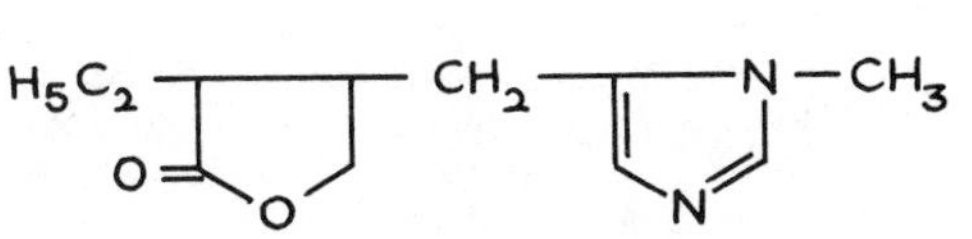

Pilocarpine

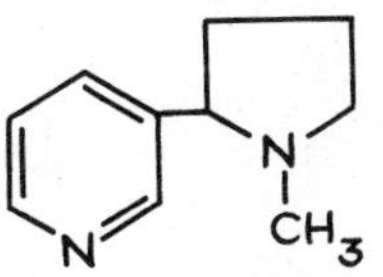

Nicotine

FIG 8–6. Chemical formulas of some additional cholinomimetic compounds.

inhibitors—ie, mild central stimulation followed by depression and culminating in convulsions. As would be expected from its similarity to acetylcholine, nicotine in larger doses causes paralysis of ganglionic transmission and of voluntary muscle. Nicotine is able to stimulate the release of antidiuretic hormone from the pituitary, an action that can influence urine volume in a hydrated subject. It is also very active in stimulating chemoreceptors of the carotid sinus; thus, initial effects on blood pressure and respiration are due to this action.

Laboratory Uses

Nicotine applied locally blocks ganglionic transmission, and the early mapping of the autonomic nervous system utilized nicotine. In addition, the systemic action of smaller doses on ganglia is used to test for the occurrence of ganglionic blockade.

Toxicology

Nicotine was at one time widely used as an insecticide. As long as it was used as an insecticide it was stored about the house and garden as a 40% solution and was responsible for serious accidental intoxications. Newer insecticides have now replaced it.

Tobacco as a Drug

Tobacco, like the many drugs discussed in Chapter 7, is subject to various degrees of use or misuse. It may be used casually or with the same compulsiveness as the socially unacceptable drugs.

One must assume that the mild central stimulant (euphoriant, awakening) properties of nicotine are important in perpetuating its usage since nicotine-free cigarettes cannot be substituted. Tolerance (except to the nauseant effect) is of a minor degree, and a withdrawal state widely claimed by tobacco smokers is not clearly established and is mostly the anxiety of an individual deprived of his compulsive act. Unfortunately, research on nicotine has until recently had an odd bias toward autonomic and cardiovascular rather than CNS pharmacology.

The clearly established carcinogenic effect of cigarette smoking is unrelated to nicotine, resulting instead from contact with the products of slow combustion (eg, tars). Unburned tobacco—eg, snuff—is also mildly carcinogenic.

OTHER GANGLION STIMULANTS

The following compounds are listed for identification rather than because of any therapeutic importance. Lobeline, an alkaloid from Indian tobacco, resembles nicotine but is even more active in stimulating chemoreceptors. It was used in the past to measure arm-to-carotid artery circulation time. Coniine (propyl piperidine) is the toxic component of hemlock and has more CNS depressant properties than nicotine. DMPP (dimethylphenylpiperazinium) and TMA (trimethylammonium) are laboratory drugs used as ganglion stimulants alternatively to electrical stimulation or to nicotine.

• • •

General References

General

Burn, J.H.: Release of noradrenaline from the sympathetic postganglionic fibre. Brit MJ 2:197–201, 1967.

Euler, U.S. von: Autonomic neuro-effector transmission. Vol 1, Chap 7, pp 215–238, in: *Handbook of Physiology.* Section 1. Field, J., Magoun, H.W., & V.E. Hall (editors). American Physiological Society, 1959.

Feldberg, W.S. (editor): Autonomic nervous system. Brit M Bull 13:153–228, 1957.

Hillarp, N.: Peripheral autonomic mechanisms. Vol 2, Chap 38, pp 979–1006, in: *Handbook of Physiology.* Section 1. Field, J., Magoun, H.W., & V.E. Hall (editors). American Physiological Society, 1960.

Ingram, W.R.: Central autonomic mechanisms. Vol 2, Chap 37, pp 951–978, in: *Handbook of Physiology.* Section 1. Field, J., Magoun, H.W., & V.E. Hall (editors). American Physiological Society, 1960.

Kuntz, A.: *The Autonomic Nervous System,* 4th ed. Lea & Febiger, 1953.

Meyers, F.H.: A critique of the concept of sympathetic-parasympathetic antagonism. J Am Geriatrics Soc 7:120–127, 1959.

Mitchell, G.A.G.: *Anatomy of the Autonomic Nervous System.* Livingstone, 1953.

Cholinomimetic Agents

Euler, U.S. von (editor): *Symposium on Tobacco Alkaloids and Related Compounds.* Pergamon, 1964.

Flacke, W., Caviness, V.S., & F.G. Samaha: Treatment of myasthenia gravis with germine diacetate. New England J Med 275:1207–1214, 1966.

Grob, D.: Myasthenia gravis: A review of pathogenesis and treatment. Arch Int Med 108:615–638, 1961.

Koelle, G.B. (editor): Cholinesterases and anticholinesterase agents. *Handbuch der experimentellen Pharmakologie.* Vol 15. Springer, 1963.

Milby, T.H.: Prevention and management of organophosphate poisoning. JAMA 216:2131–2133, 1971.

Pathogenesis of myasthenia gravis. Brit MJ 2:1–2, 1971.

Robson, J.M., & R.S. Stacey (editors): *Recent Advances in Pharmacology,* 4th ed. Little, Brown, 1968.

Root, W.S., & F.G. Hofmann (editors): *Physiological Pharmacology.* Vol 3. Academic Press, 1967. [See also general references, p 3.]

Wilson, I.B.: Molecular complementarity and antidotes for alkylphosphate poisoning. Fed Proc 18:752–758, 1959.

9...

Parasympatholytic Drugs

Atropine and many related drugs have the ability to block the parasympathomimetic (muscarinic) effects of acetylcholine. They act distal to the parasympathetic nerve ending to prevent the action of acetylcholine on smooth muscle, glands, and heart. They do not block acetylcholine liberated at the voluntary nerve-muscle junction and block only weakly at ganglia. Their ability to decrease the activity of smooth muscle and exocrine glands, along with incidental CNS effects, accounts for the wide and varied medical uses of this group of drugs.

Source, Chemistry, & Classification

The wide use of the parasympatholytics and the ease with which the chemist can synthesize analogues of the naturally occurring molecule have led to the marketing of a great number of compounds. Furthermore, other drug classes also have atropine-like actions. The need to consider each one of the many drugs individually can be largely avoided by grouping the many available preparations into 4 principal classes:

A. Natural Alkaloids: Atropine (DL-hyoscyamine) is extracted from a nightshade shrub, *Atropa belladonna.* The specific name, belladonna, is important to remember because tincture and extract of belladonna are still widely used. Scopolamine (L-hyoscine) occurs in the henbane, *Hyoscyamus niger.* Jimson (Jamestown) weed (*Datura stramonium*) must also be mentioned as a source of L-hyoscyamine because it is a rare cause of intoxication and because stramonium powder is still used.

In the structure of atropine shown below, note that it is an ester (1) and a tertiary amine (2), and that there is an asymmetric carbon at (3). Scopolamine contains the epoxy structure at (4).

The L-isomers are more potent in their effects on both the peripheral and central nervous systems.

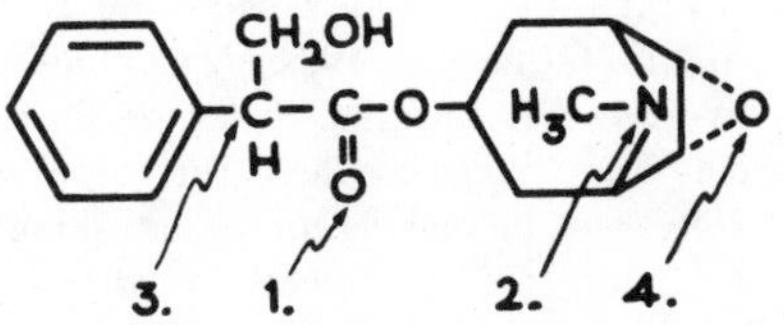

Atropine. Scopolamine contains
the oxygen shown at (4).

B. Synthetic Esters With Tertiary Amine Function in the Alcohol: A great number of synthetic esters closely related to atropine were marketed in the past. With a few exceptions (listed in Table 9–1), they have been replaced as parasympatholytics by members of the next class (C). Several drugs used in the treatment of parkinsonism, eg, benztropine (Cogentin) and caramiphen (Panparnit), are esters of this class; these drugs act on the CNS, and quaternary amines cannot, therefore, be used for this purpose.

C. Quaternary Analogues of A and B: The number of parasympatholytic compounds has been further increased by the conversion of esters of tertiary amino alcohols of the types described in paragraphs A and B above to their quaternary analogues. Thus, atropine may be converted to the methylnitrate or scopolamine to the methylbromide, and many other esters of amino alcohols may be quaternized. Examples include homatropine methylbromide (Mesopin, Novatrin) and propantheline (Pro-Banthine). Others are listed in Table 9–1.

In contrast to the tertiary amines just discussed, these quaternary amines are strong bases. The ionization of a weak base such as atropine is diagrammed in Fig 2–2. Quaternary amines are comparable to ammonium hydroxide and remain in the salt or ionized form at any pH existing in the organism. Only in strongly alkaline solutions is the free base formed:

They have no CNS actions because the charged compounds do not enter or act on neurons, ie, they do not cross the blood-brain barrier. Quaternary amines are not usually well absorbed from the intestine, but these compounds are active after oral administration. They are also slightly more active as ganglion blocking agents than is atropine itself. These drugs cannot be substituted for atropine in any situation where the central effects are important, but they are potent parasympatholytics.

A representative compound of this class is propantheline (Pro-Banthine):

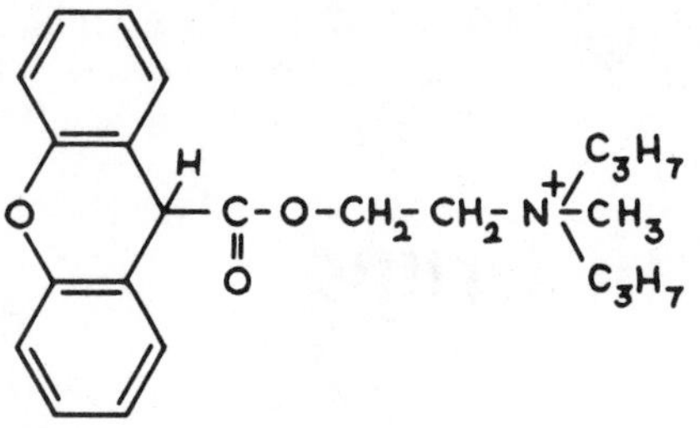

D. Antihistamines, Tranquilizers, and Antiparkinsonism Drugs: The ester structure emphasized above is not essential for atropine-like activity. The large blocking group may be connected to the amine function by a variety of connecting groups isosteric with the ester grouping, and some of the atropine substitutes listed in Table 9–1 are not esters. Chemically similar structures may be antihistamines, tranquilizers, or antiparkinsonism drugs but retain atropine-like side-effects. Similarly, the central effects of atropine may be expected to be similar to those of the tranquilizers or antihistamines.

Pharmacologic Actions

A. Mechanism of Action: Peripherally, atropine and all of the related parasympatholytic drugs are competitive antagonists to choline esters or the parasympathomimetic alkaloids discussed above at those sites where acetylcholine exerts a parasympathomimetic or muscarinic effect. Thus, following the administration of atropine, acetylcholine—whether injected or neurally liberated—still exerts its sympathomimetic or nicotinic effects and still acts at voluntary muscle. However, the effect of the acetylcholine that acts beyond parasympathetic postganglionic endings is blocked. Heart rate, for example, is ordinarily slowed by vagal stimulation or by the injection of methacholine or a similar parasympathomimetic. When atropine is acting, the bradycrotic effect is blocked and tachycardia reflects the now unopposed sympathomimetic action.

Acetylcholine release is not altered. Atropine acts beyond the nerve ending on the acetylcholine receptors of the effector organ. Nerve function, including liberation of the mediator, is not altered, but—the receptor now being occupied by atropine—acetylcholine can no longer act to depolarize the cell and initiate contraction or secretion. Atropine then has a greater affinity for the receptor site than does acetylcholine but much less efficacy in initiating activity.

The atropine-acetylcholine relation is competitive—ie, when acetylcholine and atropine are present, the resultant effect depends upon the ratio between the concentrations of the agonist and antagonist. Atropine block can be overcome by increasing the concentration of acetylcholine, eg, by administering a cholinesterase inhibitor. That fraction of atropine attached to the effector cell is in equilibrium with the atropine in the extracellular fluid. As atropine is

excreted, the unaltered receptor again responds to the relatively larger concentration of acetylcholine present. Equilibrium block of this type contrasts with the situation in which the antagonist reacts to irreversibly alter the receptor or enzyme.

Atropine acts only where acetylcholine is being liberated or when a parasympathomimetic has been injected. The effect of atropine on some tissues can be demonstrated only by the altered response to a challenge of injected acetylcholine, since no cholinergic influence is present physiologically. Most blood vessels, for example, are not under a tonic cholinergic influence and do not dilate following atropine administration. Yet they are dilated by injected acetylcholine, and such dilatation is blocked by prior administration of atropine. This example also demonstrates that muscarinic receptors are distributed independently of parasympathetic innervation.

Atropine has specificity of action in the usual doses. The response of smooth muscle to acetylcholine can be blocked with amounts of atropine that do not block the response to histamine or other stimulant. This specificity of action has led to the concept of specific and separate receptors for different agonists and their antagonists.

The action of atropine is also specific in the sense that it has no blocking action at voluntary nerve-muscle junctions except in special experimental situations. It has a transient and quantitatively minor action in blocking acetylcholine at ganglionic synapses. In therapeutic dosage, the quaternized analogues do have some ganglion blocking action. Because the parasympathomimetic (muscarinic) actions of cholinomimetic drugs are blocked but the effect on ganglia and adrenal medulla persists, the sympathomimetic effects of such drugs will become much more apparent after atropine administration.

The mechanisms underlying the effects of atropine on the CNS are not established. Acetylcholine is certainly one central transmitter, and some of the central effects of atropine are reversed by physostigmine, a cholinesterase inhibitor; but the temptation to relate the central effects of atropine, the tranquilizers, and the antiparkinsonism drugs to a central cholinolytic effect cannot yet be justified by any direct evidence.

B. Effects:

1. Cardiovascular—

a. Heart rate is determined by the balance between vagal slowing and sympathetic accelerator influences acting on the intrinsic rate and is one of the very few examples where the concept of control of function by the balance between sympathetic and parasympathetic influences holds. Vagal blockade with atropine would be expected to cause tachycardia. Tachycardia does appear when the dose is large enough. However, in smaller doses, atropine causes bradycardia before cardioacceleration, or bradycardia may be the sole reaction. The effect of atropine on the unanesthetized human is unpredictable unless dosage and route of administration are stipulated. Bradycardia has been shown by vagal nerve and brain stem section experiments to be due to the stimulation of medullary vagal centers.

The tachycardia that atropine induces in dogs is greater than that which follows vagal section and can only be abolished by sympathectomy, adrenal medullectomy, and vagal section. This indirect sympathomimetic effect of atropine has not been demonstrated in humans, but the extremely rapid rates seen after toxic doses of atropine suggest that it does occur.

b. Blood pressure in the recumbent patient may be slightly elevated after the injection of atropine because of a minor increase in cardiac output accompanying the tachycardia. Postural hypotension may occur with the patient in the erect position. These changes may occur after injection of atropine but are negligible in the patient receiving chronic oral medication.

2. Smooth muscle—All nonvascular smooth muscle is relaxed, ie, its motility is decreased, by atropine or other parasympatholytics. It is an oversimplification to relate this effect to blockade of the influence of extrinsic parasympathetic nerves since section of these nerves does not have the same effect of smooth muscle relaxation and since atropine demonstrates a similar action on the spontaneous activity on isolated smooth muscle tissues and on noninnervated tissue. The acetylcholine that is antagonized must be that responsible for the intrinsic motility of the involved organ—perhaps that related to the intrinsic ganglia contained in every automatic tissue.

Large doses of atropine depress the response of smooth muscle not only to acetylcholine but to all stimuli.

The claim is still made that some of the atropine substitutes, even in small doses, depress activity of the intestinal or urinary tract by a "musculotropic" effect, ie, an effect on smooth muscle independent of acetylcholine antagonism. Experimentally, this conclusion was based on the ability of the drug to reduce the contractions of isolated muscle caused by barium ion as well as those caused by acetylcholine. However, barium acts in isolated preparations by stimulating ganglionic transmission, and its effect is equivalent to the addition of acetylcholine. Because of the frequency of smooth muscle dysfunction, the parasympatholytics are still often referred to as "spasmolytics."

3. Secretions—The secretory activity of the exocrine glands is decreased. The effect is marked on the glands of the respiratory tract, the gastric and salivary glands, and on sweat glands (except those of the apocrine type). Experimentally, the effect on pancreatic secretion, control of which is largely humoral, is minimal.

4. CNS—The quaternary amine type of compounds described as class C above and listed in Table 9—1 does not act on the CNS. If the quaternaries are excluded, the behavioral and neurophysiologic effects of atropine, scopolamine, and all of their synthetic congeners can be discussed together.

Drugs of this class are depressants insofar as manifest behavioral change is concerned, ie, they cause a particular kind of sedation or slowing. However, the depression is accompanied by signs that the underlying neurophysiologic mechanism is stimulation. The same statement will have to be repeated in the discussions of the antihistamines and of the antipsychotic tranquilizers. The parasympatholytics cause excitement and hallucinations more commonly, but the behavioral effects of the 3 drug groups are otherwise very similar.

If a series of increasing doses of a parasympatholytic drug are given to a human subject, the following successive changes occur: (1) Sedation—not of the pleasant alcohol or barbiturate type, but rather a slowing apt to be described as unpleasant and accompanied by dizziness and fatigue. (2) Excitement or delirium—ie, hyperreactivity or misinterpretation of stimuli. Hallucinations occur with large doses. (3) Profound depression or coma. (4) Amnesia for the period of intoxication. (5) Convulsions. (6) Respiratory depression only with very large doses.

Scopolamine and atropine are often said to have different behavioral effects, but the manifestations of the action on the CNS of these drugs vary greatly with the dose. The conclusion that atropine is a "stimulant" (causes excitement) but scopolamine a sedative was originally suggested because these drugs were not compared over a wide range of doses but only at randomly selected—ie, clinically used—dosages. Scopolamine (L-hyoscine) is 3—10 times more potent than atropine in its CNS effects. At the usual nontoxic doses, scopolamine is more apt to cause sedation. If the drugs are compared over a range of doses, the above changes occur with atropine, scopolamine, and the related synthetic drugs.

The parasympatholytics cause EEG changes similar to those seen during normal or drug-induced sleep, ie, bursts of high-voltage, slower frequency activity. These changes persist even when behavioral excitement occurs.

5. Respiration—The parasympatholytic drugs are bronchiolar dilators even in normal, ie, nonasthmatic, subjects. In addition, atropine and scopolamine have in the past had central respiratory stimulating properties ascribed to them. Atropine was formerly used in the treatment of depression induced by morphine, and scopolamine was favored in preanesthetic medication because it was thought to partially antagonize the respiratory depression caused by morphine. Scopolamine, like the phenothiazine tranquilizers, can cause additional sedation without causing additional respiratory depression when combined with morphine, but neither atropine nor scopolamine is a respiratory stimulant in clinically applied doses. The control of respiration does involve cholinergic paths; thus, the respiratory arrest caused by toxic doses of cholinesterase inhibitors can be delayed by atropine.

Absorption, Metabolism, & Excretion

The natural alkaloids are completely absorbed across all mucosal surfaces. Absorption across the cornea is limited, but any fraction of a dose instilled into the eye that traverses the nasolacrimal duct into the pharynx will be completely absorbed. The quaternary analogues are less completely (about 25%) and less regularly absorbed.

In the human, hydrolysis of these esters is an unimportant factor in the termination of their activity. Most of the natural alkaloid appears in the urine unchanged. Their maximal effect is reached about 1 hour after oral administration and is dissipated in 3–4 hours after single doses. With large or repeated doses, the effect is prolonged. Pupillary changes are the last to diminish and may outlast the other effects of atropine and related drugs by hours or, after large doses, days.

Clinical Uses

The clinical uses of atropine and its relatives are based either upon their effects on smooth muscle and secretions or upon their CNS effects. The parasympatholytic effects described above can all be demonstrated in humans if large doses are used. However, in evaluating the uses listed below and in comparing the many compounds available, it must be borne in mind that these drugs must often be used for extended periods. Therefore, the results observed following a single large dose are not necessarily of value in determining the usefulness of much smaller doses that can be given 3–4 times daily without producing disturbing or disabling side-effects.

A. Peptic Ulcer: The belladonna alkaloids have been widely used for many years as part of the treatment of peptic ulcer. There is a theoretical basis for this practice, but no benefit from treatment with chronically tolerated doses has ever been satisfactorily demonstrated. Gastric, duodenal, or marginal ulcer does not occur in the absence of free acid in the gastric secretion, and a part of the pain is related to smooth muscle contractions. All of the parasympatholytic drugs that we have listed can suppress basal (fasting) secretion, although the secretion stimulated by the presence of food in the stomach is much less altered by well tolerated doses. Thus there is a clear rationale for the use of parasympatholytic drugs in the treatment of peptic ulcer. However, the question whether atropine has a favorable effect on the rates of healing or recurrence of peptic ulcer can be answered only by observing the results of a controlled clinical trial. The process has a variable course and responds to other drugs and to nonspecific treatment, and the clinical trial must, therefore, include control groups. If reports of uncontrolled experience are eliminated, the clinical trials published to date do not validate the use of parasympatholytics in the ulcer regimen. Nevertheless, most physicians add small doses of an atropine-like drug to the regimen of a patient with ulcer. A few reject this use and another group prescribes only a dose at bedtime each day; this dose can be slightly larger than the amount used 4 times a day and is more likely to be effective against the basal, overnight acid secretion. If gastric retention is present, the possibility of pyloric obstruction outweighs any possible benefits.

B. Functional Gastrointestinal Disturbances: A wide variety of symptoms of disturbed motor function of the gastrointestinal and biliary tract are treated with the parasympatholytic drugs, and usually with sedatives and explanation as well. Cramping pain, pylorospasm, eructation, epigastric discomfort, and diarrhea are examples of such complaints which are not associated with any underlying organic disease. The parasympatholytics do appear to be effective in the short-term relief of these symptoms. The treatment of serious diarrheas associated with irritative lesions is discussed in the chapter on narcotic analgesics.

C. Relax Other Smooth Muscle: Parasympatholytics decrease the strength of contraction of the bladder wall and relieve the pain and tenesmus that accompany cystitis. Contraction of the ureter and of the bile ducts can be inhibited in the investigative situation. Clinically, however, ureteral and biliary colic usually require narcotic analgesics for their relief.

D. Acute Pancreatitis: There are several reasons why atropine might be useful in treating acute pancreatitis. A reduction of gastric acid secretion with consequent reduction of acid stimulation of the duodenum should prevent the release of secretin and stimulation of pancreatic secretion. Nasogastric suction can also prevent the entry of acid gastric contents into the duodenum and is evidently much more useful. Blockade of the vagal stimulus to pancreatic secretion and relaxation of the sphincter of Oddi are other theoretical reasons for the use of atropine, but its use in acute pancreatitis must be regarded as unestablished or controversial.

E. Ophthalmologic Uses of Autonomic Drugs: The parasympatholytic drugs have important uses deriving from their effects on pupillary diameter, on accommodation, and on intraocular pressure. The effects of other autonomic agents on these functions will also be introduced at this time.

1. Pupillary size—The iris contains circularly arranged, parasympathetically innervated smooth muscle that responds to cholinomimetic and cholinolytic drugs. Contraction of this sphincter muscle by parasympathomimetic drugs causes pupillary constriction, whereas relaxation by parasympatholytic drugs causes dilatation.

Some investigators describe a pupillary dilator muscle, a minute amount of radially arranged muscle on the posterior surface of the iris, that dilates the pupil by its contraction when it is stimulated by sympathomimetics. The radially coursing blood vessels of the iris also influence pupillary size by their constriction or by internal pressure changes. Whether the effect of the dilator muscle or the blood vessels is predominant has no practical significance since both act to dilate the pupil in response to sympathetic influences.

Mydriasis (pupillary dilatation) occurs following systemic or topical application of atropine and other parasympatholytic drugs that relax the sphincter muscle. The effect is useful in facilitating ophthalmoscopic examination and when prolonged dilatation of the pupil is desired—eg, in iritis, to prevent adhesions of the iris to the lens (synechias). When only a brief effect is needed, sympathomimetics may be used to achieve dilatation, as for ophthalmoscopy, without interfering with accommodation.

Miosis (pupillary constriction) is utilized in the treatment of glaucoma (see below) to facilitate the outflow of aqueous from the anterior chamber.

2. Accommodation—The ciliary muscle has only parasympathetic innervation and responds solely to parasympathomimetic and parasympatholytic drugs. When relaxed or when paralyzed by parasympatholytics (cycloplegics), the ciliary body is distended by the turgidity resulting from its vascularity and by its natural elasticity. The relaxed ciliary body moves away from the visual axis of the eye, exerting tension on the suspensory ligament of the lens, and thus flattens the lens to accommodate for distant vision. To emphasize—in the relaxed state of the ciliary muscle, the eye is accommodated for distant vision.

When the ciliary muscle contracts, the radial fibers shorten toward the attachment at the scleral spur and the circumferential fibers also move the ciliary body toward the lens (Fig 9–1). The reduced tension on the suspensory ligament allows the lens to become rounded by its own elasticity and thus accommodate for near vision.

Cycloplegic drugs (atropine and its relatives) permit the measurement of refractive error without interference by the accommodative ability of the eye. With age, the lens loses much of its elasticity and cycloplegic drugs are not necessary for an accurate refraction.

Ciliary spasm is produced by the parasympathomimetic drugs as a toxic effect or as a consequence of the use of miotics. The effect is blurring of distant vision.

3. Intraocular pressure—Glaucoma or increased intraocular pressure is not only treated with drugs, but its presence provides a contraindication to the use of parasympatholytic drugs.

Aqueous humor is formed by filtration and by active secretion at the ciliary processes (shown at 1 in Fig 9–2). Fluid passes through the pupil into the

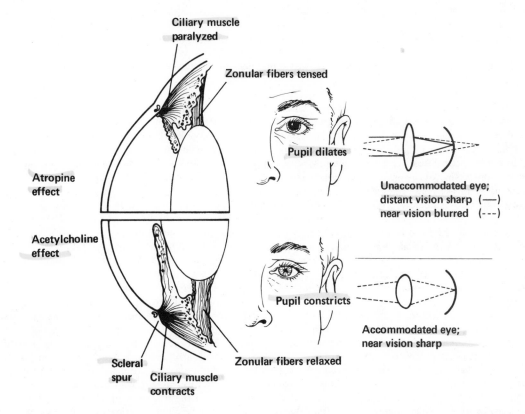

FIG 9–1. Accommodation and pupillary size. In the upper half of the figure the eye is shown with the ciliary muscle and the sphincter muscle of the pupil relaxed by atropine. Below, these muscles are contracted by a cholinergic drug or by parasympathetic nerve activity. Contraction of both the circular and radial fibers of the ciliary muscle moves the ciliary body toward the optical axis, loosening the fibers of the suspensory ligament and allowing the lens to become more convex. The radial fibers are fixed to the scleral spur, and shortening (contraction) has the same effect as contraction of the circular fibers. Under parasympathetic influence, the eye is thus accommodated for near vision. The pupil is constricted by the contraction of the sphincter muscle of the pupil. Constriction of the pupil—ie, movement of the iris toward the optical axis—pulls the structures away from the angle and facilitates drainage of aqueous.

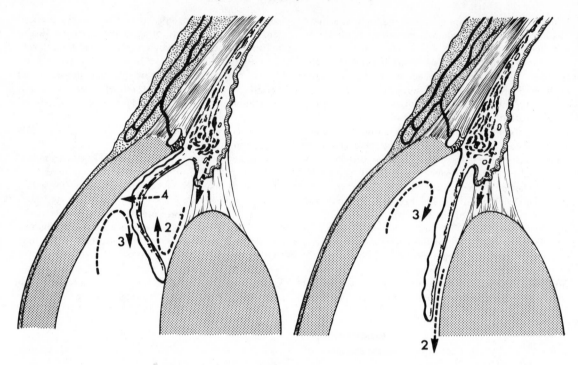

FIG 9–2. Circulation of aqueous in acute (closed-angle) and chronic (open-angle) glaucoma.

anterior chamber and is reabsorbed through the trabecular meshwork, a specialized area of the cornea at the angle.

Primary glaucoma, ie, glaucoma that is not secondary to other ocular disease, is most commonly of the chronic simple or open-angle type. Degenerative changes occur in the reabsorbing area, and, with continued production of aqueous, a destructive increase in pressure develops. Miotics—eg, pilocarpine or physostigmine—increase the outflow of aqueous. The effect is probably due to the ciliary muscle pulling on the scleral spur and opening outflow paths in the meshwork. Sympathomimetics may also be used, and the formation of aqueous may be reduced by the use of acetazolamide.

In acute or angle-closure glaucoma, the anterior chamber is shallow and the trabecular area at the angle appears to be occluded by the sharply angulated iris. However, the factor that makes the treatment situation so urgent is that some initial pressure change bulges the iris in such a way that the passage of aqueous through the pupil is blocked. The process may be precipitated by locally applied parasympatholytics. Immediate treatment utilizes pilocarpine or other miotic and an osmotic diuretic such as glycerol. If a response is not apparent within a few hours, the pupillary block must be surgically corrected (shown at 4 in Fig 9–2).

The following are the drugs referred to above that lower intraocular pressure:

a. Miotics—Pilocarpine, 2%, is still the most widely used topical miotic. The therapeutic effect on pressure lasts for about 4 hours, although pupillary constriction may persist for 24 hours after a single application. Physostigmine (0.1–1%) is a tertiary amine that is well absorbed and longer acting. Like the other less popular cholinesterase inhibitors (DFP, echothiophate, demecarium), it causes more ciliary spasm with discomfort and blurred vision and also blepharospasm because of the effect on striated muscle.

b. Carbonic anhydrase inhibitors—eg, acetazolamide (Diamox) and others—are usually classed as diuretics and are discussed in Chapter 17. They greatly suppress the formation of aqueous.

c. Sympathomimetics (epinephrine) act both by increasing aqueous outflow and by inhibiting the formation of aqueous.

d. Hypertonic solutions of osmotic diuretics given intravenously will withdraw fluid from the eye as from other tissues. Glycerol, mannitol, or urea may be used in acute glaucoma. (See Chapter 17.)

F. Treatment of Parasympathomimetic Toxicity: The use of atropine as a partial antagonist to the effects of the organic phosphates and other parasympathomimetics has already been discussed. A variation of this use is in the management of the side-effects associated with the administration of cholinesterase inhibitors given for their effect on voluntary muscle—eg, during the treatment of myasthenia gravis or when a cholinesterase inhibitor is used to abolish residual curarization postoperatively. The undesired parasympathomimetic effects may be eliminated with atropine without blocking the desired effect on voluntary muscle, emphasizing that atropine antagonizes acetylcholine at smooth muscle and glands but not at skeletal muscle.

G. The Common Cold: The traditional cold powders and some modern over-the-counter cold remedies contain belladonna alkaloids. The drying effect does provide some symptomatic relief, and this is probably the explanation of any minor effectiveness that over-the-counter remedies that contain antihistamines may have in the treatment of colds. The sympathomimetics are much more effective nasal decongestants.

H. Asthma: Atropine is not used in the treatment of asthma by the physician because the drying of secretions may add an obstructive element to the bronchiolar constriction. However, proprietary asthma remedies—especially those based on the inhalation of fumes from burning stramonium powder—are effective in the judgment of many patients.

I. Preanesthetic Medication: Preanesthetic medication with atropine or scopolamine is used prior to all but a few general anesthetics. The reduction in secretions thus accomplished prevents obstruction by the secretions in the airway and also, by preventing droplets of secretion from stimulating the larynx, helps to prevent laryngeal spasm. Other aspects of preanesthetic medication are discussed in Chapter 20.

J. Over-the-Counter Sleeping Pills: Over-the-counter sleeping pills may legally contain small amounts of scopolamine plus certain antihistamines. Because "sleeping pills" are supposed by the laity to be suitable suicidal agents, a number of cases of scopolamine intoxication have occurred as a result of excessive ingestion of these proprietary preparations.

K. Obstetric Analgesia and Amnesia: Scopolamine in combination with morphine or other narcotic analgesics was at one time widely used to provide analgesia during labor. Many patients became excited rather than sedated by the medication, but the scopolamine did produce amnesia for the experience.

L. Parkinsonism and Other Pathologic Extrapyramidal States: See Chapter 30.

M. Motion Sickness: Scopolamine is the prototype of drugs active in preventing motion sickness and, with lesser effectiveness, it is used to reduce nausea due to other causes. Drugs more closely related to the antihistamines have largely replaced the parasympatholytics in this use. This indication is therefore discussed with the antihistamines. (See Chapter 19.)

Adverse Reactions

A. Side-Effects: Dry mouth (with thirst or difficulty in swallowing), blurred vision, urinary retention in older men, dizziness or light-headedness, and fatigue are common side-effects that limit the amount of parasympatholytics tolerated during chronic use.

B. Toxicity: A patient is easily made uncomfortable with these alkaloids but it is very difficult to cause truly dangerous toxicity except in children. Eye drops that traverse the nasolacrimal duct and are absorbed from the nasopharyngeal mucosa are an occasional cause of the signs of acute toxicity described below. Jimsonweed, proprietary sleeping medications, and the use of belladonna as a hallucinogen are rare causes of poisoning.

Intoxication results in the expected parasympatholytic signs: pupillary dilatation, dry mouth, tachy-cardia, urinary retention, constipation, and blurred vision. The sequence of behavioral changes described above is seen: sedation, delirium, hallucinations, coma, and, with huge doses, convulsions or respiratory depression. An effect of toxic doses not predicted by the pharmacologic effects outlined above is a dry flushed skin, especially in the blush area. A great rise in body temperature may occur because of the inhibition of sweating. Children are especially vulnerable to this action. Such hyperpyrexia can be controlled by maintaining a low environmental temperature and by the application of cold baths and sponges.

The manifestations of acute toxicity may persist for a few hours or several days. Treatment includes control of environmental temperature, catheterization if necessary, protection of exposed mucosal surfaces, support of respiration when indicated, and avoidance of overtreatment of the convulsions. Experience with the treatment of organic phosphate intoxication and with a now obsolete form of therapy for psychotic patients has established that the lethal dose in adults is more than 0.5 gm of atropine and more than 0.2–0.3 gm of scopolamine.

Cholinesterase inhibitors—eg, neostigmine—and other parasympathomimetic drugs are not often used in the treatment of poisoning with atropine-like drugs. A miotic—eg, physostigmine or pilocarpine—may be used if photophobia from pupillary dilatation is a prominent complaint. However, the actions on the CNS rather than the peripheral effects are the dangerous actions in poisoning in adults.

A cholinesterase inhibitor that is able to enter the CNS will antagonize the CNS effects of atropine. Physostigmine (eserine) is a tertiary amine and is active; quaternary amines such as neostigmine are not. The effectiveness of physostigmine was established because of interest in a potent, synthetic atropine analogue as a potential chemical warfare agent ("BZ"). Such agents cause delirium and hallucinations and are potential incapacitating agents.

Contraindications & Cautions

Parasympatholytic drugs should not be used in the presence of glaucoma except for single, small doses such as are used in preanesthetic medication. In addition, cycloplegics instilled into the eye can precipitate glaucoma. They should not be used in patients over 35 years of age unless the existence of a shallow anterior chamber is excluded. Pupillary dilatation for routine ophthalmoscopic examination can be accomplished with sympathomimetics.

Gastric retention and acute urinary retention secondary to prostate hypertrophy are more commonly encountered contraindications to the use of these drugs.

Selection of Drug

When parasympatholytics are used for clearly established indications and when a potent effect is necessary, atropine or scopolamine will usually be used rather than one of the synthetic substitutes. After

TABLE 9–1. Parasympatholytic drugs: Dosages and preparations available.

	Suggested Initial Oral Dose (3–4 Times a Day)*	Preparations Available
Natural alkaloids		
Atropine (DL-hyoscyamine)	0.5 mg	Tablets, 0.3, 0.4, and 0.6 mg Injectable (IM, subcut, or IV): 0.3, 0.4, 0.5, 0.6, 1, and 1.2 mg/ml, 1, 20, and 30 ml Ophthalmic ointment, 1 and 2%, 1/8 oz Ophthalmic solution, 0.5%, 15 ml; 1%, 1, 2, and 15 ml; 2%, 15 ml; 3%, 1 ml; 4%, 15 ml
Belladonna extract (mostly L-hyoscyamine)	15 mg	Tablets, 8 and 15 mg
Tincture of belladonna	10–20 drops	As such
Scopolamine (L-hyoscine)	0.5 mg	Tablets, 0.3, 0.4, and 0.6 mg Injectable (IM, subcut, or IV): 0.3, 0.4, 0.5, 0.6, and 1 mg/ml, 1, 2, and 20 ml Ophthalmic solution, 0.5%, 1 ml
Synthetic esters analogous to natural alkaloids (tertiary amines)		
Homatropine hydrobromide	†	Powder, 1 gm, 1/8 oz, and 1 oz Ophthalmic solution, 2%, 1, 4, 7.5, and 15 ml; 5%, 1, 4, and 15 ml
Eucatropine	†	Ophthalmic solution, 2 and 5%
Cyclopentolate (Cyclogyl)	†	Ophthalmic solution, 0.5%, 15 ml; 1%, 2 and 15 ml; 2%, 2 and 7.5 ml
Tropicamide (Mydriacyl)	†	Ophthalmic solution, 0.5 and 1%, 15 ml
Dicyclomine (Bentyl)	20 mg	Tablets, 20 mg Capsules, 10 mg Syrup, 10 mg/5 ml Injectable (IM), 10 mg/ml, 2 and 10 ml
Flavoxate (Urispas)	200 mg	Tablets, 100 mg
Methixene‡ (Trest)	1 mg	Tablets, 1 mg
Oxyphenonium (Antrenyl)	10 mg	Tablets, 5 mg
Oxyphencyclimine (Daricon)	10 mg (twice daily)	Tablets, 10 mg
Piperidolate (Dactil)	50 mg	Tablets. 50 mg
Thiphenamil (Trocinate)	100 mg	Tablets, 100 mg
Synthetic esters that are quaternary amines		
Homatropine methylbromide (Mesopin, Novatrin)	5 mg	Tablets, 5 and 10 mg Elixir, 5 mg/5 ml
Methscopolamine (Pamine)	2.5 mg	Tablets, 2 and 2.5 mg Syrup, 1.25 mg/5 ml, 120 ml Injectable (IM, subcut), 1 mg/ml, 1 ml
Glycopyrrolate (Robinul)	1–2 mg	Tablets, 1 and 2 mg Injectable (IV, IM, subcut), 0.2 mg/ml, 1 and 5 ml
Pentapiperium (Quilene)	10–20 mg	Tablets, 10 mg
Pipenzolate (Piptal)	5 mg	Tablets, 5 mg
Propantheline (Pro-Banthine)	15 mg	Tablets, 7.5 and 15 mg Sustained action tablets, 30 mg Injectable (IM or IV), 30 mg ampules
Mepenzolate (Cantil)	25 mg	Tablets, 25 mg
Diphemanil‡ (Prantal)	50–100 mg	Tablets, 100 mg Sustained action tablets, 100 mg (2 every 8 hours)
Hexocyclium‡ (Tral)	25 mg	Tablets, 25 mg Sustained action tablets, 50 and 75 mg
Isopropamide‡ (Darbid)	5 mg (twice daily)	Tablets, 5 mg
Tridihexethyl‡ (Pathilon)	25 mg	Tablets, 25 mg Sustained action capsules, 75 mg Injectable (IM, IV, subcut), 10 mg/ml, 1 ml ampules

*Exceptions noted.
†For ophthalmic use.
‡Not an ester. See paragraph D under Source, Chemistry, & Classification.

rejecting claims based upon uncontrolled experience and assays that are not necessarily applicable to the clinical situation, it would seem that many of the synthetic modifications are potent drugs but that none have any demonstrated superiority over atropine or scopolamine.

The matter of drug selection should be simplified by avoiding the many mixtures of atropine substitutes with phenobarbital or other sedatives. Both parasympatholytic and sedative drugs require dosage adjustment on an individual basis, and a mixture with a fixed proportion of ingredients makes this impossible.

Some of the preparations available are listed in Table 9–1.

The maximum tolerated dose must be determined for each patient during chronic administration of a parasympatholytic drug. This is more easily accomplished with the natural products because of the more flexible and varied dosage forms available. In fact, one of the oldest preparations, tincture of belladonna, permits the most accurate titration of dose. An initial dose of 10–20 drops in water 4 times a day—0.5–1 ml, equivalent to 0.15–0.3 mg of atropine—can be increased or decreased by small amounts. The liquid preparation is, however, inconvenient for many patients. Atropine itself or extract of belladonna may also be used.

One of the quaternary derivatives should be used if CNS effects—eg, dizziness or tiredness—rather than a peripheral effect limits the tolerated dosage.

The suggested doses of the synthetics listed in Table 9–1 are merely the tablet sizes available and usually provide less than optimal dosage. Experience with many of the atropine substitutes is limited, and the studies have not usually been critical. The suggested doses of different drugs are not necessarily equivalent.

The dosage for children more than 1 month of age may be calculated on the basis of weight.

●   ●   ●

General References

Bachrach, W.H.: Anticholinergic drugs: Survey of the literature and some experimental observations. Am J Digest Dis (New Series)3:743–799, 1958.

Crowell, E.B., & J.S. Ketchum: The treatment of scopolamine-induced delirium with physostigmine. Clin Pharmacol Therap 8:409–414, 1967.

Eger, E.I.: Atropine, scopolamine, and related compounds. Anesthesiology 23:365–383, 1962.

Galin, M.A., & M.D. Zweifach: Glaucoma. New England J Med 267:237–242, 291–295, 1962.

Johnston, D., Goligher, J.C., & H.L. Duthie: Medical vagotomy: An assessment. Brit MJ 2:1481–1485, 1966.

Langer, E.: Chemical and biological warfare (II): The weapons and the policies. Science 155:299–303, 1967.

Leopold, I.H. (editor): *Ocular Therapy.* Mosby, 1968.

Longo, V.G.: Behavioral and electroencephalographic effects of atropine and related compounds. Pharmacol Rev 18:965–996, 1966.

Miller, R.D., & others: Measurement of atropine-induced vascular pooling. Circulation 10:423–429, 1954.

10 . . .

Sympathomimetic Drugs

Drugs that partially or completely mimic the effects of sympathetic nerve stimulation or adrenal medullary discharge make up a group that is very complex. This complexity is due to the great amount of investigative effort that these drugs have received and to the great number of compounds included in the group. The intense research activity in this area is a reflection of the interest in the naturally occurring neurotransmitters that are the prototypes of the drugs. Epinephrine and norepinephrine (arterenol, levarterenol) would be of great interest even if they had no therapeutic usefulness because of their physiologic importance and their relationship to the action of other drug types. Interest is increased by the fact that the sympathomimetics are therapeutically useful in a variety of common clinical disorders.

The introduction of ephedrine from Chinese folk medicine in 1924 provided an orally active agent and suggested the synthesis of compounds in which various effects could be selectively increased or decreased. In contrast with some drug groups, these differences in effect are real and clinically significant, permitting individual sympathomimetic drugs to be selected for particular clinical purposes.

The classification used in this discussion (summarized in Table 10-1) hardly seems a simplification, but it does organize the many drugs available into a manageable few pharmacologic categories. Each of the classes of sympathomimetics is discussed separately below.

THE CATECHOLAMINES: EPINEPHRINE, LEVARTERENOL, & ISOPROTERENOL

These 3 amines differ qualitatively from each other only in that individual drugs may cause pure vasoconstriction (levarterenol, norepinephrine), pure vasodilatation (isoproterenol), or a mixture of vasodilatation and vasoconstriction (epinephrine).

Chemistry (Table 10-2)

These drugs are phenylethylamines that act directly on the effectors. The phenylisopropylamines introduced below exert their effect indirectly through epinephrine and norepinephrine present in the organism. The 3 common amines have 2 phenolic hydroxyl substituents and are grouped together as catecholamines.

Dopa and dopamine (Fig 10-4) are also catecholamines. In this chapter they will be considered only as precursors of norepinephrine and epinephrine. Their importance in the CNS in relation to the action of major tranquilizers and the treatment of parkinsonism will be discussed in later chapters.

Epinephrine (adrenaline is a generic name in most countries, but Adrenalin is a protected name in the USA) was originally an extract of adrenal medulla consisting of approximately 80% epinephrine and 20% norepinephrine. It is now prepared from pure synthetic (L)-epinephrine. The other 2 are also synthetic. The L-isomer is the active form in each case.

TABLE 10-1. Summary classification of the sympathomimetics.

1. **Catecholamines:** Phenylethylamines that act directly on the effector cells. Levarterenol (norepinephrine) is a pure vasoconstrictor. Isoproterenol is a pure vasodilator. Epinephrine causes mixed dilatation and constriction. All are similar in cardiac stimulant and smooth muscle relaxant effects.

2. **Ephedrine and other phenylisopropylamines:** Orally active, long-acting compounds that act indirectly through catecholamines of the body.

3. **Amphetamine and related CNS stimulants:** Variants of ephedrine which are selectively more potent as CNS stimulants and comparatively less active on cardiovascular function. (See Chapter 28.)

4. **Indirect-acting vasodilator amines:** Phenylisopropylamines with indirect action. Effects are similar to those of isoproterenol but of longer duration, eg, nylidrin or isoxsuprine.

5. **Incomplete sympathomimetics:** Varied chemical types used as vasoconstrictors on nasal mucosa but otherwise lacking many properties of the true sympathomimetics listed above.

6. **Tyramine:** Acts entirely by liberating norepinephrine from labile pool in nerve and chromaffin tissue.

TABLE 10–2. Formulas of the catecholamines and phenylephrine.

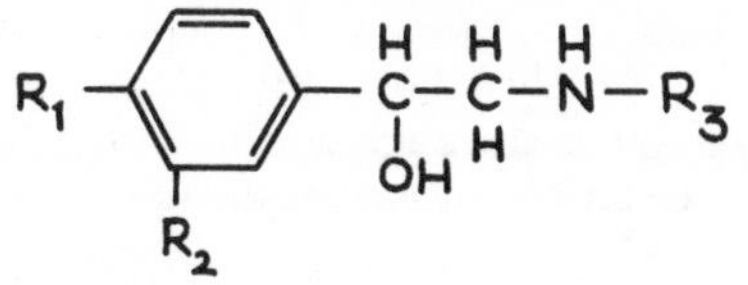

	R_1	R_2	R_3
L-Epinephrine (Adrenalin)*	HO–	HO–	–CH₃
Levarterenol (Levophed, L-norepinephrine)	HO–	HO–	–H
Phenylephrine (Neo-Synephrine)*	H–	HO–	–CH₃
Isoproterenol (Isuprel)*	HO–	HO–	–C₃H₇

*Trade names of these old drugs are provided for identification only. They are available from many suppliers under their generic names.

Phenylephrine is not a catechol but is a direct-acting amine comparable to norepinephrine.

Pharmacologic Actions

A. Mechanisms of Action: The catecholamines act directly on receptors on the effector tissues (smooth muscle, gland, or heart). Sympathetic innervation is not necessary for their action; on the contrary, denervation increases the sensitivity of effectors to these direct-acting amines.

The various effects of the sympathomimetics can be placed into 2 categories and described as being due to an action of the drug on hypothetical alpha and beta receptors in the effector tissue, alpha receptors mediating vasoconstriction and beta receptors initiating vasodilatation, cardiac stimulation, and relaxation of the nonvascular smooth muscle of gut, bronchioles, etc.

The concept of receptors is suggested by the fact that a given tissue may respond to closely related sympathomimetic amines by either relaxation or contraction, and each of these opposing effects can be selectively eliminated by appropriate blocking agents. Thus, the blood vessels within voluntary muscle respond to norepinephrine by contraction, and the vasoconstriction is blocked by alpha-adrenergic blocking agents such as phenoxybenzamine. Epinephrine or isoproterenol causes vasodilatation in the same vascular bed, and the response is prevented by propranolol or other beta blocking agents but is not altered by phenoxybenzamine.

The ability of the same cell to respond oppositely to closely related molecules suggests that some process or structure intervenes between the drug and the contractile mechanism. The concept of receptors is strongly supported by the availability of compounds that selectively block one agonist and leave the effector tissue able to respond to the related agonist and to

other unrelated drugs. For example, propranolol will block the dilatation caused by epinephrine but leaves unaltered not only the vasoconstrictor response to norepinephrine but also the dilating effects of histamine or acetylcholine (which can, however, be blocked by other specific agents).

The important and possibly the only effect of alpha receptor activation is vasoconstriction. There are 3 other excitatory effects, of which pupillary dilatation is the one seen clinically. In addition, in the laboratory situation, alpha agonists cause retraction of the nictitating membrane and contraction of smooth muscle organs such as the uterus and genitourinary tract. The contraction in intact animals is brief and precedes inhibition. In isolated tissues, the stimulation may be persistent under conditions that increase vascularity or increase the effect of vascular contraction in proportion to the effect of relaxation of nonvascular smooth muscle—ie, alpha agonistic effects may all be due to vasoconstriction.

All of the other sympathomimetic actions are due to activation of the "beta receptor" and are blocked by propranolol or other beta-adrenergic blocking drugs. These "inhibitory" actions include vasodilatation, stimulation of cardiac rate and force of contraction, and relaxation of nonvascular smooth muscle. The alpha and beta receptor concept cannot be applied to the metabolic and CNS effects of the sympathomimetic amines.

Some amines, notably isoproterenol, are pure beta agonists. Phenylephrine and methoxamine (Vasoxyl) are almost pure alpha agonists. Most sympathomimetic drugs—eg, epinephrine, norepinephrine, ephedrine, and amphetamine—have mixed effects.

B. Effects:

1. On blood vessels—The basic difference between the catecholamines (from which the other differences in cardiovascular effects derive) is that levarterenol constricts all blood vessels; isoproterenol causes no vasoconstriction but is a pure vasodilator; and epinephrine constricts blood vessels in the skin and splanchnic area but dilates arterioles in voluntary muscle. Because the vascular effect of epinephrine that is most easily observable is blanching of the skin, this drug is often thought of as a vasoconstrictor. Actually, however, epinephrine exerts both constrictor and dilator effects, and in its net effect the dilatation is greater. The teleologic concept of Cannon that sympatho-adrenal discharge prepares for "fight or flight" is a useful device for remembering that epinephrine constricts the blood vessels of the skin and splanchnic area but dilates those of muscle (thus shunting blood from the noncritical to the active organs).

The vasoconstrictor action of epinephrine on the superficial vessels is easily apparent from the skin blanching that follows its administration and is verified by the fall in skin temperature. Direct quantitation of constriction or dilatation in other vascular beds is more difficult and is usually inferred from the resistance to flow, ie, R = P/F (resistance equals pressure divided by flow), a relation that is valid only over a narrow range of change since the relation of flow to pressure is not linear over a wide range of pressures and flows. "Total peripheral resistance" (TPR), obtained by dividing mean arterial blood pressure by cardiac minute volume, is an index, however approximate, of the sum of vasomotor changes in all beds in either direction. TPR falls when epinephrine is infused—ie, it is a net vasodilator, and pressure falls even though cardiac output is increased. Levarterenol or norepinephrine increases TPR, ie, an increase in pressure occurs even though minute volume does not change significantly.

2. On the heart as a pump—Each of the catecholamines increases the force of ventricular contraction. The effect is demonstrable in isolated hearts which are independent of other hydrodynamic influences (Fig 10–1). It is demonstrable in the intact subject with a strain gauge attached to the ventricle and by other technics. The increased force of contraction following the administration of epinephrine or isoproterenol results in a great increase in minute volume. However, although the force of contraction is increased by levarterenol, the cardiac output (minute volume) is unaltered or even slightly decreased.

The different effects of the amines on cardiac output are explained by their different vasomotor effects. Because levarterenol is a potent vasoconstrictor, it increases resistance to ejection, ie, increases the amount of work required to elevate intraventricular pressure to the level of aortic diastolic pressure and the work necessary to accelerate and move a given volume of blood against the higher pressure. Levarterenol is thus stimulating the heart to more forceful contraction and the heart is performing more work, but this action is not manifested as increased cardiac output because the increase is in "pressure work" rather than "volume work."

3. On blood pressure—Blood pressure is a derived function that depends upon peripheral resistance, cardiac output, and cardiac rate. In general, the pulse pressure reflects stroke volume, and diastolic pressure is altered by vasoconstriction and vasodilatation.

Levarterenol, therefore, does not alter pulse pressure greatly because it does not significantly affect stroke volume. (Stroke volume will be increased and pulse pressure widened if reflex slowing of the heart

rate occurs, which is usually the case.) Diastolic and systolic pressures will rise proportionately.

Epinephrine acts to widen the pulse pressure and to elevate systolic pressure by increasing stroke volume. The vasodilatation that it also causes may actually lower diastolic pressure or, if diastolic pressure rises, the elevation will be less than the rise of systolic pressure.

(The differences described above are demonstrable only if the drugs are infused or otherwise slowly administered. Following an instantaneous intravenous injection, as in some laboratory exercises, the distinctions between epinephrine and levarterenol will not be apparent.)

Beginning with the fact that isoproterenol is a pure vasodilator, its other cardiovascular effects may be accurately predicted. The heart is greatly stimulated, and a resultant increase in cardiac output is possible because total peripheral resistance has been decreased. Pulse pressure is increased. Diastolic pressure is decreased because more run-off of blood from arteries to tissues can take place through the dilated arterioles. Systolic pressure is maintained to some degree by the increased stroke volume, rising slightly or falling less than does the diastolic.

In discussing epinephrine and levarterenol, the term vasomotor was used without careful definition. Arteriolar constriction was the predominant factor, but venous constriction, by increasing return to the heart, would also elevate blood pressure by increasing cardiac output. In the case of isoproterenol, venous dilatation can lead to peripheral pooling with a consequent decrease in venous return, leading to a decrease in cardiac output which in turn leads to a decrease in blood pressure. This is the sequence of events in some asthmatics taking isoproterenol sublingually while reclining in bed who become dizzy or faint when they arise suddenly because of venous pooling and postural hypotension.

The differential effect on blood pressure of the 3 amines, again assuming a constant heart rate, can be diagrammed (Fig 10–2).

4. On heart rate—The effect of epinephrine and levarterenol on the heart rate is the resultant of their

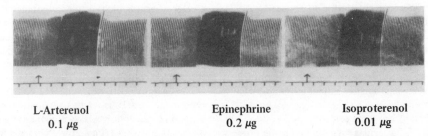

| L-Arterenol | Epinephrine | Isoproterenol |
| 0.1 μg | 0.2 μg | 0.01 μg |

FIG 10–1. The effect of epinephrine, L-arterenol, and isoproterenol on the ventricular kymogram of the isolated perfused rabbit heart. Time in 10-second intervals. The drug was injected at arrow (↑). (Reproduced, with permission, from Lands & Howard: A comparative study of the effects of L-arterenol, epinephrine, and isopropylarterenol on the heart. J Pharmacol Exper Therap 106:71, 1952.)

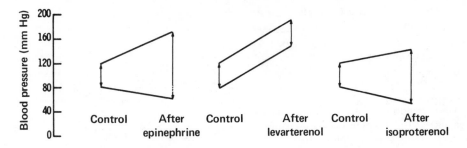

FIG 10–2. Effect of epinephrine, levarterenol, and isoproterenol on blood pressure.

direct action (increasing the rate) and of reflex slowing due to the rise in blood pressure. This direct action can be demonstrated in isolated hearts (Fig 10–1) or in intact animals or humans following abolition of the efferent arm of the bradycrotic reflex by vagal section or by atropine.

The net effect depends upon the dosage and other circumstances. We have all been alarmed by slow, very forceful beats attending fright or anger only to note a furiously rapid rate a moment later. After injection of levarterenol, reflex bradycardia almost invariably predominates. (A consistent explanation for the reflex slowing due to catecholamines depends upon demonstrating the effect of the amines on the walls of the pressure-sensitive areas.)

Isoproterenol can only lead to tachycardia since the direct and reflex influences act in the same direction.

Tachycardia will narrow the pulse pressure and bradycardia will widen it and disturb the idealized blood pressure responses described above.

5. On smooth muscle–In general, nonvascular smooth muscle is relaxed by the sympathomimetic drugs. The effect–eg, reduced force of bladder contraction–is more easily demonstrated with long-acting sympathomimetics such as ephedrine than with the catecholamines.

There are many situations in which smooth muscle organs react like vascular smooth muscle–ie, they contract in response to sympathomimetic drugs and the contraction is blocked by alpha-adrenergic blocking agents. The pupillary dilator muscle of the eye (if it exists distinct from blood vessels of the iris) is contracted, causing wider dilatation of the pupil than that achieved by relaxation of the circular muscle of the iris by atropine. The nictitating membrane in animals is also contracted and retracted to the inner canthus by sympathetic or sympathomimetic activity. The closely related smooth muscle that inserts into the lids is also contracted. This change explains the widened palpebral fissure or lid slit, or the staring eyes, of the sympathetically stimulated subject.

Levarterenol is relatively less potent than epinephrine in its effect on smooth muscle. Isoproterenol causes more prominent effects on smooth muscle not because of greater absolute potency but because of its slightly longer duration of action.

6. On exocrine glands–These effects are discussed to add physiologic rather than therapeutic information.

a. Salivation–The salivary glands contain 2 cell types and functionally respond as 2 separate organs. One type, comprising the parotid gland and the serous cells of the submaxillary gland, receives only parasympathetic innervation. The mucus-secreting cell type of the submaxillary and sublingual glands receives only sympathetic innervation. Epinephrine and the longer-acting amines such as ephedrine would not be expected to alter the secretion of serous saliva but to increase the amount of viscid saliva secreted. Such an effect can be demonstrated in man. However, the vasoconstriction and reduction in blood flow caused by the sympathomimetics usually decreases secretion, and dry mouth is a common side-effect. Atropine decreases the volume of secretion from both types of glands by acting on the intrinsic mechanism of the glands.

b. Sweating–Sweating also involves 2 types of glands. Apocrine sweat glands open onto hairs in the axillas and genitocrural region. The humoral mechanism controlling these glands has not been clarified. Although they are not stimulated by sympathetic nerve stimulation or by sympathomimetic amines, sympathomimetic influences may give the impression of transient stimulation by emptying the glands. This emptying is brought about by contraction of myoepithelial cells and is equivalent to pilo-erection.

Eccrine sweat glands produce a watery rather than a cellular sweat and are stimulated in the human by sympathetic postganglionic fibers that are, however, cholinergic. Thus, any stimulus leading to sympathetic nervous system activation–eg, hypotension or anxiety –will cause sweating but sympathomimetic amines will not, although they may also empty the eccrine glands as described above for apocrine glands. The situation may be quite different in other species.

7. Metabolic effects–The catecholamines (levarterenol is less potent than epinephrine and isoproterenol) increase liver glycogenolysis and thereby elevate blood glucose levels. Increased muscle glycogenolysis, which generates glucose-6-phosphate but not glucose, elevates blood lactic acid. Plasma potassium also rises.

The mechanism by which epinephrine elevates blood glucose is important because it may also explain the action of epinephrine at other sites of action. Epi-

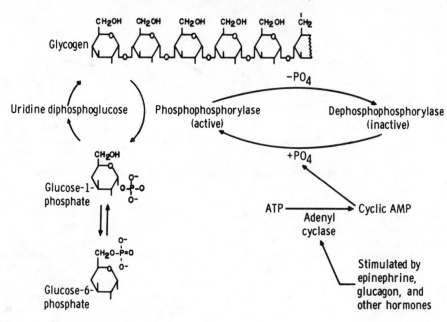

FIG 10–3. Glycogen formation and breakdown. Cyclic AMP phosphorylates phosphorylase, and a number of hormones increase the formation of cyclic AMP by increasing the activity of adenyl cyclase, the enzyme complex catalyzing cyclic AMP formation from ATP. (Reproduced, with permission, from Ganong: *Review of Medical Physiology*, 5th ed. Lange, 1971.)

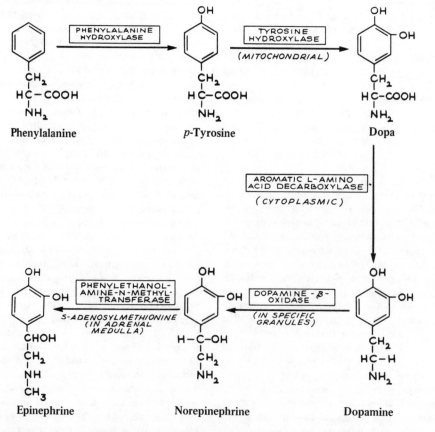

FIG 10–4. Biosynthesis of catecholamines. DOPA, dihydroxyphenylalanine; dopamine, dihydroxyphenylethylamine.

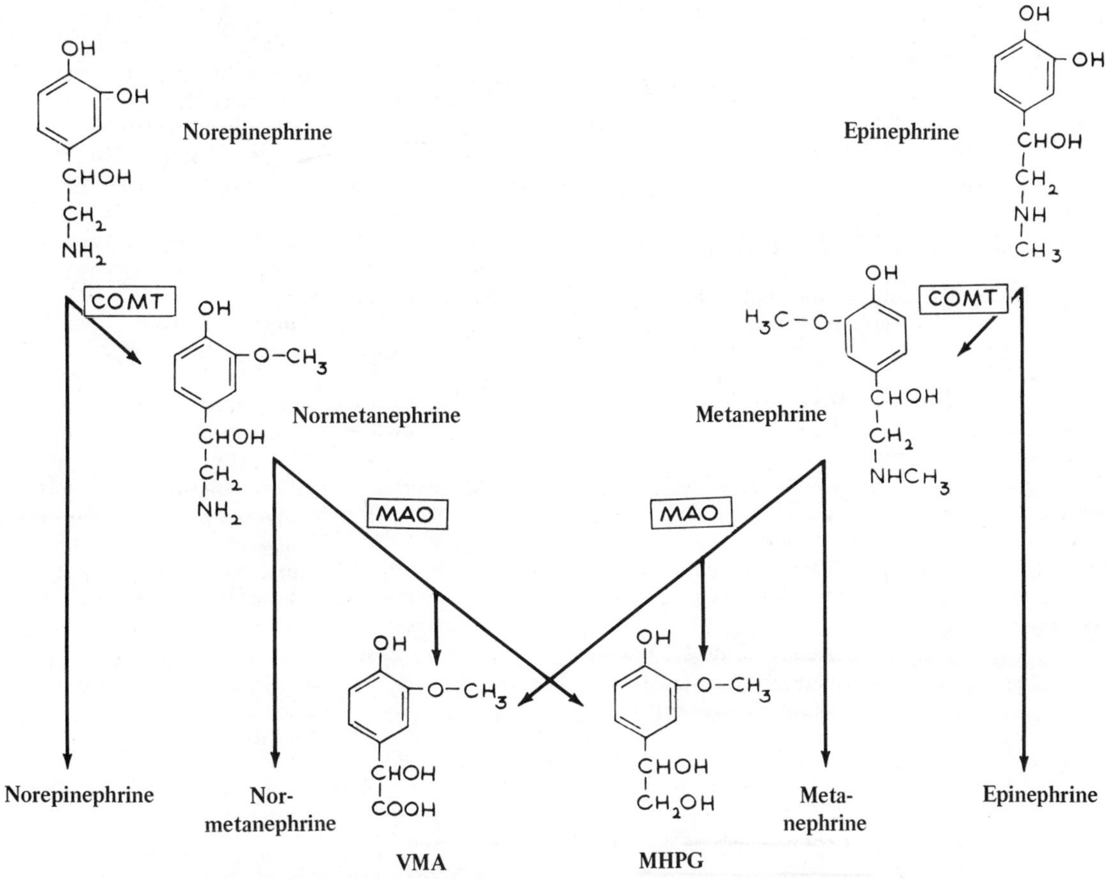

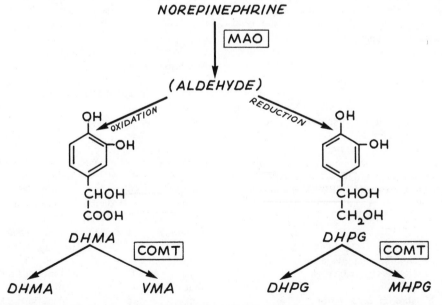

FIG 10–5. **Metabolism of free catecholamines.** Urinary excretion products appear on the lowest line. Excretion products may be conjugated with glucuronide or sulfate. COMT, catechol-O-methyltransferase; VMA, 3-methoxy-4-hydroxymandelic acid; MHPG, methoxyhydroxyphenylglycol; MAO, monoamine oxidase.

FIG 10–6. **Metabolism of norepinephrine of storage pool and CNS.** Urinary excretion products are shown in lowest line. Excretion products may be conjugated with glucuronide or sulfate. MAO, monoamine oxidase; DHMA, dihydroxymandelic acid; DHPG, dihydroxyphenylglycol; COMT, catechol-O-methyltransferase; VMA, 3-methoxy-4-hydroxymandelic acid; MHPG, methoxyhydroxyphenylglycol.

Adenine   Ribose   Cyclic phosphate

Cyclic adenosine-3′,5′-monophosphate
(cyclic AMP)

nephrine stimulates or activates adenyl cyclase, thus accelerating the formation from ATP of cyclic AMP, an activator of phosphorylase (Fig 10–3).

Cyclic AMP is probably involved in the action of many other drugs and hormones and is further discussed in Chapter 33. The xanthines discussed in Chapter 13, for example, inhibit phosphodiesterase, the enzyme that removes cyclic AMP. Accumulation of AMP results.

FFA (unesterified or free fatty acids) are released from adipose tissue by sympathomimetic drugs, causing the level of FFA in the blood to be elevated.

The number of eosinophils in peripheral blood decreases after catecholamine administration. In man at least, the eosinopenia provides no reliable information about pituitary or adrenal function.

The catecholamines also have a "calorigenic" effect, ie, oxygen consumption is increased. This action is the sum of many of the above effects and not due to a general increase in the metabolic rate of all cells.

8. CNS stimulation—Endogenous epinephrine or exogenous epinephrine or isoproterenol in sufficient amounts can lead to alerting, tremulousness, and respiratory stimulation. (Rapid epinephrine injections in the laboratory may inhibit respiration by acutely elevating blood pressure.) Manifest anxiety and tremulousness appear as side-effects during the use of epinephrine and isoproterenol. Levarterenol is so much less active in this respect that blood pressure may be greatly elevated by infusion of the drug without subjective complaints of anxiety.

The apparent CNS stimulation is, however, largely if not entirely due to a peripheral action of epinephrine. The amount of afferent activity reaching the reticular activating system (RAS) is augmented by the changes in blood pressure, and the alerting effect of epinephrine is reduced by denervating pressure-sensitive areas.

Central stimulant effects are more clearly seen when the longer-acting compounds such as ephedrine are used. Their effect is clearly central in origin.

Absorption, Metabolism, & Excretion

A. Synthesis and Storage: The synthesis and storage of the catecholamines not only have important

implications for their own pharmacologic activity; they are also important to an understanding of the mechanism of action of some sympathomimetic drugs that are not catecholamines and the mechanism of action of the drugs that decrease sympathetic activity.

The synthetic pathway is summarized in Fig 10–4. Most synthesis takes place at the storage sites; however, sympathetic nerves and chromaffin cells can take up preformed norepinephrine, an important process in terminating the action of norepinephrine. Preformed norepinephrine cannot reach the intracellular storage sites in the brain; synthesis must occur from precursors that can enter the parenchymal cells of the CNS.

Epinephrine and norepinephrine are stored within the granular vesicles and the cytoplasm of postganglionic sympathetic neurons; chromaffin cells of the adrenal medulla, heart, and arterioles; and specific areas of the CNS. In sympathetic nerve, norepinephrine is held in 2 functional pools: a labile pool from which it is liberated by nerve stimulation, and a storage pool in equilibrium with the labile fraction. Stored norepinephrine is held within the specific granules protected from enzymatic degradation by the limiting membrane of the vesicle and by combination with other substances. The norepinephrine of these storage granules is in equilibrium with that in similarly appearing granules that are part of the labile pool equilibrating with cytoplasmic norepinephrine. Tyramine acts to deplete only the labile pool, but reserpine acts on both pools.

B. Termination of Catecholamine Action: The process most important in terminating the action of catecholamines liberated from nerve or chromaffin tissue or injected is reentry or uptake by the sympathetic nerve, a process elucidated by following the disposition of tritium-labeled amine. At the same time, the metahydroxyl group may be methylated through the action of catechol-O-methyltransferase (COMT) and both reentry and activity terminated (Fig 10–5). A significant amount of norepinephrine enters the blood stream unchanged and, together with adrenal medullary epinephrine, causes the diffuse effects of sympatho-adrenal discharge. As a later process, occurring at a distance from the site of action (principally in the liver), either the unaltered catecholamines or the methylated metabolites may be oxidatively deaminated by monoamine oxidase (MAO), a mitochondrial enzyme. Only the small fraction of circulating or urinary catecholamines that escapes unaltered by either COMT or MAO is an index of sympathetic nerve activity. The other metabolites may be derived from the storage pool as well as from neuronal activity. If both MAO and COMT act on epinephrine or norepinephrine, the substance formed is 3-methoxy-4-hydroxymandelic acid or vanillolformic acid. The clinical laboratory analysis most commonly available for assay of catecholamine liberation determines the amount of this substance in urine. It is conventionally if confusingly referred to as vanillylmandelic acid or VMA.

Re-uptake of norepinephrine is an active process inhibited by cocaine, phenoxybenzamine and desipramine, chlorpromazine, and, presumably, all of the related tranquilizers and antidepressants.

C. Metabolism of Storage Catecholamines: The pool of catecholamines resistant to liberation is slowly metabolized and replaced. Intracellular MAO acts prior to any other process. The aldehyde formed as the first product of oxidative deamination may subsequently be reduced or oxidized to an alcohol or acid, and these products may or may not be methylated by COMT before excretion (Fig 10–6). Catecholamines in the CNS are metabolized in the same way.

Clinical Uses

A. Allergic Reactions: Some immediate allergic reactions are due to the liberation of histamine from stores within the body. The antihistamine drugs act as competitive antagonists to histamine much as atropine acts as a competitive antagonist to acetylcholine. They can therefore prevent the further effects of histamine in some situations but cannot reverse histamine effects already established. The sympathomimetics are not "antihistamines" in the same sense but are physiologic antagonists to histamine, ie, the effects of the sympathomimetics are opposite in direction to those of histamine. For this reason, they can actively reverse the bronchiolar constriction, vasodilatation, and edema that accompany an immediate allergic reaction.

The primary treatment of an anaphylactic reaction (Chapter 6) is the injection of epinephrine (0.3–0.5 mg [0.3–0.5 ml of 1:1000] IM or IV). Other immediate allergic reactions such as urticaria, angioneurotic edema, or serum sickness may be more effectively treated by the administration of ephedrine and the antihistamines (Chapter 19). The delayed type of allergic reaction cannot usually be treated with the sympathomimetics or antihistamines, but the anti-inflammatory steroids suppress such allergic inflammations.

B. Asthma: Bronchial asthma (in contrast to cardiac asthma) is due initially to bronchiolar constriction, but inflammatory edema and inspissated secretions may intensify the obstruction as the process continues. Treatment involves more than one drug group, but the sympathomimetics are probably the most important. Aminophylline, a xanthine type of smooth muscle relaxant, may be useful as an alternative to the sympathomimetics. Expectorants such as potassium iodide or water are also often used. The anti-inflammatory steroids may be used in persistent and difficult cases.

Acute asthmatic attacks—those requiring emergency medical care—will usually occur in patients who have already used maximal dosages of the sympathomimetic asthma medication that they keep on hand and will resist the action of epinephrine. The treatment that is usually effective is the slow intravenous injection of aminophylline.

The treatment of chronic asthmatic wheezing involves choosing among many drugs, and their relative popularity is based as much on patient acceptance as the preference of the physician. Epinephrine or isoproterenol may be used by inhalation of an aerosolized solution or of microcrystals. Isoproterenol is also available for sublingual administration, but side-effects such as anxiety and palpitation are usually more prominent. Ephedrine may be given chronically by mouth, usually combined with a small dose of phenobarbital to counteract the central stimulant effects of chronic administration.

Aminophylline and other xanthines may be given chronically, but only a few patients tolerate chronic medication without nausea. The anti-inflammatory steroids are reserved for use when the drugs with fewer untoward actions have been tried without success.

C. Hypotension: By reducing the intensity of sympathetic outflow, spinal anesthesia and many drugs may cause a hypotension that is predominantly postural. Since vascular smooth muscle is still responsive to the mediators in this situation, any sympathomimetic can be used to restore blood pressure. It should be emphasized that hypotension is not necessarily the same as shock. If cardiac output and tissue perfusion are well maintained, hypotension does not require vigorous treatment. Preventing the pooling of blood (by keeping the patient recumbent) which is responsible for hypotension is a more rational and satisfactory way of combating hypotension than adding another drug.

D. Shock: Since about 1950, the treatment of shock by blood volume replacement and other means has been supplemented in some areas by the use of vasodilators. Adoption of the practice in this country was delayed by a period of wide (and ill-advised) use of infusions of levarterenol (Levophed).

Shock differs from hypotension in that in shock the hypotension leads to greatly augmented sympathetic activity. (The hypotensive drugs to be discussed as treatments for hypertension all block sympathoadrenal discharge and do not cause shock.) Increased sympathetic activity is initially useful in maintaining perfusion pressure to the brain. However, if it is long continued, it reduces the perfusion of the tissues and leads to additional loss of plasma volume as plasma-rich blood is sequestered in the splanchnic area. In a few patients, plasma reexpansion is not achieved after large volumes of fluid are given—ie, the added blood or other fluid is sequestered and the effective plasma volume is not increased. These patients may benefit from vasoactive drugs.

Vasoconstrictors appear illogical since infusions of norepinephrine and other pressor amines further reduce plasma volume and since animals can be driven into lethal shock by infusing an adequate dose. Thus, shock and norepinephrine toxicity are simply different points of entry on the same cyclic process:

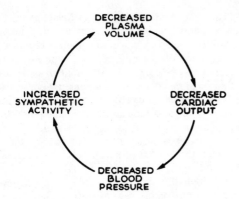

A large volume of experimental and clinical data has suggested that vasodilators are useful in the treatment of shock. The same investigators whose work led to the concept of antipsychotic tranquilizer drugs and the consequent progress in therapy reported good results in treating shock on the assumption that blockade of the sympathetic system was necessary. They used a mixture of chlorpromazine and promethazine, which drugs—like isoproterenol—have beta agonist effects (see Chapter 25). Isoproterenol is now used in those few patients who do not respond to blood volume replacement in all forms of shock except cardiogenic shock. (There is no consensus on the treatment of cardiogenic shock.) Phenoxybenzamine (Dibenzyline), by blocking the vasoconstrictor effects of endogenous epinephrine and norepinephrine, also acts as a vasodilator and has been used as an investigative drug.

E. Complete AV Block: The slow idioventricular rate that accompanies the usual atherosclerotic heart block is not necessarily symptomatic, but it, or a shift in cardiac rhythm, may cause syncope. Ephedrine given orally—usually in combination with phenobarbital to minimize central stimulation—is the usual treatment. In children with heart block secondary to surgical repair of a septal defect, isoproterenol is more commonly used. In either situation, an implanted pacemaker is occasionally necessary.

F. Nasal Congestion: Vasodilatation and edema of the nasal mucosa ("nasal congestion") is an inflammatory reaction that is commonly infectious in origin although it may be due to allergy or may be of unknown etiology (eg, when it accompanies chronic sinusitis). Regardless of the cause, the vasoconstrictor action of the sympathomimetics provides transient relief. If the complaint is due to an immediate allergic reaction (hay fever), the antihistamines will also be effective.

The sympathomimetics can be applied topically in the form of nose drops or spray or by the inhalation of a volatile salt of an amine. The addition of corticosteroids or antibiotics to the spray does not add to its effectiveness. The antihistamines are better given systemically.

Effective systemic use of vasoconstrictors as nasal decongestants is more difficult. The dosage of phenyl-

ephrine (Neo-Synephrine, etc) usually given for this purpose is certainly far below the amounts needed. Other sympathomimetics, if given in adequate doses, cause frequent side-effects but are effective. Ephedrine, pseudoephedrine, and other drugs shown in Table 10–3 cause, in addition, a pleasurable subjective response because of their euphoriant effect.

G. Other Uses: The following applications of the sympathomimetics are either infrequent or are discussed more fully in other parts of this book.

1. With local anesthetics—(See Chapter 22.) The superficial vasoconstriction caused by the addition of epinephrine to solutions of injected local anesthetics delays absorption and thereby decreases toxicity and prolongs the action of the local anesthetic.

2. Topical hemostatic—Epinephrine may be applied locally to a traumatized surface to reduce bleeding from small vessels. It is occasionally still so used in dental surgical practice and in professional sports.

Adverse Reactions

A. Side-Effects: Epinephrine and isoproterenol induce feelings of anxiety, tremulousness, and a frightening awareness of a forceful or rapid heart beat. Following epinephrine administration, the patient will appear pallid and sweaty; in contrast, after isoproterenol he may be flushed. Levarterenol causes less anxiety, and, as it is ordinarily used, side-effects are not common.

B. Overdosage Toxicity: The most common reported cause of epinephrine toxicity is the accidental injection of a dose 10 times larger than that ordered. Such a dose given subcutaneously usually causes the side-effects listed above in an intense form plus headache and substernal pain. Fatal cases have usually shown acute pulmonary edema due to the extremely high arterial and left atrial pressures. Isolated cases of intracranial bleeding have also been reported. When no cause of death is apparent, it is presumed to be due to ventricular fibrillation. Serious arrhythmias are a more common problem if the epinephrine is injected (or liberated during excitement or asphyxia) in a patient sensitized by prior administration of a halogenated hydrocarbon type of anesthetic.

Isoproterenol does not cause the same extreme hypertension, and its acute toxicity in animals is less than that of epinephrine. Nevertheless, the number of sudden, unexpected deaths among young asthmatics has increased as isoproterenol aerosols have come into wide use, and the trend was reversed (in England and Wales) by making them prescription drugs. Isoproterenol given by inhalation exerts an effect for at least 1 hour. The patient should be cautioned against repeating inhalation too often, especially from pressurized aerosols.

The serious toxicity of prolonged infusion of levarterenol was mentioned under the treatment of shock. In addition, the intense vasoconstricting effect of levarterenol can cause local necrosis when a continuous infusion does not enter a rapidly flowing venous channel. If extravasation occurs or ischemic changes are apparent, an alpha-adrenergic blocking agent such as phentolamine should be infiltrated into the area (see Chapter 11).

Contraindications & Cautions

The catecholamines should be used with great care in patients with angina, hypertension, and hyperthyroidism.

Preparations Available

Epinephrine:

Injectable (subcut, IM, IV, intracardiac), 1:1000, 1 ml ampules and 30 ml vials; 1:500 suspension (IM only), 1 ml ampules (in oil)

Topical solution, 1:100, 5 ml ampules and 30 ml vials

Inhalation:

Solution, 1:1000 (1%) and 1.25% (as 2.25% of racemate, Vaponephrin)

Aerosol (Medihaler-Epi), 7 mg/ml. Delivers 0.16 mg/dose.

Levarterenol:

Injectable (IV infusion), 0.2%, 4 ml ampules; 0.02%, 2 ml ampules

Phenylephrine:

Capsules, 10 and 25 mg

Elixir, 1 mg/ml

Injectable (subcut, IM, IV), 1% in 1 and 5 ml

Topical and intranasal:

Jelly, 0.5%, 5/8 oz

Nasal spray, 0.25% (pediatric), 20 ml; and 0.5%, 20 ml

Solution (isotonic), 0.25%, 1, 4, and 16 oz; 0.5%, 1 oz; 1%, 1, 4, and 16 oz

Solution (aromatic), 0.25%, 1 oz

Ophthalmic use:

Viscous solution, 10%, 5 ml Mono-Drop bottles

Low surface tension solution, 0.125%, 15 ml bottles; 2.5%, 15 ml bottles; 10%, 5 ml dropper bottles

Isoproterenol:

Tablets, 10 and 15 mg

Sublingual tablets, 10 and 15 mg

Injectable (subcut, IM, IV infusion, intracardiac), 1:5000 solution, 1 and 5 ml ampules

Inhalation:

Solution, 1:100 and 1:200

2 mg sulfate per ml (Medihaler-Iso), delivers 0.075 mg/dose, in 15 and 22.5 ml

0.25% hydrochloride (Norisodrine), delivers 0.125 mg/inhalation, in 15 ml

Powder, 10 and 25% (Norisodrine), in 100 mg cartridges

Isuprel Mistometer, 15 ml, delivers 0.125 mg per dose

Suppositories, 5 mg

EPHEDRINE & OTHER PHENYLISOPROPYLAMINES

The clinically important properties of ephedrine and the many related phenylisopropylamines are their longer duration of action and the fact that they can be given orally. The effects of ephedrine resemble those of epinephrine and levarterenol, but CNS stimulant properties are more prominent. Some phenylisopropylamines—eg, amphetamines—are used for their CNS stimulant effects. The CNS stimulant drugs are discussed in Chapter 28, but the present section describes their cardiovascular pharmacology.

Chemistry

The mechanisms described above for terminating the action of the catecholamines are not available for this group. The phenylisopropylamines are poor substrates for monoamine oxidase—in fact, they are inhibitors of that enzyme. Ring substituents may be introduced to increase the reactivity and thus reduce the duration of action, but in the absence of ring substituents the duration of action is prolonged. Ephedrine and many of its analogues are stable enough to be active after oral administration for a period of many hours.

In all drugs of this group the alpha carbon is asymmetric. If, in addition, the beta carbon bears a hydroxyl group, it also is asymmetric and 2 pairs of isomers are possible. Thus, a D- and an L-ephedrine and a D- and an L-pseudoephedrine exist, as shown below:

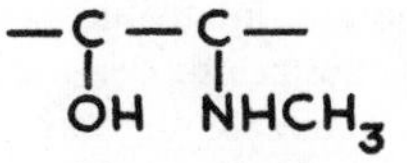

(−) Ephedrine 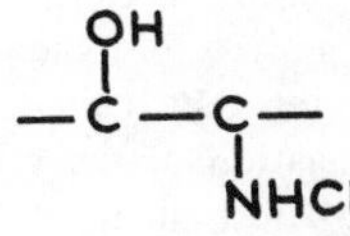   (+) Pseudoephedrine

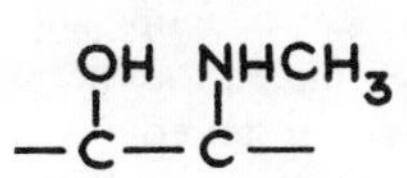

(+) Ephedrine 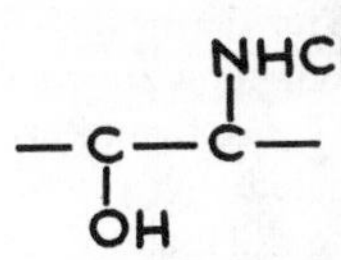   (−) Pseudoephedrine

Ephedrine as used clinically is now a synthetic form of the naturally occurring L-ephedrine. These bases are dispensed as the water-soluble salts of some simple acid, ie, as the hydrochloride or sulfate.

TABLE 10–3. Formulas of ephedrine, amphetamine, and related drugs.*

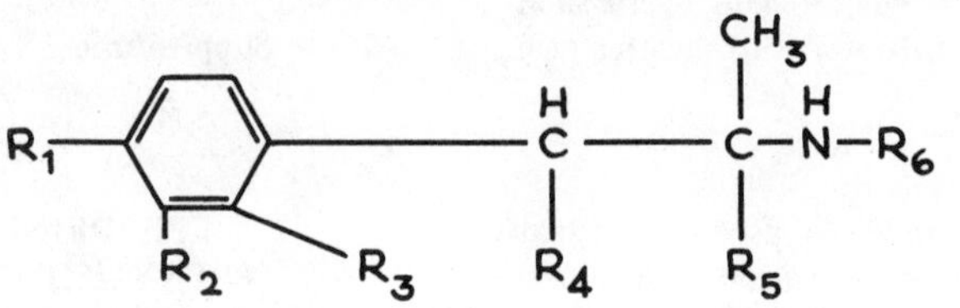

	R_1	R_2	R_3	R_4	R_5	R_6
Ephedrine, pseudoephedrine				HO–		–CH$_3$
Amphetamine						
Methamphetamine						–CH$_3$
Mephentermine (Wyamine)					–CH$_3$	–CH$_3$
Phenylpropanolamine (Propadrine, norephedrine)				HO–		
Hydroxyamphetamine (Paredrine)	HO–					
Metaraminol (Aramine)		HO–		HO–		
Methoxamine (Vasoxyl)		H$_3$C–O–†	H$_3$C–O–†	HO–		

*When no group is indicated as substituted for R, it is assumed that it is an H atom.
†Methoxy substituents are in 2, 5 positions.

Pharmacologic Actions

A. Mechanisms of Action: The ephedrine molecule does not itself act upon smooth muscle or other effector. Its effect is indirect through the action of endogenous epinephrine and norepinephrine present in the organism. Two separate mechanisms are present.

The first mechanism is the liberation of norepinephrine from storage sites in nerve and chromaffin tissue. However, if the source of these intrinsic amines is eliminated by prior treatment with reserpine, the effects of ephedrine persist and may, as in the case of the blood pressure response, be augmented. Elimination of the ephedrine effect requires not only pretreatment with reserpine but denervation of the organ or tissue being studied.

The second (and quantitatively more important) mechanism, therefore, depends upon sympathetic nerve activity but cannot be more clearly defined than by saying that it depends upon an intensification and prolongation of the effect of amines that are already acting. Both in the laboratory and in the clinic, the intensity and duration of response to injected or liberated epinephrine or norepinephrine are increased by prior treatment with ephedrine.

This discussion of mechanism of action applies to the peripheral effects of ephedrine but not necessarily to its CNS stimulating actions. Central effects are not eliminated by reserpine pretreatment sufficient to deplete the brain of catecholamines and serotonin.

B. Effects:

1. Cardiovascular—The cardiovascular effects of ephedrine cannot be equated with those of either epinephrine or norepinephrine. The response is variable, and a degree of controversy therefore exists. If ephedrine acts through epinephrine or norepinephrine already acting in the organism, the variability becomes understandable. In the laboratory, using animal preparations with high epinephrine levels due to barbiturate anesthesia, asphyxia, or shock, the similarity between the effects of ephedrine and those of epinephrine is demonstrable. In unanesthetized, calm humans, the response is closer to that of norepinephrine, ie, cardiac output increases very slightly and vasodilatation is minimal.

2. Other effects—The other effects of ephedrine are qualitatively similar to those described for the catecholamines (above) but are of longer duration. Smooth muscle is relaxed and the pupils dilated. The manifestations of CNS stimulation may be marked.

Absorption, Metabolism, & Excretion

Ephedrine and related phenylisopropylamines are not substrates for COMT. Only a small amount is oxidatively deaminated in the human. A large fraction of a dose of ephedrine, amphetamine, etc is excreted unchanged or with minor chemical change. Since they are slowly metabolized and well absorbed, they are active after oral administration.

Clinical Uses

Ephedrine is substituted for epinephrine in those situations where its longer duration of action or activity after oral administration are advantageous—eg, the nonemergency treatment of allergic reactions, asthma, hypotension during spinal anesthesia, AV block, and as a nasal vasoconstrictor or decongestant. Ephedrine may also be added to the treatment regimen of a patient with myasthenia gravis to improve voluntary muscle function.

Adverse Reactions

A. Side-Effects: The side-effects of ephedrine are similar to those of epinephrine but longer acting. Anxiety, tremulousness, palpitation, and insomnia are common when ephedrine is given 3 or 4 times each day as in the treatment of asthma. Difficulty in initiating urination may be experienced by an older man due to relaxation of the bladder musculature.

B. Overdosage Toxicity: Ephedrine is capable of causing the behavioral changes described after large doses of amphetamine. However, the feelings of anxiety and awareness of heart action are so much more intense after ephedrine that it is not misused. Acute toxicity is seldom encountered because single large doses do not maintain the blood pressure at greatly elevated levels for the entire period of drug action. Vasoconstriction persists, but cardiac output is lowered and plasma volume is decreased as during levarterenol infusions. The acute tolerance that develops to the pressor effects of ephedrine is called tachyphylaxis.

Side-effects and overdosage effects of ephedrine are treated by sedation with barbiturates.

Preparations & Dosages
A. Oral: When a continued effect is necessary, ephedrine sulfate (or, uncommonly, the hydrochloride) is given 3 or 4 times daily. The usual initial dose is 25 mg. Side-effects are common, but ephedrine may be administered in combination with phenobarbital to minimize CNS stimulation. Local application of other sympathomimetics, as by nose drops or inhalation of an aerosol, is substituted for oral ephedrine whenever possible.

Ephedrine is available as tablets or capsules containing 15, 25, 30, 50, and 60 mg; as a syrup containing 20 mg/5 ml; and as nasal drops, 0.5–3%.

B. Injection: 25–50 mg of ephedrine may be injected intramuscularly or subcutaneously. Ampules containing 25 or 50 mg of ephedrine sulfate in 1 ml are available.

Congeners of Ephedrine
Many compounds chemically related to ephedrine have been synthesized and studied. It is possible to exaggerate or diminish some of the pharmacologic properties of ephedrine in these new molecules and to alter the duration of action. In amphetamine and related drugs, the CNS stimulant properties are more prominent and the cardiovascular actions slightly less. In others, the potency as vasoconstrictors is increased, and the resulting pressor agents are suggested as substitutes for levarterenol in the treatment of shock. Methoxamine (Vasoxyl) is practically a pure alpha agonist, but the usefulness of such drugs in shock and hypotension is now questioned. It has also been possible to synthesize indirect-acting amines that lack vasoconstrictor effects—ie, act only on beta receptors. These are listed separately below.

The theoretical optimum for a patient with asthma—a bronchodilator drug devoid of CNS stimulant and cardiovascular effects—is not available.

A. Hydroxyamphetamine (Paredrine): This compound is prepared synthetically for use as a drug but is also a (para-hydroxylated) metabolite of amphetamine. It is almost lacking in CNS stimulating effects and, in

general, is a poor vasoconstrictor although it acts on the heart as ephedrine does. It has been suggested for systemic use in complete heart block, but its common use is as a nasal decongestant and mydriatic. For these last purposes hydroxyamphetamine (Paredrine) is supplied as a 1% nasal solution and 1% ophthalmic solution.

Hydroxyamphetamine is available in tablets containing 20 mg and as ophthalmic solution, 1%, 15 ml bottles.

B. Phenylpropanolamine (Propadrine): Similar to ephedrine but possibly with less CNS stimulant effects at the usual dosages, this drug is available without prescription, usually in combination with an antihistamine, in many cold remedies. It is available as 25 and 50 mg capsules and as an elixir containing 20 mg/5 ml should there be an occasion to prescribe it.

C. Mephentermine (Wyamine): This compound has a long duration of action and is predominantly a beta agonist. Inhalers containing the free base and 0.5% nasal solution are available for use as nasal decongestant, showing that it is not devoid of vasoconstricting ability. Even though mephentermine is said to be a weak CNS stimulant, the contents of the inhaler are sometimes used in lieu of amphetamine. Tablets are available, but no applications are apparent. It is available as the sulfate in ampules containing 1, 2, and 10 ml (15 and 30 mg/ml) for subcutaneous or intramuscular injection of 10–30 mg.

D. Metaraminol (Aramine, Pressonex): This drug must be separated from other phenylisopropylamines because of the important information on its mechanism of action. Studies with isotopically labeled metaraminol show that it is taken up by granules in sympathetic nerve endings, replacing norepinephrine. Subsequent sympathetic nerve activity does not liberate norepinephrine but metaraminol or an active metabolite, the false mediator. The concept of a false mediator has important application to other drugs and is further discussed in Chapter 12 in relation to methyldopa.

The effects of metaraminol are similar to those of norepinephrine, and its use is as a pressor agent. It may be given intramuscularly in doses of 5 or 10 mg, or diluted and given as an intravenous infusion at a rate sufficient to attain the desired blood pressure. Since its duration of action (1 hour) is much longer than that of norepinephrine, intravenous infusion must be started slowly. It is supplied as 1 and 10 ml ampules containing 10 mg/ml.

INDIRECT-ACTING INHIBITORY AMINES

Nylidrin and isoxsuprine are similar to ephedrine in that they are phenylisopropylamines, but the nitrogen bears a substituent which is bulkier than the usual methyl group.

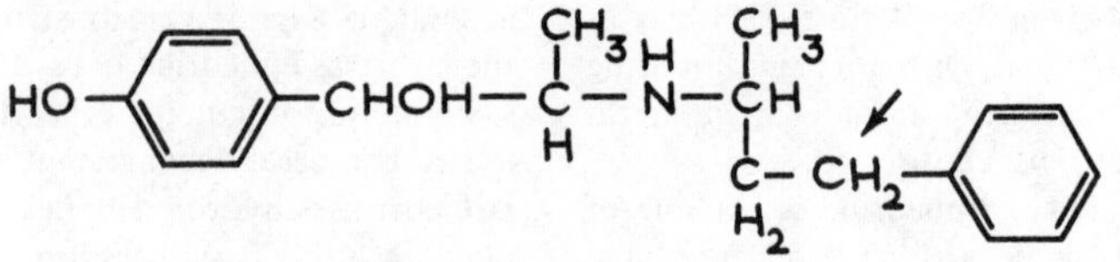

Nylidrin (Arlidin)
(Isoxsuprine [Vasodilan] has an oxygen in
place of the CH$_2$ group shown by the arrow.)

Qualitatively, the effects of these compounds are similar to those of isoproterenol. They are potent stimulators of cardiac rate and force of contraction and are pure vasodilators. They are effective in relaxing smooth muscle and as central stimulants. Their net effect, therefore, is as described above for isoproterenol.

However, these drugs have a much longer duration of action than isoproterenol and may be given orally. In addition, their mechanism of action is indirect, ie, they act to increase the cardiac stimulant and vasodilating properties of epinephrine already acting in the organism.

Nylidrin and isoxsuprine are vasodilators, but they are not useful in chronic arterial insufficiency (see Chapter 13). They have been used as investigational drugs to suppress uterine contractions and defer labor.

INCOMPLETE SYMPATHOMIMETICS

The amines listed below are used only as topical vasoconstrictors of the nasal mucosa or conjunctivas. For these reasons they are usually discussed with the sympathomimetic drugs, but they have few other properties in common with this group. The imidazole derivatives, for example, are vasoconstrictors but have no effect on the myocardium, and, although they relax the intestine, they do not act on the smooth muscle of the bronchioles.

These drugs are familiar in the form of nose drops, inhalers, or in plastic spray bottles. When the latter form is used in children who are reclining rather than upright, a stream rather than a spray may be ejected. In such cases a toxic reaction can occur with hypotension and central depression rather than the expected epinephrine-like effects.

Preparations Available
   Imidazole derivatives:
      Naphazoline* (Privine):
         Nasal solution, 0.05%, 1 oz
         Nasal spray, 0.05%, 20 ml
         Nasal jelly, 0.05%, 20 gm
         Ophthalmic solution, 0.5%, 15 ml

Tetrahydrozoline* (Tyzine):
   Nasal solution, 0.05%, 15 ml; 0.1%, 1
      and 1 oz
   Nasal spray, 0.1%, 15 ml
Xylometazoline* (Otrivin):
   Nasal solution, 0.05 and 0.1%, 30 ml
   Nasal spray, 0.05 and 0.1%, 15 ml
Oxymetazoline* (Afrin):
   Nasal solution, 0.05%, 30 ml
   Nasal spray, 0.05%, 15 ml bottle

Arylisopropylamines:
   Cyclopentamine (Clopane):
      Nasal solution, 1%, 30 ml
      Nasal spray, 0.5%, 15 ml
   Propylhexedrine (Benzedrex):
      Inhaler only

Alkylamine:
   Tuaminoheptane (Tuamine):
      Inhaler
      Nasal solution, 1%, 30 ml
   Methylhexamine (Forthane):
      Inhaler only

TYRAMINE

Tyramine originates physiologically from the decarboxylation of tyrosine. It has no therapeutic applications, but its mechanism of action is important in understanding certain other drugs and drug interactions.

Tyramine acts as a sympathomimetic by displacing norepinephrine from the labile pool in sympathetic nerve and other chromaffin cells without blocking uptake or synthesis. Its effects are therefore exactly like those of norepinephrine, but may be more persistent if the amount of tyramine is large or continuously present. The action of tyramine is completely prevented by pretreatment with agents such as reserpine known to deplete the organism of norepinephrine.

*Generic preparation available. Trade name included for identification only.

*Generic preparation available. Trade name included for identification only.

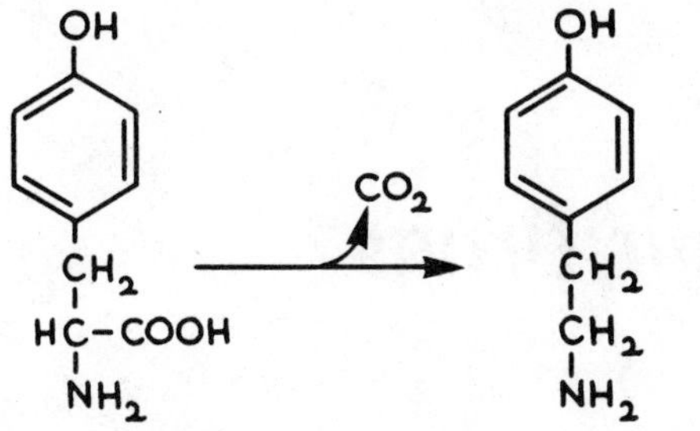

OH

CH$_2$

HC—COOH

NH$_2$

p-Tyrosine

$\xrightarrow{\quad CO_2 \quad}$

OH

CH$_2$

CH$_2$

NH$_2$

Tyramine

Tyramine is inactivated entirely by MAO. If this enzyme is inhibited by an MAO inhibitor type of central stimulant, the tyramine response is prolonged and intensified. Tyramine ingested in cheese or other fermented foods by patients receiving an MAO inhibitor has caused serious hypertensive episodes leading in a few cases to cerebral hemorrhage.

•   •   •

General References

Axelrod, J.: Noradrenaline: Fate and control of its biosynthesis. Science 173:598–606, 1971.

Bayer, O., Blumberger, K.J., & S. Effert: Ueber Kreislauf- und Herzwirkungen des Noradrenalins (Arterenol) beim Menschen. Cardiologia 16:145–168, 1950.

Cohn, J.N.: Comparative cardiovascular effects of tyramine, ephedrine, and norepinephrine in man. Circulation Res 16:174–182, 1965.

Collier, H.D., Meyers, F.H., & G.H. Schmitt: Hemodynamic effects of infusions of epinephrine and arterenol in normal and shocked dogs. Am J Physiol 189:224–228, 1957.

Gilbert, R.P., & R. Hohf: Hemodynamic basis of norepinephrine shock. Proc Soc Exper Biol Med 116:43–46, 1964.

Greiss, F.C., Jr., & D.L. Crandell: Therapy for hypotension induced by spinal anesthesia during pregnancy. JAMA 191:793–796, 1965.

Inman, W.H.N., & A.M. Adelstein: Rise and fall of asthma mortality in England and Wales in relation to use of pressurized aerosols. Lancet 2:279–284, 1969.

Himms-Hagen, J.: Sympathetic regulation of metabolism. Pharmacol Rev 19:367–461, 1967.

Kardos, G.G.: Isoproterenol in the treatment of shock due to bacteremia with gram-negative pathogens. New England J Med 274:868–873, 1966.

Moore, J.I., & N.C. Moran: Cardiac contractile force responses to ephedrine and other sympathomimetic amines in dogs after pretreatment with reserpine. J Pharmacol Exper Therap 136:89–96, 1962.

Schmutzer, K.J., Rasschke, E., & J.V. Maloney: Intravenous L-norepinephrine as a cause of reduced plasma volume. Surgery 50:452–457, 1961.

Smith, H.J., & others: Hemodynamic studies in cardiogenic shock: Treatment with isoproterenol and metaraminol. Circulation 35:1084–1091, 1967.

Speizer, F.E., Doll,R., & P. Heaf: Observations on recent increase in mortality from asthma. Brit MJ 1:335–343, 1968.

Spoerel, W.E., Seleny, F.L., & R.D. Williamson: Shock caused by continuous infusion of metaraminol bitartrate (Aramine). Canad MAJ 90:349–353, 1964.

Sutherland, E.W.: On the biological role of cyclic AMP. JAMA 214:1281–1288, 1970.

Wurtman, R.J.: Catecholamines. New England J Med 273:637–646, 693–700, 746–753, 1965.

11...
Sympathoplegic Drugs

The sympathoplegic drugs are those that block the action of sympathomimetic amines or limit sympathetic outflow. There are now many groups of drugs that decrease sympathetic activity. Their effects will be referred to as sympathoplegic since the alternative term, "sympatholytic," was used for many years to refer to just one of the drug classes which is now called, with more precision, the alpha-adrenergic blocking agents.

Summary & Classification

Below are listed all of the drug types that can reduce sympathetic influences on blood vessels and other effectors. This general classification is based on site and mechanism of pharmacologic action. The first 3 classes are discussed in this chapter. The postural hypotensive agents and reserpine are presented in Chapter 12 in the discussion of the treatment of hypertension.

A. Alpha-Adrenergic Blocking Agents: Drugs that act on the effector organ, beyond the nerve ending, to block the vasoconstricting action of epinephrine or norepinephrine. Exemplified by phentolamine (Regitine) or phenoxybenzamine (Dibenzyline).

B. Beta-Adrenergic Blocking Agents: Drugs that act on the effector organs, beyond the nerve ending, to block the cardiac and vasodilating actions of epinephrine and the cardiac effects of norepinephrine. Propranolol (Inderal) is an example.

C. Ganglion Blocking Agents: Drugs that block transmission across both the sympathetic and parasympathetic ganglia, eg, hexamethonium or mecamylamine (Inversine). They were useful postural hypotensive drugs but have largely been replaced by the postganglionic blocking drugs. They are still useful in the animal laboratory to provide chemical denervation of autonomic tissues.

D. Adrenergic Neuron or Postganglionic Blocking Agents: Guanethidine (Ismelin) and other drugs that prevent the liberation of norepinephrine from sympathetic nerve endings. They act proximal to the effector but distal to the ganglion. Guanethidine is a widely used, potent hypotensive agent.

E. Methyldopa (Aldomet): This drug is probably converted in the body to a "false mediator" liberated in place of norepinephrine. It acts peripherally like guanethidine as an adrenergic neuron blocker and centrally like reserpine to produce sedation. Methyldopa is used in the treatment of hypertension as a potent agent comparable to guanethidine.

F. Reserpine and Related Tranquilizers: Mildly hypotensive drugs that deplete or block uptake of norepinephrine and serotonin at storage sites. Sympathetic activity is reduced by a central or peripheral action.

G. MAO Inhibitors: Some members of this class have more potent hypotensive effects and less potent CNS stimulant and sympathomimetic effects than others. Pargyline (Eutonyl) is the only one used as a sympathoplegic or hypotensive drug.

H. Veratrum Alkaloids: These drugs increase afferent activity reaching the brain stem from thoracic and other chemo- and pressoreceptors. They inhibit sympathetic outflow and augment vagal influences. They are now rarely used as hypotensive agents.

I. Others: Phenothiazine type tranquilizers cause postural hypotension which is often attributed to alpha-adrenergic blockade. The vasodilatation is more probably due to an intensification of the beta-agonist effects of epinephrine. The antipsychotic tranquilizers also reduce sympathetic outflow by a central effect.

Similarly, hydralazine (Apresoline) is not a sympathoplegic drug but acts by increasing the vasodilating and cardiac stimulating effects of epinephrine.

ALPHA-ADRENERGIC BLOCKING AGENTS

Drugs of this class act on vascular smooth muscle to block the vasoconstricting effects of epinephrine and norepinephrine. Vasodilatation and other actions of the sympathetic mediators persist after alpha-adrenergic blocking agents are given. Following the administration of an adrenergic blocking agent, the hypertensive effect of epinephrine is reversed, ie, pressure falls rather than rises. Since norepinephrine lacks the vasodilating action, its effect is blocked but not reversed. The only functions other than vasoconstriction that are blocked are pupillary dilatation, lid retraction, and, in the animal laboratory, nictitating membrane contraction.

Chemistry, Classification, & Mechanism of Action (Fig 11-1)

A. Competitive, Short-Acting Antagonists: The combination of phentolamine (Regitine) with the

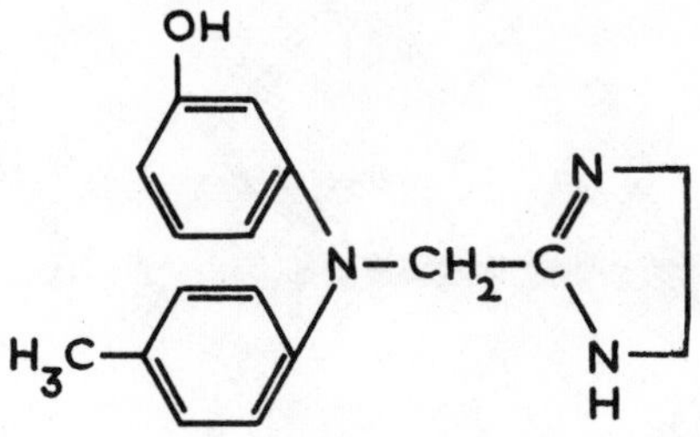

Phentolamine (Regitine)

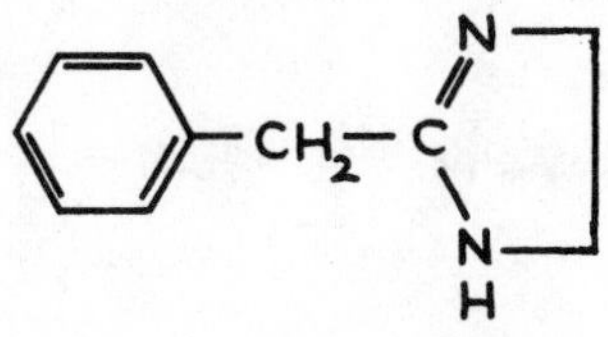

Tolazoline (Priscoline)

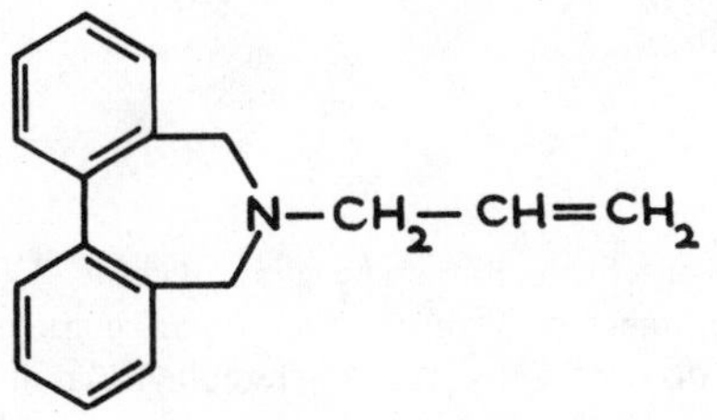

Azapetine (Ilidar)

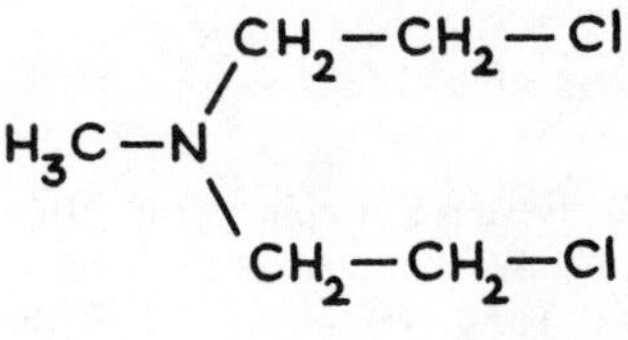

Mechlorethamine (Mustargen)

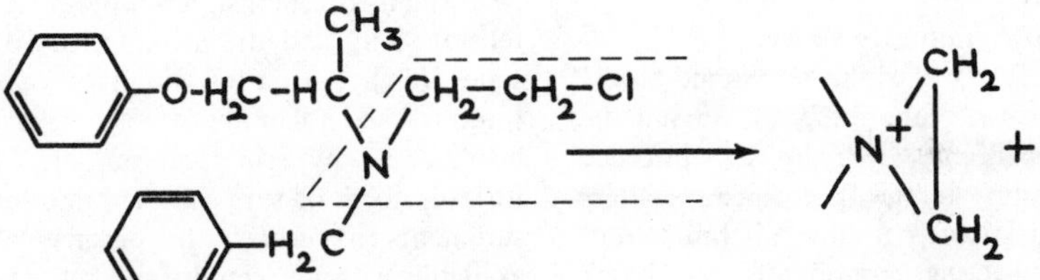

Phenoxybenzamine (Dibenzyline)

Active (ethyleneimonium) intermediate

FIG 11–1. Alpha-adrenergic blocking agents. The structure of mechlorethamine is shown for comparison with that of phenoxybenzamine, also a nitrogen mustard.

receptor that mediates vasoconstriction is reversible. This drug is therefore said to produce equilibrium blockade, ie, the free drug and drug-receptor combination are in equilibrium and the blockade disappears as the free drug is destroyed. The blockade is competitive in that it can be overcome by a large amount of epinephrine or norepinephrine.

B. Noncompetitive, Long-Acting Antagonists: Phenoxybenzamine (Dibenzyline) and Dibenamine, an earlier drug now encountered only in the experimental literature, are beta-haloalkylamines related to the other nitrogen mustards discussed later as alkylating agents in cancer chemotherapy. Their onset of action is gradual over a period of several hours, during which time the cyclization reaction shown in Fig 11–1 occurs. The receptor responsible for vasoconstriction is altered chemically. The blockade is not of the equilibrium type; it outlasts the presence of phenoxybenzamine, is noncompetitive, and persists for several days.

C. Ergot Alkaloids: Reversal of the effect of epinephrine on blood pressure was first noted after administration of ergot. Henry Dale (1906) had first rejected one lot of epinephrine as inactive on the basis of a bioassay and subsequently approved the same lot when it was resubmitted. The apparent inactivity of the first lot was due to his having used an animal that had been given ergot. For many years thereafter, the nonhydrogenated ergot alkaloids were the only alpha-adrenergic blocking agents available. The effect can be demonstrated only in anesthetized animals, however, and should no longer be regarded as an important pharmacologic action of this group of drugs. The ergot alkaloids are discussed as vasoconstrictors in Chapter 14.

D. Other Drugs With Incidental Alpha-Adrenergic Blocking Action: Tolazoline (Priscoline) and azapetine (Ilidar) are alpha-adrenergic blocking agents in the animal laboratory. They also have actions similar to those of histamine, acetylcholine, and epinephrine. Their action as vasodilators is based on their direct effect on vascular smooth muscle and is discussed in Chapter 13.

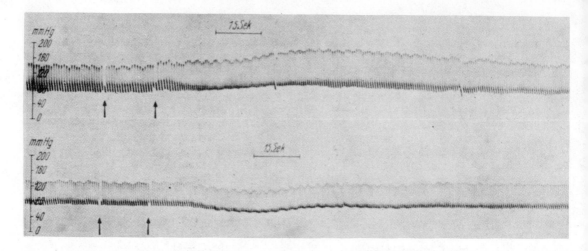

FIG 11–2. Reversal of epinephrine effect on femoral arterial pressure in the human by phentolamine. The upper record shows the control response to epinephrine, 0.2 μg/kg, injected IV during the interval marked by the arrows. The lower record shows the response to the same dose of epinephrine after phentolamine, 0.35 mg/kg, was injected IV. (Reproduced, with permission, from Bernsmeier & others: *Hemmung und Umkehr der Adrenalin-Blutdrucksteigerung am Menschen.* Z Ges Exp Med 121:435, 1953.)

Pharmacologic Actions

A. Mechanisms of Action: See above.

B. Effects: The effects of alpha-adrenergic blocking agents depend not only upon the dosage and the amount of sympatho-adrenal activity present but also on the fact that circulating amines from the adrenal are more easily blocked than neurally liberated norepinephrine. The long-acting compounds can block both circulating and neurogenic amines and cause postural hypotension in both normal and in hypertensive subjects in those few cases where an effective dose is tolerated.

Small doses of the short-acting blocking agents have little effect on the blood pressure of normal subjects or patients with essential hypertension, but lower the blood pressure when it is maintained by circulating amines liberated from a pheochromocytoma. In the presence of shock, if volume replacement is inadequate, phenoxybenzamine will further lower blood pressure.

Other effects of the sympathomimetic amines, notably tachycardia and cardiac stimulation, are usually said to be unaltered by these drugs. Actually, cardioacceleration is in part antagonized by alpha-adrenergic blocking agents, an action minimized in the pharmacologic literature but important in the management of patients with pheochromocytomas.

Clinical Uses

A. Diagnosis and Treatment of Pheochromocytoma: Tumors that arise in chromaffin tissue may release epinephrine and norepinephrine into the general circulation and cause paroxysmal or even sustained hypertension. Such tumors are rare, but essential hypertension is very common; and tests to exclude the existence of pheochromocytoma must be frequently performed to establish an etiologic diagnosis of hypertension. Any patient with a history of paroxysmal episodes of hypertension or signs of episodic or continuous catecholamine effect (anxiety, sweating, heat intolerance, hypermetabolism, etc) should be tested for this form of surgically curable hypertension. Measurements of urinary or plasma catecholamines are available in some centers and reflect the amounts liberated. The urinary metabolite of epinephrine and norepinephrine, VMA (Chapter 10), is more simply determined. It may be necessary to precipitate an increase in the amount of catecholamines liberated from the tumor as described below and to measure the change over a short period rather than determine the content in a 24-hour collection.

1. Provocative test with histamine–Liberation of catecholamines can be provoked in a patient in the interval between paroxysms by several drugs, but the histamine test is best standardized. Histamine in a dose of 0.025–0.05 mg of the base is given IV. Ordinarily, this amount of histamine–a vasodilator–will cause a fall or slight rise in the blood pressure. An increase of 60/30 mm Hg is interpreted as a positive test if that rise exceeds that caused by the cold pressor test.

2. Phentolamine test–In patients with sustained hypertension, the ability of the alpha-adrenergic blocking agents to block circulating catecholamines in smaller doses than are required to block neurally liberated norepinephrine can be utilized. Phentolamine (Regitine), 5 mg IV, usually causes only a minor fall in blood pressure in essential hypertension. A fall of 35/25 mm Hg within 2 minutes is presumptive evidence of pheochromocytoma. Frequent false-positive reactions occur with this test, and it must be supplemented by assays of urinary catecholamines or their metabolites. It is, however, a valuable screening test and may also be used to lower blood pressure following a positive histamine provocative test.

3. Preoperative management—Administration of an alpha-adrenergic blocking agent will prevent the precipitation of acute hypertensive episodes during studies undertaken to localize the tumor and will reverse the changes caused by the chronic release of the catecholamines. As is the case with patients given levarterenol infusions, these patients have a reduced plasma volume and may become seriously hypotensive when the tumor is removed. Preoperative adrenergic blockade restores blood volume. For this purpose, phentolamine by mouth every 4 hours is used. Initial doses of 12.5 mg are given, increasing to 50–100 every 4 hours as blood pressure measurements justify. Phenoxybenzamine is more convenient because only daily doses are required, but there has been less experience with this drug. Oral doses of 10–20 mg/day may be increased only after intervals of several days because of the cumulative effect of the long-acting drug.

Beta-adrenergic blocking agents may be used when tachycardia is a persistent problem. Alpha blockers usually ameliorate cardiac effects, however.

B. Other Uses: Phentolamine (Regitine) is used to prevent the local necrosis that may follow the accidental paravenous injection of norepinephrine (levarterenol, Levophed) during the treatment of shock. In the latter instance, the drug is infiltrated locally.

The limited use as vasodilators of some of the agents classified above as nominal or incidental alpha blockers is discussed in Chapter 13.

Phenoxybenzamine (Dibenzyline) is a postural hypotensive agent; its use is limited by the occurrence of emesis, however, and hypertension is treated with other agents.

In those patients in shock who remain hypotensive following more than adequate volume replacement, phenoxybenzamine is one of the vasodilators now being used on an investigative basis to mobilize sequestered fluid and restore blood pressure. (See Chapter 10.)

Preparations Available

Phentolamine (Regitine) mesylate:
Injectable (IV), 5 mg ampules

Phentolamine (Regitine) hydrochloride:
Tablets, 50 mg

Phenoxybenzamine (Dibenzyline) hydrochloride:
Capsules, 10 mg

BETA-ADRENERGIC BLOCKING AGENTS

The effects of the sympathomimetic amines (Chapter 10) are often divided into 2 groups of actions. Since the same cell—eg, some vascular smooth muscle—can respond by contraction or relaxation to the application of closely related substances, different receptors are hypothesized. The receptors are visualized as differentiated areas on the surface of the cell.

When "alpha-receptors" are activated by contact or combination with alpha-agonists–eg, norepinephrine (levarterenol) on vascular muscle—stimulation or contraction results. Vasoconstriction is the important result of alpha-receptor stimulation.

Beta-receptors mediate vasodilatation, increased force and rate of cardiac contraction, and relaxation of nonvascular smooth muscle. Isoproterenol is a pure beta-agonist. Epinephrine and norepinephrine have both alpha- and beta-stimulating actions. Norepinephrine lacks any vasodilating action but does act to stimulate the heart and relax nonvascular smooth muscle.

In part because of the inconsistent pattern of the response to norepinephrine, the concept of alpha- and beta-receptors had limited influence for many years. There are still theoretical objections to the concept, but the discovery of drugs able to selectively block one or the other groups of effects supports the formulation and, perhaps more importantly, requires a convenient terminology to differentiate the 2 types of blockers.

Alpha-adrenergic receptor blocking agents are, therefore, agents that block catecholamine-induced vasoconstriction and a few other excitatory effects such as pupillary dilatation. Beta-adrenergic receptor blocking agents block the other sympathomimetic actions, ie, vasodilatation, cardiac acceleration, increased cardiac output, bronchiolar dilatation, and hyperglycemia.

Chemistry

Propranolol (Inderal) is the only drug of this class that is now marketed in the USA. However, it is possible to synthesize compounds that are cardioselective –ie, at doses used clinically, they block the effect of sympathomimetic amines on the heart but not on the bronchioles or other noncardiac tissues. Practolol (Eraldin) is an example. Two older compounds are still encountered in the literature. Dichloroisoproterenol (DCI), the first drug of this class in which chlorine replaced the 2 ring hydroxyls, emphasizes the structural similarity of the beta-antagonists to isoproterenol, the potent beta-agonist. In fact, the use of DCI was abandoned because it caused sympathomimetic effects. The second drug, pronethalol, caused thymic tumors in rats and is no longer used.

Propranolol (Inderal)

HN

O—CH$_2$—CHOH—CH$_2$—N—C$_3$H$_7$
                                            H

Practolol (Eraldin)

Absorption, Metabolism, & Excretion

Propranolol is well absorbed after oral administration, and its onset of action is rapid. Its chemical and biologic half-life after intravenous administration to animals is reported to be only 1 hour, but oral doses given to humans 3—4 times a day maintain a constant effect.

Pharmacologic Effects

A. Mechanisms of Action: Propranolol blocks almost all of the effects of injected catecholamines except vasoconstriction. Those effects described above as due to activation of beta-receptors—cardiac acceleration, increased force of contraction, vasodilatation, and smooth muscle relaxation—are blocked (Fig 11—3). The action of the blocking agent is on the effector tissue, ie, neural function is not altered. The antagonism between propranolol and the catecholamines is probably competitive, but the kinetics of the relation have not been clarified.

The effect of administering a drug such as propranolol will depend upon the amount of constant sympathetic tone maintained on the organ or tissue observed. Thus, since the regulation of cardiac function depends upon variations in sympathetic tone, propranolol will cause marked changes in cardiac function.

B. Effects:

1. Cardiac—Blockade of the constant, excitatory sympathetic influences on the heart leads to changes in cardiac function even during the basal state. Moreover, the response of the heart to exercise or other stress is markedly decreased and the expected increase in rate and output does not occur. The effects of propranolol on the heart include the following:

a. A decrease in the rate of normal sinus pacemaker and of other atrial foci present during arrhythmia. The rate of depolarization during diastole is slowed, and a longer interval occurs before the threshold for propagated depolarization is reached. This action slows the rate of a rapid supraventricular focus, but conversion of atrial flutter or fibrillation is not ordinarily accomplished.

b. Atrioventricular (AV) conduction is slowed because the vagal action on the AV node predominates. Like digitalis, propranolol can produce a graded decrease in the rate of ventricular contraction in the presence of a rapid supraventricular rhythm.

c. The force of contraction and, therefore, the minute volume is reduced.

d. Propranolol has a quinidine-like action—ie, it suppresses an ectopic focus, especially in the ventricles —and can slow or abolish abnormal ventricular

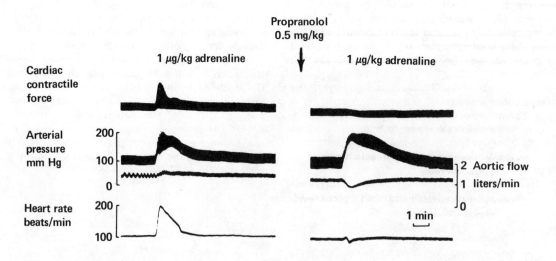

FIG 11—3. The effect in an anesthetized dog of the injection of epinephrine before and after propranolol. In the presence of a beta-receptor blocking agent, epinephrine no longer augments the force of contraction (measured by a strain gauge attached to the ventricular wall) nor increases cardiac rate. Blood pressure is still elevated by epinephrine because vasoconstriction is not blocked. (Reproduced, with permission, from Shanks: The pharmacology of beta sympathetic blockade. Am J Cardiol 18:312, 1966.)

rhythms. This action, among the most important insofar as the clinical application of propranolol is concerned, is not due to its beta-adrenergic blocking ability. The isomer of propranolol most active in correcting ventricular arrhythmias is a less active beta-blocker. The rate of intraventricular conduction is also slowed, and this action also reflects a coincidental quinidine-like effect rather than a result of sympathetic blockade.

2. Respiratory—Of the smooth muscle structures other than the blood vessels, only the bronchioles are of significance in relation to the beta-blockers. Even in normal subjects, the administration of propranolol causes bronchiolar constriction. Patients with asthma or other obstructive respiratory disease are especially susceptible and may respond to propranolol with a dangerous degree of bronchiolar constriction.

Clinical Uses

Propranolol is marketed and approved for use in the USA only for the first 3 indications listed below. Use in other situations is still investigational—ie, the drug must be used only in a planned clinical trial and after patient consent has been obtained. The chapters on the treatment of angina and the dysrhythmias contain additional information on the use of the beta-blockers.

A. Cardiac Arrhythmias: In the presence of a cardiac arrhythmia, propranolol may act either because it is a beta-adrenergic blocking agent or because of a coincidental quinidine-like action in suppressing ectopic pacemaking areas.

When given to patients with atrial fibrillation or flutter, propranolol decreases ventricular rate—especially the elevation that follows exercise. The atrial rate remains rapid, and the beneficial action on ventricular rate is presumed to be the result of prolongation of the refractory period of the AV node due to blockade of catecholamine effect.

The quinidine-like effect is more often apparent with ventricular than with atrial arrhythmias, although the rate of the ectopic focus responsible for an atrial tachycardia is slowed by propranolol.

1. Digitalis-induced arrhythmias—Arrhythmias due to digitalis toxicity appear to be better controlled by propranolol than by supplementary potassium, although any possible potassium deficit should be repaired. Propranolol may be used against digitalis-precipitated atrial tachycardia, ventricular tachycardia, or ventricular ectopic beats judged to be premonitory of a tachycardia.

2. Ventricular tachycardia—Ventricular tachycardia that is not a consequence of the use of digitalis is now most commonly treated by DC countershock (cardioversion). As an alternative treatment—eg, when equipment is not available—propranolol is as effective as quinidine.

3. Atrial flutter or fibrillation—Propranolol rarely converts these arrhythmias and offers no advantage over digitalis in slowing the ventricular rate. It will not, of course, correct any associated congestive failure. A

beta-blocking agent may be used when digitalis is discontinued in anticipation of conversion by countershock.

B. Pheochromocytoma: The importance of the use of alpha-adrenergic blocking agents in patients with a catecholamine-producing tumor before and during surgery has been discussed in the preceding section. A beta-blocker may be used in the management of the patient if persistent tachycardia requires its use. An alpha-blocking agent must always be used first lest an epinephrine-producing tumor cause even greater hypertension following blockade of the vasodilating effects.

C. Hypertrophic Subaortic Stenosis: Symptoms precipitated by exercise in patients with this rare condition are reduced by propranolol.

D. Investigative Uses:

1. Prevention of anginal pain—In controlled studies, the "beta-blockers" reduce the number of anginal attacks and increase exercise tolerance in treadmill tests. The beneficial effect is due to a reduction in the increment of cardiac work that accompanies exercise or other causes of sympatho-adrenal discharge.

2. Reduction of mortality rates following myocardial infarction—It has also been suggested that survival following a myocardial infarction is improved by the chronic administration of propranolol because the drug either prevents ventricular arrhythmias or reduces cardiac work during this critical period. The data needed to evaluate this possible use are both incomplete and conflicting.

3. Treatment of hypertension—Propranolol decreases cardiac output, and the resulting hypotension is not postural—ie, supine and standing blood pressures are lowered to an equal extent.

4. Control of signs of thyrotoxicosis—The peripheral effects of thyrotoxicosis—eg, tachycardia, elevated systolic blood pressure and widened pulse pressure, increased cardiac output, tremulousness, elevated body temperature, and the resulting increase in oxygen consumption—are strikingly similar to the effects of epinephrine and have been treated experimentally with several sympatholegic drugs. Propranolol is the most effective of these agents for this purpose.

Adverse Reactions

A. Side-Effects: Side-effects are common early in treatment with propranolol but, with continued administration, disappear or are greatly reduced within a week. They may include dizziness, tiredness and depression, gastrointestinal disturbances (nausea, diarrhea), paresthesias, muscle aching, and asthmatic wheezing. Transient falsely high responses to tests of liver (SGOT) and kidney (BUN) function occur.

B. Overdosage Toxicity: The toxic effects of propranolol are due to an extension of the effects of beta-adrenergic blockade on the heart, on bronchioles, and on glycogenolysis. They are (1) congestive failure in a patient with limited cardiac reserve, (2) hypotension, (3) AV block, (4) a dangerous degree of bronchiolar constriction, and (5) an intensified hypoglycemic response in diabetic patients receiving insulin or oral hypoglycemic agents.

Intravenous administration is especially hazardous. The drug must be given in small increments over a long period to avoid bradycardia, hypotension, and AV block with a very slow idioventricular rate.

C. Allergic Reactions: Skin rashes and thrombocytopenic purpura have been reported following propranolol administration.

Contraindications & Cautions

The reasons for the following contraindications to propranolol follow from the discussion of adverse effects: (1) Manifest or impending congestive heart failure. (2) Hypotension unless associated with an arrhythmia requiring treatment. Because of the suggestion that beta-blockers be used in the period immediately following a myocardial infarction, cardiogenic shock should be mentioned as a specific contraindication. (3) Complete heart block. (4) Asthma or other obstructive pulmonary diseases.

Propranolol should be used with special care in patients receiving any of the following: (1) insulin or oral hypoglycemic drugs, since the hypoglycemia may be intensified; (2) other sympathoplegic drugs—eg, reserpine, guanethidine or methyldopa—because the effects are additive; and (3) the MAO inhibitors, because, as in the treatment of pheochromocytomas, the augmented alpha-agonist effect may lead to hypertension.

Preparations & Dosages
Propranolol:

>Tablets, 10 and 40 mg. Give orally, 10–20 mg 3–4 times a day initially, and increase as necessary to 40 mg 3–4 times daily.
>
>Injectable (IV), 1 mg/ml, 1 ml ampules. Administration is hazardous, and the most recent package insert should be reviewed if intravenous use is contemplated. Give 1–3 mg no more rapidly than 1 mg/minute and with ECG control.

GANGLION BLOCKING AGENTS

The ganglion blocking agents are included in the group of sympathoplegic drugs even though they block transmission across both sympathetic and parasympathetic ganglia. Since they do achieve a chemical denervation of autonomic organs, the ganglion blockers are still useful laboratory tools. Until recently they were the most widely used and the most potent of the hypotensive drugs, and must be mentioned to explain their prominent place in all but the most recent literature on the treatment of severe hypertension.

Chemistry, Classification, & Metabolism

The duration of action and usefulness following oral administration of the ganglion blocking agents are correlated with their chemical structure and provide a basis for classification.

A. Monoquaternary Ammonium and Sulfonium Compounds: Tetraethylammonium (TEA) and trimethaphan (Arfonad) are both filtered and actively secreted by the kidneys, and their duration of action is brief. When trimethaphan is used to produce a controlled postural hypotension, it is, therefore, given by continuous intravenous infusion. TEA is no longer used clinically.

B. Bisquaternary Compounds: Many of these drugs were introduced for the treatment of hypertension and were of great value until replaced by newer agents—first by mecamylamine and then by guanethidine. Hexamethonium (C6) was the prototype drug, and pentolinium (Ansolysen) was probably the most widely used. Other examples are azamethonium (Pendiomid), chlorisondamine (Ecolid), and trimethidinium (Ostensin). As can be predicted by the fact that these quaternary amines are permanent cations—ie, are always in the ionized form at body pH—their absorption is incomplete and variable. The variability is increased by their action in decreasing intestinal motility.

C. Secondary Amine: Mecamylamine (Inversine) replaced the bisquaternaries and was widely and effectively used until the postganglionic blocking drugs appeared. Absorption is regular and complete.

D. Sparteine: Sparteine (Spartocin, Tocosamine) is an alkaloid isolated from broom top (*Cytisus scoparius*) (Fig 11–4).

Pharmacologic Actions

A. Mechanisms of Action: In the presence of a ganglion blocking drug, acetylcholine is still released by the preganglionic fiber. However, the postsynaptic membrane of the postganglionic fiber is not depolarized. This mechanism contrasts with the failure of repolarization caused by cholinomimetic drugs such as nicotine that can also block transmission at the ganglia (Chapter 8). The acetylcholine antagonism has been shown to be competitive and reversed by neostigmine in the case of TEA, but this relation has not actually been demonstrated for the other agents.

B. Effects: The hypotension caused by the ganglion blocking agents is similar to that described in detail for the postganglionic blocking agents. In the normal human or experimental animal, arteriolar dilatation and venous dilatation both occur as a result of decreasing sympathetic control. In the hypertensive human, venous dilatation with peripheral pooling and a failure of venous return account for the decrease in cardiac output and consequent fall in blood pressure.

In humans and in unanesthetized animals, the pulse rate increases because the high vagal tone maintaining a slow rate is removed by parasympathetic ganglion blockade. In anesthetized animals with high initial pulse rates, the rate falls after administration of a ganglion blocking agent.

A decrease in gastrointestinal motility (sometimes to the point of ileus), urinary retention, dry mouth, loss of power of accommodation, pupillary dilatation,

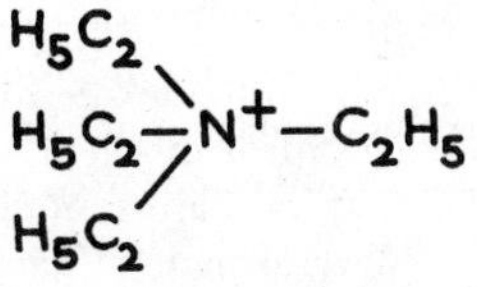

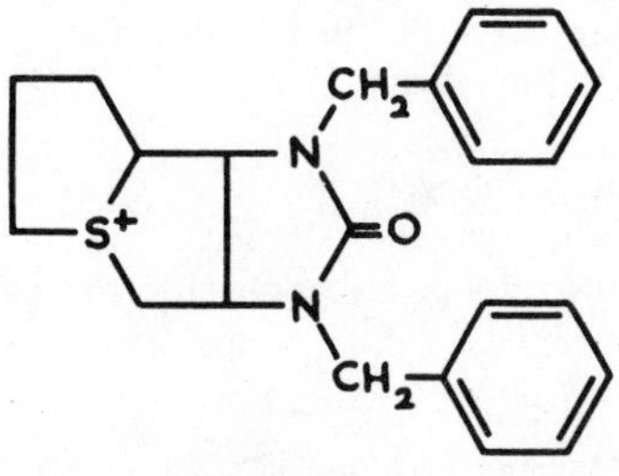

Tetraethylammonium (TEA)

Trimethaphan (Arfonad)

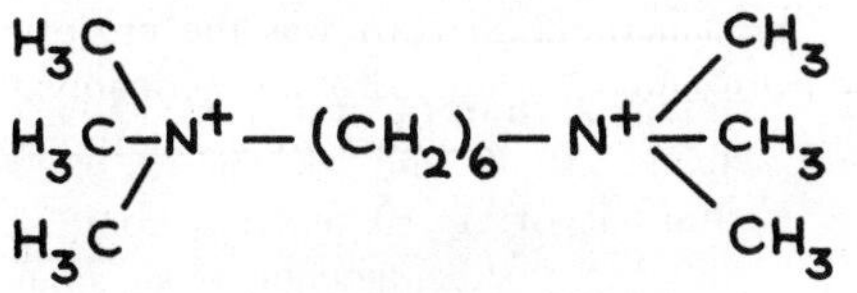

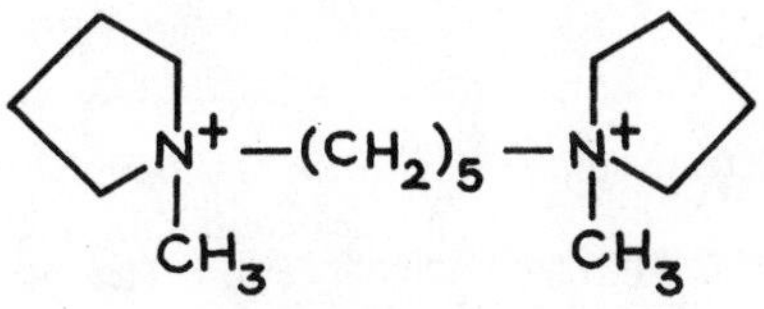

Hexamethonium (C6)

Pentolinium (Ansolysen)

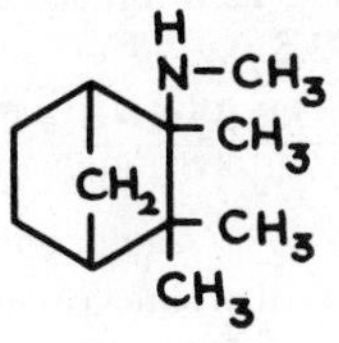

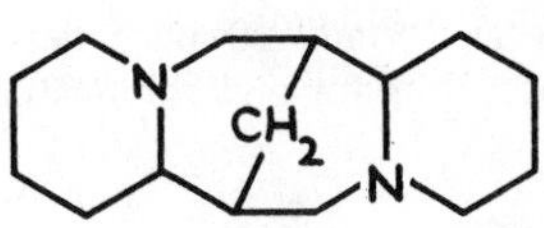

Mecamylamine (Inversine)

Sparteine (Spartocin, Tocosamine)

FIG 11-4. Structures of some ganglion blocking agents.

and impotence are side-effects due to parasympathetic blockade. The effects of blockade of the parasympathetic ganglia are different from the effects of extrinsic nerve section, the drug acting on the intrinsic ganglia present in all automatic tissues. The pylorus and bladder, for example, are relaxed by ganglion blocking agents even though they are rendered hyperactive by parasympathetic nerve sections.

The effector tissues are still able to respond to mediators, and the decrease in gastrointestinal motility, for example, may be treated with neostigmine or bethanechol.

Sparteine blocks ganglionic transmission but also has curariform effects and acts directly on the heart to slow the rate. It is used to stimulate uterine activity at term—an action that also occurs, though possibly less intensely, with the other ganglion blocking agents and with other procedures—eg, spinal anesthesia—that reduce sympathetic influences on the uterus.

Clinical Uses

A. Hypotension During Anesthesia: Trimethaphan is sometimes used by continuous intravenous infusion to induce a controlled postural hypotension and so reduce bleeding during surgical procedures on the head and neck.

B. Induction or Augmentation of Uterine Contractions: Sparteine is used as an oxytocic agent, but preferable alternative drugs—ie, oxytocin and ergonovine—are available.

C. Hypertensive Emergencies: In cases of malignant (accelerated) hypertension, when immediate treatment is judged necessary, the ganglion blocking agents are still sometimes used by injection because they do not cause the same initial release of pressor amines as do guanethidine or reserpine.

D. Investigative Uses: These agents are used investigatively to reduce or abolish all nervous influences on an autonomic tissue. Interpretation of such experiments should recognize that ganglionic synapses, intrinsic as well as extrinsic to the tissue, are blocked. In addition to blocking ganglionic transmission, TEA and, to a lesser degree, trimethaphan in large or repeated doses show effects due to the release of catecholamines from the adrenal medulla and from adrenergic nerves.

Contraindications & Cautions

The ganglion blocking agents should not be used when a precipitous fall in blood pressure would be dangerous—eg, in the presence of vascular disease. Additional contraindications to the use of sparteine are conditions when augmented uterine activity would be dangerous to the fetus or mother.

Preparations & Dosages

Trimethaphan and sparteine are the principal drugs of this group. Occasions for the use of other ganglion blocking agents (mecamylamine, pentolinium) are extremely rare.

Trimethaphan camphorsulfonate (Arfonad): Available in 10 ml ampules containing 50 mg/ml for intravenous infusion. Dilute in 500 ml of saline solution and adjust the rate of infusion to achieve the desired fall in blood pressure.

Sparteine sulfate (Spartocin, Tocosamine): Available in 1 ml ampules containing 150 mg/ml for intramuscular injection. The initial dose of 75 mg may be repeated in 30 minutes. Thereafter, give 75–150 mg at hourly intervals to a total dose of 600 mg unless the oxytocic effect appears earlier.

Mecamylamine hydrochloride (Inversine): Available as 2.5 and 10 mg tablets, and the preferred drug for oral administration. When it

is used in the treatment of hypertension, a diuretic and reserpine should also be used (as when guanethidine is used). The initial dose of 2.5 mg twice daily orally is increased by increments of 2.5 mg of the daily dose every 2–3 days until the desired response is achieved. Control of the dosage must allow for the postural nature of the hypotension and the development of a limited degree of tolerance. All of the suggestions and cautions discussed for the use of guanethidine (Ismelin) or other potent hypotensive drugs (see Chapter 12) apply to mecamylamine also.

Pentolinium tartrate (Ansolysen): Available as tablets, 20, 40, and 100 mg, for oral administration; or in 10 ml vials containing 10 mg/ml for subcutaneous or intramuscular administration. Oral administration is similar to that of mecamylamine, with initial doses of 20 mg 3 times a day, but absorption is less regular. Pentolinium can also be given in doses of 2.5 mg IM or subcut at intervals of 6 hours. The total daily parenteral dose can be increased to as much as 60 mg/day.

● ● ●

General References

Alpha-Adrenergic Blocking Agents

Goldfien, A.: Pheochromocytoma: Diagnosis and anesthetic and surgical management. Anesthesiology 24:462–471, 1963.

Nickerson, M.: The pharmacology of adrenergic blockage. Pharmacol Rev 1:27–101, 1949.

Ross, E.J., & others: Preoperative and operative management of patients with phaeochromocytoma. Brit MJ 1:191–198, 1967.

Beta-Adrenergic Blocking Agents

Amsterdam, E.A., Gorlin, R., & S. Wolfson: Evaluation of long-term use of propranolol in angina pectoris. JAMA 210:103–106, 1969.

Aström, H.: Hemodynamic effects of beta-adrenergic blockade. Brit Heart J 30:44–49, 1968.

Epstein, S.E., & E. Braunwald: Beta-adrenergic receptor blocking drugs: Mechanisms of action and clinical applications. New England J Med 275:1106–1111, 1175–1183, 1966.

Prichard, B.N.C., & P.M.S. Gillam: Treatment of hypertension with propranolol. Brit MJ 1:7–16, 1969.

Shanks, R.G., & others: Controlled trial of propranolol in thyrotoxicosis. Lancet 1:993–994, 1969.

Sloman, G., & M. Stannard: Beta-adrenergic blockage and cardiac arrhythmias. Brit MJ 4:508–512, 1967.

Ganglion Blocking Agents

Paton, W.D.M., & E.J. Zaimis: The methonium compounds. Pharmacol Rev 2:60–95, 1950; 4:219–253, 1952; and 6:59–67, 1954.

12...

Drug Treatment of Essential Hypertension

In Chapter 11, drugs that limit sympathetic influence on blood vessels and other tissues were classified according to their pharmacologic mechanism of action. In this chapter, several of the sympathoplegic drugs are discussed in greater detail, but the classification and emphasis are in terms of their therapeutic use. This apparent inconsistency conforms to common usage and emphasizes the great importance of hypertension as a problem in therapeutics.

Essential hypertension (ie, hypertension of unknown cause) is by far the most common form of elevated blood pressure. Hypertension may also be due to renal or endocrine causes for which specific surgical treatment is available. The drugs available will lower elevated blood pressure regardless of the cause, but they obviously should not be used as a substitute for specific treatment of a correctable underlying disorder.

The elevated blood pressure of essential hypertension is due to arteriolar constriction; the mortality and morbidity are not directly due to the arteriolar disorder, however, but to the effect of the sustained high blood pressure. A sustained elevation of blood pressure accelerates the rate of progression of the atherosclerotic process in larger arteries; causes additional arteriolar damage; and greatly increases the work of the heart. Consequently, essential hypertension is damaging because of the development of cardiac hypertrophy and of coronary artery, cerebrovascular, and renal arteriolar disease with subsequent congestive heart failure, myocardial infarction, strokes, renal failure, and uremia. It is important to point out that lowering blood pressure with drugs will slow the progression of all of the above processes. Some—eg, congestive failure—will regress with treatment of hypertension.

It does not follow that the lowering of blood pressure with drugs is necessarily accomplished by reversing the disease process that caused the elevation. However, if blood pressure is lowered by any mechanism, great benefits result. After the individual drugs have been discussed, the problems of clinical evaluation of the drugs used in the treatment of hypertension will be outlined and the benefits that have resulted from treatment will again be mentioned.

Essential hypertension is a process of variable course and severity. The intensity of treatment, if treatment is deemed necessary, will be correspondingly variable, and several options in treatment are available. Treatment may not require drugs—eg, weight reduction may be adequate treatment—but will usually involve the use of drugs from one or more of the following classes discussed in this chapter: (1) diuretics of the thiazide or other type; (2) reserpine and related alkaloids; and (3) potent or postural hypotensive drugs.

THIAZIDES & OTHER DIURETICS

Drugs that can reduce the total amount of sodium in the body and are suitable for chronic oral administration are used to lower blood pressure by their own action and to increase the effectiveness of other drugs. The sodium diuretics are far more effective than the prohibitively stringent restriction of dietary sodium used in the past.

The general pharmacology of the thiazide diuretics is discussed in Chapter 17, where the many compounds available are identified. In summary, they act by decreasing renal tubular reabsorption of sodium; their action is attended by significant potassium loss.

A. Hypotensive Effect of Thiazides: Thiazides do not lower blood pressure in normotensive humans. In patients with essential hypertension, blood pressure may be decreased 10% or more. For a brief period after diuretic therapy is instituted, plasma volume is decreased, and the fall in blood pressure during this period is explained by a decrease in cardiac output rather than by any decrease in total peripheral resistance. After 1–4 weeks, plasma volume and cardiac output return to control values and the fall in blood pressure is then due to arteriolar dilatation.

The mechanism by which these drugs cause arteriolar dilatation is apparently not simply a loss of either sodium or potassium but some undefined ion shift at the smooth muscle of blood vessels. Supplementary potassium does not reverse the hypotensive action, and some of the diuretics listed in Chapter 17—eg, triamterene (Dyrenium)—are hypotensive but do not increase potassium loss. Sodium loss is evidently not essential since a chemically related compound, diazoxide, is an even better hypotensive agent than the thiazides even though it is not a sodium diuretic. Unfortunately, the diabetogenic effect of diazoxide is too great to allow its general use.

B. Thiazide Diuretics in Combination With Other Drugs: The thiazide diuretics by themselves lower blood pressure slightly and prevent the progression of

UNIVERS... MEDICINA OTTAVIENSIS 99

essential hypertension in the mildest cases. When they are given concomitantly with reserpine, the effect becomes quite significant (see below). In cases requiring the use of postural hypotensive agents, the thiazides act to reduce the amount of the potent drug necessary (and, therefore, its side-effects). They act both through their inherent hypotensive action and through their ability to prevent the expansion of plasma volume which occurs when guanethidine or methyldopa is given.

A thiazide diuretic will almost invariably be the first drug used in the treatment of hypertension. Chronic administration of the thiazides is well tolerated in this situation; their toxic effects are discussed in Chapter 17. If the response to the usual doses of a thiazide—eg, hydrochlorothiazide 50 mg twice daily—is not adequate, nothing is gained by increasing the dosage and a second drug must be added to the treatment regimen.

RESERPINE

The drug that would most often be added to a thiazide is reserpine. By itself, reserpine is only a weak hypotensive drug, but it is extremely useful in combination with a diuretic or postural hypotensive agent.

Source & Chemistry

Reserpine is the purified alkaloid of Rauwolfia or snakeroot. It occurs in many plants of the genus Rauwolfia (Apocynaceae, or dogbane family), but *Rauwolfia serpentina,* the Indian snakeroot, is the usual source. A number of natural and semisynthetic alkaloids other than reserpine are available, but reserpine is the one in widest use. The chemical structures are shown in Table 12–1.

Pharmacologic Actions

A. Mechanisms of Action: Reserpine is a tranquilizer and reduces sympathetic tone. Studies stimulated by the finding that reserpine depletes the organism of norepinephrine, dopamine, and serotonin have contributed information about the mechanism of action of many drugs.

1. Amine depletion—Norepinephrine is stored in granules within sympathetic nerves; in chromaffin cells in the atria and blood vessels; and in some areas of the CNS, notably the hypothalmus. Serotonin (5-hydroxytryptamine, discussed further in Chapter 19) is stored in granules in mast cells, in platelets, in argentaffin cells distributed along the gastrointestinal tract, and in the CNS in association with norepinephrine. Dopamine occurs in association with norepinephrine and also without accompanying norepinephrine in the substantia nigra and basal ganglia. Reserpine administration is followed at first by evidence of liberation and elevated circulating levels of these 3 amines or their metabolites; subsequently, the amounts of the amines

found in brain, sympathetic nerves, and other sites of storage are reduced. Reserpine exerts a persistent effect in preventing the reaccumulation of amines in storage granules. It is tempting to conclude at once that the sympathoplegic effect of reserpine is due to depletion of norepinephrine from sympathetic nerves and that its tranquilizing effect is due to decreased levels of norepinephrine or serotonin in the hypothalamus. However, the phenothiazine tranquilizers exert behavioral effects almost identical with those of reserpine but have no effect on amine storage or metabolism. And the sympathoplegic effect of reserpine, at least in therapeutic dosages, may be central rather than peripheral in origin.

2. Central or peripheral sympathoplegic action— Early experimental work ascribed the sympathoplegic effect of reserpine to a CNS (probably hypothalamic) site of action. The consensus of pharmacologic opinion now, however, is probably that the peripheral effect on sympathetic nerve is more important.

There are practical reasons for regarding this question as unsettled. Most importantly, although reserpine does reduce sympathetic influences on blood vessels, it does not cause postural hypotension. All other drugs that effectively block sympathetic activity peripherally do cause postural hypotension. After reserpine administration, some of the reflexes responsible for maintaining blood pressure in the face of a change to the erect position remain intact, which suggests that cord or medullary centers are still able to exert an effect through sympathetic nerves.

In experimental animals, sympathetic nerve retains some functional ability after all but the very largest doses of reserpine. Perhaps the site of the sympathoplegic action of reserpine can be agreed upon only if the dosage is stipulated. In any case, in the dosages used clinically, most sympathetically mediated reflexes are retained, even when unequivocal evidence of decreased sympathetic effects on organs is also present.

3. Sympathoplegic or parasympathomimetic action—The therapeutically useful sympathoplegic effects of reserpine are accompanied by side-effects that can be interpreted as due to a loss of sympathetic inhibitory tone. Augmented parasympathetic activity has been proposed as an alternative explanation, and reciprocal action on the "ergotropic" and "trophotropic" areas of the hypothalamus has also been suggested. The experiments underlying this interpretation are all based on the idea that a side-effect blocked by atropine or by a ganglion blocking agent must originate from the action of extrinsic parasympathetic nerves. As has been discussed in earlier chapters, both atropine and the ganglion blocking agents act on intrinsic automaticity and have actions distinct from those of parasympathetic nerve section.

B. Effects:

1. Sympathetic inhibition—The sympatholytic action of reserpine results in a limited amount of vasodilatation that may be apparent as a flush, a feeling of warmth, or nasal stuffiness. The decrease in blood pres-

TABLE 12–1. Reserpine and related drugs: Chemical structures and preparations available.

R_1 ... (indole/yohimbane ring structure) ... H_3C-OOC ... R_3 ... R_2

	R_1	R_2	R_3	Usual Daily Adult Dose	Preparations Available
Reserpine	$-O-CH_3$	$-O-CH_3$	$-OOC-$ (ring with $O-CH_3$, $O-CH_3$, $O-CH_3$)	0.25 mg	Tablets and capsules, 0.1, 0.25, 0.5, and 1 mg Injectable (IM), 2.5 mg/ml in 2 and 10 ml ampules Elixir, 0.2 mg/4 ml
Deserpidine (Harmonyl)	$-H$	$-O-CH_3$	(Same as reserpine)	0.25 mg	Tablets, 0.1 and 0.25 mg
Rescinnamine (Moderil)	$-O-CH_3$	$-O-CH_3$	$-OOC-CH=CH-$ (ring with $O-CH_3$, $O-CH_3$, $O-CH_3$)	0.5 mg	Tablets, 0.25 and 0.5 mg
Syrosingopine (Singoserp)	$-O-CH_3$	$-O-CH_3$	$-OOC-$ (ring with $O-CH_3$, $OOC-O-C_2H_5$, $O-CH_3$)	*	Tablets, 1 mg
Yohimbine	$-H$	$-OH$	$-H$	†	. . .
Crude root (Raudixin, etc)				100 mg	Tablets, 50 and 100 mg
Alseroxylon fraction (Rauwiloid, etc)				2 mg	Tablets, 2 mg

*No dosage suggested since the drug is probably not absorbed after oral administration to humans.
†No therapeutic applications.

sure caused by reserpine is minor in humans and unanesthetized animals and is never postural. In the case of reserpine, then, a sympatholytic effect cannot be equated with a significant fall in blood pressure, presumably because the central site of action allows the retention of postural reflexes maintaining blood pressure. Furthermore, increasing the dosage of reserpine does not appreciably increase the hypotensive effect but does increase the side-effects.

Even though reserpine does not significantly lower blood pressure by itself, it does have a persistent sympathoplegic effect. Its usefulness lies in its ability to increase the effectiveness of other hypotensive agents, reducing the amounts of the other agents required and so reducing their side-effects.

2. Parasympathetic predominance—The side-effects of reserpine can be ascribed to loss of sympathetic inhibitory influences and consequent predomi-nance of intrinsic or parasympathetic activity. These include increased gastrointestinal motility, manifested as cramps or diarrhea; increased gastric acid secretion; bradycardia; and pupillary constriction.

3. Tranquilizer type of behavioral depression—Reserpine can be used to control psychotic behavior but was very early replaced by the phenothiazine tranquilizers in the institutional practice of psychiatry. Reserpine does, however, cause a type of sedation or depression characteristic of the antipsychotic or major tranquilizers (see Chapter 25).

4. CNS stimulation—As is true also of the drugs used primarily for their antipsychotic effect, the tranquilizing action of reserpine in high doses is accompanied by signs of CNS stimulation. Extrapyramidal signs and convulsions do not occur with the small doses of reserpine used today, but were demonstrated in the past. Even when given in the dosages used in the

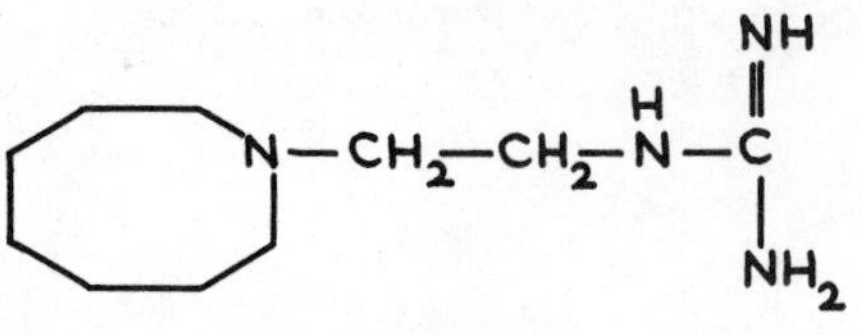

Guanethidine (Ismelin) 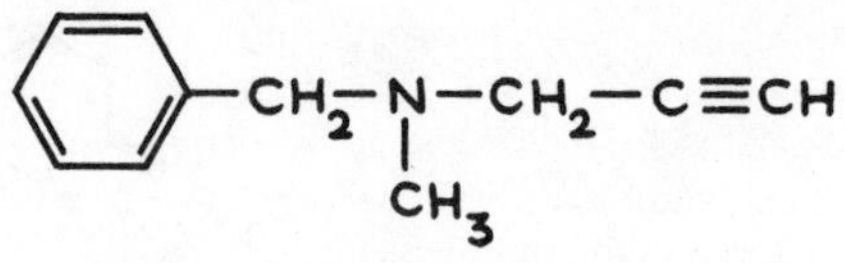   Pargyline (Eutonyl)

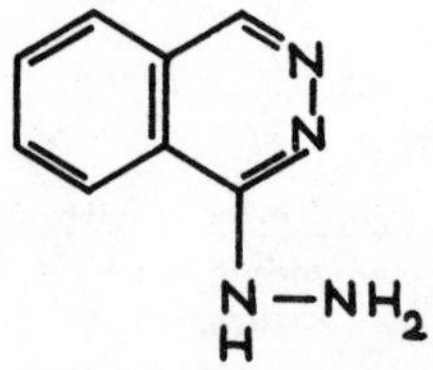

Hydralazine (Apresoline) 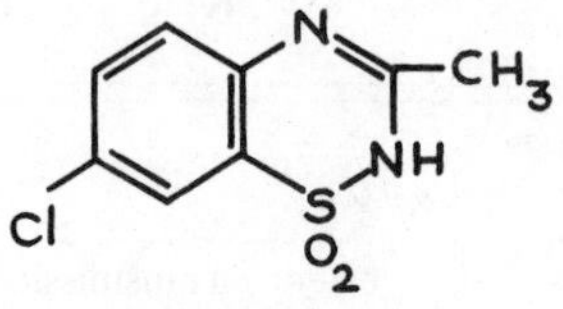   Diazoxide 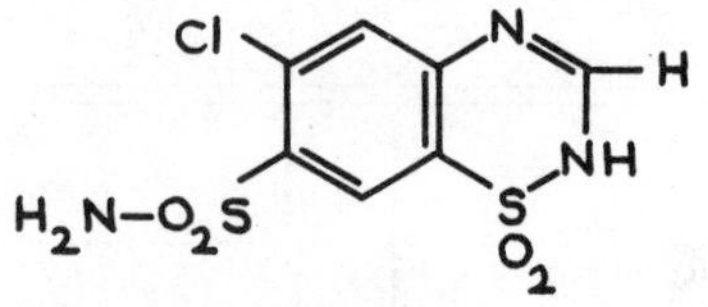   Chlorothiazide

FIG 12–1. Chemical structures of certain hypotensive drugs discussed in this chapter.

treatment of hypertension, reserpine may cause nightmares or a change in sleep pattern.

Absorption, Metabolism, & Excretion

Reserpine itself—but not necessarily all of its analogues—is well absorbed after oral administration.

Following discontinuance of reserpine medication, the tranquilizer effects persist for about 2 days and the autonomic actions for about 7–10 days. It may be a month before serotonin blood levels return to normal.

Clinical Uses

Reserpine is used in small doses—eg, 0.25 mg orally per day—in the treatment of essential hypertension. A thiazide diuretic and, in some cases, a potent hypotensive agent may be given concurrently.

Adverse Reactions

Since allergic reactions to reserpine have not been reported and since the acute toxicity is extremely low, all adverse effects can be considered side-effects. There is no advantage to increasing the dose above 0.25 mg/day, and at these dosage levels side-effects are infrequent.

Of the side-effects related to autonomic function, bradycardia, and miosis are persistent. Feelings of warmth, salivation, stomach cramps or diarrhea, and nasal congestion are usually transient complaints. Reserpine augments gastric acid secretion and can activate or initiate peptic ulcer. Even this action is minimal at daily doses of 0.25 mg or less.

Behavioral side-effects are seen even with small doses. The "tranquilizing" effect is not pleasant—as is the sedation following the use of alcohol or other sedatives, which is pleasant or euphoriant—and many patients complain of a lethargic feeling when taking reserpine. A rare patient will experience a depression in mood sufficiently severe to represent a suicidal risk,

and this risk is greatly increased with larger doses. Increased appetite and dreaming are common; nightmares are infrequent complaints. Excitement, extrapyramidal motor disorders, and convulsions occurred following the administration of the huge doses required in psychiatric practice in the past.

Sodium retention with edema occurs occasionally, and nonpuerperal lactation rarely.

Contraindications & Cautions

Reserpine is contraindicated in the presence of depression in the behavioral or psychiatric sense; during the need for electroconvulsive therapy; when, as in ulcerative colitis, increased gastrointestinal motility would be harmful; and in any patient with a history of peptic ulcer. The latter is not an absolute contraindication if the recommended small doses (0.25 mg/day or less) are used and an ulcer regimen is provided.

Administration of an anesthetic to a patient receiving reserpine may lead to hypotension. This can be avoided by discontinuing reserpine for 2 weeks before elective surgery. However, the hypotension can be reversed by sympathomimetics of both the direct-acting—eg, norepinephrine—and indirect-acting—eg, ephedrine—types.

Preparations Available (See Table 12–1.)

Reserpine, known also by many trade names, is the standard drug of this group. It is inexpensive unless ordered by certain brand names or in combination with a thiazide diuretic in fixed proportions.

No advantage has been established clinically for the alternative preparations listed in Table 12–1.

Analogous Drugs

The **dihydrogenated ergot alkaloids** (dihydroergotamine, Hydergine) discussed in Chapter 14 have properties that parallel those of reserpine. They have been used in the treatment of hypertension with limited success, possibly because they were not combined with other drugs as reserpine now is.

Yohimbine is an alkaloid chemically similar to reserpine but from a different botanical source. It is no longer used clinically. The alpha-adrenergic blocking ability of yohimbine was stressed in the past, but large doses are required to achieve this effect. In smaller doses the effects of yohimbine resemble those of reserpine. Yohimbine once had a completely undeserved reputation as an aphrodisiac.

POSTURAL HYPOTENSIVE DRUGS

The thiazide diuretics alone may suffice for the treatment of the mildest hypertensive patients. Reserpine combined with a thiazide will meet the needs of another large group. But for the more severe treatment problems a still more potent drug must be added to the regimen. The hypotension induced by the potent agents is postural or gravity assisted. The ganglion blocking agents were used with good results for a decade, but their side-effects were more intense than those associated with the drugs discussed below which block only the sympathetic part of the autonomic outflow.

ADRENERGIC NEURON
BLOCKING AGENTS

Drugs of this class are also known as postganglionic blocking agents. As these designations suggest, these drugs act to prevent the release of norepinephrine from the sympathetic nerve endings.

Chemistry

Guanethidine (Ismelin) is currently the important member of this class (Fig 12–1). Several chemically similar drugs are undergoing clinical trial but are not yet marketed in the USA. They are bethanidine (Esbatal) and debrisoquin (Declinax). Bretylium, the first drug of this class, was never marketed in the USA because of its side-effects, but is identified because of frequent published references to it.

Pharmacologic Actions

A. Mechanism of Action: Guanethidine (Ismelin) is taken up by sympathetic nerve just as norepinephrine is taken up to terminate its activity. Following its slow uptake by the nerve, guanethidine replaces norepinephrine in cytoplasm and granules and slowly accumulates in sympathetic nerve in place of norepinephrine. After 3–5 days of guanethidine administration, sympathetic nerves no longer contain and release

amounts of norepinephrine adequate to maintain normal venomotor tone. Reversal of the effect—ie, loss of guanethidine by the nerve and replenishment of norepinephrine—requires 1 week.

Blockade of norepinephrine re-uptake by guanethidine causes a transient initial sympathomimetic effect which is apparent in humans only after intravenous administration.

Amines of the CNS are not altered since the polar guanethidine does not reach parenchymal cells of the CNS.

During the guanethidine action, the effector tissue is still responsive to injected mediator, but electrical stimulation of the postganglionic fibers is without effect. Transmission across the ganglionic synapse is unimpaired. Because of the order in which the drugs were introduced, it was convenient to distinguish these postganglionic blocking agents from the ganglion blocking agents, used earlier, but the phrase "adrenergic neuron blocking agents" more clearly describes the activity that is limited to the sympathetic division of the autonomic nervous system.

B. Effects:

1. Hypotension—The fall in blood pressure caused by guanethidine can be made as intense as desired with the patient in the upright position. When the patient is recumbent, the decrease in blood pressure is much less marked.

2. Mechanism of postural hypotension—In the hypertensive human, the decrease in blood pressure induced by guanethidine is not due to arteriolar dilatation but to dilatation of veins with peripheral pooling, a decreased venous return, and consequent decrease in cardiac output.

Mean arterial blood pressure (MAP) depends upon stroke volume (V_{St}) and upon total peripheral resistance (TPR), ie, the resistance to flow provided by the arterioles as blood flows from the elastic arteries into the tissues. Stroke volume depends upon force of contraction and also upon venous return, which can vary inversely with the size of the capacitance vessels and with the plasma volume available to fill them:

$$MAP \propto V_{St} \cdot TPR$$

Following administration of guanethidine (and other postural hypotensive agents) to hypertensive humans, cardiac output (CO) falls to a degree sufficient to explain the fall in blood pressure. The ratio of MAP/CO—ie, TPR—is not significantly altered. Only in normal humans or experimental animals whose arterioles have not been damaged by hypertension does a decrease in TPR as well as a decrease in CO occur, establishing the occurrence of arteriolar dilatation.

That venous pooling is an important factor in the action of guanethidine was predicted by clinical observations on the effect of posture and the ability of bandages on the lower extremities or immersion of the patient to abolish the hypotension. Bandages and immersion would be expected to collapse veins but not to alter the caliber of the arterioles with their higher internal pressures.

3. Tolerance—A limited degree of tolerance develops early during treatment with guanethidine. To continue to achieve the same hypotensive effect, it may be necessary to slowly increase the dose to as much as 10-fold. In about 2 weeks, however, a dosage plateau is reached and no additional increase is necessary. It was observed that sensitivity to guanethidine could be restored by bleeding or by the simultaneous administration of a sodium diuretic, and that sensitivity could be decreased—ie, tolerance induced—by infusion of plasma or other fluid. Direct measurements then established that the patient's plasma volume increases concurrently with the development of guanethidine tolerance. Whatever the mechanism by which dilatation of the capacitance vessels leads to an increase in plasma volume, the increase does not continue beyond 10–12%, and the degree to which tolerance develops is correspondingly limited. Concomitant administration of a diuretic also limits tolerance.

4. Other effects—Pulse rate is slowed, and an increase in gastrointestinal motility is seen. The hypersecretion of gastric acid which occurs with reserpine does not occur with guanethidine, but diarrhea is common. The excessive motility appears most commonly after eating, and the postprandial diarrhea may be explosive and embarrassing. It can usually be controlled with atropine. With large doses, ejaculation may be delayed or prevented, but—in contrast with the action of the ganglion blocking drugs—erection is not impaired. Muscle weakness or tremor of unknown origin also appears, more commonly with the now rarely used bretylium than after the usual doses of guanethidine. Guanethidine causes a marked decrease in intraocular pressure in glaucomatous eyes.

Absorption, Metabolism, & Excretion

Guanethidine is well absorbed after oral administration, but the pharmacologic effect develops slowly. On a given daily dose, a stable, maximum effect is reached in 3–5 days, and an interval of at least that length should be allowed between changes in dosage schedule.

Guanethidine is excreted by the kidneys, mostly without chemical change.

Clinical Uses

Guanethidine is used in the treatment of severe hypertension, only after prior or simultaneous initiation of treatment with a thiazide diuretic and reserpine. It is also an investigative drug in the treatment of hyperthyroidism.

Adverse Reactions

The side-effects of guanethidine are listed above. Postural hypotension is not a side-effect but is the primary action of the potent hypotensive drugs. Faintness and fainting are undesirable effects which can be minimized by reducing the amount of guanethidine required by concomitant treatment with reserpine and a thiazide. Any vasodilating influence will intensify the postural hypotension and increase the likelihood of fainting. For example, prolonged standing, alcohol, or heat may cause fainting (especially after exercise).

Contraindications & Cautions

The patient should be instructed about factors that intensify postural hypotension and warned against getting up suddenly from a lying position.

Guanethidine and all of the drugs that decrease sympathetic outflow—ie, all those discussed in this chapter except the diuretics and hydralazine—can decrease cardiac output and cause sodium retention and edema in a patient already verging on congestive heart failure. Concurrent administration of a diuretic will prevent this effect. Edema appears early in the treatment of hypertension before the benefits of lowering blood pressure act on the heart.

Treatment with all of the hypotensive drugs should be initiated very cautiously in the presence of even early renal failure since an abruptly lowered perfusion pressure could temporarily further reduce renal function.

Guanethidine and other agents that have an initial sympathomimetic effect should not be used if pheochromocytoma is possibly present.

Guanethidine effects are reversed by antidepressants, tranquilizers of the phenothiazine type, amphetamine, and cocaine.

Preparations & Dosages

Guanethidine sulfate (Ismelin) is available as 10 and 25 mg tablets. The initial dose in combination with reserpine and a diuretic may be as small as 10 mg/day. The dosage is increased at weekly intervals, allowing for the development of tolerance, until the desired response is maintained. The dose should be adjusted on the basis of blood pressure readings taken after the patient has been in the erect position for about 10 minutes. Dosage adjustments are usually in 10 or 12.5 mg increments. The dosage is reduced if severe diarrhea occurs even if an optimal lowering of blood pressure has not been obtained. Mild diarrhea can often be controlled with atropine.

METHYLDOPA
(Aldomet)

Chemistry

Reference to the scheme in Chapter 10 (sympathomimetic drugs) showing the pathway of norepinephrine synthesis will show the relation of methyldopa (alpha-methyldopa) to the precursors of norepinephrine.

Pharmacologic Actions

A. Mechanisms of Action: Norepinephrine is synthesized through the reaction steps tyrosine → dopa → dopamine → norepinephrine. Methyldopa differs from dopa in that, like ephedrine or amphetamine, it bears an added methyl group on the carbon that adjoins the amine group. It is incorporated into the above reactions with the production of methylnorepinephrine rather than the normal mediator. Methylnorepinephrine is stored in the sympathetic endings, but when it is released by nerve stimulation it is much less effective as a sympathomimetic—ie, it is a "false neurotransmitter." Methyldopa (like dopa, which is discussed in Chapter 30 as a precursor of dopamine, used in the treatment of parkinsonism) also reaches the CNS and exerts a tranquilizing effect.

B. Effects: The effects of methyldopa can be described as combining the effects of reserpine and guanethidine. It causes postural hypotension, but cardiac output is reduced less than with guanethidine. Methyldopa lowers supine blood pressure somewhat more than guanethidine does for the same degree of postural hypotension. Expansion of plasma volume and limited tolerance develop.

In addition, methyldopa causes sedation of the tranquilizer type with complaints of tiredness or depression and cannot, therefore, be given in combination with reserpine.

Absorption, Metabolism, & Excretion

Methyldopa is well absorbed after oral administration, but the onset of its action is delayed for 4—6 hours. The effect of a single dose may last for 24 hours but it takes 2—3 days—until the response stabilizes—to determine the effect of a particular dosage regimen.

Clinical Uses

Methyldopa is used like the other postural hypotensive agents when the effect of the thiazides is not adequate. However, it is added to the thiazides alone, not combined with a diuretic and reserpine. Whether reserpine or guanethidine is combined with a thiazide or whether methyldopa is added is a matter of judgment and individual preference. Methyldopa is preferred to guanethidine in patients with impaired renal function because renal blood flow and glomerular filtration are not depressed by methyldopa. The drug also accumulates in that situation, and smaller amounts can be used. The disadvantages of methyldopa are the frequent side-effects, the cost, and the failure of many patients to respond.

Adverse Reactions

A. Side-Effects: Methyldopa causes the expected bradycardia, diarrhea, faintness, and dry mouth, and failure of ejaculation; it also causes sedation and depression comparable to that caused by tranquilizers. Tiredness and fatigability may be extreme enough to force discontinuance of the drug in 10—20% of patients.

B. Allergic Reactions: Drug fever is a rare result of treatment with methyldopa. A mild, reversible depression of liver function tests with biopsy evidence of cellular damage can also occur, often in association with drug fever or other evidence of an allergic reaction. In addition, methyldopa can lead to a positive direct Coombs test and, rarely, to hemolytic anemia.

Preparations & Dosages

Methyldopa (Aldomet) is available as 250 mg tablets. The initial dose is usually 250 mg twice daily; the average daily dose is about twice that amount. Dosage is increased at 2-day intervals until the desired effect is produced or a daily dose of 2 gm is reached. An injectable derivative, methyldopate hydrochloride (Aldomet ester hydrochloride), is supplied as 250 mg/5 ml ampules for intravenous administration. In acute situations, 500 mg can be administered IV for more rapid effect.

Like all hypotensive agents, methyldopa is also available in fixed combination with a thiazide diuretic. The dosage of methyldopa should not be adjusted using the combination since in almost every case an excess of the diuretic will be prescribed.

HYDRALAZINE
(Apresoline)

Hydralazine (Apresoline) is a hydrazine derivative (Fig 12—1) and, like many other substituted hydrazines, is an MAO inhibitor. It is not so classified, however, because it was introduced earlier than the more familiar MAO inhibitors and because, as is true for all of the MAO inhibitors, the hypotensive ability of this compound is not correlated with its enzyme-inhibiting potency.

Pharmacologic Actions

A. Mechanism of Action: Hydralazine intensifies the vasodilating action of epinephrine and isoproterenol, and in the laboratory this effect is blocked by the prior administration of propranolol. The mechanism of its hypotensive action thus appears to be similar to that of chlorpromazine (see Chapter 25) and is better described as intensification of beta-sympathomimetic effects rather than sympathoplegic.

B. Effects: Hydralazine causes vasodilatation but also tachycardia and increased cardiac output consistent with its beta-agonistic effect.

Clinical Uses

The early experience with hydralazine utilized large doses, and frequent and serious toxic effects resulted. When hydralazine is used in combination with other drugs, hydralazine can be given in smaller dosage with less toxicity. Some experienced clinicians add hydralazine to the regimen when the response to treatment with a thiazide plus reserpine is not sufficient.

It may also be given parenterally in the treatment of a hypertensive emergency until oral medication becomes effective.

Adverse Reactions

Headache (common and often persistent), nausea, weakness, palpitation, and flushing are frequent side-effects of therapeutic doses. Tachycardia and precipitation of anginal pain may occur, although this is rare with small doses and combined therapy. In toxic amounts hydralazine may also cause a reaction indistinguishable from rheumatoid arthritis and systemic lupus erythematosus. In dosages of 400 mg/day or more it causes this reaction in 10% of patients, and it may even do so rarely when given in dosages as small as 100 mg/day. The lupoid state is reversible, but irreversible damage may occur during the active process.

In one group of patients with the "hydralazine syndrome" the incidence of malignancy was disturbingly high.

Hydralazine also causes a neuropathy which may be reversed by pyridoxine. The neuropathy probably results because the hydrazine reacts with pyridoxal, as is discussed in the section on isoniazid (Chapter 52).

Skin rashes are reported occasionally.

Preparations & Dosages

Hydralazine (as a generic drug or as Apresoline) is available as tablets containing 10, 25, 50, and 100 mg, and in 1 ml ampules (20 mg/ml) for intramuscular or intravenous administration. The oral dosage is 25–100 mg as a single daily dose. The parenteral dosage of 10–40 mg is used in hypertensive emergencies and can be repeated every 4–6 hours until oral medication becomes effective.

PARGYLINE
(Eutonyl)

In Chapter 28, a group of CNS stimulants are grouped together and discussed as monoamine oxidase (MAO) inhibitors. Unlike the other MAO inhibitors discussed, pargyline is not a substituted hydrazine or hydrazide derivative but a tertiary amine (Fig 12–1).

The MAO inhibitors have CNS stimulant, sympathomimetic or pressor, and sympathoplegic or hypotensive actions in varying degrees. In pargyline the hypotensive effect is selectively increased, but the other effects may reappear as toxic actions. The mechanism of the hypotensive effect is not established, but it is not clearly related to MAO inhibition. Even the site of action is unknown, but the cardiovascular effects are in general comparable to those of the postganglionic blocking agents—ie, hypotension is postural.

The CNS stimulant properties of pargyline lead to side-effects of nervousness, insomnia, and dreaming. Transient changes in liver function tests also occur. Hypertensive reactions may occur during pargyline therapy because of the MAO inhibition it causes. Tyramine is metabolized entirely by MAO, and if it is ingested as a component of cheese, beer, some wines, or other fermented foods, the hypertensive action of tyramine may be tremendously prolonged and intensified. Other sympathomimetic amines taken, for example, as nasal vasoconstrictors may also have greatly increased pressor effect.

Pargyline should not be combined with sympathomimetics, other MAO inhibitors, or methyldopa. It potentiates the effect of meperidine (Demerol), antidepressants such as imipramine, and presumably many other drugs, as do other more completely studied MAO inhibitors also.

Pargyline is an effective postural hypotensive agent, but alternative agents are more potent and not so unpredictable in their toxic effects.

The manufacturer's labeling imposes many restrictions and obligations on the physician, and it should be reviewed for dosage and other information if the use of this drug is contemplated, rather than the use of other effective drugs that are not so unpredictable in their toxicity.

Pargyline is available in tablets containing 10, 25, and 50 mg. The dosage varies from 25–100 mg daily given as a single dose.

VERATRUM ALKALOIDS

The veratrum alkaloids are rarely used today as therapeutic agents and are included in this discussion for purposes of identification and because their mechanism of action is interesting.

Hellebores (*Veratrum viride* or *V album*) are the source of alkaloids that include (1) alkamines such as veratramine that consist of a steroid nucleus with a cyclic amine at C17, and (2) ester alkaloids in which the alkamines are esterified with organic acids. The latter type, represented by veratridine and protoveratrines A and B (Veralba), are most active on the cardiovascular system.

Veratrine is a mixture of alkaloids (mostly cevadine) from a liliaceous plant related to veratrum. It has only investigative uses and, in spite of the similar names, must be distinguished from the veratrum alkaloids. It produces contracture of voluntary muscle.

The veratrum alkaloids sensitize chemo- and pressoreceptors that lie in the distribution of the left coronary artery, in the lungs, and in the carotid sinus. The increased afferent activity that reaches the brain stem results in inhibition of sympathetic tone and augmentation of vagal efferent activity. Generalized vasodilatation with a fall in blood pressure and bradycardia result. The bradycardia is prevented by atropine.

The hypotensive and emetic doses are so similar that effective clinical use is not possible. Acute tolerance or tachyphylaxis occurs in laboratory animals, and tolerance would probably have been a problem clinically.

CLINICAL EVALUATION OF
HYPOTENSIVE DRUG THERAPY

Two separate problems must be considered in evaluating hypotensive therapy in arterial hyperten-

TABLE 12–2. Effect on average blood pressure (taken at home) of treatment with combination of drugs.*

Group	Before any drug	Last month before thiazide but receiving–		Three months after addition of–	
I	159/102	Reserpine	154/96	Chlorothiazide	145/91
II	180/116	Reserpine plus ganglion block-ing agent	161/97	Chlorothiazide (and dos-age of ganglion block-ing agent halved)	151/93
III	155/101	Placebo-1	164/104	Placebo-2	164/105

*Data from Veterans Administration Cooperative Study Group: Double blind control study of antihypertensive agents. Arch Int Med 110:230–236, 1962.

sion. One is the relatively simple matter of comparing the ability of various drugs and drug combinations to lower blood pressure. The other is to determine whether effective hypotensive therapy significantly decreased mortality and morbidity in hypertensive patients.

Effect of Drugs on Blood Pressure

Blood pressure is not a fixed and invariable measurement. In addition to the usual double blind technics, 2 special cautions must usually be observed in evaluating drugs proposed for use against hypertension: (1) A control period is necessary before medication is started. The measured blood pressure will often fall as the patient becomes accustomed to the procedure of measuring blood pressure and benefits from reassurance. A drug administered during this period will be falsely credited with effectiveness that is actually due to nonspecific factors. (2) Blood pressure must be measured regularly, not casually, and the physician is probably not the best person to take the blood pressure. Nurses, family members, or the patient himself not only record lower and less variable pressures but can take pressures at times best suited to assist in adjusting the dose of drug.

The results of studies carried out after adequate planning can be briefly summarized: Reserpine by itself lowers blood pressure more than does a placebo but no more than other mild agents such as phenobarbital. The thiazides do lower blood pressure, and the combination of a thiazide and reserpine is very useful. When a potent (postural) agent is used, blood pressure in the erect position can be lowered to any desired level. The dosage required is reduced by simultaneous use of reserpine and a diuretic.

The above conclusions can be illustrated by the results of a collaborative study imitating the usual conditions of practice. Blood pressure was measured during a period when no drug was given; then reserpine, reserpine and a postural hypotensive agent, or a placebo were given. After having become stabilized on these drugs, the patients were started on treatment with a thiazide with the results shown in Table 12–2. In the usual course of treatment, a thiazide would have been used earlier; however, these data illustrate the effect of "layering" drugs.

Effect of Hypotensive Therapy on the Course of Hypertension

The quickest method of demonstrating the effect on survival and morbidity of radically lowering blood pressure is to treat patients with the most severe (Keith-Wagener IV) hypertension. This is one situation where withholding treatment from a control group cannot be justified and the results in treated groups must be compared with mortality predicted from "literature controls." If patients with severe renal damage are not included, the predicted 5% survival after 4 years will be increased to more than 70%. Cardiomegaly, congestive failure, and retinopathy can regress.

A number of studies on patients with less severe hypertension have now given clear evidence of the benefits of treatment in deferring disabling complications and death. The following data from Veterans Administration cooperative studies are consistent with the results from at least 4 other countries using other drug regimens.

A group of 380 mildly hypertensive men (diastolic pressure 90–114 mm Hg) were divided into a placebo control group and a group treated with hydrochlorthiazide, reserpine, and hydralazine and followed for an average period of 3.3 years. The results were as follows:

	Controls	Treated
Deaths	56	22
Cardiovascular complications	19	8

Complications included, for example, strokes, congestive heart failure, renal insufficiency, and accelerated hypertension.

Groups of more severely hypertensive men (diastolic pressure 115–129 mm Hg) were followed for 16 months (70 controls) and 21 months (73 treated):

	Controls	Treated
Deaths	4	0
Cardiovascular complications	24	2

The one complication that occurred with equal frequency in both groups and has not been influenced by treatment in any of the trials was myocardial infarction. Other treatment—eg, weight reduction, proscription of cigarette smoking, and exercise—must not be neglected.

Clearly, there is now an obligation to identify those hypertensive individuals in whom treatment is justified. The exact point at which treatment of the mildest hypertensive becomes advisable is still to be defined. One generalization would suggest treatment for all men and all women below age 40 whose diastolic pressure is above 90 mm Hg. For women beyond that age, a diastolic pressure of 100 mm Hg would be tolerated.

•   •   •

General References

General

Hodge, J.V., McQueen, E.G., & H. Smirk: Results of hypotensive therapy in arterial hypertension based on experience with 497 patients treated and 156 controls, observed for periods of one to eight years. Brit MJ 1:1, 1961.

Onesti, G.: Renal pharmacodynamics of antihypertensive drugs: Clinical applications. Am J Cardiol 17:668–672, 1966.

Smirk, F.H.: Drug therapy in hypertension. Clin Pharmacol Therap 2:110–120, 1961.

Veterans Administration Cooperative Study Group on Antihypertensive Agents: Effects of treatment on morbidity in hypertension: Results in patients with diastolic blood pressures averaging 115 through 129 mm Hg. JAMA 202:1028–1034, 1967.

Veterans Administration Cooperative Study Group on Antihypertensive Agents: Effects of treatment on morbidity in hypertension: Results in patients with diastolic blood pressure averaging 90 through 114 mm Hg. JAMA 213:1143–1152, 1970.

Diuretics (See also Chapter 17.)

Green, M.A., & others: Mechanisms by which chlorothiazide potentiates the vasodepressor effect of a ganglion blocking agent. Am J Med 36:87–95, 1964.

Wilson, W.R., & R. Okun: Acute hemodynamic effects of diazoxide in man. Circulation 28:89, 1963.

Winer, B.M., Lubbe, W.F., & T. Colton: Antihypertensive actions of diuretics: Comparative study of an aldosterone antagonist and a thiazide, alone and together. JAMA 204:775–779, 1968.

Villareal, H., & others: Effects of chlorothiazide on systemic hemodynamics in essential hypertension. Circulation 26:405–408, 1962.

Reserpine

Coffman, J.D.: Persistence of reflex sympathetic nervous system activity in man on guanethidine or reserpine. Circulation 35:339–346, 1967.

Schlittler, E., & A.J. Plummer: Tranquilizing drugs from rauwolfia. In: *Psychopharmacological Agents,* vol 1. M. Gordon (editor). Academic Press, 1964.

Shapiro, A.P., & H.C. Teng: Technic of controlled drug assay illustrated by a comparative study of *Rauwolfia serpentina,* phenobarbital and placebo in the hypertensive patient. New England J Med 256:970–975, 1957.

Sheldon, M.B., & J.H. Kotte: Effect of *Rauwolfia serpentina* and reserpine on the blood pressure in essential hypertension: A long-term double-blind study. Circulation 16:200–206, 1957.

Guanethidine

Mitchell, J.R., Arias, L. & J.A. Oates: Antagonism of the antihypertensive action of guanethidine sulfate by desipramine hydrochloride. JAMA 202:973–976, 1967.

Prichard, B.N.C., & others: Bethanidine, guanethidine, and methyldopa in treatment of hypertension: A within-patient comparison. Brit MJ 1:135–144, 1968.

Well, J.V., & C.A. Chidsey: Plasma volume expansion resulting from interference with adrenergic function in normal man. Circulation 37:54–61, 1968.

Rønnov-Jessen, V.: Blood volume during treatment of hypertension with guanethidine. Acta med scandinav 174:307–310, 1963 or Lancet 2:669, 1960.

Methyldopa

Kopin, I.J.: False adrenergic transmitters. Ann Rev Pharmacol 8:377–394, 1968.

LoBuglio, A.F., & J.H. Jandl: The nature of the alpha-methyldopa red-cell antibody. New England J Med 276:658–664, 1967.

Onesti, G., & others: Pharmacodynamic effects of alpha-methyl dopa in hypertensive subjects. Am Heart J 67:32–38, 1964.

Weil, M.H., Barbour, B.H., & R.B. Chesne: Alpha-methyl dopa for the treatment of hypertension. Clinical and pharmacodynamic studies. Circulation 28:165–174, 1963.

Others

Alarcon-Segovia, D., & others: Clinical and experimental studies on the hydralazine syndrome and its relationship to systemic lupus erythematosus. Medicine 46:1–33, 1967.

Moser, M., & others: Pargyline treatment of hypertension. Experience with a nonhydrazine amine oxidase inhibitor. JAMA 187:192–195, 1964.

Schirger, A., & J.A. Spittell: Pharmacology and clinical use of hydralazine in the treatment of diastolic hypertension. Am J Cardiol 9:854–859, 1962.

13 . . .

Vasodilator Drugs:
Drug Effects on Regional Blood Flow

Those drugs discussed in Chapter 12 as useful in the treatment of hypertension have a diffuse dilating effect on all blood vessels. The additional vasodilators introduced in this chapter are sometimes alleged to have a selective vasodilator action on the coronary, cerebral, and peripheral vascular beds. They are actually also general vasodilators but, unlike the drugs used in the treatment of hypertension, they do not block the outflow of the sympathetic nervous system as part of their effect.

From our discussion of the treatment of hypertension, 2 concepts must be carried over to clarify the discussion of this group of drugs: (1) Drugs may relieve the manifestations of a disease by acting through a mechanism different from that which caused the disease; and (2) drug action in a normal subject may be different from that in a diseased subject. In addition, whereas hypertension is a disease of arterioles, the states to be discussed here involve larger vessels—the arteries. Vasodilation cannot be expected to reverse structural changes in the arteries nor to improve collateral circulation by adding a dilator influence beyond that already present due to ischemia. Anginal pain can be reduced by the reduction in cardiac work caused by venodilators, but no such mechanism exists in the case of other peripheral vascular beds.

This chapter covers the following subjects: (1) Nitroglycerin and other drugs used in the treatment of the pain of coronary insufficiency. (2) Drugs suggested for use in peripheral vascular insufficiency in the limbs. (3) Cerebral blood flow. (4) The xanthines, a group of agents with many effects other than peripheral vasodilation.

NITROGLYCERIN & OTHER "CORONARY VASODILATORS"

When atherosclerosis or other occlusive disease of the coronary arteries progresses far enough, a disproportion develops between the myocardial need for oxygen as required by cardiac work and the amount of oxygen available from coronary blood flow. Myocardial ischemia is manifested by pain of characteristic nature (pressing), intensity (severe), location (usually substernal), and radiation (usually to left shoulder and upper arm). The resulting sensation of a life-threaten-

ing, throttling pain in the chest led to the name **angina pectoris**. The unpredictability and variability of the occurrence makes the evaluation of drug treatment difficult.

Since the drugs discussed in this section have limited utility, it is important to treat causal and precipitating factors—eg, atherosclerosis, hypertension, obesity, anemia, and emotional factors. However, treatment is often symptomatic with drugs.

Chemistry & Definitions

Drugs used for the relief of angina are usually either nitrates or nitrites—ie, salts or mixed esters of either nitric or nitrous acid. They include the following:

(1) Inorganic nitrites: Sodium nitrite.

(2) Organic nitrites: Amyl nitrite.

(3) Organic nitrates: Glyceryl trinitrate.

Glyceryl trinitrate (nitroglycerin) is by far the most important drug to be discussed. Table 13–1 lists a number of other nitrated polyhydric alcohols that are often called "long-acting nitrates."

Actually, the most important difference among all of these vasodilators is in their rate of absorption. Amyl nitrite is rapidly absorbed after inhalation, and the effect of the small amounts used is quickly dissipated. Small amounts of nitroglycerin can be used sublingually. The "long-acting" nitrates such as those listed in Table 13–1 appear to be so only because they are slowly absorbed after oral administration. When they are given sublingually, as is possible for all but pentaerythritol tetranitrate, they appear to be similar to nitroglycerin similarly administered. Nitroglycerin given orally in large amounts is slowly absorbed and so becomes long-acting.

Pharmacologic Actions

A. Smooth Muscle Relaxation: Nitroglycerin relaxes all smooth muscle regardless of its location or innervation.

1. Cardiovascular effects—Generalized vasodilatation occurs, but "postarteriolar" or venous dilatation is a prominent and important factor in the blood pressure response to nitroglycerin. Plethysmographic studies established this fact before the postural hypotensive agents became available and before venous dilatation was recognized as an important factor in explaining the therapeutic effect of nitroglycerin.

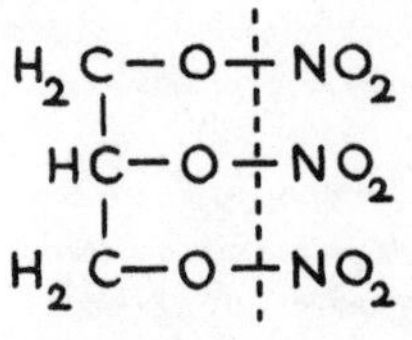

$$H_2C-O\!-\!NO_2$$
$$HC-O\!-\!NO_2$$
$$H_2C-O\!-\!NO_2$$

Glyceryl trinitrate
(nitroglycerin)

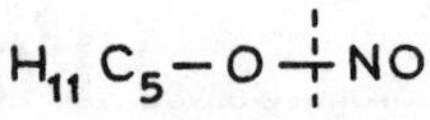

$$H_{11}C_5-O\!-\!NO$$

Amyl nitrite

$$O_2N\!-\!O-H_2C \quad CH_2-O\!-\!NO_2$$
$$C$$
$$O_2N\!-\!O-H_2C \quad CH_2-O\!-\!NO_2$$

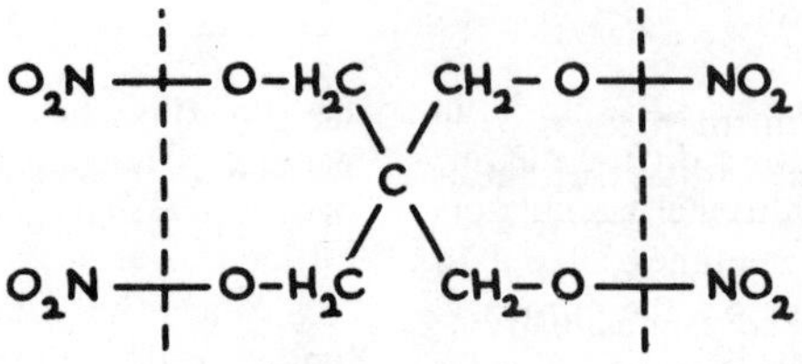

Pentaerythritol tetranitrate
(Peritrate, etc)

FIG 13–1. Examples of a nitrite and nitrates.

The vasodilator effect of nitroglycerin is more readily apparent on specific vascular beds. The blush area—the skin from the clavicles up—is particularly sensitive, and an objective flush and a subjective feeling of warmth in the area are present unless the fall of blood pressure is great enough to cause reflex release of epinephrine with vasoconstriction. Vascular smooth muscle relaxation causes the meningeal or intracranial vessels to lose their ability to resist distention, so that with each pulse they become distended and pull on receptors in the meninges. This is sensed as a throbbing headache synchronous with the pulse, a common side-effect of the vasodilator drugs. Intraocular vasodilatation leads to increased intraocular pressure which can intensify glaucoma. The coronary vessels certainly are dilated in animals and in normal humans, but whether this occurs in patients with coronary insufficiency is a question discussed in detail below.

Secondary to the generalized vasodilatation, blood pressure is decreased. The effect is similar to that of the gravity assisted or postural hypotensive agents discussed in Chapter 12 with the important difference that, since the sympathetic nervous system is not blocked, tachycardia and other evidences of sympatho-adrenal discharge may appear. The extent of the hypotensive effect thus depends not only on the dose used but also on the position of the patient. If the patient is upright and immobile, the effect will be intensified. This explains the syncope that may be induced by vasodilators and also, since the perfusion pressure to the coronary arteries may be reduced, the paradoxic effect of nitroglycerin in sometimes causing an increase in ECG signs of myocardial ischemia. If the effect is intense enough, the patient may faint or feel dizzy, but at this point the reflex activation of the sympathetic nervous system will lead to tachycardia

and the patient will appear pale, tremulous, and anxious. Nitroglycerin has no direct effect on heart rate or contractility.

2. Other smooth muscle is transiently relaxed, but this effect has no important therapeutic usefulness.

3. Mechanism of pain relief—The prototype of this drug group, amyl nitrite, was introduced (1867) by Lauder Brunton on the premise that a decrease in blood pressure would reduce cardiac work and therefore would relieve anginal pain. However, since it is easy to demonstrate dilatation of the coronary bed in animals, his theory (but not the use of the drug) was generally rejected for many years. A few investigators found good reason to reject the concept of coronary dilatation. First of all, angina is a disease of the larger coronary arteries, and at least one of the major branches is always occluded. It seemed unlikely to these early critics of the coronary vasodilatation theory that drugs could act upon these structurally abnormal arteries, and it was reasoned that ischemia severe enough to cause pain should be a maximal stimulus to dilatation of arterioles, as it probably is to the development of collateral channels also. The importance of the venous dilatation demonstrated earlier in studies of the hypotensive effect of nitroglycerin and the relief of pain afforded by standing immobile in the erect position had been noted.

Other treatments for angina, such as lowering of associated hypertension or weight reduction, are effective because they reduce the work of the heart. Cardiac catheterization technics made it possible for Gorlin & others to test the hypothesis that nitroglycerin does not act in diseased humans as a coronary dilator but acts to reduce cardiac work. These workers determined cardiac output and blood pressure by the usual methods. A catheter placed in the coronary sinus allowed them to sample mixed venous blood from the myocardium. (The coronary sinus is assumed to return a constant fraction of the coronary flow.) They also measured myocardial oxygen consumption. From cardiac output and arterial pressure, cardiac work was calculated. From coronary blood flow and central arterial pressure—ie, perfusion pressure—coronary vascular resistance was calculated. In the 10 normal patients studied, nitroglycerin was shown to double the coronary blood flow and to decrease the calculated (pressure/flow) coronary vascular resistance. In patients with angina, however, the values for coronary flow and coronary vascular resistance remained fixed. The one consistent effect of nitroglycerin in the patient with a history of angina was to decrease cardiac output and blood pressure and thereby to decrease cardiac work. The decreased cardiac output responsible for the fall in blood pressure presumably is due to venous dilatation and pooling since the subjects showed a fall in systemic and pulmonary venous pressures. Subsequent studies have confirmed and extended these observations.

Certainly, in the face of these data, any subsequent study will have to recognize the difference between animals or normal humans and humans with a disease of therapeutic interest. This fact, suggested by the experience in studying drug mechanisms in hypertension, is also important in other peripheral vascular disease.

From the concept that nitroglycerin does not act selectively on the coronary bed, it follows that many generalized vasodilators would be useful in relieving angina. Those drugs classified as useful in the treatment of hypertension, for example, should also relieve angina in the normotensive patient. They have been used primarily in hypertensive patients, and relief of angina does occur under these circumstances. It has also been reported that these drugs relieve angina in the normotensive patient with coronary disease, as would also be predicted.

Other generalized vasodilators, not necessarily of wide usefulness, have been used in treating angina—eg, alcohol, MAO inhibitors, and quinidine.

The beta-adrenergic blocking agents defined in Chapter 11 clearly act to prevent anginal attacks by reducing cardiac work. Their effectiveness has probably been important in furthering the reclassification of nitroglycerin as a general rather than a coronary vasodilator.

B. Tolerance: If a nitrite or organic nitrate is given continuously, the intensity of the effect soon declines. Increased dosage may at first achieve the same effect, but tolerance soon becomes absolute and huge doses are without effect. The mechanism of this tolerance is not understood. That the drug continues to act and that some form of adaptation occurs in the body on prolonged exposure is suggested by the fact that a rare worker exposed to nitrates in industry will have a serious or even fatal vascular reaction several days after abrupt discontinuance of exposure. Tolerance is not an important factor so long as nitroglycerin is the drug used. In the case of the "long-acting" orga-

nic nitrates, the development of tolerance must be considered in the clinical evaluation of the drugs.

Uses & Clinical Evaluation

A. Suggested Uses of Vasodilators: The following therapeutic objectives must be separately evaluated: (1) Relief of an attack of angina when it occurs. (2) Prevention of an attack of angina by administering the drug before exercise or other stimulus known to induce pain. (3) Decrease in the number of anginal attacks by chronic administration of the drug. (4) Decrease in the size of an infarct by favoring the development of collateral circulation in the period following a coronary occlusion.

B. Problems and Methods of Clinical Evaluation: The evaluation of agents designed to relieve angina is difficult for several reasons. First of all, laboratory assessment in animals or even evaluation in volunteer normal human subjects is impossible; only humans with the spontaneously occurring disease are suitable subjects for drug evaluation.

The symptom is not often regular and predictable in its occurrence. The exercise tolerance of a given patient is not fixed but varies from day to day and at different times during the same day, and angina can be precipitated or influenced by environmental factors other than activity.

A third problem in the evaluation of anti-angina drugs is the fact that the placebo response is great in this disease. This is true not only with drug treatment but with other types of treatment also. For example, to evaluate a surgical procedure (internal mammary artery ligation) alleged to be effective in relieving angina, it was necessary to compare its effects with those of a sham operation. Both procedures gave measurable but transient good results.

Any assay of an anti-anginal effect must, therefore, be conducted with placebo controls and double-blind observation. The specific technics available are the following:

1. Patient reports—A drug that is alleged to have prophylactic value in decreasing the number of attacks during chronic medication can be evaluated by asking trained patients to record and report the number of attacks experienced. An alternative method is to record the amount of nitroglycerin used to relieve pain as an indication of the number of attacks experienced—ie, a prophylactic drug should reduce the need for nitroglycerin. This is the test most immediately and confidently applicable to the actual conditions of general use.

Most of our current practices cannot be validated using this method of evaluation. Even so, studies with agents such as the beta-blockers have shown that positive results can be obtained, and it is difficult to see that a test that utilizes the usual treatment situation should be too demanding of a drug.

2. The ECG response to exercise—The ability of vasodilators to prevent ECG signs of ischemia following exercise can be used as an assay technic. Drugs can modify this response, but there are 2 important disadvantages to this assay: First, there is no fixed relation between the occurrence of pain and the ECG changes; second, only 1–2% of patients with angina are suitable for use in this procedure. The subjects used are thus not randomly selected and are not necessarily representative of the whole group of patients to be treated.

3. **Exercise tolerance tests**—Under carefully standardized conditions, the patient is exercised until pain appears. On other occasions, he is exercised after receiving a placebo or active medication, and an increase in exercise tolerance is interpreted as a useful effect. The only objection to this test, if it is done with proper attention to the experience of prior workers, is that it is difficult to translate a minor increase in exercise tolerance into a clinical response in terms of spontaneously occurring pain. Also, as in any assay, if the development of tolerance to the effect of the drug is possible, one cannot conclude from the effect of a single dose that continued administration will give equivalent effects.

C. **Conclusions:**

1. The ability of nitroglycerin to relieve an attack of angina after the pain has begun has not been demonstrated in controlled experiments on a group of unselected patients. The patient experiencing angina is forced to immobility, and the pain is likely to terminate even without the drug. A definitive trial would therefore compare the duration of an attack after nitroglycerin and after a placebo.

If, as appears likely, our knowledge of angina is incomplete and patients should be placed in several subgroups, a beneficial effect of nitroglycerin on a small fraction of the patients could be obscured by the response of the bulk of the group.

2. The value of using nitroglycerin before exercise to prevent pain is also difficult to establish to the satisfaction of all current investigators.

3. The chronic administration of a long-acting nitrate to reduce the number of attacks is of no value. The lack of potency and the development of tolerance to the nitrates must be considerable factors since at least one other long-acting drug, propranolol, has been shown to be effective. As coronary insufficiency progresses, symptomatic treatment often becomes so discouraging that the hopes of the physician for better therapy may make him unreceptive to suggestions for alternative drugs. For this reason, perhaps, the long-acting nitrates continue in wide use.

4. The claim that pentaerythritol tetranitrate was useful following coronary occlusion to reduce the size of the infarct was based on the results of a single study in which the treated and control groups were not comparable. The advertising which appeared on the basis of this study was soon prohibited, but the practice persists.

Adverse Reactions

A. **Adverse Reactions During Therapeutic Use:** The occurrence of headache and hypotension with dizziness or fainting is unusual, but ECG signs of increased myocardial ischemia are more common (10%). The hypotensive effect has in a few cases led to permanent cerebral damage. The headache is usually transient and requires no treatment, although an occasional individual may require aspirin or other mild analgesics. The hypotension should be immediately treated by placing the patient in a supine position.

B. **Methemoglobinemia:** The nitrites—only amyl nitrite and sodium nitrite of the agents mentioned thus far—are able to convert hemoglobin into methemoglobin. The hemoglobin with the iron in the ferric (oxidized) form rather than the ferrous form loses its oxygen-carrying capacity; if the process is intense enough, hypoxic anemia can result. Methemoglobinemia does not occur during the therapeutic use of any of the vasodilators thus far discussed. It may rarely occur in newborn infants following the ingestion of nitrates contained in water used for the preparation of their formula. The nitrates are reduced to nitrites in the intestine.

Amyl nitrite or even sodium nitrite may be used to deliberately induce methemoglobinemia in the treatment of cyanide intoxication. Cyanide is toxic because it inactivates cytochrome oxidase. Methemoglobin removes cyanide from solution by combining with it to form cyanmethemoglobin. Since the amount of methemoglobin is large in comparison with the amount of cytochrome oxidase, the enzyme is protected. The cyanide slowly liberated from cyanmethemoglobin is converted to thiocyanate (SCN^-) if thiosulfate has been provided by injection.

If it is necessary to treat methemoglobinemia, methylene blue, 1–2 mg/kg IV over a period of 5 minutes, is effective.

Preparations & Dosages

A. **Nitroglycerin:** Nitroglycerin is generally stipulated to be the drug to which other drugs must be compared; few physicians would take their patients off nitroglycerin to experiment with other drugs.

Nitroglycerin is available as hypodermic tablets containing 0.3, 0.4, 0.5, or 0.6 mg. The intermediate doses are most commonly used. The position of the patient is as important as dose in controlling the intensity of the effect. The tablets dissolve very rapidly, and the drug effect appears in about 30 seconds. The patient is told to place one tablet under his tongue upon the appearance of pain. After the precipitating factors have been discussed in detail, the patient may also be taught to use nitroglycerin in anticipation of angina.

Nitroglycerin tablets retain their potency for years unless stored at elevated temperatures. Supplies that are carried by the patient in such a way as to be kept near body temperature might possibly lose potency sooner.

B. **Amyl Nitrite:** Amyl nitrite is equivalent or superior to nitroglycerin in effectiveness and even more rapid in onset of action. It is a liquid dispensed in easily crushed ampules provided with a woven cover. The ampule is broken and 2–3 inhalations of the vapor are used. The use of amyl nitrite is conspicuous and the odor objectionable, and it is, therefore, virtually never used for angina.

C. Other Nitrates: The hope is for a long-acting "coronary vasodilator" to supplement or replace nitroglycerin. In view of the rapid development of tolerance to organic nitrates, it is doubtful that it will ever be possible to develop useful nitrate vasodilators; this is particularly obvious since the organic nitrates were demonstrably impotent in treating hypertension before useful hypotensive drugs became available.

The "long-acting nitrates" are listed in Table 13–1. Whether 3 or 6 alcohol groups are esterified is less important than the route of administration and whether a continuous, prolonged effect is attempted. When these drugs are given sublingually, the onset of their effect is delayed for as long as 10 minutes and the effect is dissipated in 1–2 hours–ie, with a dosage schedule of 3–4 times a day, before the next dose is taken. When these drugs are swallowed, they become long-acting because they are slowly absorbed.

Initial doses may indeed cause generalized vasodilatation. With repeated dosage, however, tolerance develops and the effect does not occur. Thus, the patient is instructed to increase the dose gradually and is simultaneously reassured that the headache which often occurs as an initial side-effect will disappear. So it will, but the therapeutic effect will disappear also despite an increase in dosage.

Cross-tolerance exists between the nitrates, and an experimental subject made tolerant to a long-acting nitrate is also less responsive to nitroglycerin.

D. Other Vasodilators: A number of nonnitrate generalized vasodilators have given some evidence of usefulness in the treatment of angina even in normotensive patients. None are suggested for use at this time; but they are of theoretical interest, and future reports may be favorable. The monoamine oxidase inhibitors appear to be useful in at least some patients with angina. Tetraethylammonium chloride (a ganglion blocking agent), quinidine, and the xanthines are similar examples.

A long series of other vasodilators less active than those used in the treatment of hypertension have been suggested as substitutes for the nitrates. Dipyridamole (Persantine) is a current example. However active this drug may be after injection or in the laboratory, it is ineffective when used as an oral anti-anginal drug. It is available in 25 mg tablets and in 2 ml ampules containing 10 mg for slow intravenous administration.

Khellin, papaverine, ethaverine, dioxyline (Paveril), heparin, and vitamin E have also been suggested for use as vasodilators but without adequate supporting data.

E. Beta-Adrenergic Blocking Agents: These drugs block the action of the sympathomimetic amines on the heart. Following their administration, the work of the heart is reduced and the cardiac response to exercise is also reduced. In the investigative situation, they are efficacious in reducing the number of attacks of angina, and are useful in those patients in whom their use does not precipitate congestive heart failure. These drugs prevent angina by reducing cardiac work (see Chapter 11).

Propranolol (Inderal) is marketed for use in the treatment of cardiac arrhythmias, but its use in the treatment of angina is still investigational in the USA.

VASODILATORS IN PERIPHERAL VASCULAR DISEASE

Generalized vasodilation can lower blood pressure, with great benefit to the hypertensive patient, and can reduce the work of the heart and thus relieve anginal pain. However, generalized vasodilatation is not helpful and may actually be harmful in the treatment of chronic arterial insufficiency of the extremities.

TABLE 13–1. Nitrates other than nitroglycerin: Dosages and preparations available.

	Initial Oral Dose (4 Times Daily)*	Initial Sublingual Dose	Preparations Available
Erythrityl tetranitrate† (Cardilate)	10 mg	5 mg	Tablets, 5, 10, and 15 mg
Pentaerythritol tetranitrate (Peritrate, PETN)	10 mg	. . .	Tablets, 10 and 20 mg Sustained release tablets, 30 and 60 mg
Isosorbide dinitrate (Isordil, Sorbitrate)	10 mg	5 mg	Tablets, 10 mg (sublingual), 40 mg Tablets (oral), 5 and 10 mg Sustained release tablets or capsules, 40 mg
Mannitol hexanitrate	30 mg	. . .	Tablets, 30 mg
Trolnitrate (triethanolamine trinitrate, Metamine)	2 mg	. . .	Tablets, 2 mg, 10 mg (sustained action)

*Initial dose given 4 times daily before meals and at bedtime. As tolerance develops (ie, as headache disappears), increase at intervals up to about 3 times the initial dose. The same holds if drugs are chronically administered sublingually. Not actually recommended for use.

†Generic preparation available. Trade name given for identification only.

Vasodilators in Chronic Atherosclerosis Obliterans

The most common type of occlusive vascular disease results from an atherosclerotic process in the large arteries. As in the case of coronary artery disease, one can anticipate certain reasons why drug therapy might be ineffective. The vessels might be structurally unresponsive, and the ischemia manifested by claudication should have already been accompanied by maximal dilatation. Most importantly, any generalized vasodilator effect that lowers systemic blood pressure (which supplies the perfusion pressure to a limb) could easily cause a reduction in regional blood flow.

However, such a priori reasoning is always inconclusive in pharmacology, and the only way of establishing or disproving the therapeutic usefulness of vasodilators in peripheral vascular disease is the clinical trial. On this basis, then, it must be emphasized that properly conducted trials designed in such a way as to discount results which may be referable to spontaneous variations in the occurrence of claudication have not established any usefulness for vasodilators in peripheral vascular disease. Indeed, in measurements of blood flow in humans with atherosclerotic disease of the limbs, vasodilators of several types have been shown to actually reduce flow through the affected region. The use of drugs to predict the usefulness of sympathectomy in producing localized vasodilatation has also not been successful.

Vasodilator drugs suggested for use in atherosclerosis obliterans can be outlined as follows:

A. Sympatholytics, or Alpha-Adrenergic Blocking Agents: These agents, discussed in Chapter 11, can block the vasoconstrictor effects of sympathetic nerve stimulation or of circulating amines. Phenoxybenzamine (Dibenzyline) has been the most carefully studied in relation to peripheral vascular disease. Like the other drugs listed below, phenoxybenzamine is active but not useful in this application.

B. Nominal Sympatholytics: Tolazoline (Priscoline) and azapetine (Ilidar) are classed as sympatholytics on the basis of animal laboratory work, but they have direct effects on blood vessels similar to those of histamine and acetylcholine. Any vasodilatation which occurs in a clinical situation following their administration is due to direct effects on vascular smooth muscle and not to their adrenergic blocking properties.

C. Smooth Muscle Relaxants: Papaverine is an alkaloid isolated from opium but differing chemically from morphine. It has no narcotic properties and is a generalized smooth muscle relaxant. Cyclandelate (Cyclospasmol) is a synthetic preparation with similar properties.

Nicotinic acid, or niacin (but not nicotinic acid amide) and a closely related analogue, nicotinyl alcohol (Roniacol), are vasodilators, but their effect may not be as generalized as that of papaverine and cyclandelate.

D. Inhibitory or Vasodilating Sympathomimetics: The availability of sympathomimetics comparable to isoproterenol but with a longer duration of action suggested that vasodilatation could be achieved and that the increased cardiac output occurring at the same time might maintain regional flows. Attractive as this possibility was, these drugs have not proved useful clinically in peripheral vascular disease.

Acute Arterial Occlusion

The occlusion caused by arterial embolism or sudden arterial thrombosis is associated with vasospasm or reflex vasoconstriction in the area. Some

TABLE 13–2. Drugs suggested as peripheral vasodilating agents.

	Recommended Doses	Preparations Available
Generalized, direct smooth muscle relaxing effect:		
Papaverine	30–60 mg IV every 3–4 hours	Tablets, 30, 60, 100, and 200 mg Injectable (IV), 30 mg/ml in 1 and 2 ml ampules and 10 ml vials
Cyclandelate (Cyclospasmol)	100–300 mg orally 4 times daily	Tablets, 100 mg Capsules, 200 mg
Cutaneous vasodilators, primarily in blush area:		
Nicotinic acid (niacin)	50–150 mg orally 3 times daily	Tablets, 25, 50, and 100 mg Sustained release capsules, 125 and 250 mg
Beta-pyridyl carbinol (nicotinyl alcohol, Roniacol)	50–150 mg orally 3 times daily after meals	Tablets, 50 mg Sustained release tablets, 150 mg Elixir, 50 mg/5 ml
Alpha-adrenergic blocking agents: (See Chapter 11.)		
Phenoxybenzamine (Dibenzyline)		
Tolazoline (Priscoline)		
Azapetine (Ilidar)		
Sympathomimetics comparable to isoproterenol: (See Chapter 10.)		
Nylidrin (Arlidin)		
Isoxsuprine (Vasodilan)		

physicians believe, probably without good evidence, that the associated vasoconstriction is relieved by vasodilators and provides a clear indication for the use of these agents. Papaverine may be given in a dosage of 60 mg IV every 2–3 hours or, preferably, 30 mg intra-arterially proximal to the site of occlusion; or tolazoline (Priscoline) may be given intra-arterially in doses of 50 mg.

More importantly, acute arterial occlusion demands the immediate institution of anticoagulant therapy. Heparin should be used not only because of its immediate effect but also because it can be immediately neutralized if surgical treatment is possible.

Vasospastic Disorders

Raynaud's phenomenon, acrocyanosis, and livedo reticularis are examples of processes that involve small cutaneous vessels rather than arterial occlusion. These conditions are ordinarily benign but may on occasion be symptoms of a serious disease such as scleroderma or may lead to ulceration of the skin. In such cases, vasodilator drugs are used with the more plausible goal of increasing blood flow through the skin rather than blood flow to muscle, as in the presence of claudication. The drugs listed in Table 13–2 are used in doses sufficient to cause a facial flush. No data are available that would permit positive statements about the usefulness of the vasodilator drugs in the more serious situations.

CEREBRAL BLOOD FLOW

The intracranial blood vessels do not respond to the same neural and humoral influences that control other vascular beds. Vascular tone is regulated by the intrinsic contractility of the vessels modified by the pressure perfusing them and by changes in CO_2 tension. They do not respond to drugs that mimic or block autonomic nervous system effects. Total cerebral blood flow thus remains constant throughout most disturbances in the circulatory system with the notable exception of reduced perfusion pressure, which results in fainting or more serious changes from hypoxia.

Because cerebrovascular disease is such an important problem, the effect of drugs on **regional** intra-

cranial blood flow is of investigative if not yet practical interest. There is no reason to expect that the chronic effects of occlusions can be modified here any more than in the coronary or limb beds. If any element of vasospasm were present, it could perhaps be modified by drugs.

Generalized vasodilators could have a deleterious effect because of the postural hypotension induced. Vasoconstrictors such as ergotamine that act on meningeal vessels rather than vessels to the parenchyma are discussed in relation to migraine in Chapter 14.

Carbon Dioxide

Carbon dioxide is a cerebral vascular dilator, and a 5% or even 10% mixture in oxygen can increase cerebral blood flow as much as 75%. (Hyperventilation has the opposite effect; when it occurs in an anxious patient, it can increase the possibility of fainting when vasodilators are used.) Other blood vessels are also dilated, so that total peripheral resistance falls even though CO_2 inhalation causes a generalized sympathoadrenal discharge. Cardiac output and pulse rate increase. Respiration, of course, is increased in rate and depth. At CO_2 concentrations of 2%, the effect is measurable; at 5%, the patient is aware of the effect but not uncomfortable; at 10%, a maximum increase occurs and the patient is dyspneic. Carbon dioxide is a general depressant at lower concentrations and a general anesthetic at great (50%) concentrations. With intermediate levels, convulsions may occur.

The uses of CO_2 are few. It has been used postoperatively to stimulate breathing and prevent atelectasis, and in the treatment of carbon monoxide poisoning and to interrupt persistent hiccup. Better alternative methods are available in each case. Continuous petit mal episodes sometimes respond favorably to CO_2 inhalations. Carbon dioxide in high concentration is used as a general anesthetic for animals by meat packers.

THE XANTHINES

Each of the 3 common xanthines has some pharmacologic importance. Caffeine and theobromine are ingredients of many popular beverages. Theophylline

Purine   Xanthine   Ethylenediamine
(2,6-dioxopurine)

(Caffeine is 1,3,7-trimethylxanthine; theobromine, 3,7-dimethylxanthine; and theophylline, 1,3-dimethylxanthine)

in combination with ethylenediamine (aminophylline) is a commonly used drug.

The xanthines have multiple effects and will be referred to in several other chapters, but the outline of their pharmacology will arbitrarily be placed here.

Chemistry

The xanthines are purine bases. The chemical structure and the close relation of the 3 xanthines of importance are shown on p 115. Caffeine is present in significant amounts in tea and coffee; theobromine is a component of cocoa. Aminophylline, the most commonly used drug form of the xanthines, is theophylline solubilized by the addition of ethylenediamine. These compounds occur naturally, but their source as drugs is synthetic. Unlike other exogenous purines, the xanthines are not metabolized to uric acid but to incompletely demethylated metabolites.

Pharmacologic Actions

The effects of each of the 3 compounds are qualitatively the same, but each affects the CNS or the cardiovascular system to a different degree. For example, the administration or ingestion of caffeine leads first to cerebrocortical stimulation, the cardiovascular and diuretic actions appearing as "side-effects." Theophylline is a less potent central stimulant than caffeine, and in therapeutic doses the cardiovascular smooth muscle and diuretic effects are exerted without significant central stimulation. The differences among the 3 xanthines are further described in the discussion of therapeutic use (below).

A. CNS Stimulation:

1. Cortical—The xanthines can produce wakefulness (or, in a fatigued patient, arousal) and improved psychomotor performance. These effects are much more difficult to demonstrate than those of amphetamine. Whether the effect is actually due to direct cortical stimulation or to indirect cortical stimulation via the reticular activating system is not known.

2. Medullary—Large doses can lead to stimulation of respiration. However, the specific effect of abolishing the Cheyne-Stokes pattern of respiration is due not to the xanthine used but to the ethylenediamine used to solubilize theophylline.

Stimulation of the vasomotor center in the medulla, causing peripheral vasoconstriction, would lead to an elevation of blood pressure were this action not usually antagonized by the direct peripheral effects described below.

Stimulation of the medullary vagal (cardio-inhibitory) center leads to a decrease in pulse rate.

In laboratory animals, the xanthines are also stimulants or facilitants of spinal cord transmission and can lead to convulsions of the spinal type.

B. Cardiovascular Effects:

1. On the myocardium—The normal sinus rate, ectopic impulse formation, and force of cardiac contraction are all increased. As a result, the vagal slowing described above will be in part masked; extrasystoles or major ventricular arrhythmias may be produced;

and cardiac output will be regularly increased. These are all direct effects on the myocardium independent of innervation.

2. Peripheral dilatation—Since the xanthines are direct smooth muscle relaxants, blood vessels will be dilated. This effect would tend to decrease blood pressure, but it is minimized by the pressor effects of medullary and cardiac stimulation.

3. Coronary circulation—The xanthines dilate coronary vessels in animals. The effect is probably due to a direct action on the smooth muscle of the arteries. However, coronary vasodilatation would also result from increased cardiac work occasioned by the direct myocardial stimulation. The xanthines were used years ago in the treatment of angina without their usefulness being clearly established. On the basis of recent studies on the mechanism of pain relief in patients with angina, the peripheral vasodilatation caused by the xanthines might be expected to act by reducing cardiac work, but the increased cardiac rate and force of contraction would act in an unfavorable direction.

C. Smooth Muscle Relaxation: The xanthines are direct smooth muscle relaxants which, as mentioned above, lead to vascular dilatation. Other smooth muscle is also relaxed, but only the effect on bronchiolar smooth muscle is of therapeutic importance. The bronchodilator effect is extremely important, and aminophylline is often effective in the treatment of bronchial asthma and acute pulmonary edema.

D. Diuresis: The xanthines block renal tubular reabsorption of sodium and were once used as diuretics in the treatment of congestive heart failure. Today, only aminophylline is used for this effect, and that rarely and only in combination with mercurial diuretics.

E. Gastric Secretion: The xanthines stimulate gastric acid secretion and enzyme production and were at one time used as a test meal to stimulate gastric secretion for diagnostic purposes until superseded by histamine. The effect remains important in the treatment of peptic ulcer, where dietary regimens exclude the use of beverages containing xanthine.

Clinical Uses

The usefulness of the xanthines is limited by 2 factors: Their potency is limited when compared with recently developed agents, and chronic oral administration of adequate doses is unsatisfactory in most patients because of the occurrence of nausea and vomiting.

A. Asthma: In the discussion of the uses of sympathomimetic agents in Chapter 10, the treatment of asthma was arbitrarily divided into 2 problems: (1) the control of chronic recurrent wheezing in the nonemergency situations, and (2) the treatment of the acute asthmatic attack that the patient is unable to control with the drugs he carries. Daily control of chronic asthma is usually most easily achieved with the sympathomimetic drugs. When aminophylline is tolerated by the patient, it is often effective. It is, therefore, commonly present in low dosage as a constituent of mixtures taken orally by the asthma patient. Theophylline has been solubilized with many agents other than ethylenediamine, and several such preparations are on the market.

Aminophylline finds its most common use in the treatment of the acute asthmatic attack. Many patients who no longer respond to epinephrine or other sympathomimetics will be promptly relieved by an intravenous injection of aminophylline.

B. Acute Pulmonary Edema: This state must first of all be carefully differentiated from chronic pulmonary edema, ie, the chronic passive congestion that occurs with congestive heart failure. The sudden transudation of fluid into the alveoli occurs in association not only with cardiac disease but with other pathologic states as well. Perhaps the state is reflex or neurogenic in origin, because the most effective treatment is the injection of morphine. Morphine cannot be used when acute pulmonary edema follows head injury or intracranial surgery, and in all cases its effect should be supplemented by the intravenous injection of aminophylline. Oxygen should be given also.

C. Cheyne-Stokes Respiration: Cyclically recurring periods of apnea and hyperpnea associated with changes in blood pressure, state of consciousness, and intracranial pressure, when due to myocardial disease or changes in cerebral circulation, can be interrupted with aminophylline. Fig 13–2 shows that the use of a xanthine in this situation merely intensifies the effect of ethylenediamine, the active component.

D. Other Uses: Several other uses of the xanthines are discussed in other sections of this book. Their use in angina pectoris has virtually disappeared, although their usefulness remains controversial. Aminophylline is still rarely used as a supplement to the diuretic effects of mercurial diuretics. Because of the ability of caffeine to constrict cerebral vessels, it is combined with ergotamine in some mixtures suggested for use in the treatment of migraine. Caffeine is added to mild analgesic mixtures but without acceptable clinical evidence of usefulness. Caffeine is also available in over-the-counter proprietaries used to maintain wakefulness.

Except as contained in beverages, the xanthines should not be considered important or useful central stimulants. In the treatment of drug intoxication, for example, they should not be allowed to interfere with more specific or more effective forms of treatment.

Adverse Reactions

In adults, oral aminophylline in chronic effective doses often causes nausea and vomiting. It should be given slowly when used intravenously to avoid headache, fall in blood pressure, and subjective awareness of a forceful heart beat. Serious cardiac arrhythmias have followed the intravenous use of the concentrated solution intended for intramuscular administration.

More serious and even fatal reactions have occurred in children, often when the dose was determined by simply using an available preparation rather than by calculation on the basis of weight. CNS effects cause agitation, convulsions, coma, and respiratory and vasomotor collapse. Regardless of the route of administration, vomiting occurs, and the vomitus often contains blood from an irritated and hypersecreting stomach.

Preparations & Dosages

The usual adult dosage of aminophylline is 200 mg orally, 250 mg IV, 250–500 mg rectally. If the dosage for children is calculated from the above doses for a 150 pound adult on the basis of the child's weight (see Chapter 4), the dosage will be within the most conservative recommendation, ie, 3 mg/lb rectally and half that amount IV. Intramuscular administration is painful and rarely used.

Aminophylline:
  Tablets (plain or enteric coated), 100 and
   200 mg
  Suppositories, 125, 250, and 500 mg

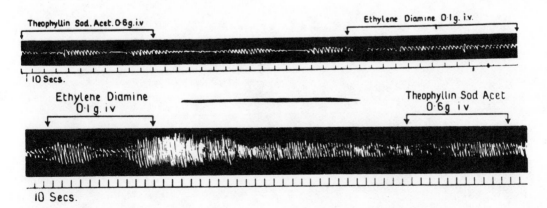

FIG 13–2. The effect of aminophylline on Cheyne-Stokes respiration in patients with left ventricular failure. Theophylline solubilized with sodium acetate is without effect. Ethylenediamine regularized respiration (above) and stimulated it (below). (Reproduced, with permission, from Marais & McMichael: Theophylline-ethylene-diamine in Cheyne-Stokes respiration. Lancet 2:437, 1937.)

Injectable (IV), 250 mg in 10 ml and 500 mg
in 20 ml
Injectable (**IM only**), 500 mg in 2 ml

Caffeine:
Tablets, 60, 100, and 250 mg

**Theophylline monoethanolamine rectal enema
(disposable):** 250 and 500 mg

Beverages Containing Xanthines

A variety of xanthine-containing beverages are
used habitually in different cultures. Drùg factors in
this habituation are present in that the drink contains
amounts of xanthine adequate to cause mild CNS stimulation.

Compared with amphetamine, caffeine effects are
mild and transient. Wide variations in individual sensitivity to alteration in the sleep pattern are established
by objective studies as well as by subjective reports.
Caffeine can in some subjects delay and lighten sleep.

Physical dependence and withdrawal have been
demonstrated in controlled experimental situations.
The habitual coffee drinker may experience mild headaches about 18 hours after being deprived of caffeine.
The occurrence of such headaches has been verified in
controlled experimental situations. The user (5 cups or
more daily) responds to morning caffeine but not to a
placebo with positive subjective feelings, whereas the
abstainer becomes dysphoric.

A single cup of coffee can elevate pulse rate and
systolic blood pressure slightly (5–10 mm Hg). Larger
amounts may cause ventricular ectopic beats. Other
arrhythmias—eg, paroxysmal atrial tachycardia—
usually appear only when the caffeine effect is reinforced by tobacco and fatigue.

The xanthine content of the drink depends upon
the method of preparation as well as the alkaloid content of the crude product. Coffee ordinarily contains
about 100 mg of caffeine per cup, although higher
values are found. Instant coffee contains only half as
much, and "caffeine-free" products a quarter or less.
Tea, especially if prepared from tea bags, rarely contains 100 mg caffeine per cup. Cola drinks contain 50
mg caffeine per 12 oz can. Cocoa drinks contain
theobromine, which is virtually devoid of CNS stimulating effects, in 200–300 mg amounts.

CROMOLYN

Cromolyn sodium (disodium cromoglycate, Intal)
is a bronchodilator that is marketed in the United
Kingdom but is an investigational drug in the USA. It
is included at this point because, like the xanthines, it
is a smooth muscle relaxant used in the treatment of
asthma.

Chemically, cromolyn is related to khellin, a
chromone plant product that is a smooth muscle
relaxant in the laboratory but not useful clinically.

The mechanism proposed for the bronchodilating
action is the interference with mast cell degranulation
by some effect on an early stage of antigen-reagin reaction. The significance of the test used to establish the
mechanism is questionable, and it is more likely that
cromolyn is a smooth muscle relaxant whose distinctiveness is in its route of administration.

It is inhaled as a dry prowder with particle sizes
small enough (2–6 μm) to reach the alveoli and to
cause an initial bronchoconstriction severe enough to
require that it be given together with isoproterenol.

There is no shortage of clinical trials, but there is
no agreement on the place of cromolyn in the treatment of asthma. It is not given during an asthmatic
state but as a prophylactic. It has been evaluated
mostly in corticosteroid-dependent asthmatics, and
there have been no claims of uniform or marked effectiveness. Cromolyn may be useful in selected patients,
but the only basis for its selection is a trial of therapy.

•   •   •

General References

Angina Pectoris

Atkinson, W.J., Jr.: Tetraethylammonium chloride in the treatment of angina pectoris. Am Heart J 39:336–352, 1950.

Gorlin, R., & others: Physiologic and biochemical aspects of the disordered coronary circulation. Ann Int Med 51:698–706, 1959.

Mason, D.T., & E. Braunwald: Effects of nitroglycerin and amyl nitrite on arteriolar and venous tone in the human forearm. Circulation 32:755–771, 1965.

Mellen, H.S., Goldberg, H.S., & H.F. Friedman: Therapeutic effects of pentaerythritol tetranitrate in the immediate postmyocardial-infarction period. New England J Med 276:319–322, 1967.

Riseman, J.E.F., Altman, G.E., & S. Koretsky: Nitroglycerin and other nitrites in the treatment of angina pectoris: Comparison of six preparations and four routes of administration. Circulation 17:22–39, 1958.

Robinson, B.F.: Mode of action of nitroglycerin in angina pectoris: Correlation between hemodynamic effects during exercise and prevention of pain. Brit Heart J 30:295–302, 1968.

Sbar, S., & R.C. Schlant: Negative results: Dipyridamole in the treatment of angina pectoris. JAMA 201:865–867, 1967.

Schelling, J.L., & L. Lasagna: A study of cross-tolerance to circulatory effects of organic nitrates. Clin Pharmacol Therap 8:256–260, 1967.

Cerebral Blood Flow

Eckenhoff, J.E. (editor): Symposium on carbon dioxide. Anesthesiology 21:585–766, 1960.

McHenry, L.C., Jr.: Cerebral blood flow studies in cerebrovascular disease. Arch Int Med 117:546–556, 1966.

Sokoloff, L.: The action of drugs on the cerebral circulation. Pharmacol Rev 11:1–85, 1959.

Peripheral Vascular Flow

Abramson, D.I.: Drugs used in peripheral vascular diseases. Am J Cardiol 12:203–215, 1963.

Barcroft, H. (editor): Peripheral circulation in man. Brit M Bull 19:97–164, 1963.

Gillespie, J.A.: The case against vasodilator drugs in occlusive vascular disease of the legs. Lancet 2:995–997, 1959.

Strandness, D.E., Jr.: Ineffectiveness of isoxsuprine on intermittent claudication. JAMA 213:86–88, 1970.

Xanthines

Colton, T., Gosselin, R.E., & R.P. Smith: The tolerance of coffee drinkers to caffeine. Clin Pharmacol Therap 9:31–39, 1968.

Goldstein, A., Kaizer, S., & O. Whitby: Psychotropic effects of caffeine in man. IV. Quantitative and qualitative differences associated with habituation to coffee. Clin Pharmacol Therap 10:489–497, 1969.

Marais, O.A.S., & J. McMichael: Theophylline-ethylenediamine in Cheyne-Stokes respiration. Lancet 2:437–440, 1937.

Cromolyn

Mathison, D.A.: Cromolyn treatment of asthma: Trials in corticosteroid-dependent asthmatics. JAMA 216:1454–1458, 1971.

14 . . .

Vasoconstrictors & Oxytocics

The vasoconstrictors already discussed—ie, the sympathomimetic amines and the facilitators of ganglionic transmission such as nicotine—have many other actions, including some degree of vasodilatation, relaxation of nonvascular smooth muscle, and cardiac stimulation. Their effects are explicable by reference to the physiology of the autonomic nervous system.

The present chapter discusses agents that stimulate the contraction of vascular or uterine smooth muscle through mechanisms unrelated to the innervation of the smooth muscle. The ergot alkaloids, the hormones of the posterior pituitary gland, the polypeptide angiotensin, and the prostaglandins are in this category.

ERGOT ALKALOIDS

History

The history of ergot over many centuries is the history of the epidemics (see Adverse Reactions, below) due to the ingestion of flour from smutted rye. The abortifacient action of toxic amounts of ergot suggested its use to hasten labor. European midwives of the 18th century adopted it and, in a crude way, standardized its dosage. An American physician, John Stearns (1770–1848), apparently learned of the use of ergot from German immigrants to New York State, and his reports (1808) led to its use by regular medical as well as folk practitioners. Used to hasten labor, it often caused excessive uterine contraction and caused ischemia damaging to the child; its present use (to prevent postpartum bleeding only) evolved slowly. The work of the British obstetrician, Chassar Moir, from 1932–1944 led to the isolation and established the use of **ergonovine**. He had noted that crude ergot had effects which were more favorable than those of pure ergotamine which had been assumed by most workers to be the single active principle.

Source, Chemistry, & Classification

The ergot alkaloids still ultimately originate in the fungus or smut, *Claviceps purpurea,* grown on kernels of rye. The growth is today carried out in fermentation vats in factories rather than in the field. Minor chemical modifications of the basic structure are possible, and the following classification separates the native or naturally occurring alkaloids from 2 chemical modifications.

A. Native Alkaloids: The important naturally occurring alkaloids are ergotamine and ergonovine. Methylergonovine and methysergide are semisynthetic derivatives (see Table 14–1 for structure). Ergotoxine is a mixture of ergocristine, ergocryptine, and ergocornine, but these natural alkaloids are not therapeutically important.

In Fig 14–1 is shown lysergic acid, the structure common to all ergots. All active alkaloids are levorotatory, inversion of the substituent (shown at 1) on C8 resulting in an inactive **iso** form. All compounds of interest are amides of lysergic acid. Ergotamine is referred to as an amino acid alkaloid because the amide nitrogen bears the condensation product of 3 amino acids. Ergonovine and the other alkaloids have simpler substituents. The amino acid alkaloids are poorly absorbed in comparison with ergonovine. However, the differences between the 2 are quantitative, and all of the natural alkaloids, the potent smooth muscle activators, retain the double bond shown at 3, ie, they are not hydrogenated.

B. Hydrogenated Alkaloids: Saturation of the double bond at C9-10 reduces the smooth muscle constricting activity of the alkaloids but intensifies their vasodilating action. Dihydroergotamine and a hydrogenated mixture of the natural alkaloids, Hydergine, are examples.

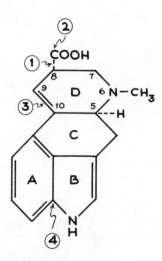

FIG 14–1. Lysergic acid. This structure is common to all ergot alkaloids.

TABLE 14–1. Chemical formulas of the ergot alkaloids.

	R_1	R_2	R_3
Lysergic acid diethylamide (LSD)	–H	$-C_2H_5$	$-C_2H_5$
Ergonovine (ergometrine)	–H	–H	CH_3 $\vert$ $-CH-CH_2OH$ (Propanol)
Methylergonovine	–H	–H	CH_2-CH_3 $\vert$ $-CH-CH_2OH$ (Butanol)
Methysergide (Sansert)	$-CH_3$	–H	Butanol
Ergotamine	–H	–H	 (Hydroxyalanine, phenylalanine, proline)

C. LSD: Lysergic acid (saure) diethylamide or LSD is also derived from ergot. The smooth muscle contracting effect of the other ergots is still present in LSD but is not always seen since very small doses produce the feelings of depersonalization or the hallucinatory state sought by the users. LSD is further discussed in Chapter 7 as one of several drugs producing a toxic psychosis. In Fig 14–1 the indole moiety formed by rings A and B is shown at 4. Such a structure suggested to a few investigators a relationship between serotonin and LSD effects, but this relationship has never been established.

Absorption, Metabolism, & Excretion

Absorption of ergotamine, the amino acid alkaloid, after oral administration is incomplete and irregular. The oral dose is approximately 10 times the parenteral dose. Onset of action is delayed for 20 minutes or longer even after intramuscular or subcutaneous injection. Intravenous or sublingual administration gives a more rapid effect. Ergonovine acts rapidly and more predictably than ergotamine.

The smooth muscle stimulating actions of ergot persist for several hours. Because toxic effects occur more frequently in patients with liver disease, metabolism is presumed to take place in the liver.

Pharmacologic Actions

A. Mechanisms of Action: These alkaloids have diverse and in part contradictory effects. What little is known about their mechanism of action is mentioned in the discussion of their effects.

B. Effects:

1. Smooth muscle stimulation—All smooth muscle, vascular or nonvascular, is contracted. The action is a direct one on smooth muscle—ie, there is no relation to innervation or to any of the chemical mediators. The actual mechanism is not known.

The smooth muscle excitant action is pronounced in the natural alkaloids but greatly reduced in the hydrogenated derivatives.

a. Oxytocic effect—Only at term is uterine muscle more sensitive to ergot than is other smooth muscle. In the absence of pregnancy or early in pregnancy, dangerous amounts of ergot are required to demonstrate the uterine stimulating effect, and even then the cervix is more affected. Ergot cannot therefore be used in any context as an abortifacient. During the third trimester the sensitivity of the uterus gradually increases, and ergonovine can be used to induce labor and contract the uterus postpartum. For the induction and stimulation of labor, it is much easier to adjust the dosage of oxytocin than that of an ergot alkaloid. For the prevention of postpartum bleeding, however, ergonovine or methylergonovine is most commonly used. The hemostasis is due to contraction of the uterine wall around the bleeding vessels of the placental site.

b. Vasoconstriction—The blood vessels in all vascular beds are constricted. Arteriolar constriction elevates systolic and diastolic blood pressures, but the effect is not great. Larger arteries are more sensitive. The dilatation of an artery by each pressure pulse is decreased while ergot is acting, and localized narrowings or even occlusion may be shown with arteriograms. The constriction of intracranial arteries is useful in the treatment of migraine, but the decreased flow through peripheral, mesenteric, or coronary arteries may cause ischemia of the tissues perfused by the artery.

2. Adrenergic blockade—Alpha-adrenergic blockade, the ability of a drug to block the vasoconstricting actions of the catecholamines, is discussed in Chapter 11. Adrenergic blockade was first produced by ergotamine and ergotoxine, and for many years these ergot alkaloids were the only such agents available for laboratory use. The blockade appears only after hypertensive doses in anesthetized animals and is unrelated to the therapeutic actions of ergot.

3. CNS actions—

a. Vasodilatation due to central sympathoplegic action—Only the dihydrogenated alkaloids produce a reduction of sympathetic outflow and a reduction of sympathetic influences on blood vessels. A minor fall in blood pressure (not postural or gravity assisted) and bradycardia are produced. This action has not proved useful in the treatment of hypertension. Dihydroergotamine does retain some smooth muscle stimulating properties and is still used occasionally in the treatment of migraine. The other hydrogenated ergots are virtually obsolete.

The sympathoplegic and tranquilizer actions of the dihydroergots closely resemble those of reserpine. Their usefulness in treating hypertension and their mechanisms of action have not been restudied since the information generated by the study of reserpine has been available.

b. Behavioral—The dihydroergots have behavioral effects comparable to those of antipsychotic tranquilizers and were used successfully in the past in the treatment of agitated psychotics before the concept of tranquilizer drugs was recognized.

Clinical Uses

A. Ergotamine in Treatment of Migraine: The clinical picture of migraine is often not classical, but a typical sequence is as follows: A patient with particular genetic and personality traits develops a headache—often in response to an environmental stimulus apparent to him. The first phase of this recurrent problem is due to intracranial vasoconstriction and is manifest as a prodrome of visual signs and malaise. If not aborted by drug therapy, the period of vasoconstriction is succeeded by a phase of vasodilatation—the intracranial vessels become dilated and flaccid, and the resulting traction on meningeal receptors with each pressure pulse is felt as a unilateral, throbbing headache accompanied by nausea, vomiting, and even prostration.

Ergot alkaloids are effective in treatment to the extent that they are vasoconstrictors and prevent the rhythmic distention of arteries (Fig 14–2). If they are given during the prodrome, the attack may be completely aborted.

Ergotamine tartrate (one of several trade names is Gynergen) is the most effective ergot alkaloid. Dihydroergotamine, a dihydroergot that retains some vasoconstrictor action, has also been suggested; however, it offers no advantage if equipotent doses are compared with ergotamine, and it can only be given by injection.

The results of ergotamine treatment may be spectacularly good, or the patient may use the amount of

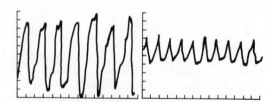

FIG 14–2. Left temporal artery pulse volume tracing during left hemicrania *(left)* **and after parenteral administration of 0.5 mg ergotamine tartrate** *(right)*. Subjective response in 8½ minutes; objective response in 10 minutes. (Reproduced, with permission, from Friedman: Studies in the pharmacology of headache. Neurology 13:27, 1963.)

drug allowed per day or week without relief. In the latter case this is often because the drug is used too late in the attack, but it may be because of reliance upon oral ergotamine, which is not dependably absorbed. Oral administration may be tried, but if relief is not obtained other routes of administration must be used before concluding that ergotamine is ineffective. Rectal suppositories are widely used, but sublingual administration or inhalation is effective and convenient. Subcutaneous injection is the most dependable route of administration of ergotamine and should be used when the drug is given as a therapeutic test.

Whatever the method of administration, a limit must be placed on the amount of drug used—eg, 1—2 mg orally may be repeated up to a total of 6 mg in 1 day and 12 mg in 1 week.

A number of proprietary mixtures are available on prescription, but their advantages over ergotamine alone given by the same route have not been demonstrated. Caffeine is added to one popular mixture (Cafergot) because it is a vasoconstrictor of intracranial vessels.

Ergotamine is not always required for the treatment of migraine. Sedatives such as phenobarbital and nonnarcotic analgesics or even codeine may be useful and preferable.

B. Methysergide (Sansert) in Preventing Migrainous Attacks: Methysergide (N-methyl-ergonovine), a less potent form of ergonovine, is completely unsatisfactory for the treatment of acute attacks of migraine, but when administered continuously it is useful in preventing headaches. This prophylactic use has been reserved for patients with "cluster headaches" or for occasions that regularly precipitate migraine in a particular patient—eg, during a menstrual period or on weekends.

Methysergide has measurable value in selected patients. However, its toxicity must be considered in judging its usefulness. The adverse reactions discussed below have occurred frequently after the use of methysergide, and the drug does not appear to be qualitatively different from ergotamine but to be merely a less potent vasoconstrictor.

C. Ergonovine as an Oxytocic: For the induction of labor, oxytocin (Pitocin) is the preferred drug. For the prevention of postpartum bleeding, either ergonovine or methylergonovine is routinely used. Ergonovine may be given prophylactically even before the delivery of the placenta, in which case one parenteral dose is given followed by repeated oral doses; or the drug may be withheld until the first sign of bleeding is seen. After complete or incomplete abortion, ergonovine becomes less effective and slightly larger doses must be used.

Hypertension is the important side-effect of ergonovine. It is especially likely to occur after vasoconstrictors have been used in conjunction with regional anesthesia or in an eclamptic patient. Oxytocin does not have this effect.

Methylergonovine (Methergine) is widely used because it is supposed to cause less elevation of blood pressure. This is probably true, although equally potent oxytocic doses have not always been compared.

Adverse Reactions

This discussion of toxicity does not apply to ergonovine, which causes a moderate elevation of blood pressure but no serious toxic reactions in the usual doses. If it were used chronically, as its methyl derivative (methysergide) is, it probably would cause more undesirable effects.

A. Side-Effects: The action of ergotamine on gastrointestinal smooth muscle may cause nausea and vomiting, abdominal cramps or epigastric discomfort, and diarrhea. Paresthesias, cold extremities, and claudication are early arteriospastic effects.

Methysergide causes the above side-effects, and its chronic administration may also cause weight gain, edema, loss of hair, and behavioral changes. Behavioral changes are similar to those associated with reserpine and include drowsiness or insomnia, restlessness, and feelings of depersonalization.

These side-effects may be severe enough to force discontinuance of the drug, a decision which is as often made by the patient as by the physician. As many as 20% of patients cannot tolerate methysergide; the rejection rate for ergotamine is probably much lower.

B. Overdosage Toxicity: Arteriospastic disease, the dangerous toxic effect of ergot derivatives, occurs in 2 forms.

1. Acute arterial occlusion—Many patients note transient coldness of the extremities after using ergotamine. In rare cases, the arteriospasm is general (rather than segmental) and persistent. Blood flow through the artery ceases completely. Blood flow may be resumed with no permanent damage, or tissue may become gangrenous before the process reverses itself. The reaction usually involves the legs; is often bilateral but not symmetrical; and the extent of damage may vary from loss of a toe to loss of an entire leg. During the reaction, blood pressure is elevated and there are ECG changes consistent with those of myocardial ischemia.

The duration of the arteriospastic state is not altered by any treatment, including the intra-arterial injection of vasodilating drugs and sympathectomy. In experimental situations, sympathectomy actually intensifies the gangrene.

The occurrence of gangrene is usually due to excessive dosages, but gangrene has occurred following therapeutic doses and even after doses that had previously been tolerated by the patient. The reaction is very rare, but the exact incidence is impossible to express. Most cases are not reported in the medical literature but do become known as the subject of litigation.

2. Retroperitoneal fibrosis—Both methysergide and ergotamine may cause acute arterial insufficiency. In addition, the chronic use of methysergide has been associated with retroperitoneal fibrosis, a previously extremely rare syndrome. In reported cases, the fibrosis has developed after use of the drug for 6 months to 4 years. Retroperitoneal fibrosis leads to ureteral obstruction with hydronephrosis and eventually loss of renal function. It is accompanied in some cases by pleural and pulmonary fibrosis and by changes in the cardiac valve rings, resulting in cardiac murmurs and disturbed dynamics of blood flow with cardiac enlargement. If the drug is discontinued in time, the process is usually reversible. Surgical intervention and retrograde urologic studies, which may precipitate complete obstruction, should therefore be delayed.

This reaction is assumed to be due to the chronic arterial constrictive action of methysergide. Reversible mesenteric artery occlusion following methysergide administration has been demonstrated by arteriography.

Patients receiving methysergide should be told to report promptly dysuria or back or pleural pain, and should be seen at least 3–4 times a year for questioning and examination. In addition, a drug-free interval should be provided periodically. The manufacturer recommends 1 month without treatment after 6 months of drug administration; some physicians experienced with the drug recommend interruption of treatment every 2 months.

C. Epidemic Ergotism: Ergot poisoning from contaminated flour is not a current problem in drug toxicity but occurred during the Middle Ages. Rye was the bread grain of the poor in continental Europe, and rye is especially susceptible to attack by *Claviceps purpurea*, the fungus that produces ergot alkaloids. Among the ripe grains of rye, sclerotia—hard, spur-shaped masses of mycelium—are formed. These may be milled with the grain or fall to the ground to germinate and produce spores that perpetuate the infestation. Ingestion of smutted grain caused 2 types of ergotism.

1. Gangrenous ergotism—This form of ergotism occurred largely in France from the 9th–14th centuries, and is comparable to thè acute arteriospastic reaction described above. A foot or leg—less commonly, an arm—became inflamed and the victim experienced feelings of cold alternating with severe burning pains (St. Anthony's fire). Numbness and dry gangrene followed, with painless loss of tissue varying in extent from nails to whole limbs. Rapidly fatal visceral gangrene also occurred.

The epidemics decreased in seriousness as wheat replaced rye and as agricultural technics such as drainage and deeper plowing developed. Rye can be cleaned of ergot, and legal standards now exist; but in the past the choice was often between eating contaminated grain or starvation. A comparatively minor outbreak was reported in France as recently as 1953.

2. Convulsive (spasmodic) ergotism—In northern Europe and Russia, another form of epidemic ergotism has occurred since the late 16th century. The most prominent sign was a painful spasmodic or spastic contraction of voluntary muscles accompanied in severe cases by convulsions. About 10–20% of those affected died, and many of those who survived suffered residual mental dullness or dementia. Primitive epidemiologic studies suggest that the occurrence of this type of ergotism was determined by a lack of dairy and meat products in the diet, and there is experimental evidence suggesting a relation to vitamin A deficiency. The last epidemic of significant extent occurred in Russia in 1926.

Contraindications & Cautions

The ergot alkaloids should not be used during pregnancy or in the presence of vascular disease (peripheral or coronary). Impaired liver function must now be considered a contraindication to the use of ergot even though ergotamine was once used to relieve the itching associated with jaundice. In view of the experience with methysergide, pulmonary and valvular disease should probably also be considered contraindications.

The drugs should be administered with careful limitation of the total dose, and intervals free of drug treatment should be provided.

Ergot alkaloids are dispensed as salts of organic acids. Both the chemical and trade names are listed to avoid the confusion arising from the trade names.

Dosages

A. Ergotamine Tartrate (Gynergen; many other trade names): Available routes of administration and one example of dose limitation in each case are as follows:

1. Subcutaneous or intravenous—0.25 mg; may repeat one time.

2. Rectal—One 2 mg suppository; may repeat same dose twice at hourly intervals.

3. Buccal or sublingual—1 or 2 mg tablet; may repeat to a total of 6 mg in 1 day and 12 mg in 1 week.

4. Inhalation (Medihaler)—A promising technic for rapid absorption which has been incompletely evaluated for safety.

5. Oral—1–2 mg; may repeat to 6 mg in 1 day and 12 mg in 1 week.

B. Methysergide (Sansert): The dosage of methysergide is 2 mg 3 (or at the most 4) times a day. Treatment should begin with a lower dose.

C. Ergonovine Maleate (Ergotrate) and Methylergonovine (Methergine): The dosage of one or the other of these drugs is usually standardized on a given obstetric service. An example is 0.2 mg IM or IV at the end of the second stage of labor; may repeat once; then 0.2–0.4 mg 2–4 times daily for 2–3 days.

Preparations Available

Ergotamine tartrate:

Tablets (Gynergen), 1 mg

Sublingual (Ergomar), 2 mg

Inhalation (Medihaler), 0.36 mg/inhalation, 2.5 ml (22.5 mg)

Suppositories (with 100 mg caffeine [Cafergot]), 2 mg

Injectable (subcut or IV), 0.25 mg/0.5 ml, 0.5 ml ampules; 0.5 mg/ml, 1 ml ampules

Methysergide (Sansert):

Tablets, 2 mg

Ergonovine maleate (Ergotrate; various others):
Tablets, 0.2 mg
Injectable (IM or IV), 0.2 mg/ml, 1, 20, and
30 ml ampules

Methylergonovine maleate (Methergine):
Tablets, 0.2 mg
Injectable (IM or IV), 0.2 mg/ml, 1 ml
ampules

ANGIOTENSIN

The physiologic role of angiotensin is of the greatest importance. It does not, however, have any established therapeutic usefulness even though a synthetic angiotensin is marketed for use as a pressor agent.

Source & Chemistry

Angiotensin amide (Hypertensin) is a synthetic octapeptide corresponding to the amide of bovine angiotensin II—ie, 1-L-asparagine-5-L-valyl angiotensin octapeptide. Angiotensin II is formed in the organism by the splitting of 2 amino acids from the decapeptide, angiotensin I. Angiotensin I in turn is a fragment split off from angiotensinogen, an α_2 globulin, by renin elaborated by the juxtaglomerular cells of the kidney.

Pharmacologic Effects

Angiotensin amide, after intravenous injection, acts as a very potent but briefly acting vasoconstrictor. Peripheral resistance is greatly elevated, but the heart is not stimulated. Consequently, a larger amount of cardiac work is expended as "pressure work" and a smaller fraction is available to pump a volume of blood—ie, cardiac output falls. Thus, even though both diastolic and systolic pressures rise, tissue perfusion is impaired rather than augmented.

The elevation of blood pressure leads to a reflex bradycardia and occasionally precipitates ventricular ectopic beats or runs of ventricular tachycardia.

In the intact organism, evidence of stimulation of other smooth muscle organs is not seen. Isolated organ preparations are contracted, but the action of angiotensin probably is on the blood vessels contained in the isolated tissue.

Angiotensin amide is suggested for use in elevating blood pressure during shock. Lacking the cardiac stimulating properties of norepinephrine (levarterenol) or other sympathomimetic amine, it is likely to reduce blood flow to all extracranial areas even more than levarterenol and is rarely used.

Adverse Reactions

Adverse reactions—other than the probability that prolonged infusion is harmful in patients with shock—are secondary to an excessive elevation of blood pressure.

Metabolism; Preparations & Dosages

Angiotensin is rapidly destroyed by peptidases and it acts for only 3–5 minutes after an intravenous dose. Like levarterenol, therefore, it is given by continuous intravenous infusion. For this purpose, angiotensin amide (Hypertensin) is supplied in vials containing 2.5 mg of the dry material. The contents of the vial are dissolved in 5 ml of water and the solution added to 500 ml of saline or glucose in water. The intravenous drip is started at the rate of 10 drops/minute and adjusted on the basis of the response of the blood pressure.

PROSTAGLANDINS

The prostaglandins are local hormones of great potential usefulness whose investigative use is just beginning.

Source & Chemistry

Prostaglandins are widely distributed in the body and derive their name from the high concentrations found in seminal fluid. There are at least 13 prostaglandins (Fig 14–3). They are very rapidly inactivated if they enter the circulation.

Effects

Vascular smooth muscle is relaxed and blood pressure is lowered because of the vasodilatation. Injected intradermally, prostaglandins cause a persistent flare. Uterine muscle is stimulated regardless of the hormonal influences present—ie, unlike oxytocin or ergot alkaloids, the prostaglandins cause contraction of the nonpregnant uterus and of the uterus throughout pregnancy. Intestinal motility is increased. The effect on bronchioles varies with the different prostaglandins.

The prostaglandins may be mediators of inflammation. In experimental inflammatory states, they are recovered from exudates and perfusates. Aspirin and, much less potently, salicylate inhibit the synthesis of prostaglandin from arachidonic acid, and such effect has been suggested as the explanation for the anti-inflammatory effect of aspirin.

Investigative Uses

The prostaglandins are being intensively investigated as abortifacients. During the first trimester, they appear less satisfactory than suction currettement simply because of the total time (10–24 hours) involved and the inconvenience of a prolonged intravenous infusion. However, after 12–14 weeks, the prostaglandins may prove preferable to the intra-amniotic injection of saline. Routes of administration being investigated include intravenous, transcervical, intra-amniotic, and intravaginal.

The prostaglandins are also used to induce labor and as a "morning-after" contraceptive.

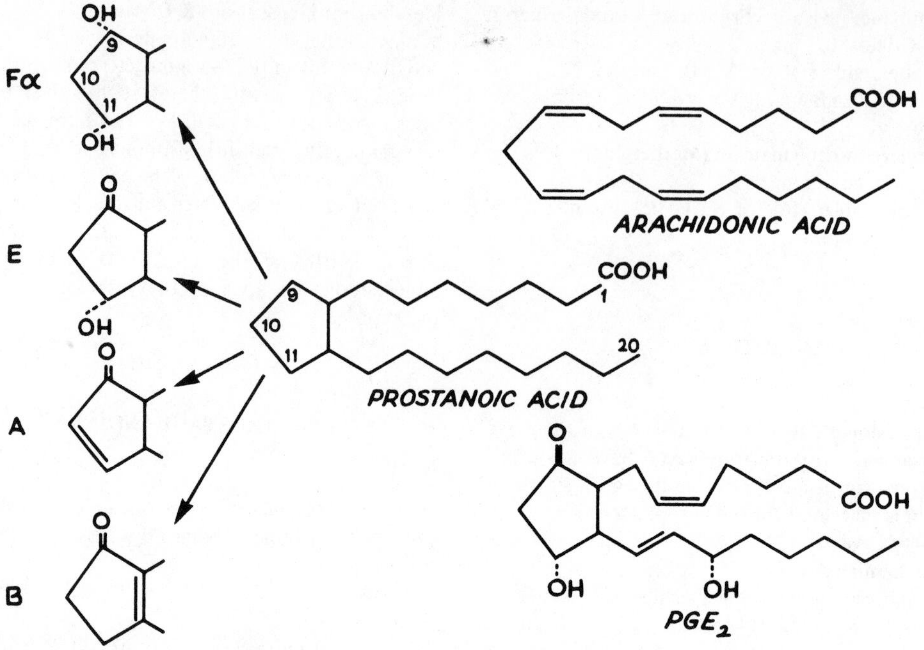

FIG 14—3. Prostaglandins synthesized in the organism from arachidonic acid or closely related fatty acids. Prostanoic acid, an intermediate, is itself inactive. The 5-membered ring is variously modified to give the 4 lettered types of prostaglandins. A subscript to the letter indicates the number of unsaturated bonds in the side chains on the cyclopentane ring.

•   •   •

General References

Ergot

Barger, G.: *Ergot and Ergotism.* Gurney & Jackson (Edinburgh), 1931.

Cahn, J., & others: Neuroplégie hypothermique dite "hibernation artificielle" par les dérivés dihydrogénés de l'ergot de seigle. Etude physiologique. Anesthésie et Analg 11:513—532, 1954.

Graham, J.R., & others: Fibrotic disorders associated with methysergide therapy for headache. New England J Med 274:359—368, 1966.

Nickerson, M.: The pharmacology of adrenergic blockade. Pharmacol Rev 1:27—101, 1949.

Pedersen, E., & C.E. Møller: Methysergide in migraine prophylaxis. Clin Pharmacol Therap 7:520—526, 1966.

Angiotensin

Nolan, J.P., Cobb, L.A., & J.I. Thompson: Circulatory responses to angiotensin in man. Clin Pharmacol Therap 8:235—242, 1967.

Udhoji, V.N., & M.H. Weil: Circulatory effects of angiotensin, levarterenol and metaraminol in the treatment of shock. New England J Med 270:501—505, 1964.

Vasoactive peptides. Symposium. Fed Proc 27:49—99, 1968.

Prostaglandins

Gillespie, A.: Prostaglandin-oxytocin enhancement and potentiation and their clinical applications. Brit MJ 1:150—152, 1972.

Karim, S.M.M.: Prostaglandins as abortifacients. New England J Med 285:1534—1535, 1971.

Prostaglandins. Ann New York Acad Sc, vol 180, 1971.

15 . . .

Digitalis

Congestive heart failure is frequently reversible even when the underlying cardiovascular disease which causes it may not be treatable; a properly managed patient may have decades of active and comfortable life after the first appearance of symptoms. The most important single part of the therapeutic regimen for congestive failure is digitalis. It often suffices for long periods before it need be supplemented by diet, diuretics, and restriction of activity. The proper use of digitalis is thus a common and important demand on the physician.

Digitalis is a difficult drug to administer. The margin between therapeutic and toxic doses is small, and in most patients there is no reliable index of optimal dosage. Toxicity is therefore frequently encountered, and many details of digitalis action thus become very important.

History

In spite of the auspicious beginning of the rational use of digitalis for congestive failure provided by the publication in 1785 of William Withering's *An Account of the Foxglove and Some of Its Medical Uses,* over a century of experience was necessary before the use of digitalis became well established and the indications clearly understood. Early in his practice in Shropshire, Withering was asked to evaluate a folk remedy containing 20 or more herbs that had been effective in relieving the edema of a prominent personage after the regular practitioners had failed. Withering (1741–1799), who became a preeminent British botanist as well as a master physician, recognized that all of the ingredients except digitalis were medically useless, and that, if the remedy were active in the treatment of dropsy (edema), digitalis must be the active ingredient. At this time he recognized the diuretic effect of digitalis but did not continue its study until he had moved to Birmingham. Here, where the industrial revolution was just beginning—and perhaps stimulated by such associates in the Lunar Club as Watt, Erasmus Darwin, Priestley, Lavoisier, and Wedgewood—Withering studied the clinical pharmacology of digitalis for 9 years before publishing his classic work. Withering standardized the collection of digitalis leaf at the time of flowering of the biennial plant and administered the dry powdered leaf much as can still be done today. He appreciated the diuretic effect and noted the action on the heart of "a degree yet unobserved in any other medicine." Withering lacked a differentiation of the types of dropsy or edema; if this limitation is recognized, his publication can be studied with great profit even today.

During his lifetime, Withering saw digitalis come into wide use. Soon thereafter, however, the indications for the use of the drug became confused and the slowing effect on heart rate began to be emphasized, leading to such characterizations as "cardiac depressant" and "opium of the heart."

The undue emphasis on the slowing of cardiac rate caused by digitalis was intensified by the work of another great physician, James Mackenzie (1853–1925). Mackenzie was a general practitioner who began to sort out for us the common cardiac arrhythmias. The guiding principle in Mackenzie's work was that, as a general practitioner, he could follow the course of his patients from the earliest signs and symptoms of a disease and measure the accuracy of the prognoses held intuitively by his preceptors. His practice included much obstetrics, and many of these patients had rheumatic heart disease with atrial arrhythmias, especially the lasting arrhythmia that he called "auricular paralysis" (fibrillation). In such cases digitalis is especially effective, and its action is accompanied by a graded slowing of ventricular rate. The emphasis upon slowing of the rate rather than correction of failure independent of an effect on rate thus became more firmly established.

Parenthetically, after 25 years of general practice, Mackenzie became a London cardiologist and, to his disappointment, became better known for the invention of a polygraph for the simultaneous recording of the venous and arterial pulse waves than for his careful studies of the natural history of the arrhythmias.

One person appreciative of Mackenzie's work was Arthur Cushny (1866–1926). Like Withering and Mackenzie, Cushny trained at Edinburgh, but he did not continue his research in the clinical tradition of the United Kingdom. He was more influenced by his experience in the laboratories of German universities. Cushny deserves credit for the development of the descriptive pharmacology of digitalis and for providing leadership in the development of modern pharmacology at Ann Arbor, London, and Edinburgh.

Early in this century, progress was made in the isolation and characterization of many cardiotonic glycosides from digitalis, and this progress in the chemical area was accompanied by progress in clinical cardiology such that by the mid 1920s the primary indication for the use of digitalis—congestive heart failure—was clear to the leaders in the profession. Additional clinical progress is mentioned later, but it will become apparent that, except for a clearer understanding of the indications for the use of digitalis and its glycosides, limited progress has occurred since the time of Withering.

Source & Chemistry

The term "digitalis" is used for convenience to include a large number of naturally occurring steroid glycosides and derived products, all of which have the same beneficial and toxic effects on the heart.

The most common source of these drugs (which cannot be synthesized) is the crimson or royal purple foxglove or the white foxglove (*Digitalis purpurea* or *Digitalis lanata*). *Strophanthus gratus* and *S Kombé* (African plants) and squill (*Urginea maritima* or *indica*) must also be mentioned as sources of glycosides. The remaining botanical sources are many, and there is even one animal source, the secretion of the glands in the skin of toads.

Each of the cardioactive principles contains the familiar steroid nucleus (Figs 15–1 and 15–2). At C17 is a lactone ring that is essential for cardioactivity. To the C3 hydroxyl is added, through a series of glycosidic links, a sequence of sugars that influence the physical properties of the compound. The steroid-lactone system freed of the sugars by hydrolysis—ie, with a free hydroxyl at C3—is called an **aglycone** or **genin**.

A. Common Glycosides: By following the stepwise hydrolysis diagrammed in Fig 15–1, the commonly used glycosides can be identified.

The leaves of *D lanata* contain a mixture of 3 glycosides. The sequence of sugars and acetyl groups is also diagrammed in Fig 15–1. One of the native glycosides, lanatoside C (Cedilanid), is used orally. If the acetyl group is removed, the resulting deslanoside (Cedilanid-D) is obtained. If the glucose is then hydrolyzed off, a "purified glycoside," digoxin, results. The properties of these 3 are quite similar. If the sequence of hydrolysis is altered and only the glucose removed, acetyldigitoxin, an uncommonly employed glycoside,

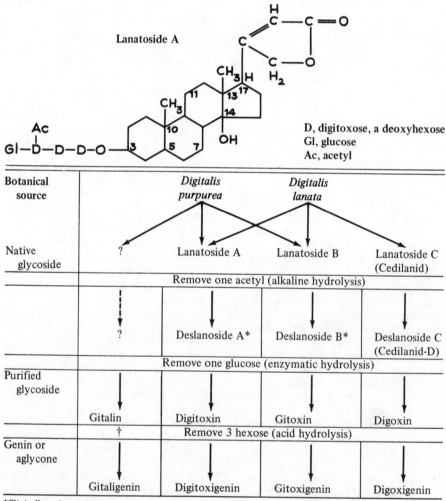

Botanical source		*Digitalis purpurea*	*Digitalis lanata*	
Native glycoside	?	Lanatoside A	Lanatoside B	Lanatoside C (Cedilanid)
		Remove one acetyl (alkaline hydrolysis)		
	?	Deslanoside A*	Deslanoside B*	Deslanoside C (Cedilanid-D)
		Remove one glucose (enzymatic hydrolysis)		
Purified glycoside	Gitalin	Digitoxin	Gitoxin	Digoxin
	†	Remove 3 hexose (acid hydrolysis)		
Genin or aglycone	Gitaligenin	Digitoxigenin	Gitoxigenin	Digoxigenin

*Clinically unimportant.

†Preparation of gitaligenin involves removal of 2 hexoses (digitoxose) by acid hydrolysis from gitalin.

FIG 15–1. Derivation of the common cardiac glycosides by progressive hydrolysis of the glycosides present in the leaf.

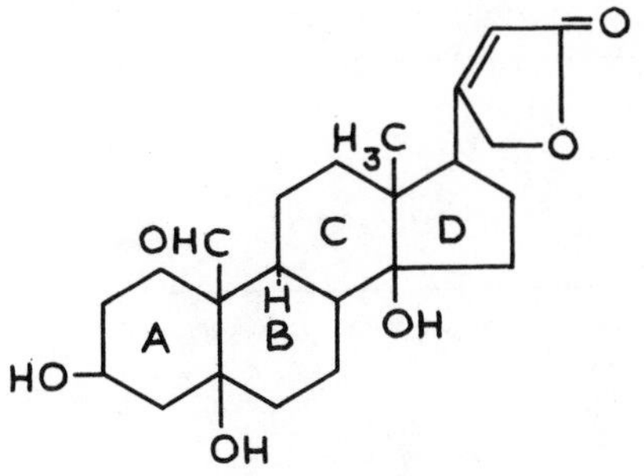

Strophanthidin-K

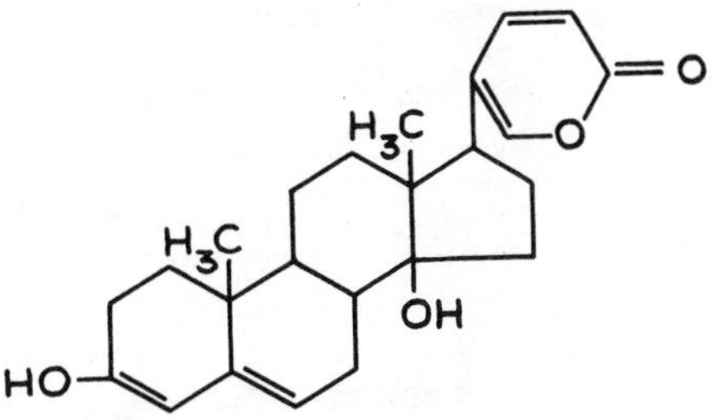

Scillaridin A

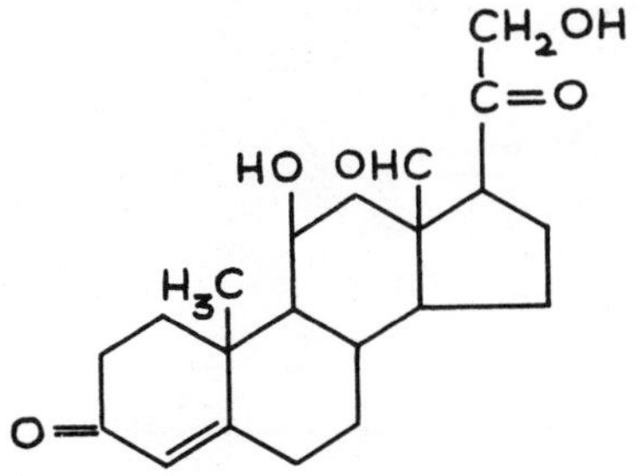

Aldosterone

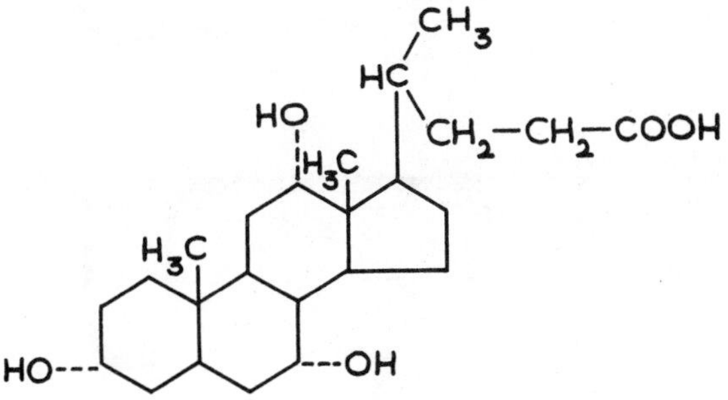

Cholic acid

FIG 15–2. Structures of 2 additional aglycones of cardiac glycosides and 2 possibly related steroids for comparison. Strophanthidin is the genin derived from a strophanthin—eg, ouabain or strophanthin G. Scillaridin A from squill contains a 6-membered lactone ring.

is prepared. From the other lanatosides, digitoxin and gitoxin are prepared.

Digoxin is 12-hydroxydigitoxin and gitoxin is 16-hydroxydigitoxin. These minor changes increase water solubility and decrease duration of action.

Digitoxin, gitoxin, and gitalin are derived from *D purpurea*. The sequence of hydrolysis is similar, but the purpurea glycosides do not bear the acetyl group. Ouabain, or strophanthidin G, is the purified glycoside from *S gratus* and must be distinguished from strophanthidin K (from *S Kombé*). The aglycone of a strophanthin is called a strophanthidin.

B. Structure-Action Relationships: The lactone ring is essential for cardiotonic activity. Digitalis contains steroid glycosides—ie, steroid plus sugars but without the lactone ring—that are not cardiotonic. The lactone ring always has an.*α,β* unsaturation but may be 5 or 6 membered (Fig 15–2). The *β*-hydroxyl at C14 is distinctive and probably essential. The stereochemistry (at C8, 9, 10, 13, and 17) is like the sterols or bile acids rather than the endocrine steroids. Unlike the sterols, however, in digitalis the orientation of the C/D rings is cis.

The several glycosides, genins, and semisynthetic modifications vary in their absolute potency and in rapidity of action. No qualitatively different variant has been identified, ie, it has not been possible to selectively increase therapeutic effect without increasing

the toxic effect. It may be that this important goal is unattainable, but it is equally likely that, since the common bioassay methods measure a toxic response, any selectively less toxic compound would be discarded as inactive.

C. Bioassay: The crystalline glycosides, being pure substances, are assayed chemically, prescribed by weight, and have a constant potency. The digitalis leaf preparations, still used to some extent, vary in the amounts of glycosides present. Each batch of the leaf must, therefore, be calibrated against an international standard of the leaf, so that a tablet of given weight will contain the same activity from batch to batch and from manufacturer to manufacturer.

The various methods that have been used all depend on the fact that a continuous infusion of a dilute tincture of digitalis will lead to cardiac arrest in systole or in ventricular fibrillation, depending upon the species. Frogs and cats were formerly used in the official assay, but the current USP recognizes the difficulty of securing enough cats and substitutes the pigeon for the assay.

A human assay method compares the T wave flattening produced by an unknown dose with the graded lowering produced by a series of standard doses of digitalis. The correlation of this assay (which uses nontoxic doses in humans) with animal assays is poor. However, the chemically determined digitoxin content

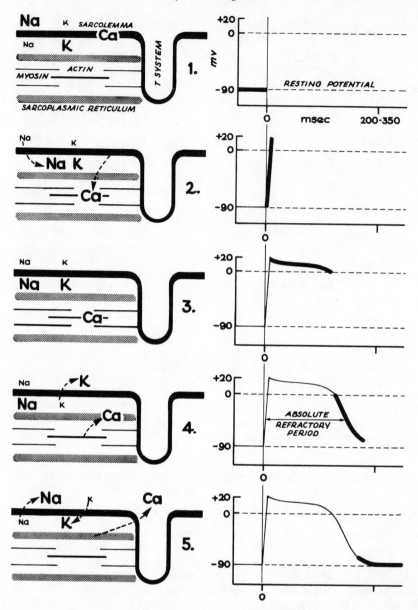

FIG 15–3. Summary of aspects of myocardial physiology on which glycosides may act. (1) Resting state. Na⁺ is in higher concentration extracellularly, K⁺ is concentrated within the cell, and Ca⁺⁺ is concentrated in the region of the sarcolemma and its invagination, the transverse tubule. Resting potential is maintained by the impermeability of cell membrane. (2) When a wave of depolarization reaches the unit or when the resting potential rises to a threshold value in pacemaker tissue, sodium rapidly enters the cell, neutralizing the resting potential. Calcium moves from storage sites, and its concentration within the cell rises. Troponin is attached to actin and inhibits actin-myosin interaction—ie, contraction. Calcium binds to troponin and removes the inhibition of bridge formation between actin and myosin. Digitalis is assumed to increase intracellular Ca⁺⁺ secondary to a change in step (5) below, and increased binding of troponin leads to a greater rate of tension development. (3) Plateau of action potential. Na⁺ entry slows and K⁺ efflux is delayed, leading to a long refractory period in comparison with nerve or skeletal muscle. (4) K⁺ efflux occurs and restoration of intracellular negativity begins. Calcium is actively transported into sarcoplasmic reticulum, allowing relaxation to occur. (5) The sodium-potassium pump returns Na⁺ to the outside and K⁺ to the inside of the cell. Calcium diffuses from sarcoplasmic reticulum to extracellular space. Digitalis appears to act by inhibiting Na⁺-K⁺ activated ATPase in the cell membrane and thus reducing the energy supply for the sodium pump. An increase in intracellular Na⁺ will force a decrease in intracellular K⁺, leading to arrhythmias and somehow an increase in delivery of Ca⁺⁺ in step (2).

of the leaf correlates well with the activity determined by bioassay in humans. For these reasons, animal assays using toxic (lethal) doses are skeptically regarded in physiologic work, although they do suffice to provide leaf preparations of constant potency. The therapeutic application of digitalis is a difficult exercise in clinical bioassay, and additional quantitative measurements in humans are mentioned below.

Pharmacologic Actions
A. Mechanism of Action:
1. Of the therapeutic effect—Studies on the effect of cardiac glycosides on intracellular potentials and ion fluxes have led to the development of plausible and attractive theories to explain the ability of the digitalis compounds to increase the force of myocardial contraction. These theories may, however, be held only tentatively if 2 conditions are imposed: (1) the effect interpreted must be demonstrable in therapeutic (low) rather than only in toxic (high) concentrations of cardiac glycosides, and (2) the effect must be demonstrable in cardiac muscle and not extrapolated from axon or erythrocyte.

The biochemical analysis of digitalis effect showed that the action is not on myocardial energy production, storage, or liberation. Neither does it have a direct action on the contractile protein.

The effect which correlates best with the cardiotonic activity of various compounds is the ability to inhibit the activity of Na^+-K^+ activated ATPase, which action would reduce the energy available to the sodium pump and lead to an increase in intracellular Na^+ (Fig 15—3). The expected increase in intracellular Na^+ and the corresponding loss of K^+ has not been demonstrated in cardiac tissue exposed to reasonable concentrations of glycoside. If the increase in intracellular Na^+ does occur, it would have the effect of increasing the amount of Ca^{++} available.

2. Of the toxic effects—The cardiac arrhythmias that occur as part of digitalis toxicity can be explained as an extension of the effect on membrane ATPase. If intracellular Na^+ is increased, K^+ must be lost to maintain an isosmotic state. The concentrations of potassium involved are smaller than the amounts of Na^+, and an important change in the ratio of K^+ inside to K^+ outside can occur. The intracellular potential would be brought closer to the threshold, and diastolic depolarization would occur.

Potassium depletion clearly favors the development of digitalis-induced arrhythmias. Potassium supplementation has an easily demonstrable effect on digitalis toxicity in the laboratory, but its clinical usefulness is limited once the patient is repleted. Potassium depletion or supplementation is unrelated to the therapeutic effect.

B. Effects:
1. Effects on the myocardium—The heart is not a homogeneous organ with a single function. Some drugs may exert directly opposite effects on the same primary function in different areas of the heart. In the case of digitalis and quinidine, it is particularly important to specify both the effect and the area of the heart in which it is manifested. Each of the essential properties of cardiac muscle—contractility, conduction, refractoriness, and automaticity—are altered by digitalis. However, the effects may be different on atrial muscle, the AV node, the SA node, Purkinje tissue, or ventricular muscle.

a. Increased force and efficiency of contraction—Digitalis enables the failing heart to contract more forcefully and more efficiently, ie, to do more work without increased consumption of oxygen or substrate. Efficiency can be measured during cardiac catheterization when blood from the coronary sinus is collected, and extractions of oxygen and metabolites can be calculated from coronary flow and coronary AV differences. The therapeutically important effect of digitalis is due to a direct action on the ventricular muscle and is demonstrable on normal as well as failing hearts (Figs 15—4 and 15—5).

As a result of the increased force of contraction, cardiac output may be increased. The cardiac output at rest of patients with congestive failure may not be greatly different from that of normals, but digitalis restores the ability to elevate output in response to need. Systolic emptying is more complete and diastolic size is decreased.

b. Slowed AV conduction—Digitalis slows conduction through the specialized tissue connecting the atria and the interventricular septum, ie, through the

MYOCARDIAL CONTRACTILE FORCE

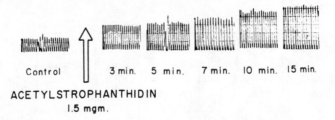

FIG 15—4. An illustration of the ability of a cardiac glycoside to increase the force of ventricular contraction in a patient not in congestive failure. A strain gauge was applied at an operation to correct an atrial septal defect. (Reproduced, with permission, from Braunwald & others: Studies on digitalis. J Clin Invest 40:52, 1961.)

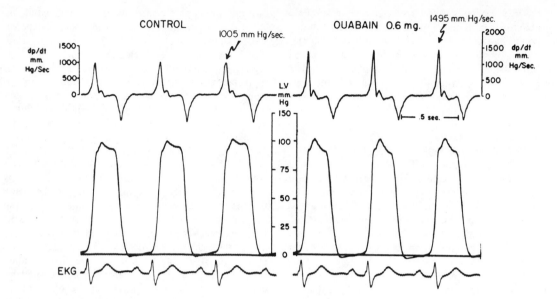

FIG 15—5. Recordings of left ventricular (LV) pressure and rate of change (dp/dt) before and 30 minutes after ouabain administration. (Reproduced, with permission, from Mason & Braunwald: Studies on digitalis. IX. Effects of ouabain on the nonfailing human heart. J Clin Invest 42:1108, 1963.)

AV node and the bundle of His. The effect is manifest as a P–R prolongation leading to increasing degrees of heart block. Intraventricular conduction (measured by QRS duration) is not affected (as it is by quinidine). This action is predominantly a direct effect, and is due only in small part to the vagal stimulation mentioned below.

c. Prolonged refractory period of AV node—The effect of digitalis in prolonging the AV nodal refractory period will not be clinically apparent so long as a slow atrial rate allows time for recovery of AV tissue between each beat. In the presence of a normal sinus rhythm, only a great prolongation of AV node refractory period will add to the effect on conduction to produce AV block.

However, in the presence of a rapid atrial rate (atrial tachycardia, flutter, or fibrillation), the prolongation of the refractory period will reduce the number of atrial impulses activating the AV node and thereby reduce the number of waves of depolarization reaching the ventricles. Digitalis will therefore slow the rapid ventricular rate associated with an atrial arrhythmia whether it alters the atrial rhythm or not.

For example, in atrial flutter with an atrial rate of 240 and a 2:1 block, the ventricular rate would be 120, the AV node responding to every second stimulus (Fig 15–6).

After digitalis, the AV node is refractory for the time occupied by 3 cycles subsequent to each response (4:1 block) and the ventricular rate would be 60 (Fig 15–7).

d. Increased ectopic impulse formation—Toxic doses of the digitalis glycosides increase the automaticity of all areas of the heart except the SA node. (By automaticity is meant the ability to initiate and propagate an impulse.)

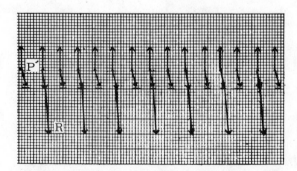

FIG 15—6. Atrial flutter before digitalis. Atrial rate 240, 2:1 block. Ventricular rate, 120.

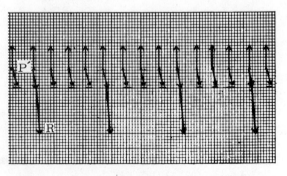

FIG 15—7. Atrial flutter after digitalis. Atrial rate 240, 4:1 block. Ventricular rate, 60.

If, as is usually the case, the effect is primarily on Purkinje fibers in the ventricles, the sequence (important in understanding the toxic signs) is (1) ventricular ectopic beats when the effect is minimal; (2) bigeminy or coupling if an ectopic beat follows each normal beat; (3) ventricular tachycardia; and (4) ventricular fibrillation terminally.

Atrial and nodal rhythms may also occur.

e. Decreased rate of SA node—The rate of the normal pacemaker—ie, the pulse rate if a normal sinus rhythm is present—is depressed by the cardiac glycosides. With smaller doses, this effect is due mostly to vagal stimulation and is reversed by atropine. With larger doses of digitalis, the effect of decreasing SA rate is direct, ie, it is not blocked by atropine. The effect of reducing the rate of the SA node appears to be inconsistent with the ability to increase automaticity. However, it is probably not due to an effect on diastolic depolarization but represents conduction failure in atrial muscle with continued rhythmicity of the SA node.

2. Effects secondary to relief of congestive failure—The increased force of cardiac contraction and the resultant increase in cardiac output relieve congestive heart failure to a degree depending upon the severity of the underlying disease. The following secondary changes are then observed: (1) Diuresis occurs, with mobilization of peripheral edema. (The glycosides have no important direct effect on the renal tubules.) (2) Venous pressure is reduced as extracellular fluid volume is contracted. (3) The tachycardia that accompanies congestive failure declines—due, probably, to the fall in pressures on the right side of the circulation. (4) Heart size decreases.

3. Resume of effects on rate—The factors that slow cardiac rate can now be summarized: (1) Correction of failure. (2) Reflex vagal stimulation. (3) Depression of SA node. (4) Prolongation of the refractory period of the AV node. (5) Slowing of AV conduction.

Action (4) is important only with a rapid atrial rate, and (5) will cause significant slowing only when complete block occurs. The vagal factors operate first; the extravagal influences, especially (3), later. Regardless of the rhythm, the slowing of the rate is not essential to the action of digitalis. This has been demonstrated by human studies in which the rate was kept elevated by atropine during digitalis administration; cardiac output increased and symptoms regressed nonetheless.

4. Electrographic effects—The electrophysiologic changes induced by the cardiac glycosides in part explain the mechanisms of the effects just described. In addition to the ECG, records from microelectrodes and surface electrodes are useful.

Microelectrodes can be placed within single cardiac fibers and the effect of cardiac glycosides on the resting and action potential observed. Fig 15–8 illustrates the results of one such experiment in which the recording was from Purkinje tissue. (Ventricular muscle responds similarly but is less sensitive.) The more rapid repolarization (decreased refractory period) explains the first group of ECG changes listed below. The appearance of diastolic depolarization—the development of pacemaker activity—is associated with ventricular arrhythmias. Atrial muscle in the laboratory situation shows a prolongation of the action potential—ie, a greatly prolonged refractory period—

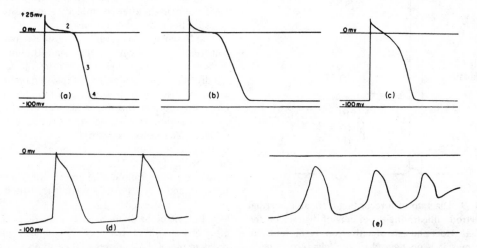

FIG 15–8. Effect of increasing concentrations of ouabain on the action potential of isolated canine Purkinje fibers. The preparation is stimulated at the rate of 30/minute. *(a)* Control record. *(b)* Initial prolongation of repolarization. *(c)* Onset of progressive decrease in duration of action potential due to shortening of duration of plateau (refractory period shortened). *(d)* Depolarization during diastole (pacemaker activity) appears. Resting potential decreases. Rate of rise and amplitude of action potential decrease. *(e)* More rapid depolarization between stimuli leads to spontaneous rather than driven activity equivalent to a ventricular rhythm. Resting potential and amplitude of action potential decrease until arrest and inexcitability occur. (Modified and reproduced, with permission, from Hoffman & Singer: Effects of digitalis on electrical activity of cardiac fibers. Progr Cardiovas Dis 7:236, 1964.)

comparable to the initial change in ventricular muscle. SA nodal tissue shows some evidence of decreased automaticity.

Electrodes may be placed on the surface of the myocardium of animals or implanted in appropriate areas. The electrograms so recorded provide information about the origin, pathway, and speed of conduction of the propagated impulse. From such studies it is seen that, in addition to causing more rapid recovery of ventricular muscle, digitalis changes the direction of that process—ie, instead of proceeding from epicardium to endocardium, it occurs in the reverse direction.

The ECG changes to be described at this point can be anticipated from the above facts.

a. ECG changes due to changes in ventricular repolarization—The wave of depolarization is rapidly distributed by Purkinje tissue through the subendocardial area. The activation of the ventricular wall proceeds from endocardial to epicardial surfaces. However, repolarization proceeds from epicardial to endocardial surface—ie, the first areas to be depolar-

ized are the last to recover (see Fig 15–9). If the ventricular complex, reflecting depolarization (negative to zero), is upright, the T wave will also be upright since the repolarization that it reflects is opposite to activation not only in electrical direction (zero to negative) but also in anatomic direction. After even subtherapeutic amounts of the cardiac glycosides have been given, the repolarization of the ventricle occurs sooner (shortened refractory period), proceeds more rapidly, and deviates from the normal epicardial to endocardial path. If recovery begins before excitation is completed, the overlapping of the 2 processes will displace the RS–T junction and the ST segment and cause ST sagging. The more rapid course will shorten the Q–T interval, and the loss of the ventricular gradient, ie, the change in order of recovery, will lower or invert the T wave.

b. ECG signs of digitalis toxicity—Digitalis toxicity is manifested by sinus bradycardia, P–R prolongation, AV dissociation, and ventricular arrhythmias (ectopic beats, bigeminy, ventricular fibrillation), and atrial arrhythmias with some degree of AV block.

The ECG does not provide an index of adequate digitalization. The changes listed in (a) above mean only that the patient has had some digitalis. The later ECG changes (b) are signs of digitalis toxicity. These changes do not appear in any predictable order, but ectopic beats and undue slowing are common early warning signs.

Among the common precipitating causes of cardiac failure is myocardial infarction. The ST segment and T wave changes which might have been helpful in the cardiographic diagnosis of a silent infarct can be obscured by similar changes due to digitalis. A preliminary ECG can serve as a base line for the later differentiation of digitalis effect or toxicity and disease.

5. Effects on other systems—

a. Vascular—The cardiac glycosides have a direct constrictor action on vascular smooth muscle. The pressor effect may be marked after the injection of the rapidly acting glycosides. In interpreting reports of the action of digitalis in shock or other hypotensive states, one must consider this direct vascular effect as well as a cardiac action. Digitalis constricts the veins of normal subjects. The venous constriction that occurs in congestive heart failure, however, decreases after treatment with digitalis. The decrease in venous tone and venous pressure follows the improvement in cardiac function and is not directly related to digitalis action, as was once suggested.

b. Gastrointestinal—Nausea and vomiting appear after absorption of toxic doses and are central and reflex in origin. Large doses of the leaf also have a local irritant action.

c. CNS—Visual and psychic toxic symptoms are central in origin. The vagal symptoms responsible for some of the action in slowing the pulse is in part due to a reflex arising in the carotid sinus area and in part to a direct central action.

d. Local—Injections other than intravenous are painful because of the local tissue irritation of the glycosides.

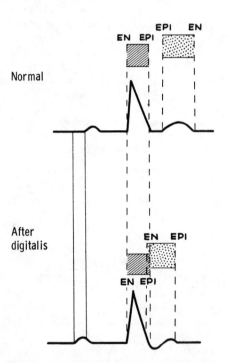

FIG 15–9. Diagram of a recording from an epicardial electrode illustrating the effects of digitalis on the ECG. Order and rate of activation of the ventricular muscle is unchanged by digitalis (cross-lined). Repolarization (stippled) is reversed from the ordinary epicardial to endocardial direction, lowering or inverting the T wave. Repolarization occurs sooner, shortening the Q–T interval or distorting the RS–T junction (J) and the RS–T segment. (Redrawn and reproduced, with permission, from Westlake & others: The effect of digitoxin on the electrocardiogram. Am Heart J 44:7, 1952.)

6. Effect on the normal heart—Whether the beneficial effect of digitalis occurs in the absence of congestive failure is an important question because it raises the possibility of prophylactic use of digitalis and because it was long questioned whether digitalis action could be analyzed using normal hearts. Digitalis is the only drug that can increase the contractility of the heart in failure; when given to a normal human, however, it slightly decreases cardiac output. Until recently, many workers had concluded that digitalis acts on a specific defect present only in congestive failure.

Now, however, the effect of digitalis on contractility can be shown on the hearts of animals and of humans without congestive failure, either by attaching a strain gauge to the ventricle or by following the rate of pressure rise within the left ventricle. These types of experiments have already been illustrated in Figs 15—4 and 15—5.

It does not follow from this that the prophylactic use of digitalis is necessarily beneficial since, in the absence of congestive failure, basal cardiac output and heart size are decreased. It does suggest that cardiac performance will not be impaired by digitalis given before cardiac surgery or before the development of overt congestive failure.

Absorption, Metabolism, & Excretion

Digitoxin is very lipid-soluble and is completely and rapidly absorbed after oral administration. Only a fraction of the other commonly used glycosides is absorbed, but the fraction is constant for a given preparation. The highly water-soluble strophanthins such as ouabain are poorly and irregularly absorbed and cannot be used orally. The ratio of the intravenous to the oral dose producing the same effect provides an indication of the absorption of a given preparation.

For metabolic studies, glycosides randomly labeled with radioactive isotopes have been prepared by tritiation or by growing the plant in an atmosphere containing $^{14}CO_2$. Tracing such preparations has shown that digitoxin disappears within a few minutes from the blood, and a concentration of water-soluble metabolites can be demonstrated in the liver and in the contents of the gastrointestinal tract. After a biliary fistula is established, digitoxin is excreted much more rapidly into the urine. These observations suggest that digitoxin undergoes an enterohepatic cycle, a water-soluble metabolite being excreted in the bile and, after hydrolysis in the gut lumen, reabsorbed as digitoxin. Digoxin is demonstrable in the blood, and a serum half-life of 30 hours has been shown.

Latent Period & Duration of Action

When an effective dose of a cardiac glycoside is given (by vein, so that there is no factor of absorption involved), there is a delay before the effect is noted. If the onset of action is rapid—ie, if the latent period is short—the duration of action is short. The long-acting compounds have a long latent period. Ouabain begins to act in 10 minutes, digoxin in about 30. Digitoxin actions begin only after 2 hours, are nearly maximal at 6 hours, persist at effective levels for 1—2 days, and are completely absent only after 2 weeks.

Adverse Reactions

Statistics on the incidence of toxic reactions and mortality are difficult to evaluate, but there is no doubt that digitalis is among the most dangerous as well as most valuable therapeutic agents employed. Because of the narrow therapeutic margin, the usual distinction between side-effects and toxic effects cannot be maintained.

The order of appearance of the toxic effects is unpredictable. A serious arrhythmia may be the first indication of toxicity. Intermittent anorexia and nausea, extrasystoles, and bradycardia are often early signs, and a patient receiving digitalis should be carefully observed for their appearance. The duration of a toxic episode when toxicity is deliberately induced for investigative purposes is usually about 2 days after discontinuance of the drug whether the toxicity is precipitated by digitoxin or the theoretically shorter-acting digoxin.

Allergic reactions to digitalis are almost unheard of.

A. Gastrointestinal: Anorexia, nausea, vomiting, and diarrhea occur. However, visceral congestion as a manifestation of congestive failure can also produce gastrointestinal discomfort.

B. Cardiac: Listed above under ECG effects.

C. Visual: Yellow or green vision, white halos around objects, snow-covered appearance of objects, and a variety of other visual symptoms have been described. They are uncommon and usually late toxic signs.

D. CNS: CNS disturbances allegedly due to digitalis toxicity often turn out to be the result of sodium depletion. However, drowsiness, headache, confusion, and toxic psychosis may be rare and late effects.

Treatment of Digitalis Toxicity

The treatment of digitalis toxicity consists first and most importantly of the discontinuance of the drug. Supplementary potassium may reverse some arrhythmias. Both mercurial and thiazide diuretics (especially the latter) can lead to a depletion of intracellular potassium, and their use should be discontinued temporarily. It has been shown by repeatedly titrating the same patient to the point of toxicity before and after decreasing total body potassium by diuretics that digitalis effects are increased by potassium depletion. Conversely, sensitivity to digitalis is lowered by potassium supplementation. Potassium should be given by mouth as potassium chloride, approximately 2 gm every 4 hours to a total of 4—10 gm daily. A slow intravenous infusion (40 mEq/hour) with constant ECG control may be used but is rarely required.

The beta-adrenergic blocking drug propranolol (Inderal), discussed in Chapter 11, is useful in the treatment of digitalis-induced arrhythmias because of an associated quinidine-like action. The use of supplemental potassium and the interest in the beta-blockers have decreased interest in other investigative treatments and in older drugs such as quinidine.

Clinical Uses

Digitalis is used in the treatment of congestive failure, atrial fibrillation, atrial flutter, and supraventricular tachycardia. The last 3 uses are discussed in the next chapter. (For dosages, see below and Table 15–1.)

Cardiac edema will usually be improved by digitalis if it is due to chronic myocardial insufficiency; digitalis is not effective when the underlying condition is mechanical in origin, as with constrictive pericarditis, congenital heart disease, and most cases of cor pulmonale.

Contraindications & Cautions

All contraindications are relative rather than absolute. There are no contraindications in the presence of failure.

A. Recent Myocardial Infarction: A common cause of death following myocardial infarction is the development of an arrhythmia. Digitalis also causes serious arrhythmias and might increase this tendency if it acts by the same mechanism. When a series of patients with recent myocardial infarctions was divided randomly into treated and untreated groups, digitalization did not increase the mortality or the incidence of arrhythmias. Failure is common after infarction, and digitalis should then be used without hesitation.

B. Ventricular Tachycardia: If ventricular tachycardia is due to digitalis, the drug should be discontinued. Tachycardia due to other causes might theoretically be converted to ventricular fibrillation by digitalis. However, digitalis has often been used to treat the failure associated with a persistent ventricular tachycardia without difficulty.

C. Partial Heart Block: Digitalis may convert partial heart block to complete block. This change may be undesirable, but, if it halts a shifting arrhythmia, it may actually prevent Stokes-Adams attacks.

D. Acute Myocardial Insufficiency: Infectious myocarditis, acute pulmonary edema, and shock following myocardial infarction are not benefited by digitalis.

E. Previous Digitalis Therapy: Before beginning digitalization, be absolutely certain that the patient is not already taking "green tablets," small white or pink "pills," "green drops," etc. A digitalized patient has already received approximately 1/3 of a lethal dose.

F. Calcium Administration: Digitalis and calcium act synergistically under experimental conditions to increase both the therapeutic and toxic effects of digitalis. Sudden deaths have been reported following the rapid intravenous administration of calcium salts to digitalized patients.

G. Potassium Depletion: Potassium depletion due to diuretics or other causes may precipitate digitalis toxicity.

TABLE 15–1. Cardiac glycosides: Dosages and preparations available.

	Digitalizing Dose		Maintenance (Oral)	Preparations Available
	Oral	IV		
Digitalis leaf	1.2–1.5 gm	. . .	0.1 gm	Tablets, 60 and 100 mg Capsules, 60 and 100 mg Enteric-coated tablets, 100 mg Pills, 30, 45, 60, and 100 mg Tincture, 100 mg/ml
Digitoxin	1.2–1.5 mg	1.2 mg	0.1–0.2 mg	Tablets, 0.05, 0.1, 0.15, and 0.2 mg Solution (oral), 10 ml of 1:1000 Elixir (pediatric), 0.05 mg/ml Injectable (IV), 0.2 mg/ml, 1 ml and 2 ml ampules and 10 ml vials
Acetyldigitoxin (Acylanid)	1.8 mg	. . .	0.1–0.2	Tablets, 0.1 and 0.2 mg
Gitalin (Gitaligin)	5 mg	. . .	0.5 mg	Tablets, 0.5 mg (equal to 1 USP unit)
Digoxin	1–3 mg	0.75–1 mg	0.25–0.75 mg	Tablets, 0.25 and 0.5 mg Elixir (pediatric), 60 ml containing 0.05 mg/ml Injectable (IV), 0.5 mg/2 ml ampule
Lanatoside C (Cedilanid)	6 mg	. . .	1 mg	Tablets, 0.5 mg
Deslanoside (Cedilanid-D)	. . .	1.2–1.8 mg (6–8 ml)	. . .	Injectable (IV), 0.2 mg/ml in 2 and 4 ml ampules
Ouabain	. . .	0.5 mg	. . .	Injectable (IV), 0.5 mg in 2 ml ampules
Acetylstrophanthidin	. . .	0.6 mg	. . .	Injectable (IV), hypo tablets containing 0.13 mg

Dosage (See Table 15–1.)

It has long been taught that, unlike most of the drugs that have been discussed thus far—which have small effects after small doses and greater effects after larger doses—digitalis must be present in the body in a certain "saturating" amount before any effect on congestive failure is noted. The effect then becomes nearly maximal all at once. The initial saturating process is accomplished by giving large initial doses or "digitalizing" doses. If smaller daily doses are given, less of the drug is metabolized each day and digitalization will only be achieved very slowly as the drug accumulates.

Recently it has been shown that small doses of digitalis glycosides do have an effect on contractility of the failing heart and that the dose-effect relationship is not nearly as "all-or-none" as had been thought. These observations have led to the use of smaller and safer digitalizing doses and more dependence upon accumulation.

After the initial dosages, digitalis must be given in amounts sufficient to replace that which is destroyed or excreted; this need is provided by daily "maintenance" doses. The size of the maintenance dose must be determined for each patient, and a less than optimal dose will not accumulate.

A. Digitalizing Dose:

No routine, either rapid or cumulative, guarantees full digitalization or freedom from toxicity. The usual doses may be too large or, what is more likely, additional small doses must be given before the maintenance dose can be started.

1. Cumulative method—If digitalis leaf is used or if digitalization with digitoxin is undertaken over a period of hours or days, the estimated digitalizing dose is given in fractions with an interval between each dose (6 hours or more) to allow the full effect of each increment to develop. If the digitalizing period extends over a period of days, allowance must be made for the drug excreted during the process. In general, giving more than 0.4 gm of the leaf at one time causes nausea.

Sample routines:

(1) Digitalis leaf, 0.1 gm 3 times daily for 5 days followed by maintenance dosage.

(2) Digitalis leaf, 0.4 gm every 8 hours for 3 doses.

(3) Digitoxin, 0.4 mg every 8 hours for 3 doses.

2. Single, average full dose (rapid) method—If the purified glycosides are used, digitalization can be accomplished quickly by giving in one dose the amount of the preparation that experience has shown is the average dose needed. (If this is attempted with digitalis leaf, the patient becomes nauseated and vomits.) This method does not allow for individual variation, but the dosages chosen are more apt to be too small than toxic. Of 1000 cases given 1.2 mg of digitoxin, for example, only 2% showed nausea, but most of them required more digitoxin before digitalization was complete. This method is rarely used.

B. Maintenance Dose: Average daily maintenance dosages are listed in Table 15–1. The most effective use of digitalis requires that an optimal dosage be determined for each patient. If the therapeutic regimen involves only digitalis, diuresis or relief of the symptoms of congestive failure can be used as the end point. If the patient is fibrillating, the heart rate is a good index. But in most patients, especially after they have been under treatment for months or years, the only method establishing with certainty that digitalization is complete is to increase the dose until the first toxic signs appear and then to select a maintenance dose slightly smaller. Withering's plan is still the best: "Let it be continued until it acts either on the kidneys, the stomach, the pulse or the bowels . . ."

Selection of a Digitalis Preparation

The factors determining the choice of cardiac glycoside have all been discussed above. The purified glycosides allow more rapid digitalization. The shorter latent period of digoxin or its equivalent is important in the treatment of atrial arrhythmias when rapid onset of action is desirable. The longer duration of action of digitoxin or digitalis leaf prevents the fluctuation of effect sometimes seen with a rapidly dissipated drug such as digoxin. Theoretically, the toxic reactions which occur following the use of digoxin should be briefer in duration than those precipitated by digitoxin. Actually, no such difference could be demonstrated in a clinical trial.

The activity of digitalis leaf is due entirely to its digitoxin content.

Ouabain has been credited on the basis of clinical impressions with being relatively more effective in stimulating the left ventricle and relatively less active in its effect on the conducting tissues. Objective studies to verify this impression are equivocal at best. Ouabain can be given only intravenously. Ouabain acts rapidly and is water-soluble and is therefore frequently used in the animal laboratory.

Gitalin has properties intermediate between digitoxin and digoxin but is not, in spite of some claims, qualitatively different from the other glycosides.

In summary, the choice among the glycosides is not of critical importance except in those situations where an immediate effect is desirable. Most physicians use the one with which they have had the most experience, often the one introduced at a critical time in their training.

General References

Balcon, R., & others: Hemodynamic effects of rapid digitalization following acute myocardial infarction. Brit Heart J 30:373–376, 1968.

Braunwald, E., & F.J. Klocke: Digitalis. Ann Rev Med 16:371–383, 1965.

Braunwald, E., Mason, D.T., & J. Ross, Jr.: Studies on the cardiocirculatory actions of digitalis. Medicine 44:233–248, 1965.

Church, G., & others: Deliberate digitalis intoxication: A comparison of the toxic effects of four glycoside preparations. Ann Int Med 57:946–956, 1962.

Fieser, L.F., & M. Fieser: Cardio-active principles. Chap 20, pp 727–809, in: *Steroids.* Reinhold, 1959.

Fogelman, A.M., & others: Fallibility of plasma-digoxin in differentiating toxic from non-toxic patients. Lancet 2:727–729, 1971.

Gilson, J.S., & F.R. Schemm: The use of digitalis in spite of the presence of ventricular tachycardia. Circulation 2:278–285, 1950.

Katzung, B.G., & F.H. Meyers: Excretion of radioactive digitoxin by the dog. J Pharmacol Exper Therap 149:257–262, 1965.

Kelly, H.G., & R.I.S. Bayliss: Influence of heart-rate on cardiac output: Studies with digoxin and atropine. Lancet 2:1071–1075, 1949.

Langer, G.A.: The intrinsic control of myocardial contraction: Ionic factors. New England J Med 285:1065–1071, 1971.

Lee, K.S., & W. Klaus: The subcellular basis for the mechanism of inotropic action of cardiac glycosides. Pharmacol Rev 23:193–261, 1971.

Lown, B., & S.A. Levine: *Current Concepts in Digitalis Therapy.* Little, Brown, 1954.

McMichael, J.: The heart and digitalis. Brit MJ 2:73–79, 1963.

Mason, D.T.: The cardiovascular effects of digitalis in normal man. Clin Pharmacol Therap 7:1–16, 1966.

Neill, C.A.: The use of digitalis in infants and children. Progr Cardiovas Dis 7:399–416, 1965.

Robertson, D.M., Hollenhorst, R.W., & J.A. Callahan: Ocular manifestations of digitalis toxicity: Discussion and report of three cases of central scotoma. Arch Ophth 76:640–645, 1966.

Rutledge, D.I., & R. Haddad: Digitalis intoxication: Gastrointestinal manifestations. M Clin North America 50:501–506, 1966.

Sciarini, L.J., & W.T. Salter: Chemical correlatives of digitalis potency in man, cat, and pigeon. J Pharmacol Exper Therap 101:167–175, 1951.

16...

Drug Treatment of Cardiac Arrhythmias

In this chapter the pharmacology of quinidine and a number of other drugs with similar effects will be introduced. Quinidine is able to suppress most cardiac arrhythmias and allow restoration of a normal sinus rhythm. However, other methods of treatment (both drug and electrical) are available, and quinidine is not often the treatment of choice for an arrhythmia. Even when indicated, it is rarely used alone. A discussion of the treatment of cardiac arrhythmias will therefore follow the discussion of quinidine and will include references to other drugs.

QUINIDINE

Quinidine is the D-isomer of quinine, and the sources and properties of the 2 naturally occurring alkaloids are similar. The effect of quinine in correcting his atrial fibrillation was noted by a Dutch Colonial who had taken it in Java for malaria. Wenckebach, an Austrian cardiologist, accepted and verified this observation, and in 1914 introduced quinine as an antiarrhythmia drug. Quinidine was introduced shortly thereafter. Quinidine and quinine are equipotent in small doses, but, when large doses are used, quinidine is more active against arrhythmias.

Quinidine

Pharmacologic Actions

A. Mechanisms of Action:

1. **Mechanism of atrial arrhythmias**—The interpretation of the effects of the antiarrhythmia drugs is conditioned by one's understanding of the origin of the atrial arrhythmias. For many years the circus movement theory of Thomas Lewis was dominant. This theory held that excitation originating in a focus close to the point of entry of the great veins into the atria could not spread uniformly but would be channeled into a circular path.

The wave of depolarization could travel this devious path at such a rate that, when it again reached the site of origin, the tissue was no longer refractory and reentry or reexcitation could occur. From the rapidly recurring, circular wave, daughter (secondary) waves would arise and spread throughout the atria. Depending upon the rate of the process, the atria might be able to respond to each impulse (flutter) or be unable to follow the rapid electrical rate (fibrillation). If a drug could prolong the refractory period, as quinidine was incorrectly alleged to do, the circus movement would be interrupted because the head of the wave would reach the tail while it was still refractory. Effects on conduction could be similarly invoked.

A circus movement and accompanying atrial arrhythmias can be experimentally produced in animals by crushing an area of the atrial wall of proper size. However, the arrhythmias that occur in man are better explained by another hypothesis.

The unitary theory of the nature of atrial arrhythmias suggests that the only difference between the arrhythmias is in the rate of firing of the ectopic focus responsible. An ectopic pacemaker with a rate of 160—180 would be described as producing atrial or supraventricular tachycardia. If the ectopic rate were somewhat more rapid—eg, 240—there would be some degree of atrioventricular block and the condition would be clinically described as atrial flutter. If the abnormal rate were raised to 300—500/minute and the atria were unable to follow each electrical stimulus, effective atrial contractions would disappear and atrial fibrillation would result. If an ectopic focus is established by the subepicardial injection of a cholinomimetic alkaloid—aconitine (to cite one experiment)—and the rate of firing controlled by cooling or with quinidine, each of the predicted arrhythmias can be produced. (Table 16—1 shows an equivalent demonstration in man.) In the clinical arrhythmias, however, the pacemakers responsible for the different atrial arrhythmias are located in different areas of the atrium.

The question of the nature of the arrhythmias as they occur in man was approached using high-speed motion pictures and ECGs at the time of commissurotomy as well as by esophageal ECG leads. In such instances, no evidence of a circular pathway or of daughter waves was seen. On the contrary, during flutter, contraction waves and electrical activity—and, during fibrillation, electrical activity—can be seen to originate from a single point.

The unitary theory of the atrial arrhythmias suggests that the ability of a drug to decrease the rate of

TABLE 16—1. Summary of the atrial arrhythmias, illustrated by portions of the continuous esophageal (E_{35}) ECG of a patient who manifested all the rhythms illustrated within a single 5-minute period.* An ectopic focus in the atrium is responsible for the development of atrial premature contractions, atrial tachycardia, atrial flutter (which can also be called atrial tachycardia with atrioventricular block), and atrial fibrillation. The rate at which this ectopic atrial focus discharges will determine the type of the atrial arrhythmia.

Rate of Discharge of Atrial Ectopic Focus	Arrhythmia
Occasional discharge at a rate slower than the basic sinus rhythm. Atrial premature contractions.	
About 160 to about 220 Atrial tachycardia (with 1:1 conduction).	
About 220 to about 350 Atrial flutter (ie, atrial tachycardia with A—V block).	
Over 350 Atrial fibrillation.	

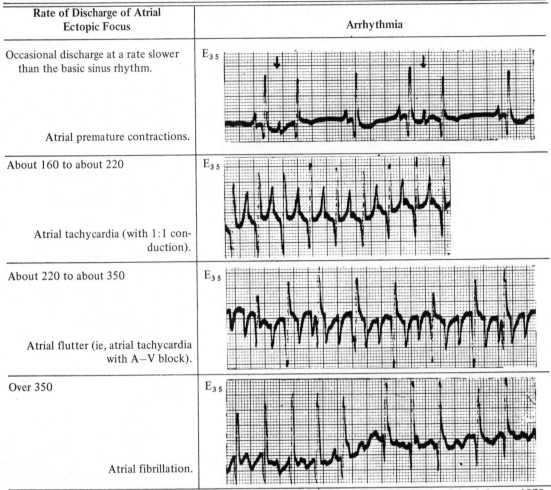

*Reproduced, with permission, from Goldman: *Principles of Clinical Electrocardiography,* 7th ed. Lange, 1970.

firing of an abnormal pacemaker would be its important effect.

2. Effect of quinidine on action potentials—The availability of microelectrode studies showing the effect of quinidine on intracellular potentials has not eliminated controversy about the mechanism of the antiarrhythmia action of quinidine. The difficulties in interpreting the microelectrode studies arise from questions about the concentration of quinidine used and about probable differences between the several areas studied.

Isolated atrial muscle can be suspended in a bath and stimulated at varying rates while a microelectrode is in place within single units. When concentrations of quinidine comparable to the therapeutic dose are added, the rate of rise of the action potential is slowed—ie, depolarization, represented by phase 0 as in Fig 16—1, is slowed. The effect is minor at slow rates

of stimulation such as might be comparable to a normal sinus rhythm, but is much more apparent at rapid rates, which simulate atrial arrhythmias.

When depolarization progresses slowly, the threshold at which complete depolarization abruptly occurs is elevated. The antiarrhythmia activity of quinidine is explained by the decreased rate of depolarization and the associated failure of the impulse to be propagated to adjacent units.

The above data appear highly relevant to the action of quinidine on the atrial arrhythmias. However, other workers point out that conducting or pacemaking tissues such as the Purkinje fibers of the ventricles might respond differently. In such tissue they feel a decrease in the rate of diastolic depolarization (represented by phase 4 in Fig 16—1) would explain the greater interval between impulses. Demonstration of

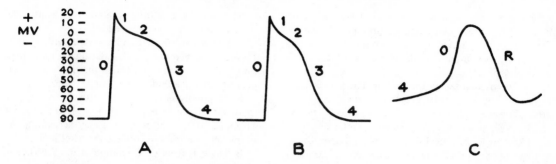

FIG 16–1. Diagrams of action potential curves. *A:* Ventricular muscle cell. *B:* Atrial muscle cell. *C:* Sino-atrial node. 0 = depolarization; 1, 2, 3 = phases of repolarization; 4 = diastolic phase = MRP (membrane resting potential); R = repolarization phase of spontaneously depolarizing tissue not divisible into phases 1, 2, and 3. (Reproduced, with permission, from Goldman: *Principles of Clinical Electrocardiography*, 7th ed. Lange, 1970.)

such an effect on diastolic leakage is difficult and requires concentrations of quinidine regarded by others as beyond the therapeutic range. Proponents of this view suggest that ectopic foci might be more sensitive to the effects of quinidine.

Quinidine in realistic concentrations has only a minor effect on the refractory period as it is derived from intracellular potential changes. Overshoot is slightly reduced. Resting potential is unchanged.

3. Effect of quinidine on cell membrane—Excitation or depolarization is due to an increase in the permeability of the cell membrane to sodium ion and the consequent rapid influx of sodium into the cell. The section immediately above suggests that this process is sensitive to the effects of quinidine.

A number of drugs impede the depolarization process without altering the resting potential and are sometimes described together as "membrane stabilizers." The drugs share the chemical pattern described in other chapters for the parasympatholytics, antihistamines, tranquilizers, local anesthetics, and here for quinidine-like drugs—ie, an amine function connected to a bulky cyclic or polycyclic group by a short chain. How the specificity seen in the actions of these drugs arises is conjectural, but all have quinidine-like actions.

B. Pharmacologic Effects:

1. On the myocardium—

a. Rhythmic function is depressed—Regardless of the mechanism—ie, whether quinidine acts by slowing the rate of diastolic depolarization in pacemaking tissue, by slowing the rate of rise after the threshold for depolarization is reached, or by some other mechanism—quinidine slows the rate of firing of the normal and of ectopic rhythmic foci. Thus, even before conversion to normal sinus rhythm, the frequency of the f (fibrillation) waves in atrial fibrillation and of the atrial rate in flutter will be slightly slowed.

The conversion of fibrillation is not all-or-none but stepwise, as the unitary theory would predict. The percentage of patients with atrial fibrillation who are seen to pass through atrial flutter en route to a normal sinus rhythm rises as the amount of ECG surveillance is increased. Examples in which atrial tachycardia occurs as an intermediate step before normal sinus rhythm are also available. Even the normal sinus pacemaker is depressed by quinidine, although—fortunately—it is relatively insensitive. Nevertheless, periods of asystole (usually brief) may on rare occasions be seen at the time of resumption of normal sinus rhythm. In the usual doses, quinidine has little effect on normal sinus rhythm.

b. Conduction velocity—Both intraventricular and atrioventricular conduction velocity is decreased or conduction time is prolonged. On the ECG the duration of both the ventricular complex and the P–R interval is increased.

c. Refractory period—The absolute refractory period as measured by intracellular recordings is not much altered by quinidine. Some older technics appeared to show that quinidine lengthened the refractory period. These methods could not distinguish between a prolongation of refractory period and a failure of the wave of depolarization to be propagated and conducted to a recording electrode. Conduction in cardiac muscle can be decremental rather than all-or-none—ie, a wave of depolarization may initially be propagated or conducted away from the excitable focus at a rapid rate but slow progressively before failing to be propagated. Quinidine exaggerates this property. Lewis himself recognized that what he had called a change in refractory period was actually conduction failure. Unfortunately, he renamed this the **"effective refractory period,"** and the term has now been applied to the inability to maintain a propagated impulse.

d. Intracardiac vagal block is the term applied to an atropine-like action of quinidine on vagal efferents reaching the atrioventricular node. There is no accompanying peripheral atropine-like effect. As a result of decreased vagal influence, the atrioventricular refractory period is shortened and, in the presence of a rapid atrial rate, more impulses pass through the node to activate the ventricles. Larger doses of quinidine are required for this effect, and the action may coincide with the conversion of fibrillation to flutter, resulting in a very rapid ventricular rate. To prevent this adverse result, quinidine is given in the presence of a rapid atrial rate only after the administration of adequate doses of digitalis.

e. Ventricular tachycardia—Quinidine may be used in the treatment of ventricular tachycardia. As a toxic effect, however, quinidine may cause ventricular tachycardia. (Ventricular tachycardia does not refer simply to a rapid ventricular rate but to a specific arrhythmia arising from one or more rapidly firing ventricular foci.)

f. Depression of myocardial contractility—In the animal laboratory, quinidine depresses contractility of the myocardium. There is no evidence that this action is measurably present during its clinical use.

2. Vasodilatation—Quinidine has a direct relaxing effect on vascular smooth muscle, and the resulting vasodilatation can lead to hypotension.

3. On skeletal muscle—Quinidine has a very weak curare-like ability to weaken skeletal muscle response. It is used to relieve the muscle hypertonicity present in the rare case of congenital myotonia. Intensification of effect of curare has been noted in postsurgical patients.

Absorption, Metabolism, & Excretion

Quinidine is completely but slowly absorbed from the gastrointestinal tract and from the injection site following intramuscular administration. The maximum blood level is reached about 2 hours after each dose, and, after 24 hours, a perceptible amount (10% of maximum) remains. Either ring of the quinidine molecule can be hydroxylated in the liver, and these metabolites, together with much unchanged quinidine, are excreted in the urine to account for approximately 90% of an ingested dose.

Adverse Reactions

The dose-related toxic effects of quinidine can be divided into those that may occur in any patient—whether a normal sinus rhythm or some abnormal rhythm is present—and those that occur only in the presence of an abnormal rhythm.

A. Toxic Effects of Quinidine Not Necessarily Associated With an Arrhythmia:

1. Gastrointestinal—Nausea, vomiting, abdominal cramps, and diarrhea are common local irritant effects of quinidine.

2. Cinchonism—Symptoms of quinidine toxicity similar to those caused by other cinchona alkaloids or by salicylates include giddiness, light-headedness, tremulousness, tinnitus, impaired hearing, and blurred or double vision.

3. QRS prolongation—If the effect on intraventricular conduction leads to an increase of more than 25% in the duration of the ventricular complex (or a duration greater than 0.14 seconds), further administration of the drug should be carried out very cautiously. A 50% widening of the QRS complex is often followed by ventricular fibrillation.

4. Ventricular tachycardia, if it occurs after the administration of quinidine, is, of course, an indication

for discontinuing the drug. Premonitory ventricular premature beats may be observed.

5. Ventricular fibrillation may occur with or without a preceding period of ventricular tachycardia. Brief periods or paroxysms of fibrillation may cause syncope, just as may periods of asystole.

6. Hypotension, which can occur after oral administration but is more common after the parenteral administration of quinidine, may necessitate discontinuance of efforts to convert an arrhythmia.

B. Toxic Effects of Quinidine in the Presence of an Arrhythmia:

1. Rapid ventricular rate—The intracardiac vagal block and consequent decrease in refractory period of the AV node caused by quinidine may lead to a sudden increase in the number of waves of excitation that reach the ventricles. This may occur with either atrial fibrillation or flutter. To prevent the increase in ventricular rate, digitalis should always be given before quinidine is used in the treatment of an atrial arrhythmia unless electrical conversion is contemplated.

2. Asystole—The normal pacemaker is depressed by quinidine as well as the ectopic sites. When a stubborn arrhythmia has finally been suppressed, there may be a delay before the slower pacemaker takes over. This period of asystole may be recognized on the ECG or may appear as syncope or convulsions due to cerebral ischemia.

C. Allergic Reactions: Fever, urticaria, other skin rashes, asthma, and, rarely, thrombocytopenic purpura may result from acquired sensitivity to quinidine.

Contraindications & Cautions

In the presence of complete atrioventricular dissociation, the effect of quinidine in slowing the ventricular focus could be disastrous. The effect of quinidine on atrioventricular conduction could convert an incomplete block to complete atrioventricular block. Quinidine should not, therefore, be used in the presence of any degree of block other than that usually associated with the atrial arrhythmias. Similarly, bundle branch block or intraventricular conduction defect is a contraindication to the use of quinidine. Active rheumatic fever, bacterial endocarditis, pregnancy, and untreated thyrotoxicosis are relative contraindications to the use of quinidine.

Digitalis should always be used in optimal amounts before quinidine is given, except when the prompt treatment of an arrhythmia is necessary or when cardioversion is planned. Congestive heart failure should be corrected to the greatest extent possible before quinidine is used.

A test dose should be given if the situation permits (see below).

Dosages

Much larger doses of quinidine are required to convert an arrhythmia than to prevent recurrence or occurrence of an arrhythmia. Dosage is therefore divided into dosage for conversion and dosage for maintenance.

A. Conversion:

1. Oral—Unless the need for treatment is immediate, a test dose of 0.1 or 0.2 gm orally of quinidine is given and the patient observed for at least 2 hours to eliminate the rare patient who is allergic to quinidine or unusually sensitive to its toxic effects.

The dosage of quinidine is determined by the therapeutic objective and is reached by a preselected plan. The plan must take into consideration that the disappearance of the drug from the body occurs slowly and that nearly 10% of the dose may remain after 24 hours.

The usual or anticipated dosage varies depending upon the arrhythmia being treated. The treatment of the specific arrhythmias is outlined below.

Quinidine is a hazardous drug and, since other methods of treatment are available, the tendency is to use even greater caution than in the past.

The following 2 schemes or regimens used to attempt the conversion of atrial fibrillation to a normal sinus rhythm are given as examples:

a. One common method which requires hospitalization and close observation is as follows: On the first day, give quinidine, 0.2 gm every 2 hours, until therapeutic response or toxicity is noted or until 4–5 doses have been given. The amount of quinidine excreted depends in part upon the amount in the body, and after 4–5 doses on this schedule no further cumulative effect on blood levels is seen. On the second day, give 0.4 gm of quinidine every 2 hours for 5 doses. On subsequent days, the dosage may be increased to 0.6 gm every 2 hours for 5 doses. There is a residual level in the morning following the above dosages, and ECG control and clinical observation are necessary before each dose is given.

b. An alternative method is to give a fixed dose—eg, 0.2 gm–4 times a day and, in the absence of toxicity or a response, increase the dose every 4–5 days.

2. Intramuscular—The same doses by the intramuscular route can be used if the patient is unable to take the medication orally and the situation is not critical. Quinidine gluconate, 0.8 gm in 10 ml ampules, is available.

3. Intravenous—The intravenous route should be used only when the urgency is great. Quinidine gluconate, 0.8 gm in 10 ml ampules, can be diluted with 50–100 ml of 5% glucose and given slowly intravenously at a rate of 1 ml/minute with frequent ECGs and blood pressure measurements. Procainamide (Pronestyl) or lidocaine is perhaps more often used when intravenous antiarrhythmia therapy is necessary.

B. Maintenance or Prevention: Dosages of 0.2–0.4 gm orally 4 times a day are used to prevent recurrence of the arrhythmia. The reliability of the sustained-release preparations available for prolonged action has not been completely confirmed.

Preparations Available

Quinidine sulfate:
    Tablets, 120, 200, and 300 mg
    Capsules, 200 mg
    Injectable (IM or IV), 200 mg/1 ml ampules

Quinidine hydrochloride:
    A parenteral (IV) preparation is available but never used.

Quinidine gluconate:
    Sustained-action tablets (Quinaglute), 330 mg
    Injectable (IM or IV), 80 mg/ml, 10 ml vials

OTHER ANTIARRHYTHMIA DRUGS

What has been said about the cardiac effects of quinidine applies also to the drugs discussed below unless a specific exception is made.

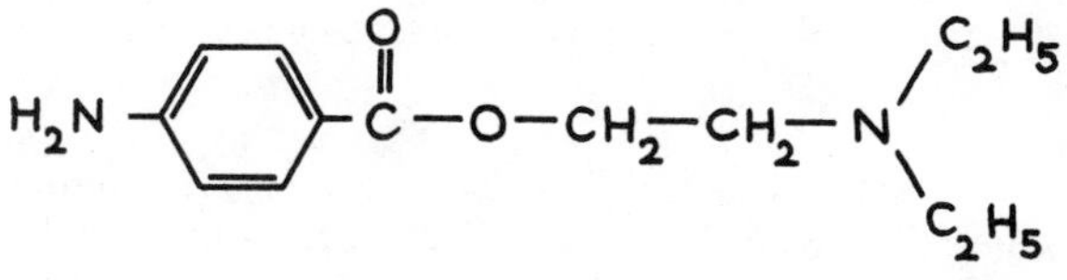

Procaine

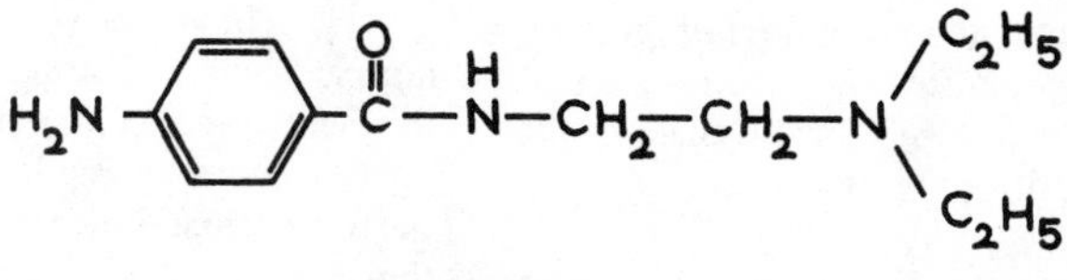

Procainamide
(Pronestyl)

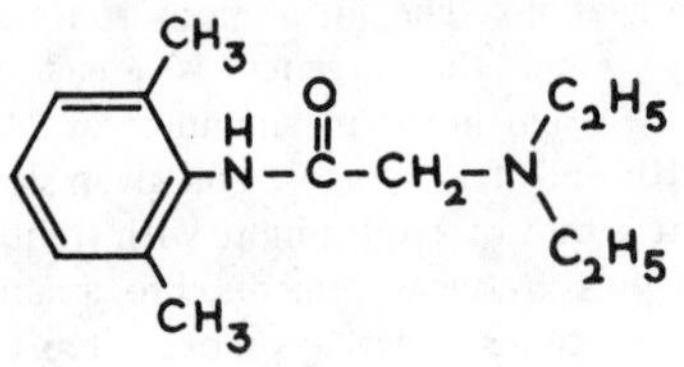

The structural diagram shows:

CH₃ — (benzene ring) — N(H) — C(=O) — CH₂ — N(C₂H₅)(C₂H₅), with CH₃

Lidocaine
(Xylocaine)

PROCAINAMIDE
(Pronestyl)

The local anesthetics have quinidine-like action in addition to their primary effect. Procaine has been shown to be active in suppressing ventricular arrhythmias, but its action is very brief since it is an ester and is rapidly hydrolyzed. Procainamide is the amide analogue of procaine. It retains the quinidine-like actions of procaine but is not rapidly hydrolyzed, and its action persists long enough so that it is active after oral as well as parenteral administration.

Pharmacologically, procainamide is the equivalent of quinidine. It causes the same toxic effects except that cinchonism does not occur and allergic reactions are more frequent. A series of patients have developed a reversible but potentially damaging form of disseminated lupus erythematosus as a result of long-term procainamide therapy; a larger fraction show antinuclear antibody without symptoms.

When procainamide was first introduced, its parenteral dosage form was superior to the then available forms of injectable quinidine. At that time it was also claimed that procainamide acted selectively upon ventricular arrhythmias, but it is active against atrial arrhythmias if enough is given. Its use as an equivalent or alternative to quinidine when a parenteral drug was needed in the treatment of ventricular tachycardia has decreased with the advent of electrical treatment and other drugs and dosage forms. In the prevention of ventricular arrhythmias in the period immediately following myocardial infarction, the usefulness of procainamide is better established than that of other drugs.

Dosages & Preparations

Procainamide hydrochloride (Pronestyl) is available for oral administration as 0.25 gm (equivalent to 0.2 gm of quinidine) and 0.5 gm capsules. Ampules containing 1 gm/10 ml are available for intramuscular or intravenous injection. If given intravenously, procainamide should be diluted and given no more rapidly than at a rate of 50 mg/minute. Blood pressure and ECG changes should be monitored for the changes discussed under adverse reactions to quinidine.

LIDOCAINE
(Xylocaine)

Lidocaine is another local anesthetic used to treat ventricular arrhythmias. In its brief duration of action and need to be given by constant intravenous infusion, it resembles procaine more than procainamide. The advantage claimed is that in small doses it causes less hypotension. In the usual doses it causes drowsiness, but larger doses may cause muscle twitching, confusion, and focal or generalized convulsions. Its other effects, including the ability to precipitate as well as to suppress ventricular arrhythmias, are similar to those of procainamide or quinidine.

Lidocaine is currently finding increasing use in intensive care units in patients who are postoperative or who have a recent myocardial infarction. It is used to treat ventricular arrhythmias or to prevent their occurrence either as routine prophylaxis or in the presence of ventricular ectopic beats possibly premonitory of tachycardia. Controlled studies do not verify the superiority claimed for lidocaine in this situation nor establish its safety. Reports of the "recurrence" of ventricular arrhythmias during the continued administration of the drug or the progression of an arrhythmia in the face of increasing dose may as easily be interpreted as toxic reactions.

Lidocaine exerts an immediate effect but its action persists only 10 minutes. For this reason it is most often given as a single large initial intravenous dose—eg, 1–2 mg/kg in 30 seconds—followed by a continuous intravenous infusion (1–3 mg/minute) to maintain the effect.

BETA-ADRENERGIC BLOCKING AGENTS

The beta-receptor blocking agents—eg, propranolol (Inderal)—are discussed in Chapter 11 as one class of drugs that decrease the effect of sympathetic mediators on the heart and other tissues. They happen —coincidentally, and independently of their beta-blocking property—to be quinidine-like.

Because they block the effect of norepinephrine or epinephrine on atrioventricular nodal tissue, nodal refractory time is prolonged. In the presence of a rapid atrial rate—eg, atrial flutter or fibrillation—fewer of the waves of depolarization from above will reach the ventricles after propranolol administration. Propranolol will, like digitalis, slow the ventricular rate even though the rapid atrial rate continues.

The beta blockers also slow the rate of firing of normal sinus and other atrial pacemakers by reducing the sympathetic accelerator influence.

Propranolol can be used in lieu of digitalis to slow the ventricular rate when conversion by DC countershock is planned since it does not predispose to ventricular arrhythmias as digitalis does.

The beta blockers are more useful than quinidine and its congeners in treating arrhythmias that are due to digitalis toxicity. The arrhythmias are suppressed, and a normal rhythm is established.

OTHER QUINIDINE EQUIVALENTS

The antipsychotic tranquilizers—eg, chlorpromazine or other phenothiazine derivatives, the closely related antidepressants such as imipramine—and many of the antihistamines have antiarrhythmia actions in the laboratory and clinically. These drugs probably act by the same mechanism as does quinidine, but the available data are insufficient to be certain. The slightly greater frequency of sudden, unexplained deaths in patients treated with large doses of tranquilizers and some aspects of the acute toxicity of the antidepressants are apparently related to the quinidine-like cardiac effects.

Diphenylhydantoin (Dilantin), an anticonvulsant, is also able to suppress ventricular arrhythmias both in the experimental animal and clinically. Some investigators, on the basis of laboratory studies open to conflicting interpretations, conclude that it is qualitatively different from quinidine. It does not lower blood pressure or depress cardiac contractility unless given with propylene glycol, the solvent usually supplied. However, after intravenous administration it has demonstrated most of the actions of quinidine, including changes in conduction and the production of fatal ventricular arrhythmias.

TREATMENT OF CARDIAC ARRHYTHMIAS

The treatment of the common cardiac arrhythmias not only involves several drug groups—ie, digitalis, quinidine, beta-adrenergic blockers, and sympathomimetics—but also a physical technic, direct current (DC) countershock. DC countershock (cardioversion) applies a high-voltage direct current of brief duration (2.5 msec) through the chest at the level of the heart. The externally applied charge is sufficient to depolarize the entire heart, and a normal sinus rhythm is often established upon recovery. The shock is electrically triggered by the R wave of the ECG to avoid the vulnerable period of the myocardium. Quinidine used prior to DC countershock increases the number of successful conversions, and maintenance doses are given to prevent recurrence of the arrhythmia. Digitalis is dis-

continued for at least 48 hours before cardioversion because it increases the risk of ventricular tachycardia and fibrillation. A beta-adrenergic blocking agent may be used prior to cardioversion in place of digitalis to maintain a slow ventricular rate in the presence of a continued rapid atrial rate.

PAROXYSMAL ATRIAL TACHYCARDIA

The paroxysmal supraventricular tachycardias are usually self-limiting disorders but may be recurrent. Treatment is both immediate (to terminate the paroxysm) and prophylactic in those few patients with frequent recurrences.

Treatment of Acute Episode

Assuming that paroxysmal atrial tachycardia is not due to digitalis toxicity, it will probably occur in an otherwise healthy individual and treatment should involve minimal hazard. Sedation and the removal of precipitating factors (fatigue, tobacco, alcohol) may suffice.

A. Augment Vagal Influences on the Heart: This can be done in various ways: (1) by applying carotid sinus pressure; (2) by inducing vomiting by stimulation of the pharynx or with syrup of ipecac, 8–15 ml; (3) with pressor drugs; or (4) with digitalis. Methacholine and neostigmine have also been used but cause strong and unpleasant side-effects.

B. Anti-arrhythmia Drugs: Oral doses of digitalis, quinidine, or propranolol may be used if needed. Digitalis should not be selected if it has been recently administered and the arrhythmia may be a manifestation of digitalis toxicity.

C. DC Countershock: This procedure is effective but rarely justified.

Prevention of Attacks

Attempt to identify and treat or remove the cause, eg, emotional stress, fatigue, or excessive use of alcohol or tobacco. Quinidine sulfate, 0.2–0.6 gm 3–4 times daily, may be used to prevent frequent and troublesome attacks. Begin with small doses and increase if the attacks are not prevented and toxic effects do not occur.

If quinidine is not effective or not tolerated, full digitalization and maintenance may prevent or decrease the frequency of attacks. Propranolol is also effective.

ATRIAL FIBRILLATION

Atrial fibrillation may be due to any of several causes, and the need for treatment and response to treatment are correspondingly diverse. Atrial fibrillation associated with rheumatic mitral valve disease involves the great hazard of repeated emboli arising from thrombi that form on the walls of the noncontracting atrial appendages. If the fibrillation is associated with atherosclerotic heart disease, the hazard of emboli is virtually negligible. In either case, only a slight increase in cardiac efficiency is attained by conversion of the fibrillation to normal sinus rhythm beyond the effect achieved by merely slowing the ventricular rate with digitalis, and the need for conversion is seldom urgent.

Digitalis is the first drug used in the treatment of atrial fibrillation. Digitalis corrects any congestive fail-

ure present and slows the ventricular rate through the additional mechanism of prolonging the refractory period of the atrioventricular node (Fig 16–2). Propranolol will also slow the ventricular rate but will reduce cardiac output and cannot be used if congestive failure is present. If it is then judged advisable, attempts can be made to correct the atrial fibrillation to a sinus rhythm. DC countershock is now probably most frequently used to accomplish conversion, but quinidine may be used. This achieves only a minor additional increase in cardiac efficiency but protects against embolization.

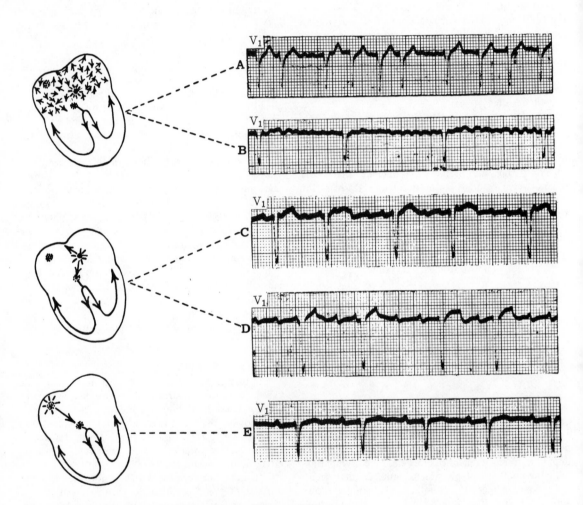

A. Before therapy: Atrial fibrillation; ventricular rate = 120.

B. After digitalization: Atrial fibrillation; ventricular rate = 50.

C. During initial quinidine therapy: Atrial flutter; atrial rate = 300. There is a varying atrioventricular block (3:1 to 5:1), resulting in a ventricular rate of 75.

D. During continued quinidine therapy: Atrial flutter persists, but the atrial rate has been reduced to 210. There is a varying atrioventricular block, resulting in a ventricular rate of 65.

E. Further quinidine therapy: Regular sinus rhythm; rate = 68.

FIG 16–2. Atrial fibrillation: Response to digitalis and quinidine. (Reproduced, with permission, from Goldman: *Principles of Clinical Electrocardiography,* 7th ed. Lange, 1970.)

ATRIAL FLUTTER

The first (and often the only) drug used in the treatment of atrial flutter is digitalis. Digitalis will increase the degree of atrioventricular block and thereby slow the ventricular rate and make the patient comfortable; in addition, in at least half of cases it converts the flutter to atrial fibrillation. Such a recently established atrial fibrillation is not stable and will often convert to a normal sinus rhythm whether digitalis is continued or discontinued and whether quinidine is given or not (Fig 16–3). The dose of digitalis required may be a little larger than that used for congestive heart failure.

DC countershock is effective and convenient in terminating atrial flutter and is usually used in preference to digitalis or quinidine.

If quinidine is used to convert the flutter or a digitalis-induced fibrillation, the patient should be fully digitalized to avoid a sudden increase in ventricular rate.

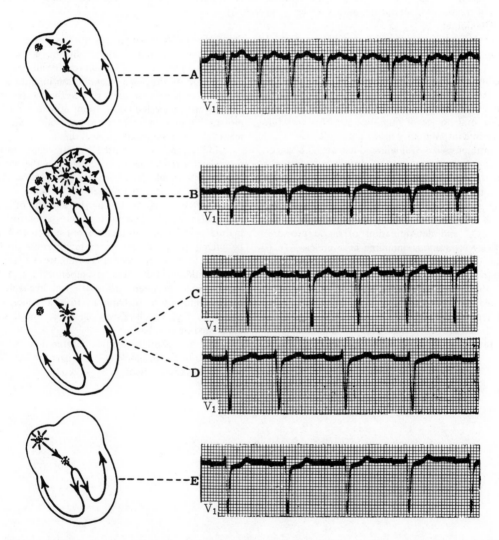

A. Before therapy: Atrial flutter with 2:1 atrioventricular block. Atrial rate = 272; ventricular rate = 136.

B. After digitalization: The rhythm is now atrial fibrillation; the ventricular rate has been slowed to 80.

C. During initial quinidine therapy: Quinidine has changed the atrial fibrillation to atrial flutter. The atrial rate is 272 (as in A), but because of the blocking action of digitalis on the atrioventricular node there is 3:1 and 4:1 atrioventricular block, resulting in a ventricular rate of 85.

D. During continued quinidine therapy: Atrial flutter persists, but the atrial rate has been reduced to 200. There is 2:1 and 3:1 atrioventricular block, resulting in a ventricular rate of 75.

E. Further quinidine therapy: The rhythm has reverted to regular sinus rhythm.

FIG 16–3. Atrial flutter: Response to digitalis and quinidine. (Reproduced, with permission, from Goldman: *Principles of Clinical Electrocardiography,* 7th ed. Lange, 1970.)

VENTRICULAR TACHYCARDIA

Ventricular tachycardia is a rapid idioventricular rhythm that constitutes a medical emergency. Treatment is selected from among the following options:

A. Propranolol (Inderal): If the ventricular tachycardia is due to digitalis toxicity, the beta-adrenergic blocking agent propranolol (Inderal) can be used. For dosage, see Chapter 11.

B. DC Countershock: When the arrhythmia is clearly not due to digitalis toxicity, DC countershock (when available) is rapidly replacing pharmacologic methods of treatment in all but the mildest cases.

C. Quinidine:

1. Oral—Give quinidine, 0.4 gm orally every 2 hours for 3 doses, if the attack is well tolerated and the patient is not in shock. If the attack continues and there is no toxicity from the quinidine, increase the dose to 0.6 gm orally every 2 hours for 3 doses or use DC countershock. If countershock is not available and the larger oral dosage of quinidine is not successful, give quinidine intravenously or intramuscularly.

2. Intramuscular—Quinidine gluconate, 0.8 gm or 0.5 gm of quinidine base, may be given intramuscularly and repeated every 2 hours for 2–3 doses.

3. Intravenous—Quinidine may be given intravenously as quinidine gluconate, 0.8 gm diluted with 50 ml of 5% glucose **slowly** (1 ml/minute), with continuous ECG and determination of blood pressure. When giving intravenous quinidine in severe cases (particularly when the previous rhythm was complete atrioventricular block), the physician should be alert to the possibility of precipitating ventricular fibrillation or asystole.

D. Procainamide:

1. Oral—Give 0.5–1.5 gm every 4–6 hours.

2. Intramuscular—Give 0.5–1 gm and repeat in 4 hours.

3. Intravenous—Give procainamide hydrochloride (Pronestyl), 1 gm **slowly** IV (at a rate not to exceed 100 mg/minute). During the infusion, continuous ECG or, at least, repeated blood pressure determinations are essential. Severe hypotension may result from this medication.

E. Lidocaine: Lidocaine is probably more frequently used than quinidine or procainamide. (See above for dosage.)

F. Vasopressors: If shock is present as a result of ventricular tachycardia or results from the drugs given intravenously, it can be treated with levarterenol (Levophed) or other vasopressor drugs (see Chapter 10).

Prevention of Ventricular Arrhythmias

In the hours immediately following a myocardial infarction, continuous ECG monitoring will show some disturbance of rhythm or conduction in almost every patient. Coronary care units reduce the mortality during this critical period (from about 30% to about 20%) mostly by preventing or providing immediate treatment for major ventricular dysrhythmias.

Lidocaine is widely used by intravenous infusion to prevent arrhythmias even though it is the one drug of those available that has not been shown to be superior to a placebo infusion in reducing the incidence of tachyarrhythmias or the amount of serious ventricular ectopic activity. It suppresses unifocal premature ventricular contractions but not those held to be premonitory of ventricular tachycardia—ie, those that are closely coupled or alternating from 2 foci.

Quinidine given orally is superior to a placebo. Comparisons between drugs are not available, but procainamide by mouth appears to be the most effective drug if plasma levels are measured and dosage is controlled on that basis.

The depression of cardiac contractility caused by the beta-adrenergic blockers outweighs the benefits of its antiarrhythmia effects.

•   •   •

General References

Blomgren, S.E., & others: Antinuclear antibody induced by procainamide. New England J Med 281:64–66, 1969.

Bloomfield, S.S., & others: Quinidine for prophylaxis of arrhythmias in acute myocardial infarction. New England J Med 285:979–986, 1971.

Cheng, T.O.: Atrial flutter during quinidine therapy of atrial fibrillation. Am Heart J 52:273–289, 1956.

Chopra, M.P., & others: Lignocaine therapy for ventricular ectopic activity after acute myocardial infarction: A double-blind trial. Brit MJ 3:668–670, 1971.

Conn, H.L., & R.L. Luchi: Some cellular and metabolic considerations relating to the action of quinidine as a prototype antiarrhythmic agent. Am J Med 37:685–699, 1964.

Gibson, D., & E. Sowton: Use of beta-adrenergic receptor blocking drugs in dysrhythmias. Progr Cardiovas Dis 12:16–39, 1969.

Hoffman, B.F., & P.F. Cranefield: The physiological basis of cardiac arrhythmias. Am J Med 37:670–684, 1964.

Koch-Weser, J., & others: Antiarrhythmic prophylaxis with procainamide in acute myocardial infarction. New England J Med 281:1253–1260, 1969.

Koch-Weser, J., & S.W. Klein: Procainamide dosage schedules, plasma concentrations, and clinical effects. JAMA 215:1454–1460, 1971.

Paine, R.: Procainamide hydrochloride and lupus erythematosus. JAMA 194:23–26, 1965.

Prinzmetal, M., & others: The nature of spontaneous auricular fibrillation in man. JAMA 157:1175–1182, 1955.

Sokolow, M., & D.B. Perloff: The clinical pharmacology and use of quinidine in heart disease. Progr Cardiovas Dis 3:316–330, 1961.

Stannard, M., Sloman, G., & L. Sangster: Hemodynamic effects of lignocaine in acute myocardial infarction. Brit MJ 2:468–472, 1968.

Unger, A.H., & H.J. Sklaroff: Fatalities following intravenous use of sodium diphenylhydantoin for cardiac arrhythmias: Report of two cases. JAMA 200:335–338, 1967.

Way, W.L., Katzung, B.G., & C.P. Larson, Jr.: Recurarization with quinidine. JAMA 200:153–154, 1967.

Vaughan-Williams, E.M.: The mode of action of antifibrillary drugs. Pages 119–132 in: *Pharmacology of Cardiac Function*. O. Krayer (editor). [Proceedings of the 2nd International Pharmacological Meeting, Vol 5.] Pergamon, 1964.

17 ...

Diuretics

Congestive heart failure was mentioned in Chapter 15 as a disease process characterized by sodium retention resulting in expanded extracellular fluid volume or edema. The same process of increased renal tubular reabsorption of sodium may accompany cirrhosis of the liver, renal disease, toxemia of pregnancy, the side-effects of drugs, and other states of fluid retention. In all of these situations, treatment directed at the cause is desirable, but treatment of the sodium retention must often also include inhibiting renal tubular function to decrease reabsorption of sodium. The usefulness of diuretics in the treatment of essential hypertension (Chapter 12) is also correlated with their ability to increase the excretion of sodium. It is, therefore, sodium diuresis (natriuresis) rather than merely an increase in urine volume that is the important therapeutic effect of most of the drugs discussed in this chapter.

The sequence in which the diuretics are discussed in this chapter is not, as may first appear, based simply on the chronologic order of their introduction. The thiazide diuretics, the most widely used group, combine properties of 2 obsolescent groups and are more easily discussed following consideration of the 2 groups of older diuretics.

The following types of compounds and effects are discussed in this chapter:

(1) Mercurial diuretics: The organic mercurials act strongly on the proximal tubule to produce sodium diuresis with only a minor depletion of potassium. However, the mercurial diuretics can be used only by injection.

(2) Carbonic anhydrase inhibitors: Inhibition of carbonic anhydrase by certain sulfonamides interferes with the ion exchange mechanisms of the distal tubule responsible for acidification of the urine. The resulting sodium diuresis is transient and accompanied by a disproportionate loss of potassium.

(3) Thiazide diuretics: The most widely used class of diuretics are orally active sulfonamides that have an action similar to that of the mercurials on the proximal tubules but retain some of the properties of the carbonic anhydrase inhibitors from which they were derived.

(4) Two very potent diuretics: Furosemide and ethacrynic acid have a greater effect on the loop of Henle than the thiazides.

(5) Miscellaneous potassium-sparing diuretics: The thiazide diuretics cause increased excretion of potassium as well as of sodium and may cause potassium depletion as a toxic effect. Diuretics that do not cause a loss of potassium or may even cause potassium retention are available. These are the aldosterone antagonists and some miscellaneous compounds that act directly on the renal tubules.

(6) Acidifying salts such as ammonium chloride are weak diuretics.

(7) Osmotic diuretics are not used to increase sodium loss but to maintain a high volume of urine or to withdraw water from overhydrated cells.

MERCURIAL DIURETICS

The diuretic effect of inorganic mercury in the form of calomel (mercurous chloride) was noted 4 centuries ago, but the effective use of mercury as a diuretic was an outgrowth of observations made in 1919 during the treatment of syphilis with an organic mercurial drug. The use of the mercurials increased only slowly thereafter as understanding of the role of sodium in the production of edema grew. Until the introduction (in 1957) of the orally active thiazides, the injected mercurials were widely used in the treatment of congestive heart failure and some other forms of edema.

Chemistry

Mercuric ion (Hg^{++}) is essential for the action of these diuretics, but it must be provided in the form of a weakly dissociated organic compound.

The general chemical structure of a mercurial diuretic can be represented as follows:

$$R_1-CH_2-CH-CH_2-Hg^+$$
$$\underset{CH_3}{\overset{O}{|}}$$

R_1 represents a variety of organic substituents. The dissociation of mercuric ion from such a compound is favored in an acid medium and inhibited in an alkaline medium, a possible explanation for the decrease in activity of this class of drugs in the presence of systemic alkalosis.

The organic mercurials, in contrast to inorganic mercuric salts, react less with proteins at the site of injection and are less strongly bound to plasma proteins after absorption. They are therefore distributed to tissue cells, especially in the renal cortex, in higher concentrations.

The mercurials are dispensed as solutions containing equimolar amounts of theophylline, a xanthine base, or, in the case of mercaptomerin (Thiomerin), of thioglycollate (mercaptoacetate). The structure is, therefore, better shown by including the additional substituent:

$$R_1-CH_2-CH(O-CH_3)-CH_2-Hg-R_2$$

Addition of the theophylline reduces systemic and local toxicity and increases the rate of absorption.

Absorption, Route of Administration, & Excretion

The major limitation of the mercurial diuretics is their poor absorption after oral administration and the almost invariable gastrointestinal irritation that they cause. They are, therefore, given by intramuscular injection, following which their action begins in about 2 hours, becomes maximal in 5–6 hours, and is dissipated in less than 24 hours. Intravenous administration offers no advantage and adds the risk of ventricular fibrillation.

The mercurial diuretics are concentrated in the renal cortex, where there is a high concentration of sulfhydryl groups with which they react. The mercury is excreted mostly by the renal tubules. Smaller amounts are excreted into the colon and mouth. Excretion is rapid and is nearly complete in 24 hours.

Pharmacologic Effects

A. Site and Mechanism of Action: The mercurials act to inhibit many enzymes, and the effect is not discretely localized. However, the primary effect is on the proximal convoluted tubule to reduce sodium reabsorption. Other functions known to be localized in the proximal segment are depressed by the mercurials (glucose reabsorption, PAH secretion), and stop-flow analysis is confirmatory. Early studies had eliminated the possibility of an extrarenal action in mobilizing fluid.

B. Pattern of Electrolyte Loss: To the extent that active sodium reabsorption is reduced in the proximal tubule, the passive reabsorption of chloride and water is similarly decreased. The volume of isotonic fluid and, therefore, the total amount of sodium delivered to the distal tubule is increased. At the cation exchange site of the distal tubule, an increased amount of sodium is reabsorbed and an increased number of potassium and hydrogen ions are excreted. Since the mercurials act on the 70–80% of the filtered sodium ion and water that is ordinarily reabsorbed at the proximal tubule, the minor increase in sodium exchange at the distal tubule does not weaken the therapeutic effect of the mercurials. The increased exchange does explain the increase in potassium excretion that occurs. Furthermore, the increased excretion of cations other than sodium (H^+, K^+) explains the excess of chloride loss over sodium loss and the production of hypochloremic alkalosis by the continued use of mercurial diuretics.

C. Potentiation of Effect: In the presence of hypochloremic alkalosis, the effect of the mercurials is reduced. Activity after repeated doses is restored, and even the effect of initial doses is increased, by pretreatment with ammonium chloride. The effect is not due entirely to a change in intracellular pH and increased dissociation of the mercurial since it is not duplicated by the acidosis that follows breathing 10% CO_2.

Clinical Uses

The mercurials are now used in only an occasional hospitalized patient with edema resistant to other drugs or when the intense action is desirable. They should not be used in the presence of renal failure.

Adverse Reactions

During the period of intensive use of the mercurials, toxic reactions were exceedingly rare. A few deaths from ventricular fibrillation followed intravenous injections, and a rare case of renal tubular necrosis was reported.

Sodium depletion—ie, low plasma concentrations of sodium in the face of continuing edema—occurred following intensive use, especially with the patient taking a restricted diet. Potassium depletion was rarely symptomatic.

Dosages & Preparations Available

The following preparations are available as injectable solutions providing approximately 80 mg of mercury in each 2 ml. The dosage is 1–2 ml (usually 2 ml) IM. Mercaptomerin and mercuhydrin can be given subcutaneously.

Mercaptomerin (Thiomerin): 1, 2, 10, and 30 ml;
  and dry powder, 1.4 and 4.2 gm/vial
Meralluride (Mercuhydrin): 1, 2, and 10 ml
Mersalyl (Salyrgan): 1, 2, 10, and 30 ml

CARBONIC ANHYDRASE INHIBITORS

Inhibitors of carbonic anhydrase are no longer used clinically as diuretics. However, they are used in the treatment of one form of glaucoma and in the present context permit the description of the effect of carbonic anhydrase inhibition in uncomplicated form in anticipation of the discussion of the thiazide diuretics.

Chemistry

Some of the earlier, unsubstituted bacteriostatic sulfonamides caused, paradoxically, a systemic acidosis and the production of a large volume of alkaline urine. This action was shown to be due to inhibition of carbonic anhydrase activity and a consequent decrease in the ability to acidify the urine. More potent inhibitors have since been synthesized, and all, like the thiazide diuretics, bear a free sulfonamide (sulfamyl) group. The structure of 2 representative carbonic anhydrase inhibitors is shown in Fig 17–1.

Pharmacologic Actions

　　A. Mechanism of Diuretic Action: The hydration of carbon dioxide takes place very slowly unless accelerated by the enzyme carbonic anhydrase. Carbonic anhydrase is a metalloprotein, and its inhibitors combine with the zinc in the molecule of enzyme to cause a noncompetitive inhibition. The rate of production within cells of hydrogen and bicarbonate ion is greatly reduced and the amount available for active transport into secretions decreased.

$$CO_2 + H_2O \rightleftharpoons H_2CO_3$$
$$\rightleftharpoons H^+ + HCO_3^-$$

　　In the kidney, the consequences of carbonic anhydrase inhibition are apparent at the ion exchange site of the distal tubule. The reactions shown in Fig 17–2 accompany the following changes in the composition of the urine:

　　1. Reduced reabsorption of sodium—Most of the sodium in the distal tubular urine is reabsorbed by an active process, and, during this reabsorption, an equivalent amount of easily diffusible anion, chloride, is also reabsorbed. This process is not altered by inhibition of carbonic anhydrase. Sodium that accompanies a less easily diffusible anion, bicarbonate, is reabsorbed only by exchange for hydrogen or potassium ions secreted into the lumen of the tubule by the renal cells. If the amount of available hydrogen ion is reduced, there will

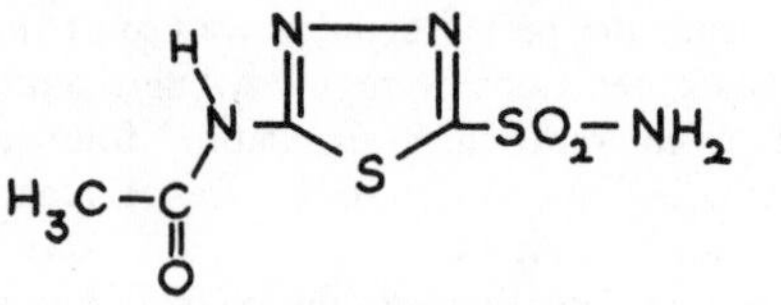

Acetazolamide
(Diamox)

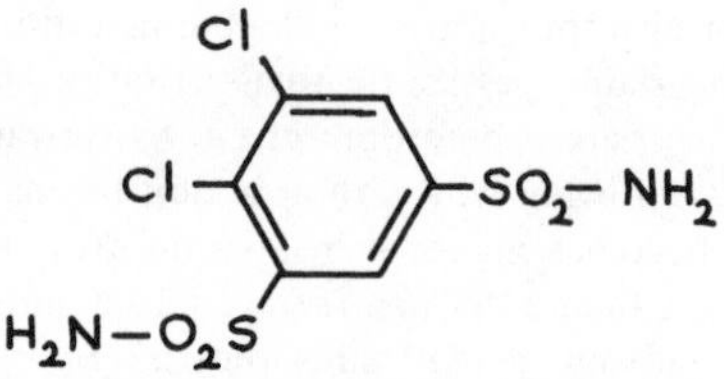

Dichlorphenamide
(Daranide)

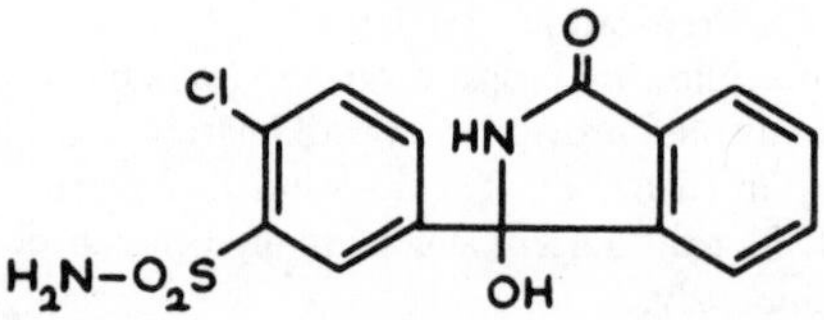

Chlorthalidone
(Hygroton)

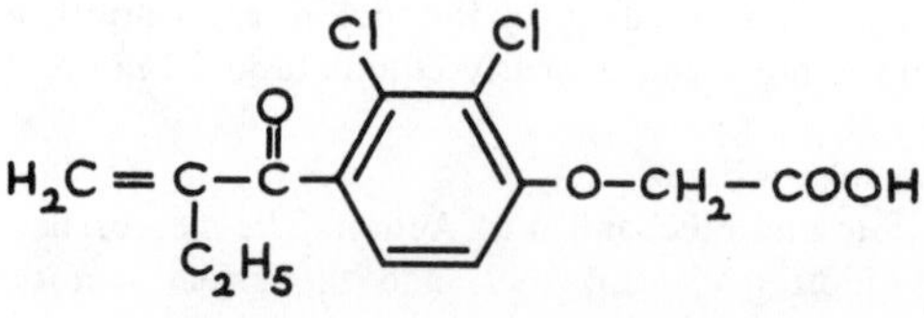

Ethacrynic acid
(Edecrin)

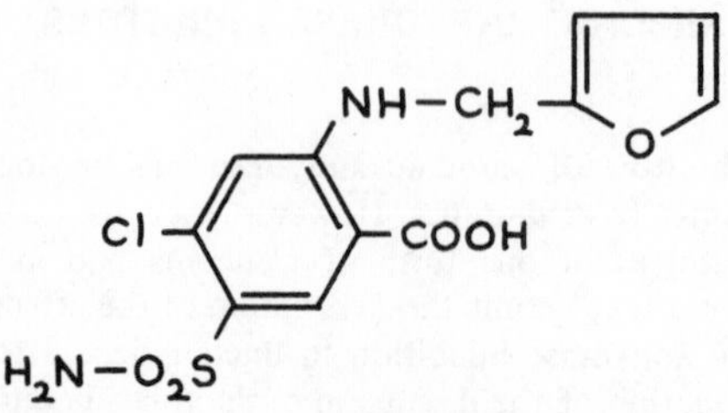

Furosemide
(Lasix)

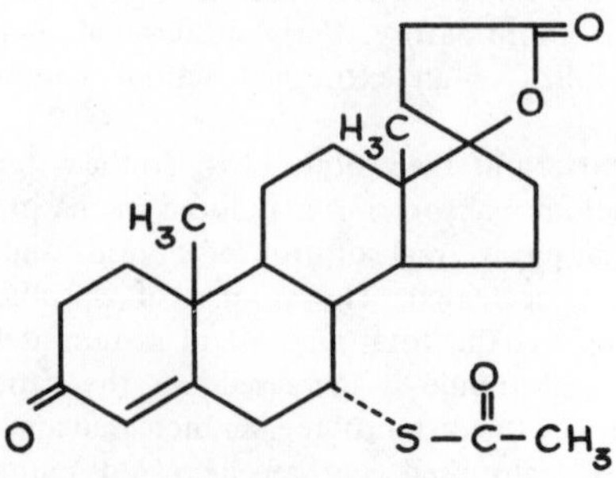

Spironolactone
(Aldactone)

FIG 17–1. Chemical structures of 2 carbonic anhydrase inhibitors and of several diuretics discussed in the text.

be less reabsorption of this small fraction of the total sodium reabsorbed by the kidney.

2. Bicarbonate excretion increased—Ordinarily, the secreted hydrogen ion combines with bicarbonate ion provided by the glomerular filtrate, and the carbonic acid thus formed is mostly reabsorbed as CO_2. In effect, then, the bicarbonate ion is normally reabsorbed almost completely. If carbonic anhydrase is inhibited and hydrogen ion is lacking, bicarbonate will remain in its poorly diffusible form and will be excreted in unusually large amounts. The urine will thereupon become alkaline. Plasma bicarbonate will fall, and, as plasma chloride is elevated, a mild systemic acidosis will appear.

3. Increased potassium excretion—Potassium competes with hydrogen ion for the limited capacity of the same transport system. If the amount of H^+ available is reduced, a larger amount of K^+ will be exchanged for Na^+. Carbonic anhydrase inhibitors, therefore, cause a loss of potassium.

4. Ammonia retained—The availability of hydrogen ion normally allows the conversion of ammonia to ammonium ion, which remains in tubular and bladder urine. After carbonic anhydrase inhibition, uncharged ammonia diffuses back into the renal cells and into the blood.

B. Limitation of Usefulness as Diuretics: The carbonic anhydrase inhibitors cannot cause a great sodium diuresis because the amount of bicarbonate and, therefore, the amount of sodium reabsorption tied to the excretion of that poorly diffusible ion is small.

More important, even the small sodium diuresis caused by carbonic anhydrase inhibition lasts for only a day or two. As the bicarbonate load presented to the renal tubules decreases—ie, as systemic acidosis develops—sodium excretion is again restored to normal.

Even though the natriuretic effect is transient, inhibition of carbonic anhydrase can be maintained for long periods and effects other than sodium diuresis will persist.

C. Other Consequences of Carbonic Anhydrase Inhibition: Many secretory processes other than those in the kidney involve the active transport of H^+ or HCO_3^-. However, carbonic anhydrase inhibition is clinically important only in the case of the aqueous humor.

1. Aqueous humor—The aqueous contains a high concentration of bicarbonate ion, and inhibition of carbonic anhydrase decreases the rate of formation of aqueous, reducing intraocular pressure.

2. Carbon dioxide transport—It is possible that carbonic anhydrase inhibition leads to a transient elevation of tissue pCO_2, but the CO_2 transport mechanisms are generally resistant.

3. CNS—Carbonic anhydrase inhibition decreases the rate of spinal fluid formation. However, the CNS effects of the inhibitors—eg, somnolence and an anticonvulsant action—cannot be explained on this basis.

Absorption, Metabolism, & Excretion

All of the carbonic anhydrase inhibitors are well absorbed after oral administration. Effects on the pH

TABLE 17–1. Carbonic anhydrase inhibitors used in treatment of glaucoma: Dosages and preparations available.

	Usual Oral Dose (1–4 Times Daily)	Preparations Available
Acetazolamide (Diamox)	250 mg	Tablets, 125 and 250 mg
Dichlorphenamide (Daranide)	50 mg	Tablets, 50 mg
Ethoxzolamide (Cardrase)	62.5–125 mg	Tablets, 62.5 and 125 mg
Methazolamide (Neptazane)	50 mg	Tablets, 50 mg

of the urine are apparent within 30 minutes, are maximal in 2 hours, and persist for 12 hours after a single dose. Excretion, as for other organic acids, is by tubular secretion.

Clinical Uses

These drugs are no longer used as diuretics. They are used as a supplement to other drugs or surgery in the treatment of glaucoma.

Adverse Reactions

Paresthesias and drowsiness are common. The low urinary citrate that accompanies the alkaline urine can lead to the precipitation of calcium phosphate crystals or stones.

Dosages & Preparations Available

See Table 17–1.

THIAZIDE DIURETICS

The thiazide diuretics emerged from efforts to synthesize more potent carbonic anhydrase inhibitors. Some disulfonamides (see dichlorphenamide in Fig 17–1) were highly active, but no more useful as diuretics until ring closure involving one of the sulfonamide groups was carried out. The resulting compounds retain a minor ability to inhibit carbonic anhydrase. Unexpectedly, however, they have the added effect of blocking sodium reabsorption very much as the mercurials do. They have the great advantage over the mercurials of being suitable for chronic oral administration.

Chemistry

The drugs shown in Table 17–2 are variously called thiazide, benzothiadiazide, or sulfonamide diuretics. The sulfamyl group is essential to their activity. The last compound in the table, for example, does not contain the thiadiazine ring, but is qualitatively similar

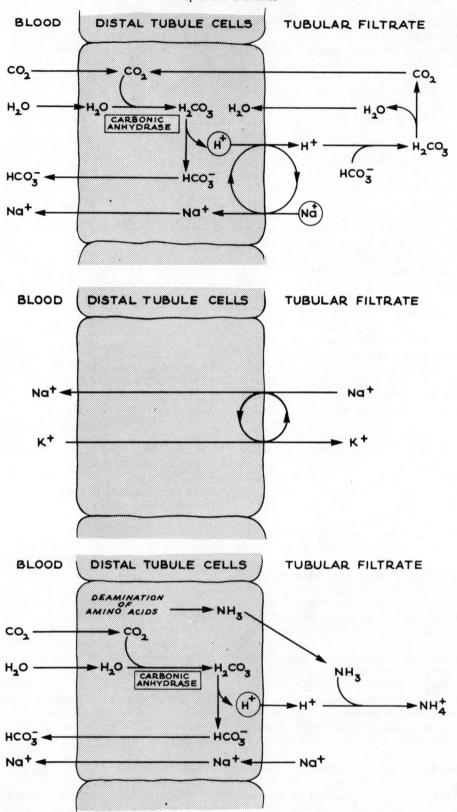

FIG 17–2. Summary of reactions occurring at the level of the distal renal tubule. See text for explanation.

to the others which are benzothiazides. Furosemide (Fig 17–1) is a sulfonamide that has a stronger action on the loop of Henle than the thiazides and is discussed separately at the end of this section.

Absorption, Metabolism, & Excretion

All of the thiazides are useful after oral administration, but there are some differences among them in their metabolism. Chlorothiazide (Diuril), the prototype of this group, is less lipid-soluble than the remaining thiazides; it is poorly absorbed and must be given in large doses. Chlorthalidone (Hygroton) is slowly absorbed and, therefore, has a longer apparent duration of action.

All of the thiazides are excreted to at least some extent by the same mechanism responsible for the secretion of uric acid and compete for some of the limited capacity of that system. The excretion of uric acid may therefore be reduced following thiazide administration.

At least some of those thiazides with a substituent on C3 undergo hydrolytic opening of the thiadiazine ring. The resulting disulfamyl metabolites are stronger carbonic anhydrase inhibitors than the parent drug.

Pharmacologic Actions

A. **Mechanisms of Action**: The mechanisms of the diuretic effect of the thiazides can be partially clarified by outlining the sites in the kidney at which the thiazides and other drugs can act:

1. **Proximal tubule**–About 70% of the water and sodium ion filtered at the glomerulus is reabsorbed at this site. The thiazides and mercurials both act on this general function. The active process by which sodium is transported from tubular fluid to interstitial fluid and then to blood is inhibited; the passive diffusion of the accompanying water and chloride is correspondingly reduced.

The exact functional site at which the thiazides act is different from that altered by the mercurial diuretics since even maximal effects of the 2 drugs are additive to each other–ie, 2 separate functions are saturated.

2. **Distal tubule**–The properties of the cation exchange mechanism located in the distal segment of the renal tubule are discussed in detail in relation to the carbonic anhydrase inhibitors.

Dosages of the thiazides large enough to produce a useful degree of sodium diuresis by an action on the proximal tubule also decrease carbonic anhydrase activity in the distal tubule. The potassium loss produced by the thiazides is greater than that produced by the pure carbonic anhydrase inhibitors–eg, acetazolamide–because the action on the proximal tubule results in the delivery of a greater amount of sodium to the ion exchange site for exchange with potassium.

TABLE 17–2. Chemical structures of thiazide (benzothiadiazide, sulfonamide) and similar diuretics.

	R_1	$\Delta 3 = 4$	R_2	R_3
Chlorothiazide (Diuril)	Cl–	Yes	–H	–H
Hydrochlorothiazide (Esidrix, Hydrodiuril, Oretic)	Cl–	No	–H	–H
Hydroflumethiazide (Saluron)	F_3C–	No	–H	–H
Methyclothiazide (Enduron)	Cl–	No	$–CH_2–Cl$	$–CH_3$
Trichlormethiazide (Metahydrin, Naqua)	Cl–	No	$–CH–Cl_2$	–H
Benzthiazide (Aquatag, Exna)	Cl–	Yes	$–CH_2–S–CH_2–$phenyl	–H
Bendroflumethiazide (Benuron, Naturetin)	F_3C–	No	$–CH_2–$phenyl	–H
Polythiazide (Renese)	Cl–	No	$–CH_2–S–CH_2–CF_3$	$–CH_3$
Cyclothiazide (Anhydron)	Cl–	No	$–CH_2$⬡	–H
Quinethazone* (Hydromox)	Cl–	No	$–C_2H_5$	–H

*A quinazolinium derivative–ie, at position 1 there is C=O rather than SO_2.

TABLE 17-3. Thiazides and other diuretics: Dosages and preparations available.

	Daily Oral Dose	Preparations Available
Bendroflumethiazide (Benuron, Naturetin)	2.5–10 mg	Tablets, 5 mg (Benuron)
		Tablets, 2.5 and 5 mg (Naturetin)
Benzthiazide (Aquatag, Exna)	25–100 mg	Tablets, 25 and 50 mg (Aquatag)
		Tablets, 50 mg (Exna)
Chlorothiazide (Diuril)	0.5–1 gm	Tablets, 250 and 500 mg
		Syrup, 250 mg/5 ml
		Injectable sodium salt (IV), 500 mg/vial
Chlorthalidone* (Hygroton)	50–100 mg	Tablets, 50 and 100 mg
Cyclothiazide (Anhydron)	1–2 mg	Tablets, 2 mg
Furosemide* (Lasix)	40–80 mg	Tablets, 40 mg
		Injectable (IV), 20 mg/2 ml ampule
Hydrochlorothiazide (Esidrix, Hydrodiuril, Oretic)	25–100 mg	Tablets, 25 and 50 mg
Hydroflumethiazide (Saluron)	25–100 mg	Tablets, 50 mg
Methyclothiazide (Enduron, Aquatensen)	2.5–10 mg	Tablets, 2.5 and 5 mg
Polythiazide (Renese)	1–4 mg	Tablets, 1, 2, and 4 mg
Quinethazone* (Hydromox)	50–100 mg	Tablets, 50 mg
Trichlormethiazide (Metahydrin, Naqua)	2–8 mg	Tablets, 2 and 4 mg

*Not a thiazide but a sulfonamide qualitatively similar to the thiazides.

Bicarbonate excretion is slightly increased, and the urine becomes alkaline. Systemically, however, the effect of potassium depletion in causing an alkalosis is prepotent over the tendency toward acidosis caused by bicarbonate loss—ie, administration of the thiazides causes a minor hypokalemic (extracellular) alkalosis.

3. Loop of Henle—Drugs that act on the distal tubule are weak diuretics and add little but adverse effects to the results of inhibition of sodium transport in the proximal tubule. To achieve a diuretic effect even more potent than that of the mercurials, a drug would have to act on the active transport of sodium across the wall of the ascending arm of the loop of Henle. At this site about three-quarters of the sodium remaining after passage through the proximal tubule is reabsorbed.

B. Effects: Several extremely powerful diuretics—eg, furosemide (Lasix) and ethacrynic acid (Edecrin)—clearly do act on the loop of Henle, and it is probable that the thiazides also have some action at that locus.

Sodium reabsorption by the loop of Henle maintains the hyperosmolality of the interstitial fluid in the deep or papillary portion of the medulla. If the osmotic gradient is destroyed by administration of a drug, the ability to finally dilute or concentrate the urine is lost. Such an effect is achieved at least briefly with ethacrynic acid.

The thiazides are able to reduce the volume of urine in patients with diabetes insipidus. For that reason, it has been suggested that the thiazides also act on the distal portion of the loop of Henle and reduce the ability of the tubule to form dilute urine.

Clinical Uses

The thiazides are not only the most widely used diuretics but are among the most widely used of all prescription drugs.

A. Essential Hypertension: (See Chapter 12.) A thiazide diuretic is usually the first drug used in the treatment of hypertension. By itself, it causes only a limited (10%) reduction in blood pressure and is suitable for the control of only the mildest cases. However, it potentiates the effect of other hypotensive agents and is almost always the first "layer" of treatment.

The mechanism of the hypotensive effect is not known. The arteriolar dilatation that occurs is not due to sodium or potassium depletion but, presumably, to some undefined ion shift at the wall of the vessel.

The hypotensive action has not been demonstrated for furosemide.

B. Fluid Retention States: The thiazides are very useful as part of the treatment of the edema of congestive heart failure. Nephrotic edema is also reduced, but less regularly, and other methods of treatment are available. Patients with edema secondary to cirrhosis react unpredictably and are especially endangered by potassium loss and ammonia retention. Sodium retention due to steroids—whether oral contraceptives, other estrogens, androgens, or endogenous steroids responsible for premenstrual edema—is easily treated with any of the sodium diuretics.

Whether the thiazides, when used during pregnancy, reduce the incidence of toxemic states or are useful in their treatment is controversial, and few data are available on which to base an informed opinion. There is no question but that they are useful if the cardiovascular disease existed before the pregnancy.

C. Diabetes Insipidus: The thiazide diuretics can be used to reduce the volume of urine elaborated by a patient with diabetes insipidus whether of the usual vasopressin-sensitive type or the nephrogenic type. The ability of a thiazide to decrease the ability of the kidney to produce a dilute urine argues for an action on the loop of Henle.

Adverse Reactions

A. Side-Effects: Weakness, fatigability, and paresthesias (as described for the carbonic anhydrase inhibitors) occur. Mild gastrointestinal symptoms—eg, nausea, cramps, and epigastric discomfort—are also common.

B. Dose-Related Toxicity:

1. Potassium depletion—The potassium loss described above is most intense early in treatment when diuresis is most profound and the diet is most likely to be restricted. Serum potassium levels are poor indices of changes in total exchangeable potassium in the body but will usually reflect the decrease in total body potassium if the patient is depleted sufficiently to experience symptoms such as anorexia, nausea, weakness, and drowsiness.

Supplementary potassium chloride should be given if symptoms of depletion appear or when a diuretic response and dietary restriction are present. Later, the dietary sources of potassium—eg, fruit, fruit juice, and vegetables—will usually be adequate. Supplementary potassium is not without its own dangers; in one epidemiologic study of therapeutic misadventures, it was the most common cause of lethal reactions.

2. Impaired carbohydrate tolerance—Glucose tolerance is impaired by the thiazides even though certain other sulfonamides are antidiabetic agents. This adverse reaction is unimportant in patients with normal carbohydrate tolerance; but the hyperglycemia of overt diabetes may be intensified, and some patients with abnormal glucose tolerance tests or a family history of diabetes may develop glycosuria when given a thiazide. The effect is dose-related, and continued treatment with smaller doses is often possible. However, a diuretic that does not alter glucose tolerance (eg, triamterene; see below) can be substituted. This toxic effect is rapidly reversible upon discontinuance of the thiazide.

3. Increased blood levels of uric acid—The thiazides, like uric acid, are weak acids secreted by the cells of the proximal tubules and can interfere with the excretion of uric acid. An elevation of plasma uric acid may occur which is unimportant in normal subjects but may precipitate or intensify gout in susceptible patients.

The usual uricosuric agents (see Chapter 40) act at a more distal level of the nephron to block reabsorption—ie, increase urinary excretion—of uric acid. They are still effective during the administration of thiazides.

4. Other toxic effects—The decreased renal excretion of ammonia may be dangerous in the presence of impaired liver function.

One test of thyroid function—protein-bound iodine—will often be decreased to less than normal levels, but ^{131}I uptake is uninfluenced. The size of the iodine pool is probably decreased by the iodide diuresis that accompanies chloride loss.

Enteric-coated tablets that contained both a thiazide and supplemental potassium chloride caused toxic reactions in the past but are no longer available. These preparations released the potassium chloride in the jejunum, and the high local concentration of potassium caused ulceration and subsequent scarring and stenosis in the upper small intestine.

C. Allergic Reactions: Skin rashes are seen occasionally. Serious allergic reactions must be extremely rare considering the wide use of the thiazides. Thrombocytopenic purpura has been reported several times.

Contraindications & Cautions

The thiazide diuretics should be used with caution in the following situations:

(1) Renal insufficiency may be intensified by a contraction of plasma volume.

(2) The arrhythmias of digitalis toxicity are intensified by potassium depletion. Administration of a thiazide may precipitate toxicity in a patient previously stabilized on digitalis.

(3) The reasons have already been given for cautious administration in the presence of diabetes, gout, cirrhosis, and during the administration of corticosteroids or other potassium-losing states.

Dosages & Preparations Available

The preparations listed in Table 17–3 (with the exception of furosemide) differ only in their absolute potency. Chlorthalidone is slowly absorbed, and its action is, therefore, more prolonged.

TWO VERY POTENT DIURETICS

Two diuretics act to block sodium transport in the ascending arm of the loop of Henle as well as in more proximal sites. Consequently, a greater fraction of filtered sodium can escape reabsorption.

1. FUROSEMIDE
(Lasix)

This agent is a sulfonamide and retains some of the properties of the thiazides—eg, the diabetogenic effect—but it is not effective in the treatment of hypertension. However, its potency approaches that of ethacrynic acid. The onset of diuresis after the administration of furosemide is rapid, but, in contrast to the other sulfonamide diuretics, its effect persists for only about 4 hours.

See Table 17–3 for dosage and preparations available. The structure of furosemide is shown in Fig 17–1.

2. ETHACRYNIC ACID
(Edecrin)

Ethacrynic acid is a synthetic drug chemically unrelated to any of the other diuretics so far discussed and remarkable for its potency.

Ethacrynic acid acts to inhibit the active transport of sodium in the proximal tubule and throughout the loop of Henle. For a brief period after its administration, 40–50% of the sodium and water filtered at the glomerulus escapes reabsorption. In hydropenic subjects, the ability to concentrate tubular urine is lost when ethacrynic acid is given; and in hydrated patients the urine cannot be as well diluted during its passage through the loop of Henle—ie, the loop loses its ability to dilute or concentrate the urine and its ability to maintain the osmotic gradient in the medulla.

Potassium and hydrogen ion excretion are also increased, presumably because of the increased amount of sodium reaching the distal tubule. Supplementary potassium chloride must be given.

Ethacrynic acid has been used in patients with refractory edema of various causes. There is no doubt about its potency.

However, its toxicity, especially with chronic use, is also greater than that of the thiazides. Most of the toxic reactions are a consequence of its potency—eg, dehydration, hypotension, hypokalemia, alkalosis, deafness—since essential as well as excess sodium may be lost. As would be predicted from its structure (Fig 17–1), ethacrynic acid may cause elevated levels of plasma uric acid. Alterations in glucose tolerance have also been reported. Gastrointestinal bleeding has occurred after its use. The incidence of hepatic damage and agranulocytosis needs to be defined.

The onset of action of ethacrynic acid is rapid. Maximum activity is reached in about 2 hours, and diuresis persists for 6–8 hours.

Ethacrynic acid (Edecrin) is supplied as 25 and 50 mg tablets and as vials containing 50 mg of the sodium salt for intravenous use. The initial dose is 50 mg every 2–3 days. The maximum daily dose is 150–200 mg.

POTASSIUM-SPARING DIURETICS

1. SPIRONOLACTONE
(An Aldosterone Antagonist)

Spironolactone (Aldactone) is a synthetic steroid resembling aldosterone. Its structure is shown in Fig 17–1.

Aldosterone acts on the distal tubule to enhance the sodium-potassium exchange mechanism—ie, to cause sodium retention and potassium loss. An aldosterone antagonist causes sodium diuresis and potassium retention. The intensity of action of such an antagonist depends upon the amount of aldosterone acting on the kidney—ie, it would not show any diuretic action in an adrenalectomized animal but would be unusually active in those cases in which edema is accompanied by hyperaldosteronism.

Spironolactone is a weak diuretic and is usually used in combination with a thiazide or other diuretic. Its effect develops very slowly, requiring 2–3 days of administration for a maximal effect.

Spironolactone is occasionally used in the treatment of patients with cirrhosis and edema when other diuretics are toxic or ineffective.

It is relatively nontoxic but may cause gynecomastia and, when given by itself, hyperkalemia. When given in combination with a thiazide, it does not usually completely antagonize the potassium loss caused by that drug.

Spironolactone (Aldactone) is supplied in 25 mg tablets. The dosage is 25–50 mg 3–4 times daily.

2. TRIAMTERENE
(Dyrenium)

Triamterene is a pteridine derivative that has actions (sodium diuresis, potassium retention) similar to those of the aldosterone antagonist. It acts, however, directly on the distal tubule, and its action persists after adrenalectomy. Like spironolactone, it is usually used in combination with a thiazide.

Triamterene produces an elevation in blood urea levels with chronic administration. Other side-effects are minor, and the toxic reactions described for the thiazides do not occur when it is administered as such. It is, however, usually used as a proprietary mixture with a thiazide, in which case the effects of the thiazide predominate and triamterene contributes only a minor reduction in potassium loss.

Triamterene (Dyrenium) is supplied as 100 mg capsules. Initial dosage may be 100 mg twice daily, but when a response occurs the dosage should be decreased to 100 mg daily or every other day.

Triamterene
(Dyrenium)
(2,4,7-triamino-6-phenylpteridine)

ACIDIFYING SALTS

Acidifying salts are no longer used as diuretics, but they may still be encountered when used to potentiate the mercurial diuretics or for uses unrelated to renal function.

Ammonium chloride is the common acid salt. Following absorption, the ammonium ion is converted to urea by the liver, leading to an excess of chloride which is retained in the plasma at the expense of bicarbonate. Even in a normal subject, the acidosis that follows the administration of 10–15 gm of ammonium chloride may cause increased ventilation at rest and exertional dyspnea. In a patient with congestive heart failure, the increased respiratory activity may not only be uncomfortable but may also place an additional demand on his limited cardiac reserve.

On the first day of administration, the excess chloride is excreted with an equivalent amount of sodium. The sodium diuresis decreases after the first day, and compensation is complete in less than 5 days if administration of ammonium chloride is continuous. Of the several mechanisms restricting sodium loss, the most important is the increased production of ammonia by renal tubular cells; the excess chloride is thus excreted as ammonium chloride, and only a negligible osmotic diuretic action persists.

Ammonium chloride may be used to increase or restore sensitivity to mercurial diuretics. In this context it may be given with potassium chloride.

Ammonium chloride is supplied as 0.5 gm enteric-coated tablets. The minimal dose is 1–1.5 gm 4 times daily.

Ammonium chloride is also an expectorant—ie, it is able to increase the volume and decrease the viscosity of the secretions of the respiratory tract secondary to its local gastric irritant effect. For this purpose it obviously must not be coated but used as a syrup, usually containing 0.3 gm/5 ml. Ammonium chloride as an expectorant is inferior to the iodides.

OSMOTIC DIURETICS

Osmotic diuretics are used to induce water diuresis rather than natriuresis, and their applications are totally different from those of the sodium diuretics so far discussed.

Two concepts or uses included in the term osmotic diuretic are discussed below.

Maintenance of High Urine Volume

If a drug that is not metabolized—eg, mannitol—appears in the glomerular filtrate but is not reabsorbed by the renal tubules, it will hold in the lumen of the tubule enough water to maintain it in an isosmotic solution. Since mannitol and other osmotic diuretics are not reabsorbed in the proximal tubule, a greatly increased volume of isotonic tubular fluid reaches the loop of Henle. The sodium transporting capacity of the ascending loop is limited, and sodium cannot be reabsorbed rapidly enough to maintain the hyperosmolality of the medullary interstitium—ie, some isotonic fluid diffuses out of the tubule and weakens the countercurrent mechanism by reducing the osmotic gradient along the pyramids. Because of this lesser gradient, less water leaves the collecting ducts and urine volume is increased.

This action is used to maintain a high urine volume but not to extract abnormal amounts of fluid from the body. Thus, the osmotic diuretics can be used to prevent anuria following a hemolytic reaction, extensive surgery, or trauma and hemorrhage; and to maintain a very high urine volume during the treatment of intoxication by barbiturates, salicylates, or other agents excreted in the urine.

In oliguric patients, a test dose of 12.5 gm of mannitol is administered intravenously over a period of 3–5 minutes. Unless urine output increases during the next 3 hours to 40–60 ml/hour, the condition is probably unresponsive to mannitol. If urine volume does increase, mannitol is given by intravenous infusion to produce a urine flow of about 100 ml/hour. If mannitol is used prophylactically or to promote the excretion of a poison, an initial intravenous loading dose of 25 gm can be given followed by infusion to maintain the desired urine output.

Dehydrating Action

If a substance that does not enter the cells or does not enter a particular anatomic area such as the brain or anterior chamber of the eye is given as a very strong solution, water will leave the cells or anatomic area to dilute the drug to isotonicity pending its excretion. This "dehydrating" action is used in 2 situations:

A. To Reduce Intracranial Pressure: Increased intracranial pressure (eg, in brain tumor, head injury, brain swelling) may be reduced for 3–10 hours by intravenous administration of urea. Give urea as 30% solution (in 10% invert sugar) in a dosage of about 1 gm/kg at a rate of about 60 drops/minute. Poor renal function and active intracranial bleeding are contraindications.

B. To Reduce Intraocular Pressure: Three different agents (urea, mannitol, and glycerol) have been used to lower intraocular pressure preoperatively in angle-closure glaucoma. Urea and mannitol are administered intravenously. Glycerol may be given orally. The dosage of all 3 of these osmotic drugs is 1.5 gm/kg.

•　•　•

General References

General

Cafruny, E.J.: Renal pharmacology. Ann Rev Pharmacol 8:131–150, 1968.

Earley, L.E.: Current concepts: Diuretics. New England J Med 276:966–968, 1023–1025, 1967.

Milne, M.D.: Diuretics and electrolyte balance. Chap 7, pp 214–260, in: *Recent Advances in Pharmacology.* Robson, J.M., & R.S. Stacey. Churchill, 1962.

Mercurials

Kessler, R.H.: The clinical pharmacology of the mercurial diuretic compounds. Clin Pharmacol Therap 1:723–734, 1960.

Levitt, M.F., & M.H. Goldstein: Mercurial diuretics. Bull New York Acad Med 38:249–263, 1962.

Thiazide Derivatives

Boley, S.J., & others: Potassium-induced lesions of the small bowel. JAMA 193:997–1006, 1965.

Kessler, R.H.: Clinical pharmacology of chlorothiazide compounds. Clin Pharmacol Therap 3:109–118, 1962.

Moser, R.H.: Bibliographies on diseases of medical progress: Modern oral diuretics. Clin Pharmacol Therap 8:755–765, 1967.

Others

Flanigan, W.J., & G.L. Ackerman: Site of action of ethacrynic acid. Arch Int Med 118:117–122, 1966.

Galin, M.A., Davidson, R., & N. Shachter: Ophthalmological use of osmotic therapy. Am J Ophth 62:629–634, 1966.

Gantt, C.L., Ecklund, R.E., & J.M. Dyniewicz: Significance of aldosterone antagonism in the treatment of edema and ascites. Am J Med 33:490–500, 1962.

Healy, J.J., & others: Body composition changes in hypertensive subjects on long-term oral diuretic therapy (furosemide in hypertension). Brit MJ 1:716–719, 1970.

Hutcheon, D.E., Mehta, D., & A. Romano: Diuretic action of furosemide. Arch Int Med 115:542–546, 1965.

Maren, T.H.: Carbonic anhydrase: Chemistry, physiology, and inhibition. Physiol Rev 47:595–781, 1967.

Rosomoff, H.L.: Adjuncts to neurosurgical anesthesia. Brit J Anaesth 37:246–261, 1965.

Russell, R.P., Lindeman, R.D., & L.F. Prescott: Metabolic and hypotensive effects of ethacrynic acid: Comparative study with hydrochlorothiazide. JAMA 205:11–15, 1968.

Stason, W.B., & others: Furosemide: A clinical evaluation of its diuretic action. Circulation 34:910–920, 1966.

18 . . .

Anticoagulants & Vitamin K

The clotting of blood and the action of drugs on the clotting process are best understood as problems in enzyme chemistry. This chapter is included in the section on cardiovascular agents because the common and important uses of the drugs to be considered—to prevent the formation or extension of intravascular clots—are related to cardiovascular disease.

Two classes of anticoagulant drugs are discussed: heparin, which acts directly on the clotting mechanism; and the indirectly acting anticoagulants, which act on the liver to inhibit the synthesis of prothrombin by acting as analogues of vitamin K.

INHIBITORS OF PROTHROMBIN SYNTHESIS

Source & Chemistry

The first inhibitor of prothrombin synthesis, bishydroxycoumarin, was originally isolated from fermented clover that was causing hemorrhagic disease in cattle. Drugs of this class are now synthetically prepared and inexpensive compared with a natural product such as heparin. They can be grouped into 2 classes: the coumarin derivatives, and the appreciably more toxic indandiones (Table 18–1 and Fig 18–1).

Warfarin sodium and dicumarol (bishydroxycoumarin), examples of the first class, are the 2 most commonly used prothrombin depressants. The indandiones are exemplified in Fig 18–1 by phenindione. Warfarin is the only agent that is soluble in water and available for injection. All drugs of this class are, however, well absorbed after oral administration. Other available derivatives are listed in Table 18–1.

The structure of a vitamin K is shown in Fig 18–1 to suggest the competitive relation between vitamin K and these inhibitors. Salicylates are also weak inhibitors of the liver synthesis of clotting factors and may add to the anticoagulant effect of more potent drugs.

Absorption & Metabolism

Unlike heparin, the prothrombin depressants are active after oral administration.

Following administration of these drugs, there is a latent period; when the drug is discontinued, there is a period of many days before prothrombin concentra-

tion returns to normal. The period that elapses until activity is maximal and the period necessary for recovery vary somewhat with the different drugs. However, the latent period is due in part to the need to metabolize prothrombin already present, and the long duration of action reflects the time needed for resynthesis of prothrombin rather than the persistence in the body of the inhibitors of synthesis.

The variation of the maintenance dose between patients is due in part to variations in the rate of biotransformation.

Pharmacologic Actions

A. **Clotting Mechanism:** In this and subsequent sections it may be helpful to refer to Fig 18–2, a tentative scheme of the clotting mechanism that includes the presently characterized factors but omits many details of the sequence of events. Most of the coagulation factors exist in an inactive or precursor form so that blood remains fluid until its clotting is initiated by contact with injured tissue or lysed platelets or by contact with a wettable surface such as glass. Phase 1 of clotting results in the formation of active thromboplastin. Three of the factors involved—VII (proconvertin), IX (PTC), and X (Stuart-Prower factor)—are synthesized in the liver, and the synthesis is dependent upon adequate vitamin K. Phase 2 is the conversion of prothrombin to thrombin. Prothrombin is a protein similarly synthesized. Phase 3 is the proteolytic action of thrombin on fibrinogen to form a fibrin unit that can then further polymerize to form the blood clot.

B. **Inhibition of Prothrombin Synthesis:** Vitamin K is necessary for the synthesis in the liver not only of prothrombin (factor II) itself but also of proconvertin (VII), PTC (IX), and Stuart-Prower (X) factor. Vitamin K is not incorporated into any of these proteins, but their synthesis is deficient in the absence of vitamin K and is prevented by the administration of any of the coumarin drugs. The relationship between vitamin K and the coumarins is competitive, larger doses of one overcoming the effect of the other. It is convenient and not greatly misleading to refer to these antagonists as if prothrombin were the only protein whose synthesis was affected.

The lowering of plasma prothrombin concentration will develop slowly following administration of any one of these inhibitors. In part, the length of the delay depends upon the drug used; even with the most rapidly acting drugs, however, time must be allowed

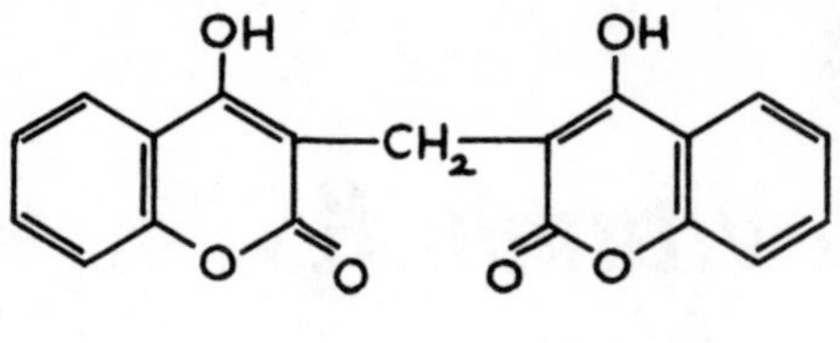

Dicumarol (bishydroxycoumarin) 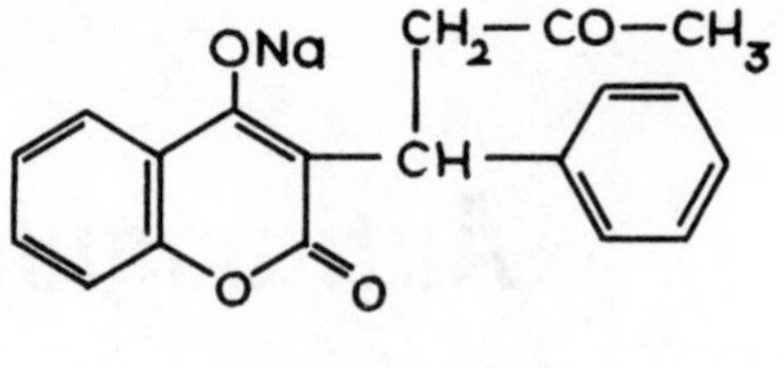   Warfarin sodium

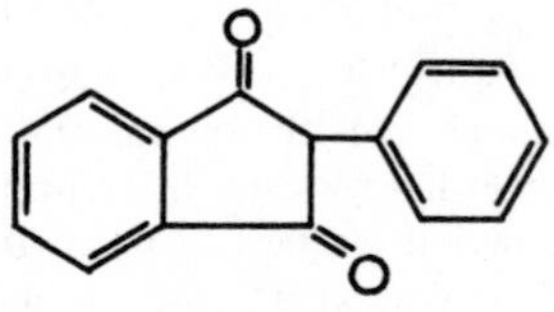

Phenindione 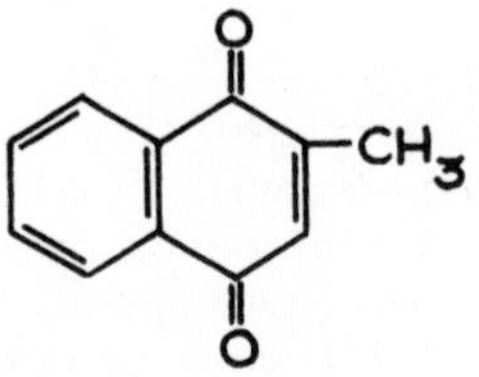   Menadione 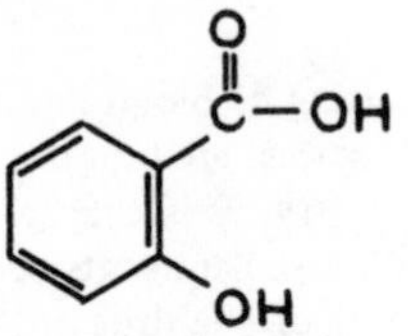   Salicylic acid

FIG 18–1. Anticoagulant drugs. The structural formulas of the 2 most commonly used coumarin type anticoagulants (dicumarol and warfarin) and a representative of the indandione type (phenindione) are shown. The structure of menadione, a synthetic vitamin K, is shown because the above anticoagulants are antagonists of vitamin K. Salicylic acid also has minor prothrombin depressant effects.

for the disappearance of prothrombin already synthesized. Similarly, the duration of action reflects the time necessary for resynthesis of prothrombin as well as upon the duration of action of the particular drug used.

It is also obvious that the addition of bishydroxycoumarin to drawn blood will not prevent clotting since the action of the drug is on the synthesis of clotting factors in the liver.

Clinical Uses

A. Prevention or Treatment of Venous Thrombosis: Enforced bed rest in elderly patients, prescribed most commonly during the weeks after a myocardial infarction, involves a great hazard of venous thrombosis. Blood flow in the deep veins of the calf or pelvis may be so slow that intravascular clotting occurs. The process is noninflammatory, and the clot is not bound to the walls of the veins. The thrombus may grow or be propagated by the accretion of additional material, and either the original clot or an extension that reaches a more rapidly flowing channel may be broken loose. The embolus thus formed will be impacted in a pulmonary vessel with results depending upon the size of the infarct. The most important use of the oral anticoagulants is to prevent (1) the occurrence of venous thrombosis during a period of unusual risk or (2) the propagation of a clot once it has been formed, and thus to prevent embolization until the clot has been bound to the wall of the vein.

When a venous thrombosis has already occurred, the use of anticoagulants is obligatory. The patient should receive the immediately effective heparin intravenously and administration of the slower acting oral anticoagulants begun at the same time.

The usefulness of routine anticoagulant therapy during the period immediately following a coronary

occlusion is less certain. Patients vary in the severity of their illness during the early period, and other means of reducing the incidence of venous thrombosis are used. These other methods (elastic bandages, bed exercises, ambulation) are effective in proportion to the quality of nursing care available. The results of clinical trials evaluating anticoagulants in the period immediately following coronary occlusion therefore vary depending upon the institution and patient selection. In some trials, thromboembolic complications were halved in incidence and a resulting increase in survival of perhaps 5% achieved. In other trials in other institutions, no difference could be demonstrated between treated and control groups. At this time, therefore, the decision whether to use anticoagulants or not is made on the basis of the severity of the illness, the care available, and the experience of the physician in the particular setting.

Pulmonary embolism is still the most common cause of death after fractures of the hip in the elderly. Anticoagulant therapy is not regularly prescribed in this country for these aged patients even though the results of controlled studies are impressive. In a recent careful study, for example, thromboembolic complications occurred in 22 of 83 control patients and only 7 of 83 treated patients.

B. Acute Arterial Occlusion: The effects of acute arterial occlusion (eg, by an embolus) are intensified by thrombosis in the area. Anticoagulation with heparin is initiated at once for its immediate effect, and an inhibitor of prothrombin synthesis is given for its persistent effect.

C. Prevention of Thrombus Formations in Fibrillating Atria: Mural thrombi may form on the noncontracting walls of the atrial appendage during atrial fibrillation. Emboli from the atria are an important complication of rheumatic mitral valve disease. Long-

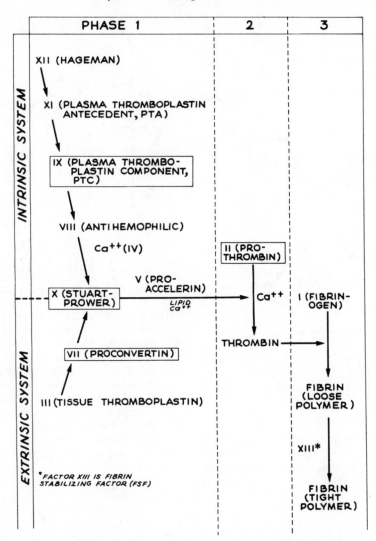

FIG 18–2. The coagulation mechanism (simplified). The conversion of prothrombin to thrombin is accomplished by 2 series of reactions that converge on factor X. The synthesis of coagulation factors shown within the boxes is inhibited by the dicumarol type of anticoagulant. *Phase I:* The system intrinsic to the blood begins with the activation of factor XII by contact with a proper surface. A cascade of reactions successively converts the factors shown to an active form which acts on the next substance in the sequence until activated factor X is generated. In the extrinsic system, tissue components act on factor X after activation by proconvertin. *Phase 2:* Stuart-Prower factor acting on prothrombin in the presence of calcium produces thrombin. *Phase 3:* Thrombin combines with fibrinogen to form fibrin. (Modified, with permission, from Deykin: Thrombogenesis. New England J Med 276:623, 1967.)

term anticoagulant therapy will prevent the formation of new thrombi and allow old thrombi to become fixed in place as scar tissue develops. Such treatment is usually preparatory to more definitive treatment of the mitral valve deformation or conversion of the arrhythmia.

D. Prevention of Coronary Thrombosis: The atherosclerotic process may gradually occlude a coronary artery, especially in older patients. Usually, however, the occlusion is due to formation of a clot on the surface of an atherosclerotic plaque. The question

arises whether reducing coagulability by continuous, long-term anticoagulant therapy will prevent or defer the final episode. The answer to this current and important question requires laborious clinical evaluation of impeccable design. Unfortunately, many available studies must be ignored.

To shorten the period of study and reduce the number of subjects needed, high-risk groups can be used—eg, patients who have experienced one myocardial infarction or who have angina. The control group must not only receive placebo medication but also

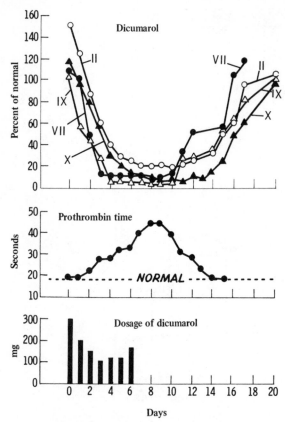

FIG 18–3. Typical effect of dicumarol on factors VII, IX, X, and II. (Redrawn and reproduced, with permission, from Kazmier & others: Effect of oral anticoagulants on factors VII, IX, X, and II. Arch Int Med 115:668, 1965.)

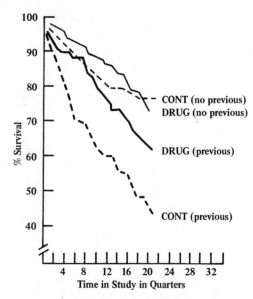

FIG 18–4. The effect on survival of long-term treatment with dicumarol sufficient to prolong prothrombin time to 2–2½ times normal. The men followed in this collaborative study were separated into a group that had had a myocardial infarction prior to the one for which they were hospitalized (80 treated, 72 controls) and a group without a history of infarction (305 treated, 278 controls). (Reproduced, with permission, from Ebert & others: Long-term anticoagulant therapy after myocardial infarction. JAMA 207:2266, 1969.)

placebo laboratory tests. Patients must be selected for random assignment to test or control groups in such a way that the resulting groups are comparable in sex, age, intensity of present disease, occurrence of associated disease, and economic status or other determinants of patient cooperation. The intensity of the anticoagulant effect must be carefully established.

A few cautious conclusions may be made from the results of some acceptable trials: (1) The prothrombin levels often accepted during the general use of anticoagulants are ineffective. (2) Those who benefit most (or, according to some observers, the only beneficiaries) are male and under 60 years of age. (3) The benefit–ie, lower incidence of second occlusions–occurs in the first 6 months of therapy. (4) Patients with angina benefit if the angina is of recent origin. (5) Where the pain of "acute coronary insufficiency" is premonitory of infarction, anticoagulant therapy is of established value.

There is a possibility that the danger of thrombosis is greater immediately after anticoagulants of this type are discontinued. Treatment is therefore continued for several years and slowly discontinued over a period of weeks or months.

Control of Dose

Administration of coumarin anticoagulants requires a large initial dose in order to achieve rapid therapeutic effect; the maintenance dose is then determined on an individual basis. Because of the wide variability in patient response, the required initial amount is often given in divided doses over a period of 2 days. It is possible to give a single very large dose–eg, warfarin, 75 mg–on the first day and begin a maintenance dose on the second day. The maintenance dose is determined for each patient on the basis of prothrombin times. Early in the therapeutic period, prothrombin times must be determined daily in order to adjust the dose. The prothrombin time on a given day will reflect the action of the dose of anticoagulant given 2 days previously except when the more rapidly acting warfarin is used. The prothrombin time is usually maintained at 10–30% of normal for the first few weeks of treatment. What constitutes an adequate level of prothrombin depression thereafter is arguable, but the level is usually allowed to rise to between 30 and 40%, probably with a decrease in therapeutic effectiveness.

The usual (Quick) prothrombin time is sensitive to changes in the concentration of factors VII and X in

TABLE 18–1. Prothrombin depressants: Dosages and preparations available.

	Dosage (Oral)*			Approximate Time to Peak Effect	Approximate Duration of Effect	Preparations Available
	1st Day	2nd Day	Usual Maintenance Dose and Range			
Coumarin derivatives						
Dicumarol (bishy-droxycoumarin)	200–400 mg	100–200 mg	75 mg (25–150)	2–3 days	4–5 days	Tablets, 25, 50, and 100 mg Capsules, 25 and 50 mg
Warfarin (Coumadin, Panwarfin, Athrombin-K)	30–50 mg	10–15 mg	7.5 mg (5–15)	1–2 days	2–3 days	Tablets, 2, 2.5, 5, 7.5, 10, and 25 mg Vials, 50 mg/2 ml and 75 mg/3 ml
Phenprocoumon (Liquamar)	30 mg	10 mg	3 mg (1.5–6)	1–2 days	4 days	Tablets, 3 mg
Acenocoumarol (Sintrom)	16–28 mg	8–16 mg	6 mg (2–10)	1–2 days	2 days	Tablets, 4 mg
Indandione derivatives†						
Diphenadione (Dipaxin)	40–60 mg	10–20 mg	7 mg (2.5–10)	.2–4 days	10 days	Tablets, 5 mg
Phenindione (Danilone, Hedulin)	100–250 mg twice daily	25–75 mg twice daily	50 mg (12.5–75) twice daily	1–2 days	2–4 days	Tablets, 20, 50, and 100 mg
Anisindione (Miradon)	300 mg	200 mg	75 mg (25–250)	1–2 days	4 days	Tablets, 50 mg

*Only warfarin may be given intravenously. Dosages are single daily doses unless otherwise specified.
†Allergic reactions, including agranulocytosis, occur. Phenindione may cause hepatitis.

addition to prothrombin (II). Which of these is important in determining the therapeutic effect or in determining whether bleeding occurs is not known. The sensitivity or lack of specificity of the prothrombin time is generally regarded as adequate, and it is the commonly used test. It is, however, not altered by changes in the concentration of IX (PTC), whereas one alternative test (Thrombotest) is sensitive to changes in the concentration of all 4 factors lowered by dicumarol.

In the experience or judgment of some investigators, bleeding may occur early in the use of anticoagulants because factor X is reduced to dangerous levels but prothrombin times are at apparently therapeutic levels.

In judging the results of different clinical trials, the comparison of the anticoagulant effect must take into consideration the test used.

Adverse Reactions

Side-effects are minor, consisting of mild diarrhea or soft stools.

A. Hemorrhage: The important toxicity of the anticoagulants is hemorrhage, which may be significant because of the amount of blood lost or because the bleeding is into a critical area. The occurrence of hemorrhage is not exactly predictable on the basis of prothrombin time determinations. Hemorrhage may occur when prothrombin times are within "safe" limits, and it does not always occur when prothrombin times greatly exceed the desired values. Hemorrhage usually occurs in an area of previous vascular damage; following myocardial infarction, for example, intracardiac bleeding or hemopericardium is a hazard. Bleeding may be renal (hematuria), gastrointestinal, rectal, intracranial, retroperitoneal, into the skin, and in many other sites. The reported incidence of bleeding will depend upon the intensity of therapeutic effect achieved and upon the care with which bleeding is sought. If microscopic hematuria is considered significant bleeding, the complication of bleeding may be said to be present in as many as 1/3 of patients receiving the drug. Serious hemorrhage may occur in as many as 2% of patients.

Treatment of overdosage: Vitamin K is the antagonist to the coumarins, and the administration of phytonadione (emulsion of vitamin K_1) will restore the prothrombin level. However, the action even of this most potent vitamin K preparation requires hours for significant clinical effect. When an immediate effect is desired, prothrombin must be given. Prothrombin is available in the form of fresh blood or of plasma preserved by freeze-drying so that prothrombin activity is preserved. The prothrombin complex itself has been prepared for investigative use and shown to be active.

B. Possible Risks of Abrupt Cessation of Therapy: A number of investigators noted an increase in the incidence of coronary occlusion and thromboembolic episodes during the 1- to 3-month period following abrupt cessation of long-term anticoagulant therapy. An increase in the concentration of factor VIII is reported to be present at this time. Not all groups of patients have shown this "rebound" hazard—ie, its existence is questionable, and the differences between groups in reported studies merely reflect differences in the severity of the underlying disease. Another view is that complications deferred by the benefits of anticoagulant therapy appear when therapy is discontinued too soon. If practice is based on changes in the laboratory tests of coagulability, the drug should be withdrawn over a period of at least 2 months after long-term (but not short-term) treatment.

C. Allergic Reactions to the Indandiones: The indandiones cause frequent and serious allergic toxicity. For example, allergic toxicity occurs in as many as 3% of patients receiving phenindione. It may be manifested as rash, fever, neutropenia or agranulocytosis, and hepatic or renal damage. Since the coumarin derivatives lack this potential, there are few occasions for the use of the indandiones.

Contraindications & Cautions

The contraindications to the use of anticoagulants cannot be reduced to a list satisfactory to every physician and applicable to every patient. Factors to be considered include the following:

A. Bleeding or Potential Bleeding From Any Site: Active peptic ulcer, hematologic disease, possible cerebral hemorrhage, active bacterial endocarditis, or any other intercurrent disease with a hemorrhagic potential are contraindications to the use of anticoagulants. Any local factor such as a catheter, Wangensteen drainage, or a drain in a wound will increase the danger of bleeding. Anticoagulants are usually discontinued before a major surgical procedure. However, with prothrombin levels of 15–20%, all but CNS and eye surgery can be done. Minor procedures can be carried out without great hazard. Many of the procedures in dental surgery, for example, including open and closed extractions, have been performed on patients receiving continuous anticoagulant therapy. Bleeding can be avoided by careful hemostasis and packing to provide optimal mechanical factors for clotting and avoiding cavities in the socket.

Anticoagulant therapy can be initiated soon after obstetric delivery.

Coumarin anticoagulants should not be used if laboratory facilities for the determination of prothrombin times are unavailable or inadequate.

B. Other Contraindications: The dosage of an anticoagulant should be adjusted with great care in the presence of hepatic or renal disease. Untreated, severe hypertension is a contraindication in the opinion of some physicians, as is advanced age or debility also.

C. Interaction With Other Drugs: The anticoagulants are often given for long periods of time, and their very use implies that the patient has a serious primary problem that will require the use of other drugs. Drug interactions are therefore likely to be common, and their consequences may be disastrous.

It is also true that the interactions with other drugs have been widely studied because technics for the determination of plasma levels of coumarin anticoagulants and of their biologic effects (in the form of prothrombin times) are more easily available than is true for most drug groups. Many of the suggested interactions are based on studies in animals or on studies of binding to plasma albumin in glass. Many of the hypothesized reactions have not had their clinical significance established and are not included in the examples below. (See also Chapter 2.)

1. Stimulation of metabolism—The administration of many lipid-soluble drugs in continued dosages can increase the amount and activity of the hydroxylating enzymes contained in liver microsomes. An anticoagulant given after such enzyme induction may be metabolized with unusual rapidity with a reduction in the anticoagulant effect. More dangerous is the possibility of an increase in anticoagulant effect if the inducing drug is discontinued.

The administration of phenobarbital and other long-acting barbiturates, glutethimide (Doriden), and griseofulvin reduces both plasma levels and the hypoprothrombinemic effect of the coumarin drugs. All barbiturates cause the same effect but must be given at proper intervals if they are short-acting.

With adequate dosage of the inducing drug, all patients will show a change after a week of treatment, but the extent of the change is highly variable. Recovery requires 2–3 weeks. If prothrombin times and dosage adjustment are done at proper intervals, no mishap need occur; in fact, epidemiologic studies (rather than anecdotal evaluations) do not incriminate drug interactions in many bleeding episodes.

2. Displacement from binding sites—The coumarins in plasma are bound to albumin to a large extent (97%) and are protected from metabolic change or excretion until they dissociate to replace the unbound drug that leaves the vascular compartment. Phenylbutazone, sulfinpyrazone, and norethandrolone (Nilevar) displace warfarin and dicumarol from binding sites on plasma protein and increase the amount of anticoagulant delivered to its site of action in the liver. An intensification of anticoagulant effect is maximal after 3–5 days of administration of the second agent.

Displacement from bound to free form also increases the rate of metabolism and excretion; after 1–2 weeks, a new steady state is established during which the original dose will again give the same blood levels and achieve the same anticoagulant effect.

3. Inhibition of metabolism—All purinol administration greatly prolongs the half-life of dicumarol, but the effect on prothrombin time is not yet established. Disulfiram (Antabuse) has a similar effect.

4. Others—Clofibrate (Atromid-S) markedly potentiates the effect of anticoagulants, but the mechanism is not clearly established. Quinidine has a lesser effect.

Cholestyramine interferes with the absorption of the anticoagulants (and many other drugs) unless an interval of several hours elapses between administration of cholestyramine and the other agent.

5. Effects of anticoagulants on other drugs—When dicumarol and, presumably, warfarin are added to the regimen of a patient receiving chlorpropamide, tolbutamide, diphenylhydantoin, or phenobarbital, the effect of these drugs is greatly prolonged and intensified by mechanisms that have not yet been established.

HEPARIN

Source & Chemistry

Heparin, together with histamine and serotonin, occurs in the granules of mast cells or tissue basophils. It is a strongly acidic mucopolysaccharide made up of recurring units of glucuronic acid and sulfated glucosamine.

Heparin for drug use is extracted from beef lung and liver. Some variation in its properties still occurs, and the dosage of heparin is measured in USP units. The bioassay is based on its ability to prevent clotting of sheep plasma under standardized conditions, and 1 mg is equivalent to at least 120 USP units.

Pharmacologic Actions

A. Anticoagulant: Heparin acts directly to neutralize any thrombin formed and also inhibits the action of activated factors XI (PTA) and IX (PTC). (Fig 18-2.) The study of its action is complex and incomplete, but the important point is that it acts as an anticoagulant immediately, both in vivo and in vitro. The duration of the effect is dependent on the dose, but it is brief. After intravenous injection of ordinary doses, the effect is about 50% dissipated in 1 hour and clotting time is again normal in less than 4 hours. Heparin and the coumarin anticoagulants are compared in Table 18-2.

B. Other Effects: Plasma that is turbid from chylomicrons is "cleared" more rapidly if heparin is injected postprandially. The effect does not occur in vitro but only in vivo after the injection of heparin. The "clearing factor" thus produced is increased "lipoprotein lipase" activity. There is no evidence that this action is related to the normal mechanism of chylomicron metabolism, nor have efforts to demonstrate a therapeutic role for this action of heparin been successful.

Clinical Uses

A. Acute Anticoagulant Effect: The most common use of heparin is to provide an anticoagulant effect during the interval required for the effect of a coumarin compound to develop and stabilize. It is also used when it may become desirable to rapidly terminate the anticoagulant effect, as during cardiac surgery or in the treatment of acute arterial occlusion when surgical treatment may become advisable.

Table 18-2. Comparison of heparin and coumarin anticoagulants.

	Heparin	Coumarin Derivatives
Onset of action	Immediate	Gradual to peak at 48 hours
Duration	< 4 hours	2-5 days
Route of administration	Parenteral	Oral
Laboratory control of dose	Clotting time	Prothrombin time
Treatment of overdose	Protamine	Fresh blood, plasma, vitamin K
Cost	Expensive (dollars/day)	Inexpensive (pennies/day)
Active in vitro	Yes	No

B. Long-Term Anticoagulant Effect: Heparin may be used for an extended period in the same situations listed in the discussion of inhibitors of prothrombin synthesis. However, it is no more efficacious than dicumarol or warfarin during chronic treatment, and its cost and the need for repeated injection are important disadvantages.

Control of Dose

Heparin effect is quantitated by clotting time only. (Clotting time is a specific test, not a general description. The Lee-White tube method is used.) Heparin prolongs prothrombin time for at least 2 hours after its administration and can interfere with the adjustment of dicumarol dosage.

Adverse Reactions

The important toxic effect of heparin is hemorrhage as discussed in detail in the above section on coumarin derivatives. Rare allergic reactions have been reported.

Patients receiving 15,000 units or more per day of heparin during long-term therapy develop osteoporosis. This effect is also demonstrable in animals. The mechanism of the osteoporosis is unknown but is not related to the anticoagulant properties of heparin.

Treatment of overdosage: Because heparin is so short-acting, it is rarely necessary to neutralize its effect. The most common situation requiring a heparin antagonist is postsurgical management when an extracorporeal pump has been used.

Protamine, a strongly basic protein, will neutralize the acid heparin on approximately a milligram per milligram basis. A 1% solution of protamine sulfate is available for slow intravenous injection.

Toluidine blue and hexadimethrine, a synthetic base, are obsolete heparin antagonists that have been withdrawn from the market.

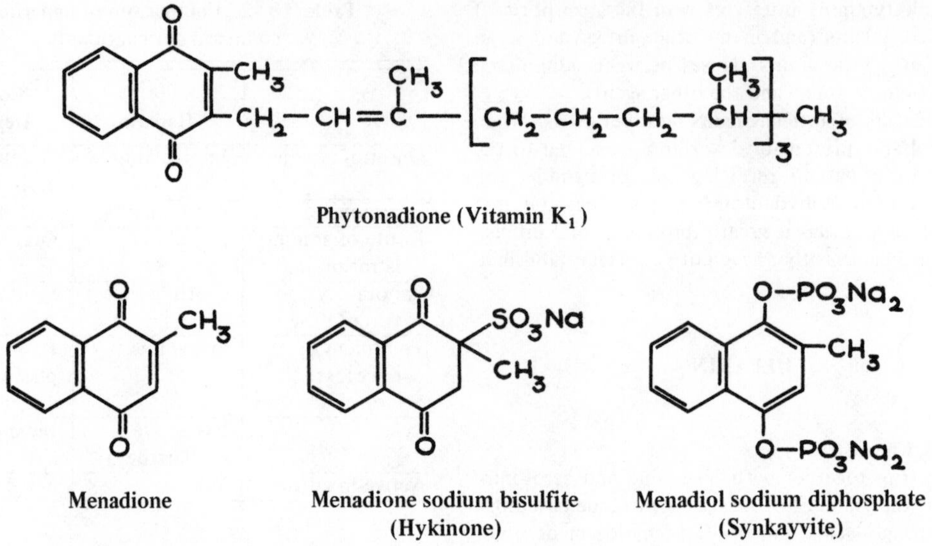

Phytonadione (Vitamin K_1)

Menadione   **Menadione sodium bisulfite**   **Menadiol sodium diphosphate**
                              (Hykinone)   **(Synkayvite)**

FIG 18—5. **Chemical structure of a natural vitamin K_1; menadione, a lipid-soluble synthetic analogue; and 2 water-soluble derivatives of menadione.**

Contraindications & Cautions

Present or potential bleeding from any site, as listed above for the hypoprothrombinemic agents, is the only contraindication to the use of heparin.

Preparations & Dosages

Heparin is given only by injection. Sodium heparin solutions for injection contain 1000–40,000 units/ml.

For immediate effect, administer 3000–9000 units IV every 4–6 hours or until subcutaneously injected heparin is effective.

For prolonged effect, inject a concentrated solution (20,000 units/ml) slowly through a small needle into the subcutaneous fat below the posterior iliac crest. A dose of 10,000–15,000 units is usually given every 12 hours, but clotting time should be determined to adjust the dose.

Heparin may also be given as a continuous intravenous infusion.

K VITAMINS

Chemistry

The naturally occurring K *(Koagulation)* vitamins are fat-soluble and are not absorbed from the gut lumen unless bile is also present. The important pharmacology of the K vitamins centers about this fact.

Vitamin K_1 is called phytonadione when used as a drug, either orally or as an injectable emulsion. Its structure is shown in Fig 18–5. Menadione is not active as such but is transformed by the liver into active vitamin K_2. Menadione is itself lipid-soluble, but

the 2 derivatives shown are water-soluble and have therefore had some use not only as injectable preparations but also as oral agents absorbed in the absence of bile acids, ie, during jaundice.

Pharmacologic Actions

Vitamin K is necessary for the liver synthesis of prothrombin and factors VII, IX, and X. Deficiency, whether dietary, drug-induced, or accompanying liver disease, leads to hypoprothrombinemia and hemorrhage. Disturbances in the absorption of vitamin K from the gastrointestinal tract are common in humans, but dietary deficiency is so rare that the possibility can almost be ignored. No minimum dietary requirements have been established, and it is usually held that synthesis by intestinal bacteria provides a supply of vitamin independent of the diet. Certainly this is true for coprophagous species, but the response of normal and warfarin-treated humans suggests that absorption from the colon does not occur and that the dietary source is the important one. In any case, the wide occurrence of K vitamins makes dietary deficiency states unimportant except possibly in explaining some variability in the response of patients receiving anticoagulants.

Additional aspects of the pharmacology of vitamin K are discussed with the uses of the drug.

Clinical Uses

A. In Obstructive Jaundice: Unlike other fat-soluble vitamins, vitamin K is stored in only small amounts in the body. In the absence of the bile necessary for continued absorption, hypoprothrombinemia will develop in a few days. If bile deficiency is due to obstructive jaundice and not to hepatocellular damage, injected vitamin K will rapidly restore prothrombin

TABLE 18–3. Vitamin K: Dosages and preparations available.*

	Post-natal	Pre-natal	Drug-Induced Hypoprothrombinemia		Obstructive Jaundice, etc	Preparations Available
			Minor	With Bleeding		
Phytonadione (Mephyton, Aqua-Mephyton, Konakion, Mono-Kay)	0.5–1 mg IM, IV, or orally	1 mg IM on admission	2.5–10 mg IM or orally	10–50 mg IM or IV	2.5–25 mg IM or orally	Tablets and capsules: 5 mg Injectable (IM or IV): 1 mg/0.5 ml 2 mg/0.5 ml 10 mg/1, 2.5, 5, and 10 ml 25 mg/2.5 ml 50 mg/1 ml 50 mg/5 ml
Menadione sodium bisulfite (Hykinone)	1 mg IV or IM	. . .	. . .	. . .	5 mg IM or orally daily	Tablets, 5 mg Injectable (IM or IV): 2.5 mg/0.5 ml 5 mg/0.5 and 1 ml 10 mg/1 ml 72 mg/10 ml
Menadiol sodium diphosphate (Synkayvite, Kappadione)	. . .	5 mg IM or IV on admission	. . .	. . .	5 mg IM or orally daily	Tablets, 5 mg Injectable (IM or IV): 1 mg/0.5 ml 2.5 mg/0.5 ml 5 mg/1 ml 10 mg/1 ml 75 mg/2 ml

*Phytonadione (vitamin K_1) is less toxic and acts more rapidly than the other preparations available. The other 2 drugs are absorbed in the absence of bile.

levels to normal. Preoperative administration of vitamin K in patients with surgically correctable obstructive jaundice has reduced hemorrhagic complications during the procedure. If the jaundice is due to hepatocellular damage and the hypoprothrombinemia is due not to failure of absorption but inability of liver cells to synthesize prothrombin, the hemorrhagic tendency cannot be reversed with vitamin K.

B. Possible Prevention of Hemorrhagic Disease of the Newborn: Prothrombin levels are low at birth and fall further during the first few days after birth. The fall during the neonatal period is terminated, it is usually said, when the intestinal tract is contaminated and bacterial synthesis provides vitamin K. There are reasons to question this explanation and to look instead for a dietary explanation. In any case, neonatal hypoprothrombinemia can be minimized either by the prenatal administration of vitamin K to the mother or by postnatal administration to the newborn. The prothrombin levels certainly are elevated by such treatment, but the routine use of prenatal vitamin K for many years has not resulted in any decrease in the incidence of bleeding during the neonatal period other than postcircumcision bleeding. Because of the risk of kernicterus, the administration of vitamin K to a premature infant should be limited to a single dose of 0.5–1 mg of phytonadione parenterally.

C. Treatment of Anticoagulant Toxicity: The rapid reversal of drug-induced hypoprothrombinemia requires the use of a source of prothrombin such as fresh blood or plasma as discussed above. Vitamin K may be used if the situation is not urgent or as a supplement to one of the immediate sources of prothrombin. Phytonadione acts more rapidly than the water-soluble menadione derivatives, a significant effect developing in 3–6 hours after the intravenous administration of 50–150 mg.

Adverse Reactions

Vitamin K is a nutritional factor but nevertheless has some toxicity when used as a drug.

A. Hyperbilirubinemia: The newborn and, especially, the premature infant is unusually susceptible to some toxic effects of drugs because of his immaturity. Rapid hemolysis in the immediate postnatal period leads to an increase in the amount of bilirubin that must be conjugated with glucuronide and excreted into the bile. After needlessly large doses of vitamin K postnatally and even after very large maternal doses of menadione sodium bisulfite in the immediate prenatal period, the elevation of serum bilirubin has been great enough to resu.. in kernicterus. Which of the possible mechanisms that can cause hyperbilirubinemia is responsible in the case of vitamin K is not established.

B. Impaired Liver Function and Hypoprothrombinemia: In a few cases, repeated, large intravenous doses of any of the vitamin K drugs have caused liver damage and hypoprothrombinemia.

C. Hemolytic Anemia: Menadione and its water-soluble analogues are among those drugs that can precipitate hemolysis in patients with a genetically determined deficiency of glucose-6-phosphate dehydrogenase (G6PD).

Contraindications & Cautions

Vitamin K should be used only in the presence of hypoprothrombinemia—not indiscriminately in the presence of all bleeding. As is mentioned above, it should not be used as a substitute for blood or plasma if bleeding occurs after anticoagulant drugs, and newborns should receive only a single 1 mg dose.

If phytonadione is given intravenously, as it often is, the rate of administration should not exceed 5 or 10 mg/minute to prevent hypotensive episodes. The emulsion may be diluted with isotonic saline or glucose solutions.

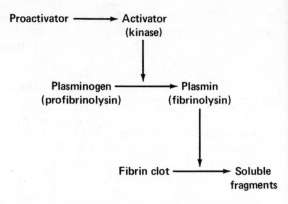

FIG 18—6. Summary of the fibrinolytic system.

acknowledged. Urokinase is an investigative drug now being evaluated. Effectiveness in the treatment of pulmonary emboli is claimed for streptokinase following preliminary studies.

FIBRINOLYTIC SYSTEMS

PLASMIN (FIBRINOLYSIN) & PLASMIN ACTIVATORS

Agents that could act on thrombi and emboli after their formation—ie, to dissolve them rather than prevent their extension as the anticoagulants do—would be of great usefulness. Efforts to reach this goal have so far stemmed from a study of the natural clot-removing or fibrinolytic mechanism.

This mechanism is summarized in Fig 18—6.

Activators or kinases involved in the first step may be found in urine (urokinase) and some tissues in an active form. The physiologically important kinase exists as an inactive proactivator until activated by various stimuli including streptokinase, an enzyme formed during the growth of hemolytic streptococci.

An activated kinase converts plasminogen, a plasma globulin, to plasmin or fibrinolysin, a proteolytic enzyme that acts on fibrin and other proteins at lysine-arginine bonds.

The drugs suggested by studies of the fibrinolytic system for trial as thrombolytic agents are (1) **fibrinolysin,** prepared by the action of streptokinase on human or bovine blood; (2) **bacterial streptokinase,** which would act following administration to increase the concentration of plasmin within a clot; and (3) **urokinase,** derived from human urine.

Human fibrinolysin (Thrombolysin) is still available for use as an adjunct in the treatment of venous thrombosis, but its lack of efficacy is now generally

AMINOCAPROIC ACID
(Inhibitor of Fibrinolysis)

Aminocaproic acid (Amicar, epsilon-aminocaproic acid, $H_2N-C_5H_{10}-COOH$) is a synthetic compound related to lysine. It acts as a competitive antagonist to activators of plasminogen—ie, it prevents the generation of plasmin.

Aminocaproic acid has been used in specific situations when unusually great fibrinolytic activity has been established. Primary hyperfibrinolysis is extremely rare. Secondary hyperfibrinolysis is a compensatory mechanism that follows widespread intravascular clotting—eg, after abruptio placentae or surgical procedures utilizing cardiac bypass. The exact indications for the use of aminocaproic acid in these situations depend upon the response to other therapy—eg, transfusion and heparin.

This drug has also been used when fibrin formation—as in hemophilia—is so deficient that inhibition of even the normal fibrinolytic process may be beneficial.

The systemic toxicity, including the possibility of thrombotic complications, has not been completely evaluated in humans.

Aminocaproic acid (Amicar) is available in tablets containing 500 mg; as a syrup containing 250 mg/ml; and, for intravenous use, in vials containing 5 gm/20 ml. Each preparation bears a warning limiting use of the drug to acute, life-threatening situations.

The suggested oral and intravenous dose (in the USA) is 5 gm initially followed by 1.25 gm/hour.

TABLE 18—4. Proteolytic and other enzymes: Sources and suggested uses.

	Source	Action	Suggested Uses
Chymotrypsin (Chymoral, Zolyse, Avazyme, Alpha Chymar)	Beef pancreas	Proteolytic	Cataract extraction, anti-inflammatory agent, liquefaction of respiratory secretions
Streptokinase-streptodornase (Varidase)	Streptococcus	Fibrinolytic Deoxyribonuclease	Anti-inflammatory, topical debridement
Fibrinolysin and deoxyribonuclease (Elase)	Beef blood Beef pancreas	Fibrinolytic Deoxyribonuclease	Topical debridement
Pancreatic dornase (Dornavac)	Beef pancreas	Deoxyribonuclease	Liquefaction of respiratory secretions
Trypsin (Tryptar, Parenzyme)	Beef pancreas	Proteolytic	Topical debridement
Plant protease concentrate (bromelains, Ananase)	Pineapple	Proteolytic	Anti-inflammatory
Proteolytic enzymes from *Carica papaya* (Papase)	Papaya	Proteolytic	Anti-inflammatory
Alpha-amylase (Buclamase)	Bacterial	Amylase	Anti-inflammatory

OTHER ENZYMES

A number of other enzymes are used as drugs. Some of these—eg, penicillinase, pancreatin, and hyaluronidase—are discussed in other chapters. Several proteolytic enzymes, deoxyribonuclease (which depolymerizes DNA), and amylase are suggested for several uses, but only one of these (zonulolysis) is well established. The preparations are listed in Table 18—4.

Intraocular Use of Chymotrypsin

Pancreatic chymotrypsin injected into the posterior chamber of the eye dissolves the zonular fibers and facilitates lens extraction in the surgical treatment of cataract.

Anti-inflammatory Uses

Many of these enzymes are suggested for use in hastening the resolution of inflammation due to various forms of trauma. The theory apparently is that the enzymes will (even after oral administration) reach the site of injury and hasten dissolution of fibrin clots. No clinical trials have supported the suggested use. Injected enzymes—eg, chymotrypsin—have caused several deaths from anaphylactic shock.

Topical Debridement

Enzymes can be applied to the skin as solutions or ointments, injected into empyema cavities or other accumulations of exudate, or inhaled as an aerosol to act on the surface of the respiratory tract. They are probably active in some of these situations, but studies to evaluate their efficacy have usually included other forms of treatment also. Only fibrinous clots and exudates of inflammatory cells are liquefied. Bone and dead tissues are not affected.

•   •   •

General References

Anticoagulants

An assessment of long-term anticoagulant administration after cardiac infarction. Second report of the working party on anticoagulant therapy in coronary thrombosis to the Medical Research Council. Brit MJ 2:837–843, 1964.

Assessment of short-term anticoagulant administration after cardiac infarction. Report of the working party on anticoagulant therapy. Brit MJ 1:335–342, 1969.

Behrman, S.J., & I.S. Wright: Dental surgery during continuous anticoagulant therapy. JAMA 175:483–488, 1961.

Ebert, R.V., & others: Long-term anticoagulant therapy after myocardial infarction. Final report of the VA cooperative study. JAMA 207:2263–2267, 1969.

Griffith, G.C., & A. Silverglade: Symposium on heparin. Am J Cardiol 14:1–54, 1964.

Gurewich, V., Thomas, D.P., & R.K. Stuart: Some guidelines for heparin therapy of venous thromboembolic disease. JAMA 199:152–154, 1967.

Koch-Weser, J., & E. M. Sellers: Drug interactions with coumarin anticoagulants. New Eng J Med 285:487–498, 547–558, 1971.

Rebound thrombosis after stopping anticoagulants. Brit MJ 2:1343–1344, 1966.

Salzman, E.W., Harris, W.H., & R.W. DeSanctis: Anticoagulation for prevention of thromboembolism following fractures of the hip. New England J Med 275:122–130, 1966.

Vitamin K

Finkel, M.J.: Vitamin K_1 and the vitamin K analogues. Clin Pharmacol Therap 2:794–814, 1961.

Potter, E.L.: Effect on infant mortality of vitamin K administered during labor. Am J Obst Gynec 50:235–247, 1945.

Udall, J.A.: Human sources and absorption of vitamin K in relation to anticoagulation stability. JAMA 194:127–129, 1965.

Enzymes

Colman, R.W.: Proteolytic enzymes in clinical medicine. Clin Pharmacol Therap 6:598–630, 1965.

Elase and other proteolytic enzyme drugs. Med Lett Drugs Ther 9:17–18, 1967.

European Working Party: Streptokinase in recent myocardial infarction: A controlled multicentre trial. Brit MJ 3:325–331, 1971.

Hirsh, J., & others: Streptokinase therapy in acute major pulmonary embolism: Effectiveness and problems. Brit MJ 4:729–734, 1968

Pechet, L.: Fibrinolysis. New England J Med 273:966–973, 1024–1034, 1965.

19...
Histamine, Antihistamines, Serotonin

A great amount of information of physiologic or pathologic significance has originated in the study of substances extracted from the body. Some workers have even introduced the term autopharmacology to describe this research area, postulating that a potent substance which is widely distributed in large amounts in the body will eventually be shown to have a physiologic role. Histamine and serotonin are 2 such substances for which no physiologic function has yet been established. However, they are important in a number of pathologic states and in the explanation of the action of other drugs, especially the antihistamines.

HISTAMINE

Chemistry, Occurrence, & Metabolism

Histamine is formed by the decarboxylation of histidine. The reaction may occur within the lumen of the intestine (the enzymatic activity deriving from coliform organisms) or within many types of cells. Histamine formed within the intestine or ingested preformed is absorbed, but it is rapidly metabolized by the intestine and liver and probably does not contribute to the histamine stored in the body.

Histamine occurs in at least 3 pools or types of storage sites. One fraction is held in the granules of mast cells and of basophils, the equivalent cells in peripheral blood. In these granules, histamine is bound with heparin and cannot exert an effect nor be metabolized. The mast cells are degranulated and the histamine released by the antigen-antibody complex formed as the first step in an immediate allergic reaction and by the histamine-liberating chemicals listed below.

Histamine also occurs in the mucosal layer of the gastrointestinal tract, where it is not contained in mast cells and not depleted by histamine liberators. The hypothalamus and area postrema contain histamine that reacts still differently, being depleted by reserpine.

The metabolism of histamine is summarized in Fig 19-1. Its activity is terminated principally by methylation and subsequent deamination by monoamine oxidase. A second histaminase, diamine oxidase, also acts to deaminate histamine.

Pharmacologic Actions

A. Mechanisms of Action: In humans, at least, the effects of histamine can be summarized as direct stimulation of glands and contraction of nonvascular smooth muscle but relaxation of vascular smooth muscle. The action is directly on the gland or smooth muscle, ie, it is unrelated to innervation. Since specific antagonists are known which block the actions of histamine without blocking the actions of agents such as epinephrine or acetylcholine, it is possible to speak of specific histamine receptors.

In the preceding chapters a number of other drugs that act directly on smooth muscle have been discussed. They are reviewed in Table 19-1.

B. Effects:

1. On blood vessels—Our understanding of the effects of histamine is still incomplete. Histamine acts on the smallest vessels, which are difficult to study. In addition, there are important variations between species in the response to histamine; the rat and rabbit, for example, respond with arteriolar constriction rather than the dilatation seen in humans. In the human, histamine acts to dilate arterioles, capillaries, and venules. Blood pressure is lowered in part by arteriolar dilatation, but the postural nature of the hypotension and studies of the change in distensibility of veins suggest that venous pooling of blood is a more important mechanism. The face is flushed, and the subject may experience a throbbing vascular headache.

The hypotension caused by histamine leads to sympatho-adrenal activation and tachycardia. With

TABLE 19-1. Summary of drugs acting directly on smooth muscle.
(+ denotes stimulation or constriction; − denotes relaxation or dilatation.)

	Effect On	
	Vascular Smooth Muscle	Other Smooth Muscle
Nitroglycerin Quinidine Papaverine	−	−
Ergot alkaloids Vasopressin	+	+
Histamine Bradykinin Prostaglandins	−	+

large doses, the combined venous pooling and arteriolar constriction lead to shock.

2. Capillary permeability—Permeability of the walls of capillaries and small venules is increased by the action of histamine. If the effect is local and circumscribed, the accumulation of extravascular extracellular fluid is apparent as a wheal (hive, urticarial lesion). A more generalized effect is demonstrated by the abnormal ease with which a large trypan blue molecule leaves the blood vessels and stains tissues and by the hemoconcentration and elevation of the hematocrit. The increased capillary permeability is usually said to be a consequence of capillary and venular dilatation.

3. Contraction of nonvascular smooth muscle—Bronchiolar constriction and increased intestinal motility are the clinically important manifestations of the generalized smooth muscle stimulation caused by histamine.

4. Stimulation of gastric secretion—Histamine causes maximal secretion of acid and pepsin, and is the standard stimulus applied in the study of gastric secretion. It is found in high concentrations in the gastric mucosa and appears in gastric secretion. However, no role in the normal control of gastric secretion has yet been established for this substance.

The antihistamines decrease histamine-induced hypersecretion only when they are given in doses large enough to have an atropine (acetylcholine blocking) effect. The direct effect of histamine on the parietal and chief cells is decreased but not eliminated by vagotomy. (This is in contrast to the response to insulin, which, unlike histamine, can be used to test for the completeness of a vagotomy.)

Except for an increase in salivation, the action of histamine on other glands is unimportant. The sympatho-adrenal discharge initiated by the hypotension resulting from histamine administration will, of course, cause sweating.

5. Local action—If histamine is injected intradermally or is released by trauma, a "triple response"

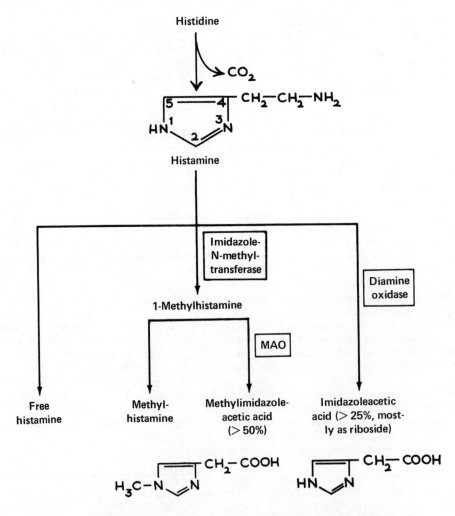

FIG 19–1. Synthesis, metabolism, and common urinary metabolites of histamine.

is seen: (1) Capillary dilatation results in a small red area at the site of injection. This area soon becomes slightly bluish or is obscured by blanching due to edema. (2) Arteriolar dilatation causes redness ("flare") over a wider area. The flare is mediated through an axon reflex—ie, the afferent impulse initiated by histamine travels in the expected direction toward the neuronal cell body, at the same time initiating an antidromic vasodilator impulse that travels centrifugally down another branch of the same sensory neuron. (3) A wheal of localized edema forms in the area of capillary dilatation.

These changes are accompanied by transient pain and itching.

Clinical Uses
A. Gastric Analysis:
1. Histamine test—Gastric analysis is necessary to establish or eliminate the existence of achlorhydria. If acid is demonstrated in a fasting sample aspirated through a gastric tube, no stimulus to secretion is necessary. If, however, the fasting specimen contains no acid, histamine, 0.5 mg, is injected subcutaneously and samples are collected for the following hour or until acid is shown to be present. Achlorhydria is by definition the absence of acid following histamine stimulation.

In the doses needed for stimulation of gastric secretion, histamine often causes flushing, sweating, tachycardia, and hypotension, and sometimes a throbbing headache. These side-effects can be only partially prevented by prior treatment with an antihistamine. Betazole (Histalog), an alternative drug to histamine, also causes maximal stimulation of gastric secretion but without the high incidence of side-effects that occurs with histamine. Betazole is an isomer of histamine, a pyrazole rather than an imidazole derivative. A subcutaneous injection of 50 mg of betazole is equivalent to 0.3 mg of histamine.

2. Azuresin test—A "tubeless" method of gastric analysis can be performed by giving azuresin (Diagnex Blue) orally. In this diagnostic preparation a dye, azure A, is combined with an exchange resin. In the presence of acid—ie, hydrogen ion—the dye is displaced from the resin and can be detected in the urine by its bluish-green color. A positive test is reliable, but a negative test must be confirmed by passing a gastric tube; for this reason, the less pleasant intubation procedure is still used.

B. Diagnosis of Pheochromocytoma: (See Chapter 11.) When pheochromocytoma is suspected but the patient has a minimal blood pressure elevation, histamine will cause the release of catecholamines from the tumor if one is present. Paroxysmal hypertension rather than the usual fall in blood pressure will then follow the administration of histamine.

Adverse Reactions
Even with the small doses (0.01 mg/kg subcut) used in gastric analysis, a flush, headache, and precipitous fall in blood pressure may be seen. The hypotension is predominantly postural and usually requires no treatment other than the recumbent position. If treatment is required, epinephrine (0.3 mg subcut) is an effective physiologic antagonist.

Pain and itching at the injection site are also common.

Contraindications & Cautions
Histamine should not be used in asthmatics or when hypotension may be especially dangerous—eg, in the presence of angina.

Preparations & Dosages
Histamine is dispensed as solutions of the diphosphate or dihydrochloride salts. However, doses and labeling are expressed in terms of the equivalent amount of free base.

For gastric analysis, the dose is 0.01 mg/kg subcut or IM. Solutions containing 1 mg/ml of the base in 1 and 10 ml vials are available.

Betazole (Histalog) is given subcut or IM, either 0.5 mg/kg or as a total dose of 50 mg. In either case the dose is equivalent to about half the standard dose of histamine.

For use in the diagnosis of pheochromocytoma, histamine is available in 1 ml ampules containing only 0.1 mg/ml of the base. In this application, 0.05 mg is diluted to 5 ml with saline and injected rapidly intravenously.

Histamine Liberation by Drugs & Toxins
No function has been established for histamine in any physiologic process. Many hypotheses have been tested and rejected. Current suggestions are as yet unconvincing.

There are several pathologic processes involving histamine that have a relation to drug therapy. Anaphylaxis and probably other immediate allergic reactions result when basophilic granules disgorge histamine, heparin, serotonin (in some species), kinins, and slow-reacting substance (SRS), a poorly characterized long-acting bronchial constrictor.

In addition, a number of drugs and toxins act to degranulate basophils. Histamine liberation explains some of the effects of a few therapeutic and toxic agents, and histamine liberation can be used to deplete an organism of histamine for investigative purposes.

A. Classes of Histamine Liberators:
1. Compounds that cause general tissue damage—Trypsin, peptone, snake and bee venoms, detergents.

2. Large molecules—PVP, horse serum, some dextrans.

3. Endotoxins.

4. Bases—Some simple amines (epinephrine, morphine, codeine, meperidine), but especially diamines (stilbamidine, propamidine, D-tubocurarine, dimethyltubocurarine, succinylcholine, 1,10-diaminodecane, and 48/80).

The last substance (48/80) is a polymer made up of units of a substituted phenylethylamine connected through methylene groups. It is the agent commonly used in the laboratory to deplete histamine stores in an animal.

B. Effects: Histamine liberators actually release all of the constituents of basophilic granules. The immediate effects are, therefore, comparable to anaphylaxis in the species being studied. The late effects do not involve serotonin or heparin but are due to histamine depletion and exhaustion of those responses due to histamine liberation. For example, repeated small doses of 48/80 can be given to an animal. After the liberated histamine is metabolized, another drug may be given and that part of its action due to histamine release will no longer occur. The histamine contained in the CNS is not released by the above compounds but is released by treatment with reserpine.

THE ANTIHISTAMINES

History

Reasoning from the atropine-acetylcholine type of antagonism, Bovet concluded that there should be compounds with the ability to block the actions of histamine. The first such compound, reported by Bovet and Staub in 1937, was not clinically efficacious, but useful drugs were developed in France during World War II.

Chemistry & Classification

In the discussion of the chemistry of atropine and its congeners (Chapter 9), the members of a large group of drugs were characterized as chemically similar in being made up of a large blocking group connected by a group of proper length to a tertiary amine function.

The antihistamines, parasympatholytics, and tranquilizers have this chemical configuration and can be expected to share some of the same pharmacologic properties. Nevertheless, it is possible to selectively emphasize one property or another in choosing compounds for a specific therapeutic purpose. Thus, the antihistamines are more potent as histamine antagonists than as acetylcholine antagonists but will retain atropine-like side-effects and cause sedation of the tranquilizer type.

The antihistamines are often classified chemically on the basis of the nature of the connecting group. Examples are given below.

1. Ethers or ethanolamine derivatives—

Diphenhydramine hydrochloride (Benadryl) or dimenhydrinate chlorotheophyllinate (Dramamine)

2. Ethylenediamine derivatives—

Tripelennamine (Pyribenzamine)

3. Phenothiazine derivatives—The phenothiazines used as antihistamines and antinauseants are often considered a separate chemical class, but the relation to the other antihistamines is clearer if they are regarded as ethylenediamine derivatives.

Promethazine (Phenergan)

4. Alkylamine derivatives—

Chlorpheniramine (Chlor-Trimeton)

The foregoing provides examples rather than a complete chemical classification. The chemical type is not ordinarily considered in selecting an antihistamine for use in a specific situation. The alkylamines (4) are in widest use because they are effective but less likely to cause depression than other types.

The chemical classification does reemphasize that there is considerable arbitrariness in classifying drugs within the tranquilizer-antihistamine-parasympatholytic group. Diphenhydramine hydrochloride (Benadryl), for example, is classed an "antihistamine" because of its most common clinical usage, but it has important atropine-like actions and causes sedation like a "tranquilizer." It is also a more potent local anesthetic than procaine and has been used in the treatment of parkinsonism and cardiac arrhythmias. A different salt, the chlorotheophyllinate (Dramamine), is widely used to prevent motion sickness.

Absorption, Metabolism, & Excretion

The antihistamines are all well absorbed after oral administration. This action begins as soon as they are absorbed—ie, 10–30 minutes after an oral dose. They are metabolized by both liver and kidney. Most antihistamines act for about 4 hours and are administered 4 times daily. Some antihistamines—eg, promethazine or chlorcyclizine—are excreted more slowly, and may be given at 12-hour intervals.

Pharmacologic Actions

A. Mechanisms of Action: The antihistamines have multiple effects and may act through several mechanisms. Their primary effect is competitive antagonism to histamine. The antigen-antibody reaction or other histamine-liberating stimulus is unaltered, but histamine is prevented from acting on the effector organ. The relation is competitive, ie, enough histamine can overcome the blockade of a given amount of antihistamine. In combating an acute allergic reaction (eg, laryngeal edema or bronchiolar constriction), an antihistamine may block any further effect of histamine, but, lacking any effect of its own, it cannot immediately repair the damage. In contrast to this competitive antagonism of histamine is the action of a physiologic antagonist which, by an action of its own that is opposite in direction to that of histamine, can immediately repair the lesion and reverse the clinical course. Epinephrine and other sympathomimetics are physiologic antagonists of histamine.

When dosage is controlled, the histamine-antagonizing effect can be specific—ie, the response of smooth muscle or other effector to histamine is blocked by concentrations of an antihistamine that do not block the action of acetylcholine or other agonists. With larger concentrations, the acetylcholine blocking action interferes and the even greater concentrations possible in laboratory experiments block the reaction of smooth muscle to almost all stimulants.

B. Effects:

1. Histamine antagonism—With the exception of the stimulation of gastric acid secretion, the effects of histamine described above are prevented or reduced when an antihistamine is administered. After pretreatment with an antihistamine, the organism no longer responds to injected histamine (or histamine derived from mast cell disruption) by a fall in blood pressure, bronchiolar constriction, or laryngeal or other edema. In theory, the relation being competitive, the histamine effects could be completely blocked. In practice, the amount of antihistamine that can be administered is limited by side-effects and toxic reactions, and protection may not be absolute.

• **2. CNS effects**—In the usual therapeutic doses, the antihistamines cause the specific kind of depression or sedation described for the antipsychotic tranquilizers (see Chapter 25). Unlike the euphoriant effect of alcohol or other sedative-hypnotics, the behavioral change is generally perceived as unpleasant by the patient.

In a few patients, even therapeutic doses cause restlessness and hyperactivity—evidence that the underlying neurophysiologic change is stimulation rather than depression. With toxic doses, signs of stimulation (including convulsions) accompany the sedation more frequently than is the case with the tranquilizers. Extrapyramidal signs are not seen. They are thus exactly comparable to atropine or other parasympatholytic agents. The CNS effects are unrelated to their histamine-antagonizing properties.

3. Other effects—The antihistamines are topically active local anesthetics, atropine-like or parasympatholytics, and have quinidine-like effects that are used investigationally in the treatment of cardiac arrhythmias.

Clinical Uses

A. Some Immediate Allergic Reactions: The antihistamines are useful against only a few of the many manifestations of the allergic reaction. They are most consistently effective in some of the allergic reactions that are immediate in the immunochemical sense and acute in the clinical sense. Vasodilatation and edema, similar to the effects described for histamine, are prominent in the immediate allergic reaction.

1. Anaphylaxis—Anaphylaxis is important not only because it presents an acute treatment problem but also because it provides an experimental analogue of clinical acute allergic reactions. Anaphylaxis occurs when the antigen-antibody complex acts to liberate histamine, serotonin, and heparin from (tissue) mast cells or (circulating) basophils and from platelets. The signs of the anaphylactic reaction vary among different species depending upon their reaction to histamine and upon the amounts of histamine or serotonin available for release. In humans, histamine and heparin (but not serotonin) are released and urticaria, bronchial spasm, laryngeal edema, and hypotension are prominent.

The antihistamines can completely protect experimental animals against anaphylaxis, and anaphylaxis in the human could presumably be prevented or modified by adequate prior doses of an antihistamine. However, the treatment of this emergency is not with antihistamines but with the sympathomimetics that are physiologic antagonists to histamine. The antihistamines could only prevent further histamine effects, but respiratory obstruction and shock would be lethal before the histamine effects already present had dissipated. An acute anaphylactic reaction, therefore, is treated by injection of epinephrine in doses of 0.3–0.6 mg IM or IV. When there is reason to fear that an anaphylactic reaction may occur when medical care is not available, the patient may be provided with isoproterenol to be used sublingually or by inhalation.

2. Urticaria and angioneurotic edema—The swelling, redness, and itching of hives are reduced by the antihistamines. It may be desirable to reinforce these effects with a sympathomimetic such as ephedrine.

3. Serum sickness—Serum sickness today is as often a reaction to a nonprotein drug such as penicillin as to a biologic product such as tetanus antitoxin. The reaction occurs after a sensitization period of 1 to nearly 3 weeks. The signs and symptoms—ie, urticaria, fever, adenopathy, arthralgia, and vasculitis—may be transient or may persist for a week or more until all of the antigen is utilized. The antihistamines modify the severity of reaction in many cases, but supplementary treatment—eg, ephedrine or corticosteroids—is usually required.

4. Hay fever—Acute allergic rhinitis, especially if it is seasonal or otherwise clearly related to a specific antigen, usually responds dramatically to the antihistamines. Chronic nasopharyngeal congestion—eg, chronic sinusitis—is not often allergic in origin and, when it is, an infection secondary to the initial allergic process may also be present; therefore, it is much less likely to respond. A trial of antihistamine treatment may be justified, but the continued use of an antihistamine without evidence of therapeutic response or the routine combination of an antihistamine with a nasal decongestant of the sympathomimetic type is not rational.

5. Other immediate reactions—Precipitating antibodies cannot be demonstrated in association with atopic allergic reactions. The circulating antibodies (reagins) in this group are skin-sensitizing and can be demonstrated by passive transfer. Acute allergic rhinitis (see above) responds to treatment with the antihistamines, but other reactions in this group do not. These include atopic dermatitis and autoimmune or collagen diseases.

A rare patient with asthma that is an episodic reaction to a specific antigen is comparable to the patient with hay fever and is benefited by treatment with the antihistamines. In general, asthma is felt to be a contraindication to the use of antihistamines because of the atropine-like effects that cause drying of bronchial secretions.

The anti-inflammatory steroids will suppress all inflammatory reactions, including both immediate and delayed allergic reactions. The mechanism of this effect (see Chapter 35) is not related to histamine antagonism.

6. Reactions of the delayed type—Reactions of the delayed type are associated with cellular immunity rather than serum antibodies. The reaction is delayed after contact with the allergen, and the pathologic reaction is one of infiltration by immune cells and chronic inflammation. Histamine is in no way involved. Examples of this type of reaction are the reaction to skin test antigens or to the sensitizing substance of poison ivy. The antihistamines do not influence any of those conditions. The anti-inflammatory steroids suppress this type of inflammation.

B. Motion Sickness: The parasympatholytic drugs, the antihistamines, and the phenothiazine tranquilizers all have a central depressant action that is useful in preventing or treating motion sickness. The

discussion is placed in this chapter because the agents most commonly used in treatment or prevention are antihistamines or are chemically related to them.

Motion sickness occurs when changes in acceleration continuously stimulate the hair cells of the maculae and, to a lesser extent, the cristae of the semicircular canals. The afferent activity, conditioned by individual and environmental factors, results in malaise, nausea, and vomiting.

The ability of a drug to prevent motion sickness is not correlated with its potency as a peripheral antihistamine or parasympatholytic nor with its potency as a tranquilizer. The most widely used drugs, therefore, are selected because they have few atropine-like or sedative side-effects.

Owing to the interest of the armed forces, many field studies and clinical trials evaluating drugs against motion sickness are available. The studies vary in their control of the variables involved, but Fig 19–2 illustrates that, when the principles of bioassay are applied, the data are as precise as in most laboratory evaluations. Unfortunately, such data are available only for scopolamine.

The effectiveness of drugs will vary with individual susceptibility, the intensity and duration of the motion, the interval between medication and onset of motion, dosage, and whether effectiveness is measured by a subjective report or the objective occurrence of vomiting. Percentage figures for effectiveness are, therefore, meaningful only if the situation is carefully described. In general, the following drugs are effective in the dosages listed:

1. Cyclizine (Marezine),* 50 mg 3 times daily.
2. Meclizine (Bonine),* 50 mg 1–3 times daily.
3. Dimenhydrinate (Dramamine),* 25–50 mg 3–4 times daily. (High incidence of sedation.)
4. Promethazine (Phenergan), 25 mg 3 times daily, is effective if the first dose is given 2–4 hours before motion begins.
5. Scopolamine, 0.6–1 mg in 1 dose at onset of motion. In many studies involving motion of brief duration, scopolamine appears most effective. If the dose must be repeated 2–3 times daily—ie, for long-continued motion—it is relatively less effective and causes more side-effects than other available drugs.
6. Amphetamine may be given with any of the above to counteract sedation. In some experimental situations (human centrifuge), it is active by itself.

C. Ineffective Against the Common Cold: Though the efficacy of the antihistamines in the common cold has never been shown, it is obvious from sales figures of both prescription and nonprescription preparations that it is the advertising agencies rather than the clinical pharmacologist who endorse the use of these preparations.

Beginning in 1947, there appeared a series of poorly controlled studies reporting that antihistamines cured the common cold in 85–100% of cases. These

---

*Available without prescription and usually more expensive if ordered by prescription.

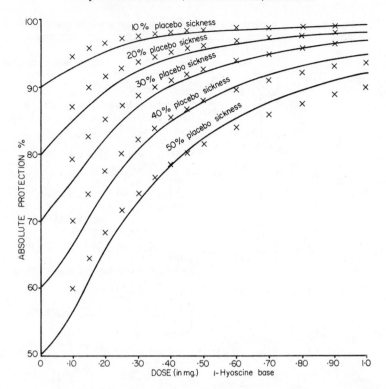

FIG 19–2. Illustration of the protection against motion sickness afforded by the prior administration of scopolamine. This figure also illustrates the great precision achieved in a clinical trial if the principles of bioassay are followed. Data from various published studies utilizing several different situations are combined to provide a dose/effect curve. An objective quantal response is recorded—ie, vomiting or no vomiting. Crosses represent the change in pattern when only the data from trials in small ships are plotted. (Reproduced, with permission, from Brand & Perry: Drugs used in motion sickness. Pharmacol Rev 18:905, 1966.)

trials were not double-blind; assignments to control or treated groups were not random; and the diagnosis was established on the basis of the patient's statements. Subsequent studies that utilized the most elementary controls were unable to verify any action of the antihistamines on the duration, severity, or incidence of colds.

The common preparations are mixtures containing not only the antihistamine but also a sympathomimetic which, depending upon the amine chosen and the dose, may or may not be effective as a nasal decongestant (see Chapter 10). Aspirin or aspirin compound and cough suppressants may also be included in the mixture. The current PDR lists over 60 such preparations as "cold preparations" or "cough-cold preparations," and other mixtures of such "expensive aspirin" are available without prescription.

D. Over-the-Counter Sleeping Tablets: Several antihistamines and belladonna alkaloids may be included in proprietary medications sold without a prescription. Several of these preparations are sold as bedtime sleeping medications, and some are as effective as the usual 100 mg of a short-acting barbiturate when used to induce sleep. The sedation that is judged unpleasant during the day is not a problem at night.

There is no justification for use of the tranquilizer-like properties of the antihistamines to relieve anxiety.

Adverse Reactions
A. Side-Effects: The most common side-effect is "drowsiness" or "sedation." This sedation is similar to that caused by the phenothiazine tranquilizers rather than that caused by the barbiturates or other sedative-hypnotic agents. Depending upon the patient, the antihistamine selected, and the dose or preparation used, the incidence of "drowsiness" may vary from 2–50% of patients. Most patients find the sensation unpleasant and may complain of tiredness or dizziness. This drowsiness may be ignored or may even be advantageous when the medication is given at bedtime or when it is desirable to reduce activity.

Very rarely, a symptom of CNS stimulation—eg, nervousness or insomnia—may be reported.

Of the atropine-like side-effects, dry mouth is the most common. Blurred vision, urinary retention, palpitations, and constipation are rare but do occur with higher doses.

B. Acute (Overdosage) Toxicity: Serious toxicity in the adult is rarely encountered. Children may be attracted to the colorful tablets found in many homes

TABLE 19–2. Antihistamines: Dosages and preparations available.

	Single Adult Dose	Preparations Available
Potent; sedation infrequent		
Chlorpheniramine (Chlor-Trimeton, Teldrin)	4 mg	Tablets, 4 mg Sustained action tablets, 8 and 12 mg Injectable (IM or IV), 10 mg/ml, 1, 10, and 20 ml; 100 mg/ml, 2 and 10 ml
Dechlorpheniramine (Polaramine)	2 mg	Tablets, 2 mg Sustained action tablets, 4 and 6 mg Syrup, 2 mg/5 ml
Brompheniramine (Dimetane)	4 mg	Tablets, 4 mg Sustained action tablets, 8 and 12 mg Elixir, 2 mg/5 ml Injectable, 10 mg/ml (IM, subcut, or IV), 1 ml; 100 mg/ml (IM or subcut only), 2 ml
Dexbrompheniramine (Disomer)	2 mg	Sustained action tablets, 4 and 6 mg
Carbinoxamine (Clistin)	4 mg	Tablets, 4 mg Sustained action tablets, 8 and 12 mg Elixir, 4 mg/5 ml
Triprolidine* (Actidil)	2.5 mg	Tablets, 2.5 mg Syrup, 1.25 mg/5 ml
Chlorcyclizine*	50 mg	Tablets, 50 mg
Dimethindene (Forhistal, Triten)	2 mg	Tablets, 1 mg Sustained action tablets, 2.5 mg Syrup, 1 mg/5 ml Pediatric drops, 0.5 mg/0.6 ml
Cyproheptadine (Periactin)	4 mg	Tablets, 4 mg Syrup, 2 mg/5 ml
Pyrrobutamine (Pyronil)	15 mg	Tablets, 15 mg
Potent; sedation often prominent		
Diphenhydramine (Benadryl)	50 mg	Capsules, 25 and 50 mg Elixir, 10 mg/4 ml Injectable (IV or IM), 10 mg/ml, 10 and 30 ml; 50 mg/ml, 1 ml
Bromodiphenhydramine (Ambodryl)	25 mg	Capsules, 25 mg Elixir, 10 mg/4 ml Injectable (IM or IV), 5 mg/ml, 10 ml
Tripelennamine (Pyribenzamine)	50 mg	Tablets, 25 and 50 mg Sustained action tablets, 50 and 100 mg Elixir, 30 mg/4 ml Injectable, 25 mg/ml, 1 and 10 ml
Pyrilamine, mepyramine (Neo-Antergan)	50 mg	Tablets, 25 and 50 mg Timed release capsules, 75 mg
Promethazine*† (Phenergan)	25 mg	Tablets, 12.5, 25, and 50 mg Syrup, 6.25 mg/5 ml; 25 mg/5 ml Suppositories, 25 and 50 mg Injectable (IM or IV), 25 mg/ml, 1 and 10 ml; 50 mg/ml, 1 and 10 ml
Less potent; less sedative		
Antazoline (Antistine)	. . .	Ophthalmic, 0.5%, 15 ml
Phenindamine (Thephorin, and in many proprietaries)	25 mg	Tablets, 25 mg
Thonzylamine (Anahist, and in many proprietaries)	50–100 mg	Tablets, 25 and 50 mg
Methapyrilene (Histadyl, and in many proprietaries)	50–100 mg	Capsules, 25 and 50 mg Syrup, 20 mg/5 ml Drops, 16 mg/ml, 25 ml Injectable, 25 mg/ml, 10 ml; 20 mg/ml, 10 ml

*These longer-acting drugs are given twice daily; the others, 3–4 times daily.

†Phenothiazine derivatives (see also Table 25–3).

and are more susceptible. A recent review collected 17 fatal cases of antihistamine toxicity, 13 of which were in children. What fraction of the total cases of deaths due to antihistamines this represents is not known.

The expected drowsiness may progress to coma, often with a period of restlessness or excitement at some time. The coma may—unexpectedly, unless one recalls that these drugs are related to the tranquilizers—be preceded by preconvulsant jerks or progress to actual convulsions. Respiratory depression may also occur with huge doses. Atropine-like effects are also seen: dilated pupils, tachycardia, and a red, hot, dry skin.

There is no specific treatment, and symptomatic treatment should not be too vigorous. The convulsions are probably not so threatening as the additional depression caused by efforts to control the convulsions with thiopental or similar drugs.

C. Allergic Reactions: These drugs, used in the treatment of allergic reactions, may act as sensitizing agents and cause dermatitis when applied to the skin as creams or ointments. Only isolated reports of serious systemic reactions—eg, agranulocytosis—have appeared.

Contraindications & Cautions

The labeling of antihistamines sold without a prescription must bear a warning against driving or operating machinery while using the drugs since they may cause drowsiness. The patient receiving antihistamines by prescription should perhaps receive the same warning. However, many patients using antihistamines chronically do drive and work and there is no epidemiologic evidence that this group is involved in an unusual number of accidents. Anecdotal evidence from individual cases is undependable because of the tendency to use any prescribed drug retrospectively as an excuse for a mishap or as a cover for the effect of alcohol or other clearly dangerous drugs. The effects of the antihistamines are additive to those of other tranquilizers or other sedative-hypnotics.

If a patient reports undue sedation, the dosage should be reduced or a different antihistamine tried. If necessary, amphetamine or a related sympathomimetic stimulant may be given to combat the sedation.

Preparations & Dosages

A. Therapeutic Classification: (Table 19–2.) The antihistamines can be classified according to the degree of sedation anticipated as a side-effect, their potency, and their duration of action. Patients vary in their reaction to the antihistamines but generally prefer one of the less sedating drugs—eg, chlorpheniramine, the most widely prescribed antihistamine, or related compound. The advantage of the longer-acting drugs (8 rather than 4 hours) is most apparent when they are given at bedtime.

B. Topical Application: None of the available antihistamine creams or ointments are active when applied to the intact skin. Applied to the denuded skin, they act more because of their local anesthetic effect and the physical properties of the preparation (cream or other base) than because they are antihistamines.

C. Cyproheptadine: Cyproheptadine (Periactin) is promoted as a serotonin antagonist (see below) as well as a histamine antagonist. Several other antihistamines have the same limited antiserotonin property, and there is no evidence that this is related to their therapeutic effects. Unlike chlorpheniramine, the other antihistamine with which it was compared, cyproheptadine does increase appetite and leads to increased weight gain and linear growth in children. Unfortunately, comparison with a tranquilizer is not available.

SEROTONIN

Serotonin (5-hydroxytryptamine, 5-HT, enteramine) is not a therapeutic agent but is important in relation to the action of other drugs and several disease states. Important physiologic functions have been suggested for it, but the establishment of any one of these roles awaits additional experimental analysis.

Chemistry

A. Synthesis: Serotonin is synthesized from dietary tryptophan by hydroxylation and decarboxylation (Fig 19–3). The synthesis occurs at all of the storage sites except the platelets, which take up preformed serotonin.

B. Distribution: The largest fraction (90%) of serotonin in the body is synthesized and stored in the argentaffin or enterochromaffin cells of the mucosa of the gastrointestinal tract. It is also stored in platelets and released by platelet disintegration and is, therefore, found in serum and in the spleen. In some species (but not man), it is found in the granules of mast cells and liberated concurrently with histamine. Serotonin occurs in some invertebrates and is a chemical mediator in some molluscs. One banana contains several milligrams of serotonin—enough to elevate urinary levels of its metabolite, 5-hydroxyindoleacetic acid (5-HIAA), and interfere with diagnostic tests for carcinoid.

However, the fraction of serotonin that has occasioned most current interest is that in the CNS. Here its occurrence parallels that of norepinephrine—ie, concentrations are greatest in the hypothalamus and mesencephalon. However, even here the concentration does not exceed 1 μg/gm, compared with 2–15 μg/gm in the gastrointestinal tract, 0.1–0.2 μg/ml of blood, and 2 mg/gm of carcinoid tissue.

C. Metabolism: Serotonin is oxidatively deaminated to 5-HIAA. No alternate pathway comparable to the methylation of catecholamines is present to cooperate in terminating the action. However, in the pineal gland, N-acetylation and 5-methylation produce melatonin.

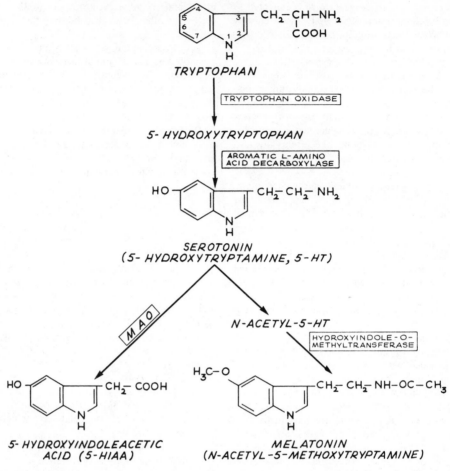

FIG 19–3. Synthesis and metabolism of serotonin. Note that the same enzyme catalyzes the decarboxylation of 5-hydroxytryptophan to serotonin and dopa to dopamine.

Pharmacologic Effects

A. Mechanisms of Action: As is true of many drugs, serotonin has multiple and sometimes conflicting actions. These include the augmentation of afferent activity from chemoreceptors, 2 direct actions on smooth muscle, and an excitatory or stimulant effect on the CNS. Serotonin may have multiple mechanisms of action, or these effects may all be due to the demonstrated depolarizing action on cell membranes.

B. Effects:

1. Cardiovascular and respiratory—Serotonin can cause an immediate fall in blood pressure accompanied by bradycardia; a rise in blood pressure accompanied by tachycardia; and a prolonged fall in blood pressure. Which of these effects is predominant depends upon the method of administration (rapid intravenous injection or infusion), dosage, and other factors. The use of blocking agents allows each effect to be demonstrated in each species.

a. Reflexly generated effect—The rapid intravenous injection of serotonin is followed by a fall in blood pressure; a paradoxical bradycardia—ie, slowing rather than the tachycardia expected to accompany a fall in blood pressure; and a complex change in respira-

tion. This combination of changes, often referred to as the Bezold or Bezold-Jarisch triad, was mentioned above (Chapter 12) in explaining the action of the veratrum alkaloids. The drug sensitizes peripheral chemo- and pressoreceptors, and the increased afferent activity reaching the brain stem augments vagal and decreases sympathetic tone. In the case of serotonin, 3 areas are sensitized or 3 reflexes initiated. The **coronary chemoreflex** depends upon receptors located in the distribution of the left coronary artery. These receptors are not necessarily within the myocardium but may lie in relation to the pulmonary artery dorsal to the heart. The bradycardia and hypotension are blocked by severing the afferent pathway (by vagal section) or the efferent arm of the reflex by hexamethonium or other ganglion blocking agents. Atropine will block only the bradycrotic effect. A **pulmonary depressor reflex** due to stimulation of chemoreceptors in the pulmonary circulation augments the fall in blood pressure. A **pulmonary respiratory chemoreflex** inhibits respiration, but stimulation of carotid sinus receptors may cause hyperpnea. The change in respiration is thus variable but consists typically of brief apnea followed by an increased respiratory rate.

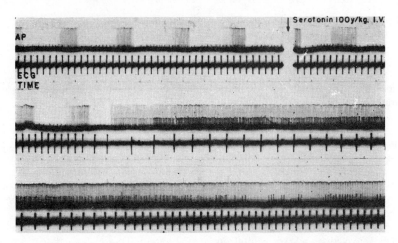

FIG 19–4. Effect of serotonin on action potentials recorded from a single afferent vagal fiber active with inspiration. The record is from a cat maintained with artificial respiration. Time is in seconds. Eight seconds after the intravenous injection of serotonin (at arrow), bradycardia started abruptly. Simultaneously, additional, smaller action potentials of undetermined origin appeared. Nine seconds after the injection of serotonin, a continuous flow of action potentials occurred on pulmonary afferent vagus fibers. As the bradycardia subsided, the smaller spikes disappeared whereas pulmonary afferent fibers still showed a continuous flow of action potentials. (Reproduced, with permission, from Schneider & Yonkman: Action of serotonin [5-hydroxytryptamine] on vagal afferent impulses in the cat. Am J Physiol 174:131, 1953.)

The receptors adapt rapidly, and the reflex effect is usually followed in a fraction of a minute by a pressor effect.

b. Pressor effect—Following the period of hypotension, or if the above reflex effects are abolished by pretreatment with hexamethonium, serotonin causes an epinephrine-like pressor effect. The rise in blood pressure is accompanied by an increase in heart rate, cardiac output, and blood glucose levels and is prevented by alpha-adrenergic blocking agents. Serotonin is also qualitatively similar to epinephrine in elevating pressures on the right side of the circulation, but is relatively more potent. Tachyphylaxis (acute tolerance) to the pressor effect develops after only a few injections.

c. Prolonged fall in blood pressure—A constant intravenous infusion of serotonin, perhaps the experimental situation most closely analogous to release of endogenous serotonin, causes a prolonged fall in blood pressure due to vasodilatation. Cardiac output is increased during the infusion. The exact mechanism is not known.

2. Other smooth muscle—Nonvascular smooth muscle is stimulated by serotonin. The bronchiolar constriction and increased intestinal motility that result are clinically important. The action on other smooth muscle—eg, the uterus—is not important in the intact animal, but the stimulation of isolated tissue provides a basis for assaying this effect of serotonin.

3. CNS—See below.

Relation to Physiologic & Pathologic Processes

A. Possible Chemical Mediation in CNS: The demonstration that serotonin is found in the hypothal-

amus and a few other areas of the brain and the finding that the effect of reserpine is accompanied by a decreased concentration of serotonin in those areas led to the plausible hypothesis that serotonin is a mediator of transsynaptic conduction in the CNS or, at least, a modulator of transmission. The evidence for this hypothesis is indirect and incomplete.

It has even been difficult to establish that the presumed mediator exerts a stimulant rather than a depressant effect. The concentrations of serotonin and norepinephrine often vary together—eg, after MAO inhibition or reserpine—and depletion experiments cannot distinguish between the effects of a decrease in the concentration of bound serotonin and the related high local concentration of free amine. Furthermore, much of the research on serotonin was done before the importance of dopamine was recognized.

Serotonin is a neurotransmitter in some invertebrate phyla, but no role has yet been established for it in the vertebrate nervous system, and the early hypotheses relating it to psychotic or other behavior have not been supported.

B. Carcinoid Tumors: Neoplasms that arise from argentaffin cells are always "functional" in the sense that they synthesize and store serotonin. The serotonin liberated by the primary carcinoid tumor of the gastrointestinal tract is small in amount and destroyed during its passage through the liver. Primary ileal tumors may metastasize to the liver, and the serotonin from the larger tumor mass enters the hepatic veins rather than the portal bed. In this situation (and in rare cases of bronchial adenoma), the circulating serotonin causes a characteristic syndrome consisting of diarrhea, asthma (bronchiolar constriction), and cutaneous flushing.

These signs occur paroxysmally and may be precipitated by eating, emotion, exertion, or pressure on a tumor mass. They can be duplicated by infusions of serotonin. In addition, subendocardial fibrosis leads to pulmonary valve stenosis and tricuspid insufficiency. The diagnosis depends in part upon the demonstration of large amounts of the serotonin metabolite, 5-hydroxyindoleacetic acid, in the urine.

Bradykinin also produces vasodilatation and a flush, and in some cases of carcinoid elevated bradykinin levels have been demonstrated during episodes of flushing.

The expectation that this syndrome could be ameliorated pharmacologically has not been realized. Of the serotonin antagonists discussed below, only phenoxybenzamine and chlorpromazine (alpha-adrenergic blockers) are active and are helpful only against the flush. Prednisolone may slow the course of the right-sided heart disease. The debilitating diarrhea can be controlled with atropine or by slowing the synthesis of serotonin by the administration of parachlorphenylalanine.

Parachlorphenylalanine (PCPA, Fenclonine) is an investigative drug and laboratory tool that inhibits tryptophan hydroxylase and interrupts serotonin synthesis by interfering with the rate-limiting step in the reactions shown in Fig 19–3. Parachloramphetamine (PCA) and parachlormethamphetamine (PCMA) are more satisfactory depletors of brain serotonin but have not yet improved the management of patients with carcinoid syndrome or contributed to the analysis of the CNS effects of serotonin.

C. Endomyocardial Fibrosis: In those areas of Africa where bananas and plantains are prominent in the diet—ie, where the diet is high in serotonin and dopamine—endocardial thickening occurs. The population affected does not metabolize serotonin as rapidly as control groups because of some coexisting chronic disease.

SEROTONIN ANTAGONISTS

An antagonist to serotonin would be potentially as important an analytical tool and therapeutic agent as atropine. This fact has perhaps generated enthusiasm for compounds and hypotheses not yet justified by the data available.

Effects

Serotonin has, as emphasized above, multiple physiologic and pharmacologic effects. In speaking of a serotonin antagonist, it is necessary to specify the serotonin action antagonized; and antagonism of one action does not imply action against all serotonin effects. It is probable that the search should be for multiple types of serotonin antagonists, just as 3 types of antagonists to acetylcholine have been defined.

The indoleethylamine, serotonin, has some effects comparable to those of a phenylethylamine such as epinephrine. Cardiac stimulation, vasoconstriction, and

the contractors of the estrogen pretreated rat uterus are blocked by phenoxybenzamine or other alpha-adrenergic blocking agents whether the stimulus is serotonin or epinephrine. These and a few other isolated tissue responses are the type of actions blocked by serotonin antagonists as currently defined.

Examples

A. Lysergic Acid Diethylamide (LSD): (See also Chapter 7.) LSD was among the first compounds other than known alpha-adrenergic blockers to be used in the laboratory as a serotonin antagonist. This action was related to its ability to cause a toxic psychosis (also called a model psychosis or hallucinatory state), and theories explaining the origin of the psychoses were propounded. However, other ergot derivatives—eg, 2-bromo-LSD—are more potent serotonin antagonists (in vitro) but lack the behavioral effects in humans.

B. Methysergide (Sansert) is discussed with other ergot alkaloids used in the treatment of migraine. It is the most potent antiserotonin of all the ergot derivatives, but is also potent enough as a vasoconstrictor to be effective (and dangerous) in the treatment of migraine.

C. Cyproheptadine (Periactin) is an ordinary antihistamine and, in tests on isolated tissues, an antiserotonin (as are many other antihistamines also). The demonstration that it is a serotonin antagonist in the intact animal is actually a demonstration of the development of tachyphylaxis to repeated injections of serotonin. It is nevertheless wrongly alleged to have special properties owing to its antiserotonin action.

OTHER DERIVATIVES OF TRYPTAMINE

Exogenous serotonin has negligible CNS effects because it does not reach the parenchymal cells of the CNS. Derivatives of tryptamine that are less polar enter the CNS more easily, and several are hallucinogenic.

Tryptamine itself is generally similar to serotonin but is a convulsant.

DMT and **DET** (N,N-dimethyl- and N,N-diethyltryptamine) are hallucinogenic if given by injection or smoked. Their action differs from that of LSD in that more sympathomimetic side-effects occur and the duration of action is less than 1 hour.

Psilocybin is derived from psilocine, or 4-hydroxydimethyltryptamine, by phosphorylation of the 4-hydroxyl group. It is isolated from a mushroom, *Psilocybe mexicana,* used by Mexican Indians for its hallucinogenic effect.

Bufotenine or **dimethylserotonin** is isolated from the secretions of toad skin and from the seeds of a plant, *Piptadenia peregrina,* used as snuff by some South American Indians. It is hallucinogenic after injection.

There is no evidence that methoxylation or N-methylation of serotonin occurs in the body to generate a psychotogenic substance.

• • •

General References

Histamine

Thompson, W.L., & R.P. Walton: Elevation of plasma histamine levels in the dog following administration of muscle relaxants, opiates and macromolecular polymers. J Pharmacol Exper Therap 143:131–136, 1964.

Weiss, S., Robb, G.P., & L.B. Ellis: The systemic effects of histamine in man. Arch Int Med 49:360–396, 1932.

West, G.B.: Studies on the mechanism of anaphylaxis: A possible basis for a pharmacologic approach to allergy. Clin Pharmacol Therap 4:749–783, 1963.

Wolstenholme, G.E.W., & C.M. O'Connor (editors): *Ciba Foundation Symposium on Histamine.* Little, Brown, 1956.

Antihistamines

Bovet, D.: Introduction to antihistamine agents and Antergan derivatives. Ann New York Acad Sc 50:1089–1126, 1950.

Brand, J.J., & W.L.M. Perry: Drugs used in motion sickness. Pharmacol Rev 18:895–924, 1966.

Burrage, W.S.: Antihistamines: Their use and abuse. New England J Med 245:532–537, 1951.

Lavenstein, A.F., & others: Effects of cyproheptadine on asthmatic children: Study of appetite, weight gain and linear growth. JAMA 180:912–916, 1962.

Serotonin

Keele, C.A., & D. Armstrong: *Substances Producing Pain and Itch.* Williams & Wilkins, 1964.

Robson, J.M., & R.S. Stacey: 5-Hydroxytryptamine. Chap 4, pp 122–155, in: *Recent Advances in Pharmacology,* 3rd ed. Churchill, 1962.

Satterlee, W.G., Serpick, A., & J.R. Bianchine: Carcinoid syndrome: Chronic treatment with *p*-chloro-phenylalanine. Ann Int Med 72:919–921, 1970.

Sjoerdsma, A.: Serotonin. New England J Med 261:181–188, 231–237, 1959.

Part III. Central Nervous System Drugs

20 . . .

General Anesthetics

Surgical anesthesia—abolition of the patient's perception of and reactions to pain—can be produced in 2 ways: **General anesthesia** is accomplished by using the drugs discussed in this chapter to produce unconsciousness; **local, regional,** or **conduction anesthesia** is induced by applying drugs to nerves or nerve roots to block the centripetal conduction of sensation from only a part or region of the body without influencing consciousness.

General anesthesia is further categorized as inhalation or intravenous. **Inhalation anesthesia** (emphasized in the present chapter) is produced by administration through the respiratory tract of gases or volatile liquids. **Intravenous anesthetics** such as thiopental are ultra-short-acting barbiturates and are similar to the barbiturates discussed in Chapter 23.

Chemical Properties

Compounds of many different chemical types can induce general anesthesia. The drugs used as intravenous anesthetics illustrate that the barbiturates and other drugs classed as sedative-hypnotics are general anesthetics. It is usual but slightly misleading to consider the inhalation anesthetics as a separate drug class because of the unusual importance of their physical rather than chemical properties.

Volatile liquids or gases are selected because administration by inhalation permits close control and easy adjustment of the dose and rapid reversibility of effect since the vapor is eliminated in expired air rather than by metabolism in the body.

The inhalation anesthetics in common use include the following chemical types:

A. Ethers: Eg, diethyl ether or methoxyflurane (Penthrane, $Cl_2HC–CF_2–O–CH_3$).

B. Halogenated Hydrocarbons: Eg, chloroform, trichloroethylene, halothane ($F_3C–CHClBr$). One of the few structure-action generalizations that is possible is that halogenated hydrocarbons are very apt to sensitize the myocardium to the ability of epinephrine to cause ventricular arrhythmias. Such a toxic effect is seen not only with inhalation anesthetics but also with compounds primarily of toxicologic interest—eg, carbon tetrachloride and the chlorinated hydrocarbon type of insecticides.

C. Alicyclic Hydrocarbons: Cyclopropane is the only example.

D. Other Hydrocarbons: Ethylene has been used as an anesthetic. Other aliphatic and aromatic hydrocarbons—eg, gasoline, toluene—are toxic or abused substances.

E. One inorganic oxide, nitrous oxide (N_2O).

Physical Properties

A. Flammability and Explosiveness: Most of the halogenated compounds—eg, halothane, methoxyflurane, and chloroform—present no hazard in this regard. Ether, cyclopropane, and other less valuable drugs can be dangerous in the presence of the electrocautery or a spark from a static discharge. Mixtures of nitrous oxide and oxygen are not explosive since both are oxidizing agents. Nitrous oxide will, however, support combustion—eg, mixtures of nitrous oxide and ether are potentially explosive and, in an atmosphere of nitrous oxide and oxygen, fires are of explosive intensity.

B. Uptake and Elimination: The initial or induction stages of anesthesia described below may pass rapidly and pleasantly for the patient or may be prolonged and unpleasant. A stormy induction period inherent in an agent to be used as the definitive anesthetic is avoided by heavy premedication or by first using a more suitable agent for induction. Nevertheless, consideration of uptake and elimination in terms of induction and recovery is a useful way to outline the physical factors involved in the transport or distribution of inhalation anesthetics.

Intravenous anesthetics establish a maximum blood level immediately upon injection and are carried in large amounts to the brain and other tissues with a high blood flow. Inhalation anesthetics are distributed in several compartments—ie, inspired air, alveolar air, blood, brain, and various other tissues. The equilibration rate between successively traversed compartments depends upon the relative solubility of the agent in the 2 compartments and blood flow through one of the compartments. The rates of equilibration determine how rapidly the partial pressure of the gas in the CNS reaches anesthetic levels—ie, equilibrates with anesthetic levels of agent in inspired air. Some physical properties of anesthetics relevant to the following discussion are shown in Table 20–1.

1. In the lung—Some agents (eg, ether) have a high blood-air partition coefficient—ie, solubility in blood is great compared with the solubility in air. Equilibration between blood and air will be slow

TABLE 20–1. Physical properties of several inhalation anesthetics.

| | Flammable and Explosive | Concentrations for Surgical Anesthesia | | Partition Coefficients | | | Clearance Rate of Blood Passing Lung* (% Alveolar Tension) |
		Inhaled Concentration (Vol%)	Blood Level (mg/ 100 ml)	Blood / Air	Brain / Blood	Oil (Fat) / Blood	
Ether	Yes	5–10	130–150	12–15	1.1	5.4	5
Halothane	No	1–3	5–25	2.3	2.6	97	26
Cyclopropane	Yes	10–25	10–20	0.42	1.3	26.7	66
Nitrous oxide	No	80–85	30–50	0.47	1.1	3	63

*Percentage equilibrium between inspired gas tension and tension in pulmonary capillary blood achieved in one passage through the lung during induction.

because the blood will quickly empty the lung; the amount of agent available for transfer to the blood is limited by the rate and depth of respiration and the concentration of drug in inspired air. If the agent is highly soluble in blood, its partial pressure in alveolar air falls rapidly to zero, but, since the blood can take up such a large amount of gas, the partial pressure in blood is elevated by only a small increment of the eventual partial pressure upon equilibration. With such an agent, induction is very slow and recovery will be correspondingly protracted.

2. **In the CNS**—Equilibration between blood and brain is rapid because solubility in the 2 tissues is similar.

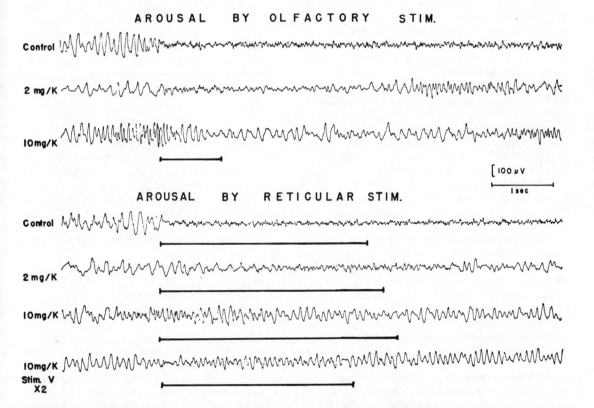

FIG 20–1. The effect of a general anesthetic on the cortical arousal that follows brief afferent stimulation that is projected diffusely to the cortex through the RAS. Electrocorticogram from a curarized rabbit. Stimulation by clove oil (above) and direct excitation of brain stem reticular formation (below). EEG arousal (lower voltage, higher frequency waves, and desynchronization) follows stimulation in the control records but is reduced by small doses of a general anesthetic. The agent used in this experiment was sodium pentobarbital, but ether and other agents act similarly. (Reproduced, with permission, from Arduini & Arduini: Effect of drugs and metabolic alterations on brain stem arousal mechanism. J Pharmacol Exper Therap 110:77, 1954.)

3. In other tissues—Other tissues with a high lipid content would be expected to take up disproportionate amounts of anesthetics with a high lipid solubility—eg, ether or halothane. Accumulation of large amounts of anesthetic in fat does occur, but blood flow through such tissue is low and the process is, therefore, slow. The longer anesthesia is continued with ether or halothane, the greater the amount sequestered in fat. During recovery, this pool of anesthetic will only slowly equilibrate with blood because of the high oil/blood partition coefficient. During induction, however, the high cerebral blood flow carries greater absolute amounts of agent to the brain.

Pharmacologic Effects

A. Mechanisms of Action:

1. Theories—Most of the substances commonly used as general anesthetics (but by no means most of the substances capable of producing general anesthesia) are not metabolized by the body and do not react chemically with any body constituents. Indeed, the inert gas xenon can produce anesthesia. Theories attempting to explain the action of anesthetics have, therefore, emphasized physical rather than chemical properties.

Early theories emphasized the general correlation of the lipid solubility of a substance with its anesthetic potency—eg, the Meyer-Overton theory. Solubility in lipid certainly determines access of an agent to specific tissues, but these theories have not led to suggestions about the actual mechanism.

More recent theories are based on the ability of even gases as inert as xenon to form gas hydrates or clathrates. Ordinarily these microcrystals form only at very low temperatures, but the current hypothesis suggests that stability is imparted by CNS proteins and that the alteration of the structure of water in the brain interferes with synaptic transmission.

2. Action on RAS—One of the effects of anesthetics, the loss of consciousness, can be explained by their action in depressing conduction within the ascending reticular activating system (RAS) or midbrain reticular formation. As the sensitivity or threshold to stimulation of the RAS is reduced, the ascending activating influence on the cortex is reduced (Fig 20–1). The electrical activity of the cortex and behavior are then both suppressed. (The EEG consequences of general anesthesia are shown in Fig 20–2.)

General anesthetics produce a generalized, graded depression of all levels of the CNS. Only the loss of consciousness is clearly related to an action on the RAS.

B. Pharmacologic Effects Related to Staging of Anesthesia: The importance of controlling the dosage of an anesthetic—ie, the depth of anesthesia—has led to the adoption of a conventionalized scale for describing the degree or stage of anesthetic action. In practice, many of the suggested observations are obscured by the presence of other drugs, but the agreed upon definitions are extremely useful in describing the effects not only of the general anesthetics but also the seda-

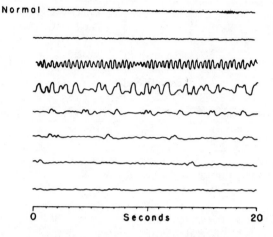

Normal

0   Seconds   20

FIG 20–2. Classification of EEG pattern changes during increasing depth of ether-oxygen or nitrous oxide, oxygen and ether anesthesia of human beings. The first and second patterns occur during induction, the third, fourth, and fifth occurring during light, moderate, and deep surgical anesthesia. The last 2 patterns are seen during excessively deep anesthesia. (Reproduced, with permission, from Faulconer: Correlation of concentrations of ether in arterial blood with electroencephalographic patterns occurring during nitrous oxide, oxygen and ether anesthesia of human surgical patients. Anesthesiology 13:361, 1952.)

tive-hypnotic drugs and alcohol (Chapters 23 and 24). This section will describe the effects involved in defining the stages of anesthesia, which is equivalent to describing the primary pharmacologic effects of the drugs. Other effects, more important in defining the differences among the several agents, are described later.

The stages of anesthesia detailed below and in Table 20–2 are as follows:

Stage 1: Analgesia
Stage 2: Excitement
Stage 3: Surgical anesthesia
Stage 4: Medullary paralysis

The details of the conventionalized description or staging apply to the effects of ether on a patient uninfluenced by premedication or adjuvant drugs. The following description will vary for different anesthetics and will be modified by adjunctive drugs.

The alteration of CNS function by anesthetics follows a pattern characterized as a combination of ascending and descending depression that spares the medulla until large doses are used. This means that depression of the caudal segments of the spinal cord and of the cortex occur earliest. With more intense effects, depression spreads upward through the cord

TABLE 20–2. **Stages and planes of anesthesia. (In = inspiration.)**

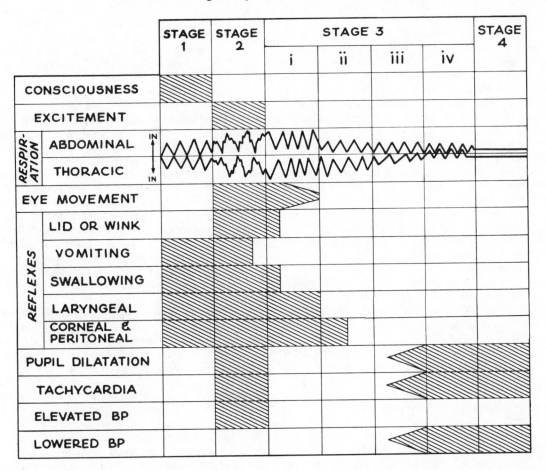

and downward through subcortical and midbrain functions until, eventually, actions on the medulla and cervical cord lead to vasomotor collapse and respiratory arrest. This pattern of depression can be applied to several functions:

1. Behavior and state of consciousness—

a. Stage 1 (analgesia)—The patient remains conscious and responsive, but, with depression of the highest centers and the beginning of disinhibition, he experiences analgesia and euphoria. The analgesia is intense enough to be useful during minor procedures—eg, dental extractions or the second stage of labor. Under certain conditions, even major surgical procedures have been carried out with ether.

Nitrous oxide, ether, and other less commonly used agents produce good analgesia. Halothane is a poor analgesic until consciousness is lost. Thiopental provides poor analgesia even during the equivalent of stage 3—ie, the patient continues to react to painful stimuli. Thiopental in small doses is even said to augment the perception of pain, but the exaggerated response to pain probably represents behavior during the excited stage.

In addition to euphoria, the patient may experience a dream-like state with disordered perceptions that are sometimes described as hallucinations. Dreams or fantasies are probably better terms. A variable degree of amnesia for the events of this stage occurs.

b. Stage 2 (excitement)—With more marked disinhibition—ie, the release of lower centers from the constant inhibitory influence of a higher center—consciousness is lost and the patient becomes excited. He may struggle and shout in a drunken, delirious manner.

Stages 1 and 2 together make up the stage or process of induction. The amount of excitement that takes place is variable depending upon (1) the amount of depressant premedication, (2) the anesthetic agent used, and (3) the amount of external stimulation present. Ether, for example, not only has a long induction period, but its irritant, unpleasant vapors further stimulate the patient. A patient may become quite excited during induction near the operating room but will remain quiet in the recovery room after the operation when the same intensity of drug effect is present.

With adequate premedication and the use of separate agents for induction and maintenance, excitement during induction is now rare. Its occurrence is, however, important in classifying and analyzing drug effects.

Beyond stage 2, responses by the anesthetized patient, even if they involve voluntary muscle, are reflexly generated.

2. Voluntary muscle—As the concentration of anesthetic in the body is increased, contraction of voluntary muscle is weakened and then abolished. The drug acts on the spinal cord or, in the case of muscles innervated by cranial nerves, on the brain stem. Polysynaptic reflexes and tonic nervous outflow to muscle are reduced. Monosynaptic reflexes are persistent and of no value in establishing the depth of anesthesia. Ether has a significant curariform activity in addition to its central effect.

Muscle relaxation determines the ease of exposure of deep structures during surgery. In addition, the pattern of ascending and descending depression of muscle activity is important in describing the changes in respiration with deepening anesthesia. Eye movement—ie, extraocular muscle activity—is also useful in judging the depth of anesthesia.

a. Respiration—

(1) Stage 1—Respiration is not altered during stage 1 unless the agent used is ether or chloroform. These irritant substances may increase the rate and cause some irregularity in pattern, including breath-holding.

(2) Stage 2—During the stage of excitement, the activity of the patient and exaggerated respiratory reflexes may cause a rapid, irregular, and rapidly changing pattern of respiration. As is true for all changes during stage 2, premedication reduces this response.

(3) Stage 3—The entry into stage 3 is marked by the onset of a regular pattern of respiration.

Stage 3 is further divided into 4 planes. In planes i and ii, respiration continues full and regular. (The border between planes i and ii is marked by disappearance of eye movements.) As depression ascends, those segments of the thoracic cord innervating the intercostal muscles are affected first. The diaphragm, which is innervated by the phrenic nerve from cervical segments 3 and 4, is not paralyzed until later.

Plane iii is characterized by incomplete intercostal paralysis. Thoracic movement is reduced and lags behind abdominal (diaphragmatic) movement upon inspiration.

Plane iv begins when intercostal paralysis is complete. The purely abdominal (diaphragmatic) breathing is rapid and shallow. Accessory muscles of respiration (scalenes, sternocleidomastoid) are used. The completely inactive intercostal muscles are not only unable to move the thorax; they are also unable to prevent its inward movement with each inspiration. The paradoxical collapse of the chest with each rising of the abdomen results in "rocking" respiration.

(4) Stage 4—Because of medullary as well as cervical cord depression, no respiratory movements occur in stage 4.

Ether is distinctive in its effect on respiration in that its irritant action stimulates respiration and delays the appearance of respiratory depression. Halothane and cyclopropane cause progressive depression of minute volume through stage 3, and their use requires that respiration be assisted to prevent CO_2 retention. Nitrous oxide does not depress respiration.

b. Extraocular muscles—When the extrinsic muscles of the eye are weakened, they no longer act in a coordinated way and the eyes rove—ie, the globes move slowly and not necessarily symmetrically. Movement is marked during stage 2 and decreases progressively during plane i of stage 3. In plane ii or beyond, both eyes are fixed in the same position but there may be slight convergence or divergence.

c. Other muscles—During stage 1 the muscles are under the usual voluntary control. Some ataxia may be present but is not ordinarily observed. Following the uncontrolled activity of stage 2, the extremities are relaxed but the abdominal and other muscles retain normal tone during plane i. Relaxation during plane ii (without the adjunctive use of curariform drugs) is sufficient for some surgical procedures, but the common intra-abdominal procedures require plane iii.

3. Changes secondary to excitement and asphyxia—

a. Pupillary size—During the excitement stage of induction, sympatho-adrenal discharge increases and the pupils dilate. Following excitement, and throughout planes i and ii, the pupils return to their initial size, which may have been influenced by morphine or atropine used as preanesthetic medication. With the appearance of intercostal paralysis (and assuming that respiration is not assisted by the anesthetist), some CO_2 retention occurs, and sympatho-adrenal stimulation again leads to pupillary dilatation.

b. Pulse rate and blood pressure—During the period of excitement, pulse rate and blood pressure are both elevated just as the pupils are dilated. However, the progressive asphyxial changes of deep anesthesia are accompanied by depression of medullary vasomotor centers. Thus, pulse rate rises but blood pressure falls progressively. Respiration ceases before the heart stops, and, if the patient can be artificially ventilated for a few breaths to remove some of the anesthetic agent, the changes of stage 4 are reversible.

4. Specific reflexes—Several specific reflexes indicate the depth of anesthesia.

a. Lid reflex—The lid "reflex" is present when retraction of the closed lid by the anesthetist evokes active closing or a resistance to opening. It disappears at the border between stages 2 and 3 when the tone of the orbicularis muscle is sufficiently reduced.

b. Swallowing and vomiting—The ability to swallow is lost in the upper part of plane i or, during recovery, is regained at that level. During recovery, vomiting does not occur until a slightly lighter stage—the border between stages 2 and 3—is reached. This order of recovery of the protective reflexes makes anesthesia much safer by reducing the problem of aspiration of vomitus.

c. Laryngeal and pharyngeal—Reaction to stimulation of the pharynx—eg, by an airway—disappears and reappears midway in plane i. Reaction to laryngeal stimulation, important when a tracheal tube is present or is to be inserted, marks the border between planes i and ii. Adjuvant drugs such as succinylcholine permit intubation at a lighter level of anesthesia.

d. Peritoneal—The reflex responsiveness of the patient to peritoneal traction or other stimulation persists until deep in plane ii. Anesthesia must be deep enough to abolish cardiovascular and respiratory responses. The corneal reflex (lid closure in response to touching the corneal conjunctiva) behaves similarly, but testing it adds the hazard of corneal abrasion.

Adverse Effects

Since the therapeutic effect of anesthetics is to produce unconsciousness and loss of perception to pain, the other pharmacologic effects are mostly undesirable. An understanding of these effects is necessary so that the adverse results of anesthesia can be minimized and is important in the selection of the anesthetic to be used from among the various agents available.

A. Cardiovascular Effects: During the stage of excitement and whenever respiratory depression with even minor hypercarbia develops, there is increased release of epinephrine from the adrenal medulla and norepinephrine from sympathetic nerve. Furthermore, as anesthesia deepens, there is vasomotor depression. The consequences of these processes—eg, tachycardia, hypertension during excitement and hypotension with deep anesthesia—have already been mentioned. Epinephrine release and other cardiovascular actions can cause other adverse effects.

1. Blood pressure—Changes in blood pressure should be described as the resultant of changes in cardiac contractility or vasomotor activity. The data needed to allow such a description are not complete or uniformly accepted, especially when mechanisms of action are proposed or the relative importance of several possible factors must be assayed. However, several descriptive statements can be made about the ability of anesthetics to maintain blood pressure or "support the circulation."

Because of the importance of medullary depression, the use of light rather than deep anesthesia is the most important factor in maintenance of blood pressure. Again, the use of a mixture or balance of agents to achieve a satisfactory degree of analgesia and muscular relation allows reduction of the dose of any one of the potent agents.

Cyclopropane is unusual in its ability to maintain or even slightly elevate blood pressure. Cardiac output is elevated—ie, there is some peripheral vasodilatation and maintained tissue perfusion.

Halothane is equally distinctive in the production of hypotension by reduced force of cardiac contractility and peripheral vasodilatation.

2. Cardiac arrhythmias—

a. Atrial rhythmicity—During induction or light anesthesia, especially with chloroform, cyclopropane, and halothane, vagal influence on the heart is greatly increased. Bradycardia, wandering atrial pacemaker, and atrioventricular nodal rhythms result. If the bradycardia is quite marked, it may exaggerate any hypotension present. Adequate premedication with atropine and avoidance of high initial concentrations of the anesthetic agent will minimize this action.

b. Ventricular arrhythmias—The production of ventricular arrhythmias is partially explained by the sensitization of the myocardium to the effects of epinephrine by cyclopropane and halogenated compounds such as halothane and chloroform. Epinephrine release during induction can be avoided by heavy premedication or by using agents that produce induction without excitement.

During deeper anesthesia, ventilation must be assisted when halothane or cyclopropane is used in order to maintain normal P_{CO_2}. Cyclopropane is currently the only agent in wide use that presents a considerable risk of ventricular arrhythmias; if the concentration of cyclopropane is great enough, arrhythmias may appear even without hypercarbia.

B. Hepatotoxicity: Transient impairment of liver function can be demonstrated in 50% of patients receiving general or spinal anesthesia even when the surgical procedure is not intra-abdominal, and is presumably due to hypoxia.

Much more important is the occurrence of fatal hepatic necrosis and the possible risk associated with the use of halothane. When the question of halothane hepatotoxicity was raised, several retrospective studies were done. One massive study concluded that hepatic necrosis within 6 weeks of surgery occurred in one out of every 10,000 administrations (82 out of 856,000) and was unrelated to the anesthetic used. Halothane, especially after repeated administrations, may on rare occasions cause an allergic hepatitis.

C. Effects on Smooth Muscle: In some patients, usually those with a history of asthma, bronchiolar constriction occurs during light anesthesia. Since it is abolished by deeper anesthesia, it is presumed to be reflex in origin.

Uterine contractions during and after delivery are inhibited by light anesthesia with halothane (and chloroform). Other agents have this action only at deeper levels.

Preanesthetic Medication

The pharmacologic preparation of a patient prior to the induction of anesthesia has 2 essential goals: the relief of anxiety and the drying of secretions. In addition, the CNS depression caused by preanesthetic medication adds to the effects of anesthetic agents and facilitates induction.

Preanesthetic medication should not be reduced to a ritual. However, a few typical methods of achieving the following goals can be outlined.

A. Relief of Anxiety: At bedtime on the night before the procedure the patient is given enough of a sedative-hypnotic to ensure a restful night—eg, 100–200 mg of sodium pentobarbital. In the morning, pentobarbital or an equivalent drug may be repeated for its effect in reducing anxiety. Morphine and other narcotic analgesics are regarded by most anesthetists as the best depressants of acute anxiety. About 45 minutes before induction or when the patient is to be moved to the surgical floor, morphine, 8–15 mg subcut, is given in combination with atropine or a similar parasympatholytic drug.

B. Decrease of Secretions: Atropine or scopolamine is an invariable part of preanesthetic medication whatever the agent used. Ether increases secretions of the respiratory tract, but even the normal volume of secretions can be dangerous. A very small amount of secretion (or any other material) can stimulate laryngospasm. Laryngospasm is associated more often with the use of thiopental. It is not a serious threat if the operator is prepared to treat it—if necessary, by giving succinylcholine to relax the larynx.

Premedication with atropine also controls the reflex bradycardia discussed above.

C. Increase of Anesthetic Effect: In the production of balanced anesthesia, the distinction between preanesthetic medication and adjuncts used during anesthesia becomes indistinct—ie, whether heavy premedication with meperidine is given or an intravenous injection of the same narcotic is given following induction, the same goals will be accomplished. These are the production of a deeper level of anesthesia with a mild agent and a reduction in the amount of the inhalation agent required.

ANESTHETIC AGENTS

The objectives of general anesthesia—obliteration of consciousness, blockade of reflex responses to surgical manipulation, and muscular relaxation sufficient for the procedure—are today rarely accomplished with a single agent. The properties of individual agents are discussed below, but they are used in various combinations and with adjunctive drugs to provide "balanced" anesthesia.

For example, induction in a premedicated patient is carried out with thiopental or, less commonly, nitrous oxide. Analgesia is augmented with narcotic analgesics given intravenously. (The availability of narcotic antagonists has made this practice safer.) Muscle relaxation is achieved with curariform or neuromuscular blocking drugs (see Chapter 21). Light anesthesia is maintained with nitrous oxide, or a potent agent—eg, halothane—is added as needed.

Factors influencing the choice of agents and technics include the following:

(1) Patient preference, eg, a bias against regional (spinal) anesthesia and an insistence on rapid induction.

(2) Patient's condition, eg, drugs used preoperatively, presence of shock or hypovolemia.

(3) Nature of the procedure, eg, need for use of electrocautery, degree of muscle relaxation required, intensity of stimulation inherent in the procedure, and estimated duration of the procedure.

Technics of Administering Inhalation Anesthesia

A. Open Drop: A volatile liquid (ethers, chloroform) is administered drop by drop onto the gauze or cloth covering of a wire frame mask applied over the mouth and nose. The inhaled concentration is controlled by the rate of drip.

B. Insufflation: This method consists of blowing anesthetic vapors or gases into the mouth, pharynx, or trachea. Some type of anesthesia machine is required for metering gas flows and vaporizing volatile agents. Insufflation has its greatest usefulness in operations for which a mask cannot be used (eg, tonsillectomy).

C. Nonrebreathing: A nonrebreathing or open technic supplies a continuous fresh supply of anesthetic agent with adequate oxygen through an apparatus which channels each exhalation to the atmosphere.

D. Partial and Total Rebreathing: These methods require anesthesia machines and are named according to the amount of exhalation the patient is required to rebreathe. A means of absorbing the exhaled CO_2 must be provided in all instances except where the rebreathing is minimal.

ETHER

Ether (diethyl ether, $H_5C_2-O-C_2H_5$) is an irritant liquid with an unpleasant odor. For over 100 years it was the safest and most widely used of the complete anesthetics.

Ether can be administered by simple technics. It is safe because its irritant properties maintain or even stimulate respiration until the deeper planes of anesthesia; because there is a wide margin between the amount needed to provide surgical anesthesia and the amount that produces medullary paralysis; and because it has no special toxic effects on the cardiovascular or other systems although it causes vasodilatation with a warm, flushed skin. It produces good muscle relaxation without adjunctive drugs. When muscle relaxants are used, the dosage—especially that of the nondepolarizing or tubocurarine type—can be reduced.

Induction with ether is slow and unpleasant, but the use of other agents for induction overcomes this disadvantage. However, ether is explosive, and recovery is prolonged and is accompanied by nausea and vomiting somewhat more often than with other agents.

DIVINYL ETHER

Divinyl ether (Vinethene, $H_2C=CH-O-CH=CH_2$) is also a volatile liquid that can be given by open drop. Induction and recovery are more rapid than with ether. Divinyl ether is still used for brief, painful procedures. It probably has hepatic effects and cannot be used for extended periods.

HALOTHANE

Halothane (Fluothane, $F_3C-CHClBr$), a heavy liquid, has become the most widely used inhalation agent because it is not explosive and only rarely causes serious adverse reactions. Postoperative nausea and vomiting is remarkably rare.

The following properties should, however, be recalled from the discussion above:

(1) Blood pressure is not always well maintained by halothane. Vasodilatation occurs, but cardiac output is only slightly decreased, and hypotension is unusual now that the concentration is controlled by adequate technic.

(2) Unlike ether, halothane causes progressive respiratory depression during stage 3.

(3) Arrhythmias occur uncommonly, but respiration should be assisted to maintain normocarbia since sensitization to epinephrine is demonstrable.

(4) Muscle relaxation is usually not adequate unless another agent is used also.

(5) The cost of the drug forces the use of a closed (total rebreathing) system in most situations.

(6) Halothane on rare occasions—usually after repeated use—causes hepatitis and massive liver necrosis through an allergic mechanism.

It was mentioned above that hepatic necrosis from all causes—shock, infection, preexisting liver disease—occurs in one out of 10,000 cases within 6 weeks of operation. To establish the relationship of a small excess of cases of acute liver atrophy to an anesthetic agent was difficult. Data showing the relationship to repeated exposure have led to general agreement that halothane causes a fatal allergic or autoimmune hepatitis in approximately one out of 800,000 administrations.

Halothane hepatitis is not dose-related. In about 75% of cases, it follows repeated use of halothane, and prior use may have been accompanied by evidence of a reaction—eg, fever occurring after an initially afebrile postoperative period, or jaundice. Deliberate reexposure can induce changes in liver function in sensitized subjects. It is difficult to explain why only 2 of the many anesthetists and others exposed repeatedly to halothane in the operating room have shown reactions.

METHOXYFLURANE

Methoxyflurane (Penthrane, $Cl_2HC-CF_2-O-CH_3$) is an ether that is a liquid with a comparatively high boiling point. It is the most potent agent available (0.5% concentration will maintain surgical anesthesia), but induction may require 20 minutes. Respiration must be assisted. Cardiovascular effects are less than with halothane, and muscular relaxation is better.

Methoxyflurane is metabolized in the liver, and both inorganic fluoride and nonvolatile organic fluorides are demonstrable after its use. The amounts of inorganic fluoride generated are probably sufficient to explain the "fluoride diabetes insipidus" seen to some extent in all patients after the use of methoxyflurane. The process is characterized by varying degrees of unresponsiveness to ADH (vasopressin), with polyuria, dehydration, and thirst, hyperosmolality of the plasma, and nitrogen and uric acid retention. Slow recovery usually occurs, but the number of reported fatalities is excessive considering the limited use of the drug.

FLUROXENE

Fluroxene (Fluoromar, $F_3C-CH_2-O-CH=CH_2$), is an ether that must be considered flammable, although the hazard is minor. Induction is rapid and pleasant, and recovery is very rapid. Cardiovascular changes are less than with halothane.

Fluroxene can be administered by all technics and appears to be useful for brief procedures.

CYCLOPROPANE

Cyclopropane $\left(\begin{array}{c} H_2C-CH_2 \\ \backslash \, / \\ C \\ H_2 \end{array}\right)$ is a gas given by the closed (total rebreathing) method for reasons of economy and safety. The explosive hazard of cyclopropane use is real but can be guarded against, and it perhaps unduly restricted the use of this very good agent during the period when it had to be compared with ether, which is also explosive. Now, of course, it must be compared with nonexplosive halothane.

Induction is extremely rapid, and so also is the progression through the stages of anesthesia. Respiration is progressively depressed. Blood pressure and cardiac output are well maintained during anesthesia, and cyclopropane is still selected for use in patients in shock or in whom shock is impending.

CHLOROFORM

Chloroform ($CHCl_3$) is a volatile liquid that is more potent than ether. It is easily administered, but care is required. Initial concentrations that are too great will cause cardiac arrest by augmenting vagal tone. This effect is avoided by adequate premedication with atropine. (An alternative opinion ascribes accidents during induction to ventricular fibrillation due to sensitization of the myocardium to the effects of epinephrine.) With deep anesthesia, and a degree of hypercarbia, ventricular arrhythmias may occur. Chloroform is also hepatotoxic.

The use of chloroform was a matter of great controversy. Undoubtedly the dangers inherent in its use were exaggerated, but it is at least slightly more dangerous than other potent agents even when used for brief procedures, and alternative drugs are available.

TRICHLOROETHYLENE

Trichloroethylene ($HClC=CCl_2$) is a complete anesthetic but is not so used by itself because of the rapid, shallow respiration and cardiac arrhythmias that it causes. It produces analgesia rapidly and is suggested for use in providing analgesia during delivery.

NITROUS OXIDE

Nitrous oxide (N_2O, gas, laughing gas) is not a complete anesthetic. Used by itself, it cannot take the patient to stage 3 even when the maximum safe concentration (85% N_2O, 15% O_2) is administered. Combined with oxygen in the usual ambient concentration (80% N_2O, 20% O_2) and in the absence of preanesthetic medication or other depressant, it will ordinarily produce only analgesia and euphoria. If higher concentrations are given—eg, a "few" breaths of 100% gas or continued inhalation of 85% nitrous oxide in oxygen—the patient can be carried to stage 2, with analgesia, euphoria, a dreamy or fantasizing state sometimes described as hallucinatory, giddiness, a pounding or ringing sensation in the head, and altered perceptions.

Nitrous oxide does not cause respiratory depression nor add to the respiratory depression of more potent agents.

Its effects appear after a few inhalations, and recovery is equally rapid.

Adverse Reactions

Nitrous oxide is not toxic to any organ system. In the past, it was responsible for many adverse reactions when it was used with inadequate oxygen—ie, 100% N_2O. Nitrous oxide is nonexplosive but will support combustion. Systems for administering nitrous oxide and oxygen in dental offices have recently caused several fires of great intensity. The danger is easily controlled by proper equipment, maintenance, and use.

Clinical Uses

Nitrous oxide can be used as an agent for induction after heavy premedication with narcotic analgesics and barbiturates. Its greatest usefulness, however, is as a component of balanced anesthesia. It is also used for production of intermittent analgesia during delivery.

For many years nitrous oxide has been almost entirely replaced in dentistry by local anesthesia. The abandonment is not entirely rational, being due in part to a reaction to the abuses of nitrous oxide and thiopental by inexperienced operators and in part to some confusion between the goals of analgesia and anesthesia. "Gas" is now coming into wide use in dentistry again. This time, however, it is being given by nose mask so that administration can continue throughout the procedure. Local anesthesia is added if required, suggesting that the goal is not so much analgesia as euphoria or the relief of anxiety, which has been attempted (usually unsuccessfully) with preprocedural barbiturates.

KETAMINE

Another incomplete anesthetic that can be given intravenously or intramuscularly to produce effects slightly more profound than those of N_2O is ketamine (Ketaject, Ketalar).

Chemistry

Ketamine (2-chlorophenyl-2-methylaminocyclohexanone) is chemically and pharmacologically related to phencyclidine (phenyl-cyclohexyl-piperidine, PCP, Sernylan), an agent used in veterinary practice to immobilize primates and a drug commonly if illegally used by ingestion or smoking to produce euphoria and a fantasizing state.

Ketamine

**Phencyclidine
(PCP, Sernylan)**

Pharmacologic Effects

Following the administration of ketamine, the patient rapidly passes into a fugue or trance: The eyes remain open, but the patient does not respond. Some movement may continue, and muscle tone and resistance to movement may be markedly increased. Good analgesia is produced, and there is later amnesia for the experience.

Respiration is not depressed except by large or too-rapidly administered doses. Whether laryngeal and pharyngeal reflexes are depressed sufficiently to make aspiration a danger is still arguable. Blood pressure and pulse rate are increased significantly.

The onset of action after intravenous administration is about 1 minute. The useful effect lasts 5–10 minutes after intravenous administration and 10–20 minutes after intramuscular administration. Complete recovery takes much longer.

For longer procedures, the dose can be repeated or the agent given intramuscularly.

Adverse Reactions

During recovery, adults frequently (incidence > 15%) experience vivid dreams that may be unpleasant and accompanied by excitement. Children are much less susceptible. (In considering the similarity of ketamine and nitrous oxide, recall the usual caution that nitrous oxide never be administered unless a third person is in the room to protect the operator from accusations based on dreaming or fantasizing.)

Clinical Uses

Ketamine is used by itself and mostly in children to provide analgesia during painful procedures—eg, burn dressings, cystoscopy.

INTRAVENOUS OR FIXED ANESTHETICS

Thiopental and similar ultra-short-acting barbiturates are shown in Table 23–2 and discussed in that chapter.

●   ●   ●

General References

Artusio, J.F., Jr. (editor): *Halogenated Anesthetics.* Clinical Anesthesia Series. Davis, 1963.

Atkinson, R.S.: Trichloroethylene anaesthesia. Anesthesiology 21:67–77, 1960.

Black, G.W.: A review of the pharmacology of halothane [Fluothane]. Brit J Anaesth 37:688–705, 1965.

Catchpool, J.F.: Effect of anesthetic agents on water structure. Fed Proc 25:979–985, 1966.

Dobkin, A.B., & J.P. Su: Newer anesthetics and their uses. Clin Pharmacol Therap 7:648–682, 1966.

Dundee, J.W.: Clinical pharmacology of general anesthetics. Clin Pharmacol Therap 8:91–123, 1967.

Eastwood, D.W. (editor): *Nitrous Oxide.* Clinical Anesthesia Series. Davis, 1964. [Note chapter on ethylene.]

Fairlie, C.W., & others: Metabolic effects of anesthesia in man. IV. A comparison of the effects of certain anesthetic agents on the normal liver. New England J Med 244:615–622, 1951.

Halothane hepatitis. [For debate.] Brit MJ 1:448–450, 4:96–100, 1971.

Keys, T.E.: *The History of Surgical Anesthesia.* Schuman, 1945.

Klatskin, G., & D.V. Kimberg: Recurrent hepatitis attributable to halothane sensitization in an anesthetist. New England J Med 280:515–522, 1969.

Magoun, H.W.: *The Waking Brain,* 2nd ed. Thomas, 1963.

Mazze, R.I., Shue, G.L., & S.H. Jackson: Renal dysfunction associated with methoxyflurane anesthesia. JAMA 216:278–288, 1971.

Price, H.L., & P.J. Cohen (editors): *Effects of Anesthetics on the Circulation.* Thomas, 1964.

Robinson, V.: *Victory Over Pain. A History of Anesthesia.* Schuman, 1946.

Taves, D.R., & others: Toxicity following methoxyflurane anesthesia. II. Fluoride concentrations in nephrotoxicity. JAMA 214:91–95, 1970.

Trey, C., Lipworth, L., & C.S. Davidson: The clinical syndrome of halothane hepatitis. Anesth Analg 48:1033–1042, 1969.

21...

Curariform or Neuromuscular Blocking Drugs

Drugs that paralyze voluntary muscle are used primarily as adjunctive agents during anesthesia. The pharmacology of these drugs has already been implied in previous chapters in the discussions of other drugs which act by blocking or intensifying the action of acetylcholine. Curare and related synthetic drugs act as competitive antagonists to acetylcholine and share properties with the ganglion blocking agents. In mechanism of action they are comparable to the parasympatholytics. The other large group of neuromuscular blocking drugs are similar to the cholinomimetic drugs (Chapter 8); the initial stimulating (depolarizing) effect is minimized and the action in preventing repolarization of the motor end plate is increased.

History

Indians in the farthest reaches of the Amazon and Orinoco Valleys and in the rain forests of Guiana used crude curare as an arrow and dart poison in hunting. They prepared a gummy aqueous extract from huge creeping vines or "bushropes" (probably *Chondodendron tomentosum* in Ecuador and Peru and *Strychnos lethalis* in the more eastern area). Before the resinous mass was rubbed into the grooves in arrow tips, it was stored in gourds, clay pots, or bamboo tubes—thus the name tubocurarine for the alkaloid finally isolated from tube curare.

During the centuries following the Spanish conquest, many reports on the properties of curare were returned to the Old World along with actual samples of tube, pot, and calabash (gourd) curare. One of these samples from the greatest of naturalist explorers, Humboldt, was given to Magendie, characterized in Chapter 1 as the man who first systematically applied the experimental method to physiology. Magendie used curare to immobilize experimental animals and transferred an interest in arrow poisons to his successor, Claude Bernard. Bernard demonstrated that, in an animal poisoned with curare, a muscle could still be directly stimulated even though it would not respond to stimulation of its nerve. This experiment was the first demonstration of the independent excitability of muscle and localized the action of curare at a site between nerve and muscle. He recognized that curare had no CNS effect and speculated that the apparently peaceful death it caused might actually be horrible to "an intelligence finding itself still living in an unresponsive body."

Not until 1935 were reasonably standardized extracts of curare available, and the introduction of curare into the practice of anesthesia followed the work of Griffith in 1942.

Chemistry

The 2 major groups of curariform drugs—those that prevent depolarization and those that prevent repolarization or maintain depolarization—have certain similarities in chemical structure (Fig 21–1). For both groups, optimal activity is found in compounds that contain 2 quaternary nitrogens separated by a distance of about 14 A or the distance established by 10 intervening atoms. As with other agonists and antagonists discussed earlier, it is helpful to explain the similar structural requirements by using the concepts of affinity and intrinsic activity. A molecule with great affinity for the receptor at some postsynaptic site on the motor end plate but lacking some additional property essential for initiating depolarization—eg, tubocurarine—will act as a competitive antagonist. A compound that combines affinity for the receptor with great intrinsic activity in initiating a response—eg, succinylcholine—will act like a great excess of the physiologic mediator, acetylcholine.

A. Nondepolarizing Agents: Tubocurarine, the semisynthetic derivative dimethyltubocurarine, and gallamine, a synthetic drug, are examples of this group. The curarines are still derived from the plant source, but it is no longer necessary that they pass through the hands of an Indian witch. Agents of this class are also known as pachycurares because of their compact rather than linear molecular configuration; as stabilizing agents because they prevent the depolarizing effect of acetylcholine on the postsynaptic membrane; and as competitive agents because the effect can be overcome by the accumulation of an excess amount of acetylcholine.

B. Depolarizing Agents: Agents of this class which cause persistent depolarization are exemplified by succinylcholine or decamethonium (Fig 21–1). They are also occasionally referred to as leptocurares because of the apparent linear or thread-like configuration of the molecule.

Absorption, Metabolism, & Excretion

The available neuromuscular blocking agents are all quaternary amines and are not suitable for oral administration. They are well absorbed from injection

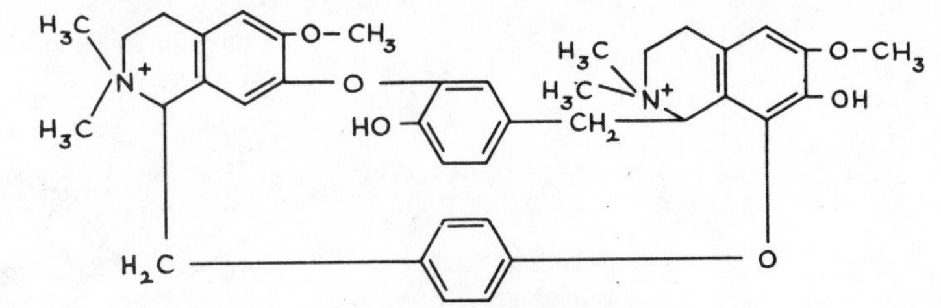

Tubocurarine

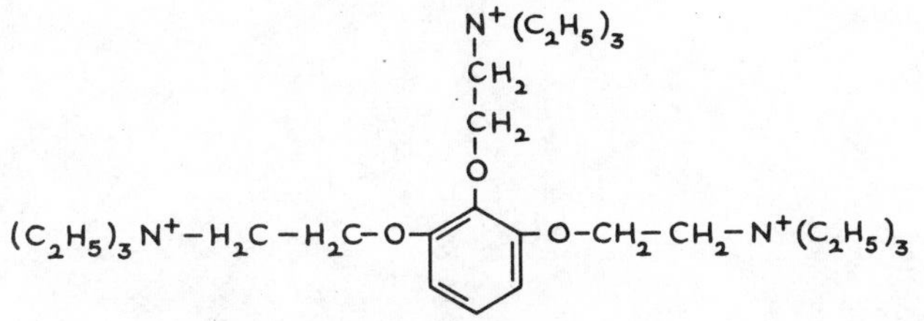

Gallamine

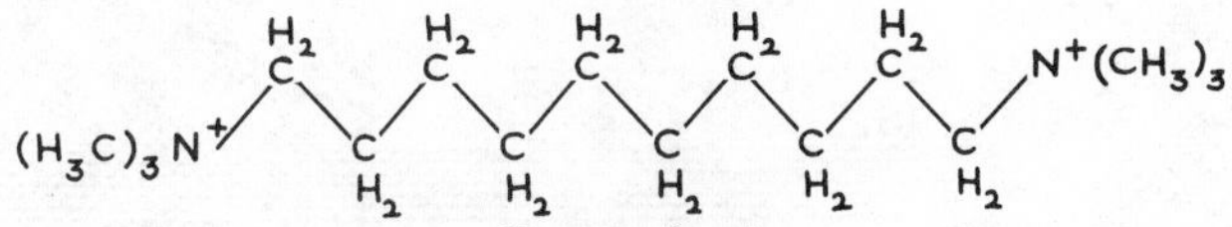

Decamethonium

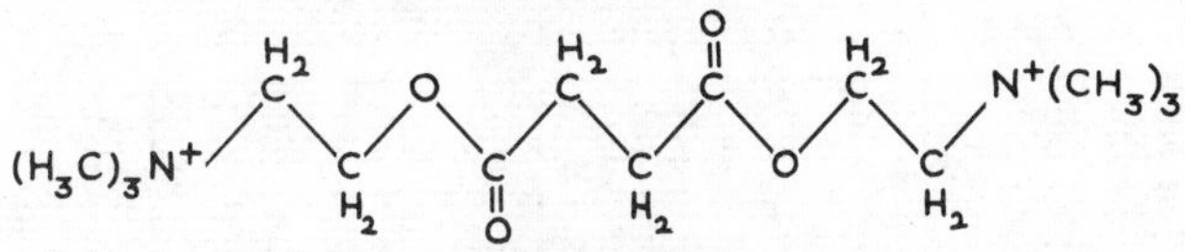

Succinylcholine

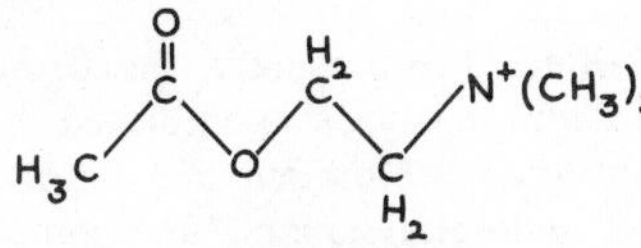

Acetylcholine

FIG 21–1. Above are shown the chemical structures of 2 nondepolarizing pachycurares. Below, the structures of 2 depolarizing blocking agents are compared with acetylcholine.

sites, but the established uses all utilize the intravenous route.

Tubocurarine is rapidly removed from plasma. Its metabolic fate is not known. It appears that the comparatively rapid termination of its action is due to redistribution rather than destruction or excretion.

Succinylcholine is hydrolyzed stepwise to succinylmonocholine and then to succinate and choline. Pseudocholinesterase governs the first step of the hydrolysis.

Pharmacologic Effects

A. Mechanisms of Action: The acetylcholine liberated by somatic nerve does not act diffusely or directly on striated muscle to depolarize it but acts first on the membrane of an intermediate structure, the motor end plate. The axon of the motor nerve divides as it approaches its termination on muscle, and branches (5–300) go to each fiber in the motor unit.

At the neuromuscular junction, the axonal branch loses its myelin sheath and expands and branches into a folded end foot with a great surface area (Fig 21–2). The underlying sarcoplasm is thickened and elevates the sarcolemma. The sarcolemma, in this area called the end plate membrane, is complexly folded and closely applied to the end foot of the axonal branch. However, an ultramicroscopic cleft separates the 2 structures, and, upon stimulation of the nerve, acetylcholine is liberated into the synaptic cleft to depolarize the end plate membrane—ie, to generate an end plate potential. Depolarization of the motor end plate is propagated to the muscle mass.

1. Nondepolarizing agents—Tubocurarine and analogous compounds act at the motor end plate in a manner comparable to atropine at parasympathetic neuro-effector junctions. Acetylcholine is still liberated, but, in the presence of the blocking agent, depolarization of the postsynaptic membrane does not

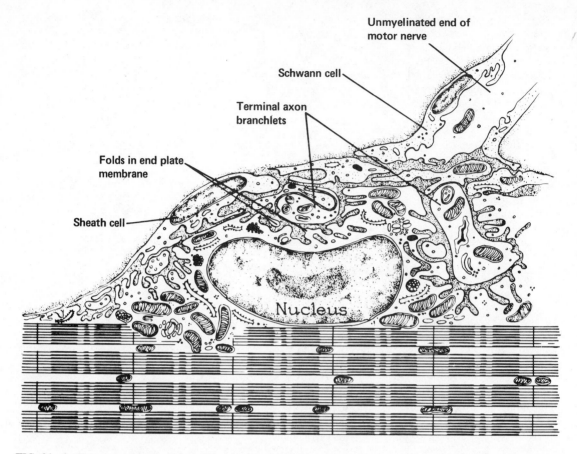

FIG 21–2. Neuromuscular junction. The drawing is based on electronmicrographs of tissue from mice, and shows the terminal ends of a motor neuron axon buried in the end plate cytoplasm, with the much folded end plate membrane around them. (Modified and redrawn, with permission, from Anderson-Cedergren: Ultrastructure of motor end plate and sarcoplasmic components of skeletal muscle fiber. J Ultrastructure Res, Suppl 1, 1959.)

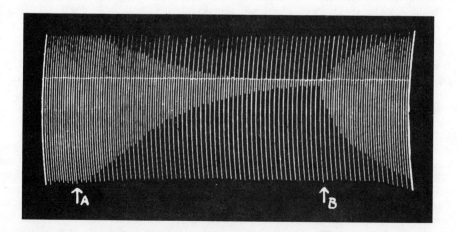

FIG 21–3. The action of tubocurarine on a preparation of rat diaphragm in an isolated tissue bath. Alternate stimuli are applied to the phrenic nerve and directly to the muscle. At A, 20 μg of D-tubocurarine chloride were added. Direct stimulation of the muscle continues to cause contraction, but indirect stimulation through the nerve loses its effect until, at B, the curare is washed out. (Reproduced, with permission, from Holems & others: The analysis of the mode of action of curare on neuromuscular transmission. J Pharmacol Exper Therap 103:383, 1951.)

take place. The action is purely one of blockade, and no initial stimulation occurs (Fig 21–3). The relation between tubocurarine and acetylcholine is competitive and can be overcome by the increased amounts of acetylcholine that accumulate following the administration of a cholinesterase inhibitor such as neostigmine. Drugs that have themselves a strong acetylcholine-like action—eg, succinylcholine or other drugs of the depolarizing class discussed next—also antagonize the effects of curare.

2. **Depolarizing agents**—Succinylcholine and decamethonium act like a great excess of acetylcholine to depolarize the membrane of the motor end plate and to prevent its repolarization. The initial phase of their activity, therefore, involves a dissolution of the resting potential or the appearance of an action potential and is accompanied by stimulation of muscular contraction prior to the development of a flaccid paralysis. The persistent depolarization involves only the region of the motor end plate. The adjoining muscle has its usual resting potential but is inexcitable—a familiar if unexplained observation in electrophysiology called cathodal block. At least theoretically, the effect of these drugs is antagonized by blocking agents of the nondepolarizing type.

In the case of both classes of neuromuscular blocking drugs, direct stimulation of muscle causes contraction even though stimulation through the nerve is ineffective.

In the laboratory and evidently in some clinical situations, the above classification does not hold for large doses of succinylcholine or decamethonium. In this special case, the depolarizing effect (phase I) may be followed by a stage (phase II) during which the motor end plate is repolarized but protected against the effects of acetylcholine, much as if curare had been used. If this second phase of "desensitizing block" is reached, the action of succinylcholine may be prolonged rather than brief.

B. **Effects:**

1. **Skeletal muscle weakness and paralysis—**

a. **Nondepolarizing agents**—After the intravenous injection of tubocurarine or related drugs, muscle weakness or flaccid paralysis, depending upon the dose, begins in less than 2 minutes and a maximal effect is reached within 5 minutes. Muscles of the face, neck, eyes, and pharynx are weakened first—leading, in the conscious patient, to difficulty in speaking, accumulation of secretions in the throat, and diplopia. Other small muscles such as those of the hand and the intercostal muscles are next affected, followed by action on muscles of the limbs, abdomen, chest, and, finally, the diaphragm. The ability to maintain a sustained contraction is altered before the strength of a single contraction is weakened. The effect is first apparent upon sustained effort. In the anesthetized patient, the effect is seen after applying both single and rapidly repetitive (tetanizing) stimuli when the nondepolarizing block is characterized by a decreasing response to repeated, single stimuli (fading) and poorly sustained tetanus.

b. **Depolarizing agents**—The initial stimulating effect of the depolarizing agents leads to incoordinated contraction of muscles. The stimulating effect causes fasciculations of groups of muscle fibers, apparent as rapid worm-like movements beneath the skin. The contractions may occasionally cause elevation of an arm or arching of the back. The stimulated contractions are equivalent to exercise to which the patient is unaccustomed and are followed during the postoperative period by muscle soreness in the neck, back, or pharynx.

During electrical stimulation, depolarizing block is seen to cause a weakening of contraction to a degree dependent upon dose. Additional fading after single stimuli is not seen, however, and tetanus is sustained but at a reduced level.

2. **Other effects**—Other pharmacologic effects must be related to the individual compounds rather than to groups of compounds. Tubocurarine, for example, causes some ganglionic blockade and is a weak histamine liberator. It may, therefore, cause a fall in blood pressure and bronchiolar constriction. Gallamine lacks those actions but antagonizes acetylcholine at cardiac vagal endings and may cause tachycardia. Succinylcholine has some cholinergic effects on the heart and may cause bradycardia.

Clinical Uses

A. **Augmentation of Muscle Relaxation During Anesthesia:** In addition to rendering the patient unconscious and preventing his perception of and reaction to painful stimuli, optimal anesthesia provides enough voluntary muscle relaxation to permit the exposure needed (or deemed necessary) by the surgeon. If muscle relaxation is achieved by a curariform drug, less potent anesthetics can be used or smaller amounts of the complete anesthetics are needed during the procedure. Thus, "balanced anesthesia"—eg, thiopental-nitrous oxide-tubocurarine, as defined in the preceding chapter—can be used rather than deep anesthesia with ether. Furthermore, tracheal intubation can be carried out without or before deep anesthesia if the jaws and deeper structures are relaxed with succinylcholine.

This theory is widely accepted and is the basis for the almost invariable use of muscle relaxants. Nevertheless, when the practice was coming into use, study of over half a million anesthesias in 10 separate hospitals suggested an increase in deaths during the interval prior to actual surgery if curare had been used.

B. **Modification of Convulsions Due to Electroconvulsive Therapy:** The convulsions of electroshock therapy, still advisable for some depressed or schizophrenic patients, can collapse a vertebral body or even break a long bone. The muscular contractions can be weakened or even prevented by muscle relaxants without interfering with the therapeutic effect of the CNS discharge. For this purpose, the patient is given a single intravenous dose of succinylcholine after a few inhalations of oxygen. Thiopental anesthesia is usually also provided.

C. **Other Suggested Uses:** Curariform drugs have also been tried in various spastic and convulsive states, including tetanus. In each case, the drug is either not useful or better alternate treatments are available.

Contraindications & Cautions

The neuromuscular blocking drugs are ordinarily used by anesthetists who have the requisite experience and equipment. In other applications—eg, prior to electroconvulsant therapy—facilities for intubating and ventilating the patient should be available in the event of apnea.

The dosage of neuromuscular blocking agents is modified by interaction with other drugs and disease states.

A. General Anesthetics: When diethyl ether is used, the dosage of curare type agents is reduced about 65%; halothane and cyclopropane reduce the requirement by 20% or less.

B. Antibiotics: The effect of tubocurarine is intensified in some situations by neomycin, streptomycin, kanamycin, gentimicin, polymyxin B, and colistin.

C. Quinidine and Lidocaine: Isolated reports have appeared of recurarization when antiarrhythmic therapy is given during the postoperative period. The interaction is easily demonstrable in the laboratory.

D. Glaucoma: Succinylcholine, presumably by the initial contraction of extraocular muscles, elevates intraocular pressure and could be dangerous in the presence of acute glaucoma or a puncture wound of the globe. The effect can be prevented by the prior administration of a small (3 mg) dose of tubocurarine.

E. Myasthenia Gravis: These patients are very sensitive to nondepolarizing agents and very resistant to the depolarizing type.

Adverse Reactions

Apnea following the use of curariform drugs may extend into the postoperative period and may require assisted ventilation for extended periods. The unexpectedly prolonged action may follow overdosage or, in the case of succinylcholine only, may be due to a defect in the patient's ability to metabolize the drug.

A. Antagonists to Tubocurarine and Related Drugs: The nondepolarizing agents such as tubocurarine, dimethyltubocurarine, and gallamine can be antagonized by cholinesterase inhibitors of the type discussed in Chapter 8.

The cholinesterase inhibitors such as neostigmine and edrophonium (Tensilon) act predominantly by allowing the accumulation of acetylcholine liberated at the neuromuscular junction. They have, however, a direct action in strengthening the force of muscle contraction—ie, an effect that can be demonstrated on muscle following denervation when acetylcholine is not present.

Neostigmine (1–3 mg IV) or edrophonium (10–30 mg IV) will terminate the action of tubocurarine. They will intensify the action of the depolarizing type of blocking agent. They can be given combined with atropine to minimize parasympathomimetic effects on secretion. The effect of edrophonium lasts for only about 10 minutes.

B. Prolonged Apnea After Succinylcholine: In an occasional patient the duration of action of succinylcholine following a single intravenous dose or following termination of a continuous infusion will not be the expected 2–4 minutes but 1–4 hours or more. This has not been completely explained. Most patients who experience apnea have adequate plasma cholinesterase levels and probably have developed a nondepolarizing block rather than the initial depolarizing block. The more persistent action may be due to succinylmonocholine, the first metabolic product of the hydrolysis of succinyldicholine.

A few apneic patients may show a deficiency of plasma cholinesterase or pseudocholinesterase. This enzyme is differentiated from true cholinesterase by its ability to hydrolyze benzoylcholine and the ability of dibucaine to inhibit the reaction. There are few studies using succinylcholine itself as the substrate. Most individuals (96%) are homozygous for the gene determining the activity of this enzyme. At least 2 other genes occur at this locus, and a few individuals are homozygous for one of the mutants and are then grossly deficient in benzoylcholinesterase.

Dosages

A. Tubocurarine (D-Tubocurarine): In addition to its neuromuscular blocking action, tubocurarine can act weakly as an acetylcholine antagonist at ganglia and, like many other diamines, can act as a histamine liberator. These effects can cause a fall in blood pressure, and histamine release will on rare occasions lead to bronchiolar constriction.

The effect of tubocurarine, as of all of the drugs of this class, is almost immediate after intravenous injection. About 10 minutes after a single dose, the effect diminishes rapidly, and muscle strength is completely normal after about 40 minutes.

The dosage is variable and not predictable on the basis of weight or other apparent factors. The dose is, therefore, given fractionally or in increments until the desired effect is achieved. The average dose is about 6–9 mg IV. Ether anesthesia reduces the amount of curare required to about one-third of the usual dose.

Quinidine, lidocaine, and a number of antibiotics (neomycin, streptomycin, polymyxin B, colistin, kanamycin, and viomycin) may intensify the effects of curare.

B. Dimethyltubocurarine Chloride (Mecostrin) and Dimethyltubocurarine Iodide (Metubine): These preparations are equivalent to tubocurarine but are about 3 times as potent.

C. Gallamine Triethiodide (Flaxedil): Gallamine has cholinolytic actions at the vagal as well as voluntary nerve endings and can cause tachycardia. Its duration of action is somewhat shorter than that of tubocurarine.

D. Pancuronium (Pavulon): In this compound the 2 quaternary ammoniums are separated by the steroid nucleus. It is generally similar to the other nondepolarizing relaxants, but the ganglion blocking and histamine liberating actions of tubocurarine and the consequent hypotension and bronchiolar constriction are virtually absent. The advantage claimed over gallamine is that there is no difficulty in reversing the action of large doses. Pancuronium is 5 times as potent as D-tubocurarine.

E. Succinylcholine (Anectine): In addition to the brief initial stimulation of voluntary muscle mentioned above, succinylcholine has other acetylcholine-like effects. These may result in bradycardia and a fall in blood pressure (parasympathomimetic effect) followed by tachycardia and a rise in blood pressure (sympathomimetic or nicotinic effect).

A single injection of about 30 mg IV given over a period of 10–20 seconds produces transient apnea. A sustained effect is accomplished by a continuous intravenous infusion of 2–4 mg/minute.

F. Decamethonium (Syncurine): This depolarizing agent is now rarely used. It has a more sustained action than succinylcholine. Maximal effect after a single injection persists for 4–8 minutes and is completely dissipated in 20 minutes, when it is excreted into the urine.

Preparations Available

Tubocurarine:
Injectable (IV), 3 mg/ml, 10 ml vials; 15 mg/ml, 1 ml ampules

Dimethyltubocurarine chloride (Mecostrin):
Injectable (IV), 1 mg/ml, 10 ml vials

Dimethyltubocurarine iodide (Metubine):
Injectable (IV) 1 and 2 mg/ml, 20 ml vials

Gallamine triethiodide (Flaxedil):
Injectable (IV), 20 and 100 mg/ml, 10 ml vials

Succinylcholine (Anectine):
Injectable (IV), 20, 50, and 100 mg/ml, 10 ml vials; powder, 0.5 and 1 gm vials

Decamethonium (Syncurine):
Injectable (IV), 1 mg/ml, 10 ml vials

•   •   •

General References

Beecher, H.K., & D.P. Todd: A study of the deaths associated with anesthesia and surgery. Ann Surg 140:2-34, 1954.

Eckenhoff, J.E. (editor): A symposium on muscle relaxants. Anesthesiology 20:407–549, 1959.

Foldes, F.F.: The pharmacology of neuromuscular blocking agents in man. Clin Pharmacol Therap 1:345–395, 1960.

Hunter, A.R.: Suxamethonium apnea. Anaesthesia 21:325–336, 1966.

Katz, R.L.: Clinical neuromuscular pharmacology of pancuronium. Anesthesiology 34:550–556, 1971.

Rumble, L., & others: Observations during apnea in conscious human subjects. Anesthesiology 18:419–438, 1957.

Taylor, D.B., & O.A. Nedergaard: Relation between structure and action of quaternary ammonium neuromuscular blocking agents. Physiol Rev 45:523–524, 1965.

Way, W.L., & R.D. Miller: Clinical pharmacology of neuromuscular blocking agents. GP 38:100–108, December 1968.

22 ...

Local Anesthetics

Local anesthetics can block conduction along the axon and can prevent the sense organ from initiating an afferent impulse. They are, therefore, applied to nerve roots or trunks or infiltrated into an area of the body to provide local, regional, or conduction anesthesia—ie, anesthesia of an area without the loss of consciousness that attends general anesthesia. Motor and autonomic fibers are also blocked. Some of the local anesthetics may also act to anesthetize mucous membranes after topical application, and all have potentially dangerous systemic toxic effects after absorption.

History

The application of cocaine as the first local anesthetic grew out of the interest in its CNS stimulating effect. The history of such use is discussed together with that of amphetamine in Chapter 28.

Following a period of personal and professional use of cocaine as a euphoriant, Sigmund Freud and his chief, Joseph Breuer, invited a young ophthalmologist, Carl Koller, to collaborate in further study. Freud was primarily interested in the systemic effects of cocaine, but Koller had previously tested many drugs as local anesthetics in the eye without success. Credit is generally accorded Koller (1884) for introducing the concept of local anesthesia, especially since the experiments were done while Freud was away visiting his fiancée. William Halsted probably deserves credit for first defining and using regional anesthesia (1885).

Cocaine is an ester of benzoic acid, and synthetic substitutes that were esters of para-aminobenzoic acid soon appeared. In 1904 Fourneau introduced butethamine, but procaine, the compound synthesized by Einhorn, was unchallenged as the standard drug for 40 years. Drugs active after topical application to mucous membranes and some with a duration of action exceeding that of procaine were added. In 1943, lidocaine was introduced following the work of Löfgren and Lundquist and has come into wide use.

Chemistry

A. **Structure-Action Relationships:** Certain generalizations about the structural requirements for local anesthetic activity are frequently made. A secondary or tertiary amine is linked through a connecting group of proper length to an aromatic residue (Fig 22–1). The same generalization about structure has been applied to other "membrane stabilizers," and the para-

sympatholytics, antihistamines, tranquilizers, and quinidine-like drugs generally are potent local anesthetics even though tissue irritation or other effects may preclude their use as local anesthetics. However, the compounds selected for use as local anesthetics do have some specificity in their action—ie, except for quinidine-like actions, they share few properties with the above classes of drugs.

Many substances are local anesthetics even though their chemical structure does not conform to the above generalization.

B. **Chemical Classes:** The commonly used local anesthetics can be classified on the basis of the connecting group between the amine function and the hydrocarbon residue. Thus the common local anesthetics may be esters, amides, ethers, or ketones. (See Fig 22–1 and Preparations Available.) The esters may be further classified on the basis of the acid contributing to ester formation—eg, esters of benzoic acid or of para-aminobenzoic acid. An example of the variations and proliferation of compounds possible within just one of the general chemical classes is shown in Table 22–1.

Perhaps the only practical significance of this classification arises in the rare situation of a patient or doctor allergic to a local anesthetic. Since cross-sensitivity to agents of the different classes does not occur, a substitute drug can be selected—eg, for a patient sensitized to procaine or other ester of para-aminobenzoic acid, an amide can be substituted.

Note that the suffix "caine" does not identify any one of the chemical groups.

C. **Properties as Weak Bases:** The local anesthetics (with the exception of a few topically active agents) are amines and are weak bases—ie, acceptors of hydrogen ion. The free base is an oil or amorphous solid, lipid-soluble but insoluble in water. Suspensions of the free base may be used, but the drugs are usually dispensed as crystals or aqueous solutions of a salt, almost always the hydrochloride. Solutions of the salts are acid (pH 4.0–6.0) and stable.

The salt of a weak base $R-NH_2$ and a strong acid hydrolyzes:

$$R-NH_3^+ + Cl^- + H_2O \rightleftharpoons$$

$$R-NH_2 + Cl^- + H_3O^+$$

TABLE 22–1. Structures of esters of para-aminobenzoic acid.

$$\text{H}\!-\!\underset{R_1}{\overset{R_2 \quad R_3}{N}}\!-\!\!\!\!\!\!\!\!\!\overset{O}{\underset{}{C}}\!-\!O\!-\!CH_2\!-\!CH_2\!-\!\underset{R_5}{\overset{R_4}{N}}$$

	R_1	R_2	R_3	R_4	R_5
Procaine				$-C_2H_5$	$-C_2H_5$
Chloroprocaine			$-Cl$	$-C_2H_5$	$-C_2H_5$
Butethamine					$-C_4H_9$
Naepaine					$-C_5H_{11}$
Proparacaine		$-O-C_3H_7$		$-C_2H_5$	$-C_2H_5$
Benoxinate		$-O-C_4H_9$		$-C_2H_5$	$-C_2H_5$
Propoxycaine			$-O-C_3H_7$	$-C_2H_5$	$-C_2H_5$
Tetracaine	$-C_4H_9$			$-CH_3$	$-CH_3$

In an acid solution (greater concentration of H^+), the local anesthetic will be present as the charged, salt form, which is water-soluble and less diffusible. At body pH or if alkali is added—ie, hydronium ions removed—the reaction will move to the right and a larger fraction of the local anesthetic will exist as the lipid-soluble, uncharged free base, which will partition more readily into the lipid material of the cell membrane. The drugs penetrate nerve in the form of the free base but are dispensed as clear solutions of the salt.

D. Pharmacologic Classification: Most of the local anesthetics listed below can be used either by injection or by topical application; a few are suitable only for topical application, and some, notably procaine, act only after injection. This property merely reflects the necessity of dispensing procaine in acid solutions, in which it is stable. In alkaline solutions, the lipid solubility and topical activity of procaine is greater. Cocaine has sympathomimetic properties and a potential for abuse, and must be considered as a special case.

Absorption & Metabolism

The rate of absorption from the common sites of injection depends upon the vascularity and blood flow to the area and is similar to absorption after other intramuscular or subcutaneous injections. After application of local anesthetics to the mucosa of the pharynx or respiratory tract, blood levels may be almost as high and almost as rapidly attained as after intravenous injection.

Metabolism of the local anesthetics does not take place at the site of application but in the plasma or liver. Reducing blood flow to the site of injection and slowing absorption by the addition of a vasoconstrictor to the local anesthetic solution will, therefore, reduce systemic toxicity. Esters such as procaine are hydrolyzed by pseudocholinesterase of plasma. Amides such as lidocaine are hydrolyzed more slowly in the liver.

Pharmacologic Effects

A. Mechanism of Local Anesthetic Action: The local anesthetics act on all types of nerve fibers to block conduction. (Not all of the many compounds in use have been studied, but the properties of all are similar enough that it seems safe to generalize from the data acquired for procaine and a few other prototypes.)

1. Effects on electrophysiologic events—Conduction in segments of an axon proximal and distal to an area exposed to a local anesthetic is normal. In the segment exposed to concentrations of anesthetic above a certain threshold value, an action potential is not generated—ie, depolarization and propagation of the impulse stops when the wave of excitation reaches that part of the nerve exposed to the anesthetic. The resting potential is practically unchanged.

The changes in the electrical events and in conduction time are graded rather than all-or-none—ie, the earliest changes are a slowing of the rate of depolarization and of conduction, very much like those already described for quinidine.

If the Hodgkin-Huxley model of the cell is accepted, one can only conclude that the increase in permeability of the cell membrane to Na^+, which is the first event in depolarization, is prevented by procaine and related agents. How the membrane is stabilized is not established.

2. Site of action and active molecular form—The potency of local anesthetics applied topically or to intact nerves is increased in alkaline solutions—ie, with more of the drug in the form of the free base. However, experiments on desheathed nerves suggest that the unchanged form merely diffuses to the axonal membrane more rapidly but that most of the local anesthetics are more active as cations in a neutral solution. Significant amounts of procaine are found in the axoplasm—ie, enter the cell—when the drug is applied to the (large, squid) axon.

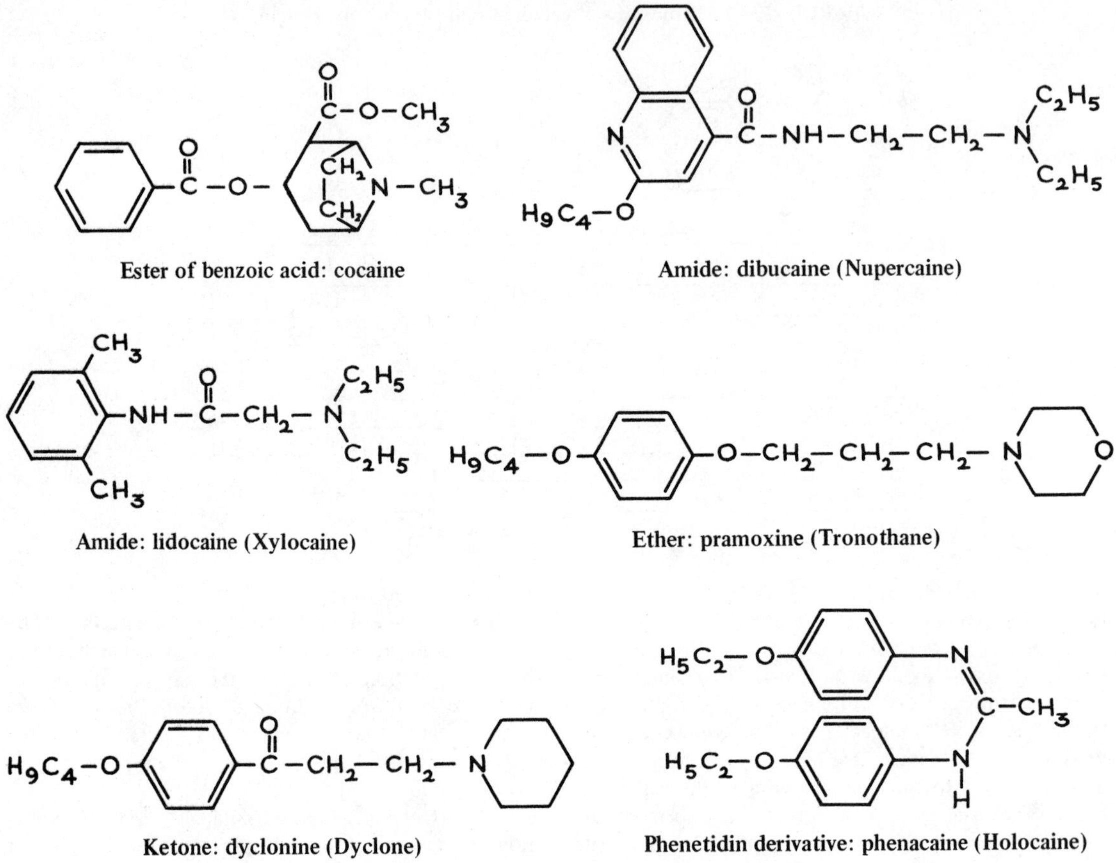

Ester of benzoic acid: cocaine

Amide: dibucaine (Nupercaine)

Amide: lidocaine (Xylocaine)

Ether: pramoxine (Tronothane)

Ketone: dyclonine (Dyclone)

Phenetidin derivative: phenacaine (Holocaine)

FIG 22–1. Chemical classes of local anesthetics.

A local anesthetic must reach the plasma membrane of the axon before it can act. In the case of spinal anesthesia, the drug acts on nerve roots, and mixing and diffusion in the spinal fluid rapidly bring the local anesthetic into contact with the neuron. As the nerves course distally, they are surrounded more heavily by connective tissue structures (sheath, epineurium, perineurium) and the perilemma that is continuous with the pia-arachnoid. These structures slow access to the axon even if the local anesthetic is deposited exactly on the nerve. Using a stronger solution of anesthetic will hasten diffusion and the onset of anesthesia and also increase the chance of a toxic reaction. The popularity of some agents—eg, lidocaine—is based on their greater diffusibility and more rapid onset of action.

All axons are embedded in the cytoplasm of Schwann cells, but the covering is interrupted by a continuous cleft, and in nonmyelinated nerves Schwann cells are not an important barrier to diffusion or to ion transport at the surface of the axon. In myelinated nerves, the Schwann cells have encircled the axon with layers of dense lipid which are barriers to the diffusion of drugs and also to ion transport. Local anesthetics act on myelinated fibers only at the nodes of Ranvier, where the myelin is interrupted.

Depolarization also jumps from node to node, and the speed of conduction is greater in myelinated nerves.

B. Effects:

1. **Local effects on neural transmission**—The local anesthetics block transmission through all nerve fibers whether they are sensory, motor, or autonomic in function. The effect on specialized sensory receptors is either to prevent their depolarization by stimuli or to produce the equivalent effect by blocking conduction in their axon close to the sense organ.

Since all fiber types are ordinarily blocked, regional anesthesia will produce changes other than the primarily desired loss of sensation. The motor paralysis produced may have the desirable effect of producing good muscle relaxation during surgery but may limit patient cooperation, as during delivery; or may be dangerous, as when the level is high enough to weaken respiratory movements. Blockade of sympathetic transmission may be used to produce a kind of reversible sympathectomy of a region; but during spinal anesthesia, with a high enough level, it may lead to hypotension.

Local anesthetics may have a differential effect when applied to a mixed nerve because the smaller the fiber (axon), the more sensitive it is to the action of local anesthetics. (Table 22–2 summarizes the fiber

TABLE 22-2. Nerve fiber types in mammalian nerve.*

Fiber Type		Function	Fiber Diameter (μm)	Conduction Velocity (m/sec)
A	α	Proprioception; somatic motor	12–20	70–120
	β	Touch, pressure	5–12	30–70
	γ	Motor to muscle spindles	3–6	15–30
	δ	Pain, temperature	2–5	12–30
B		Preganglionic autonomic	<3	3–15
C	dorsal root	Pain	0.4–1.2	0.5–2
	sympathetic	Postganglionic sympathetics	0.3–1.3	0.7–2.3

*Modified and reproduced, with permission, from Ganong: *Review of Medical Physiology,* 5th ed. Lange, 1971.

types found in nerve. A fibers are myelinated; B fibers are lightly myelinated; C fibers are unmyelinated.) As regional anesthesia develops following the application of a local anesthetic to a nerve or nerve root, the first modalities affected are those mediated by small, non-myelinated (C) fibers—ie, pain and vasoconstrictors maintained by sympathetic postganglionic activity—and those carried by small, myelinated (Aδ) fibers—ie, pain and temperature. Other sensation disappears next, and motor function last.

The differential effects are most apparent during the development of the effect or during recovery, but it is possible to achieve a persistent differential anesthesia—ie, sensory loss without muscle paralysis—by applying a suitably low concentration of the agent.

During recovery, the least sensitive fibers recover first. After motor function returns, sensation returns as the more sensitive, small fibers regain function.

The least sensitive fibers are those with the thickest myelin sheath, but the differential sensitivity is not related to the direct influence of the myelin sheath as a barrier since the local anesthetics act only at the nodes of Ranvier.

Another differential effect is seen during the appearance and recovery from a nerve block. Block of both motor and sensory function begins proximally and progresses distally because fibers from the more proximal sites are added to the outer mantle of the nerve covering the fibers in the core that originate in the more distal part of the limb. During the onset of anesthesia, an effective concentration of drug reaches the outer layers first. During recovery, diffusion lowers the concentration most rapidly in the same area so that recovery will proceed from the proximal to the distal part of the limb.

2. CNS stimulation—All of the local anesthetics have, under certain conditions, CNS stimulating effects comparable to those of other convulsant stimulants discussed in Chapter 28. Medullary stimulation may cause bradycardia, hypertension, and respiratory stimulation. Stimulation of a higher level can cause anxiety, tremulousness, excitement, and convulsions. The

mechanism and site of the last action is not known, but convulsions can still be produced in animals following decerebration.

3. CNS depression—If the CNS stimulating effect progresses to convulsions, a period of postconvulsive depression can occur. In addition, however, the local anesthetics have a primary depressant effect on the medulla and on higher centers. The depressed stage may occur without a prior excited stage or after only a transient period of stimulation. The depression of CNS function results in hypotension due to loss of vasomotor control, severe respiratory depression, and stupor or coma. The period of depression is far more dangerous to the patient than the stimulated state, and is intensified by barbiturates or similar drugs.

4. Cardiovascular effects—

a. Hypotension—The local anesthetics can alter blood pressure by several mechanisms. During the period of CNS stimulation, blood pressure may be elevated. It is, however, the later profound hypotension that occurs as a toxic effect during the period of CNS depression that is more dangerous. The hypotensive effect is intensified by the direct vasodilator effect of the local anesthetics—comparable to that described for quinidine and procainamide. A direct depressant effect on the heart can be demonstrated in the laboratory although its clinical significance in toxic reactions to local anesthetics is not established.

b. Quinidine-like effects—In addition to a direct vasodilating action, the local anesthetics possess those cardiac actions described for quinidine and related antiarrhythmia drugs in Chapter 16. Lidocaine is used in the treatment of cardiac arrhythmia, and all are capable of producing the same changes in conduction as those described for quinidine.

5. Additional effects of cocaine—Cocaine has 2 general effects not shared with the other local anesthetics. It can be used by injection, ingestion, or as snuff to produce a long-acting CNS stimulating effect generally comparable to that of amphetamine. Because of the feeling of euphoria at the time of injection and the stimulation produced, cocaine may be misused.

In addition, cocaine has sympathomimetic properties that are due to its ability to prevent the reentry into sympathetic nerve of norepinephrine liberated at the nerve ending. Of the norepinephrine liberated by sympathetic nerves as a chemical mediator, about half is not chemically destroyed but its action is terminated by its reentry into the terminal portion of the sympathetic nerve. Cocaine decreases the reentry and, therefore, possesses norepinephrine-like properties. It will potentiate injected sympathomimetics, dilate the pupil, and, most important in relation to its use as a local anesthetic, act as a vasoconstrictor either after injection or when applied topically to a mucous membrane.

6. Other effects—Procaine and related drugs are weak antihistamines and even weaker parasympatholytics. They are curare-like only in large doses in the laboratory, but clinically may be additive to the action of curare.

Clinical Uses & Technics of Administration

The technic by which regional anesthesia is produced influences the choice of the local anesthetic preparation and its toxicity and is, therefore, summarized at this point.

A. Topical Application: Not even those local anesthetics classified as topically active can penetrate the keratinized surface of the intact skin. It is conceivable that the free base in a proper oily vehicle or solvent could act on the skin, but no useful preparation is now available. The local anesthetics will act on grossly denuded skin, but far more important is their ability to anesthetize mucosal surfaces that are not keratinized. The corneal surface or the mucosa of the. mouth, oral and nasal pharynx, larynx, trachea, and urethra are easily anesthetized. The discomfort of an endoscopy or other procedure and pain (eg, the pain of a herpetic lesion) can be reduced.

Absorption of the agent from a mucosal surface is extremely rapid, and the total dose used should be no more than one-quarter the maximum allowed for injection. Preparation for endoscopy is probably the most common source of local anesthetic toxicity.

Procaine and closely related compounds are not topically active. Many of the agents listed in the section on Preparations Available are marketed only for topical use either in the eye or, with little justification, on the skin.

B. Infiltration: In all of the remaining technics of administration, the anesthetic agent is injected. The site of injection may be anywhere along the course of the nerve from the peripheral receptor to the entry of the nerve root into the CNS.

Infiltration anesthesia is produced by injecting the agent throughout the area to be rendered insensitive. Infiltration along the line of an incision or infiltration of the edges of a laceration to be sutured are the most common examples. As is true for most of the injection technics, this procedure usually begins with the production of a wheal in the overlying skin using a small needle. A larger needle is then introduced through the insensitive area in the skin. The needle advances along an area of decreased sensitivity provided by injections of agent through the advancing needle.

C. Field Block: In producing a field block, the anesthetic agent is not injected into the area to be dissected but into an area surrounding it. Field blocks are applicable to the scalp and anterior abdominal wall where nerves course superficially to reach the area to be anesthetized.

D. Nerve Block: Local anesthetics may be deposited close to a mixed nerve—eg, the palatine, inferior alveolar, pudendal, a cord of the brachial plexus, and many others—and the area innervated will become anesthetic.

E. Spinal (Subarachnoid) Anesthesia: The term spinal anesthesia denotes subarachnoid or intrathecal injection of a local anesthetic agent. For the production of spinal anesthesia, a lumbar puncture is done—ie, the point of the needle enters the dural sac lower than the most caudal extension of the spinal cord. A previously prepared solution of the local anesthetic is injected, or the crystalline agent is dissolved in CSF and reinjected. The local anesthetic solution may be made heavier (hyperbaric) by using 10% dextrose as the solvent.

Following the injection, functions disappear in the order described above, and a level of anesthesia is established. The level must be high enough to permit performance of the desired procedure without pain but should not be needlessly high in order to prevent respiratory weakness or undue hypotension subsequent to vasodilatation. The level is controlled by altering the volume of solution injected, the rate of injection, the amount of local anesthetic, and the position of the patient. The anesthetic agent is rapidly removed from the CSF and fixed in the nerve roots and sensory ganglia, and the height of the level does not vary after about 15 minutes.

Spinal anesthesia produced by tetracaine, probably the currently most commonly used agent, lasts for 1−2 hours. Procaine is a shorter-acting agent. The duration of spinal anesthesia can be increased about 1/3 by the addition of 0.2 mg (0.2 ml of 1:1000) of epinephrine.

A variation of spinal anesthesia commonly used for obstetric analgesia is called saddle block. With the patient in a sitting position, a hyperbaric solution is injected and settles to the lowest portion of the dural sac where it anesthetizes those nerve roots that originate from the most terminal segments of the cord, ie, those that innervate the body segments that would be in contact with a saddle. In this application, where prolonged duration is a great advantage, dibucaine may be used although its systemic toxicity is great enough that its use in spinal anesthesia is ordinarily contraindicated.

F. Epidural Spinal Anesthesia: In this technically more difficult procedure, the point of the needle rests in the epidural space which is not fluid-filled and which extends from the foramen magnum to the sacral hiatus. The concentration and total dose of the local anesthetic is very large, and care must be taken to prevent its subarachnoid injection. Since the subarachnoid space is not entered, spinal headaches are less common and patients are less likely to object to the procedure.

Caudal anesthesia is a technically simpler variation of epidural anesthesia in which a needle enters the epidural space through the sacral hiatus below the termination of the dural sac. Anesthesia of only the most caudal segments can be achieved, making the method suitable for obstetric analgesia. A catheter can be inserted through the lumen of the needle and left in place for periodic supplementation of anesthesia, in which case the method is known as continuous caudal anesthesia.

Adverse Reactions

A confusing variety of reactions can occur just after the injection of a local anesthetic, and they may or may not be related to the effect of the drug used. Conventionalized definitions and terms must be used accurately to minimize confusion. Overdosage toxicity can occur, and one patient may be affected by a smaller dose than another. Such a response should never be described as "hypersensitivity," a term preempted by the immunochemist and denoting true allergy. Allergic reactions to the local anesthetics are extremely rare. Anxiety is very common during the procedure and culminates in vasovagal syncope just after the needle is withdrawn. The assumption that the sympathomimetic vasoconstrictor added to the anesthetic solution may reach toxic amounts further complicates the discussion. For these reasons, reactions not directly related to the anesthetic agent as well as direct toxic reactions are discussed below.

A. Overdosage Toxicity: Dose-related toxic reactions occur when the precautions outlined below are not followed and an excessive amount of drug enters the systemic circulation in a brief time. These incidents occur most often prior to endoscopy when a mucosal surface is flooded with solution, giving poor control of the total amount. Toxic reactions are also seen during obstetric procedures and other situations in which multiple or repeated injections may be given. Dentists are responsible for very little overdosage toxicity, however many faints they may induce.

The reaction may involve transient or persistent CNS stimulation followed by CNS and cardiovascular depression, or the depressed stage may appear without apparent prior CNS stimulation.

Stimulation may first be apparent as excitement, apprehension, or nausea. At this time, the pulse rate will usually be slightly slowed and blood pressure slightly elevated. Respiration will be increased in rate and depth. The skin will be pale, cool, and moist, and the total picture will resemble an epinephrine effect or severe anxiety.

More profound CNS stimulation will lead to preconvulsive muscular twitchings and then to convulsions. At this time blood pressure and pulse rate will be elevated, and even between convulsions the patient may be dyspneic and cyanotic with rapid, shallow respirations.

Following the period of excitement (or without going through a period of excitement), the patient will be depressed and in shock due to the mechanisms mentioned above—ie, medullary depression, vasodilatation, and postconvulsant depression. Areflexia and coma, extreme hypotension, and respiratory failure may follow.

Treatment of overdosage: Treatment differs depending upon whether it is given in the early (convulsive) or late (shock) stage. Vigorous treatment of the convulsive stage may intensify the difficulties of the shock stage.

(1) Convulsions: The period of convulsions is so alarming that the patient is likely to be overtreated. The convulsions are actually tolerated well if the patient is kept oxygenated with oxygen and assisted respiration. Whenever the risk of overdosage with local

anesthetics is appreciable, oxygen together with masks and bag should be available. (Such equipment is critically important in other situations also and probably should be available whenever local anesthesia is given.) If the patient is oxygenated between convulsions, he can be carried through the period of excitation without being subjected to the hazard of receiving CNS depressant drugs that add to the postictal depressed state or the primary depression.

A variety of further treatment methods have been suggested to control the convulsions. If an anesthetist is in attendance and prepared to give intravenous injections and assist respiration, the peripheral manifestations of the convulsant activity may be blocked with succinylcholine. Various intravenous barbiturates are suggested, but even the shortest-acting barbiturates add a hazard to the later course of the patient. Administering a rapidly reversible inhalation anesthetic would probably be more rational, but this practice is no longer commonly suggested.

(2) Shock: Treatment of the depressed or shock stage is the same as for any other form of shock, but the prognosis is much less favorable. Because of the respiratory depression, the need for assisted respiration is greater in this than in other forms of shock. Vasopressors have been used, but the results are unimpressive. The effectiveness of vasodilators in this form of shock has not been evaluated.

B. Allergic Reactions:

1. Systemic reactions—Anaphylactic reactions following the use of local anesthetics are theoretically possible but must be extremely rare. Dentists occasionally observe facial swelling in their patients several hours after the injection of a local anesthetic. The swelling is not due to hemorrhage and is suggestive of angioneurotic edema.

2. Dermatitis—Topical sensitization to local anesthetics requires frequent contact. It is occasionally seen in dentists who repeatedly get the drug on their fingers.

C. Sequelae of Spinal Anesthesia:

1. Hypotension—Spinal anesthesia may lead to hypotension due to blockade of sympathetic vasoconstrictor fibers. The higher the level of spinal anesthesia, the more intense the hypotension may become. Vasopressor drugs—eg, ephedrine or other sympathomimetic amine—may be injected prior to spinal anesthesia when hypotension is anticipated, or they may be given to treat hypotension when it develops.

2. Trauma of lumbar puncture—The anesthetist is generally more skilled in performing a lumbar puncture than most practitioners, but even he may traumatize the area, causing a transient backache. Whenever the dural sac is punctured, there is always the risk of postspinal headache due to leakage of CSF fluid.

3. Neurologic damage—Spinal anesthesia does not differ appreciably from general anesthesia in the incidence of serious complications or less dangerous sideeffects. Rare cases of lasting spinal cord or nerve root damage have occurred, but these episodes have been less frequent since the methods of handling and sterilizing the ampules of the drug were changed. The necessary precautions involve not only the physician and pharmacist but also the administrators responsible for drug storage and distribution. The assumption now is that neurologic damage due to spinal anesthesia is caused by the introduction of chemical or bacterial contaminants with the agent or the use of improper concentrations of the local anesthetic. Such contamination leads to meningitis (aseptic, purulent, or chronic adhesive) with signs varying from a minor cauda equina syndrome to transverse myelitis.

The following precautions should be observed: (1) Ampules containing the local anesthetic should be sterilized by autoclaving either on the spinal tray or in glass tubes from which they can be dumped onto the open spinal tray without introducing contamination or being themselves contaminated in the process. The ampules must not be sterilized by immersing in any germicidal solution since imperceptible cracks in the glass may admit the irritant solution to the inside of the ampule. (2) Syringes and needles must be rinsed with special care after cleaning so that detergents or other chemical irritants do not adhere. Disposable equipment offers an advantage in this respect. (3) Skin preparation and sterile technic should be carried out with great care. (4) If the lumbar puncture is extremely difficult, plans for the anesthesia should be modified. (5) If paresthesias, indicating contact with nerve tissue, persist after insertion of the needle, the anesthetic should not be injected.

Neurologic complications are even more rare after epidural anesthesia than after subarachnoid spinal anesthesia.

D. Other Adverse Effects: Prolonged use of any of the local anesthetics in the eye can lead to keratitis comparable to that which follows sensory denervation.

Following paracervical block with mepivacaine, fetal bradycardia or tachycardia may occur. Studies of concurrent maternal and fetal blood levels suggest that the drug reaches the placenta and fetus by direct entry from the injection site rather than by transfer from maternal to fetal circulations.

E. Reactions Not Due to the Local Anesthetic Agent:

1. Vasovagal syncope—The common faint (sometimes called primary shock or neurogenic fainting) must be differentiated from drug reactions. This type of fainting occurs in patients who react with great anxiety to the impending procedure and especially to the ordeal of the needle. During the period of anxiety, the patient shows the usual signs of epinephrine release. With the sudden release of anxiety when the injection is completed and the needle withdrawn, some additional stimulus initiates an intense vagal surge with resultant bradycardia and peripheral pooling of blood, leading to hypotension, which causes, in turn, cerebral ischemia and fainting. At the moment of fainting the pulse is slow and bounding, but the patient has the appearance of one in shock. The faint is benign unless the patient is kept erect or has cerebral or coronary

vascular disease, in which case the occurrence of a cerebral or myocardial infarct is not impossible.

2. Reaction to epinephrine—Anesthesia for dental procedures requires injection into highly vascular areas, and the duration of anesthesia is often unsatisfactory unless epinephrine is added to the solution. The epinephrine could conceivably precipitate anginal pain in a patient with coronary artery disease.

The interprofessional groups that have made recommendations in this area emphasize that the amounts of epinephrine provided are small compared to the amounts endogenously liberated by an anxious patient and especially by a patient experiencing pain due to inadequate anesthesia. Slow injection, the use of the smallest amounts of solution possible, and perhaps premedication to minimize anxiety permit the use of epinephrine-containing solutions, even in patients with angina.

Contraindications & Cautions

The only absolute contraindication to the use of local anesthetics is injection into an infected area. A number of precautions are important.

A. Control Total Dose: The lowest effective concentration and the smallest effective total volume of a local anesthetic should be used. The need to increase the concentration or volume above accepted levels often suggests inadequate technic.

The package inserts for each local anesthetic preparation establish a maximum total dose for various technics. These assume that there will be no difficulty such as inadvertent intravascular administration. If repeated injections are necessary for extensive procedures or because an initial injection was unsuccessful, an interval of even a few minutes between applications greatly increases safety.

B. Add Vasoconstrictors to Injected Anesthetics: The addition of epinephrine to all but topically applied anesthetics reduces blood flow through the infiltrated area and slows absorption of the local anesthetic. The duration of the anesthetic effect is prolonged, and, since biotransformation can keep pace with a slower rate of absorption, blood levels do not rise as high and toxicity is decreased.

The addition of epinephrine is especially indicated when injection is into a very vascular area or when more concentrated solutions of the anesthetic are used.

Epinephrine should not be added to solutions to be injected into the fingers, ears, or penis since vasoconstriction can lead to tissue necrosis.

C. Premedication: In the laboratory, sedation with a barbiturate provides protection against convulsions and the immediate lethality of local anesthetics. The effect on total mortality—ie, early and late—is less. Adequate premedication of the human subject with barbiturates would presumably provide similar protection, but the effectiveness of the small doses usually used is probably very limited.

D. Avoid Intravascular Injection: The most important precaution in avoiding intravenous injection is to give the injection slowly so that pressure does not build up locally and force the solution into vessels. Aspirating before injection may draw blood into the syringe if the needle is in a vessel or if a vessel has been opened by the point of the needle—providing the needle is not too small. If blood is aspirated, the needle should be repositioned, but failure to aspirate blood does not protect against intravascular injection as well as does very slow injection.

Selection of Drug

A. How Available Drugs Differ: It has already been emphasized that not all of the marketed local anesthetics are active after topical application and that others, because of local irritative effects or because limited investigative work has been performed, are suitable only for topical application. Those local anesthetics intended for use by injection do differ considerably among themselves. However, the properties of potency, toxicity, and duration of action generally change together, and an advantage gained by altering one property is often lost by a correlated change in another. The evaluation of a compound, therefore, is dependent upon the intended use.

1. Potency and systemic toxicity—Potency can be evaluated in the laboratory in many ways, eg, by determining the concentration necessary to abolish the corneal reflex in rabbits or to block conduction in an isolated nerve trunk. Ultimately potency is measured as the least concentration required to consistently produce a particular block in humans.

Systemic toxicity in the human is accurately predicted by determinations of median lethal doses in animals. The LD_{50} is not an absolute value but depends upon species, route of administration, concentration of the injected solution, and many other variables. The toxicity of local anesthetics can be compared only if the determinations are made under identical conditions.

In the compounds now available for use, anesthetic potency and systemic toxicity have not been separated, and the more potent drugs are also the more toxic.

2. Duration of action—The duration of action generally correlates well with potency and systemic toxicity. When a longer duration of action is an important consideration in the intended use, a more toxic drug must be selected. Thus, tetracaine is widely used in spinal anesthesia because of its somewhat longer duration of action, but it is uncommonly used for other technics. Dibucaine may be used for the production of saddle block for obstetric analgesia because in such cases the duration of the need for anesthesia is unpredictable and may be quite long. Dibucaine may be used even though its greater toxicity virtually contraindicates its use in any other situation except topical application.

3. Onset of action—The interval between deposition of the local anesthetic and appearance of complete anesthesia is a property that is also correlated with the above 3.

4. Diffusibility—Some agents have a latent period that is shorter than would be predicted by their potency. The same drugs appear to produce a good block more dependably than other agents when they are deposited slightly distant from the intended site. This decreased latent period and increased tolerance for minor errors in technic is probably related to the greater diffusibility of the particular drug. This property has been important in establishing the wide use of lidocaine.

B. Injectable Local Anesthetics: The many local anesthetics available are listed below. Those with distinctive properties have already been mentioned. Many are advertised for specific applications—eg, dental anesthesia—without any established superiority over older, unprotected compounds.

A few local anesthetics suggested for use by injection can be categorized as follows:

1. Procaine is the standard drug to which other members of this group are compared. Chloroprocaine (Nesacaine) is more rapidly hydrolyzed than procaine; it acts for a shorter period but is less toxic. Hexylcaine (Cyclaine) is an example of a related drug of intermediate potency and duration of action; in a situation in which procaine produces anesthesia for 1 hour, the action of the intermediate drugs may persist for 1½–2 hours.

2. Lidocaine and related amides have the advantages inherent in their greater diffusibility and intermediate duration of action. Mepivacaine (Carbocaine) is slightly longer-acting than lidocaine. Prilocaine (Citanest) has intermediate properties but can produce methemoglobinemia.

3. Tetracaine (Pontocaine) and dibucaine (Nupercaine) are mentioned above because of their long duration of action.

C. Topical Anesthetics:

1. Cocaine—Of the topically active agents, cocaine is distinctive in its ability to cause vasoconstriction when applied to mucous membranes. Its use is now limited to application to the mucosa of the nose and pharynx. In other applications it has been replaced by less irritant and more easily dispensed drugs.

2. Benzocaine—Benzocaine (ethyl aminobenzoate) is a substance with very low solubility in water that is present in proprietary sprays, powders, and creams. It acts briefly—ie, only for as long as it is in contact with a mucosal surface.

Preparations Available

Esters of para-aminobenzoic acid:

Procaine (Novocain, etc):

Injectable (infiltration, nerve block, spinal, epidural, caudal), 0.1%, 500 and 1000 ml; 0.5%, 30 ml; 1%, 1, 2, 5, 6, 10, 30, 50, and 100 ml; 2%, 2, 3, 5, 10, 30, 50, and 100 ml; 10%, 2 ml; 20%, 5 ml

Chloroprocaine (Nesacaine):

Injectable (infiltration, nerve block), 1 and 2%, 30 ml; 2 and 3%, 50 ml

Butethamine (Monocaine)*:
  Injectable (infiltration, nerve block),
    1% (with epinephrine, 1:75,000),
    5 ml; 1.5% (with or without epi-
    nephrine, 1:30,000 or 1:100,000),
    5 ml
Naepaine (Amylsine):
  Ophthalmic solution, 4%
Proparacaine (Ophthaine):
  Ophthalmic solution, 0.5%, 15 ml

Esters of benzoic acid:
Cocaine:
  Topical (solution), 1, 2, 5, 10%.
Piperocaine (Metycaine):
  Topical (mucous membranes), 150 mg
    tablets and bulk powder for mak-
    ing solution
  Injectable (infiltration, nerve block,
    and caudal), 1.5%, 200 ml
Hexylcaine (Cyclaine):
  Topical, 5%, 60 ml solution
  Injectable (infiltration, nerve block),
    1%, 30 and 100 ml
Meprylcaine (Oracaine)*:
  Injectable (infiltration, nerve block),
    2% (with epinephrine, 1:50,000),
    2, 2.5, and 20 ml
Benoxinate (Dorsacaine):
  Ophthalmic solution, 0.4%, 15 ml
Propoxycaine (Blockain):
  Injectable (infiltration, nerve block),
    0.5%, 20 ml
Tetracaine (Pontocaine):
  Topical, 0.5% (ophthalmic), 1, 15, and
    60 ml; 2% (nose and throat), 30
    and 120 ml; tablets, 100 mg, for
    making solution; 1% (cream), 30
    and 450 gm; 0.5% (ointment, with
    0.55% menthol), 30 gm
  Injectable (infiltration, nerve block,
    caudal, spinal), 0.15% (in Ringer's
    solution), 100 ml; 0.2% (in 6%
    dextrose), 2 ml; 0.25% (in 6% dex-
    trose), 2 ml; 0.3% (in 6% dex-
    trose), 5 ml; ampules (crystals),
    10, 20, and 250 mg

Esters of meta-aminobenzoic acid:
Metabutethamine (Unacaine)*:
  Injectable (infiltration, nerve block),
    3.8%
Isobucaine (Kincaine)*:
  Injectable (infiltration, nerve block),
    2% (with epinephrine, 1:65,000),
    1.8 ml

Cyclomethycaine (Surfacaine):
  Topical, 4% (aerosol), 60 ml; 0.5%
    (cream), 30 and 450 gm; 0.75%
    (jelly), 3.75 and 30 gm; 1% (oint-
    ment), 30, 450, and 2250 gm

Amides:
Dibucaine (Nupercaine, Nupercainal):
  Topical, 0.5% (cream), 30 gm; 1%
    (ointment), 30 and 450 gm
  Injectable (infiltration, nerve block,
    peridural, spinal), 0.5% (with or
    without epinephrine, 1:200,000),
    50 ml; 1% (with or without epi-
    nephrine, 1:200,000), 30 ml; 1%
    (with or without epinephrine,
    1:200,000), 20 and 50 ml; 1%,
    100 ml; 1.5%, 20 ml; 1.5% (with
    epinephrine, 1:200,000), 30 ml;
    2% (with or without epinephrine,
    1:100,000), 2, 20, and 50 ml; 2%,
    10 ml; 2% (with epinephrine,
    1:200,000), 20 ml
Lidocaine (Xylocaine, etc):
  Topical, solution, 4%, 5 and 50 ml;
    ointment, 2.5 and 5%, 15 and 35
    gm; jelly, 2%, 35 ml; viscous, 2%,
    100 and 450 ml
  Injectable (infiltration, nerve block,
    spinal, epidural), 0.5% (with or
    without epinephrine, 1:200,000),
    50 ml; 1% (with or without epi-
    nephrine, 1:100,000 or
    1:200,000), 2, 20, 30, and 50 ml;
    1.5% (with or without epineph-
    rine, 1:200,000), 20 and 30 ml;
    2% (with or without epinephrine,
    1:50,000, 1:100,000, or
    1:200,000), 2, 20, 30, and 50 ml;
    4%, 5 ml; 5%, with glucose, 7.5%,
    2 ml
Mepivacaine (Carbocaine):
  Injectable (infiltration, nerve block,
    spinal, caudal, peridural), 1%, 30
    ml (in modified Ringer's solution)
    and 50 ml (in saline solution);
    1.5%, 30 ml (in modified Ringer's
    solution); 2%, 20 ml (in modified
    Ringer's solution) and 50 ml (in
    saline solution); 4%, 2 ml
Prilocaine (Citanest):
  Injectable (infiltration, nerve block,
    epidural, caudal), 1%, 30 ml; 2%,
    30 ml; 3%, 20 ml

Ethers:
Pramoxine (Tronothane):
  Topical, 1% (cream), 30 and 450 gm;
    1% (jelly), 30 gm; 1% (solution),
    60 and 120 ml

*Marketed for use in dentistry.

Dimethisoquin (Quotane):
  Topical, 0.5% (ointment), 30 gm; 0.5%
    (lotion), 60 ml

Ketones:
  Dyclonine (Dyclone):
    Topical, 0.5% (solution), 30 and 240
      ml

Phenetidin derivative:
  Phenacaine (Holocaine):
    Ophthalmic ointment, 1 and 2%, 3.75
      gm

● ● ●

General References

Adriani, J.: The clinical pharmacology of local anesthetics. Clin Pharmacol Therap 1:645–673, 1960.

Adriani, J.: Reactions to local anesthetics. JAMA 196:405–408, 1966.

Adriani, J., & R. Zepernick: Clinical effectiveness of drugs used for topical anesthesia. JAMA 188:711–716, 1964.

American Dental Association and American Heart Association: Management of dental problems in patients with cardiovascular disease: Report of a joint conference. J Am Dent A 68:333–342, 1964.

de Jong, R.H.: *Physiology and Pharmacology of Local Anesthesia.* Thomas, 1970.

Johnson, H.A.: Infiltration with epinephrine and local anesthetic mixture in the hand. JAMA 200:990–991, 1967.

Kennedy, B.R., Duthie, A.M., & G.D. Parbrook: Intravenous regional analgesia: An appraisal. Brit MJ 1:954–957, 1965.

Lane, C.G., & R. Luikart II: Dermatitis from local anesthetics: With a review of 107 cases from the literature. JAMA 146:717–720, 1951.

Phillips, O.C., & others: Neurologic complications following spinal anesthesia with lidocaine: Prospective review of 10,440 cases. Anesthesiology 30:284–289, 1969.

Sharrey-Schafer, E.P., Hayter, C.J., & E.D. Barlow: Mechanism of acute hypotension from fear or nausea. Brit MJ 2:878, 1958.

Shnider, S.M., & others: High fetal blood levels of mepivacaine and fetal bradycardia. New England J Med 279:947–948, 1968.

Smith, B.E., Hehre, F.W., & O.W. Hess: Convulsions associated with anesthetic agents during labor and delivery. Anesth Analg 43:476–482, 1964.

Vandam, L.D., & R.D. Dripps: Long-term follow-up of patients who received 10,098 spinal anesthetics. IV. Neurologic disease incidental to traumatic lumbar puncture during spinal anesthesia. JAMA 172:1483–1487, 1960.

23...

Sedative-Hypnotics

The sedative-hypnotic drugs have pharmacologic properties which are quite similar to those of the general anesthetics. When large doses are used, as in a suicidal attempt or when a barbiturate such as thiopental is used to induce general anesthesia, the difference between a sedative-hypnotic and a general anesthetic disappears. General anesthetics are gases or volatile liquids selected from among the general CNS depressants because their physical properties allow rapid onset and ready reversibility of action. The sedative-hypnotics are solid or liquid substances that cause generalized depression of the CNS for a longer period than do the rapidly exhaled gases. They are thus more conveniently compounded and more suitable for oral administration for the induction of sleep or the relief of anxiety.

These 2 uses—the induction of sleep and the symptomatic relief of anxiety—represent a huge need and market, and the proliferation of compounds is correspondingly great. Loose application of the term "tranquilizer" has led to additional confusion. Before the many individual compounds in this general class of drugs are identified, a preliminary discussion of the classification of drugs is required.

Classification of Drugs

It is not necessary or feasible for the individual physician to evaluate separately each of the many drugs available and suggested for use to him. The more recently introduced and vigorously promoted drugs provide the greatest challenge to the confidence of a physician. Genuinely new drug effects are in fact discovered at intervals of several years, usually with great impact on medicine; but most new drugs are selected for marketing not because they are essentially different from other drugs but because they are similar to drugs which have already been marketed successfully. It is, therefore, usually possible and efficient to study the effects of a large group of drugs or of a prototype drug and then look for smaller variations within the group. Classifications in general break down at the borders between categories, but for drugs this is not usually true because drugs are usually selected prior to marketing to conform to the classification. This chapter will emphasize data that justify including the many drugs listed in the broad class of sedative-hypnotics.

A Further Note on Terminology

These preliminary cautions are necessary because it has been difficult to integrate the new antipsychotic tranquilizers and a large number of recently marketed sedatives into medical practice.

The sedative class of drugs, exemplified by the barbiturates, has been used for the relief of anxiety and the induction of sleep since about 1903. After 1950, the antipsychotic tranquilizers were recognized as a separate class of drugs, and their use revolutionized the institutional practice of psychiatry. The physician in noninstitutional practice, dealing regularly with anxious rather than psychotic patients, believed that this important advance should have an impact on his practice also. However, when the tranquilizers were used in the treatment of anxiety, the results were disappointing. At this point the physician should have concluded that a drug of the sedative-hypnotic class rather than of the tranquilizer class was indicated (as in the past) for this group of patients. But he was offered a series of sedative drugs advertised as "tranquilizers," "minor tranquilizers," "successors to the tranquilizers," etc. The physician then adopted one of these mislabeled sedatives and concluded that it was "the only tranquilizer that worked for him." Recognition of the fact that meprobamate was merely an expensive variant of an intermediate-acting sedative required 10 years. The influence of advertising and ambiguities in the use of the term "tranquilizer" continue to be confusing in relation to some recently introduced sedatives.

What Is a Sedative-Hypnotic? What Is a Tranquilizer?

Table 23–1 summarizes the differences between the sedatives and the antipsychotic tranquilizers.

Each of the drugs listed in this chapter as a sedative-hypnotic will, if given in progressively larger doses, lead to sedation, excitement or disinhibition, hypnosis, general anesthesia, and ultimately medullary depression with death. With repeated or continuous administration, the sedatives are anticonvulsant, habituating, cause a withdrawal state, and are spinal cord depressants.

In contrast, the tranquilizers (represented by any of the phenothiazine compounds discussed in Chapter 25 or by reserpine) do not cause general anesthesia, ie, the patient can be aroused even after huge doses. They are convulsant in their action, not habituating, and

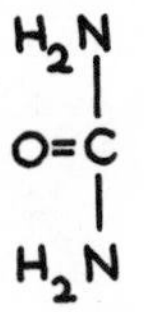

Urea 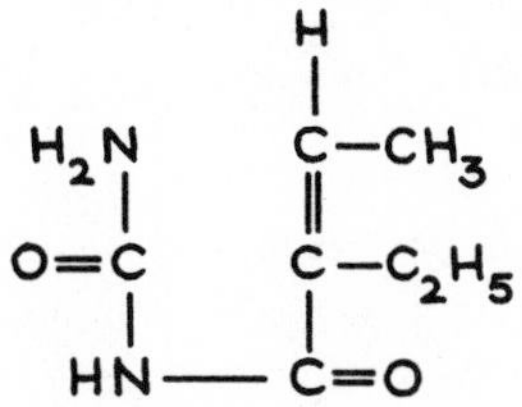   Ectylurea (Levanil) 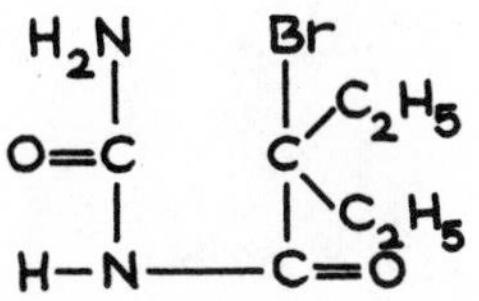   Carbromal 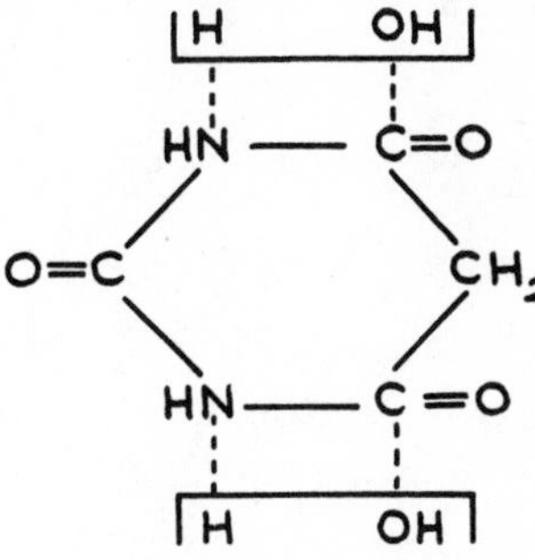   Malonylurea (barbituric acid)

their therapeutic usefulness is in the treatment of psychotic rather than anxious patients.

Chemical Classification & Identification

The most useful classification of the sedative-hypnotics is based on their duration of action. There are, however, advantages to beginning with a chemical classification. The most important of these advantages is to predict classification in the sedative group. The most recent modification of a barbiturate, a urethane, or an alcohol may, as a first approximation, be expected to act quite similarly to the other drugs in each class. The metabolism of a drug and its physical and chemical properties are also more easily understood as characteristics of a chemical class of drugs. (For example, all barbiturates are weak acids; all urethanes are neutral compounds.)

The following classes of chemical compounds include most of the sedatives used in therapy or encountered in the environment.

A. Monoureides: The monoureides—eg, ectylurea or carbromal—are mentioned to show their relationship to the diureides (barbiturates) and urethanes. These newer compounds have replaced the monoureides.

B. Barbiturates (Diureides):

1. Chemistry—The barbiturates are cyclic diureides. The ring is formed when urea (on the left in the diagram above) reacts with a dicarboxylic acid, malonic acid.

Barbituric acid itself is not a hypnotic. Barbiturates with longer or shorter durations of action are made by substituting various groups for the hydrogens on the CH_2 shown above or by preparing thiobarbiturates. In the thiobarbiturates a sulfur replaces the

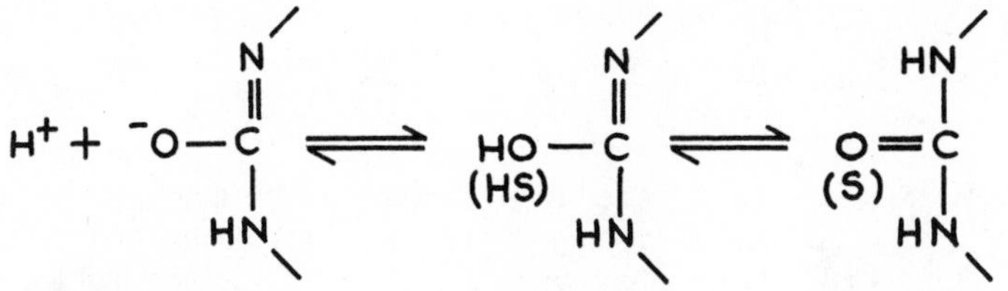

Ionized or salt form   Lactim (enol) acid form   Lactam (keto) form

TABLE 23–1. Comparison of actions that differentiate sedatives and tranquilizers.

Sedatives (eg, barbiturates, meprobamate, alcohol)	Tranquilizers (eg, phenothiazines, reserpine)
With increasing doses:	Control of psychotic behavior
Relief of anxiety	Easy arousal
Sedation	Extrapyramidal signs: parkinsonism, dystonias
Ataxia	Convulsions
Excitement, drunkenness, disinhibition	Autonomic effects (atropine-like, sympathoplegic)
Anesthesia	
Respiratory and vasomotor depression and death	
With continued administration:	
Anticonvulsant action	
Physical dependence (withdrawal state)	
Habituation	
Voluntary muscle relaxation	

TABLE 23-2. Formulas of barbiturates.

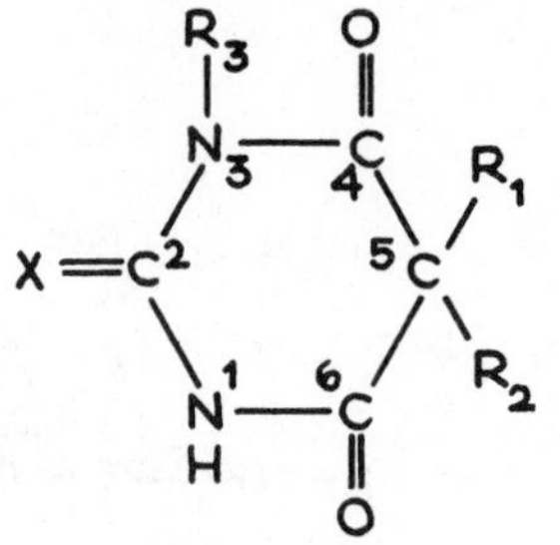

	X	R_3	R_1	R_2
Short-acting barbiturates				
Pentobarbital* (Nembutal)	O	–H	$–C_2H_5$	$–C_5H_{11}$
Secobarbital* (Seconal)	O	–H	–allyl†	$–C_5H_{11}$
Intermediate-acting barbiturates				
Amobarbital* (Amytal)	O	–H	$–C_2H_5$	$–C_5H_{11}$
Long-acting and anticonvulsant barbiturates				
Phenobarbital	O	–H	$–C_2H_5$	–phenyl
Mephobarbital* (Mebaral)‡	O	$–CH_3$	$–C_2H_5$	–phenyl
Metharbital (Gemonil)‡	O	$–CH_3$	$–C_2H_5$	$–C_2H_5$
Primidone (Mysoline)‡	H⟩H	–H	$–C_2H_5$	–phenyl
Ultrashort-acting barbiturates				
Thiopental* (Pentothal)	S	–H	$–C_2H_5$	$–C_5H_{11}$
Thiamylal (Surital)	S	–H	$–C_3H_5$	$–C_5H_{11}$
Hexobarbital (Sombucaps)	O	$–CH_3$	$–CH_3$	–cyclohexenyl

*Generic preparation available. Common trade names are included for identification only. These old drugs are available from many suppliers under their generic name.
†Allyl: $–CH_2CH=CH_2$.
‡Converted to phenobarbital or barbital in the body.

oxygen in the urea moiety. (See Table 23-2.) Whether a barbiturate has a slow onset of action and long duration of action or a rapid onset and short duration of action is a function of its lipid solubility.

2. Absorption, metabolism, and excretion—Lipid solubility varies as an intrinsic property of different barbiturates but is also related to the strength (degree of dissociation or pK) of the acid form of a barbiturate. The barbiturates exist in 2 tautomeric or prototropic (isomeric) forms:

The lactim form is a weak acid. In the un-ionized form it is lipid-soluble and will cross cell boundaries easily. Thus it is well absorbed, enters nerve tissue quickly, and is reabsorbed from renal tubular urine. In the charged or salt form that exists in a more alkaline solution, it is water-soluble and differently distributed.

The ultra-short-acting barbiturates used as general anesthetics—eg, thiobarbiturates such as thiopental— are intrinsically extremely lipophilic and also exist in the same tautomeric forms as the oxybarbiturates. Their distribution depends upon the lipid content of the tissue and the blood flow through it. After injection, they are quickly concentrated in the brain because of its lipid content and great vascularity, reaching a maximal concentration within 1 minute. As blood levels fall, thiopental leaves the nerve tissue and is redistributed to the other tissues. The brief duration of action of thiopental is thus due to rapid redistribution. Because of its poor blood supply, adipose tissue or depot fat is unimportant in this process unless repeated or large doses are given. After redistribution, thiopental is slowly metabolized in the liver.

The long-acting barbiturates—eg, phenobarbital— are only slowly distributed to the brain because they are partially ionized at body pH, ie, in the plasma. They also are metabolized in the liver, principally by oxidation at C5, but as much as 35% of a dose appears unchanged in the urine.

The short-acting and intermediate-acting barbiturates have properties in between those of the thiobarbiturates and phenobarbital. They are entirely metabolized in the liver—ie, a negligible amount is excreted unchanged in the urine.

C. Piperidinedione Derivatives, "Nonbarbiturate" Sedatives: The formulas below suggest that the substituted piperidinediones are structurally related to the

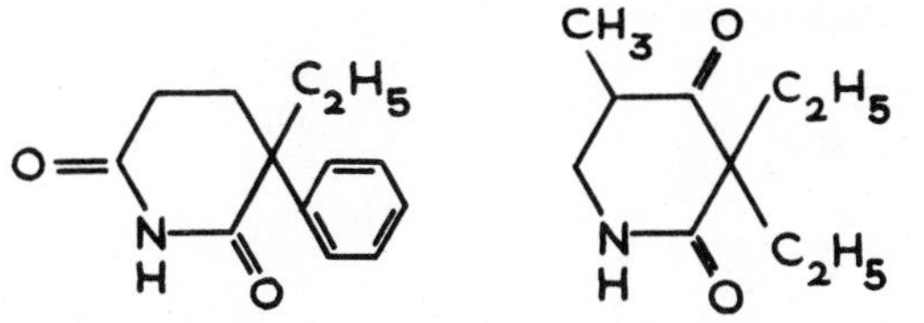

Glutethimide
(Doriden)

Methyprylon
(Noludar)

FIG 23−1. Piperidinedione derivatives.

barbiturates. The same structure-action generalizations hold. Thus glutethimide, the phenylethyl derivative, is equivalent in its actions to phenobarbital, the phenyl-ethyl substituted barbiturate, although it is somewhat shorter acting and may cause convulsions as a toxic effect. Methyprylon is a short-acting hypnotic.

D. Carbamates and Dicarbamates: (Table 23−3.) A carbamate or urethane is an ester of carbamic acid. If both hydroxyl groups on a dihydric alcohol are esterified with carbamic acid, a dicarbamate is formed. Ethyl urethane, commonly called by the class name, urethane, is a laboratory anesthetic. Other carbamates have been used clinically as sedatives and even as fixed (intravenous) anesthetics. The dicarbamates (Table 23−4) also have all of the effects discussed below as characteristic of the sedative-hypnotic group. However, they were introduced close to the time that the effects of the major tranquilizers were characterized, and special properties were claimed for some years. Several carbamates and dicarbamates included in Tables 23−3 and 23−4 are also alleged without substantial basis to act selectively as spinal cord depressants and, there-fore, as voluntary muscle relaxants.

E. Benzodiazepines and a Quinazolone: (Table 23−5.) The drugs of this group are the most recently introduced sedatives, and the tremendous popularity of chlordiazepoxide (Librium) and diazepam (Valium) is due in large part to the confusion in terminology

that obscures the fact that they are pharmacologically equivalent to the barbiturates and other sedatives.

Oxazepam (Serax) is the metabolite into which chlordiazepoxide and diazepam are transformed.

The first benzodiazepine was the result of an unsuccessful effort to synthesize a quinazolone. When the quinazolone (methaqualone) was successfully synthesized, it was found to be a short-acting sedative.

F. Alcohols: Ethanol is the important example of a sedative-hypnotic that is an alcohol. Special aspects of its pharmacology and the properties of other alco-hols of toxicologic importance are discussed in Chapter 24.

Chloral hydrate is converted rapidly to trichloro-ethanol after absorption. Other therapeutically useful alcohols are chlorobutanol (Chloretone), ethchlorvynol (Placidyl), and phenaglycodol (Ultran). Methylpara-fynol (Dormison) is virtually inactive.

G. Bromides: Bromides—ie, sodium, potassium, or ammonium bromide or mixtures of these salts—are regarded as obsolete drugs but are still present in sev-eral proprietary over-the-counter drugs, including Bromo-Seltzer.

H. Ethers, Hydrocarbons, Esters, Ketones: Several ethers and hydrocarbons are useful general anesthetics. Paraldehyde, a cyclic ether formed by the polymeriza-tion of acetaldehyde, is the only additional therapeu-tically useful member of this group. The toxicity of many others that are commonly encountered is due in part to their hypnotic properties. Many industrial sol-vents, including those deliberately inhaled by "glue sniffers," have no effects other than acute CNS depres-sion. Others cause, in addition, even more dangerous chronic toxicity—eg, benzene may cause aplastic anemia, carbon tetrachloride is hepatotoxic, and petro-leum distillates cause chemical pneumonia.

Pharmacologic Actions

A. Mechanism of Action: Discussion of the mech-anism of action of the sedative-hypnotics would require repetition of the theories proposed for the action of the general anesthetics, with no more defini-

TABLE 23−3. Carbamates (urethanes).

$$R-O-\overset{\displaystyle O}{\overset{\displaystyle \|}{C}}-NH_2$$

	R	Hypnotic Dose	Preparations Available
Ethinamate (Valmid)	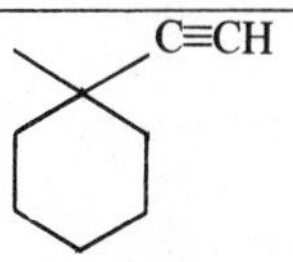 (C≡CH cyclohexane structure)	0.5 gm	Tablets, 0.5 gm
Methocarbamol (Robaxin)	*	*	*
Chlorphenesin carbamate (Maolate)	*	*	*

*See discussion of spinal cord depressants and Table 23−7. These nominal cord depressants are listed here to show the chemical similarity with sedatives.

TABLE 23–4. Dicarbamates.

$$H_2C-O-\underset{\underset{O}{\|}}{C}-NH_2$$
$$R_1-\underset{\underset{H_2C-O-\underset{\underset{O}{\|}}{C}-N-R_2}{|}}{C}-CH_3 \quad H$$

	R_1	R_2	Sedative Dose*	Preparations Available
Meprobamate† (Equanil, Miltown)	$-C_3H_7$	$-H$	400 mg	Tablets, 200 and 400 mg
Mebutamate (Capla)‡	$-C_4H_9$	$-H$	. . .	Tablets, 300 mg
Carisoprodol (Rela, Soma)‡	$-C_3H_7$	$-C_3H_7$	. . .	Tablets, 350 mg Capsules, 250 mg
Tybamate (Solacen, Tybatran)	$-C_3H_7$	$-C_4H_9$	350 mg 3–4 times daily	Capsules, 250 and 350 mg

*These intermediate-acting drugs are not recommended for continuous sedation. See text.
†Generic preparation available. Trade names included for identification only.
‡Not suggested for use as sedative or hypnotic. Possible use is discussed in text.

tive conclusions. The barbiturates and the few other sedatives that have been studied are selective depressants of the ascending reticular activating system (RAS), and this action can explain the loss of consciousness induced. If 2 conditions are imposed on the biochemical studies of barbiturate action—that reasonable concentrations must be used and that the CNS must be unusually sensitive to the effect—all of the voluminous work can be called exploratory at best.

B. Effects: Several precautions must be observed if the description of the effects of sedative-hypnotics is to be accurate and the classification of the drug valid. The drug must be studied over a wide range of doses if the complete sequence of effects described below is to be observed—or, if different drugs are being compared, equally potent doses must .be used before a claim of selectivity of effect for one or the other drugs is made. Furthermore, many of the effects to be described are subjective, and drug effects may therefore seem to vary unpredictably. Actually, the drugs themselves, which can act only on the organic substrate of behavior, are quite consistent. However, the content and intensity of the reaction are conditioned by individual factors and the setting in which the drug is given. The varied reactions to alcohol in different individuals and in different situations are common examples of this fact.

1. Gross behavioral changes—

a. Sedation—Sedation results from small doses of drugs of this class. It may be defined as decreased responsiveness to a constant level of stimulation or a decrease in spontaneous activity and ideation. It is not quite equivalent to drowsiness but may progress to sleepiness.

b. Disinhibition—Disinhibition occurs following the use of larger amounts of a sedative. This effect is presumed to be due to depression of a higher cortical center and release of a lower or phylogenetically older level from constant inhibitory control. It may be

minor in degree and may appear as euphoria. This feeling will be accompanied by impaired judgment and a loss of self-control, both of which are in contrast with the euphoria seen after the use of the narcotic analgesics. With larger doses, or in the presence of continuous stimulation such as pain, the disinhibition may result in drunkenness and excitement. This excitement is a manifest behavioral change due to depression or disinhibition and is not equivalent to stimulation in the physiologic sense.

c. Relief of anxiety—This effect is probably not separable from the sedative and euphoriant effect, but it is mentioned separately because of its therapeutic importance.

d. Ataxia and nystagmus—These signs appear at the stage of disinhibition and persist until anesthesia supervenes.

e. Sleep (hypnosis)—Sleep is induced by all of these drugs if sufficiently large doses are administered. Small (sedative) doses suffice if the patient is ready for sleep. The dose required will vary with the physiologic and psychologic state of the individual and the environmental situation in which the drug is given. The resulting sleep is equivalent to normal or physiologic sleep, but with larger doses it can be deeper, ie, less time is spent in the REM (dreaming, light sleep, rapid eye movement) phase.

f. Anesthesia—Stage III of general anesthesia as defined in Chapter 20 can be induced in animals and in humans. Demonstration of this effect in humans often depends upon a suicidal attempt with the drug, although short- and ultra-short-acting barbiturates are used as anesthetic agents. All of the agents classified as sedatives in this chapter have been used in successful suicidal attempts or in attempts that resulted in anesthesia. The production of anesthesia in the human as well as in animals has been established.

TABLE 23−5. Benzodiazepines and methaqualone.

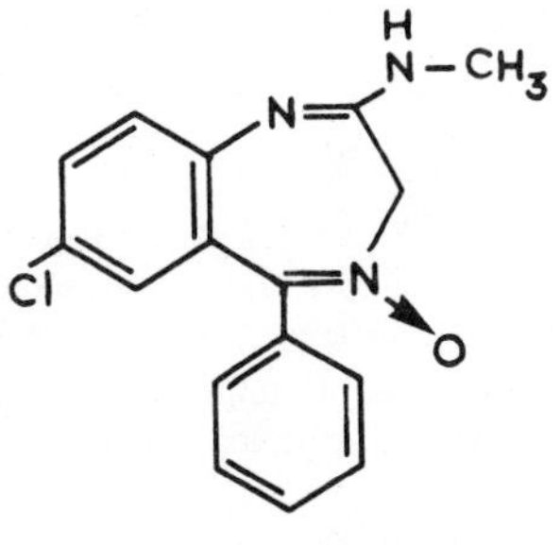

Chlordiazepoxide

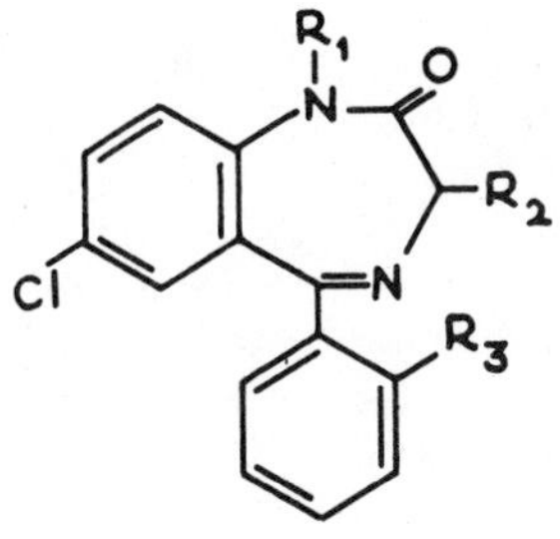

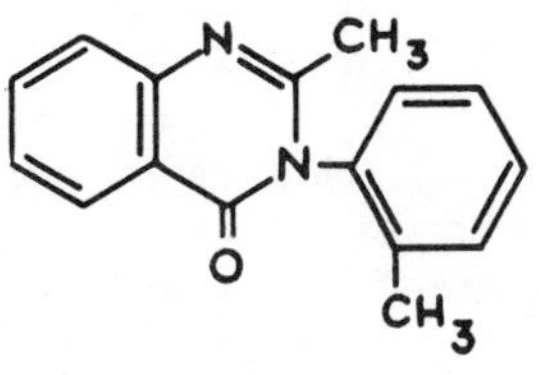

Methaqualone

	R_1	R_2	R_3	Sedative Dose (3−4 Times Daily)	Hypnotic Dose	Preparations Available
Short-acting Methaqualone*	See above			. . .	150−300 mg	Tablets, 150 and 300 mg Capsules, 200 and 400 mg
Flurazepam (Dalmane)	$-C_2H_4-N(C_2H_5)_2$		−F	. . .	15−30 mg	Capsules, 15 and 30 mg
Intermediate-acting Diazepam (Valium)	$-CH_3$			5−10 mg	. . .	Tablets, 2, 5, and 10 mg Ampules, 5 mg/ml, 2 ml
Long-acting Oxazepam (Serax)		−OH		15−30 mg	. . .	Capsules, 10, 15, and 30 mg Tablets, 15 mg
Chlordiazepoxide (Librium)	See above			10−20 mg	. . .	Tablets, 5, 10, and 25 mg Capsules, 5, 10, and 25 mg Ampules, 100 mg powder, with diluent in separate ampules

*Available as Optimil, Parest, Quaalude, Somnafac, Sopor.

2. Effect on the EEG−The effect of a graded series of doses of a sedative on the EEG is exactly what would be predicted from similar observations on general anesthetics and from studies on sleep. Small doses of sedatives, producing a state of disinhibition or light sleep, lead to an increase in fast activity. With larger doses or when sleep is induced by smaller doses, the pattern is that of slow wave activity equivalent to the normal sleep pattern. Still larger doses, as with general anesthetics, cause a progressive decrease in amplitude with "burst suppression" or periods of inactivity. Finally, all activity disappears.

3. Analgesia−The barbiturates are said to be poor general anesthetics because the patient may respond reflexly to pain during surgical anesthesia. Deeply anesthetized patients, however, are totally unresponsive.

The analgesic activity of the barbiturates has been tested on patients with postoperative (incisional) pain. These drugs were found to be effective, although less so than the narcotic analgesics. However, in the presence of pain, the excitement of the disinhibited (stage II) period may be greatly intensified. This inappropriate response to an intense stimulus appears to be equivalent to that seen during induction with general anesthetics. When the barbiturates are used alone for their analgesic effect, the possibility of a paradoxic excitement should be kept in mind.

4. Anticonvulsant effect−All of the sedative-hypnotics are anticonvulsants both in the laboratory and clinically. Phenobarbital and other long-acting drugs such as chlordiazepoxide are selectively more effective in this regard, and their use in the treatment of epilepsy is discussed in Chapter 29. At this time the anticonvulsant action is emphasized for the purpose of classifying drugs into the sedative category. The tranquilizers will be contrasted in that they are convulsants during their administration but not upon withdrawal.

5. Withdrawal state—When large doses of any of these drugs are given chronically, continued administration may be necessary to prevent a withdrawal state—ie, physical dependence is present. Physical dependence to the opiates also develops, but the symptoms of withdrawal are different. The withdrawal state after abrupt cessation of sedative administration is characterized by hyperexcitability that may progress to convulsions. (See below under Adverse Reactions.)

6. Habituation—The relief of anxiety and the euphoria provided by these drugs has led to the casual or compulsive misuse of every member of this group. This problem is discussed elsewhere (Chapter 7) but is mentioned here as a basis for classifying the drugs. The similarity to the general anesthetics does not disappear at this point, since ether frolics and chloroform habitués were well known in the past.

7. Spinal cord depression (voluntary muscle relaxation)—Monosynaptic spinal reflexes are depressed by the barbiturates and the other sedative-hypnotics that have been studied only by very large doses. The simple myotatic reflexes persist until deep anesthesia.

The effect of depressing polysynaptic reflexes or internuncial transmission in the cord is of greater interest because of the claim that some sedatives, notably meprobamate and diazepam, are unusually potent in this effect and are potentially useful in relaxing abnormally contracted voluntary muscle associated with joint disease or tension. This effect on spinal cord function, actually of no therapeutic importance, is mentioned here to emphasize that it is a property of all drugs of this class. In fact, if the cord depressant action is assayed in animals by the ability of a drug to antagonize strychnine convulsions (which are due to spinal cord facilitation), phenobarbital is seen to be more active than meprobamate.

The hypnotic effect does not correlate well with the ability to depress internuncial transmission. The depression is demonstrable in purer form by compounds that are only weak anesthetics and are discussed below.

8. Cardiovascular and respiratory effects—The cardiovascular, respiratory, and autonomic effects of the sedatives are indirect and are due either to decreased activity or to the sympathomimetic effects during the occasional periods of excitement that may appear.

With larger doses, respiration is progressively depressed. The peripheral chemoreceptors are less sensitive to the barbiturates and other sedatives than is the respiratory center, and respiration is therefore maintained by the stimulation of hypoxia rather than by an increase in P_{CO_2}. Later, medullary depression occurs and respiration is further depressed.

In the deeply anesthetized patient, shock may occur as a result of vasomotor depression.

Pentobarbital is a common anesthetic for laboratory animals, and when so used it causes a sympathomimetic effect with elevated blood pressure and tachycardia.

Clinical Uses

A. Induction of Sleep: There are some situations where the physician can anticipate the need for medication at the hour of sleep. It is considerate, for example, to offer sedation to a patient attempting to sleep in the strangeness of a hospital or to someone who has undergone an anxiety-engendering day. However, the indication for sleep-inducing medication is usually established by the complaint of the patient who is dissatisfied with the pattern of his sleep. The nature of his complaint—ie, the pattern of his insomnia—is the important factor in determining the drug selected for use. A few patients, because of anxiety or other reasons, have trouble going to sleep but once asleep have no further difficulty. For such patients a rapidly acting hypnotic with a short duration of action is adequate. Other individuals have no difficulty going to sleep but awaken after a few hours to spend a restless night and arise unrefreshed. Others have both problems. For these individuals an intermediate-acting drug with its attendant risk of hangover may be used, or a short-acting drug is prescribed at bedtime with instructions to repeat it one time if necessary.

The effectiveness of the hypnotics in initiating and maintaining sleep cannot be assumed on the basis of uncontrolled observations in the clinic or by extension to humans of the effects of larger doses upon animals. It is easy to overvalue the effectiveness of a sleep-inducing agent given at bedtime when the subject is physiologically and psychologically prepared for sleep. Careful clinical assays not only establish effectiveness but provide a basis for comparing the potency, duration, and other properties of the many compounds available.

One general method of clinical evaluation is to make EEG records throughout the period of drug action. The amount of time spent by the patient in a wakeful state, in deep sleep, and in dreaming (REM) sleep can be determined.

However, the largest volume of data useful for comparing various compounds has been derived from double-blind studies in which the observations of a technician and the reports of the patient are used to determine the onset and duration of sleep and the occurrence of residual effects (hangover) in each subject.

B. Relief of Anxiety; Sedation:

1. Situational anxiety—Anxiety may be an appropriate reaction to some circumstances. If the situation does not recur too regularly, a barbiturate or other sedative may be used over short periods to minimize anxiety. Many people use alcohol in this way, and the risks associated with the use of other sedatives are similar. Relief of anxiety may occur, but with a corresponding decrease in manual proficiency and judgment. In some situations (eg, a critical school examination), sedation may impair performance even though the subject is deceived by the euphoria into believing that he has performed well. There are, however, situations in which mild sedation may improve both performance and mood.

2. Preprocedural medication—The anticipation and experience of a painful or frightening medical or dental procedure is a special instance of situational anxiety. The difficulty is that the patient must remain cooperative and not unduly anxious even when the procedure involves pain or other frightening stimulus. Sedative drugs alone may be satisfactory, but ordinary doses given to a rested but anxious patient during the day probably have little effect. If the dose of a barbiturate or other sedative is increased, the risk of excitement with pain is increased, and the effect on the behavior of an outpatient following the procedure must also be considered. The combination of a phenothiazine tranquilizer and a small dose of a narcotic analgesic—eg, half doses of meperidine and promethazine intramuscularly—is an alternative often used in situations where preprocedural medication is called for.

C. Neurotic Anxiety: Situational anxiety is anxiety generated by an immediately present external threatening or fearful situation. Neurotic anxiety is anxiety in response to an insufficient environmental stimulus or no apparent adequate stimulus at all.

Neurotic anxiety may be manifested as subjective fear or tension; as any of a variety of psychophysiologic disorders; as obsessive or phobic behavior; or as depression. Of an unselected group of ambulatory patients, probably more than half will have solicited help because of complaints related to anxiety.

The sedative-hypnotics often provide partial symptomatic relief of anxiety and decrease the intensity of associated organic symptoms. Drugs should certainly not be used to the exclusion of psychotherapy, and the occasional hazards attending their use must be borne in mind.

There are few objective measurements of the results of treatment with sedatives alone. However, subjective patient reports and evaluations by physicians under carefully controlled conditions have established the effectiveness of each of the drugs classified in this chapter as sedatives. In controlled studies, the placebo effect on this most subjective of responses is not so great as might be supposed. In the noninvestigative situation, however, the nonspecific factors are amplified and merge with psychotherapeutic technics such as reassurance.

The long-acting sedatives—phenobarbital is the reference standard—are preferable to short- or intermediate-acting drugs for the relief of anxiety. If short-acting preparations are used, the effect appears quickly and decays rapidly (as with alcohol). The patient soon associates these cyclic changes (3–4 times each day) with his medication, and may tend to take additional doses or larger doses. The less intense, more constant effect of the long-acting cumulative sedatives is safer and more satisfactory.

When drugs are used in this way, adequate explanation is always necessary so that the patient will not fix upon his organic symptom and its relief and thus fail to understand the real origin of his problem.

Anxiety may also occur as a symptom attending other more serious if less common psychiatric illnesses (psychosis, sociopathic disorders). Here also, anxiety may be controlled by sedatives, but effective treatment requires far more than sedation.

D. Depression: Drugs used in the treatment of depressions are discussed in Chapter 28. It will be noted that depression (and fatigability) are among the most common manifestations of anxiety. Treatment of this symptom or type of depression with sedatives may be effective. Major (psychotic) depressions may be intensified by sedatives.

E. Excitement Due to Drugs or Disease: The sedative-hypnotics can be used to reduce the excitement associated with hyperthyroidism or to counteract the stimulant effects of ephedrine in an asthmatic patient.

F. Reduction of Spontaneous Activity: Enforced bed rest may be made more tolerable by sedation. Marked excitement cannot be controlled by sedatives in less than anesthetic doses. Maniacal excitement is now an indication for the use of a phenothiazine tranquilizer.

G. Other Uses: The anticonvulsant and preanesthetic uses of the sedatives are discussed elsewhere in this book. Sleep may be induced with these agents during an EEG recording in the attempt to activate latent abnormalities.

Adverse Reactions

The undesirable effects common to all of the sedative-hypnotic drugs listed in this chapter will be discussed here. Additional toxic effects which are specific for a single agent are mentioned as properties of the individual preparations (below).

A. Side-Effects and Chronic Toxicity:

1. Drowsiness—All of the sedatives listed in this chapter cause drowsiness if enough is given, and some patients will be made drowsy even by small doses. Some claims to the contrary are made. Obviously, therapeutically equipotent doses of the drugs being compared must be given before a claim of fewer side-effects can be accepted.

Whether drowsiness is regarded as an undesirable effect or not depends upon physician expectations, the personality of the patient, and the patient's need for and expectations from therapy. To some patients, the feeling of being slowed down may be threatening; to others, it and the associated relief of anxiety are quite welcome.

2. Impaired performance and judgment—A person need not be rendered staggering drunk before his motor performance and, probably more important, his judgment are significantly impaired. The most common offending agent in this regard is alcohol, and the problem of the impaired driver is discussed in the next chapter.

At this time it should be emphasized that all sedatives are equivalent to alcohol in their effects; that all are additive in their effects with alcohol; and that their effects persist longer than might be predicted. Some simple psychomotor tests—eg, key tapping, auditory reaction time, and memory for digits—are impaired for as long as 8 hours after a dose of pentobarbital, as is pilot performance during a simulated flight also. In the carefully controlled studies of athletic performance referred to in Chapter 28 in relation to amphetamine, pentobarbital was shown to have a deleterious effect on performance, but the euphoric swimmer or runner felt that he had done well and underestimated his time.

3. Hangover—The effect of the sedatives may extend beyond a period judged by the patient to be desirable. After a bedtime dose of even a short-acting sedative, the patient may on the following morning complain of feeling dizzy, lethargic, or exhausted. Long-acting agents occasion more complaints of this type.

4. Drug abuse or habituation—No other sedative (or any other drug) is abused so widely and with such great social and individual harm as alcohol. However, every one of the therapeutic and several of the toxic agents—eg, gasoline, freons—listed above have been misused because of the euphoria and suppression of anxiety that they provide.

The short- or intermediate-acting drugs are more apt to be misused because of their rapid onset and intense effect. Smoking a drug such as marihuana or inhaling a hydrocarbon offers the same advantage to an even greater degree because of the rapid absorption of active components across the alveolar membrane.

Sedatives may, like alcohol, be abused continuously and compulsively. More commonly they are used as spree drugs or as a substitute for other drugs when the preferred drug (alcohol, methamphetamine, or heroin) is not available. In some subjects the distinction between therapeutic use and misuse becomes blurred—eg, in the patient whose physician provides a large supply of a sedative to use daily or several times daily prior to anticipated anxiety-inducing situations.

Except for alcohol and some of the hydrocarbons, none of the commonly used sedatives cause chronic toxicity other than sedation, drunkenness, and the possibility of a withdrawal state.

5. Withdrawal state—All of the therapeutic agents listed, including those most recently introduced, have caused a withdrawal state. Withdrawal of therapeutic doses may result only in a disturbed pattern of sleep with restlessness and dreaming objectively established by EEG changes showing excessive (rebound) REM sleep. After discontinuance of larger doses, there may be a hyperexcitable state with associated weakness, tremor, anxiety, and elevated blood pressure, pulse, and respiratory rate. Following even larger doses, convulsions may occur and a toxic psychosis may appear with agitation, confusion, and hallucinations. If the drug is alcohol, the state is called delirium tremens.

In experiments on humans given pentobarbital or secobarbital for many weeks, it was shown that withdrawal after daily doses of 0.4 gm resulted in only minor symptoms. Withdrawal after doses of 0.5 gm/day caused pronounced tremor and anxiety. Following 0.8 gm/day, 75% of the subjects had at least one convulsion and 60% had a toxic psychosis. Meprobamate may pose a special hazard in this regard since doses of 800 mg 4 times a day result in pronounced withdrawal signs in many patients who have taken these therapeutic doses for weeks.

The symptoms of withdrawal following abuse of a short- or intermediate-acting sedative appear in 18–24 hours and increase to a maximum at 2–3 days. When phenobarbital, chlordiazepoxide, or a similar long-acting depressant is withdrawn, symptoms may not appear for a week. A withdrawal state is very rare after the use of these slowly eliminated compounds which, in effect, accomplish their own slow withdrawal. Epileptic patients are especially susceptible to increased seizures upon withdrawal or abrupt decrease in the dose of a sedative or anticonvulsant.

Treatment consists of readministration of a sedative-hypnotic followed by planned gradual withdrawal. Once a toxic psychosis has developed, it is difficult to shorten the withdrawal syndrome.

B. Acute Toxicity Due to Overdosage: In large doses the hypnotics produce a state of prolonged, deep anesthesia. Respiration is depressed. If a stage of severe medullary depression is reached, circulatory shock occurs. Tendon reflexes persist until the deepest stages. Nystagmus is seen until the equivalent of plane 2 of stage III anesthesia is reached. Pupillary size is not a consistent sign of intoxication since initial constriction may be replaced by dilatation due to asphyxia.

The diagnosis is usually made on circumstantial evidence: a suicide note, a phone call, or an empty prescription container. Simple chemical tests on urine are useful, but treatment must be instituted before the results of blood tests are available.

The lethal dose of a barbiturate or other hypnotic varies tremendously depending upon the circumstances of ingestion. If the person arranges not to be discovered for some time after ingestion of the drug, as little as 8–10 times the hypnotic dose may be fatal. If he reaches medical care in time, ingestion of many times that amount may be consistent with survival.

The variability in lethal dose reflects the fact that the causes of death differ if death occurs before rather than after hospitalization. Uncared for, the deeply anesthetized patient may die of respiratory depression or obstruction. With appropriate treatment, these need not occur; and if the patient dies, he will usually die from shock, acute renal insufficiency, or pulmonary changes resulting from immobilization—eg, pneumonia, acute pulmonary edema, atelectasis.

Barbiturate blood levels do not correlate well with mortality rates. Coroners' cases—ie, patients who die without medical care—have lower blood levels than do patients who are not judged to be dangerously intoxicated in the hospital. In general, blood levels of a short-acting barbiturate greater than 3–3.5 mg/100 ml are serious. Phenobarbital blood levels of 8–10 mg/100 ml are dangerous, but recovery has been reported after levels of 18.8 mg/100 ml.

C. Treatment of Acute Intoxication: We are indebted to a group of physicians in Copenhagen for the development of a plan of treatment for acute intoxication with hypnotics based on examination of the causes of death in these anesthetized patients. In 1949 the treatment of all cases of drug depression was centralized in a single Copenhagen hospital. After establishment of what we would now call an intensive care unit and the introduction of a physiologic (often called "conservative") treatment rationale, the death rate in comparable groups of patients fell from 12% to 1%. Treatment of the hospitalized patient is not standardized, but would be based on some of the following considerations.

1. Observe continuously—Treatment is best carried out in an intensive care unit, where observation can be continuous and carefully recorded.

2. Support respiration—The airway is kept open by an oropharyngeal airway, intubation, or by tracheostomy if necessary. Secretions are aspirated frequently. If necessary, respiration is mechanically assisted. Continuous mechanical respiration is avoided if possible since it often leads to alkalosis and confusion of the neurologic signs.

3. Prevent or treat shock—A fall in blood pressure or narrowing of the pulse pressure should be treated without waiting for the development of shock. Blood or plasma substitutes should be given. Pressor amines such as levarterenol have previously been widely used, but the same objections apply as those discussed under the treatment of shock (Chapter 10). The use of isoproterenol infusions is now becoming more common.

4. Maintain renal function—Whether or not exaggerated diuresis is induced to hasten elimination of the drug, adequate water (in the form of 5% glucose in water) and saline must be provided. Prevention of prolonged shock protects against acute renal insufficiency.

5. Increase rate of excretion of drug—In profoundly depressed patients, efforts to hasten excretion may be justified—eg, osmotic and alkaline diuresis, peritoneal dialysis, or hemodialysis.

Osmotic diuretics are used to increase urine volume to 10 or more liters of urine per day. Since the duration of coma is shortened, it is reasonable to assume that the substances whose excretion is hastened are active, sedating compounds. Mannitol is probably the most commonly used osmotic diuretic. It is not free of renal toxicity, and urea is sometimes used instead.

If the urine is kept alkaline (pH $>$ 8.0) with Ringer's lactate (Hartmann's) solution or with half-normal saline to which is added one 50 ml ampule of $NaHCO_3$ containing 45 mEq, renal tubular reabsorption of phenobarbital is decreased. The barbiturates are weak acids, and reabsorption is less if they are present in the renal tubular urine in the salt (charged) form. Phenobarbital has a long half-life in the blood (3 days), is present in high concentration, and its ionization can be easily influenced—ie, it has a favorable pK. Alkalinization of the urine is not useful if intoxication is due to the shorter-acting barbiturates or the other hypnotics. The urine can be kept alkaline with the carbonic anhydrase inhibitor acetazolamide more easily than with alkaline fluids. Experience with this technic is limited but promising.

Peritoneal dialysis and hemodialysis are both effective in removing practically all of the hypnotics, but, since recovery rates are already good, dialysis is not often needed. Dialysis adds a hazard of its own and should not be considered in lieu of the above treatment.

6. Prophylactic penicillin—In general, prophylactic antibiotic therapy is not often indicated. However, prophylactic penicillin during the treatment of a drug depression has reduced the incidence of pneumonia.

7. Nursing care—The critical importance of the nursing service need not be belabored. Aspiration of secretions, regular movement of the patient, and packing of pressure points to prevent ulcers are necessary. If the period of anesthesia is prolonged, the eyes should be covered to protect the cornea from drying and dust.

8. Aftercare—Most of these patients will have ingested drugs in a suicidal attempt. Obviously, the need for care does not end when they regain consciousness. Each patient should be considered a psychiatric problem and challenge.

9. Measures that *should not be used*—

a. Gastric lavage—If the patient is reached promptly, gastric aspiration may be advisable. Introduction of additional lavage fluid, however, has repeatedly been shown to hasten gastric emptying and to lead to aspiration even in conscious patients. A depressed patient should not be aspirated. Some physicians feel that lavage is permissible if a cuffed endotracheal tube is first inserted. Others withhold lavage because it imposes added risks of cardiac arrhythmias and respiratory arrest.

b. Central stimulants—The use of central stimulant drugs in hypnotic intoxication is still sometimes treated as if it were a controversial issue yet to be decided. It is not so regarded by those who have reported the most favorable survival experience, who regard the stimulants as contraindicated. The convulsant stimulants or analeptics discussed in Chapter 28—eg, pentylenetetrazol (Metrazol) and picrotoxin—were used in the past. Since respiratory arrest is not a common cause of death in hospitalized patients, the brief and weak action of the analeptics is of doubtful benefit. The hazards associated with their use are convulsions followed by fatal postconvulsion depression and hyperpyrexia.

Amphetamine is not a convulsant stimulant and perhaps could be useful in the treatment of drug depression. Experience with the very large doses needed is limited.

D. Allergic Reactions: Serious allergic reactions to those hypnotics that are still marketed are very rare. A morbilliform rash sometimes occurs as an allergic response to barbiturates (especially phenobarbital) and most of the other sedatives.

TABLE 23–6. Dosages and preparations available of some commonly used
sedative-hypnotics not provided in prior charts.*

| | Oral Dose | | |
	Hypnotic (Single Dose)	Sedative (3–4 Times Daily)	Preparations Available
Short-acting			
Pentobarbital sodium† (Nembutal)	100–200 mg	30 mg‡	Tablets, 50 and 100 mg (sustained release) Capsules, 30, 50, and 100 mg Elixir, 20 mg/5 ml Suppositories, 30, 60, 120, and 200 mg Injectable (IV), 50 mg/ml, 2, 5, 20, and 50 ml; 150 mg/ml, 2 ml; 300 mg/ml, 10 ml
Secobarbital sodium† (Seconal)	100–200 mg	30 mg‡	Tablets (enteric-coated), 50 and 100 mg Capsules, 30, 50, and 100 mg Elixir, 20 mg/5 ml Suppositories, 30, 60, 120, and 200 mg Injectable (IV), 50 mg/ml, 1, 20, and 30 ml; 100 mg/ml, 1 ml; 250 mg dry powder
Methyprylon (Noludar)	300 mg	. . .	Tablets, 50 and 200 mg Capsules, 300 mg Elixir, 50 mg/5 ml
Ethchlorvynol (Placidyl)	500 mg	100–200 mg‡	Capsules, 100, 200, 500, 750, and 1000 mg
Paraldehyde	12–16 ml	. . .	Vials containing 2, 5, 10, and 30 ml
Chloral hydrate	1 gm	. . .	Capsules, 250 and 500 mg Syrup, 500 mg/5 ml Elixir, 267 mg/5 ml Suppositories, 300, 500, and 975 mg
Intermediate-acting			
Amobarbital† (Amytal)	100–200 mg	15–30 mg‡	Tablets, 15, 30, 50, and 100 mg Capsules, 50, 65, and 200 mg of sodium salt Elixir, 20 and 40 mg/5 ml Suppositories, 200 mg Injectable sodium salt (IV), ampules containing 65, 125, 250, 500, and 1000 mg of dry powder; vials containing 0.5 and 1 gm
Glutethimide (Doriden)	500 mg	125–250 mg‡	Tablets, 125, 250, and 500 mg Capsules, 500 mg Suppositories, 8, 15, 30, and 60 mg
Long-acting			

Phenobarbital	100 mg	15–30 mg	Tablets, 8, 15, 30, 65, and 100 mg
			Sustained action tablets, 50 mg
			Sustained action capsules, 65 and 100 mg
			Elixir, 20 mg/5 ml
			Suppositories (sodium salt), 15, 30, and 65 mg
			Injectable sodium salt (IM or subcut):
			    Hypodermic tablets, 60 mg
			    Powder (dry, sterile), 65, 130, 160, 200, 325, and 500 mg
			Injectable sodium salt (IM or IV), aqueous solution in propylene glycol, 65 mg/ml, 2 ml; 120 mg/ml, 1 and 10 ml; 160 mg/ml, 2 and 10 ml; 325 mg/ml, 2 ml

Phenaglycodol (Ultran)	. . .	200–400 mg	Tablets, 200 mg Capsules, 300 mg

*Other less widely used barbiturates (and single hypnotic doses) are as follows: **Long-acting**: Aprobarbital (Alurate), 80–160 mg; barbital (Veronal), 300–600 mg; diallylbarbituric acid (Dial), 100–300 mg. **Intermediate-acting**: Butabarbital (Butisol), 50–200 mg; cyclobarbital (Phanodorn), 200–400 mg; heptabarbital (Medomin), 200–400 mg; hexethal (Ortal), 200–600 mg; probarbital (Ipral), 200–400 mg; talbutal (Lotusate), 120 mg; vinbarbital (Delvinal), 100–200 mg.

†Generic preparation available. Trade name included for identification only.

‡Short- and intermediate-acting drugs are not recommended for continuous sedation.

Contraindications & Cautions

A patient with a history of an allergic reaction to one of the sedatives should be given a sedative of a different chemical type. Porphyria or a family history of porphyria contraindicates the use of the barbiturates.

In the presence of hepatic or renal insufficiency, sedatives should be ordered in small initial doses to allow for slower biotransformation and excretion. Actually, patients with cirrhosis with ascites and marked BSP retention do not show either prolonged sedation or elevated blood levels after administration of short-acting barbiturates. Hepatic damage must evidently be massive before the precaution becomes important.

The effects of the sedatives are additive with each other. Since alcohol is so commonly used, its effects are often added to those of both prescribed and illegally obtained sedative drugs. The combined misuse of a sedative—commonly amobarbital or meprobamate—and alcohol may result in a seriously impaired driver with a blood alcohol level below that accepted as defining intoxication in the legal sense. The lethal dose of a barbiturate is much less following the ingestion of alcohol—ie, in evaluating the state of a patient who has attempted suicide, the total amount of depressant taken must be considered.

"Sleeping pills" have in most countries become the favorite agent for suicide attempts, but suicide is too complex a problem to be discussed as a simple matter of drug availability. It is inconvenient and impractical to routinely limit all prescriptions to less than a lethal dose, and patients can accumulate drugs or acquire them from more than one source. The physician as well as the laity should be discreet with drugs, but the best hope for the prevention of suicide is to recognize warning signs ("cry for help") and take appropriate action.

It is often suggested that under the influence of small doses of barbiturates—or alcohol plus barbiturates—a person may without suicidal intent ingest a potentially lethal dose of a hypnotic. Emotional and legal factors impinging on the certification of cause of death make investigation of this "automatism" hypothesis difficult. Studies of the circumstances surrounding such deaths and interviews with people who have survived such episodes suggest that automatism is rare if it ever occurs.

Preparations, Dosages, & Selection of Drug

In classifying the sedatives in relation to their use, duration of action is the most important property. As explained above, the long-acting sedatives are preferable to the short- or intermediate-acting drugs in the prolonged treatment of anxiety. For the induction of sleep, the short-acting compounds are usually most useful, although the sleep patterns of some patients may suggest the use of a drug with intermediate properties.

Some of the commonly used sedatives are reviewed below. Of the many drugs available, the physician need select only one or perhaps 2 from each class for his use.

A. Dosage: The dosages of many of the sedatives are listed in Table 23–6. The hypnotic dose is given at bedtime, often with permission to repeat once before 1 a.m. if necessary.

For sedation, the longer-acting, cumulative drugs are given 3–4 times a day. Actually, 2 doses per day of a cumulative drug such as phenobarbital or chlordiazepoxide will in a few days give a constant blood level throughout the 24 hours.

The effective and tolerated dose varies with the individual and must be determined for each patient. Doses should be changed only at intervals of 3–4 days unless the first dose proves to be excessive. The dose can often be increased when the patient becomes accustomed to the effect. As an example, phenobarbital, 15 mg 3–4 times a day, is a common initial dose. A fourth daily dose is usually tolerated, and some patients may require and tolerate 30 mg 3–4 times a day. Others may complain of the effects unless the dose is reduced to 8 mg. Still others may take the daytime doses in addition to 100 mg at bedtime without complaint.

B. Ultra-Short-Acting Hypnotics: The ultra-short-acting barbiturates are generally used only as intravenous anesthetics. The rapid termination of their activity suggests that they would not be useful oral agents even though their great lipid solubility would lead to rapid absorption from the gastrointestinal tract. Given in an investigative situation when the stomach is empty, thiopental, hexobarbital, and methohexital all rapidly induce sleep of brief duration. Hexobarbital (Sombucaps) is available as 250 mg capsules. The recommended dose of 500 mg is less than the 10 mg/kg used in the above investigation.

C. Short-Acting Hypnotics: Pentobarbital is the standard drug of this category. Secobarbital does not differ from it in its properties. Others selected from those identified earlier in this chapter are the following:

1. Chloral hydrate and equivalents—Chloral hydrate is a very rapidly acting hypnotic. It was for many years available only as a salty solution and was, therefore, largely replaced by the more easily dispensed barbiturates. It is now available in a capsule of 0.5 gm. The hypnotic dose is 1 gm. It occasionally causes gastric irritation.

Chloral betaine (Beta-Chlor) is a solid complex that liberates chloral hydrate after ingestion. It is easier to dispense than liquid chloral hydrate. Tablets are labeled in terms of their chloral hydrate content.

2. Chlorobutanol (Chloretone)—This alcohol has all of the advantages of chloral hydrate but is an easily dispensed solid and does not cause gastric irritation. The dosage is 0.5–1 gm.

3. Paraldehyde—Paraldehyde is a liquid with an unpleasant taste and an odor that is more offensive to other people than to the patient himself. Paraldehyde acts rapidly. It is primarily metabolized by the liver, but some appears in the expired air, accounting for the odor and the pulmonary irritation that sometimes occurs. Paraldehyde has been a traditional remedy for the excited or inebriated person, but it has no special advantage in this context. Like other drugs dispensed as liquids or solutions, it is more rapidly absorbed than solids in tablets or capsules.

Paraldehyde is a cyclic ether formed by the polymerization of acetaldehyde. The reaction is slowly reversible, and the liberated acetaldehyde may be oxidized to acetic acid. Old supplies of paraldehyde may become strongly acid. As paraldehyde stocks are now only slowly utilized, the chance of encountering a deteriorated solution has increased. Paraldehyde from a previously opened bottle should not be used unless it has been kept in a refrigerator.

4. Flurazepam (Dalmane)—The claim is made that the short-acting benzodiazepine causes less suppression of REM sleep than do other hypnotics, inducing a more normal sleep pattern and causing less of a rebound increase in REM sleep and dreaming upon withdrawal. The same claim is made for chloral hydrate used in certain dosages. When attempts are made to compare equipotent doses of several hypnotics, it appears that there is a threshold dosage for each drug above which REM sleep suppression occurs.

D. Intermediate-Acting Sedative-Hypnotics: Amobarbital (Amytal) is the prototype of this class. Two analogous compounds are as follows:

1. Meprobamate (Miltown, Equanil)—This carbamate is merely another intermediate-acting sedative without any special attributes. The drug was advertised as a "tranquilizer" but used for the treatment of anxiety without the caution that is exercised in the use of amobarbital, its nearest equivalent. Misuse, withdrawal states, and euphoric states have been produced more commonly than with the barbiturates. Direct comparisons in double-blind tests on anxious patients, both institutionalized and ambulatory, have shown that neither the patient nor the physician can distinguish meprobamate from amobarbital. The cost of meprobamate is no longer as high as it once was, but the objection to using an intermediate-acting drug for continuous sedation remains.

2. Glutethimide (Doriden)—This drug was widely used because it was an early "nonbarbiturate sedative." When used at bedtime, it causes hangover the next morning in many patients. Like other short- and intermediate-acting sedatives, it has greater potential for misuse than do the long-acting drugs. If it has any distinctiveness, it is in its toxicity. A few patients have had convulsions, sometimes accompanied by a toxic psychosis, not only after withdrawal but during continued administration of the drug.

3. Diazepam (Valium)—This heavily promoted drug is not subject to the same prescribing regulations as apply to other intermediate-acting sedatives, and it is often prescribed as if it were somehow distinctive from them. Much of the drug now prescribed is misused as the patient increases the dosage and shortens the interval between doses to maintain the euphoriant effect.

E. Long-Acting Sedatives:

1. Phenobarbital—Phenobarbital is still the most widely used drug of this category. Its repute has suffered unjustifiably because it was developed and used long before the period of enthusiasm for psychopharmacology and before the reintroduction of drugs into psychiatry.

2. Chlordiazepoxide (Librium) and oxazepam (Serax)—These drugs are currently very widely used. Their only distinctiveness is that they are excreted over a period of several days and have a duration of action that may be somewhat longer than that of phenobarbital. A cumulative effect may be seen, and the appearance of withdrawal effects may be delayed for a week or more after the drug is discontinued.

Each of these drugs is an effective sedative if given in adequate doses. The claim that anxiety can be relieved without the occurrence of drowsiness as a side-effect is based on experience with small doses.

No deaths from the use of these long-acting benzodiazepine sedatives by themselves have yet been reported. This may in part reflect the distribution of small doses and the failure of the layman to identify these drugs as "sleeping pills" suitable for suicide.

The cost to the patient of treatment with one of these newer drugs is considerably greater than equivalent treatment with phenobarbital.

3. Bromides—Bromide ion is distributed and excreted exactly as is chloride ion. Given over a period of many days, it accumulates and acts as a long-acting sedative. Bromides are no longer prescribed but are still present in some proprietary remedies—eg, Bromo-Seltzer contains potassium bromide, 2½ gr per capful, and Miles Nervine, 9½ gr per capful of triple bromides. Prolonged use results in characteristic toxic effects: an acneiform rash, increased oral, nasal, and lacrimal secretions, and, occasionally, toxic psychosis. Treatment of overdosage is based on increasing the excretion of chloride and, therefore, of bromide by giving sodium chloride or, preferably, ammonium chloride and maintaining a high urine volume with a diuretic.

THALIDOMIDE; THE POSSIBILITY OF A PURE SOMNIFACIENT

A drug that could relieve anxiety or induce normal sleep without the adverse effects and dangers associated with the available sedative-hypnotics would be of obvious value. There is no reason to expect great changes in the treatment of anxiety, but the experience with thalidomide suggests that a drug with no actions beyond the induction of normal, quickly reversible sleep is possible.

Thalidomide is without demonstrable acute toxicity. In animals and humans, sleep occurs after its administration if the subject is undisturbed, but, except for a minor anticonvulsant effect, it has none of the other actions described for the sedatives or tranquilizers. It cannot cause anesthesia or be used as a suicidal agent. It is ineffective in the chronic, symptomatic treatment of anxiety.

Because of these advantages, thalidomide quickly came into wide use as a hypnotic, and in some countries it was available without prescription. A particularly unfortunate circumstance was that it was widely recommended and used early in pregnancy. Then followed the terrible epidemic of a specific and rare congenital defect, phocomelia. About 500 of these children with flipper-like limbs and other defects were born in Germany and other countries. Thalidomide was not marketed in the USA because of concern about a peripheral neuritis that it caused in adults.

The embryopathic effect of thalidomide is due to its chemical nature rather than to its somnifacient action. At least 2 chemically different compounds have pharmacologic properties similar to thalidomide. A drug lacking both the acute toxicity of the barbiturates and the special toxicity of thalidomide is theoretically possible.

DEPRESSANTS OF INTERNUNCIAL TRANSMISSION

The sedative-hypnotics depress polysynaptic reflexes involving the spinal cord and brain stem. In the laboratory, this action decreases voluntary muscle hyperactivity when it is due to hyperactivity of such multineuronal reflexes. It is possible to find compounds in which the sedative properties are minimized and the more specific cord depressant action emphasized, and the depressants of internuncial transmission could, therefore, be discussed as a separate drug class. However, the clinical efficacy of the "central muscle relaxants" was never established. The drugs still suggested for use are sedatives, and such usefulness as they have is due to their ability to relieve anxiety.

Chemistry & Classification

A. Glycerol Ethers: Mephenesin, in the laboratory at least, acts with considerable specificity—ie, it depresses polysynaptic reflexes in dosages that cause only minimal sedation. No evidence of clinical usefulness was ever provided.

B. Monocarbamates: As the limitations of mephenesin became apparent, a number of esters of carbamic acid with one of the remaining hydroxyl groups of mephenesin were prepared. The 2 carbamates listed in Table 23–7 are very similar chemically, and are stronger sedatives and less specific cord depressants than mephenesin.

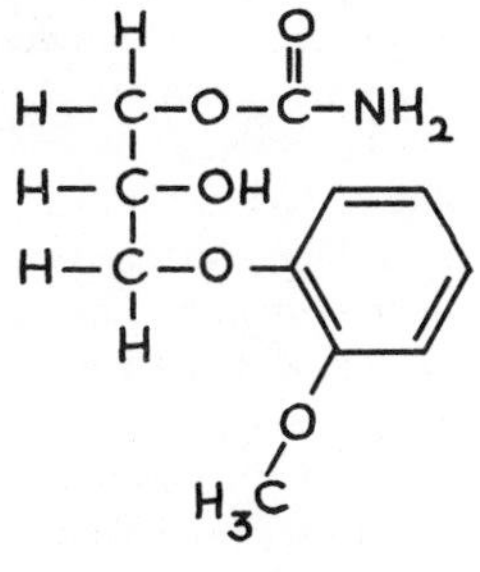

Methocarbamol
(Robaxin)

C. Oxazole: The one oxazole still marketed has not been shown to be useful clinically.

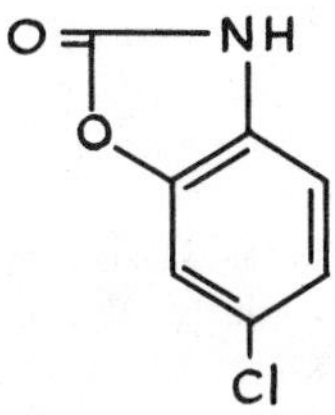

Chlorzoxazone
(Paraflex)

D. Sedative-Hypnotics: All drugs that are sedatives also depress internuncial transmission. When a voluntary muscle relaxant of this category is indicated, a long-acting sedative is probably the best choice. Phenobarbital should be considered the prototype of this group, but newer drugs such as chlordiazepoxide (Librium) and diazepam (Valium) are more vigorously promoted for use.

TABLE 23–7. Spinal cord depressants: Dosages and preparations available.

	Usual Adult Dosage (3–4 Times Daily)*	Preparations Available
Monocarbamates Methocarbamol (Robaxin)	1.5–2 gm	Tablets, 500 and 750 mg Injectable (IM or IV), 100 mg/ml, 10 ml vials
Chlorphenesin carbamate (Maolate)	400 mg	Tablets, 400 mg
Oxazole Chlorzoxazone (Paraflex)	250–500 mg	Tablets, 250 mg

*Doses suggested by manufacturer. Not actually recommended for use.

Meprobamate was said (unjustifiably) to be more effective than other sedatives in relaxing striated muscle. Much was made of its relations to "propanediols" such as mephenesin, although no free hydroxyl group remained.

Pharmacologic Effects

A. Mechanisms of Action: Polysynaptic reflexes of the spinal cord or analogous reflexes involving the brain stem are inhibited or made less responsive to stimuli. (These reflexes are also called multineuronal or are said to involve internuncial or connecting neurons between the primary afferent and efferent neurons.) Some descending influences from the reticular formations are also depressed, and after very large doses depression comparable to that caused by the sedative-hypnotics appears.

B. Effects: Only the tendon jerk or phasic muscle stretch reflex is monosynaptic. Therefore, a variety of reflexes and reflex activity are reduced. In animals, the effects are most easily demonstrated in some experimental hypertonic state. After cord section, for example, flexion and crossed extension are suppressed by doses that are without effect on the patellar or other tendon reflexes. Ventral root potentials are altered correspondingly. Decerebrate rigidity is relieved. Strychnine facilitates polysynaptic reflexes; the convulsions so generated are antagonized.

In man, the effects that can be demonstrated are much less striking.

Clinical Uses

A. Skeletal Muscle Spasm: Trauma or inflammation in or around a joint may lead to muscular splint-ing or guarding that may add to the pain and disability. Muscle relaxants are widely used in the treatment of sprains, bursitis, arthritis, and similar problems. Their use is based on the assumption that the spasm originates through cord reflexes that can be depressed by drugs of the mephenesin type and that effective dosage levels of the muscle relaxants can be administered. Controlled clinical trials have not established any usefulness for orally administered spinal cord depressants in these common situations. In fact, even when given intravenously, methocarbamol was no more effective than a placebo injection in aiding in the reduction of shoulder dislocations.

Sedative-hypnotic drugs may act by relieving anxiety rather than through any specific effect on the spinal cord. When muscle tension is a manifestation of anxiety—eg, tension headache—drugs that suppress anxiety may have demonstrable usefulness.

B. Spastic States: In chronic states of spasticity—eg, paraplegia, cerebral palsy—only the long-acting sedatives show any activity. Definition of their areas of usefulness is incomplete.

C. Strychnine Toxicity: Strychnine is now rarely encountered as a toxic agent but is an interesting laboratory drug. The alkaloid is isolated from the seeds of an Asian tree, *Strychnos nux vomica.* It has no remaining therapeutic uses but is used as a rodenticide.

Strychnine antagonizes one of the inhibitory mediators of the spinal cord (Fig 23–2). Reflex activity is thereby greatly augmented, and the slightest stimulus may result in a "convulsion" which is actually more comparable to an intense decerebrate rigidity. Unlike most convulsions, strychnine spasms are intense and sustained enough to cause death from asphyxia.

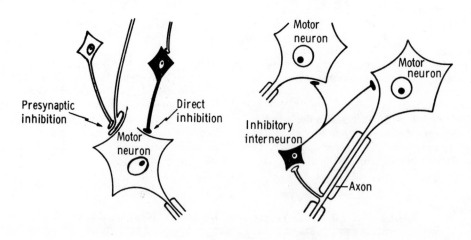

FIG 23–2. Left: Two types of inhibition demonstrated in the spinal cord. **Direct inhibition:** A chemical mediator released from an inhibitory neuron acts to cause hyperpolarization (inhibitory postsynaptic potential) of motor neuron. Strychnine blocks the action of the inhibitory mediator; tetanus toxin prevents its release. **Presynaptic inhibition:** A second chemical mediator is released onto the ending or axon of an excitatory neuron. The size of the postsynaptic excitatory potential is reduced. Picrotoxin blocks the action of this inhibitory mediator. **Right:** Diagram of a specific inhibitory system involving an inhibitory interneuron or Renshaw cell. (Reproduced, with permission, from Ganong: *Review of Medical Physiology,* 5th ed. Lange, 1971.)

Strychnine intoxication is treated by the induction of general anesthesia, either with thiopental or other barbiturate or with an inhalation agent.

In the laboratory, the ability of a compound to antagonize strychnine toxicity can be used to assay its ability to depress multisynaptic reflexes. With large doses, strychnine also facilitates monosynaptic reflexes and acts on the brain stem.

D. Tetanus: Tetanus toxin prevents the release of a second inhibitory chemical mediator in the spinal cord and brain stem and produces muscular rigidity and spasms. It also acts predominantly on polysynaptic reflexes.

Drugs can be used to control the convulsions of tetanus and to supplement the benefits of general care, early tracheostomy, antitoxin, and penicillin. Cord depressants of the mephenesin type are not used. The choice is between a variety of sedative-hypnotics and chlorpromazine. Comparative studies are few, most authors merely advocating the use of the newest drug.

Chlorpromazine appears to many investigators in geographic areas where tetanus is more common to be the preferable drug. Chlorpromazine does not protect against strychnine convulsions but depresses both mono- and polysynaptic reflexes in the intact animal. It decreases outflow in the gamma efferents to muscle.

In large doses, chlorpromazine intensifies rather than reduces spinal cord activity. The dosage, for example, should be 50–150 mg every 4–8 hours for adults or 4–12 mg for neonates.

Adverse Reactions

If a sedative-hypnotic is used as a centrally acting muscle relaxant, it will have the expected side-effects —eg, drowsiness, ataxia, or paradoxical excitement.

Chlorzoxazone (Paraflex) is a metabolite of zoxazolamine (Flexin), a drug no longer marketed that caused fatal hepatitis. Chlorzoxazone is probably also hepatotoxic in rare instances.

Preparations & Dosages

See Table 23–7.

●   ●   ●

General References

Sedative-Hypnotics

Beecher, H.K.: *Measurement of Subjective Responses: Quantitative Effects of Drugs.* Oxford Univ Press (New York), 1959.

Bloomer, H.A.: Limited usefulness of alkaline diuresis and peritoneal dialysis in pentobarbital intoxication. New England J Med 272:1309–1313, 1965.

Bunn, H.F., & G.D. Lubash: A controlled study of induced diuresis in barbiturate intoxication. Ann Int Med 62:246–251, 1965.

Bush, M.T., Berry, G., & A. Hume: Ultra-short acting barbiturates as oral hypnotic agents in man. Clin Pharmacol Therap 7:373–378, 1966.

Essig, C.F.: Addiction to nonbarbiturate sedative and tranquilizing drugs. Clin Pharmacol Therap 5:334–343, 1964.

Fraser, H.F., & others: Degree of physical dependence induced by secobarbital or pentobarbital. JAMA 166:126–128, 1958.

Kelley, W.N., & others: Acetazolamide in phenobarbital intoxication. Arch Int Med 117:64–69, 1966.

Lasagna, L.: A comparison of hypnotic agents. J Pharmacol Exper Therap 111:9–20, 1954.

Lasagna, L.: A study of hypnotic drugs in patients with chronic diseases. J Chronic Dis 3:122–133, 1956.

Litman, R.E., & others: Investigations of equivocal suicides. JAMA 184:924–929, 1963.

Mellin, G.W., & M. Katzenstein: The saga of thalidomide. New England J Med 267:1184–1194, 1238–1244, 1962.

Oswald, I., & R.G. Priest: Five weeks to escape the sleeping-pill habit. Brit MJ 2:1093–1095, 1965.

Price, H.L., & others: The uptake of thiopental by body tissues and its relation to the duration of narcosis. Clin Pharmacol Therap 1:16–22, 1960.

Raymond, M.J., & others: A trial of five tranquilizing drugs in psychoneurosis. Brit MJ 2:63–66, 1957.

Root, W.S., & F.G. Hofman: Sedatives and hypnotics. Vol 1, part A, pp 185–273, in: *Physiological Pharmacology.* Academic Press, 1963.

Setter, J.G., Maher, J.F., & G.E. Schreiner: Barbiturate intoxication: Evaluation of therapy including dialysis in a large series selectively referred because of severity. Arch Int Med 117:224–236, 1966.

Shideman, F.E.: Clinical pharmacology of hypnotics and sedatives. Clin Pharmacol Therap 2:313–344, 1961.

West, E.D., & A.F. da Fonseca: Controlled trial of meprobamate. Brit MJ 2:1206–1209, 1956.

Wikler, A.: Relationships between clinical effects of barbiturates and their neurophysiological mechanisms of action. Fed Proc 11:647–652, 1952.

Spinal Cord Depressants

Berger, F.M.: Spinal cord depressant drugs. Pharmacol Rev 1:243–278, 1949.

Diamond, S.: Double-blind study of metaxalone. Use as skeletal-muscle relaxant. JAMA 195:479–480, 1966.

Laurence, D.R., & R.A. Webster: Pathologic physiology, pharmacology, and therapeutics of tetanus. Clin Pharmacol Therap 4:36–72, 1963.

Payne, R.W., & others: Diazepam, meprobamate, and placebo in musculoskeletal disorders. JAMA 188:229–232, 1964.

Shaftan, G.W., & H. Herbsman: Negative results: Intravenous methocarbamol in reduction of shoulder dislocations. JAMA 188:69, 1964.

24...

Alcohols

ETHYL ALCOHOL
(Ethanol)

The pharmacologic effects of ethyl alcohol and a few other alcohols of toxicologic interest are very similar to those of the sedative-hypnotics discussed in the preceding chapter. Alcohol is an important special case because it is a social rather than a therapeutic drug and its wide use and misuse lead to damage to the individual user and to irresponsible or antisocial behavior.

Source & Chemistry

The growth of a ubiquitous yeast in a sugar-containing medium forms alcohol and CO_2. Since paleolithic times, in one culture or another, virtually every fruit juice, plant sap, tuber, honey, and grain have been fermented in order to produce an alcoholic drink. If grain is used as the source of carbohydrate, the simpler sugars must be made available for utilization by the yeast. This is accomplished by first adding malt, a powder made from sprouted barley which contains diastase. Yeast ceases its growth when the concentration of ethanol in the medium reaches 14–16%. Stronger liquors can then be obtained by distilling the wine or distiller's beer formed from fruit juice or grain.

In addition to ethanol, fermentation produces higher alcohols, a variety of aldehydes, acids, esters, and ketones. Most of these "congeners" are volatile and appear in the distilled beverage as well as in wine. The higher alcohols, mostly isoamyl alcohol, are referred to as fusel oil. Isoamyl alcohol and ethyl acetate, the congeners present in greatest concentrations, are long-acting depressants and may add to the effects of alcoholic beverages.

Beer ordinarily contains no more than 2–4% alcohol, although some beers may contain up to 6%. Wines contain approximately 12% alcohol. Fortified wines (sherry or port) are prepared by adding brandy to wine, and their alcohol content may be in excess of 20%. A variation of the fortified wines are the sweet wines popular among the alcoholics in the Skid Rows of most cities. In the preparation of these sweet wines, fermentation is halted by the addition of concentrated alcohol before much of the sugar has been consumed. These strong, sweet wines provide a large number of calories but no other nutritive factors. In the lives of some people they may almost completely take the place of food. Whisky, brandy, rum, gin, and other distilled liquors contain 35–50% alcohol.

Absorption

The discussion of the absorption and metabolism of alcohol has special importance because of the need to define, for legal purposes, the degree of intoxication of an individual. The judgment must usually be made retrospectively, after the subject has been arrested for some offense.

Alcohol requires no digestion or dissolution and is a small, neutral, water-soluble molecule. It is, therefore, rapidly absorbed by simple diffusion over the entire gastrointestinal tract. Absorption from the stomach occurs promptly, but at a rate slower than that in the upper small intestine. In the fasting state, about 20% of a single dose of alcohol is absorbed from the stomach; the remainder is absorbed from the small intestine as rapidly as it leaves the stomach. After a single dose of alcohol, absorption is 90% complete in 1 hour, the peak blood level being reached in approximately 40 minutes. The blood alcohol level returns to zero in 8–10 hours. (Fig 24–1.)

Food in the stomach slows the absorption of alcohol by prolonging the emptying time and, since it covers some of the mucosal surface, by slowing diffusion. Dilute alcoholic solutions—eg, beer or tall drinks—are absorbed more slowly than moderately concentrated (30%) solutions such as cocktails.

Distribution

The distribution of alcohol throughout the body is in proportion to the water content of the various tissues.

Small amounts of alcohol (2–4% of the total dose) are lost into the urine and into the alveolar air by diffusion. The alcohol in alveolar air is in equilibrium with the alcohol in the blood passing through the lungs; a determination of the alcohol concentration in respiratory air can therefore be used to estimate blood concentrations for medicolegal purposes. The concentration of alcohol in the urine is less precisely proportionate to the average blood concentration during the period of urine collection. Urine specimens are, therefore, less useful for legal purposes. The total amount of alcohol lost in the urine also depends upon the volume of urine excreted.

Metabolism

A. Steps in Oxidation: Ethanol is converted in the liver to acetaldehyde, which is oxidized to acetate or acetyl-Co A, which in turn enters the tricarboxylic acid (TCA) cycle for further oxidation to CO_2 and water.

The first step occurs, practically speaking, only in the liver.

$$H_3C-CH_2-OH \xrightarrow[NAD^+ \quad NADH+H^+]{\boxed{\text{ALCOHOL DEHYDROGENASE}}} H_3C-\overset{\overset{\displaystyle H}{|}}{C}=O$$

The second step, the oxidation of acetaldehyde, occurs in the liver and other tissues that contain aldehyde dehydrogenase. The oxidation of acetaldehyde takes place more rapidly than its production from alcohol, but acetaldehyde levels rise after the administration of alcohol. When aldehyde dehydrogenase and, therefore, the metabolism of acetaldehyde are inhibited by the prior administration of disulfiram (Antabuse), acetaldehyde blood levels are higher and symptoms of acetaldehyde toxicity occur. (Fig 24–2.)

The above pathway accounts for 90–95% of ingested labeled (^{14}C) alcohol.

B. Maximal Rate of Metabolism: The rate of metabolism of alcohol does not rise continuously as the amount in the body is increased. The rate of conversion of alcohol to acetaldehyde in the liver reaches a maximum when the dehydrogenase system is saturated. This occurs with blood levels of about 0.1%. The maximum rate is fairly constant for a given individual. Variation between individuals and among experimenters is greater, but one common generalization is that the typical 70 kg human can metabolize 10 ml (8 gm) of alcohol per hour, or about 2/3 oz of 100 proof (50%) whisky per hour. Other estimates are closer to 1 oz of whisky per hour. Since ethanol provides 7 cal/gm, a persistent drinker can derive 1800 cal/day from alcohol.

C. Alteration of Rate of Metabolism: Insofar as the practical goal of hastening the treatment of acute intoxication is concerned, it can be said that there is no way of increasing the rate of metabolism of alcohol. The administration of fructose in the investigative situation does have such an effect both in animals and in humans.

Pharmacologic Effects

A. Mechanisms of Action: The mechanisms of action of alcohol, like its effect in general, are similar to those of the short-acting barbiturates discussed in the previous chapter. Alcohol diffusely depresses the CNS, but the mechanism of this effect is as obscure as it is in the case of the sedative-hypnotics. The loss of consciousness eventually induced is explicable on the basis of depression of the RAS.

Alcohol does have effects on organ systems other than the CNS, and these actions are not present in the other sedative-hypnotics. The vasodilating, local, and nutritional effects of alcohol are discussed below.

B. Effects:

1. CNS depression—

a. Behavioral—Alcohol is simply one example of a short-acting sedative-hypnotic, and the description of the CNS effects of the sedatives presented in Chapter 23 is entirely applicable to alcohol and need not be repeated here in detail. The actions of the sedatives were, in turn, related to the stages of general anesthesia, and the distinctiveness of alcohol is most easily made clear by reference to these stages. Ether and other useful general anesthetics quickly carry the patient through stages 1 and 2 (induction) and cause a prolonged stage 3, ie, there is a wide margin between the anesthetic dose and the lethal or stage 4 dose. The dose-effect relation for alcohol is such that stages 1 and 2 are prolonged, but, once anesthesia is achieved, only a small additional amount can lead to the stage of medullary paralysis.

Small amounts of alcohol lead to sedation and the relief of anxiety. Larger amounts cause more pronounced disinhibition with ataxia, impaired psychomotor performance, faulty judgment, and uninhibited or irresponsible behavior.

The manifest effects of the ingestion of alcohol in amounts sufficient to cause drunkenness may appear at first glance to be different from the effects of the barbiturates. However, if barbiturates or other sedatives are taken in sufficient amounts in a situation where

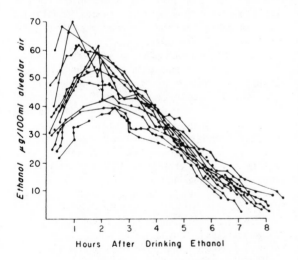

FIG 24–1. The rate of absorption and metabolism of ethanol, 0.5 ml/lb body weight, in 10 tests on the same subject over a 2-month period. The level of alcohol in alveolar air reflects the blood level. (Reproduced, with permission, from Freund & O'Hollaren: Acetaldehyde concentrations in alveolar air following a standard dose of ethanol in man. J Lipid Research 6:473, 1965.)

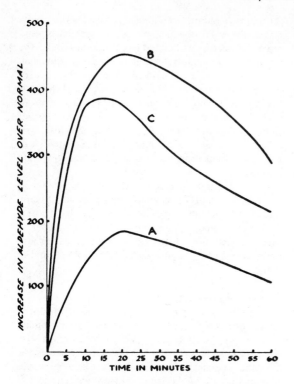

FIG 24–2. The effect of pretreatment with disulfiram on acetaldehyde blood levels (μg/100 ml). A: Levels after 0.5 ml/kg of 45% alcohol in 10 patients. **B:** Levels after the same dose of alcohol in 44 patients pretreated with disulfiram. **C:** Levels after half the previous dose of alcohol in 29 pretreated patients. (Reproduced, with permission, from Hine & others: Human pharmacology of Antabuse-alcohol reactions. J Clin Invest 31:319, 1952.)

stimulation persists, the same excited or disinhibited behavior is seen. Alcohol is a social drug, and is not taken at bedtime with the expectation of sleep but in a setting that requires continued functioning. The apparently paradoxical excitement is therefore more commonly seen after alcohol.

The manifest effects of the depression caused by alcohol on behavior will vary with the individual and with the setting. Whether alcohol is ingested at a party or at bedtime in the home will influence the kind of behavioral change it causes. Similarly, the individual reaction will depend upon whether alcohol unmasks an underlying ebullience or depression. Most importantly, alcohol, in our culture, is taken at times and in situations that require continued functioning of the individual. Embarrassing or criminal behavior, eg, drunken driving or the commission of other crimes, is thus a major problem.

The excitement or uninhibited behavior that occurs after the use of alcohol is a manifestation of depression, not stimulation. This distinction between the manifest behavioral change and the underlying

pharmacologic mechanism must always be made, especially since alcohol is still often called a stimulant.

It is, of course, possible to drink to the point of unconsciousness or anesthesia. It is also possible to ingest a lethal amount of alcohol, although this is difficult unless other depressant drugs are also used.

b. Withdrawal–The compulsive user of alcohol who ingests large amounts for extended periods, when forced by some circumstance to discontinue or reduce his alcohol consumption, will experience the same withdrawal state described in Chapter 23 for the sedatives. This state is characterized by hyperexcitability that may progress to convulsions and, sometimes, by a toxic psychosis with hallucinatory behavior. This state, called delirium tremens when the agent is alcohol, is further discussed below.

c. Tolerance–There are several ways in which a limited degree of tolerance to the effects of alcohol can develop during its chronic use. One form of tolerance can be demonstrated when, in the same individual, a larger dose or higher blood level of alcohol is required to produce the same pharmacologic effect following continued administration. This kind of tolerance can be established, but, as is also true of the barbiturates, it is small in degree. Only small changes in the metabolism of alcohol occur during the development of this form of tolerance, and it is presumed to be an adaptation of the CNS to the effect of alcohol.

A quantitatively more significant form of tolerance can be demonstrated by comparing the effects of alcohol on experienced and inexperienced drinkers. In this case, the presumption is that tolerance is due to a behavioral adaptation, ie, the user learns to control his manifest behavior following repeated experience of the depressant or disinhibiting effect.

2. Vasodilatation–The primary cardiovascular effect of alcohol administration is vasodilatation. The cardiovascular effects are best understood in comparison with the actions of other direct smooth muscle relaxants such as nitroglycerin. The vasodilating action of alcohol is often said to be secondary to central depression, but this conclusion is based largely on the difficulty of demonstrating a vasodilating action of alcohol in isolated preparations. Central depression of comparable degree induced by other depressant drugs does not cause the same amount of vasodilatation, and it appears quite likely that the vasodilatation ascribed to alcohol is in fact due to the action of the active metabolite, acetaldehyde, an extremely potent vasodilator. Since the blood levels of alcohol and acetaldehyde rise and fall almost synchronously, it is impossible to separate their effects in the intact organism. Infusions of acetaldehyde or the accumulation of endogenous acetaldehyde following the administration of disulfiram (Antabuse) lead to vasodilatation and other effects ordinarily described as due to alcohol. Similarly, the bradycardia and fall in blood pressure mentioned below may be due in part to the depletion of norepinephrine from its stores within the body, and this effect also is brought about by acetaldehyde administration.

The vasodilatation causes a warm, flushed skin and a subjective feeling of warmth. Loss of heat from the body is increased. Cerebral blood flow is not changed. Anginal pain is sometimes relieved, but, since the relief of pain is not accompanied by ECG evidence of a decrease in myocardial ischemia, the effect is usually explained as analgesia due to central depression. For reasons elaborated in the discussion of the treatment of angina, it is now probable that alcohol ingestion relieves anginal pain because it is a generalized vasodilator and reduces cardiac work.

The effects on heart rate and on blood pressure are secondary to the decrease in peripheral resistance or to the reflex sympathetic activation caused by the vasodilatation and aborted fall in blood pressure. Heart rate and stroke volume may increase, and only with huge doses is bradycardia seen. The change in blood pressure varies widely with the dose of alcohol. With small or extremely large doses, a decrease in blood pressure is usual. Moderate doses may actually increase blood pressure.

3. Respiration—Very large doses of alcohol cause the respiratory depression predictable on the basis of the central depressant effect. Small or moderate amounts of alcohol cause a stimulation of respiration. This action is also more easily explained as due to acetaldehyde.

4. Gastrointestinal—The CNS depressant effect of alcohol and the accompanying relief of anxiety or euphoriant effect can increase the appetite. The bitter taste of sherry or other alcoholic beverages is also said, on less substantial grounds, to be useful in this regard.

Gastric acid secretion is increased by the ingestion of alcohol in all but the most concentrated forms. A local effect on the antrum to release gastrin explains at least a fraction of the hypersecretion, but an action on the upper small intestine is also present. Alcohol obviously should be avoided by the patient with an active peptic ulcer, and either avoided or used only with the protection of antacids and atropine by the ulcer patient wishing to avoid recurrences.

Alcohol ingested in a concentrated form even in the presence of food will cause gastric irritation with hyperemia, prolonged emptying time due to pylorospasm and decreased gastric motility, increased mucus and decreased acid secretion, and, eventually, vomiting and bleeding.

Chronic atrophic gastritis occurs in a small fraction of chronic alcoholics.

5. Diuresis—Initially, alcohol suppresses the release of ADH and causes diuresis independent of the volume of fluid taken in as a beverage. Later, urine volume again reflects fluid intake.

Clinical Uses

A. Sedative: Alcohol used as a sedative has the same disadvantages as any other short-acting sedative, ie, the patient quickly associates the production of euphoria with the medication and, noting also the brief duration of the effect, may, personality and situation permitting, assume control of the dose himself. For continuous sedation, a longer-acting compound is preferable. Whether the physician prohibits, permits, suggests, or prescribes alcohol in the form of a social beverage usually depends upon nonpharmacologic factors.

B. Antiseptic: Ethyl alcohol is germicidal. In order to achieve a germicidal effect on dried surfaces or matter, its concentration should be close to 70%. It, or the equivalent (but nontaxed and nonpotable) isopropyl alcohol, is still used to prepare the skin at the site of an injection or for similar purposes. In this application the cleansing properties are probably more useful than the germicidal effect. Alcohol is not active against spores and viruses. Hexachlorophene or quaternary ammonium chlorides have replaced alcohol to a large extent for skin preparation or wet sterilization.

Adverse Reactions

In 1966, in the USA, alcohol consumption amounted to 2.43 gallons of hard liquor for every person over 21 plus 3 billion gallons of beer and 185 million gallons of wine. The cost at retail of these social drugs was 15 billion dollars. Approximately 70% of American adults drink, but half of the production is consumed by less than 10% (perhaps as few as 6%) of the adult population. The consequent toxicity dwarfs all but a few other problems of public and individual health.

A. Acute Behavioral Changes:

1. Acute alcoholic intoxication—In small doses the disinhibiting effect of alcohol relieves anxiety and facilitates social behavior. It is suitable and accepted as a social or recreational drug.

Alcohol also impairs measurable psychomotor performance, and impairs judgment by reducing conscious self-control during the period of disinhibition. The drinker is the person least able to judge the degree of impairment, and he continues to drive cars and interact with other individuals without appreciating his disability.

The duration of action of alcohol, especially in the face of continued absorption, is long enough so that the intoxicated individual becomes responsible for a significant fraction of the total of antisocial and criminal acts. For example, when special studies rather than routine accident reports are considered, it is established that approximately 3 out of 5 fatally injured drivers had been drinking and that 60% of these had blood alcohol concentrations above 0.1% (100 mg/100 ml).

The physician is not often called upon to treat acute alcoholic states, but occasionally he will be asked to quiet an excited drunk. For this purpose, chlorpromazine, 25–50 mg IM or orally, is often used. If a sedative is used instead of a major tranquilizer, it should be a long-acting one such as phenobarbital or chlordiazepoxide. Short-acting sedatives act exactly as alcohol does. They may quiet the patient for a time, but he will soon return to the excited level.

2. Quantitative measures of intoxication—The relation between blood alcohol concentration and pharmacologic effect is variable in different individuals, and the effect of the same level is greater when the level is rising than during recovery. The following generalizations can be made:

> **50 mg/100 ml**: (The level produced by 2 oz of whisky in 2 hours.) Euphoria and minor motor disturbances.
>
> **60 mg/100 ml**: Nystagmus. More errors on simple tests.
>
> **80 mg/100 ml**: (3 oz whisky.) Impaired driving ability. First EEG changes.
>
> **100–150 mg/100 ml**: Gross motor incoordination.
>
> **200–300 mg/100 ml**: Amnesia for the experience.
>
> **300–350 mg/100 ml**: Coma.
>
> **355–600 mg/100 ml**: May cause or contribute to death.

Commission of an act such as robbery is defined and punished as a crime whether the individual was intoxicated at the time of the act or not. On the other hand, whether driving a car or being responsible for an accident is a crime may depend upon whether the individual is under the influence of alcohol or not. The measurement of blood alcohol levels and the study of the relation between blood levels and behavior have consequently been emphasized in this context. No absolute definition of the degree of intoxication that constitutes drunk driving is acceptable to all groups at this time. Impairment of performance of real or simulated driving provides an index acceptable to most investigators, and is the basis for the British definition of drunk driving as driving with a blood alcohol of 80 mg/100 ml or more, ie, after drinking 3 or more 1 oz whiskies within an hour. However, some laboratory tests of motor performance are not impaired until higher blood alcohol concentrations are reached and provide a basis for setting a higher level—eg, the ridiculously high level defended in courts, in the USA by some experts of 150 mg/100 ml. Still another group argues persuasively that judgment is impaired before psychomotor tests, and blood levels of 50 mg/100 ml are penalized in some countries.

In most states of the USA, there is no statutory definition of the blood alcohol concentration defining drunkenness, and in each case the analysis must be interpreted for the court by an expert witness. Some states have defined drunk driving by law—eg, in California, a blood level over 100 mg/100 ml. In Britain it is an offense to drive with a blood alcohol concentration of 80 mg/100 ml or above.

In some jurisdictions—eg, California, New York, Britain—an "implied consent" law is in effect. In accepting a license to drive, the citizen consents to the collection of blood or other specimen for alcohol determination if detained by the police; if he refuses, his license to drive can be taken away.

3. Alcoholic coma—Acute overdosage toxicity may, under special circumstances, progress to a stage of anesthesia. This usually requires that someone already quite drunk take in an additional huge increment of alcohol over a short period of time.

The problem and the treatment are similar to those of barbiturate overdosage. However, the margin between the anesthetic dose and the lethal dose is narrower in the case of alcohol than with the barbiturates, and the differential diagnosis is more difficult because of the greater likelihood that some disorder such as head injury or pneumonia may be superimposed on a comparatively minor toxic state.

Treatment is as described for barbiturate intoxication (see p 221) except that neither alkaline nor osmotic diuresis is used.

4. Hangover—The occurrence of hangover is more common after alcohol ingestion than after use of the other short-acting sedative-hypnotics discussed in Chapter 23, in part because of the metabolic effects of alcohol but also because so many more doses of alcohol are consumed. Hangover is in part simply a manifestation of withdrawal less completely developed than the severe state described below. Using sleep patterns as an index, it can be established that the first half of a night's rest after alcohol may be deeper than usual, but that after 4 hours a disturbed sleep pattern reflecting increased excitability is seen. Nondrug factors are certainly involved in the production of alcoholic hangover—eg, remorse or at least regret, loss of sleep, unaccustomed activity, and anxiety—but some of the symptoms are demonstrable under conditions that control these factors.

The signs and symptoms of hangover include tremors, fatigue, vertigo, throbbing headache, labile blood pressure, gastritis with nausea and vomiting that is partly local and partly central in origin, acidosis, weakness, and dehydration with persistent thirst.

Treatment logically begins the night before, with restraint. Failing this, prophylactic measures can be carried out at bedtime. Emesis can be induced, usually with no difficulty, to get rid of some of the unabsorbed alcohol. Fluids, aspirin, and sodium bicarbonate can be taken at this time to anticipate the dehydration, malaise, and acidosis.

The quickest and most effective treatment for alcoholic hangover is to terminate the acute withdrawal state with alcohol, but the danger of this in establishing or maintaining a pattern of drinking is apparent.

Other methods of treatment include fluids, aspirin, a systemic alkali such as sodium bicarbonate for the systemic acidosis, and a nonabsorbed antacid if gastritis is prominent. The amphetamines are widely used by those to whom they are available; there is no reason to doubt that they make people feel better.

B. Withdrawal State; Delirium Tremens: The "DTs" or shakes of alcohol withdrawal are closely comparable to the withdrawal syndrome described for the sedative-hypnotics, but the alcohol withdrawal syndrome is both more common and more severe and occurs in patients whose general health tends to be poor.

After a binge of 2 weeks or more a patient may be forced by lack of money or urged by his own judgment to discontinue or taper off. He may then ask a physician for treatment when his symptoms are still very minor. His subsequent course will vary in severity depending upon how heavily he has been drinking and the rapidity of withdrawal. In mild cases the symptoms may last for only 2 days; in other instances the symptoms may increase in severity for several days and culminate in a period of delirium lasting 3–4 days. The symptoms are those of hyperexcitability that may progress to a typical toxic psychosis characterized by marked alterations in perception with auditory, visual, and tactile hallucinations.

Specific signs and symptoms may include anxiety, tremors, restlessness, agitation, insomnia, irritability, sweating, nausea, vomiting, exaggerated reflexes, tachycardia, slight elevation of temperature in moderately severe cases ($< 38°$), convulsions (often before delirium), delusions, hallucinations, and, in severe cases, temperature $> 38°$. The mortality rate in various recent series ranges from 1% to 37%.

Treatment: These patients usually need fluids, but not necessarily parenterally. If they are able to take fluids by mouth, sodium chloride (2 gm every 4 hours) can be added. Vitamins are probably needed in most cases, but they are not required immediately and repeated administration is not necessary.

Even when most seriously disturbed, these patients are responding in a distorted way to stimuli that are truly present. Explanation, lighted rooms, and attendants with supportive attitudes will minimize their reaction. Jail or other threatening environments will usually intensify the excitement and paranoia.

Replacing the short-acting sedative, alcohol, with a long-acting sedative makes slow withdrawal possible. This policy has come into widespread use because of interest in a newer drug, chlordiazepoxide (Librium). Phenobarbital in equivalantly large doses is just as satisfactory. Short-acting sedatives—eg, barbiturates, chloral hydrate, or the traditional paraldehyde—need usually be given only one time at the beginning of treatment. The major tranquilizers such as chlorpromazine have been used instead of the sedatives; they are probably equally satisfactory in mild cases, and may even return the patient to a normal status more quickly. However, antipsychotic tranquilizers increase the likelihood of convulsions, and reported experience establishes that the mortality rate is higher if they are used.

C. Nutritional Toxicity: Alcohol is easily available for chronic use and is ingested in large absolute amounts—ie, in doses of many grams as compared with the milligram doses of other abused drugs. When such large amounts of alcohol are ingested, it is not added to the diet but replaces a part or most of the normal diet. The calories derived from alcohol are unaccompanied by vitamins or protein, and one or more of the following deficiencies or disease states may result.

1. Folic acid and iron deficiency.

2. Pellagra, or at least the dermatitis characteristic of that disease.

3. Nutritional polyneuropathy—Peripheral nerve degeneration with muscle wasting is only slowly revers-

ible, and the specific deficiency has not been identified.

4. Cardiac beriberi—High output cardiac failure due specifically to thiamine deficiency is a rare occurrence.

5. Wernicke's syndrome—Wernicke's encephalopathy (ataxia, oculomotor palsy, confusion) is an acute disorder due to thiamine deficiency.

6. Korsakoff's psychosis—Following Wernicke's encephalopathy or other signs of acute thiamine deficiency, there may occur a chronic, degenerative change characterized by poor memory for recent events often covered by confabulation.

7. Portal cirrhosis—There is a clear correlation between the consumption of alcohol and the incidence of cirrhosis in a community or group. A direct toxic effect of alcohol is present as well as an undefined nutritional deficiency.

CHRONIC ALCOHOLISM

The magnitude of the problem of alcohol misuse forces its consideration as a separate entity. It is, however, a variation of the general problem of drug abuse discussed in Chapter 7 and should be considered in the same general terms of drug, individual, and social factors.

The importance of individual susceptibility and the spectrum of misuse is more apparent with alcohol than with other drugs because it is used openly. Many individuals, perhaps 30%, actively avoid the experience of drinking. Others accept it when the social situation suggests or almost imposes it. A large group uses alcohol intemperately but episodically, and a few find that its use has become a compulsion dominating their entire lives. Estimates of the incidence of chronic alcoholism vary depending upon where along this continuum a division is made. It is probable that a million people in the USA are drug-driven, chronic alcoholics by everyone's definition and 4–6 million qualify as problem drinkers. Most definitions of chronic alcoholism emphasize the compulsive nature of the behavior—often, however, using another term or description. Sociologic factors involved in the problem of alcoholism are most apparent in the general approval of the use, possession, and sale of alcohol. The compulsive alcoholic will, like other compulsive drug users, subordinate all other activities to maintain a supply of his drug. In addition, however, the acute effects of the drug prevent his functioning effectively, and alcohol has significant chronic toxicity. Society is damaged not only by the dependency of the individual but also by his irresponsible acts.

An explanation for the fact that only some individuals compulsively misuse alcohol has been sought by some in a biochemical rather than a personality defect. The several suggestions for individual need or intolerance for alcohol have transiently influenced treatment but have no basis. The emphasis on the importance of the first drink reflects the danger of disinhibition by alcohol, which encourages further intake, and the traditional proscription against the first drink acknowledges the vulnerability of the compulsive user.

Treatment

The general approach to the treatment of alcoholism is the same as for other problems of drug misuse. The penal or punitive approach is not effective and lacks public support. The psychotherapeutic approach (including variations provided by the churches and by Alcoholics Anonymous) is effective in those individuals who acknowledge that they are sick and themselves solicit help. The percentage of a randomly selected group of alcoholics assigned to any treatment program that are helped is small until the patient accepts the need to change. Group therapy with major responsibility assigned to former users is then perhaps most profitable.

In the face of general social approval and widening individual use, no efforts at abatement by education are likely to be effective, especially since such efforts are in competition with the proselytizing efforts of a huge advertising outlay.

A. Pharmacologic Blockade With Disulfiram: Disulfiram (Antabuse, Alcophobin) is used industrially in the vulcanization of rubber. It was studied as an anthelmintic, and its ability to produce alcohol intolerance was observed fortuitously.

Disulfiram
(Antabuse, Alcophobin, tetraethylthiuram disulfide)

1. **Pharmacologic action**—Disulfiram acts by inhibiting aldehyde dehydrogenase. Alcohol is then oxidized at the usual rate to acetaldehyde, which accumulates and causes toxic effects that render the patient extremely uncomfortable (Fig 24—2).

Disulfiram thus has few effects unless the patient ingests alcohol. He then experiences warmth, a flush, a throbbing headache, nausea and vomiting, drowsiness, and a hangover. His blood pressure falls to a degree determined mostly by his posture. The reaction is reproduced by acetaldehyde infusions in humans.

2. **Technic of administration**—The patient must agree to accept the drug daily and must understand that drinking will lead to a most unpleasant experience. The drug must not be administered surreptitiously.

Disulfiram (at first, 0.5 gm, and later 0.25 gm) is given daily. After a few days, the patient is given a test dose of alcohol by the physician (½ oz of whisky followed in 30 minutes, if necessary, by an additional ½ oz) and experiences a didactic reaction. The test experience may be repeated at a later date or may be deferred or foregone.

The fear of the reaction is the deterrent to drinking, and the drug must be taken indefinitely. If possible, the prescribed drug is dispensed to a member of the family or other person who can witness its ingestion each day.

At least 12 hours are required for the effect of disulfiram to develop. The patient cannot drink for 3—10 days after discontinuing the medication. The reaction occurs within 20 minutes after the ingestion of alcohol and lasts for 30—120 minutes. Nonbeverage alcohol—eg, inhaled after-shave lotion—has caused mild reactions.

3. **Adverse reactions**—Disulfiram itself causes drowsiness, nausea, headache, cramps, fatigability, and a metallic taste in some patients. The most serious reaction, uncommon with the doses now used, is a confusional state.

Giving up the use of alcohol may lead to indirect adverse results such as anxiety, hostility, and experimentation with other drugs.

The acetaldehyde reaction itself has not been dangerous. One case has been reported of myocardial infarction developing during the reaction. The reaction is treated by recumbency and ephedrine.

4. **Contraindications**—Disulfiram is contraindicated in serious cardiovascular disease, epilepsy, and cirrhosis. The drug should not be given if the subject has been drinking or taking paraldehyde.

5. **Effectiveness**—Disulfiram was introduced at a time when drug treatment was unfashionable in psychiatry and when the lowering of blood pressure with drugs was a frightening novelty. Some adverse judgments were not based on experience. On the other hand, few controlled evaluations are available. The more carefully selected the patient group and the shorter the follow-up, the better the results. Nevertheless, some workers report complete success in 50% of their group.

B. Related Compounds:

1. **Calcium carbimide (Temposil)**—This compound ($N \equiv C-N=Ca$) has properties similar to those of disulfiram, but the action develops rapidly and is dissipated in 12—24 hours. This disadvantage is balanced by the occurrence of fewer side-effects in the usual dosage of 50—100 mg daily.

2. **Metronidazole (Flagyl)**—This drug, of established usefulness as a trichomonacide, is an investigational drug in the treatment of chronic alcoholism. It does inhibit aldehyde dehydrogenase. The additional claim that it causes an aversion to alcohol independent of an acetaldehyde reaction has not been established.

OTHER TOXIC ALCOHOLS

A number of alcohols—eg, trichloroethanol, phenaglycodol (Ultran), and others listed in Chapter 23—are more potent than ethanol and are used as sedatives.

Other monols are used industrially and are occasionally inhaled or mistakenly ingested. Most of these have the same acute toxicity as ethanol—ie, they are general anesthetics. In general, the potency of the alcohols increases as the length of the carbon chain increases. Unsaturation or chlorine substitution adjacent to the hydroxyl group also increases activity.

Methanol must be discussed separately because it has specific toxic effects in addition to the expected CNS depressant action. Isopropyl alcohol is widely available and is occasionally used as an ethanol substitute. It is in part oxidized to acetone and causes some reversible impairment of renal function.

1. METHYL ALCOHOL
(Methanol)

Methanol (wood alcohol, H_3C-OH) is encountered as duplicating machine fluid, as an adulterant in illegal liquor, in canned heat, and as an industrial solvent. It is ingested mistakenly or in desperation by individuals who want ethanol. The lethal dose of methanol is 2–8 oz.

Methanol is metabolized, in large part to formic acid, only at 1/5 the rate of ethanol, and its effects are, therefore, of long duration and are cumulative. More of a given dose appears in the urine and expired air than in the case of ethanol. Methanol is much less active as a central depressant than ethanol, but it produces a severe acidosis only partially explicable by the amount of formic acid generated. The optic nerve is especially vulnerable to either the acidosis or the formic acid.

Following ingestion of methanol, the individual becomes drunk. Six to 36 hours later (an interval allowing the ingestion of more methanol), headache, dizziness, nausea, blindness, excitement, coma, and acidosis appear. Blindness or impaired vision may persist if the patient recovers.

Treatment
Treatment, other than supportive, includes the following:

A. Ethanol: Simultaneously administered alcohols compete for the limited capacity of the organism to metabolize alcohols. Ethanol is metabolized preferentially over methanol, and the conversion of methanol to formic acid is delayed. Give 50% alcohol or equivalent beverage, 1 ml/kg orally, followed by 0.5 ml/kg every 2 hours for 4 days.

B. Sodium Bicarbonate: Give sodium bicarbonate orally or intravenously in amounts large enough to restore normal plasma bicarbonate or maintain an alkaline urine.

C. Dialysis: Dialysis should be considered early if it is available.

2. GLYCOLS

Ethylene glycol (HOH_2C-CH_2OH) is a component of antifreeze and an industrial solvent. It is a CNS depressant, but chronic exposure also causes renal tubular necrosis. It is oxidized to oxalate, crystals of which are deposited in the kidney. As little as 100 ml has been fatal.

Diethylene glycol ($HOH_2C-H_2C-O-CH_2-CH_2OH$) is similar to ethylene glycol but less toxic. It can cause hepatic necrosis in addition to renal damage.

Propylene glycol ($H_3C-CHOH-CH_2OH$) and **polyethylene glycols** ($HOH_2C[H_2C-O-CH_2]_x-CH_2OH$) are much less toxic and may be used in oral and injectable drug preparations and in cosmetics.

•   •   •

General References

Davis, V.E., & others: Alteration of endogenous catecholamine metabolism by ethanol ingestion. Proc Soc Exper Biol Med 125:1140–1143, 1967.

Gillespie, J.A.: Vasodilator properties of alcohol. Brit MJ 2:274–277, 1967.

Isselbacher, K.J., & N.J. Greenberger: Metabolic effects of alcohol on the liver. New England J Med 270:351–356, 402–410, 1964.

Lieber, C.S.: Hepatic and metabolic effects of alcohol. Gastroenterology 50:119–133, 1966.

Lowenstein, L.M., & others: Effect of fructose on alcohol concentrations in the blood in man. JAMA 213:1899–1901, 1970.

Mardones, J.: The alcohols. Pages 99–183 in: *Physiological Pharmacology*, vol 1. Root, W.S., & F.G. Hofmann (editors). Academic Press, 1963.

Mendelson, J.H.: Ethanol-1-C^{14} metabolism in alcoholics and nonalcoholics. Science 159:319–320, 1968.

Murphree, H.B., Greenberg, L.A., & R. Carroll: Neuropharmacological effects of substances other than ethanol in alcoholic beverages. Fed Proc 26:1468–1473, 1967.

Romano, C., Meyers, F.H., & H.H. Anderson: Pharmacologic relationship between aldehydes and arterenol. Arch Int Pharmacodyn 99:378–390, 1954.

Roueche, B.: *The Neutral Spirit: A Portrait of Alcohol.* Little, Brown, 1960.

Waller, J.A.: Chronic medical conditions and traffic safety: Review of the California experience. New England J Med 273:1413–1420, 1965.

Waller, J.A.: Use and misuse of alcoholic beverages as factor in motor vehicle accidents. Pub Health Rep 81:591–597, 1966.

Yules, R.B, Lippman, M.E., & D.X. Freedman: Alcohol administration prior to sleep: The effect on EEG sleep stages. Arch Gen Psychiat 16:94–106, 1967.

6. Convulsant effect—Huge doses of any tranquilizer may cause convulsions, although this is rare clinically. Epileptics are far more susceptible.

7. Effect on conditioned responses—Conditioned avoidance can be extinguished by reasonable doses of phenothiazine, whereas barbiturates are without effect in this situation until the response is prevented by motor impairment.

8. Effects not present—Habituation to the antipsychotic tranquilizers does not occur, and physical dependence or tolerance does not develop. A withdrawal state does not occur. Supposed withdrawal symptoms must be distinguished from reemergence of a psychosis following discontinuance of the drug.

Absorption, Metabolism, & Excretion

The absorption of those tranquilizers that have been studied is slow and incomplete. The effect after intramuscular or intravenous injection is immediate, but after oral administration the maximum effect does not develop for several hours. The effect then persists for about 24 hours. Fig 25–1 demonstrates the more complete absorption of both intramuscular and liquid

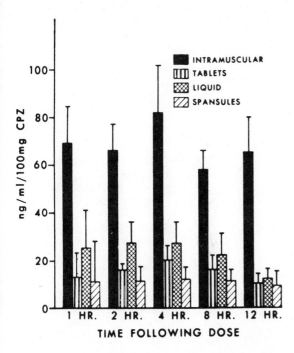

FIG 25–1. Plasma levels following the administration of chlorpromazine in 4 dosage forms. Patients had been receiving the same dosage form prior to the test dose but initial plasma levels were low. Levels are adjusted to reflect the difference in dosage between the 13 subjects and the smaller (50–100 mg) IM dose. (Reproduced, with permission, from Hollister, L.E., & others: Studies of delayed action medication. Clin Pharmacol Therap 11:54, 1970.)

preparations compared with ordinary tablets and especially with a "prolonged release" capsule.

The principal metabolic pathways involve oxidation to a sulfoxide and hydroxylation of the rings at several sites. The metabolites can be demonstrated in the urine by simple color tests for phenols.

The first step in oxidation to the sulfoxide involves formation of a free radical that may participate in the abnormal pigment deposition discussed below (see Adverse Reactions).

Clinical Uses

A. Treatment of Schizophrenic Reaction: The phenothiazines can reduce excitement and control hostile and aggressive behavior in psychotic patients. This effect has had a tremendous impact on the institutional practice of psychiatry by reducing the amount of restraint needed.

Further than this, however, the tranquilizers suppress symptoms, particularly psychotic ideation, in a manner that cannot be explained easily by the depressant effect of the drugs. To some observers—especially those who tend to accept the hypothesis that schizophrenia is due to some biochemical abnormality—the normalization of behavior suggests that the phenothiazines exert a specific antipsychotic effect. Others point out that patients are anything but normal while taking the large doses of phenothiazines required even though they may be able to return to the community on maintenance doses.

That the phenothiazines have decreased the duration of hospitalization required for severe psychosis and may even prevent (or at least delay) hospitalization has been demonstrated by many studies. The number of patients in mental hospitals in the USA increased steadily to a maximum of 555,000 in 1955. The number decreased by 100,000 during the next decade as tranquilizers came into wide use. Fig 25–2 shows the improvement in release rates since the availability of the tranquilizers in one selected group: male Caucasian patients age 25–44 admitted to California state hospitals for the first time with a diagnosis of schizophrenic reaction.

However, factors other than the introduction of tranquilizers could have caused the changes since 1950—eg, increased funds for institutional care or the trend toward community centered care. Only controlled studies can establish the efficacy of the drugs and permit comparison with other available drugs. One well designed study from the same California hospitals permits correlation of short-term drug effects with the eventual gain described in Fig 25–2. This investigation utilized patients age 20–50 who had been hospitalized in a large state institution for 2–10 years before treatment. In a double-blind manner, they were given one of 4 phenothiazines and the dosages were gradually increased to the optimal level over a period of 30 days. One group received an inactive placebo, but another control group received an active placebo of atropine and phenobarbital to mimic in part the side-effects of the phenothiazines and maintain a more truly blind

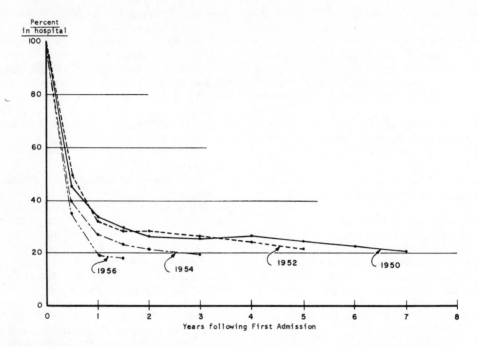

FIG 25–2. Retention curves for first-admission male patients with the diagnosis of schizophrenic reaction,
demonstrating the shorter periods of hospitalization as antipsychotic tranquilizers came into wider use.
(Reproduced, with permission, from Epstein & Morgan: Trends in release rates of schizophrenic patients.
Comprehensive Psychiat 2:199, 1961.)

situation. The active drugs used and the mean modal
doses of each were as follows:

Chlorpromazine, 1800 mg
Perphenazine, 182 mg
Prochlorperazine, 338 mg
Triflupromazine, 621 mg

Fig 25–3 shows the degree of improvement as
measured by a rating scale. The apparent lag in the
effect of one phenothiazine is probably due to masking
of improvement by side-effects. The meaning of this
improvement in scores is shown by the fact that at the
end of the treatment period only 5 out of 96 patients
who received placebos were ready for discharge, whereas 70 of 192 treated patients were ready to leave the
institution.

One collaborative study utilized 409 newly
admitted patients from psychiatric hospitals of several
types. Three phenothiazines and a placebo were given
in a double-blind manner for 6 weeks. Symptoms were
rated and the overall state and degree of improvement
judged. On a 7-point scale of severity of mental illness,
for example, drug-treated patients were judged to have
changed from markedly or severely ill ("5.5") to
mildly ill ("3"). The mean of the placebo group
changed to moderately or markedly ill ("4.5").

This kind of evaluation has its limitations but
permits some conclusions. The 3 active drugs—chlorpromazine (600 mg average daily dose), fluphenazine
(6 mg/day), and thioridazine (700 mg/day)—did not
differ in therapeutic effectiveness. Fluphenazine, of

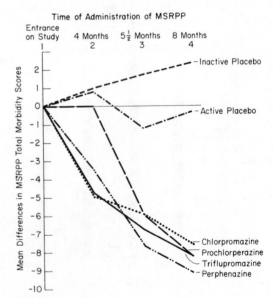

FIG 25–3. Effectiveness of antipsychotic tranquilizers. Groups of 48 hospitalized psychotic
patients were studied on each of 6 treatments.
The initial score on a rating scale is plotted at
zero; a decrease in total morbidity score indicates
improvement. (Reproduced, with permission,
from Adelson & Epstein: A study of phenothiazines with male and female chronically ill schizophrenic patients. J Nerv Ment Dis 134:547,
1962.)

the piperazinylpropyl group, caused more extrapyramidal side-effects but less drowsiness. Thioridazine caused less muscle rigidity but appreciably more vomiting.

Drugs that appear equivalent when tested on groups of patients (as above) might have different effectiveness if tested on patients further segregated by symptoms, ie, different tranquilizers might be selectively more effective against paranoia, motor retardation, or the behavior patterns. Such is probably the case, but only fragmentary data are available even in patients with depression.

B. Depression: The present discussion will conform to a questionable and changing convention that classifies and separately discusses certain drugs as antidepressants even though differentiation from tranquilizers is not possible pharmacologically (see Chapter 28). Both tranquilizers and the drugs listed in Table 28–1 are effective in the treatment of the major endogenous depressions. When an antidepressant or a tranquilizer is used in treating depression, the dosage is not progressively increased to an effective level as in the treatment of other psychoses but a ceiling dose is observed.

C. Other Psychiatric Problems: Emotional instability and odd behavior in aged patients with "chronic brain syndrome" may be controlled with phenothiazines. Usefulness in other situations cannot be assumed. Disturbed mentally retarded patients, for example, are not improved by phenothiazine treatment.

D. Pruritus: Itching associated with an allergic reaction of the immediate type—eg, urticaria—may be relieved by antihistamines, some of which are phenothiazines. The antihistamines are not usually effective in other pruritic states, and, if they are, it is not because of their antihistaminic effects. Tranquilizers have only limited usefulness against itching in general. Some studies fail to show any superiority over a placebo, which gives the expected 40% favorable responses. Some studies do show a superiority over a placebo but not over a sedative. Tranquilizers may be preferable in this condition to sedatives in children because of the lower incidence of excitement due to disinhibition which sometimes follows the administration of sedatives. Selective antipruritus action is claimed without good basis for 2 phenothiazines. One is trimeprazine (Temaril), which, however, causes sleepiness in the usual dose of 2.5 mg 4 times a day. The sleepiness is not objectionable at bedtime, and a larger dose may be used; but the other phenothiazines are equivalent to trimeprazine. Methdilazine (Tacaryl) is another phenothiazine, often classed as an antihistamine, suggested for this special use.

E. Antiemetic: See Chapter 19.

F. Preprocedural Medications In Combination With Narcotic Analgesics: Narcotic analgesics and tranquilizers both cause sedation, but the effect of injecting a mixture of the 2 is more than additive. Such mixtures—eg, meperidine and promethazine—are therefore used as preoperative medication. The potentiating effects on sedation do not extend to the analgesic action in the opinion of some investigators, but this conclusion is still uncertain. For additional discussion, see Chapter 26.

G. Analgesia: Methotrimeprazine (Levoprome, Nozinan) is a phenothiazine similar in structure and effects to the other tranquilizers. However, the analgesic properties that are present to a negligible degree in chlorpromazine are greatly increased in this compound. When given by injection, it is nearly as potent as morphine. Huge doses must be given orally, but this compound is of great interest because it is the most potent nonaddicting analgesic so far studied.

Adverse Reactions

In those situations in which a few small doses of a tranquilizer are used, it might be possible to differentiate side-effects and overdosage toxicity. However, because these drugs are most commonly used in large doses for prolonged periods, this differentiation is usually not possible.

A. Dose-Related Toxicity:

1. Behavioral—

a. Somnolence—Again it must be emphasized that taking an antipsychotic tranquilizer is not a subjectively pleasant experience. The feelings of lassitude and fatigability are unpleasant. With continued administration, patients become somewhat tolerant or accustomed to this effect, but it limits their function to some extent and decreases the dependability with which they will take their medication without supervision—ie, as an outpatient. The incidence of suicide is greater among psychotics receiving drug therapy than in groups receiving only institutional care. The greater freedom of activity permitted the patient controlled by drugs is probably a factor, but so probably is the behavioral depression caused by the tranquilizers.

b. Others—A few patients may experience feelings of excitement and restlessness. These feelings are more common early in treatment and after the administration of those piperazine or piperazinylpropyl derivatives characterized as "stimulant" tranquilizers.

Early in treatment, a patient depressed by a tranquilizer may at the same time develop a toxic psychosis with confusion and hallucinations. Such a reaction is more common with those drugs that resemble the antihistamines and atropine substitutes.

2. Extrapyramidal effects—Disturbances of the extrapyramidal motor system appear in 4 general patterns.

a. Parkinsonism equivalent—As the phenothiazines are given to institutionalized schizophrenic patients—ie, to therapeutic response or the maximum tolerated dose—parkinsonism is among the most frequent side-effects. It consists of akinesia, muscular rigidity, and fine resting tremors and may vary in severity from slight impairment of facial mobility to completely disabling rigidity.

To minimize the development of muscular rigidity, many physicians administer an antiparkinsonism drug—eg, benztropine (Cogentin)—when large

TABLE 25-1. Chemical structures of antipsychotic tranquilizers.

	R_1	R_2	Names
Dimethylaminopropyl derivatives	$-Cl$		Chlorpromazine (Thorazine)
	$-H$		Promazine (Sparine)
	$-CF_3$		Triflupromazine (Vesprin)
Dimethylaminoisopropyl derivatives			Promethazine (Phenergan)
	$-\overset{\displaystyle O}{\overset{\displaystyle \|}{C}}-C_2H_5$		Propiomazine (Largon)
Piperazinylpropyl derivatives	$-Cl$	$-CH_3$	Prochlorperazine (Compazine)
	$-CF_3$	$-CH_3$	Trifluoperazine (Stelazine)
	$-S-C_2H_5$	$-CH_3$	Thiethylperazine (Torecan)
	$-Cl$	$-CH_2-CH_2-OH$	Perphenazine (Trilafon)
	$-CF_3$	$-CH_2-CH_2-OH$	Fluphenazine (Prolixin, Permitil)
	$-\overset{\displaystyle O}{\overset{\displaystyle \|}{C}}-CH_3$	$-CH_2-CH_2-OH$	Acetophenazine (Tindal)
	$-\overset{\displaystyle O}{\overset{\displaystyle \|}{C}}-C_2H_5$	$-CH_2-CH_2-OH$	Carphenazine (Proketazine)
	$-\overset{\displaystyle O}{\overset{\displaystyle \|}{C}}-C_3H_7$	$-CH_3$	Butaperazine (Repoise)
Piperidyl derivatives	$-S-CH_3$		Thioridazine (Mellaril)
	$-\overset{\displaystyle O}{\overset{\displaystyle \|}{S}}-CH_3$		Mesoridazine (Serentil)
	$-\overset{\displaystyle O}{\overset{\displaystyle \|}{C}}-CH_3$	$-CH_2-N\!\!<\!\!\rangle\!-C_2H_4OH$	Piperacetazine (Quide)
Thioxanthene derivatives	$-Cl$	$-N(CH_3)_2$	Chlorprothixene (Taractan)
	$-SO_2-N(CH_3)_2$	$-N\!\!<\!\!\rangle\!N-CH_3$	Thiothixene (Navane)

doses of a phenothiazine tranquilizer are being used. Only limited data are available to evaluate this practice, but it is probably better to use the antiparkinson agents after the side-effect occurs. The prophylactic effect is not marked, and the drugs have effects that can add to the side-effects of the tranquilizer.

b. Dystonias—Dystonias are most commonly seen in children and young adults either early in treatment or immediately following the injection of a phenothiazine or the accidental ingestion of a single large dose. The muscles of the shoulder girdle and jaws are most likely to be involved. Violent dystonias with movements of the arms and head that can be mistaken for convulsions may occur, or there may be athetoid movements or persistent oculogyrate movements. Since they occur in a depressed, unresponsive patient, these reactions may be misdiagnosed and therefore overtreated and overstudied.

This toxic reaction is well tolerated and should be treated conservatively. Of the drugs that may relieve the dystonia, diphenhydramine (Benadryl) has apparently been most used in children.

c. Akathisia—Akathisia is a feeling of restlessness or of compelling need for movement. The patient may walk about impatiently, tap his foot incessantly, or complain of "restless legs."

d. Tardive dyskinesia—The drug-induced extrapyramidal states described above are completely reversible upon discontinuation or reduced dosage of the tranquilizer. Another dyskinesia, however, is not only irreversible; it is usually intensified when the phenothiazine is withdrawn.

The late dyskinesia occurs, usually in patients above 40 years of age, after exposure to large doses of tranquilizers for periods of 6 months to 2 years or longer. In contrast to the acute dystonias, the onset is insidious and the movements are rhythmic and coordinated rather than spasmodic. The tongue, lips, face, and jaws are most commonly involved, resulting in a picture suggestive of Huntington's chorea or the toxic effect of levodopa. The state may be suppressed with high doses of tranquilizer, presumably with additional risk. Other treatments—eg, amantadine or reasonable doses of reserpine—are being evaluated. Estimates of the incidence of this toxic effect vary—peculiarly—from a denial of its existence to 10% of certain groups of patients.

3. Convulsions—Precipitation of convulsions is possible but quite rare during the use of the antipsychotic tranquilizers unless some additional factor is present—eg, if the patient is an epileptic or if another convulsant drug is being used.

4. Atropine-like effects—Parasympatholytic side-effects may be quite prominent. They include dry mouth, blurred vision, and constipation or even paralytic ileus. The expected tachycardia and pupillary dilatation may appear, especially with large doses, but these measurements may be little changed or bradycardia and pupillary constriction may be observed. This variability in the response of the heart rate and pupillary size suggests that a central sympatholytic effect is also present.

5. Postural hypotension—The intensification of the beta-agonist effects (vasodilatation) of the sympathomimetic amines was described above as the basis for the fall in blood pressure. This side-effect is especially troublesome after injection of the tranquilizer and early in treatment. It may be intense enough to cause dizziness or fainting.

6. Metabolic and endocrinologic changes—Weight gain is a common side-effect of prolonged administration of tranquilizers, including reserpine. The increase in caloric intake cannot be explained by changes in the behavioral state—ie, it does not merely reflect an elevation of mood, as is true for the similar effect of the antidepressant drugs.

The endocrinologic side-effects are due to hypothalamic depression and consequent decrease in some of the tropic hormones of the anterior pituitary. Decrease in gonadotropin liberation leads to menstrual irregularities which usually become less with continued treatment. Lactation may occur for the reasons discussed above.

7. Oculocutaneous pigmentation—For some patients, the continued use of large doses of a phenothiazine is the only alternative to grossly disturbed behavior or recurrent hospitalization. In some patients, especially women, the exposed parts of the skin (face, neck, back of hands) take on a mauve or slate color after years of therapy with chlorpromazine. Pigment deposits in the anterior lens capsule and posterior surface of the cornea can be seen by slit lamp examination in a third or half of some groups receiving prolonged chlorpromazine therapy. Visual acuity is not reduced, but some blurring of vision may be reported. At autopsy, the pigment is also seen in macrophages throughout the body.

Thus far, chlorpromazine and thioridazine are the only phenothiazines that have caused this state. The daily dosage of chlorpromazine must exceed 500 mg/day. Experimentally, a single large dose followed by exposure to ultraviolet or visible light causes an unusual degree of erythema, but in clinical practice this occurs only after treatment for 3 years or longer. Women are far more susceptible.

The dense granules that accumulate are not identical with melanin or unchanged chlorpromazine ultramicroscopically, but they may be a combination of melanin and a photooxidation product of chlorpromazine.

The process is very slowly reversible over a period of several months. Treatment consists of protection from light and substitution of a phenothiazine that requires a smaller absolute dose or of a combination of chlorpromazine with such an agent.

8. Pigmentary retinopathy—Deposition of pigment in the retina with impaired vision occurs rarely and by a process separate from the more common oculocutaneous pigmentation. Smaller doses and brief periods are involved. Thioridazine (Mellaril) has caused most of the few reported cases.

B. Acute Intoxication: The acute overdosage toxicity of the tranquilizers is very low in adults, and the possibility of a fatal outcome following attempted suicidal or accidental ingestion is negligible unless a second depressant drug is also involved.

These drugs are only slightly more dangerous in children; however, children are especially susceptible to the dystonic state described above, and such states are occasionally seen following accidental ingestion of one of the drugs or its therapeutic use in the treatment of vomiting.

C. Allergic Reactions:

1. **Cholestatic jaundice**—Chlorpromazine and a few other drugs such as methyltestosterone and erythromycin estolate can cause jaundice or less marked degrees of liver dysfunction by causing intrahepatic biliary obstruction rather than by direct liver cell damage. The obstruction is at the level of the smallest biliary radicles, and initially the usual clinical laboratory tests give results consistent with obstructive jaundice. As in other forms of jaundice, the laboratory tests may later give evidence of hepatocellular damage, but the process is benign and completely reversible although many weeks may be required. In the early days of chlorpromazine use, the incidence of this adverse reaction was very high, perhaps 3–5%. The number of cases then decreased rapidly, and for the past few years chlorpromazine jaundice has been rare. The reaction was apparently due to an unidentified impurity which was removed as methods of preparing the drug were improved. The reaction is often assumed, without immunochemical evidence, to have been allergic in origin. Prior sensitization is not a factor since the jaundice appeared in almost every case within the first 6 weeks of treatment.

2. **Other allergic reactions**—The rare occurrence of agranulocytosis appears to reflect the extent of use of the individual drugs except in the case of promazine, which is unusually hazardous in this regard. Contact dermatitis can occur when the situation permits, as in nurses who handle the drug. Other cutaneous reactions also occur, including a photosensitivity reaction that resembles eczema.

Contraindications & Cautions

The antipsychotic tranquilizers should not be used in comatose patients and should be given with care and in reduced doses if CNS depressant drugs have been taken. These include alcohol as well as the barbiturates and narcotics.

Selection of Drug

From the discussion above of the major tranquilizers, the following ideas should be repeated: (1) The antipsychotic tranquilizers are not effective anti-anxiety drugs. (2) In the treatment of schizophrenia, no differences in effectiveness among the potent drugs have yet been established. (3) Most psychotic patients

TABLE 25–2. Antipsychotic tranquilizers—chlorpromazine and related compounds: Dosages and preparations available.

	Equivalent Adult Oral Dose (3–4 Times/Day)	Preparations Available
Chlorpromazine (Thorazine)	25–50 mg	Tablets, 10, 25, 50, 100, and 200 mg Sustained action capsules (Spansules), 30, 75, 150, 200, and 300 mg Concentrate, 30 mg/ml, 120 ml and 1 gal Syrup, 10 mg/5 ml, 120 ml Suppositories, 25 and 100 mg Injectable (IM, IV*), 25 mg/ml, 1 and 2 ml ampules and 10 ml vials
Promazine (Sparine)	50–200 mg	Tablets, 10, 25, 50, 100, and 200 mg Concentrate, 30 mg/ml, 120 ml; 100 mg/ml, 30 ml Syrup, 10 mg/5 ml, 120 ml Injectable (IM, IV*), 50 mg/ml, 1 and 2 ml ampules; 25 and 50 mg/ml, 10 ml vials; 25 and 50 mg/ml, 1 and 2 ml Tubex
Triflupromazine (Vesprin)	10–20 mg	Tablets, 10, 25, and 50 mg Suspension, 10 mg/ml, 120 ml Injectable (IM, IV*), 10 mg/ml, 10 ml vials; 20 mg/ml, 1 ml ampules
Thioridazine (Mellaril)	10–25 mg	Tablets, 10, 25, 50, 100, and 200 mg Concentrate, 30 mg/ml, 120 ml
Mesoridazine (Serentil)	10–25 mg	Tablets, 10, 25, 50, and 100 mg Injectable (IM), 25 mg/ml, 1ml ampules
Chlorprothixene (Taractan)	25 mg	Tablets, 10, 25, 50, and 100 mg Concentrate, 100 mg/5 ml, 16 oz Injectable (IM), 25 mg in 2 ml ampules

*All intravenous injections should be given with great caution because of the possibility of precipitous hypotension.

will require maintenance doses of tranquilizers after discharge from the hospital. The dosage required may be very large and should not be arbitrarily reduced by the physician in the community. The drug can be discontinued when the illness has run its course—a time that can be defined only by trials at intervals. (4) The duration of action of the major tranquilizers is such that administration once or twice daily provides a sustained effect. (5) Liquid preparations were introduced for convenience in institutional practice and to prevent the hoarding of tablets by patients, but they also provide for more complete absorption.

The available drugs, whether phenothiazines or not, can therefore be discussed using the classification suggested in the section on the chemistry of the phenothiazines: (1) chlorpromazine and similar drugs; (2) the "stimulant" tranquilizers, which cause less somnolence but more extrapyramidal side-effects; (3) those that cause more sedation; (4) those with limited potency; and (5) those suggested for special application against vomiting and itching.

A. Chlorpromazine and Comparable Agents: Chlorpromazine (Thorazine) no longer causes jaundice with the distressing frequency that it once did, and the consensus would clearly name it as the standard drug of the tranquilizer class. With the expiration of the patent on it, it is also less expensive than other tranquilizers. In the treatment of psychotics, it is often combined with one of the piperazinylpropyl compounds such as trifluoperazine (Stelazine) because of the unquantitated impression that a balance of sedation and stimulation is thus achieved.

Promazine (Sparine) has caused a high incidence of agranulocytosis. With so many alternative drugs available, there is no need to use it.

Thioridazine (Mellaril) is favored by some physicians because it probably causes less parkinsonism. However, it is also more likely to cause vomiting and retinopathy.

B. "Stimulant" Tranquilizers: There is little basis for differentiating among the piperazinylpropyl derivatives shown in Table 25–1.

Haloperidol (Haldol) is not a phenothiazine but one of a group of butyrophenones. It causes many extrapyramidal reactions but little sedation and perhaps fewer autonomic side-effects. Droperidol (Inapsine) is also a butyrophenone chemically and pharmacologically similar to haloperidol. Rarely used by itself, it is encountered as a component of Innovar, a tranquilizer-narcotic mixture.

Fluphenazine (Prolixin) is provided in a form slowly absorbed after injection and can be given in doses of 25 mg every 2 weeks. The advantages claimed are the savings in nurses' time and less dependence upon patient cooperation after discharge.

C. Tranquilizers That Cause More Somnolence: Promethazine (Phenergan) is not used in the treatment of psychotic patients because of the sedation that it causes.

Propiomazine (Largon) is similar to promethazine and offers no advantage over the more widely used compounds. It is available only in an injectable dosage form, and experience has been limited to adjunctive uses in anesthesia.

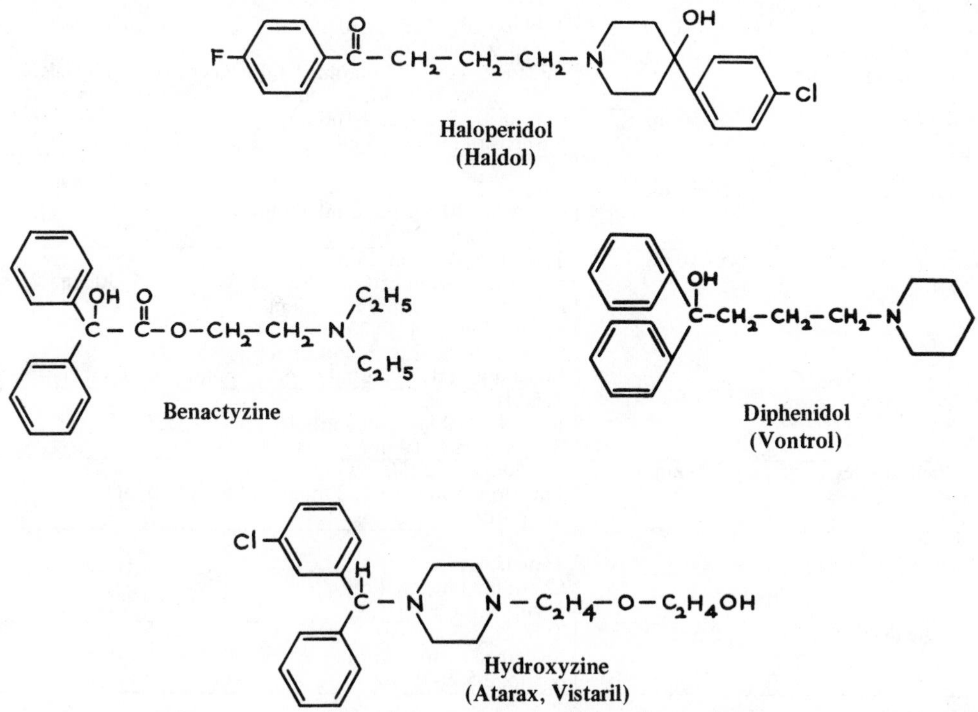

FIG 25–4. Chemical structures of some nonphenothiazine tranquilizers.

TABLE 25-3. Antipsychotic tranquilizers with special properties:
Dosages and preparations available.

	Equivalent Adult Oral Dose (3–4 Times/Day)	Preparations Available
Stimulant-tranquilizers		
Trifluoperazine (Stelazine)	1 mg	Tablets, 1, 2, 5, and 10 mg Concentrate, 10 mg/ml, 60 ml Injectable (IM), 2 mg/ml, 10 ml vials
Perphenazine (Trilafon)	2–4 mg	Tablets, 2, 4, 8, 8 (Repetabs), and 16 mg Concentrate, 16 mg/5 ml, 120 ml Syrup, 2 mg/5 ml, 120 ml Suppositories, 2, 4, and 8 mg Injectable (IM, IV), 5 mg/ml, 1 ml ampules and 10 ml vials
Fluphenazine (Permitil)	1 mg	Tablets, 0.25, 1, 2.5, 5, and 10 mg Concentrate, 5 mg/ml, 120 ml
(Prolixin)	1 mg	Tablets, 1, 2.5, and 5 mg Elixir, 0.5 mg/ml, 60 and 480 ml Injectable (IM), 2.5 mg/ml, 10 ml vials
(Prolixin Enanthate)	. . .	Injectable (subcut, IM), 25 mg/ml (in sesame oil), 5 ml vials
Acetophenazine (Tindal)	20 mg	Tablets, 20 mg
Butaperazine (Repoise)	5–10 mg	Tablets, 5, 10, and 25 mg
Piperacetazine (Quide)	10 mg	Tablets, 10 and 25 mg
Carphenazine (Proketazine)	25–50 mg	Tablets, 12.5, 25, and 50 mg Concentrate, 50 mg/ml, 120 ml
Thiothixene (Navane)	1–2 mg	Capsules, 1, 2, 5, and 10 mg Concentrate, 5 mg/ml Injectable (IM), 2 mg/ml in 2 ml ampules
Haloperidol (Haldol)	0.5 mg	Tablets, 0.5, 1, 2, and 5 mg Concentrate, 2 mg/ml, 15 ml Injectable (IM), 5 mg/ml
Tranquilizers with prominent sedation		
Promethazine (Phenergan)	25 mg	Tablets, 12.5, 25, and 50 mg Syrup, 6.25 mg/5 ml and 25 mg/5 ml Suppositories, 25 and 50 mg Injectable (IM, IV), 25 and 50 mg/ml, 1 ml ampules, 1 ml Tubex, and 10 ml vials
Propiomazine (Largon)	20 mg	Injectable (IM, IV), 20 mg/ml, 1 and 2 ml ampules
Tranquilizers of limited potency		
Hydroxyzine hydrochloride (Atarax) hydrochloride (Vistaril)	25–50 mg	Tablets, 10, 25, 50, and 100 mg Syrup, 10 mg/5 ml Injectable (IM), 25 mg/ml, 1 ml Isoject and 10 ml vials; 50 mg/ml, 1 and 2 ml Isoject and 2 and 10 ml vials
pamoate (Vistaril)	25–50 mg	Capsules, 25, 50, and 100 mg Suspension, 25 mg/5 ml
Antiemetics		
Diphenidol (Vontrol)	25–50 mg	Tablets, 25 mg Injection, 20 mg/ml, 2 ml ampules Suppositories, 25 and 50 mg
Prochlorperazine (Compazine)	5–10 mg	Tablets, 5, 10, and 25 mg Sustained action capsules (Spansules), 10, 15, 30, and 75 mg Concentrate, 10 mg/ml, 120 ml Syrup, 5 mg/5 ml, 120 ml Suppositories, 2.5, 5, and 25 mg Injectable (IM), 5 mg/ml, 2 ml ampules and 10 ml vials
Thiethylperazine (Torecan)	10 mg	Tablets, 10 mg Injection, 10 mg/2 ml ampule Suppositories, 10 mg
Trimethobenzamide (Tigan)*	250 mg	Capsules, 100, 250 mg Injection, 100 mg/ml, 2 ml ampules and 20 ml vials Suppositories, 200 mg
Antipruritics		
Methdilazine (Tacaryl)	8 mg	Tablets, 8 mg Chewable tablets, 4 mg Syrup, 4 mg/5 ml
Trimeprazine (Temaril)	2.5 mg	Tablets, 2.5 mg Sustained action capsules, 5 mg Syrup, 2.5 mg/5 ml

*Not a tranquilizer.

D. Less Potent Tranquilizers: Nonphenothiazine compounds may be potent and useful tranquilizers—eg, haloperidol or chlorprothixene. However, the non-phenothiazine tranquilizers listed below are much less useful. They are often called "diphenylmethane derivatives"; and they resemble the clinically similar anti-histamines and synthetic substitutes for atropine, and their dosages and effectiveness are limited by their atropine-like side-effects. They are listed here for identification only and are not suggested for any of the uses discussed above. These "minor tranquilizers" should not be used in the treatment of anxiety.

Hydroxyzine (Atarax, Vistaril) is closely related chemically to the familiar antihistamines and anti-nauseants.

Benactyzine differs from one of the earliest synthetic atropines, adiphenine (Trasentine), only in the hydroxyl group on the benzilic acid moiety. It is not used much by itself (as Suavitil), but is present in Deprol in combination with meprobamate.

· · ·

LITHIUM

Lithium ion, administered in the form of lithium carbonate, is used as an alternative or supplement to the major tranquilizers in the control of the manic stage of manic-depressive illness.

Pharmacologic Effects

Therapeutic doses of lithium do not have gross effects comparable to those of either the tranquilizers or the sedatives, and its mechanism of action is not known. The onset of action is delayed for several days after the drug is started, and 6–10 days elapse before the peak effect is reached.

Absorption, Metabolism, & Excretion

The drug is well absorbed after oral administration and is distributed throughout the body water. It is excreted by the kidneys and at therapeutic dosages has a half-life of 24 hours. Of the lithium in glomerular filtrate, about 80% is reabsorbed by the tubules, but this fraction is not influenced by diuretic drugs.

Clinical Uses

Lithium carbonate is approved for marketing in the USA only for use in the control of mania, and the drug has been remarkably successful for this purpose. Its use in any other clinical conditions is still investigative.

A. Control of Manic Episodes: A violent manic state is best controlled by the injection of chlor-promazine or other antipsychotic tranquilizer. In this situation, when the long latent period of lithium is disadvantageous, it may be started simultaneously with chlorpromazine or a similar tranquilizer. The patient

entering the manic phase of a manic-depressive illness is more likely to be hypomanic, and a delay of a few days is not critical if the patient can be protected from the consequences of his expansiveness. Some psychiatrists prefer to use lithium at such a time because it is usually effective and causes less impairment of function than chlorpromazine.

B. Prophylaxis Against Affective Illness: Lithium is clearly not effective in the treatment of an established depression, but it has been claimed that it can prevent cyclic changes in mood and thus prevent not only manic attacks but also the development of depression and of the depressed stage of the manic-depressive syndrome. Some of these reports have been quite enthusiastic, and it may be that this use will ultimately be justified by adequately controlled double-blind studies. At present, however, the consensus is that the value of lithium in the prevention of depression is unestablished. If the effect is present, it requires 6–12 months for its appearance.

Adverse Reactions

Toxic effects during chronic administration are predicted by serum levels, which must be determined during treatment with lithium. Side-effects are generally mild if the serum level is kept below 1.5 mEq/liter. When serum levels exceed 2 mEq/liter, dosage should be decreased or the drug withheld temporarily. Serum lithium decreases by half every 24 hours.

Acute toxic effects may be graded as follows:

A. Mild: Nausea which passes after a few days. A fine tremor of the hands or jaw may interfere with the patient's function and is not relieved by antiparkinson agents.

B. Moderate: Anorexia, vomiting, diarrhea, thirst and polyuria, coarse tremor, muscle weakness and twitching, sedation, and ataxia.

C. Severe: Chorea, athetosis, confusion, stupor, and convulsions.

D. Terminal: Coma.

Chronic administration often leads to the development of a goiter that can be reduced by treatment with thyroid substance. Only in isolated cases has hypothyroidism developed. Sodium retention may occur. T-wave depression is seen but with no accompanying evidence of cardiac dysfunction.

Contraindications & Cautions

Lithium should not be used in the presence of impaired renal function or cardiovascular disease or in any other situation that involves a restricted diet or diuretic drugs, since sodium restriction or increased loss leads to lithium retention. Excessive loss of fluid or inadequate intake also leads to higher than expected lithium levels.

Lithium is probably safe for use during pregnancy, but its use should be avoided until definitive data are available. It should not be used when facilities for the determination of serum lithium levels are not available.

Preparations & Dosages Available

Dosage is controlled by the regular determination of lithium blood levels.

Manic patients are given initial doses of 600 mg of lithium carbonate 3 times each day, but the serum level should not exceed 1.5 mEq/liter. As excitement subsides, the maintenance dose—usually 300 mg 3 times a day—should give serum levels of 0.5–1 mEq/liter.

Lithium carbonate (Eskalith, Lithonate, Lithane) is available in tablets or capsules of 300 mg.

•   •   •

General References

General

Davis, J.M.: The efficacy of tranquilizing and antidepressant drugs. Arch Gen Psychiat 13:552–572, 1965.

Dundee, J.W.: A review of chlorpromazine hydrochloride. Brit J Anaesth 26:357–379, 1954.

Fischer, R.W.: Comparison of antipruritic agents administered orally. JAMA 203:418–419, 1968.

Gokhale, S.D., Gulati, O.D., & H.M. Parikh: An investigation of the adrenergic blocking action of chlorpromazine. Brit J Pharmacol 23:508–520, 1964.

Hollister, L.E.: Clinical use of psychotherapeutic drugs: Current status. Clin Pharmacol Therap 10:170–198, 1969.

Klein, D.F., & J.M. Davis: *Diagnosis and Drug Treatment of Psychiatric Disorders.* Williams & Wilkins, 1969.

National Institute for Mental Health Collaborative Study Group: Effectiveness of phenothiazine treatment of acute schizophrenic psychoses. Arch Gen Psychiat 10:246–261, 1964.

National Institute of Mental Health Collaborative Study Group: Differences in clinical effects of three phenothiazines in "acute" schizophrenia. Dis Nerv System 28:369–383, 1967.

Adverse Reactions

Chlorpromazine melanosis. Leading article. Brit MJ 2:630–631, 1967.

Crane, G.E.: High doses of trifluoperazine and tardive dyskinesia. Arch Neurol 22:176–182, 1970.

DeWied, D.: Chlorpromazine and endocrine function. Pharmacol Rev 19:251–288, 1967.

Hollister, L.E.: Complications from psychotherapeutic drugs—1964. Clin Pharmacol Therap 5:322–333, 1964.

Mathalone, M.B.R.: Eye and skin changes in psychiatric patients treated with chlorpromazine. Brit J Ophth 51:86–93, 1967.

Pisciotta, A.V.: Agranulocytosis induced by certain phenothiazine derivatives. JAMA 208:1862–1868, 1969.

Satanove, A., & J.S. McIntosh: Phototoxic reactions induced by high doses of chlorpromazine and thioridazine. JAMA 200:209–212, 1967.

Methotrimeprazine

Beaver, W.T., & others: A comparison of the analgesic effects of methotrimeprazine and morphine in patients with cancer. Clin Pharmacol Therap 7:436–454, 1966.

De Kornfeld, T.J., Pearson, J.W., & L. Lasagna: Methotrimeprazine in the treatment of labor pain. New England J Med 270:391–394, 1964.

Lithium

Baldessarini, R., & J. Stephens: Lithium carbonate for affective disorders. Arch Gen Psychiat 22:72–77, 1970.

Council on Drugs: Evaluation of lithium carbonate for treatment of manic-depressive psychosis. JAMA 215:1486–1488, 1971.

Luby, E.D., Schwartz, D., & H. Rosenbaum: Lithium-carbonate-induced myxedema. JAMA 218:1298–1299, 1971.

Lynn, E.J., Satloff, A., & D.C. Tinling: Mania and the use of lithium: A three-year study. Am J Psychiat 127:1176–1180, 1971.

Prophylactic lithium. Brit MJ 3:479–480, 1970.

26...
Narcotic Analgesics & Narcotic Antagonists

NARCOTIC ANALGESICS

Ideally, drugs should relieve pain by acting on a specific pathologic state. If specific drug therapy is not available—or during the interval between the start of therapy and effective control—it is often necessary to give drugs for the pain itself rather than for the underlying disease.

In this section are discussed the narcotic analgesics or narcotics—ie, morphine, codeine, and other alkaloids derived from opium and some equivalent synthetic analogues. In therapeutic doses these drugs relieve pain without causing general CNS depression as the general anesthetics do. In larger doses the narcotics are more general depressants, and all are subject to misuse or addiction. The nonnarcotic or antipyretic analgesics such as aspirin are discussed in the next chapter.

History

The opium poppy is indigenous to Asia Minor, and awareness of the euphoriant effect of some part of the poppy plant is implicit in the Sumerian records of 4000 BC. Clear accounts exist of its use in the Egyptian, Greek, and Roman cultures. Paracelsus was aware of its usefulness and prepared the first tincture of opium (laudanum), subsequently simplified by Sydenham.

Friedrich Sertürner (1783–1841) isolated morphine from opium and demonstrated for the first time that a single purified chemical substance could account for the pharmacologic effects of a natural product. Sertürner, a reluctant apprentice to a pharmacist in Prussia, was disturbed by the variable potency of available opium preparations and set out to purify and standardize it. Working at a time when neither experimental pharmacology nor the chemistry of natural products were recognized fields of endeavor, Sertürner succeeded in isolating morphine from opium. Using a bioassay in dogs, he established that morphine, as he named the alkaline substance, was the somnifacient principle of opium. His early reports (1803) were either rejected by editors or ignored after publication. He eventually tested his purified preparation on himself and 3 friends, administering 3 doses of 30 mg in 45 minutes and observing the vomiting, flush, and near coma. This work was finally published in 1817 and attracted the interest of the influential French chemist Gay-Lussac. The work of Sertürner influenced Pelletier and Caventou, and in the same year other pure principles from plant sources were successfully isolated.

The addicting properties of opium have also been important in its history. In China, opium was used only for the treatment of dysentery until the mid-1700's. The English, Portuguese, and Dutch built up a large trade supplying opium to China, and addiction had become so much of a problem by the early 1800's that the Chinese government acted to bar the importation of opium and reduce the amount of opium smoking. These acts precipitated a 3-year war terminated by the Treaty of Nanking (1842), which gave England Hong Kong, opened 5 ports to British traders, and specifically authorized continued trade in opium.

The risk of addiction was probably underestimated in the West for some time thereafter. Opium and morphine were widely prescribed and easily available in many patent medicines. Misuse was common until about 1920, but the predominant pattern was one of oral use. Since the laws were changed at that time, the number of people involved has become comparatively small but the narcotic is injected. The compulsion based on the experience at the time of injection is very difficult to treat, and associated criminal activity has greatly increased.

Source & Chemistry

A. Source: Morphine and other naturally occurring narcotics and their semisynthetic modifications are isolated from opium. Opium is collected from only one variety of poppy, *Papaver somniferum.* A few days after the petals fall, the unripe, still succulent seed pod is lightly incised. A day later the sticky brown gum that has collected is scraped from the surface of the pod. As much as 25% of this crude opium may be made up of alkaloids. The content of morphine varies from 9–14% and is adjusted to 10% in the standardized preparations.

The legal production of opium is regulated by the United Nations. India, Turkey, and Russia are the largest producers of opium from which morphine and other alkaloids are isolated. Morphine is used as such; however, a larger amount is converted chemically into codeine, which occurs in opium in amounts insufficient to meet the needs of medicine.

TABLE 26-1. The naturally occurring opium alkaloids and some semisynthetic opiates.

	R_1	R_2	$\Delta 7=8$*	R_3	R_4
Morphine	–OH	–OH	Present	–H	–H
Oxymorphone (dihydrohydroxymorphinone, Numorphan)	–OH	=O	Absent	–OH	–H
Hydromorphone (dihydromorphinone, Dilaudid)	–OH	=O	Absent	–H	–H
Methyldihydromorphinone (Metopon)	–OH	=O	Absent	–H	–CH$_3$
Codeine (methylmorphine)	–O–CH$_3$	–OH	Present	–H	–H
Dihydrocodeine (Paracodin)	–O–CH$_3$	–OH	Absent	–H	–H
Hydrocodone (dihydrocodeinone, in Hycodan)	–O–CH$_3$	=O	Absent	–H	–H
Oxycodone (dihydrohydroxycodeinone, in Percodan)	–O–CH$_3$	=O	Absent	–OH	–H
Heroin (diacetylmorphine)	$\overset{O}{\overset{\|}{-O-C-CH_3}}$	$\overset{O}{\overset{\|}{-O-C-CH_3}}$	Present	–H	–H
Thebaine	–O–CH$_3$	–O–CH$_3$	†	–H	–H

*$\Delta 7=8$ indicates double bond between C7 and C8.
†Double bonds between C6 and C7 and between C8 and C14.

The illegal production of opium is huge. The large amounts of opium still used in the Orient are produced mostly in Southeast Asia. The illegal heroin that reaches the West apparently originates as opium grown in Turkey. It reaches France and Italy, usually through Lebanon or Syria, and the morphine is converted by a simple chemical process to heroin, which is more potent and perhaps more satisfying to the user.

The naturally occurring narcotic analgesics–eg, morphine and codeine–may be used as such or they may be modified chemically to form the many semisynthetic opiates listed in Table 26–1. In addition, purely synthetic compounds have been prepared that have pharmacologic properties similar to those of the naturally occurring drugs.

B. Chemical Classification of Narcotic Analgesics: The chemical classification serves to identify the large number of drugs available prior to a discussion of their biologic effects. The chemical classification does not correlate well with the more useful pharmacologic classification based on the intensity of the pain that can be relieved by the narcotic, which ability is closely correlated with addiction liability. Thus, the first class

listed below (the opiate alkaloids) includes morphine, a potent and strongly habituating analgesic, and codeine, which will not relieve severe pain but has much less potential for misuse. In the second group are methadone, a potent analgesic, and dextropropoxyphene (Darvon), a compound that is not legally classed as a narcotic.

1. Natural and semisynthetic opiates–The alkaloids that occur in opium are placed in 2 general chemical classes: benzylisoquinoline alkaloids and phenanthrene derivatives.

The benzylisoquinoline alkaloids are not narcotics or analgesics, nor are the legal controls as strict as for other opiates. Papaverine (see Chapter 13) is a smooth muscle relaxant or vasodilator. Noscapine is similar to papaverine but is suggested for use in the control of cough.

The analgesic alkaloids are called phenanthrene derivatives because of the tricyclic system they contain. The general structure is shown in Table 26–1, and the critical changes occur at R_1 and R_2. In morphine, hydroxyl groups are present at both R_1 (phenolic) and R_2 (alcoholic).

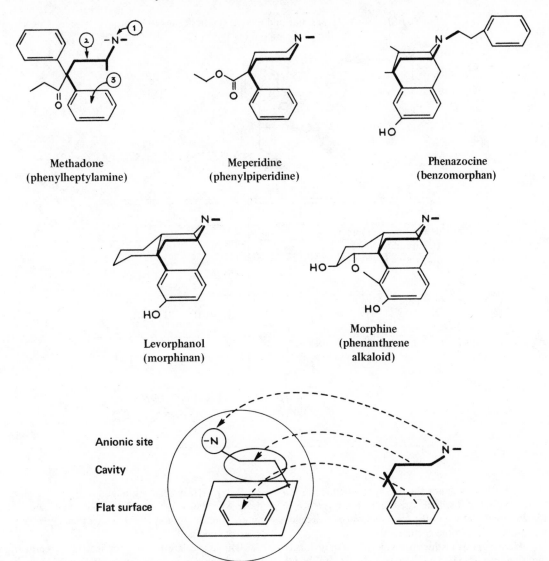

FIG 26-1. *Above:* The chemical structures of an opium alkaloid and 4 examples of synthetic narcotic analgesics written to emphasize the structure common to all: (1) a tertiary nitrogen; (2) a short hydrocarbon chain held in a plane perpendicular to the page; (3) a flat aryl group held in the plane of the page. *Below:* The skeleton structure is shown next to a hypothetical receptor surface (Beckett and Casy) which can accept the narcotic agent but not its mirror image isomer. Narcotic antagonists can attach to the receptor, but the N-substituent reduces their potency as agonists.

Methylmorphine (codeine) contains a methyl ether or methoxy group at R_1. All such methylmorphine derivatives are named as codeine derivatives even though some—eg, oxycodone—may be more potent pharmacologically than codeine. If the free phenolic hydroxyl remains, the compound is named as a derivative of morphine.

The alcoholic hydroxyl at R_2 can be oxidized to a keto group with subsequent saturation of the double bond between C7 and C8. Such derivatives are named morphones or codones. A hydroxyl group may be added at R_3 to form hydroxymorphone or hydroxycodone.

Heroin (diacetylmorphine) is rapidly hydrolyzed in the brain and liver to morphine.

As is true for all of the compounds discussed in this chapter, the opiate alkaloids are dispensed as the water-soluble salts.

2. Methadone—A large number of synthetic compounds have been tested in an effort to improve on the properties of the natural alkaloids of opium and especially to separate the analgesic and addicting properties. Whether any of these drugs offer advantages over the older alkaloids is questionable, but some have come into wide use and are of theoretical importance and promise.

TABLE 26–2. Meperidine and related synthetic analgesics of the phenylpiperidine type.

	R_1	R_2
Meperidine (Demerol)	–H	–CH$_3$
Alphaprodine (Nisentil)	–CH$_3$	–CH$_3$
Anileridine (Leritine)	–H	–CH$_2$–CH$_2$–⟨⟩–NH$_2$
Piminodine (Alvodine)	–H	–CH$_2$–CH$_2$–CH$_2$–NH–⟨⟩
Diphenoxylate (in Lomotil)	–H	–CH$_2$–CH$_2$–C–C≡N

Methadone was not the first synthetic narcotic to be prepared, but it will be listed first since reference to Fig 26–1 will show that the phenylheptylamines represent the simplest of the chemical classes.

Methadone is distinct from morphine in its longer duration of action. The withdrawal state following methadone administration is more prolonged but of lesser intensity than that following withdrawal from other narcotics, and methadone may be substituted for heroin prior to withdrawal. Propoxyphene (Darvon) is generally regarded as an analogue of methadone even though it is an ester rather than a ketone (Fig 26–2).

The analgesic and euphoriant properties of methadone are in the levorotatory form, although the drug is dispensed as a racemic mixture. In the case of dextropropoxyphene, it is claimed that the dextro isomer possesses analgesic potency comparable to that of codeine without measurable addiction liability. This doubtful claim is discussed below (see p 262).

3. Meperidine and other phenylpiperidines— Meperidine (Demerol), the first of the synthetic analgesics to be prepared, was synthesized in the belief that it would have atropine-like properties. Reference to Fig 26–1 will show how it can be considered as resulting from ring closure (piperidine ring formation) of the alkylamine of methadone. The belief that meperidine is nonaddicting and parasympatholytic has been difficult to discredit. It and the analogues listed in Table

26–2 have effects that are qualitatively identical with those of the other narcotic analgesics, and their potency and potential for abuse are much greater than those of codeine.

Diphenoxylate is a weaker analogue exempt from some of the narcotic regulations and available in a proprietary mixture (Lomotil) for the control of diarrhea. Ethoheptazine (Zactane) contains a 7-membered ring in place of the piperidine ring and is virtually inactive.

4. Morphinans–The morphinans (Table 26–3) can be considered as derived from the natural alkaloids by the removal of the oxygen or of one ring–ie, they are tetracyclic rather than pentacyclic. However, they are prepared synthetically. Levorphanol (Levo-Dromoran) is a drug of this class that is equivalent to morphine. Methorphan can be considered as related to levorphan in the same way codeine is related to morphine. Its dextro isomer, dextromethorphan, is devoid of analgesic or habituating abilities but is widely used in proprietary cough medicines.

5. Benzomorphans–(Table 26–4.) One member of this group, phenazocine (Prinadol), is available as a morphine substitute. However, the major interest in this chemical class is generated by the claim that pentazocine is a potent analgesic to which dependence does not develop because it is also a narcotic antagonist. Actually, the drug is misused but is not subject to regulation.

TABLE 26–3. Synthetic analogues of the opiates that are morphinan derivatives.

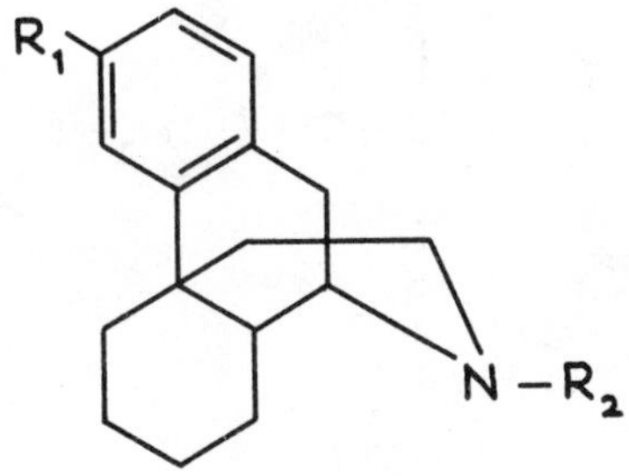

	R_1	R_2
Levorphanol (Levo-Dromoran)	–OH	–CH$_3$
Methorphan	–O–CH$_3$	–CH$_3$
Levallorphan (Lorfan)	–OH	–CH$_2$–CH=CH$_2$ (allyl)

6. Narcotic antagonists–An allyl group (–CH$_2$–CH=CH$_2$) is substituted for the methyl group attached to the basic nitrogen of morphine, levorphanol, or oxymorphone to form N-allyl-normorphine (nalorphine or Nalline), levallorphan (Lorfan), and naloxone (Narcan). These specific antagonists are able to reverse all of the depressant effects of all of the narcotics, natural and synthetic, mentioned in this chapter. Nalorphine and levallorphan retain weak morphine-like effects; naloxone is a pure antagonist. In pentazocine (Talwin), the 5-carbon substituent confers weak antagonistic properties and a significant agonistic (analgesic) effect is retained.

The uses of the antagonists to treat acute intoxication and in the diagnosis and treatment of opiate abuse are discussed at the end of this chapter.

Pharmacologic Effects

The qualitative differences among the many narcotic analgesics are minor. If the narcotic antagonists and the dextro isomers of some of the compounds are excluded, the actions of all of the drugs listed above can be described together. Important differences between the drugs are summarized below when the choice of a preparation is discussed.

A. Mechanism of Action: The effects of morphine and related drugs are due to a mixture of depression of some specific CNS functions but stimulation of others and a mixture of sympathomimetic and parasympathomimetic influences. Some specific mechanisms–eg, cholinesterase inhibition or histamine liberation–have been established. In general, however, not even the studies localizing the site of specific action within the CNS are conclusive.

B. Effects:

1. Analgesia–The essential pharmacologic effect of the strong analgesics is to relieve pain following the administration of doses so small that they do not cause general CNS depression with sedation, respiratory depression, or other disabling results.

Pain is not the result of a precise neurophysiologic process but is the highly subjective interpretation of certain sensory stimuli by a specific individual in a given situation. Pain is usually said to involve 2 components: the sensation reaching the CNS and the perception of the stimulus–ie, the individual ("psychic") processing and reaction. Morphine alters the second of these processes, so that the patient may report that the pain is still present but is less distressing.

The subjective nature of pain introduces intricate problems in the evaluation of the effectiveness of analgesic drugs. The evaluation, discussed in more detail below, can be carried out only in humans enduring real–ie, pathologic or spontaneously occurring–pain, and not in any laboratory preparation nor even in humans undergoing experimentally induced pain.

The narcotic analgesics relieve pain almost regardless of its origin or intensity. In fact, the more intense the pain, the easier it is to demonstrate the effectiveness of the drug.

2. On behavior–The opiates are commonly said to produce euphoria, but this is an oversimplification. When given to a subject who has not previously experienced the effects of the drug and who is not in pain, morphine and codeine will more commonly produce a subjectively unpleasant reaction. A barbiturate and, even more dependably, amphetamine will evoke euphoric responses in the same subject under double-blind conditions. In the presence of pain or fear, the reaction of a patient to an opiate may be much less dysphoric, and, in some people, the relief from anxiety

TABLE 26–4. A narcotic (phenazocine) and a mixed agonist-antagonist (pentazocine) that are benzomorphan derivatives.

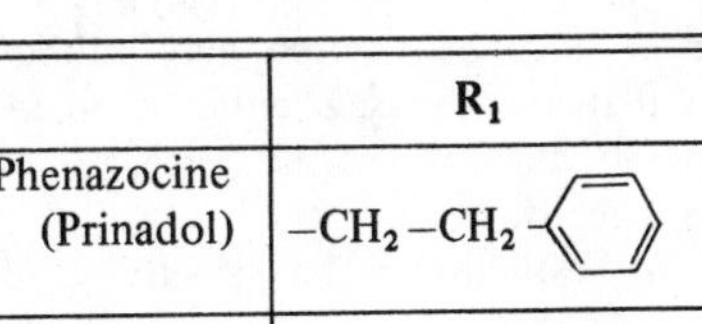

	R_1
Phenazocine (Prinadol)	–CH$_2$–CH$_2$– 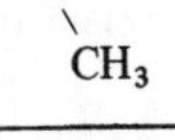 ⬡
Pentazocine (Talwin)	–CH$_2$–CH=C(CH$_3$)(CH$_3$)

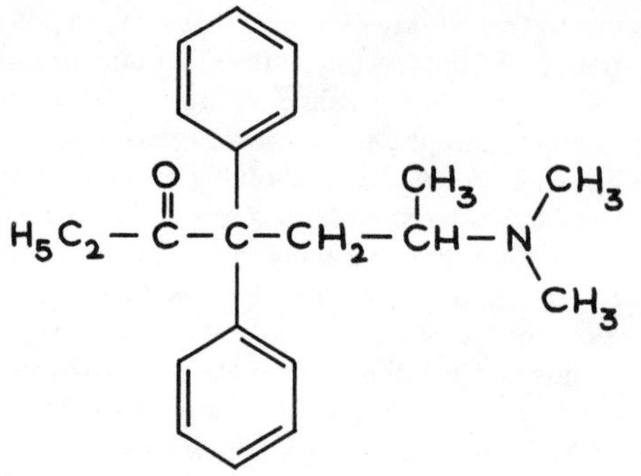

Methadone

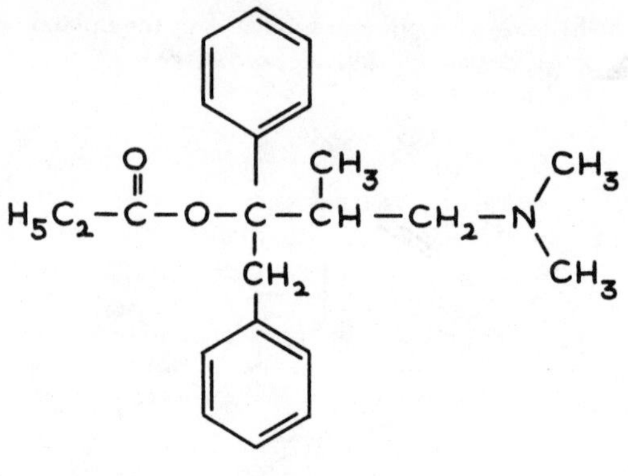

Propoxyphene
(Darvon)

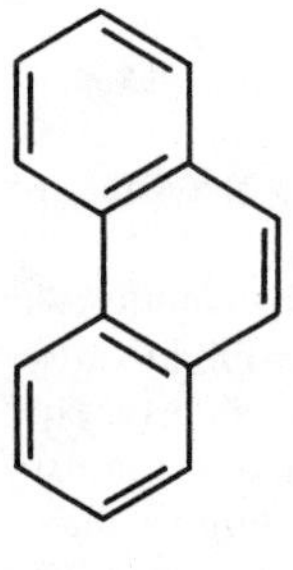

Phenanthrene

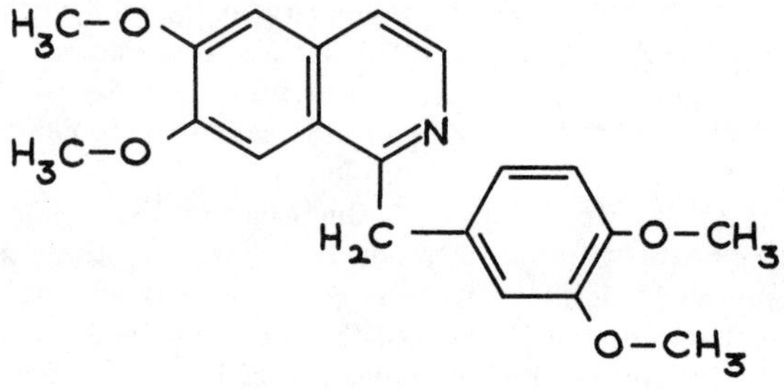

Papaverine (a benzyliso-
quinoline alkaloid)

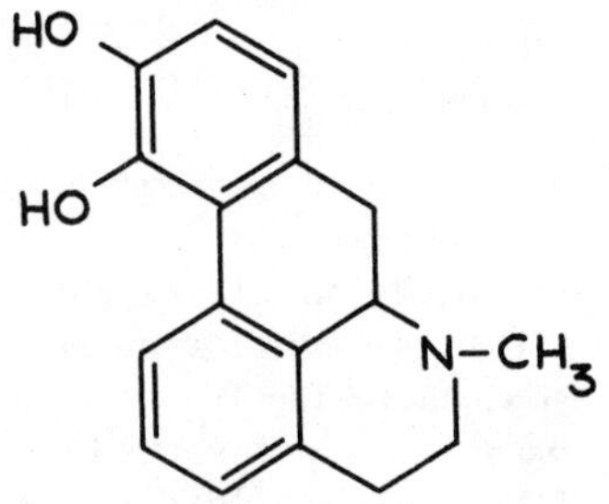

Apomorphine

FIG 26-2. The chemical structures of several compounds not included in the tables above and mentioned in the text.

and aggressive feelings may be pleasurable enough to provoke a desire for repetition of the experience.

In therapeutic doses, the sedative effects are minimal, the patient being quiet but responsive and functional. After increasingly larger doses, the subject will become drowsy, inattentive, and inefficient and fall into a sleep from which he may still be easily aroused. Very large doses induce coma.

Excitement rather than depression is rarely seen in humans unless a combination of drugs is used—eg, morphine and scopolamine in obstetric analgesia. The various members of this drug group vary in their ability to cause excitement, however, and toxic doses of codeine, meperidine, or propoxyphene may cause excitement and their action may culminate in convulsions that are suprasegmental in origin. Some species, notably the cat and the horse, respond regularly with excitement.

3. On respiration—The sensitivity of medullary centers to CO_2 is reduced and respiration correspondingly depressed. After therapeutic doses, the decrease in rate and volume may be no more than that which can be explained by the decreased activity. However, even after such therapeutic doses, a decreased responsiveness to increased concentrations of CO_2 in the inspired air is demonstrable. With larger doses, respiratory rate falls progressively and finally becomes not only slow but shallow and irregular in pattern.

The respiratory depression and CO_2 retention have 2 further important consequences. Intracranial vessels are dilated by the elevated level of CO_2. Cerebral blood flow and intracranial blood volume increase, and intracranial pressure is thereby elevated. The asphyxial changes also cause hyperglycemia, which in humans is usually minor. The hyperglycemia can be prevented by controlling the respiration or, in animals, by adrenalectomy, establishing that it results from the sympatho-adrenal discharge caused by asphyxia.

While medullary sensitivity to CO_2 is reduced, the sensitivity of the chemoreceptors in the carotid sinus and aortic arch areas is increased and the respiratory center is still able to respond to the stimulus of hypoxia. Increasing the concentration of oxygen in the inspired air may reduce this stimulus and further depress respiration.

4. On other areas of CNS—Nausea and vomiting are caused by a stimulating action of morphine on the chemoreceptor trigger zone of the medulla. However, movement intensifies and recumbency reduces the emetic effect, suggesting that vestibular factors are also involved. Following the initial stimulation, the vomiting center is depressed, so that vomiting does not result from closely spaced doses.

Coughing is suppressed by the narcotic analgesics, and this is the one action that can be separated from the analgesic potency of these drugs.

5. On the cardiovascular system—The skin is warm and flushed. The heart rate is slowed only by large doses. Postural hypotension severe enough to cause dizziness or fainting can occur even after therapeutic doses of narcotics if the patient arises suddenly or is studied on a tilt table. The hypotensive effect is intensified by the simultaneous administration of phenothiazine tranquilizers or atropine-like drugs.

The cause of the hypotension is not clear but is probably central in origin—ie, due to medullary vasomotor depression. Many of the strong analgesics have been shown to be histamine liberators of significant potency. Such action adequately explains the itching and urticaria that appear after the administration of these drugs. However, the hypotension is longer lasting and probably too intense to be explained by this mechanism.

6. On the gastrointestinal tract—The important observation is that the net effect of the opiates or their surrogates is constipating. Constipation is a frequent side-effect of repeated doses, and diarrhea can be effectively treated with narcotics.

The explanations for this fact introduce confusion and some conflict. Most laboratory investigators have concluded that these drugs increase intestinal contraction to such an extent that propulsive or effective activity is decreased. They have, however, used very large doses in animals and have made their observations only for a short period after administration; furthermore, their technic of measurement has often added the stimulating effect of distending the intestine. Clinical investigators using roentgenologic technics and those laboratory investigators who have used smaller doses and followed their animals for extended periods have described a phase of markedly inhibited activity following the transient stimulation. An exception to this generalization is the occurrence of a persistent pylorospasm that prolongs gastric emptying time. Despite the various interpretations, there is no argument with the observation that the ultimate effect is one of constipation.

7. On the biliary tract—The smooth muscle of the biliary tract, including the sphincter of Oddi, is stimulated—at least acutely. This is true for all of the narcotics studied, including meperidine. One of these drugs may nevertheless be used to relieve the pain of biliary colic.

The impaired drainage from the common duct into the intestine has several metabolic consequences. Serum amylase and lipase levels are elevated by the administration of morphine whether pancreatitis is present or not. SGOT and alkaline phosphatase levels are unchanged following the administration of morphine if a functioning gallbladder is present. In the presence of biliary tract disease or following cholecys-tectomy, the levels may rise—due, presumably, to contraction of the sphincter of Oddi with reflux.

8. On pupillary size—The decrease in pupillary size is of considerable practical importance in recognizing narcotic intoxication and is also the basis for a test for drug misuse described below. The miosis is replaced by pupillary dilatation when epinephrine liberation is provoked either by excitement or by respiratory depression and asphyxia.

9. Tolerance and physical dependence—These problems are discussed in detail below in relation to drug misuse or dependence. However, they do occur during the therapeutic use of narcotic analgesics and should be defined here. As **tolerance** develops, larger and larger doses of the drug must be administered in order to achieve the same effect. **Physical dependence** exists when drug administration must be continued to maintain normal function—ie, to prevent the withdrawal state.

Absorption, Metabolism, & Excretion

All of the opiates and synthetic equivalents are well absorbed from injection sites. However, their suitability for oral administration varies between compounds. Morphine itself has a greatly delayed onset of action after oral administration, and the oral dose must be several times the injected dose. It appears that absorption is complete, although variable in rate, and that rapid conjugation, either in the liver or the intestinal wall, occurs. Many of the alternate drugs listed in Table 26–5 are preferable for oral administration.

Morphine is inactivated for the most part by conversion to the 3-monoglucuronide in the liver. A small amount is demethylated to normorphine. Both free and conjugated morphine are excreted into the urine. A small fraction (10%) is excreted in the feces following excretion into bile.

The conversion of all injected heroin and a small fraction of a dose of codeine to morphine is discussed in relation to those drugs below.

Clinical Uses

A. Relief of Pain: Morphine or one of its less potent surrogates can be used to relieve pain almost regardless of its nature. Isolated, sharp pains—eg, those generated by movement or touching a sensitive area—are probably less effectively suppressed than constant pain. The pain of trauma, myocardial infarction, biliary or ureteral colic, inflammation, infiltration or pressure by a neoplasm, etc are examples of situations in which a narcotic analgesic is used.

Contraindications to the use of narcotics are listed below, and the hazard of addiction precludes the use of all but the least potent agents in chronic or recurrent pain that threatens to be of long duration—eg, arthritis, migraine, or trigeminal neuralgia. However, the narcotic analgesics should be used as a general rule to relieve pain for which the antipyretic analgesics such as aspirin are ineffective or until specific treatment becomes effective.

TABLE 26–5. Narcotic analgesics: Dosages and preparations available.

	Dose		
	Subcut*	**Oral**	**Preparations Available**
Most potent			
Morphine	8–15 mg	. . .	Hypodermic tablets, 8, 10, 15, and 30 mg Injectable (subcut, IM, IV), 8, 10, 15, and 30 mg/ml
Heroin	. . .	. . .	. . .
Hydromorphone (dihydro-morphinone, Dilaudid)	2 mg	2 mg	Hypodermic tablets, 1, 2, 3, and 4 mg Suppositories, 3 mg Injectable hydrochloride salt (subcut, IM, IV), 2, 3, and 4 mg, 1 ml ampule and 2 ml disposable syringe; sucrate, 2 mg/ml, 10 and 20 ml vials
Oxymorphone (Numorphan)	1.5 mg	. . .	Injectable (subcut, IM, IV), 1 mg/ml, 1 and 1.5 ml ampules and 15 ml vials; 1.5 mg/ml, 1 and 2 ml ampules and 10 ml vials
Levorphanol (Levo-Dromoran)	2 mg	2 mg	Tablets, 2 mg Injectable (subcut, IM, IV), 2 mg/ml, 1,and 10 ml
Phenazocine (Prinadol)	2 mg (IM)	. . .	Injectable (IM, IV), 2 mg/ml, 1 ml ampule (IM); 2 mg/ml, 10 ml vials
Methadone (Dolophine, various others)	5 mg	5 mg	Tablets, 5 and 10 mg Syrup, 1.67 mg/5 ml Injectable (subcut or IM), 10 mg/ml, 1, 20, and 30 ml
Intermediate potency			
Meperidine (Demerol, various others)	75–150 mg (IM)	75–100 mg	Tablets, 50 and 100 mg Elixir, 50 mg/5 ml Injectable (subcut, IM, or IV), 50 mg/ml, 0.5, 1, 1.5, 2, 10, and 30 ml; 100 mg/ml, 1, 2, and 30 ml; 50, 75, and 100 mg, 1 and 2 ml disposable syringes
Alphaprodine (Nisentil)	40–60 mg	. . .	Injectable (subcut or IV), 40 mg/ml, 1 and 10 ml; 60 mg/ml, 1 ml
Anileridine (Leritine)	25–50 mg	25–50 mg	Tablets, 25 mg Injectable (subcut, IM, IV), 25 mg/ml, 1, 2, and 30 ml
Piminodine (Alvodine)	10–20 mg	25–50 mg	Tablets, 50 mg Injectable (subcut, IM, IV), 20 mg/ml, 1 ml ampules
Pentazocine (Talwin)	30 mg	50 mg	Tablets, 50 mg Injectable (subcut, IM, IV), 30 mg/ml, 1, 1.5, 2, and 10 ml
Dihydrocodeinone (in Hycodan)	. . .	. . .	. . .
Oxycodone (in Percodan)	. . .	. . .	. . .
Least potent			
Codeine	30–65 mg	30–65 mg	Hypodermic tablets, 8, 15, 32, and 65 mg Injectable phosphate salt (subcut, IM, IV), 32 mg/ml, 1 ml ampules and 20 ml vials; 32 and 65 mg, 1 ml disposable syringes
Dihydrocodeine (Paracodin)	65 mg	65 mg	. . .

*Recommended single dose. The "nonnarcotic analgesics" and the narcotic antagonists are discussed in the text. Give subcutaneously except as noted. Most preparations can also be given intravenously in emergencies (see Preparations Available).

B. Problems of Clinical Evaluation: Relief of pain is the prototype of a subjective response to a drug whose clinical evaluation is difficult. There is no question about the effectiveness of the familiar agents, but the problem of clinical evaluation becomes important and difficult when comparisons must be made between available drugs; when new compounds must be evaluated; when precise information about dose is required; or when the nature of pain is studied.

The subjective nature of pain emphasized above becomes even more apparent when the action of drugs on pain is studied. The nature of the pain associated with a particular disease can be quite accurately described (quality, radiation, etc), and the stimulus and afferent pathways can be defined. None of these factors nor the threshold for perception of a particular stimulus, however, constitute an adequate definition of pain, since they do not consider those subjective factors that alter the individual reaction. Pain originates not only from the original sensation but also from the meaning that the individual attaches to the stimulus. The significance of this "meaning of the stimulus" is shown by studies comparing the amount of analgesic drug needed by patients sustaining roughly comparable injuries in 2 different situations. The civilian, threatened by the consequences of the accident, suffers more pain and requires more morphine than the soldier whose almost identical injury may promise relief from combat duty. The narcotic analgesics alter the anxiety engendered by the anticipation of pain and other factors constituting the "psychic processing" of the original sensation.

Because of the subjective nature of pain, it is unlikely that any available experimentally induced pain in laboratory animals or in humans has significant value in the clinical evaluation of analgesics. The common technics for measuring the alteration of response to pain in animals involve measuring the intensity of a reflex response initiated by a stimulus presumed to be painful. For example, a source of heat may be focused on the tail of a rodent (blackened to absorb heat) and the time until the response (tail flick) measured. This response is a spinal reflex that can still be modified by drugs in the cord sectioned animal.

Experimental pain may be produced in humans by stimulation with heat, pressure, electricity, or ischemia. This is equivalent to measuring the pain threshold, which is not only not constant in different subjects or at different times in the same subject but also bears no dependable relation to the clinical actions of analgesics.

Consequently, the consensus today is that pain can be studied and analgesic drugs assayed only in the human experiencing pathologic or spontaneously arising pain—ie, nonexperimentally induced pain. The group of patients available in sufficient numbers and experiencing generally comparable pain are those suffering postoperative or incisional pain. The responses of these patients to drugs is studied following the general pattern described for an acceptable clinical trial in Chapter 3. A comparison of the drug under study

with either a placebo or a standard analgesic must be included, and the patients must be randomly assigned to groups or the order of drug administration randomly determined. The double-blind technic must, of course, be employed. At intervals before and after the administration of the drug, the patient is queried by a disinterested technician or other observer about the intensity of his pain and the presence of side-effects. When these subjective responses are converted to an arbitrary descriptive scale and the data properly organized, remarkably fine discrimination and reproducibility are possible. There is no question of the applicability to the clinical situation since the assay situation is simply the clinical situation organized to permit quantitative, controlled observations.

C. Sedation or Relief of Anxiety: Sedative-hypnotics of the barbiturate type produce a disinhibited, euphoric state more dependably than the narcotics and are clearly more suitable for the treatment of most anxiety states. However, the more potent narcotic analgesics alter the reaction of the patient to stimuli other than pain and relieve anxiety in the most acute and distressing situations—eg, bereavement.

This property is relevant to the problem of selecting a preanesthetic or preprocedural medication. As has been discussed in Chapter 20, some anesthetists have argued that in a patient free of pain the barbiturates are a more rational drug for the relief of anxiety preoperatively. However, morphine or another potent narcotic, especially when combined with other depressant drugs, is generally regarded as a more dependable drug for producing indifference to the impending events.

D. Acute Pulmonary Edema: Morphine is the drug of first choice in the treatment of acute pulmonary edema, and its effectiveness is such that it is often described as a "specific" treatment. Aminophylline and oxygen may also be administered. The mechanism by which morphine brings about relief is not clear. Its effectiveness is one of several pieces of data suggesting that acute pulmonary edema, which occurs in association with other than cardiac disease, should not be thought of as a consequence of acute left ventricular failure but as a reflexly generated state which can be interrupted by this central depressant.

E. Cough: The narcotics depress the cough reflex, and this action can be separated from the analgesic effect. For example, the dextrorotatory isomer of some compounds is devoid of analgesic effects but may be used to suppress coughing.

For control of coughing, the ordinary narcotics can be given by mouth in doses approximately half the analgesic doses listed in Table 26–5. The least potent agent that is effective should be used—ie, codeine in most cases.

F. Diarrhea: The constipating effects of the narcotics, ordinarily a troublesome side-effect, may be used in the symptomatic treatment of acute diarrhea. The traditional preparation often selected for this application is paregoric (camphorated opium tincture), which acts because of the morphine that it contains.

All narcotics possess constipating activity in proportion to other analgesic effect. Again, codeine (15 mg orally 3 times daily) is the most common alternative to paregoric.

Adverse Reactions

A. Side-Effects: One or more of the side-effects listed below occur in most patients receiving narcotics in therapeutic doses. The potent drugs cause more intense side-effects, but the weaker analgesics such as codeine given chronically lead to side-effects with equal or greater frequency.

1. Behavioral—Even in the presence of pain, the subjective reaction is not invariably pleasant. Feelings of anxiety, lethargy, or confusion may make the experience unpleasant. Agents such as codeine or propoxyphene which possess the excitant properties to a greater extent may cause restlessness, tremulousness, and hyperactivity.

2. Nausea and vomiting—This action has been discussed under Pharmacologic Effects.

3. Constipation—The ability of the narcotic analgesic to decrease propulsive activity in the intestine can lead to a constipating effect that may outlast the analgesic effect by a day or more. The same effect of morphine or a similar agent given preoperatively contributes to the development of paralytic ileus or a delayed return of intestinal activity postoperatively. All patients are distended by air swallowed during general anesthesia, as can be shown by simple measurements of their girth pre- and postoperatively, and preoperative narcotics prolong the effect of this distention.

4. Urinary retention—The incidence of postoperative urinary retention is similarly increased by narcotics.

5. Itching, urticaria—The histamine liberating abilities of the narcotic analgesics, apparent after injection more commonly than after oral administration, may lead to itching, especially in the skin about the nose, or even to the appearance of wheals.

6. Cardiovascular—The acute postural hypotension already described is most often seen when a patient quickly arises while the drug is acting, when he may experience dizziness, faintness, or even syncope.

7. Respiratory—Therapeutic doses of the narcotics do not usually cause alarming respiratory depression unless other depressant drugs are also acting. General anesthesia is, of course, the common situation in which their use is combined with the use of other respiratory depressant drugs. Postoperatively, the depression of respiration, the depression of cough reflexes, and the suppression of the occasional deep breath that is part of the normal pattern of respiration can predispose to atelectasis.

B. Acute Toxicity: Acute opiate toxicity is seen following suicidal or accidental ingestion of prescribed medication and after therapeutic accidents, but drug users provide most of the cases seen. The diagnosis depends upon the history or evidence (such as needle marks) of narcotic misuse. The comatose patient will have slow, shallow, irregular respiration. The decrease in rate is usually more marked than is the case after barbiturate intoxication. The pupils may be constricted, but asphyxial changes obscure this change more often than not. Blood pressure may be slightly reduced. The pulse rate is also slowed until the tachycardia of shock supervenes.

The treatment of acute opiate intoxication depends upon the use of narcotic antagonists. These drugs (discussed in detail below) are competitive antagonists to all of the natural and synthetic narcotics and rapidly reverse all of the depressant effects of the narcotics. Nalorphine (Nalline), levallorphan (Lorfan), and naloxone (Narcan) are examples of narcotic antagonists. They can also be used to reverse unexpected reactions to therapeutic doses.

C. Habituation and Misuse: The problem of the abuse of central depressant and central stimulant drugs involves not merely the pharmacologic properties of the drug but psychiatric and sociologic factors as well. Misuse of the opiates should not be set off as a separate problem but should be considered as part of a general medical problem involving several drug types (see Chapter 7).

1. Tolerance—Tolerance to the effects of the narcotics develops more quickly and to a much greater degree than tolerance to other drugs subject to abuse. Animals given repeated and progressively larger doses and humans who have access to large amounts of heroin or other narcotics are soon able to tolerate many multiples of the usual lethal doses. Tolerance develops to all of the effects listed above except constipation and pupillary constriction. Tolerance can thus be defined as a state when larger doses are required to elicit the same effect or when a fixed dose exerts a decreasing effect.

The rate at which tolerance develops depends upon several factors, including especially the interval between doses and the amount of drug provided. The development of tolerance in heroin addicts today is limited by the difficulty and expense involved in obtaining the drug, and many are able to continue more or less indefinitely on a fixed dose, continuing to experience the "rush" at the time of injection but showing little depression later. In the therapeutic situation, if constant and severe pain forces the administration of potent narcotics at 4–6 hour intervals, the analgesic effect may decrease within a few days. If the interval between therapeutic doses can be lengthened well beyond the duration of action of the drug—ie, given 2 times per day—tolerance may not be apparent after several weeks.

2. Physical dependence and withdrawal—Parallel to the development of tolerance and independent of any psychologic dependence, the organism develops a need for the continued administration of the narcotic in the sense that continued administration is necessary to prevent the development of the physiologic disturbances known as the abstinence or withdrawal syndrome. Or, to restate the definition in the same terms used in the discussion of alcohol and barbiturates, if narcotic administration is abruptly discontinued following the administration of the drug for an adequate period, a withdrawal state is seen.

The onset of the withdrawal state follows the last dose after an interval that varies with the amount of narcotic used and with the specific compound used. In the case of morphine or heroin, symptoms appear 8–16 hours or more following the final dose and increase in intensity for 48–72 hours, after which the symptoms slowly subside. The most persistent symptom, insomnia, may last 4 weeks or longer. The figures are somewhat smaller in the case of the shorter-acting meperidine, and the duration is prolonged after the administration of methadone.

The mechanism or mechanisms underlying tolerance and the abstinence syndrome are not known. The signs and symptoms can be remembered by considering that the body adapts to the continued presence of a depressant drug by activating excitatory systems whose activity persists after the drug is withdrawn. The abstinence syndrome will thus bear close similarity to the effects of large doses of amphetamines.

The signs and symptoms can be organized as follows: (1) **Autonomic hyperactivity**: Sympathetic effects are lacrimation, rhinorrhea, sweating, piloerection ("gooseflesh" or "cold turkey"), dilated pupils, elevated blood pressure and pulse rate, and hyperpyrexia. Parasympathetic hyperactivity causes emesis, abdominal pain, and diarrhea. (2) **Behavioral hyperexcitability**: Anxiety, restlessness, yawning, tremor, insomnia. In the most severe states (unusual at this time), the hyperexcitability may progress to convulsions or a toxic psychosis. (3) **Muscle and joint pains.** (4) **Anxiety** that is not due to physical withdrawal but occurs because the compulsive act is not performed. This anxiety is the therapeutically important problem in treating heroin abuse as well as cigarette smoking, overeating, or other compulsion.

In the therapeutic situation, especially if the narcotics are used only as required, withdrawal is mild and not usually related by the patient to the analgesic. The person who uses illegal opiates experiences and recognizes the withdrawal state whenever the routine of use that he usually maintains is interrupted. Dangerously severe withdrawal states are uncommon in the compulsive heroin user today because of the restraint placed upon the amounts available by the cost and the dilution of the illegal drug. The actual discomfort and the fear of the physical effects of withdrawal is, nevertheless, an important initial barrier to the treatment of the heroin user and presents a situation during which he deserves support by drugs and other means.

Withdrawal is, however, the least difficult part of treatment of this compulsion. The typical heroin user withdraws and returns to the drug many times during his career, demonstrating that factors other than "junk sickness" are operating.

3. Patterns and effects of misuse—Narcotics, whether injected, swallowed, or smoked, are subject to varying degrees of misuse. One individual may use single doses sporadically and another may use them compulsively 4 or more times a day regardless of the consequences. The damage to the individual is variable but may be quite minor. The sporadic user may be unaffected in his general social behavior, but the compulsive user usually loses interest in everything but the need to maintain his habit, which inevitably forces him into criminal activity. It is this associated criminal activity rather than any inherent action of the drug that is damaging to society and to the individual.

4. Treatment—Some general ideas apply to the treatment of drug misuse regardless of the specific agent involved (see Chapter 7). The individual may be handled as a criminal; therapy in various forms may be provided; or the drug may be provided under controlled conditions. Only 2 special aspects of treatment are discussed here.

a. Withdrawal—Withdrawal is not often supervised by a physician but occurs in the room of the user or in jail. Humane and safe withdrawal is best accomplished by substituting methadone for heroin, the dosage depending upon the degree of tolerance and dependence. The dosage of methadone can then be reduced or the drug withdrawn, whereupon a mild withdrawal state occurs. The dosage of methadone required can be reduced by sedation and autonomic blocking agents. The use of methadone in the treatment of addiction is restricted in many states.

b. Methadone maintenance—Rather than provide the individual with heroin for intravenous use, a currently expanding treatment concept offers him large oral daily doses of methadone. As he becomes tolerant to the large doses of methadone used (80–160 mg/day), he can no longer achieve any effect from reasonable amounts of heroin. Methadone maintenance or blockade thus frees the patient from the need to engage in criminal activity to support his habit and makes it possible for him to leave the drug culture. The disadvantages are that the individual on methadone is not free of depressant drug effects and that other drugs may be misused since he is deprived of the anxiety-relieving action of intravenous narcotics.

Methadone in this use is technically an investigative drug subject to regulation by federal and state authorities. It may be shipped only to programs approved by federal and state agencies for use in maintenance or withdrawal or to hospital pharmacies for use as an analgesic or for inpatient withdrawal. The patient selected for maintenance treatment must be 18 years of age or older; must have a verified history of heroin abuse for at least 2 years; and must show evidence from urinalysis of current use. Initially, the patient must appear daily at the clinic to receive his allocation of the drug; later, he may be allowed "take-home doses" and need appear only twice weekly. Methadone must be dissolved in juice so that it cannot be injected. Weekly urinalysis to detect morphine (the metabolite of heroin) is required.

5. Diagnosis and detection of narcotic use—There are 2 general screening methods for establishing that an individual has or has not been using opiate drugs. In the "Nalline test," an injection of the narcotic antagonist nalorphine is given and the pupillary response followed. If the subject is using a significant amount of a narcotic, the pupil will dilate when the opiate is antagonized. The subject will also experience a mild heroin-like effect which is countertherapeutic and, as the test is usually administered, will be ·brought into contact with a large number of other users. A second method involves collecting a urine sample and analyzing an extract chromatographically in order to demonstrate metabolites of narcotics and other drugs subject to misuse such as methamphetamine. These technics cannot be used as a screening test on a suspect population or individual, but they may be made a condition of probation or parole following conviction or commitment. They are thus a police or social function, and the interest of the physician is more likely to be in therapy rather than detection.

Contraindications & Cautions

Morphine and the other more potent narcotic analgesics are potentially very dangerous drugs in some patients. Nevertheless, the contraindications are, in general, relative rather than absolute, calling for a great reduction in dose or the use of a less potent agent such as codeine rather than a more depressant drug of this group. Obviously, opiates should not be used unless there is an indication for their use—eg, a patient in traumatic shock may be apathetic rather than complaining of pain, and the use of analgesics should then be deferred. The following precautions should be observed.

A. Increased Intracranial Pressure From Head Injury or Other Cause: If administration of a narcotic causes even a minor degree of respiratory depression, the CO_2 retention can cause dilatation of intracranial vessels and a further increase in intracranial pressure. The increase can be controlled during anesthesia by assisting the respiration.

B. Chronic Pain: Some types of chronic pain—eg, that associated with the terminal stages of malignancy—require the chronic use of narcotics. The smallest amount of the least potent agent is used, with the longest interval possible between doses, in order to minimize side-effects and tolerance and to maintain the benefit to the patient—but not because of any legal concern about habituation. Pain such as that of migraine or arthritis that recurs over a period of many years should be treated with narcotics with great caution. Codeine is virtually free of addiction liability in a situation of this kind unless the patient has had experience with more potent narcotics, in which case codeine may be used to maintain a habituation established primarily with another agent.

C. Asthma: Morphine and meperidine have been effective in interrupting an otherwise resistant attack of asthma. However, it appears that bronchiolar smooth muscle, like other smooth muscle, may respond in 2 ways to morphine. A very rare patient, instead of responding with bronchiolar dilatation, may show greatly increased respiratory distress and die suddenly after the administration of morphine or meperi-

dine. The narcotics are not essential in the treatment of asthma and should not be used.

D. Other Pulmonary Disease: In the presence of cor pulmonale, emphysema, kyphoscoliosis, or other conditions in which no reserve of respiratory function exists, the slightest additional depression may lead to respiratory decompensation.

E. When Narcotics Might Delay or Obscure Diagnosis: This caution is perhaps more theoretical than real. It may be necessary to use morphine in the presence of acute abdominal pain, and even when pancreatitis is suspected (in which case the narcotic may elevate the serum enzyme levels that are useful in diagnosis).

F. Grossly Impaired Liver Function: As would be predicted from other tests of the metabolic function of the liver, the response to morphine is not altered until liver function is greatly decreased. However, in the presence of cirrhosis accompanied by encephalopathy, jaundice, or ascites, the risk of hepatic coma is increased by the administration of an opiate. The mechanism by which coma is precipitated is not known.

G. Hypothyroid State: Myxedematous patients are said, on the basis of clinical observations, to be unusually sensitive to narcotics.

H. Combination With Other Drugs: The respiratory depressant effects of the barbiturates or alcohol are additive to those of the narcotic.

Dosages & Selection of Drug
A. Differences Among Drugs of This Class:

1. Potency—The potency of the various members of this drug group should not be defined by the number of milligrams used but in terms of the intensity of the pain that can be relieved. Very intense pain, such as that occurring early in the course of a myocardial infarction or the pain of ureteral colic, may not be relieved by codeine no matter how much is used but responds well to morphine. It has not yet been possible to separate potency from the addiction liability inherent in the narcotic. Therefore, the most important and most useful classification of narcotics is the one that places them in 3 groups depending upon their ability to relieve pain (see Table 26—5). Morphine and its congeners relieve the most severe pain but are also most potent in causing euphoria. Codeine will not relieve all types of pain, but the hazard of primary addiction is negligible. Meperidine and its analogues form an intermediate class.

2. Other qualitative differences—The narcotics can differ in the balance between sedative and excitant effects that each causes. This difference is most apparent in the side-effects that occur. Morphine rarely causes excitement; codeine only rarely causes sedation.

3. Duration of action—Methadone has been repeatedly mentioned above as a narcotic with a distinctively long duration of action. Meperidine and related compounds have a duration of action only half that of morphine.

4. Prescription regulations—See Chapter 4.

B. Most Potent Narcotics: Drugs of this class relieve the most severe pain but have a correspondingly high addiction liability and cause a high incidence of the more uncomfortable side-effects.

1. Morphine is the most important drug in this category. It is most often given subcutaneously. The technics described in the section on clinical evaluation are sufficiently sensitive to permit accurate determination of the relation of dosage to effectiveness, duration of action, and incidence of side-effects. The optimal subcutaneous dose is 10 mg. An increase to 15 mg provides a minor increase in duration of effect but a significant increase in the number of side-effects and degree of respiratory depression.

The intravenous dose, used in situations of great urgency such as acute pulmonary edema or very severe pain, is 4–8 mg. The oral dose is 8–20 mg, but morphine is less dependable by mouth than by other routes of administration.

2. Pantopon is a mixture of all of the alkaloids of opium. The mixture is 50% morphine, and the other alkaloids do not have significant actions.

3. Paregoric (camphorated tincture of opium) is an antidiarrheal preparation containing 1.6 mg of morphine in each 4 ml of an unpleasantly flavored vehicle. More pleasant solutions of morphine alone could be prepared, but paregoric is an official preparation and its standard concentration causes less confusion. The now official name "paregoric" minimizes the possibility of confusion with the much stronger tincture of opium (laudanum), which is practically never used.

4. Heroin is slightly more potent than morphine and is a dense rather than fluffy powder. It is therefore preferred as a smuggled commodity and is more easily "cut" or diluted with lactose or other substance. Drug users can differentiate it from morphine after intravenous administration and prefer heroin because of its more intense immediate effect—ie, the orgasm-like sensation that accompanies injection. Heroin is deacetylated stepwise and excreted as morphine. 6-Monacetylmorphine enters the brain rapidly. Because of the problem of heroin misuse, the drug has been outlawed as a therapeutic agent in all countries.

5. Methadone has been mentioned above because of its long duration of action and its use in withdrawing patients from other narcotics and in the blockade of heroin effect in the treatment of heroin users. The potential for misuse of methadone is very great, and it is not used as an analgesic. The effects of therapeutic doses persist for 6–8 hours. With very large doses—eg, the 80–160 mg dosage used in the methadone maintenance treatment of heroin abuse—the effects last for 24 hours or longer.

6. Hydromorphone (Dilaudid) has a slightly shorter duration of effect than morphine and may cause less sedation.

7. Oxymorphone (Numorphan) is more potent than morphine but causes more euphoria and more nausea and vomiting.

8. Levorphanol (Levo-Dromoran) is a well absorbed synthetic.

9. Phenazocine (Prinadol) causes more respiratory depression than morphine.

C. Narcotics of Intermediate Potency:

1. Meperidine (pethidine BP; Demerol) is the prototype of this group of analgesics that are more potent than codeine but less effective than morphine. Meperidine is like codeine in that its excitant properties are prominent. Its duration of action is about half that of morphine (approximately 2 rather than 4 hours), an advantage for brief procedures or when used prior to delivery. It is injected intramuscularly rather than subcutaneously because of its irritant properties. It is well absorbed from the gastrointestinal tract.

Early claims were that meperidine had low or even no addicting properties. Perhaps because of this claim and because of factors of availability, it soon became and has remained the narcotic which doctors and nurses are most likely to misuse.

Meperidine was originally synthesized as an atropine substitute and was marketed with claims that, in contrast to morphine, it relaxed smooth muscle. Whenever meperidine has been compared with morphine for its effects on intestine, biliary tract, bronchioles, etc, no difference has been demonstrated when equipotent doses were used. The original claim has been difficult to dispel and is still influential.

2. Alphaprodine (Nisentil), anileridine (Leritine), and piminodine (Alvodine) are equivalent to meperidine although their duration of action may be even briefer.

3. Oxycodone has been used in proprietary mixtures, especially Percodan. The suggestive similarity of the name of this mixture to codeine was allowed to suggest to many a therapeutic equivalence with codeine. It is actually more potent and more addicting but, until recently, was subject to less legal discipline in prescribing. The laws were recently changed to reflect its similarity to other narcotics of intermediate potency.

D. Least Potent Narcotics:

1. Codeine is the most commonly used narcotic analgesic, and whenever possible, when narcotics are necessary, treatment should begin with and be limited to this weak analgesic. Primary addiction to codeine—ie, misuse without prior experience with a more potent drug—is virtually unheard of. Side-effects are common but minor in nature compared with morphine or meperidine. Sedation is unusual. Excitement may occur, and large doses may even cause convulsions in children. Respiratory depression is negligible.

Codeine is demethylated to form small amounts of morphine and normorphine. These substances probably have no role or only a minor role in producing the effects of codeine.

Codeine is given orally in doses of 30 or 65 mg (½ or 1 gr). If it is dispensed in combination with another active drug—eg, aspirin or aspirin compound (APC)—fewer legal restraints on prescribing exist (see Chapter 4). In such mixtures it is the codeine that determines the analgesic effectiveness of the mixture.

2. Dihydrocodeine is given in smaller doses than codeine but is otherwise equivalent.

3. Ethylmorphine (Dionin) is not used as an analgesic. It is identified because of occasional references to its use as a corneal irritant.

4. Diphenoxylate is contained in a proprietary mixture (Lomotil) used in the treatment of diarrhea. The presence of another ingredient (atropine) exempts the mixture from some of the rules governing narcotic prescriptions, but the mixture is not superior to codeine, 15 mg 3–4 times each day.

5. Dextromethorphan is the dextro isomer of a derivative of levorphanol (Table 26–3). It is almost completely free of analgesic and respiratory depressant properties, and is a component of many over-the-counter and prescription medications for cough.

6. Thebaine (Table 26–1) has no therapeutic applications but is of theoretical interest because it possesses the excitatory but none of the depressant properties of morphine. It causes behavioral excitement and convulsions that originate in the spinal cord comparable to those that occur after toxic doses of strychnine.

7. Apomorphine (Fig 26–2) is prepared by heating morphine with strong acid. It very dependably induces emesis by stimulating the chemoreceptor trigger zone of the medulla. It is a depressant like morphine, and its action is terminated by the narcotic antagonists. Its use in acute intoxications as an emetic agent is discussed in Chapter 64.

E. Propoxyphene (Darvon, Dextropropoxyphene): Propoxyphene is rarely used as such but is in extremely wide use as a combination with aspirin compound (APC). Its prescription is not governed by the regulations controlling narcotics, and for this reason it is often referred to as a nonnarcotic analgesic.

Propoxyphene was characterized chemically above as the D-isomer of a compound related to methadone, and in structure and action is best regarded as an extremely weak narcotic analgesic.

Propoxyphene with aspirin compound (Darvon Compound) is a popular prescription medication because it is "nonnarcotic" and because of the claim that it is equivalent in potency to codeine. This claim is not substantiated by such clinical evaluations as are available. Obviously, Darvon Compound must be compared with aspirin compound as well as with codeine with aspirin to establish its relative potency. The analgesic effect of 32 mg of propoxyphene is not greater than that of aspirin compound. Propoxyphene in doses of 65 mg does have an effect somewhat greater than that of the aspirin compound with which it is mixed, but it is much less potent than codeine.

Frequent side-effects are dizziness, drowsiness, nausea, vomiting, and constipation. The acute toxic effects that follow accidentally ingested overdoses include, in addition, coma, convulsions, and respiratory depression. One death has been reported. Nalorphine antagonizes the respiratory depression and probably all of the other toxic effects except convulsions.

Propoxyphene is not classified as a narcotic by federal authorities but is regarded as equivalent to codeine by the WHO. The possibility of primary addiction can be safely ignored, but an occasional person who has experienced the effects of other narcotics will use propoxyphene to maintain his habituation. Some patients recognize a euphoriant effect, and very large doses provide some relief from the withdrawal state following strong opiates.

NARCOTIC ANTAGONISTS

Some references to the narcotic antagonists have already been made. Their properties are discussed in this section with repetition of some material.

Chemistry
Most of the narcotic analgesics have an N-methyl substituent (Tables 26–1 and 26–3). The common antagonists to the narcotics are made by substituting the allyl group ($-CH_2-CH=CH_2$) for the methyl group. The structure of pentazocine is shown in Table 26–4.

Pharmacologic Effects
A. Mechanism of Action: The antagonists exert narcotic actions by the same undefined mechanism as morphine and other drugs of this group—ie, they can produce analgesia and respiratory depression.

In addition, if any one of the narcotic analgesics, natural or synthetic, is acting, the antagonists will immediately terminate the effect. The relation is competitive, and the action is most commonly explained by the displacement of the agonist from the receptor.

B. Effects:

1. Morphine-like—By themselves, nalorphine and levallorphan produce all of the effects described above for the potent analgesics. With small doses, euphoria may be experienced, but misuse is not a problem because larger doses lead to subjectively unpleasant feelings or to a toxic psychosis. In the case of nalorphine and levallorphan, not even large doses cause the same degree of respiratory depression and analgesia as morphine. Pentazocine, however, can be used to produce anesthesia comparable to that following the use of morphine. Naloxone lacks any morphine-like action.

2. Narcotic antagonism—All of the depressant effects of the opiates are immediately reversed, but the stimulant effects (excitement, convulsions) are not modified. Not only are respiratory and other depressant effects antagonized, but, in a tolerant subject, the withdrawal state is promptly induced.

Clinical Uses
A. Treatment of Acute Poisoning Due to Narcotics: Acute poisoning of major or minor degree induced in the course of the therapeutic or other use of the narcotics can be dramatically treated with the narcotic antagonists. However, a beneficial effect appears only if the depression is due to a morphine-like drug—ie, the effect is specific and the narcotic antagonist would

only add to the respiratory depression such as that caused by a barbiturate or other depressant.

Nalorphine, 2.5–5 mg IV, can be given as an initial dose. No more than 10 mg IV should be given to ascertain the response. Nalorphine, 2.5–5 mg IV, can then be repeated every 2 hours if needed. Levallorphan, 1 mg IV, may be substituted for 5 mg of nalorphine.

An abstinence syndrome or withdrawal reaction can be precipitated in an addict intoxicated by an overdose. The necessary dose of the antagonist should be reached by increments even in the very depressed subject since the sudden precipitation of withdrawal symptoms by a large dose can be dangerous.

A special situation is the use of narcotic antagonists in the mother who has been given narcotics during delivery and the degree of her respiratory depression predicts a depressed infant. The *mother* should be given nalorphine 10–15 minutes before delivery. If the neonate shows dangerous respiratory depression due to narcotic administration to the mother, the antagonist can be given into the umbilical vein.

B. As a Nonaddicting Analgesic: Theoretically, a proper balancing of agonist-antagonist effects should result in a compound that is an effective analgesic at low doses but produces dysphoria with larger doses. The early antagonists could not be used as analgesics because the dysphoria and alterations of perception were common and intense.

Pentazocine (Talwin) is an analgesic of low or intermediate potency and also a very weak narcotic antagonist. Given to a heroin-dependent patient within 12–18 hours after the last dose of the narcotic, it may precipitate mild discomfort. Thereafter it will partially relieve the withdrawal state. Its continued use may lead to a mild withdrawal state when it is discontinued. Examples of misuse, especially by people with prior experience with narcotics, are now common.

During its therapeutic use, pentazocine may cause side-effects similar to those of other narcotic anal-gesics. It may also cause dizziness, distortion of visual perception, and hallucinations, especially if the dosage is rapidly increased. The use of pentazocine is not governed by the narcotic laws.

C. Detection of Narcotic Use: It was mentioned above that testing for narcotic use is often made a condition for parole or probation. Tests of excretion products in the urine offer advantages—notably, that other commonly used drugs can be detected. However, the "Nalline test" is still very popular among certain groups.

Under constant lighting conditions and with the patient fixing his vision on the same spot at each determination, the pupillary size is measured before and 20, 30, and 40 minutes after the subcutaneous injection of 3 mg of nalorphine or 1.5 mg of levallorphan. The pupil in the normal subject will constrict 0.5 mm or more. Pupillary dilatation of 0.5 mm or more is considered a positive response. Minor abstinence symptoms often occur.

Nalorphine can be used to precipitate the withdrawal state, but the indication for this is purely investigative. The test is uncomfortable and potentially hazardous to a dependent subject. To precipitate withdrawal, the 3 mg initial dose was followed in 20 minutes by 5 mg. The results are of interest when compared with ordinary withdrawal. Signs and symptoms of withdrawal appear in 5–15 minutes, reach a peak in 30–45 minutes, and last only a few hours but are very intense.

Preparations Available

> **Nalorphine (Nalline):** Adult preparation, 5 mg/ml, 1 and 2 ml ampules; neonatal preparation, 0.2 mg/ml, 1 ml ampules

> **Levallorphan (Lorfan):** 1 mg/ml, 1 and 10 ml

> **Naloxone (Narcan):** 0.4 mg/ml, 1 and 10 ml

● ● ●

General References

General

Reynolds, A.K., & L.O. Randall: *Morphine and Allied Drugs.* Univ of Toronto Press, 1957.

Vandam, L.D.: Clinical pharmacology of the narcotic analgesics. Clin Pharmacol Therap 3:827–838, 1962.

Way, E.L., & T.K. Adler: The pharmacologic implications of the fate of morphine and its surrogates. Pharmacol Rev 12:383–446, 1960.

Wikler, A.: Sites and mechanisms of action of morphine and related drugs in the central nervous system. Pharmacol Rev 2:435–506, 1950.

Clinical Effects & Evaluation

Beaver, W.T., & others: A comparison of the analgesic effects of pentazocine and morphine in patients with cancer. Clin Pharmacol Therap 7:740–751, 1966.

Beecher, H.K.: *Measurement of Subjective Responses. Quantitative Effects of Drugs.* Oxford Univ Press (New York), 1959.

Bellville, J.W., & J.C. Seed: A comparison of the respiratory depressant effects of dextropropoxyphene and codeine in man. Clin Pharmacol Therap 9:428–434, 1968.

Gary, N.E., & others: Acute propoxyphene hydrochloride intoxication. Arch Int Med 121:453–457, 1968.

Katz, K.H., & H.L. Chandler: Morphine hypersensitivity in kyphoscoliosis. New England J Med 238:322–324, 1948.

Keats, A.S., & J.C. Mithoefer: The mechanism of increased intracranial pressure induced by morphine. New England J Med 252:1110–1113, 1955.

Laidlaw, J., Read, A.E., & S. Sherlock: Morphine tolerance in hepatic cirrhosis. Gastroenterology 40:389–396, 1961.

Lasagna, L., & H.K. Beecher: The optimal dose of morphine. JAMA 156:230–234, 1954.

Lasagna, L.: The clinical evaluation of morphine and its substitutes as analgesics. Pharmacol Rev 16:47–83, 1964.

Miller, R.R., Feingold, A., & J. Paxinos: Propoxyphene hydrochloride: A critical review. JAMA 213:996–1006, 1970.

Mossberg, S.M., & others: Serum enzyme activities following morphine. A study of transaminase and alkaline phosphatase levels in normal persons and those with gallbladder disease. Arch Int Med 109:429–437, 1962.

Abuse (See Chapter 7.)

Antagonists

Foldes, F.F.: Human pharmacology and clinical use of narcotic antagonists. M Clin North America 48:421–443, 1964.

27 . . .

Antipyretic Analgesics

Aspirin and the other drugs of this class are usually designated antipyretic or nonnarcotic analgesics to separate them from the more potent narcotic analgesics. They relieve mild pain of diverse causes, including some of the most common complaints—tension headache, joint and muscle pain, the malaise of viral infections, etc. They lower an elevated body temperature and reduce the inflammation of rheumatoid arthritis and rheumatic fever.

Aspirin is by far the most important and most commonly used drug of the group. Other antipyretic analgesics offer an advantage over aspirin in a few situations, but most are far more toxic. Most are available without a prescription, and a large number of combinations and preparations are advertised.

In this chapter, the salicylates will be discussed in detail first. The other groups will be discussed in part by reference to the properties of the salicylates, and their distinctive toxicities will be described.

Classification of Antipyretic Analgesics

A. Salicylates: Aspirin and sodium salicylate.

B. Para-aminophenol Derivatives: Phenacetin and acetaminophen. These aniline derivatives are equivalent to the salicylates except that they are not uricosuric and are not quite as safe as the salicylates for chronic use; however, they cause less acute gastric irritation.

C. Pyrazolone Derivatives: Aminopyrine, phenylbutazone, etc. The use of the older drugs of this group has declined because of their serious allergic toxicity. The newer compounds in greater current use also have much greater acute and chronic toxicity than the salicylates.

D. Quinoline Derivatives: Quinine was the first antipyretic analgesic, but is no longer used as such. Neocinchophen is a quinoline used at one time for its uricosuric effect. Methopholine (Versidyne) is a recently developed isoquinoline derivative. It was withdrawn from the market because its use was associated with corneal opacities. This class will not be further discussed below.

E. Nonaddicting Opioids: Propoxyphene (Darvon) and ethoheptazine (Zactane) are often classed with the drugs discussed in this chapter. Chemically and pharmacologically, they are much more similar to the narcotics discussed in the previous chapter, and their limited usefulness has already been mentioned.

F. Other Organic Acids:

1. Indomethacin (Indocin) is discussed below, but its toxicity and limited efficacy suggest that it will never be widely used.

2. Mefenamic acid (Ponstel) is an antipyretic analgesic marketed with the conditions that it not be used for more than 1 week and that it not be used in children. The usual adult dose is 250 mg (1 capsule) every 6 hours for not more than 1 week. The drug is probably less effective than aspirin and is clearly more toxic. It will not be further discussed in this chapter.

3. Ibuprofen (Brufen) is comparable in effectiveness to aspirin but causes less gastric irritation. It is suggested for use when the patient must take an antirheumatic drug in the morning on an empty stomach. It is not marketed in the USA.

History

Cinchona bark and the quinine and quinidine therein are the oldest of the drugs known to lower an elevated body temperature and relieve mild pain. The same action is exhibited by willow bark, which was shown in 1829 to contain salicin, a glucoside of salicyl alcohol. Because quinine also has a specific effect on the fever of malaria and because of confusion in the taxonomy of fevers, these old folk remedies were actually of little importance in the development of that most essential of modern remedies, aspirin.

A German chemist, Kolbe, proposed in 1873 that salicylic acid be used to treat infections because it obviously would liberate free phenol and therefore prove bactericidal. At about the time that the initially favorable reports were being modified, a Swiss physician, Carl Buss, noted its antipyretic effect and retrospectively related it to willow bark. The antirheumatic effect was described soon after. The antirheumatic effect of pure salicin was independently reported at about the same time, but this discovery was not essential to the development of the salicylates.

A second class of antipyretics was defined when another German chemist (Knorr, 1883) attempted the synthesis of a part of the quinine molecule. He discovered the effect of **antipyrine**, and only later clarified the structure and realized that no relation to quinine existed.

Then, in 1886, 2 students of the internist Kussmaul gave a patient acetanilid from a bottle with a deteriorated label, thinking that it was the naphthalene that they had been told to test as a parasiticide. Fortunately, the patient had a fever and the beneficial effect was noted.

The last error suggested to the Bayer organization that they might dispose of a huge surplus of paraaminophenol by converting it to some analogue of acetanilid, and in this way ethoxyacetanilid or phenacetin was prepared. The same laboratory, looking for an alternative to sodium salicylate, restudied acetylsalicylic acid (acetyl Spirsäure; hence the name aspirin) and demonstrated the superiority of aspirin as an antipyretic in 1899.

Finally, in 1900, the analgesic effect of these agents ·was established. Both the mistakes and the advances in research have been minor since that time.

ASPIRIN & OTHER SALICYLATES

Aspirin is so widely and often so indiscriminately used that it lacks some of the magic of prescription drugs. (The equivalent of 113 million tablets per day was manufactured in the USA in 1967.) It is, nevertheless, the standard nonnarcotic analgesic, and the physician looking for a more potent drug or one less familiar to the patient should not abandon it too quickly.

Chemistry

Aspirin (acetylsalicylic acid, ASA) probably has a pharmacologic action of its own, but it is rapidly metabolized to salicylic acid (Fig 27–1). Salicylate may be given directly as sodium salicylate, but this preparation causes more gastric irritation and is less effective. The strongly acidic properties of aspirin and salicylic acid predict many of its properties.

Salicylamide, a weak and short-acting analgesic usually discussed with the salicylates, is not converted to salicylate but acts (feebly) as the amide and is rapidly excreted as such.

Salicylic acid used as such rather than as sodium salicylate should be thought of as a topical keratolytic agent and not as a systemic drug. Methyl salicylate (oil of wintergreen) should also be considered separately as a counterirritant or liniment; it is much more toxic when taken systemically than the familiar salicylates.

Absorption, Metabolism, & Excretion

The salicylates are absorbed rapidly and completely from the stomach and upper small intestine. Providing a more acid medium in the stomach should keep a larger fraction of the salicylate in the nonionized form and promote absorption. This is true, but the acid is also more irritating than the salt, and buffered or alkaline preparations are sometimes used. (See Preparations Available, below.)

Aspirin is absorbed as such and hydrolyzed to acetate and salicylate by esterases in tissues and blood. Measurable amounts of unconverted aspirin remain in the plasma 2 hours after administration of a labeled

dose, and this, plus the fact that there is only a poor correlation between plasma salicylate level and analgesic activity, suggests that aspirin has important actions in its original form.

Ingested salicylate or that generated by the hydrolysis of aspirin may be excreted as such, but most of it is converted to water-soluble conjugates that are rapidly cleared by the kidney (Fig 27–1). Alkalinization of the urine increases the rate of excretion of the free salicylate.

Pharmacologic Effects

A. Mechanisms of Action: The nonnarcotic or antipyretic analgesics (most of what is said about aspirin applies to the other classes also) have multiple pharmacologic effects and presumably also have multiple mechanisms of action. Suggested mechanisms of action will be mentioned under the description of each effect. The important action of aspirin in relieving pain and reducing inflammation is most probably due to an action at the site of origin of the pain, probably vasodilatation. The ultimate mechanism of action is unknown, but it may be related to its action as an antagonist to bradykinin, or an inhibitor of the synthesis of prostaglandins.

Any assumption that aspirin acts predominantly on the CNS is supported only by analogies drawn from the strong analgesics and other drugs that modify the perception of all sensation rather than pain alone.

B. Effects:

1. Analgesia–Pain of many different types is relieved. It may be muscular, vascular, inflammatory (whether traumatic or irritative in origin), tension or other headache pain, arthritis, bursitis, postpartum, incisional, postextraction, and a host of others, including the pain of malignancy. The point of the extended list is to emphasize that the intensity rather than the nature of the pain determines whether aspirin will be effective.

2. Antipyretic–Normal body temperature is only slightly affected, but fever is reduced. The fall in temperature is due to dilatation of superficial blood vessels with increased dissipation of heat rather than decreased heat production. The fall may be precipitous and accompanied by profuse sweating. The cooling due to evaporation of the perspiration is not essential to the action of these antipyretics, the effect persisting even if sweating is prevented by the administration of atropine. Aspirin also lowers experimentally elevated temperature in animals with hypothalamic lesions that abolish the sweating response to heat. The antipyretic effect thus may be peripheral in origin, although other experiments suggest that its action is on the CNS and consists of a "resetting" of a hypothalamic temperature control center. The antipyretic effect can be assayed and analyzed in animals following the production of fever by the injection of bacterial endotoxin or other pyrogen.

3. Anti-inflammatory–In* addition to relieving pain and lowering temperature, the mild analgesics in large doses also reduce inflammation in situations such

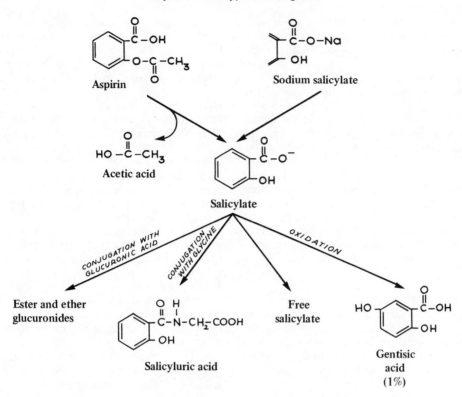

FIG 27–1. Structure and metabolism of the salicylates.

as rheumatoid arthritis or acute rheumatic fever. The injection of various foreign substances into animal tissues provides experimental inflammatory states for the study of inflammation and analysis of the effect of anti-inflammatory drugs. The anti-inflammatory action of the salicylates may be due to a vascular effect since other vasodilators—eg, beta-sympathomimetics—also reduce experimental inflammation.

4. CNS stimulation—

a. Respiration—In large amounts, the salicylates (but not the other drugs discussed in this chapter) markedly increase the rate and depth of respiration. The resulting respiratory alkalosis may be replaced by metabolic acidosis later in the period of intoxication.

b. Behavioral—Toxic doses may cause excitement, confusion, coma, convulsions, and, rarely, toxic psychosis.

c. Nausea and vomiting—Aspirin can have an irritant effect on the gastric mucosa, causing epigastric discomfort and sometimes nausea, but severe nausea and actual vomiting are usually due to CNS stimulation by the drug after absorption.

5. Metabolic and endocrine—

a. ACTH release—In animals, the adrenal cortex is stimulated by the administration of aspirin. The effect is blocked by a hypothalamic (median eminence) lesion as well as by hypophysectomy. The drug must then be acting through the hypothalamus to stimulate the liberation of ACTH. In humans, however, not even large doses of aspirin lead to evidence of adrenocortical

hyperfunction, and the anti-inflammatory action is not mediated by the corticosteroids.

b. Hypoprothrombinemia—The salicylates are weak inhibitors of prothrombin synthesis. The decrease in prothrombin concentration is not great enough to explain any bleeding episode associated with the administration of aspirin alone.

c. Platelet dysfunction—Aspirin does have an effect on hemostasis. Single doses of aspirin will produce a small prolongation of bleeding time, and a doubling if administration is continued for a week. The change is explained by the inhibitors of platelet aggregation or adhesion.

Hemostasis (and possibly arterial thrombosis) begins with the formation of a platelet plug at the site of vascular damage with subsequent deposition of fibrin through the processes described in Chapter 18. The release of adenosine diphosphate (ADP) from the platelets causes the aggregation of additional platelets following the initiation of clotting. The prior administration of aspirin partially blocks such release. There is also a failure of platelet aggregation by collagen and epinephrine in laboratory tests.

No relation has been established between platelet dysfunction and gastrointestinal bleeding; nor is the hazard of bleeding at surgery increased. The interest is not in possible toxicity but in the possibility that prolonged suppression of platelet aggregation might provide an antithrombotic technic superior to the use of inhibitors of prothrombin synthesis.

The effect of aspirin in this context is long-lasting and evidently more potent than the effect of the many other compounds that inhibit platelet aggregation—eg, clofibrate, pyrazolone analgesics, dipyridamole, tranquilizers, antidepressants, and others.

d. Other—Like other organic acids which use the same pathway, the salicylates may interfere with both the excretion and the reabsorption of uric acid by the renal tubules. The uricosuric effect of the salicylates appears only after large doses; smaller doses may have an opposite effect by interfering with uric acid secretion (excretion) by the tubule. The salicylates have been replaced as uricosuric agents by other more dependable drugs.

Glucose tolerance is slightly impaired, but ordinary doses can be used in diabetic patients without interference with the action of oral antidiabetic drugs or change in insulin requirement.

Clinical Uses

A. Pain: The antipyretic analgesics have a potency comparable in some kinds of pain to small doses of narcotics, and they should be tried in most cases where analgesia is necessary. In general, visceral cramping pain would not be expected to respond, but some types—eg, dysmenorrhea—may in fact respond to aspirin.

B. Fever: Obviously, antipyretic drugs should not replace specific therapy, but there is no reason they should not be used while the effect of the specific drug is developing or when no specific therapy is available—eg, in the case of influenza. Not only is temperature lowered, but malaise and muscular discomfort are reduced.

C. Specific Inflammatory States: These drugs are used in the treatment of rheumatoid arthritis and acute rheumatic fever. They may be given together with corticosteroids.

Adverse Reactions

A. Side-effects: The side-effects of aspirin are usually limited to epigastric discomfort, heartburn, or nausea. When larger doses must be employed, as in rheumatoid arthritis, or in a few of the most sensitive individuals, tinnitus or other symptoms of salicylism may appear.

1. Gastric irritation—One still controversial question is the importance of the irritative effect of these drugs on the stomach. The interest is a valid one but has been overemphasized by proponents of various buffered or soluble aspirin preparations.

Aspirin is a comparatively strong acid, having a carboxyl group with pKa 3.5—ie, in a solution with pH 3.5, half of the substance exists in the form of the free acid and half as the ionized salt form. Administration of aspirin in combination with an alkali would decrease the rate of absorption from the stomach by increasing the fraction of aspirin present as the charged, poorly absorbed salt (Fig 2–2). However, adequately buffered preparations reduce gastric irritation, and the brief delay in absorption is not important.

The gastric irritation manifested by epigastric pain and bleeding into the lumen of the stomach is thought, on the basis of experiments in dogs, to depend upon the presence of both aspirin and acid within the stomach. As the salicylates are absorbed, they damage the cells of the ordinarily impervious mucosal barrier. With the disruption of the junctions between mucosal cells, acid can act on the underlying tissues, and epithelial cells, red cells, plasma proteins, and ions enter the gastric contents. Administration of aspirin with an adequate amount of alkali can reduce the degree of such damage by neutralizing the acid present in the gastric contents and, by keeping the aspirin in the salt form, can delay absorption to a site beyond the vulnerable gastric mucosa. There are also observations suggesting that deposition of the insoluble acid form in comparatively large particles on the gastric mucosa intensifies the damage and that the deposition of smaller particles from soluble or buffered aspirin is less damaging.

The buffered preparations described below have been developed in an effort to circumvent the above mechanism. In evaluating the special preparations, it should be recalled that gastric irritation is only occasionally troublesome and that no one of the special preparations is superior to administering aspirin with a full glass of water. Presumably, the more rapid passage of the aspirin into the intestine and its greater dilution are responsible for the beneficial effect of the additional fluid.

2. Gastrointestinal bleeding—Not only do side-effects indicative of gastric irritation occur, but the amount of occult bleeding into the gastrointestinal tract is increased following the administration of aspirin. Blood loss is measured by labeling the red blood cells of the subject and measuring the radioactivity recovered in the feces following the administration of the drug. Normally, less than 1 ml of blood is lost in the stools each day. This figure is increased to perhaps 4 ml/day following the use of ordinary aspirin in the usual doses, but it may reach 10 ml or even 30 ml in an occasional patient. The importance of acid to the irritative effect of aspirin is called into question by the observation that patients with achlorhydria do show an increase in occult bleeding after aspirin, although less than that shown by control patients.

Aspirin does not increase acid secretion, but when it is given in isolated rather than continuous doses it does cause punctate areas of mucosal damage with exfoliation of gastric cells.

The effect of aspirin on the stomach would become extremely important if a correlation could be demonstrated between chronic administration of aspirin and anemia or an increased incidence of peptic ulcer or gastrointestinal bleeding. Only the last has been suggested, and that by retrospective studies difficult to interpret.

B. Overdosage Toxicity: Aspirin is the most common household drug, and its ingestion out of curiosity or imitativeness makes it the most common cause of poisoning in very young children. As a general rule, one may expect serious intoxication if the amount ingested exceeds 1 gr/lb or 150–175 mg/kg.

1. Salicylism–High-pitched tinnitus, vertigo, and deafness may occur at times with therapeutic doses as well as after toxic amounts. These effects are reversible.

2. Hyperthermia–In contrast to the effect of therapeutic doses, toxic doses–due to an uncharacterized CNS effect–will greatly elevate body temperature.

3. Behavioral–CNS stimulation is followed by depression. Agitation and confusion or even convulsions are followed by stupor and coma. Rarely, a toxic psychosis with paranoid and hallucinatory behavior will appear. Asterixis can be demonstrated as in hepatic failure.

4. Initial respiratory alkalosis due to respiratory stimulation.

5. Compensated respiratory alkalosis–If urine volume is maintained, renal excretion of bicarbonate, sodium, and potassium will increase, lowering plasma bicarbonate and returning pH to normal.

6. Respiratory and metabolic acidosis–If respiratory depression follows the initial respiratory stimulation, CO_2 retention will occur with a bicarbonate level already lowered by the previous compensation. Whether or not this respiratory acidosis develops, metabolic acidosis will appear. This acidosis is due in small part to the salicylic acid, to a larger extent to decreased renal function with retention of acid metabolites, and to the largest extent to the production of large amounts of organic acids (pyruvic, lactic, acetoacetic) due to an unexplained effect of salicylate on carbohydrate metabolism.

C. Treatment of Overdosage Toxicity: If the patient is seen soon enough and if the amount taken is unknown or if it is known to exceed the arbitrary guide of 1 gr/lb, gastric lavage should be performed.

Hyperthermia should be treated as vigorously as necessary with tepid water or alcohol sponges or with ice packs. Urine volume should be maintained at a high level (500 ml/hour). When urine volume or direct measurements establish that a compensated alkalosis or acidosis has developed, bicarbonate should be administered and the fluid should contain potassium ions. If the renal tubular urine is kept alkaline, the salicylate will exist in the salt (ionized) form and be less readily reabsorbed than the free acid–ie, excretion of salicylate will be hastened. If the usual treatment maintains a large volume of alkaline urine, dialysis or other radical treatment will rarely be needed. Acetazolamide (Diamox) may also be used to alkalinize the urine.

D. Allergic Reactions: Considering the large amounts involved and the varied patterns of salicylate use, it is amazing that allergic reactions are practically unheard of.

One situation often classed as allergic probably does not have an immunochemical basis and is better called analgesic-induced asthma syndrome. Young adults develop asthma preceded or accompanied by rhinitis or urticaria. Aspirin may precipitate a serious asthmatic state, but wheezing occurs even if the patient avoids aspirin. Furthermore, a number of other drugs, too varied to show cross-sensitivity, either precipitate asthma or reduce forced expiratory volume–eg, alcohol, indomethacin, amidopyrine, acetaminophen, mefenamic acid, and propoxyphene.

Contraindications & Cautions

Most aspirin is sold and used without a prescription, and the important caution should be directed to families with children: Aspirin–indeed, all medicines–should be kept out of reach of children. Colorful, flavored, and liquid preparations should be treated with special care. Aspirin should be given with great care to patients with a history of peptic ulcer.

TABLE 27–1. Antipyretic analgesics: Dosages and preparations available.

	Usual Oral Dose	**Preparations Available**
Aspirin	Adult: 0.3–1 gm Pediatric: 60 mg/kg/day in 4–6 doses	Tablets, 60, 120, 200, 250, 300, 500, and 600 mg Capsules, 300 mg Pediatric tablets, 75 mg (flavored) Enteric-coated tablets, 300 and 600 mg Buffered tablets, 300 mg Suppositories, 60, 120, 300, and 600 mg
Aspirin compound	1–2 tablets every 4–6 hours	Tablets containing aspirin, 220 mg, phenacetin, 150 mg, and caffeine, 30 mg
Sodium salicylate	0.3–1 gm every 4–6 hours	Tablets, 300, 500, and 600 mg Enteric-coated tablets, 300 mg
Salicylamide	Adult: 0.3–1 gm Pediatric: 60 mg/kg/day in 6 doses	Tablets, 220, 300, 500, and 600 mg Oral suspension (Liquiprin), 60 mg/ml
Phenacetin	300 mg every 4 hours	Tablets, 300 mg
Acetaminophen	Adult: 0.3–1 gm Pediatric: 60 mg/kg/day in 4–6 doses	Tablets, 325 mg Oral suspension, 325 mg/5 ml Oral syrup, 120 mg/5 ml Oral elixir, 120 mg/5 ml Pediatric drops, 60 mg/0.6 ml

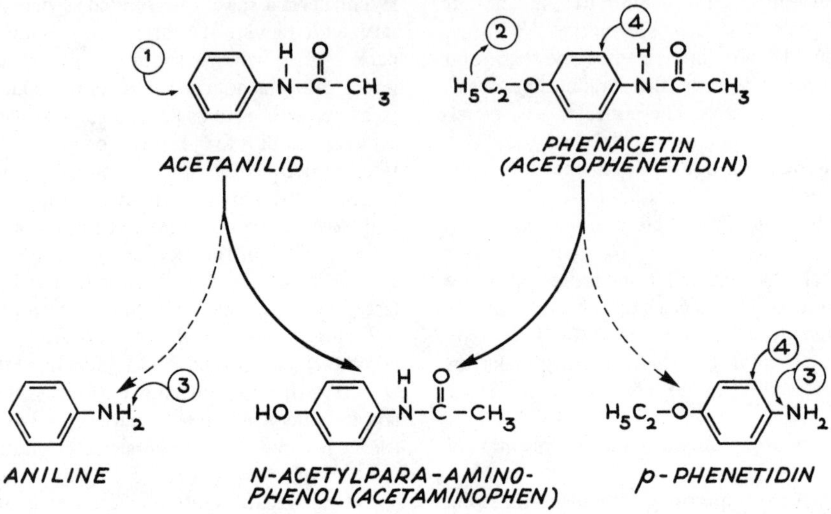

FIG 27–2. **Structure and metabolism of aminophenol analgesics.** Acetanilid is hydroxylated (1) and phenacetin deethylated (2) to the active metabolite, acetaminophen. Small amounts are hydrolyzed to aniline (3) and ethoxyaniline (3). Phenacetin may also be hydroxylated (4) to form 2-hydroxyphenacetin and 2-hydroxyphenetidin.

Dosage

The optimal analgesic or antipyretic dose of aspirin is less than the 0.6 gm commonly used. Larger doses may prolong the effect but will not increase its intensity. The usual dose may be repeated every 4 hours, and smaller doses (0.3 gm) every 3 hours.

The familiar rule that children should receive 1 gr per year of age is a safe and useful guide to pediatric dosage.

Preparations Available

A. Standard Aspirin Tablets: The official preparation of aspirin is available from many different manufacturers. These do not vary in the content of aspirin but may vary in the way in which the tablets are pressed and in the binder used. They may vary in their appearance and in the texture of the surface, but a disintegration test is part of the official standard and there is no evidence that differences among tablets are clinically significant.

B. Nominally Buffered Aspirin: The most popular buffered aspirins (Bufferin and others) do not contain enough alkali to modify the irritative process described above. Repeated studies have shown that blood levels, clinical effectiveness, and incidence of side-effects do not differ when this kind of buffered aspirin is compared with standard aspirin.

C. True Buffered Aspirin: The effervescent preparations of aspirin (Alka-Seltzer and others) contain enough alkali to solubilize the aspirin and to elevate the pH of the gastric contents. Since they are systemic antacids and since one contains bromides, they are not suitable for chronic administration.

An adequately buffered aspirin preparation or alkali separately administered in amounts sufficient to alkalinize the urine would increase renal excretion and give lower plasma levels and a lesser effect.

D. Aspirin Compound (APC): Aspirin compound is an official preparation of standard composition containing aspirin, phenacetin, and caffeine (Table 27–1).

Many popular proprietary combinations were originally similar to aspirin compound, but their composition changed following the recent recognition of the chronic toxicity of phenacetin. Since the composition of such products can be changed without changing the protected name, the label of each preparation should be consulted for its composition.

E. Enteric Coated and Sustained Release Preparations: In sensitive patients or when prolonged high dosage is required, gastric irritation can be reduced by coating the tablets with a substance that dissolves only after they have entered the small intestine. The properties of such coatings are variable, as is the rate of passage of the tablet through the stomach. With the possible exception of one preparation (Ecotrin), absorption of aspirin from enteric coated preparations appears to be incomplete.

Sustained release preparations of aspirin do not give the significant prolongation of effect claimed for them.

PHENACETIN & OTHER PARA-AMINOPHENOL DERIVATIVES

Chemistry & Metabolism

There are 2 analgesic drugs in this class: (1) Phenacetin (Fig 27–2) (acetophenetidin) is deethylated to form acetaminophen, which is actually the form of the drug responsible for the analgesic effect and those toxic effects other than methemoglobinemia. (2) Acetaminophen, the active metabolite, may be administered as such. The acetaminophen formed or ingested is conjugated and excreted in the urine. A third compound, acetanilid, is no longer used as an analgesic. It is not a phenol as administered, but is hydroxylated by the liver to acetaminophen.

Small amounts of acetanilid and phenacetin are converted to aniline and ethoxyaniline and can, therefore, cause methemoglobinemia. Acetanilid was more active in this regard.

Pharmacologic Effects

These drugs have the same analgesic and antipyretic effects as were described for aspirin. However, they are not anti-inflammatory or uricosuric, do not cause gastrointestinal tract irritation, and do not have the same effect on carbohydrate metabolism or respiration as aspirin.

Phenacetin has been said to cause drowsiness and slight euphoria after small doses in humans, and there is indirect evidence of a sedative effect in animals. The effect must be minor, but analgesics containing phenacetin have been compulsively misused by people who believe that they relieve anxiety.

Clinical Uses

A. Aspirin Equivalent: The usefulness of the aminophenol derivatives in acute rheumatic fever has not been established, and their use in chronic conditions such as rheumatoid arthritis would seem to be inadvisable because of the toxicity discussed below Phenacetin is generally used only in analgesic mixtures. As the toxicity of phenacetin is recognized, acetaminophen is used more and more by itself and in proprietary combinations. A liquid preparation is popular in pediatric practice. The effectiveness is neither greater nor less than that of aspirin, and they may be used when the gastric irritation of aspirin is a problem.

B. In Analgesic Mixtures: The most common of these mixtures is the official aspirin compound or APC tablets and equivalent proprietary mixtures. These contain aspirin, phenacetin, and caffeine. No advantage of these mixtures as analgesics has been definitely established. The effectiveness of the 2 analgesics is merely additive.

Adverse Reactions

Some of the following toxic reactions have been associated with the use of phenacetin but not acetaminophen. However, phenacetin is rapidly converted to acetaminophen and, as acetaminophen comes in to wide use, the same toxic effects can be anticipated.

A. Side-Effects: In contrast to aspirin, the side-effects of the usual doses are negligible.

B. Acute Overdosage Toxicity: The acute toxicity of phenacetin is less than that of aspirin, and it is less likely to be available for accidental or suicidal ingestion. When one of the mixtures is involved, the toxic effects of the salicylate usually predominate. Large doses of phenacetin may cause dizziness, excitement, and a toxic psychosis. Methemoglobinemia and acute hemolytic episodes can occur after phenacetin and even after huge single doses of acetaminophen. Acetaminophen has in addition a dose-related effect of causing hepatocellular damage, manifested as a change in laboratory measurements of liver function, as jaundice, or even, in a few cases, as fatal hepatic necrosis.

C. Toxicity Due to Chronic Use:

1. Methemoglobinemia and other pigmentation— Methemoglobinemia with a dusky skin color and signs of anemia may follow the chronic use of phenacetin in some susceptible individuals, possibly those with a reduced ability to transform phenacetin to acetaminophen. Larger amounts of 2-hydroxyphenacetin and 2-hydroxyphenetidin are then formed (Fig 27–2). Metabolites of the aniline derivatives cause methemoglobinemia. In addition, the skin may assume a gray appearance which is often said to be due to sulfhemoglobinemia; but the chemical evidence for this change is not conclusive, and some alternate explanation, perhaps one including pigments derived from the chronic hemolysis, is probable.

2. Hemolytic anemia—The aminophenols have a dose-related effect of decreasing erythrocyte survival time and may cause chronic hemolytic anemia. "Primaquine-sensitive" individuals whose erythrocytes are deficient in the enzyme glucose-6-phosphate dehydrogenase are unusually susceptible to hemolysis by phenacetin, but the hemolytic anemias also occur in patients with normal enzyme levels.

3. Interstitial nephritis and renal papillary necrosis—(Fig 27–3.) The recent epidemic of renal papillary necrosis associated with the habitual misuse of phenacetin is probably receding. The episode nevertheless demonstrates the difficulty of anticipating toxic effects of agents even when they have been in use for many years, and also emphasizes the caution which should attend the use of phenacetin.

Renal papillary necrosis was a rare disease until recently. Beginning in 1953, it began to appear in startling numbers and without the usual association with diabetes. The cases occurred in clusters and were associated with the habitual, prolonged use of phenacetin-containing mixtures. Factory workers in Europe were provided with the analgesic mixtures, which were taken in an effort to increase efficiency and reduce fatigue. In other countries, patients either learned or were encouraged by advertisement to take analgesics habitually for the relief of anxiety or, less commonly, to relieve headache or other minor pain.

The primary lesion is an interstitial nephritis in the inner medulla, where the local concentration of acetaminophen is greatest. The subsequent fibrotic changes in the medulla occlude the tubular vessels and compromise the blood supply to the renal papillae, which become necrotic and slough into the renal pelvis. Infection is not a necessary factor, although pyelonephritis commonly follows.

The diagnosis is suggested by the history and by renal insufficiency with loss of concentrating ability

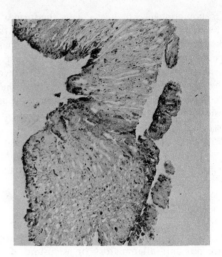

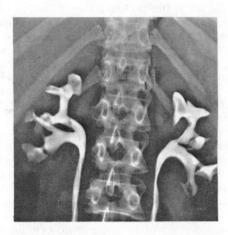

FIG 27–3. Renal papillary necrosis. *Left:* Retrograde urogram. Calyces appear enlarged because of absence of papillae. In the medial and lowest calyces on the left, the contrast medium is less dense ("negative" shadows) because of retained sloughed papillae. *Right:* Papilla passed in urine. (Reproduced, with permission, from Smith, D.R.: *General Urology,* 7th ed. Lange, 1972.)

but minor changes in urine sediment. Excretory urograms and renal biopsy can establish the diagnosis.

Phenacetin (but not aspirin) is the ingredient common to all of the mixtures that have caused serious toxicity. The compulsive self-administration of 6–8 APC's per day can cause lethal changes in 3–20 years. Larger daily doses shorten the latent period. The manufacturers of several of the proprietary mixtures responsible for many cases have now removed the phenacetin from their product. In the USA, phenacetin-containing drugs must now be labeled with a warning against chronic use.

It is difficult to argue a priori that acetaminophen should be less toxic than phenacetin. However, the anticipated nephrotoxicity has not yet appeared.

4. Carcinogenesis—In one population in which phenacetin (but not aspirin) has been misused for a long period, carcinomas of the renal pelvis have appeared in association with renal papillary necrosis. Other aminophenols can cause bladder cancer, and the presumption is that the phenacetin nephropathy makes the renal pelvis more susceptible.

PHENYLBUTAZONE & OTHER PYRAZOLONE DERIVATIVES

Analgesics of this class are longer-acting and prob-ably more potent for acute rheumatic disorders than

aspirin, but they are also more toxic. Antipyrine, the oldest and least toxic of the group, is the least used; the more toxic and more heavily advertised phenylbutazone is the most commonly used.

Chemistry

The pyrazolone derivatives are identified in Table 27–2. Aminopyrine and its sulfonate are more potent allergens than antipyrine. Phenylbutazone is hydroxylated in the body to oxyphenbutazone, and this metabolite is also available as a drug.

Antipyrine is slowly metabolized by hydroxylation at liver microsomes, with a half-life of about 8 hours. Phenylbutazone and oxyphenbutazone are even more slowly metabolized and are well reabsorbed by the renal tubules, resulting in a half-life in excess of 2 days.

Sulfinpyrazone (Anturane), the metabolite of a compound closely related to phenylbutazone, is a very useful uricosuric agent.

Pharmacologic Effects

The therapeutic effects are similar to those of aspirin—ie, these drugs are analgesic, antipyretic, and anti-inflammatory.

Clinical Uses & Dosages

The pyrazolone drugs exert an antipyretic effect in some situations in which aspirin is not completely effective—eg, Hodgkin's disease with fever unresponsive to salicylates or chemotherapy. They are probably

TABLE 27–2. Pyrazolone analgesics.

	R_1	R_2	R_3
Antipyrine	$-CH_3$	$-CH_3$	$-H$
Aminopyrine (amidopyrine)	$-CH_3$	$-CH_3$	$-N\begin{smallmatrix}CH_3\\CH_3\end{smallmatrix}$
Dipyrone (aminopyrinesulfonate, methampyrone)	$-CH_3$	$-CH_3$	$-N\begin{smallmatrix}CH_3\\CH_2-SO_3Na\end{smallmatrix}$
Phenylbutazone* (Butazolidin)	$-$phenyl	$-OH$	$-C_4H_9$
Oxyphenbutazone (Tandearil)*	$-p$-hydroxyphenyl	$-OH$	$-C_4H_9$
Sulfinpyrazone (Anturane)*†	$-$phenyl	$-OH$	$-C_2H_4-SO-$phenyl

*Note that tautomeric pairs exist.
†Uricosuric agent discussed in Chapter 40.

also more potent as analgesics and anti-inflammatory agents in arthritis, bursitis, and thrombophlebitis. There is no justification for the use of aminopyrine or dipyrone.

A. Antipyrine: Antipyrine can be used orally, 0.3–0.6 gm every 4–6 hours, as an alternative to aspirin. The volume of distribution of antipyrine or its metabolite, N-acetyl-4-aminoantipyrine, may also be used to measure total body water.

B. Phenylbutazone (Butazolidin) and Oxyphenbutazone (Tandearil): Butazolidin, Tandearil, and Butazolidin Alka are among the 200 drugs most commonly prescribed by physicians in the USA, suggesting that they are often used as first treatment drugs rather than as alternatives to aspirin. Yet the restrictions on their use and the contraindications and cautions made

a part of the labeling by the manufacturer are so stringent and comprehensive that responsibility for any adverse result of therapy would probably devolve on the physician. The drugs should not be used without reference to the package insert.

The use of these drugs is suggested or permitted in acute rheumatoid arthritis or spondylitis, osteoarthritis, psoriatic arthritis, "painful shoulder," acute superficial thrombophlebitis, and acute gouty arthritis.

The daily dose is stated to be 300–600 mg/day by the labeling. A more conservative position limits the daily dose to 200 mg. These drugs should be discontinued if no improvement is observed in 4–5 days.

Adverse Reactions

The toxicity of the pyrazolone analgesics restricts their use.

TABLE 27–3. Pyrazolone derivatives: Dosages and preparations available.

	Usual Adult Dose	Preparations Available
Aminopyrine*	300–600 mg/day	Bulk powder
Antipyrine	300–600 mg every 4 hours	Bulk powder
Dipyrone (Pyrilgin, Narone)*	325–650 mg every 4–6 hours	Tablets, 325, 500, and 650 mg Oral liquid, 500 mg/5 ml Pediatric liquid, 250 mg/ml Injection (IM), 500 mg, 2, 10, and 30 ml
Phenylbutazone (Butazolidin)	100 mg 3–4 times daily	Tablets, 100 mg Capsules (Butazolidin Alka), 100 mg, with antacids
Oxyphenbutazone (Tandearil)	100 mg 3–4 times daily	Tablets, 100 mg

*Not recommended for any use. See text.

A. Antipyrine: Antipyrine causes fewer side-effects than aspirin. Unlike aminopyrine, it has rarely been associated with agranulocytosis. It has caused an allergic erythematous rash, often about the mouth, that leaves pigmented areas when it resolves.

B. Agranulocytosis From Aminopyrine and Dipyrone: The unusually high risk of agranulocytosis following the use of these 2 analgesics is generally acknowledged. As is true for many therapeutic agents, the quantification of the risk is difficult, and the drugs continue to be used in some countries. Neither of the drugs was used recently in the USA until dipyrone reappeared during the period 1960–1964. Imports of dipyrone rose from none in 1958 to 19,000 lb in 1962. During the period 1960–1964, 18 cases of agranulocytosis associated with the use of dipyrone, 1/3 of them fatal, were reported to the AMA registry. How complete this reporting was cannot be established. The dipyrone was probably not recognized by the physician as a derivative of aminopyrine, emphasizing the need to think of drugs in terms of general classes rather than individual compounds. The use of drugs under their trade names and the prescribing of proprietary mixtures without first identifying the ingredients undoubtedly also led to the misuse.

In the USA, any preparation or mixture containing aminopyrine or dipyrone must now bear a label warning that the drug may cause agranulocytosis and that it should be used only when specifically indicated and when less toxic drugs—eg, salicylates—have proved ineffective or are not tolerated.

The characteristics of agranulocytosis are discussed in Chapter 6. The reaction is allergic in origin rather than dose-related and is due to the sudden peripheral destruction of granulocytes.

C. Phenylbutazone: Phenylbutazone and its metabolite, oxyphenbutazone, frequently cause side-effects, and serious toxic reactions are frequent enough that their use should be greatly restricted. Dose-related toxic effects include sodium retention and edema, dry mouth, nausea and vomiting, peptic ulceration and hemorrhage, and rare cases of renal tubular necrosis and liver necrosis. Allergic reactions include dermatitis, which may rarely progress to exfoliative dermatitis, and agranulocytosis.

Phenylbutazone may cause a reversible leukemoid reaction; of greater concern, however, is the possibility (not yet well established) that its chronic use may be associated with a high incidence of acute leukemia.

Administration of phenylbutazone increases the effects of tolbutamide and warfarin.

INDOMETHACIN
(Indocin)

Indomethacin is not related chemically to the above analgesics except that, like the salicylates, it is an acid.

Indomethacin (Indocin)

Indomethacin has analgesic, antipyretic, and anti-inflammatory actions and is closely comparable to phenylbutazone.

Clinical Uses

Indomethacin, like phenylbutazone, is not suggested for general use as a simple analgesic but for use only in a few special situations and after safer drugs have not given a desired effect. The doubtful justification for using it in these special situations is that indomethacin causes fewer serious toxic reactions than phenylbutazone, although the total number of all adverse reactions may be larger.

The special situations are acute gouty arthritis, rheumatoid (ankylosing) spondylitis, and osteoarthritis of the hip.

Indomethacin is also used in rheumatoid arthritis, but it is no more effective than aspirin and certainly causes more toxic reactions and side-effects. Some of the earlier studies that claimed to establish its usefulness are unacceptable or used doses that led to a prohibitive number of side-effects and toxic reactions. Recent well controlled studies that have also made an effort to make objective evaluations of the response of arthritis show no difference between drug and placebo groups. One influential study compared drug and placebo treated groups but allowed patients to take aspirin as they desired, which is what most patients with arthritis do when given other treatment. There was no difference between the groups in the amount of aspirin needed. Indomethacin, therefore, does not supplement the effect of aspirin and is probably without value in most patients.

Adverse Reactions

Indomethacin also causes frequent adverse reactions. Morning headache or migrainous daytime headaches (20%), vertigo, confusion, depression, or somnolence are common, although they may decrease with continued use or dose reduction. Nausea, blurred vision indicative of retinal damage, epigastric pain, diarrhea, activation of peptic ulcers, bleeding from any level of the gastrointestinal tract, and other reactions almost too numerous to list have been reported.

Dosage & Preparations

Indomethacin is for adult use only, at least 3 sudden deaths having occurred in children. The usual dose is 25–50 mg 3 times daily.

Indomethacin (Indocin) is available in capsules containing 25 and 50 mg. It should be taken with food or immediately after a meal.

● ● ●

General References

Salicylates

Clark, R.L., & L. Lasagna: How reliable are enteric-coated aspirin preparations? Clin Pharmacol Therap 5:568–574, 1965.

Croft, D.N., & P.H.N. Wood: Gastric mucosa and susceptibility to occult gastrointestinal bleeding caused by aspirin. Brit MJ 1:137–141, 1967.

Davenport, H.W.: Salicylate damage to the gastric mucosal barrier. New England J Med 276:1307–1312, 1967.

De Kornfeld, T.J., Lasagna, L., & T.M. Frazier: A comparative study of five proprietary analgesic compounds. JAMA 182:1315–1318, 1962.

Done, A.K.: The nature of the antirheumatic action of salicylates. Clin Pharmacol Therap 1:141–148, 1960.

Done, A.K.: Salicylate poisoning. JAMA 192:770–772, 1965.

Hollister, L.E., & S.L. Kanter: Studies of delayed-action medication. IV. Salicylates. Clin Pharmacol Therap 6:5–11, 1965.

Moser, R.H.: Bibliographies on diseases of medical progress: Salicylates. Clin Pharmacol Therap 8:333–345, 1967.

Sahud, M.A., & P.M. Aggeler: Platelet dysfunction: Differentiation of a newly recognized primary type from that produced by aspirin. New England J Med 280:453–459, 1969.

Smith, M.J.H., & P.K. Smith: *The Salicylates: A Critical Bibliographic Review.* Wiley, 1966.

Smith, P.K.: The pharmacology of salicylates and related compounds. Ann New York Acad Sc 86:38–63, 1960.

Phenacetin & Acetaminophen

Burry, A.F., De Jersey, P., & D. Weedon: Phenacetin and renal papillary necrosis: Results of a prospective autopsy investigation. MJ Australia 1:873–879, 1966.

Harrow, B.R., Sloane, J.A., & N.C. Liebman: Renal papillary necrosis and analgesics. JAMA 184:445–452, 1963.

Jacobs, L.A., & J.G. Morris: Renal papillary necrosis and the abuse of phenacetin. MJ Australia 2:531–538, 1962.

Koutsaimanis, K.G., & H.E. de Wardener: Phenacetin nephropathy, with particular reference to the effect of surgery. Brit MJ 4:131–134, 1970.

Phenacetin and bladder cancer. Leading article. Brit MJ 4:701–702, 1969.

Proudfoot, A.T., & N. Wright: Acute paracetamol poisoning. Brit MJ 3:557–558, 1970.

Reynolds, T.G., & H.A. Edmondson: Chronic renal disease and heavy use of analgesics. JAMA 184:435–444, 1963.

Ross, J.D., & R.F. Ciccarelli: Acquired methemoglobinemia due to ingestion of acetophenetidin. New England J Med 266:1202–1204, 1962.

Others

American Rheumatism Association, Cooperating Clinics Committee: A three-month trial of indomethacin in rheumatoid arthritis, with special reference to analysis and inference. Clin Pharmacol Therap 8:11–37, 1967.

Bruck, E., & others: Phenylbutazone [Butazolidin] therapy: Relation between toxic and therapeutic effects and blood level. Lancet 1:225–228, 1954.

Donnelly, P., Lloyd, K., & H. Campbell: Indomethacin in rheumatoid arthritis: An evaluation of its anti-inflammatory and side effects. Brit MJ 1:69–75, 1967.

Huguley, C.M., Jr.: Agranulocytosis induced by dipyrone, a hazardous antipyretic and analgesic. JAMA 189:938–941, 1964.

Leavesley, G.M., & others: Phenylbutazone and leukemia. MJ Australia 2:963–965, 1969.

28 . . .

CNS Stimulants & Antidepressants

The CNS stimulants and antidepressants and the therapeutic problems related to these drugs are discussed together for reasons of practicality and common usage. Any confusion generated by the grouping of several diverse classes of drugs can be minimized by emphasizing 2 preliminary ideas. First, the drugs considered here as CNS stimulants may have other important pharmacologic effects and may have been discussed in part in other chapters. Second—and this is the major source of confusion—one drug group is included because it is widely used in the treatment of major depressions but is actually not distinct from the group of antipsychotic tranquilizers already discussed.

In this chapter, therefore, the pharmacology and use of each class of CNS stimulants or antidepressants will be reviewed or introduced. The treatment of depression is discussed as an application of the antidepressants that resemble tranquilizers.

Types of CNS Stimulants & Antidepressants

A. Antidepressants That Resemble Tranquilizers: Drugs of the amitriptyline (Elavil) or imipramine (Tofranil) type are widely used antidepressants. However, their properties are similar to those of the antipsychotic tranquilizers.

B. Sympathomimetic Amines: Amphetamine and related drugs are sympathomimetics comparable to ephedrine, and their autonomic effects are discussed in Chapter 10.

C. Monoamine Oxidase (MAO) Inhibitors: The monoamine oxidase inhibitors are no longer widely used in the treatment of depression, but great interest in their mechanism of action remains. They have CNS stimulant properties which are qualitatively similar to amphetamine and also sympathomimetic and sympathoplegic effects.

D. Miscellaneous Convulsant Stimulants: These drugs, exemplified by pentylenetetrazol (Metrazol), are often called medullary stimulants but their action culminates in convulsions. It is doubtful whether any indication for their use remains.

E. Xanthines: Caffeine, aminophylline, and other xanthines are discussed in Chapter 13. The xanthines contained in beverages such as coffee or tea have a minor stimulant effect which is manifested as relief of fatigue or as wakefulness. The CNS stimulant effect of the xanthines cannot be increased to a therapeutically useful degree because of the appearance of cardiovascular side-effects. The specific effect of amino-phylline in abolishing Cheyne-Stokes respiration is due to its content of ethylenediamine.

ANTIDEPRESSANT DRUGS RESEMBLING TRANQUILIZERS

The drugs shown in Table 28–1 are commonly labeled "antidepressants" in both the professional literature and in advertisements, with the result that the pharmacology of these drugs appears confusing. They are efficacious in the treatment of depression and have provided treatment more acceptable to the patient than electroconvulsive therapy (ECT). However, they do not differ from the antipsychotic tranquilizers except that the dosage is not increased to the high levels used in the treatment of schizophrenic episodes.

When the antipsychotic tranquilizers were first evaluated, a few investigators reported a beneficial effect on patients with severe depressions—especially early in treatment, before the dosage had reached high levels. However, the use of the phenothiazines in depressed patients was generally held to be contraindicated. Imipramine, a compound synthesized as a possible analogue of the phenothiazine tranquilizers, was reported in 1958 to be effective in treating endogenous depressions. For a few years, imipramine and related compounds were generally described as a drug class distinct from the tranquilizers. Pharmacologically there was no basis for this distinction, and a few clinicians soon began to substitute mixtures of a phenothiazine tranquilizer and imipramine in treating depressions. Many antipsychotic tranquilizers have now been shown not only to be effective in certain types of depression but even preferable to the newer antidepressants. Discussion of these drugs can, therefore, be shortened by reference to the properties of the antipsychotic tranquilizers already discussed.

Chemistry

The drugs in this category are shown in Table 28–1. Imipramine and amitriptyline differ from the tranquilizers promazine (Sparine) and chlorprothixene (Taractan) in that a bridge of 2 methylene groups has been substituted for the sulfur of the older drugs and the chlorine present in chlorprothixene is not present in amitriptyline.

TABLE 28–1. Antidepressants: Formulas, dosages, and preparations available.

	R	Usual Starting Dose	Maximum Daily Dose	Preparations Available
	Imipramine (Tofranil)			
	—CH_3	25 mg 3 times daily	200 mg	Tablets, 10 and 25 mg Injectable (IM), 25 mg/2 ml
	Desipramine (Pertofrane, Norpramin)			
	—H	25 mg 3 times daily	200 mg	Capsules, 25 mg Tablets, 25 mg
	Amitriptyline (Elavil)			
	—CH_3	25 mg 3 times daily	150 mg	Tablets, 10 and 25 mg Injectable (IM), 10 mg/ml, 10 ml
	Nortriptyline (Aventyl)			
	—H	10 mg 3 times daily	100 mg	Capsules, 10 and 25 mg Solution, 10 mg/ 5 ml
	Doxepin (Sinequan) (oxygen at site shown by arrow)			
	—CH_3	25 mg 3 times daily	300 mg	Capsules, 10, 25, and 50 mg
	Protriptyline (Vivactil)			
		5–10 mg 3 times daily	60 mg	Tablets, 5 and 10 mg

When it became apparent that the antidepressants had properties similar to those of the tranquilizers, it was claimed that the demethylated metabolites were active as stimulants and that this explained the difference from the phenothiazines. The active metabolites are now available and are used, but there are no differences in effects between the parent compounds and the metabolite.

These drugs are also called imidodibenzyl, dibenzazepine, and tricyclic antidepressants. The phenothiazine tranquilizers are, or course, also tricyclic compounds.

Absorption, Metabolism, & Excretion

The pharmacokinetics of these antidepressants is similar to those described for the major tranquilizers, ie, plasma levels rise slowly after oral administration and the chemical half-life is more than 12 hours after the administration of single doses. There is a lag of several hours between ingestion and the appearance of pharmacologic effects; this must not be confused with a latent period of as long as 3 weeks before a therapeutic effect on the depressed patient develops.

The drugs are well absorbed. Demethylation of the dimethyl compounds does occur and the metabolites are active, but no new properties are conferred by the change, nor does their beneficial effect appear any sooner when the demethylated derivatives are used.

Pharmacologic Effects

The section on the pharmacologic effects of the tranquilizers in Chapter 25 can be applied without modification to the antidepressants. The differences in the relative prominence of each action are suggested below in the discussion of adverse effects.

The ability of imipramine and its relatives to prevent the uptake of norepinephrine by sympathetic nerves is currently being emphasized as a possible explanation for its mechanism of action. This action has also been demonstrated for chlorpromazine and is not distinctive for the antidepressants.

Treatment of Depressive Reactions

A. Problems in Evaluation of Therapy: The usual factors that require a controlled evaluation operate prominently during the drug treatment of depressions. The major depressions are variable in their course and are often rapidly self-limiting, so that almost any treatment may appear to be effective if it is started early. In addition, the inadequate diagnostic differentiation of depressions can result in confusion if different investigators are reporting results from different groups of depressed patients who are in fact not really comparable. One cannot assume that all depressions—reactive (situational), neurotic, involutional, or psychotic—respond similarly to drugs. Experience with severely ill, institutionalized populations is not interchangeable with experience in office practice, in which much of the depression that is seen is symptomatic of anxiety.

B. Alternative Treatments:

1. Amphetamine—Amphetamine and related sympathomimetic amines are generally said to be useful antidepressants only if the depression is mild, but there is little evidence for or against that conclusion. Tranylcypromine (Parnate), which is similar to amphetamine, is still used. Part of the resistance to the use of amphetamine is based on a fear that its therapeutic use will lead to unsupervised abuse. The danger is certainly present but must be small when the drug is taken by mouth.

2. Sedatives—The older sedatives (eg, phenobarbital) have long been used in the treatment of patients whose manifest depression is symptomatic of anxiety rather than of an endogenous depression. Recently, chlordiazepoxide (Librium), another long-acting sedative, has gained a reputation as an antidepressant. The sedatives are effective in relieving anxiety, but their use should not be extended to all categories of depression.

3. Antidepressants related to tranquilizers—The usefulness of the antidepressants as an alternative to electroconvulsive therapy (ECT) in the treatment of severe endogenous depressions in hospitalized patients is established by controlled studies. ECT is effective, and results are quickly apparent, but it is usually done only during hospitalization and is an unpleasant experience. Drugs are a less rapid means of combating depression but have the advantages that continued or maintenance treatment is possible, that they are less expensive, and that they evoke fewer objections from patients. Drug and ECT treatments can be combined.

A more precise statement of the results in the treatment of depression is difficult to formulate. Serious depressions are often episodic and self-limiting,

regardless of treatment. Assignment of depressed patients to diagnostic categories is difficult, and the use of drugs has not improved the criteria by differentiating subtypes more or less apt to respond favorably to different drugs. Because of variations in diagnostic criteria, control groups are essential for every new evaluation. The criteria of improvement also vary—eg, duration of hospitalization, a test score, or a subjective estimate of the degree of depression.

Antipsychotic tranquilizers from each of the subclasses defined in Chapter 25—chlorpromazine, perphenazine, thioridazine, and thiothixene—have been shown to be as good as or better than imipramine in the treatment of some groups of depressed patients.

4. MAO inhibitors—These drugs, discussed below, are of limited therapeutic importance.

Adverse Reactions

A. Side-Effects: Side-effects are similar to those seen after the administration of the tranquilizers. After the usual doses, atropine-like effects and postural hypotension are relatively prominent.

1. Behavioral—The distinctive kind of sedation that occurs after the administration of tranquilizers also appears after imipramine and similar antidepressants. The patient may complain of weakness, drowsiness, or additional depression of mood. Increased tension, tremulousness, visual hallucinations, and agitation are sometimes induced.

2. Autonomic—Dry mouth and constipation are common atropine-like effects; blurred vision and tachycardia are uncommon. Postural hypotension occurs frequently, and is the side-effect that most commonly limits the comfortable dose of these drugs.

3. Other—Extrapyramidal signs are rare with the doses usually employed. Weight gain, an unpleasant taste, edema, and prolonged atrioventricular conduction time occur.

B. Overdosage Toxicity: The acute toxicity of the antidepressants appears to be greater than that of the phenothiazines in that accidental deaths and successful suicides have been reported. The greater apparent toxicity arises in part at least from placing large amounts of the antidepressants in the hands of patients in whom the risk of a suicidal attempt is very great.

C. Allergic Reactions: Isolated reports of bone marrow depression and cholestatic jaundice have appeared.

D. Drug Interaction: The effects of alcohol and other depressants are additive to the sedation caused by these "antidepressants." It is generally recommended that up to 14 days elapse between the administration of an MAO inhibitor and the initiation of treatment with these drugs to avoid episodes of hypertension or excitement with convulsions. Even so, drugs of the 2 classes have often been given together without difficulty.

Preparations & Dosages

Treatment with each of the drugs is started at a low dosage level (Table 28–1). The dosage is increased at intervals of several days until a response occurs or the maximum daily dose is reached. Most patients will improve within 3 weeks of starting therapy if they are going to improve at all. The usual maximum daily dose may be exceeded in hospitalized patients. Aged patients are usually more sensitive to these drugs.

When a favorable response is achieved, the dose is slowly decreased to a maintenance level at or below the usual starting dosage. Treatment is continued for at least 3 months and the drug is gradually withdrawn.

AMPHETAMINE & RELATED SYMPATHOMIMETIC STIMULANTS

The drugs in this category are variants of the ephedrine class of sympathomimetics selected because they exhibit relatively more potent central stimulant effects and relatively less potent cardiovascular effects.

Chemistry

The structures of the sympathomimetic stimulants are shown in Table 28–2 to suggest that, like the other indirect-acting sympathomimetics, they are

TABLE 28–2. Formulas of amphetamine and related anorexigenic and stimulant amines.

	R_1	R_2	R_3	R_4
Amphetamine				
Methamphetamine			$-CH_3$	
Phentermine (Wilpo; Ionamin, a complex with a resin)		$-CH_3$		
Chlorphentermine (Pre-Sate)	$Cl-$	$-CH_3$		
Benzphetamine (Didrex)			$-CH_3$	$-CH_2-$
Phenmetrazine (Preludin)				
Phendimetrazine (Plegine)				
Diethylpropion (Tenuate, Tepanil)				
Methylphenidate (Ritalin)				
Tranylcypromine (Parnate)				

phenylisopropylamines or are isosteric with phenyl-isopropylamine.

Pharmacologic Actions

A. Mechanism of Action: As has been explained in the case of ephedrine, the amphetamines do not act directly on the effectors to bring about their peripheral sympathomimetic effects such as tachycardia or elevated blood pressure. They act indirectly through the catecholamines of the organism in part by liberating the amines and in part by a second undefined mechanism which allows their action to persist after depletion of norepinephrine with reserpine.

That the CNS stimulating effects are also mediated through catecholamines is suggested by the ability of a-methyl-p-tyrosine to block the central effects of amphetamine in animals and in man. This amino acid is an inhibitor of tyrosine hydroxylase and is assumed to deplete the brain of some specific pool of either dopamine or norepinephrine that is necessary for the action of amphetamine.

B. Effects: Refer to the discussion in Chapter 10. The duration of action of amphetamine and methamphetamine is much longer than that of ephedrine, the central effects persisting for more than 12–24 hours.

Clinical Uses

A. Obesity: The great interest in the anorexigenic effect of the sympathomimetics is based on more than the vanity of the patient; obesity increases susceptibility to a number of diseases, and life expectancy is reduced by even a minor increase in weight above an ideal weight based on insurance statistics.

The ability of ephedrine, amphetamine, and the other phenylisopropylamines to decrease appetite parallels their potency as CNS stimulants. An intense anorexigenic action can be demonstrated on animals in the laboratory, and a specific CNS effect is therefore assumed to be important rather than a change in mood, distraction, or increased activity. The amphetamines act in mentally deficient as well as normal humans.

When any of the drugs related to amphetamine is tested in obese patients under controlled conditions and is given in adequate dosage, it exerts an anorexigenic effect that is clearly beyond that of the placebo. However, after a few weeks (6–8 weeks maximum), the weight loss ceases and the patient usually resumes his previous eating and gaining habits unless other forms of treatment have been more successful. All of the controlled studies utilize a fixed dosage throughout the period of study since a progressive increase in dosage to overcome whatever process is leading to tolerance would presumably add the risk of drug misuse or habituation. Periods of treatment with amphetamines for 2 weeks alternating with equal periods without treatment are as effective as continuous treatment.

B. As Euphoriant and Antidepressant: Controlled tests show that amphetamines produce euphoria more consistently in normal humans than either morphine or

pentobarbital. This action partly explains the misuse of the amphetamines and their use in mild (usually situational or reactive) depressions. Since the amphetamines are only transiently effective in treating obesity in careful trials and probably even less effective in general use, it must be concluded that most of the 5 billion doses of diet pills made in the USA each year are actually used as euphoriants.

C. To Improve Performance: Amphetamine and its congeners are used, perhaps ill-advisedly but nevertheless effectively, to improve psychomotor performance. The deterioration of performance with fatigue can be in part prevented or reversed and a state of wakefulness maintained. This generalization applies to comparatively simple psychomotor tests; concentration in complex learning situations and judgment are not necessarily improved.

Without suggesting that the practice is anything but pernicious, it must be acknowledged that the administration of amphetamine 90 minutes before a test situation improves athletic performance (swimming, running, weight throwing) to a degree that would be highly significant in competition.

D. In Treatment of Drug Depression: The amphetamines are no longer used in the treatment of barbiturate intoxication. They are often given to patients receiving antipsychotic tranquilizers or anticonvulsant medication to minimize sedation.

E. Hyperkinetic State in Children: This syndrome was originally defined in terms of minimal brain **damage.** There has recently been a shift to brain **dysfunction,** and the syndrome is now often defined by the complaints of the parent or teacher rather than by examination of the child–ie, hyperactivity, aggressiveness, perseveration, poor performance in school. Evaluation of the results of treatment is difficult, but in controlled studies amphetamine (or methylphenidate) does appear to reduce the behavior that is impeding development in some groups. This does not appear to justify the wide extension of the treatment to less than rigorously selected groups of troublesome children in large classes. Adult doses are given each morning (or morning and noon) without causing stimulation (excitement, wakefulness, etc) until the patient reaches his early teens.

F. Convulsant States: In specific situations (often in petit mal), amphetamines are used in the management of convulsive states. (See Chapter 29.)

G. Narcolepsy: Narcolepsy is a rare condition characterized by lapses into normal sleep during periods of monotony or inactivity such as working at repetitive jobs or driving. Amphetamine prevents these lapses. A single morning dose of 10–15 mg may be adequate, or larger doses several times a day may be necessary. Cataplexy–ie, sudden loss of muscle tone without loss of consciousness at the time of an emotional expression–is often associated with narcolepsy but is not altered by treatment with amphetamine.

Adverse Reactions

This discussion applies to all of the amphetamine congeners as well as to ephedrine and related drugs.

Because some of the drugs are given only in small doses or have not become widely used, all of the reactions listed below may not yet actually have been encountered in practice.

A. Side-Effects: Common side-effects may include tremulousness, anxiety, awareness of heart action, dry mouth, and alteration of sleep habits such as insomnia or light sleep. The side-effects are usually not troublesome after a few days of continued use, but some patients are unable to tolerate the stimulation of any amphetamine.

B. Toxicity Due to Overdosage:

1. Acute toxicity—The acute toxicity of the amphetamines is low. Reported fatalities are due to a complicating coexistent disease or to the result of treatment. The lethal dose of dextroamphetamine is probably several grams. Restlessness or toxic psychosis, hypertension, and tachycardia may be prominent. Treatment consists of sedation. Maintaining a high volume of acid urine should increase the rate of excretion of the drug. In acid urine this weak base is converted to the salt form, and renal tubular reabsorption of the charged form is less and urinary excretion greater. Fig 28–1 shows such an effect. The value of acidifying the urine in acute intoxication has not actually been demonstrated. It is possible that the metabolic path is merely shifted from urinary excretion to chemical change.

2. Chronic toxicity—Continued use of large doses of amphetamines may lead to long periods of wakeful-

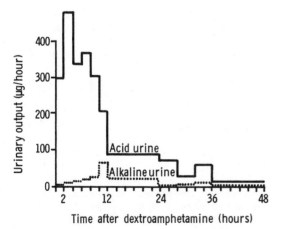

FIG 28–1. **Mean excretion of amphetamine by 3 normal subjects after ingestion of 10 mg of dextroamphetamine sulfate.** pH range of acid urine, 4.5–5.6; pH range of alkaline urine, 7.1–8.0. In an acid urine, amphetamine exists in the salt (charged) form and renal tubular reabsorption is decreased, ie, excretion is facilitated. The urine was acidified by the ingestion of ammonium chloride. (Reproduced, with permission, from Asatoor & others: The excretion of dexamphetamine and its derivatives. Brit J Pharmacol 24:295, 1965.)

ness and weight loss. Various depressants (especially barbiturates, marihuana, heroin, and alcohol) are often used by chronic amphetamine users to "turn off" the effect.

3. Toxic psychosis—Behavior is not usually greatly altered by chronic oral use of these stimulants. The subject complains of depression if he is deprived of the drug but does not acknowledge any euphoria when it is supplied. In large and repeated doses—especially intravenously—the drug becomes a psychotomimetic agent. Intense anxiety, restlessness, feelings of depersonalization, and altered perception may progress to a state similar to paranoid schizophrenia. As in other toxic psychoses, auditory and visual hallucinations are prominent, but the patient usually continues to recognize the relation between his altered perception and the drug. If paranoia or delirium is prominent, a small dose of chlorpromazine or other antipsychotic tranquilizer may be useful, but sedation with a barbiturate is usually adequate treatment.

C. Misuse and Abuse: The amphetamines, like other drugs with a potential for misuse, are abused by different individuals to different degrees, and the several patterns may vary in their hazards from minimal, as in the occasional use of a diet pill, to a totally destructive pattern, as is the case when large amounts are injected intravenously.

Cocaine is the prototype of a major CNS stimulant liable to be abused, and the history of its use parallels the recent history of methamphetamine use.

1. History of cocaine usage—When the Spanish conquistadors reached the Andean highlands, they observed the use by some of the residents of leaves from the coca plant (*Erythroxylon coca*). Leaves from the small tree or shrub were chewed, together with some alkali (lime or ashes) that liberated the free base for rapid absorption across the mucosa. At that time, coca leaves were used as a ritual drug only by the elite Incas and not by the administrators and peasants of the Inca nation. The Spaniards destroyed the structure of the society, diffused the use of coca leaves widely and encouraged their compulsive use. The enslaved people were then able to work continuously for more than a day without food or sleep even at high altitudes. Within 50 years, the population of the Inca nation was reduced from 10 million to less than 1 million.

Leaves of the Peruvian plant reached Göttingen and the laboratory of Wöhler, the first chemist to synthesize an organic compound. His student, Nieman, isolated cocaine in 1860 and noted the anesthetic effect on his tongue.

After the American Civil War, cocaine was described by some American physicians as a specific treatment for morphine addiction. Sigmund Freud was among those who used and recommended to others the use of cocaine as a euphoriant. Thus, when a colleague who had become addicted to morphine because of the pain of neuromas in an amputation stump consulted Freud, continuous use of cocaine (and cocaine addiction) was substituted for continuous use of morphine. Breuer interested Koller in the drug, and this led to application of the local anesthetic effect.

Cocaine is still misused today by the South American Indians and to a limited extent by drug "users" elsewhere, who take cocaine either as snuff or by injection—alone or in combination with heroin.

Following the isolation of ephedrine, Gordon Alles studied many amines in the search for an agent superior to ephedrine in the treatment of asthma. When he restudied phenylisopropylamine, he described its CNS stimulating effects (1933). It was promptly misused, but to a limited extent, until after World War II. Even when abuse became worldwide, the drug continued to be taken by mouth.

However, in 1957–60, several physicians repeated the error made earlier with cocaine and introduced heroin users to the intravenous use of methamphetamine. The drug was inexpensive, and many heroin users switched to methamphetamine ("speed," "crystal") to their short-term benefit.

Later (1967), a new group of younger drug users discovered methamphetamine and used huge and frequent injections of it. For about 2 years, methamphetamine was by far the most widely used "hard drug." Heroin is now once again the favored injected drug among both former speed users and new compulsive users.

2. Patterns of use—

a. Oral—Amphetamines may be used episodically as "spree" drugs to improve performance, defer fatigue, or prolong an alcoholic binge. They may be used intermittently over a long period but in moderate doses for their euphoriant or antidepressant effect.

A few people become compulsive users of one or another of the amphetamines taken by mouth. Considering the huge amounts prescribed or otherwise made available, compulsive oral use must develop in only a tiny fraction of those people who have contact with amphetamine.

b. Intravenous—The hazard of developing a compulsive pattern of use is much greater when an amphetamine is injected because of the orgasm-like "rush" at the time of injection. Following the large doses of methamphetamine ("speed") used during the recent "epidemic," the individual did not function well because of anxiety and suspiciousness. Most of the users were recent—ie, unskilled—recruits to a nominally criminal scene, and the methamphetamine subculture and marketplace lacked the social controls acting in the heroin subculture. As a result, the use of speed was associated with a large amount of violence, most of it directed toward other users.

3. Dependence and tolerance—Physical dependence manifested as withdrawal signs is difficult to establish. A depression maximal on the fourth day appears, and EEG changes and altered sleep patterns persist for days after the drug is discontinued.

The development of tolerance is also not easy to prove, although side-effects become less prominent with continued use and the abuser may use huge doses intravenously.

The principal adverse result of amphetamine misuse is the loss of productive activity imposed on the drug-dominated individual by his preoccupation with obtaining the drug. In some individuals, large doses may precipitate the toxic psychosis described above.

Misuse of the amphetamine congeners generally parallels their popularity as therapeutic agents.

An isomer of phenylpropanolamine (D-norpseudoephedrine) is contained in a plant, kat, grown in Ethiopia and habitually chewed by almost the entire population in one isolated area, Aden and Yemen.

Contraindications & Cautions

Amphetamine should not be used in the presence of hypertension, angina pectoris, hyperthyroidism, or agitation. It will greatly intensify the effects of other sympathomimetic drugs and central stimulants of the amine oxidase inhibitor type.

Preparations & Dosages

If the drugs listed in Table 28–2 are given in equipotent doses, they are generally equivalent. A few have not yet been used in doses sufficient to cause toxic psychosis, but other side-effects are similar.

Dextroamphetamine is the standard drug of the group. It is often given in doses of 5 mg 3 times daily before meals. Taking the drug before meals may serve as a reminder to the patient that he must discipline himself, but 15 mg of this long-acting drug as a single morning dose is equally effective. Some disturbance of sleep habits will be apparent 24 hours after a single dose—an observation important in interpreting the claims made for sustained release dosage forms.

Racemic DL-amphetamine (Benzedrine) causes more cardiovascular side-effects for the same amount of central stimulation.

The other isomer, L-amphetamine (Levonor), is dispensed as a salt with a large anion; if equivalent amounts of the base are given, the alleged advantages disappear.

Methamphetamine is about twice as potent as dextroamphetamine, but there are no other differences.

Phenylpropanolamine may be sold without a prescription for use as a nasal decongestant but may no longer be advertised as useful for the management of obesity since it is ineffective in permitted doses.

The other available preparations are either claimed to have fewer side-effects or a longer duration of action. The most recently introduced analogue of amphetamine, chlorphentermine (Pre-Sate), causes the same restlessness as amphetamine, but an as yet poorly defined kind of sedation is also reported. Amphetamine causes a similar side-effect, but the sedation is often interpreted as after-depression.

Fenfluramine is an amphetamine that lacks the stimulant and euphoriant effects of the other amphetamines but is still an anorexic. Chemically, it is an N-ethyl amphetamine with a meta CF_3 ring substituent. It is an investigational drug in the USA, but (as Ponderax) is in wide use in the United Kingdom.

Tranylcypromine (Parnate) is chemically and pharmacologically similar to amphetamine. It is suggested for the treatment of depression rather than obesity and is given in comparatively large doses. It is a more potent amine oxidase (MAO) inhibitor than amphetamine, and is further discussed with those drugs.

Pemoline (Cylert) is a mild stimulant similar to phenmetrazine. In the USA it is an investigative drug publicized for its effect on learning in animals and a possible effect on memory in aged humans. The early enthusiastic reports are being superseded by descriptions that emphasize the similarity of this drug to amphetamine.

Preparations Available

The first drugs listed are class II controlled substances and are subject to the restrictions described in Chapter 4. Prescriptions must bear the physician's federal registration number and cannot be refilled.

Amphetamine (Benzedrine, many others):
Tablets, 5, 10, and 15 mg
Sustained action capsules, 10 and 15 mg
Injectable (IM or IV), 20 mg/ml, 10 and 30 ml

Dextroamphetamine (Dexedrine, many others):
Tablets, 5, 10, and 15 mg
Sustained action capsules, 5, 10, and 15 mg
Elixir, 5 mg/5 ml
Injectable (IM or IV), 20 mg/ml, 10 and 30 ml vials

Methamphetamine (Desoxyn, Methedrine, various others):
Tablets, 2.5 and 5 mg
Sustained action tablets, 5, 10, and 15 mg
Elixir, 3.3 mg/5 ml
Injectable (IM, subcut, or IV), 20 mg/ml, 1, 10, and 30 ml

Methylphenidate (Ritalin):
Tablets, 5, 10, and 20 mg
Injectable (IM, subcut, or IV), 10 mg/ml, 10 ml

Phenmetrazine (Preludin):
Tablets, 25 mg
Sustained action tablets (Preludin Enduret), 50 and 75 mg

The following amphetamines are not controlled substances.

Benzphetamine (Didrex):
Tablets, 25 and 50 mg

Chlorphentermine (Pre-Sate):
Tablets, 65 mg

Diethylpropion (Tenuate, Tepanil):
Tablets, 25 mg
Sustained action tablets (Tenuate Dospan, Tepanil Ten-Tab), 75 mg

Phendimetrazine (Plegine):
Tablets, 35 mg

Phentermine:
Tablets (Wilpo), 8 mg
Capsules (Ionamin), 15 and 30 mg (as resin complex)

Pipradrol (Meratran):
Tablets, 1 and 2.5 mg

Tranylcypromine (Parnate):
Tablets, 10 mg

AMINE OXIDASE INHIBITORS

Inhibitors of monoamine oxidase (MAO) are no longer widely used in therapy. Much of the remaining interest in these drugs and much of their overenthusiastic use in the past is based on an interest in mechanism of action.

Chemistry & Classification

The drugs usually classified as MAO inhibitors are listed in Table 28-3. Iproniazid is no longer available for human use because of the liver damage that it caused, but it is still widely used in laboratory investigation because of its potency. Iproniazid and one of the other drugs still suggested for use as antidepressants are hydrazides—ie, acyl-substituted hydrazines or amides. Another is a hydrazine rather than a hydrazide. Pargyline (Eutonyl) is an amine or "nonhydrazine" MAO inhibitor already mentioned because of its use in treating hypertension (Chapter 12). Tranylcypromine is closely related to amphetamine. The ephedrine or amphetamine type of sympathomimetic drugs are MAO inhibitors, as are many other amines.

Pharmacologic Actions

A. Mechanisms of Action: The MAO inhibitors cause a long-lasting inhibition (irreversible or nonequilibrium blockade) of MAO. The action is demonstrable in humans by changes in the excretion products of amines and by actual assay of enzyme activity in biopsy specimens from the jejunum. However, it is not clear which of the pharmacologic effects are due to MAO inhibition and which are independent of enzyme inhibition.

1. Function of MAO—MAO governs the oxidative deamination of many simple primary and secondary amines. Typical reactions involving the catecholamines and serotonin have been shown in Chapters 10 and 19. The general reaction is as follows:

$$R-CH_2-NH_2 + H_2O + O_2 \longrightarrow$$

$$R-\overset{O}{\overset{\|}{C}}H + NH_3 + H_2O_2$$

The aldehyde formed is usually oxidized to an acid, but smaller amounts are reduced to the corresponding alcohol.

Whether MAO is important in relation to any of its possible substrates depends upon the existence of alternate metabolic pathways for that substrate and the accessibility of substrate to enzyme. The action of norepinephrine that is injected or liberated by nerve activity, for example, can be terminated by reentry of the norepinephrine into nerve or by its O-methylation. Inhibition of MAO does not, therefore, prolong or intensify the peripheral actions of norepinephrine. The metabolism of tyramine depends entirely upon MAO, and its pressor and CNS stimulant effects are tremendously increased by prior administration of MAO inhibitor because its effect of liberating norepinephrine continues for a longer time.

Norepinephrine and serotonin in the CNS (and the norepinephrine of peripheral nerves in the stable pool) are metabolized by MAO. These amines are deaminated by the intracellular (mitochondrial) MAO before they can leave the cell body. MAO inhibition may, therefore, have greater importance in the central than in the peripheral effects of the MAO inhibitors. The sympathomimetic actions described below are not related to MAO inhibition. The CNS stimulant action probably is a direct result of MAO inhibition.

2. Biochemical effects—MAO inhibition develops over a period of several days following therapeutic doses of these drugs. The inhibition is a nonequilibrium or noncompetitive block and persists for about 2 weeks. Reversible, brief-acting MAO inhibitors—eg, the alkaloid harmine—are available as investigative agents.

During the period of MAO inhibition, the concentration of norepinephrine, dopamine, and serotonin rises in the CNS and heart because destruction is slowed. The activity of the precursors of these amines—dopa and 5-hydroxytryptophan—is greatly augmented. An increased CNS action of the amines themselves cannot be demonstrated since they do not enter the CNS after systemic administration.

B. Effects:

1. CNS stimulation—The MAO inhibitors produce a series of changes similar to those described for amphetamine: wakefulness, euphoria, respiratory stimulation, excitement, and, after large doses, a toxic psychosis. Convulsions are rare, and the drugs are anticonvulsants in the laboratory and clinically. An increase in appetite is much more often seen than anorexia.

2. Sympathoplegic effects—The mechanism by which a decrease in sympathetic influence on the tissues is brought about is not understood. The action is slow in onset, and acute animal studies are therefore not relevant. The effects are similar to those of the postganglionic blocking agents. Postural hypotension occurs, and cardiac output is reduced; venous dilatation is therefore present.

3. Sympathomimetic effects—Drugs of this class differ in the intensity of their sympathomimetic effects, but all can produce hypertension, tachycardia, and smooth muscle relaxation after large doses.

Absorption, Metabolism, & Excretion

All of the drugs of this group are given by mouth. They are rapidly metabolized and excreted. However, their MAO inhibiting effect persists long after elimination or discontinuation of the medication.

Clinical Uses

A. Treatment of Depression: The MAO inhibitors have been almost completely superseded by the antidepressants related to the tranquilizers. In retrospect, it is doubtful whether even iproniazid had significant usefulness in major depressions. Indeed, there are many studies that question whether the hydrazines are superior to placebos.

B. Hypertension: The use of pargyline is discussed in Chapter 12.

C. Angina: The hydrazines in which the sympathoplegic or vasodilating properties predominate were investigated for possible usefulness in the prevention of anginal attacks. Clinical trials testing their effectiveness gave conflicting results, but some of the skepticism is based on objections to the use of a general vasodilator rather than a coronary dilator—a probable fallacy discussed in Chapter 13.

Adverse Reactions

A. Side-Effects: A given action of the MAO inhibitors—eg, hypotension or psychomotor stimulation—may be an undesirable side-effect or the therapeutic action, depending upon the application of the drug.

1. Sympathoplegic effects—Postural hypotension with complaints of dizziness or fainting is common. Vasodilatation may also cause a flush and a feeling of warmth, or may precipitate a vascular headache. Decreased sweating may be noted, but the sympathomimetic action may cause increased sweating, especially of the upper parts of the body. Edema may occur, as it does during the use of other postural hypotensive agents that lower cardiac output.

2. Sympathomimetic effects—These are usually limited to constipation, urinary hesitancy, and dry mouth. Hypertension may occur, but is dangerous only in the case of tranylcypromine (Parnate) or when dietary tyramine or other sympathomimetic drugs are ingested concurrently.

3. CNS effects—These include euphoria, insomnia, restlessness, and, usually, increased appetite, although the anorexia that would be expected on the basis of experience with sympathomimetic stimulants occasionally occurs. Appetite may also increase because depression is relieved.

B. Overdosage Toxicity:

1. CNS effects—Euphoria may be replaced by excitement or a toxic psychosis. After large single doses, the patient may become stuporous and unresponsive. Convulsions are rare, but fibrillary muscle jerks are common.

2. Hypertensive crises—After toxic doses, the mixture of sympathomimetic and sympathoplegic actions usually persists. Hypotension may be present but can be controlled by keeping the patient recumbent.

Serious hypertensive crises may occur if the patient ingests tyramine-containing foods during a period when his MAO activity is depressed. The absorbed tyramine is not destroyed at the usual rapid rate and so releases norepinephrine from stores augmented by administration of the MAO inhibitor. Signs of intense sympathomimetic action result, and fatal reactions due to intracranial hemorrhage have occurred. Reactions have been most often recorded during treatment with tranylcypromine (Parnate) but may occur during the use of the other MAO inhibitors also.

The most common sources of dietary tyramine, which should be avoided during treatment with MAO inhibitors, are foods prepared by fermentation, ie, some forms of cheese, beer, and red wine.

3. Hepatotoxicity—Iproniazid caused hepatocellular injury with such frequency that it was removed from the market. The diffuse cellular necrosis and inflammatory changes are comparable to those seen during infectious hepatitis, but a fatal outcome was more frequent. The occurrence of jaundice is unpredictable, but is a direct toxic effect and not an allergic reaction. The MAO inhibitors still available have also caused hepatic damage. Perhaps the incidence of hepatocellular damage is less, but the fewer cases reported may only reflect the now decreased use of these drugs.

Contraindications & Cautions

The possible hypertensive reactions to dietary tyramine discussed above should be explained to the patient, and he should be cautioned against the use of other sympathomimetic drugs, including over-the-counter cold tablets or capsules. In addition, the MAO inhibitors potentiate the effect of narcotic analgesics, tranquilizers, and sedatives such as alcohol and barbiturates. The mechanism of this potentiation is not known, but drugs of these classes should be used in smaller dosages. Both the antidepressants similar to the tranquilizers and the MAO inhibitors were likely to be tried in a patient with a depression, and frequent reactions occurred unless an interval of at least 2 weeks separated the administration of the MAO inhibitor and the antidepressant in either order.

Impaired liver function is a contraindication to the use of these drugs, and liver function tests should be done during the period of treatment.

Preparations & Dosages

Whether there are still any indications for the clinical use of MAO inhibitors is questionable. If they are used, they are given in an initial dosage (Table 28–3) that is continued for 2–6 weeks or until a

TABLE 28–3. Monoamine oxidase (MAO) inhibitors: Formulas, dosages, and preparations available.

	NH–NH R₁ ⟋ ⟍ R₂		Initial and Maintenance Doses (per day)	Preparations Available
Hydrazides				
Iproniazid (Marsilid)	(pyridine)-CO–	H₃C–CH–CH₃	. . .	. . .
Isocarboxazid (Marplan)	H₃C–(isoxazole)-CO–	–CH₂–(phenyl)	20–30 mg, then 10 mg (maximum)	Tablets, 10 mg
Hydrazines				
Phenelzine (Nardil)	(phenyl)–CH₂–CH₂–	H	30–45 mg, then 5–20 mg	Tablets, 15 mg
Amines				
Pargyline (Eutonyl)	(phenyl)–CH₂–N–CH₂–C≡CH, CH₃		25–50 mg, then 10–100 mg	Tablets, 10, 25, and 50 mg
Tranylcypromine (Parnate)	See Table 28–2.		20 mg, then 10–20 mg	Tablets, 10 mg

response is noted. The dosage is then slowly reduced to the maintenance doses listed.

Excluding pargyline (the hypotensive agent) and tranylcypromine, there is no basis for preferring one or the other of these drugs. Tranylcypromine (Parnate) is a special case. Its return to the market after the serious and lethal hypertensive episodes described above was permitted only with special restrictive labeling. It can be used only in those depressions that have failed to respond to other (not further defined) therapy. The package insert should be read by anyone contemplating the use of tranylcypromine because it is by law part of the labeling and places the responsibility for any poor result on the physician.

MEDULLARY OR CONVULSANT STIMULANTS

The CNS stimulants discussed thus far—amphetamine, caffeine, and MAO inhibitors—cause awakening and mood elevation as early effects. They are, therefore, often referred to as cortical or cerebral stimulants even though it is probable that they act on the brain stem (RAS) and only indirectly activate the cortex. The drugs listed below act on the brain stem selectively to augment its descending influences, and are often called medullary stimulants. If they are called convulsant stimulants, an important limiting property is suggested. Although they were widely used in the past, no established use for these drugs remains.

The group of medullary stimulants includes drugs of varied chemical types. Their common properties will be discussed first, and the differences between the compounds will be mentioned with the discussion of each drug.

Pharmacologic Effects

Stimulation of the respiratory, vasomotor, and vagal centers of the medulla leads to increased respiratory minute volume, a rise in blood pressure, a slowing of the pulse, and nausea and vomiting. Doses only slightly larger than those required to stimulate depressed respiration cause convulsions comparable to a grand mal seizure. The convulsions can still be precipitated in animals after decerebration. Awakening and spinal cord stimulation appear only with larger doses. Hyperthermia and cardiac arrhythmias are important toxic effects.

Suggested Uses

The treatment of severe depression due to barbiturate or other sedative-hypnotic drug has been discussed (Chapter 23). The success of the conservative or physiologic method of treating drug depression depends in part upon abandoning the use of convulsant stimulants. Possibly because the idea of using a respira-

tory stimulant in these patients is logically attractive—and because favorable results can be shown in the laboratory—the question of their use is often presented as a matter of controversy. However, it seems a fair summary to say that no investigator reporting favorable results in a significantly large experience currently uses analeptics. The action on respiration of these stimulants is brief compared to the duration of the treatment problem. The margin between the respiratory stimulant and the convulsant dose is narrow, and postconvulsant depression is disastrous. Hyperthermia, cardiac arrhythmias, and, in the awakening patient, toxic psychosis are other dangerous reactions.

Preparations Available

A. Picrotoxin: Picrotoxin is the "bitter poison" found in the berries of an Indonesian plant. The crushed berries thrown into the water poisoned fish and allowed them to be gathered. The drug is available in 20 ml vials containing 3 mg/ml.

B. Pentylenetetrazol (Metrazol): Pentylenetetrazol is of historical interest because of its use in convulsant therapy before ECT. It is used in the laboratory evaluation of anticonvulsant drugs. It is active after oral administration and is suggested, without adequate basis, for the treatment of senile confusion or memory loss. It is available in tablets, 100 mg; elixir, 100 mg/5 ml; and as a solution for injection, 100 mg/ml, in 1, 3, and 30 ml vials.

C. Nikethamide (Coramine): Diethylnicotinamide is a weak stimulant that is converted, in part, to nicotinamide in the body. It is available as an oral solution, 25% in 1, 3, and 16 oz bottles; and as a 25% solution for injection in 1.5, 5, and 20 ml vials.

D. Ethamivan (Emivan): This drug is vanillic acid diethylamide. It is, however, more potent than nikethamide, to which it is related chemically. It is available as 20 and 60 mg tablets and as a solution for injection, 50 mg/ml, in 2 and 10 ml vials.

E. Doxapram (Dopram): This drug is the agent most recently suggested for use in the postanesthetic period. It is presented as if it were in general comparable with the drugs listed in this section but with a wider range between the dose needed to stimulate respiration and the convulsant dose. It is certainly not a potent convulsant, but it causes many sympathomimetic effects and acts on the RAS much as amphetamine does. Chemically, it is somewhat similar to methylphenidate (Ritalin). It thus appears to be a sympathomimetic stimulant with a very brief duration (2–5 minutes) of action. It is available in 20 ml ampules containing 20 mg/ml.

F. Flurothyl (Hexafluorodiethyl Ether, Indoklon): Flurothyl is a convulsant agent that is a volatile liquid and can be administered by inhalation. It is suggested as an alternative to ECT. The advantage claimed is better patient acceptance. However, this advantage can operate only when ECT is given without prior thiopental or other anesthetic. It is less precisely controlled than ECT.

H. Camphor and Thujone: Characterization of these old drugs is difficult. Camphor is certainly a convulsant, but it is possible that the locus of convulsant action is cortical rather than pontile. Thujone, chemically closely related to camphor, was the constituent responsible for the habituating properties of absinthe liqueur and must, therefore, have had properties different from the medullary stimulants. Present day absinthe is flavored with anise and offers no advantage over any other 40% solution of alcohol.

● ● ●

General References

General

Klein, D.F., & J.M. Davis: *Diagnosis and Drug Treatment of Psychiatric Disorders.* Williams & Wilkins, 1969.

Amphetamine

Costa, E., & S. Garattini (editors): *International Symposium on Amphetamine and Related Compounds.* Raven Press, 1970.

Hawks, D., & others: Abuse of methylamphetamine. Brit MJ 3:715–721, 1969.

Hollingsworth, D.R., & T.T. Amatruda, Jr.: Toxic and therapeutic effects of EMTP in obesity. Clin Pharmacol Therap 10:540–542, 1969.

Jönsson, L.-E., Änggåro, E., & L.-M. Gunne: Blockade of intravenous amphetamine euphoria in man. Clin Pharmacol Therap 12:889–896, 1971.

Kosman, M.E., & K.R. Unna: Effects of chronic administration of the amphetamines and other stimulants on behavior. Clin Pharmacol Therap 9:240–254, 1968.

Lewis, S.A., Oswald, I., & D.L. F. Dunleavy: Chronic fenfluramine administration: Some cerebral effects. Brit MJ 3:67–70, 1971.

Sleep disorders and highway accidents. Editorial. New England J Med 274:906–907, 1966.

Smith, G.M., & H.K. Beecher: Amphetamine sulfate and athletic performance. JAMA 170:542–557, 1959; 172:1502–1541, 1623–1629, 1960; 177:347–349, 1961.

Towbin, A.: Organic causes of minimal brain dysfunction. JAMA 217:1207–1214, 1971.

Weiss, B., & V.G. Laties: Enhancement of human performance by caffeine and the amphetamines. Pharmacol Rev 14:1–36, 1962.

Antidepressants

Blinder, M.G.: Differential diagnosis and treatment of depressive disorders. JAMA 195:8–12, 1966.

Clinical Psychiatry Committee of the Medical Research Council: Clinical trial of the treatment of depressive illness. Brit MJ 1:881–885, 1965.

Crimson, C.: Chlorpromazine and imipramine: Parallel studies in animals. Psychopharmacology Bull 4(2):1–151, 1967.

Herr, F., Stewart, J., & M.-P. Charest: Tranquilizers and antidepressants: A pharmacological comparison. Arch Int Pharmacodyn 134:328–342, 1961.

Hollister, L.E.: Clinical use of psychotherapeutic drugs: Current status. Clin Pharmacol Therap 10:170–198, 1969.

Overall, J.E., & others: Nosology of depression and differential response to drugs. JAMA 195:946–948, 1966.

Poussaint, A.F., Ditman, K.S., & R. Greenfield: Amitriptyline in childhood enuresis. Clin Pharmacol Therap 7:21–25, 1966.

Rickels, K., & others: Drug treatment in depression. Antidepressant or tranquilizer? JAMA 201:675–681, 1967.

Rose, J.T.: Treatment of depression: A comparative trial of imipramine and desipramine. Brit J Psychiat 113:659–665, 1967.

Steel, C.M., O'Duffy, J., & S.S. Brown: Clinical effects and treatment of imipramine and amitriptyline poisoning in children. Brit MJ 3:663–667, 1967.

Other Drugs

Atkinson, R.M., & K.S. Ditman: Tranylcypromine: A review. Clin Pharmacol Therap 6:631–655, 1965.

Goldberg, L.I.: Monoamine oxidase inhibitors. Adverse reactions and possible mechanisms. JAMA 190:456–462, 1964.

Hahn, F.: Analeptics. Pharmacol Rev 12:447–530, 1960.

Karliner, W.: Present status of Indoklon convulsive treatments. Dis Nerv System 27:470–473, 1966.

29...

Anticonvulsant Drugs

The anticonvulsant drugs are used primarily in the treatment of epilepsy but are also effective in controlling convulsions due to other causes—eg, intracranial tumor or trauma or uremia. The types of seizures will be defined below after the properties of the several classes of anticonvulsant drugs have been discussed. Because most patients who are treated for epileptic states receive more than one drug and because treatment is continuous for many years, the chronic toxicity of the anticonvulsant drugs is of particular importance.

The anticonvulsant drugs are classified as follows: (1) long-acting barbiturates, (2) diphenylhydantoin and related hydantoin derivatives, (3) trimethadione and other oxazolidinediones, (4) succinimides (equivalent to trimethadione), (5) phenacemide, a drug both unusually effective and unusually toxic, and (6) adjunctive drugs that are not primarily anticonvulsant.

LONG-ACTING BARBITURATES

All of the drugs defined in Chapter 23 as sedative-hypnotics are anticonvulsant drugs and may be used acutely to terminate a convulsive state. Large doses are required, however, and for chronic administration only the long-acting sedatives are satisfactory. Phenobarbital and related barbiturates are the standard drugs, but other long-acting sedatives—eg, chlordiazepoxide (Librium)—are efficacious. Intermediate-acting sedatives such as meprobamate and diazepam (Valium) have been used, but the rapidly changing level of activity of the short- and intermediate-acting sedatives makes them less suitable for continued use.

Chemistry & Metabolism

Phenobarbital was characterized in the discussion of sedative-hypnotics as the standard long-acting sedative. It is also the most commonly used anticonvulsant barbiturate.

Table 23–2 shows the structures of 3 other compounds that are occasionally used as anticonvulsants. Mephobarbital (Mebaral) is demethylated rapidly to phenobarbital, and metharbital (Gemonil) is demethylated to barbital, a long-acting barbiturate which has been replaced in therapeutic use by phenobarbital. Primidone (Mysoline) is not actually a barbiturate as ingested but is oxidized to phenobarbital. The blood levels of phenobarbital that follow ingestion of these compounds are adequate to explain their actions.

Aminoglutethimide (Elipten) is a sedative related chemically to glutethimide (Doriden). It was used as an anticonvulsant until withdrawn from the market because of doubtful efficacy and possible toxicity. Aminoglutethimide has investigational uses as an inhibitor of adrenocortical function.

Pharmacologic Effects

A. Mechanisms of Action: Unlike the short-acting barbiturates, phenobarbital and related compounds are anticonvulsant in doses that are not anesthetic or even markedly sedative. One point of view holds that this establishes a specific anticonvulsant action for phenobarbital. Another view, however, is that the usefulness of these drugs derives from their sustained, constant level of effect. The basis for the anticonvulsant action of these general CNS depressants remains conjectural. It can be said, however, that the well established effect of the sedatives on the ascending RAS is not related to their anticonvulsant activity since amphetamine, which facilitates transmission within the RAS, can be used to counteract the sedation without abolishing the anticonvulsant action.

B. Effects: The effects of phenobarbital have been discussed in Chapter 23.

Clinical Uses

Phenobarbital and similar drugs are useful in grand mal epilepsy and in the control of symptomatic convulsions. They are less often effective in psychomotor epilepsy, petit mal epilepsy, and other clinical types of epilepsy.

Adverse Reactions

A. Side-Effects: The most common adverse reactions to the sedatives during anti-epileptic treatment are those related to sedation and disinhibition—ie, drowsiness, dizziness, ataxia, diplopia (with or without nystagmus), and behavioral (personality) changes. These effects are minimized by using combinations of anticonvulsant drugs, each in less than disturbing doses. Phenobarbital is usually well tolerated.

B. Withdrawal: Epileptic patients are unusually susceptible to the hyperexcitable state induced by withdrawal or too rapid reduction of dosage not only of sedatives but other anticonvulsants also. To avoid precipitating convulsions, the dosage should be reduced by small decrements with, if possible, intervals of several weeks between adjustments. In the event that toxicity specific for one compound appears—eg, drug rash or other allergic reaction—another anticonvulsant drug in equipotent dosage should be substituted.

C. Effects of Chronic Treatment: Long-continued treatment with phenobarbital is not dangerous, and habituation is not a problem. The learning and intelligence of epileptic children are not impaired by chronic treatment with the usual doses, but prolonged treatment with combinations of anticonvulsant drugs may be damaging.

Primidone, like diphenylhydantoin, can interfere with folic acid absorption and cause macrocytosis. A similar but weaker effect is demonstrable with phenobarbital.

Dosages

A. Phenobarbital: The usual adult dose is 100–200 mg daily. Doses as large as 400 mg daily may sometimes be necessary and are often well tolerated. The long-acting sedatives are usually given in 3–4 divided doses daily, but there is no need to do so. Larger doses can be divided into 2 daily doses, and the smaller doses usually required are often given as a single dose each day. In children, the initial dosage can be based either on weight or on age, but the tolerated dose may be more than predicted by weight or age and is determined by the response and tolerance of each patient.

B. Mephobarbital (Mebaral): The daily dose is twice that of phenobarbital given in divided doses—ie, 200–400 mg daily.

C. Metharbital (Gemonil): The usual dose is 100 mg 2–3 times daily.

D. Primidone (Mysoline): Dizziness and sedation are sometimes severe at the beginning of treatment with primidone. The initial small doses—50 mg 3 times daily—can be increased to 250 or even 500 mg 3 times daily. Experience with metharbital and primidone has been less than with phenobarbital and mephobarbital.

DIPHENYLHYDANTOIN
& CONGENERS

Chemistry

The chemical structures of diphenylhydantoin (Dilantin) and 2 related hydantoin derivatives are shown in Table 29–1. The hydantoins can be considered as ureides and are related to the barbiturates. In fact, one hydantoin no longer marketed was at one time used as a hypnotic drug. Nevertheless, diphenylhydantoin is a specific rather than a general depressant—ie, it is able to control convulsions without causing general sedation. It was suggested for clinical trial because of its ability to modify electroshock convulsions in the laboratory.

Pharmacologic Effects

A. Mechanisms of Action:

1. Origin of convulsions—Any speculation about the site of action of an anticonvulsant drug must be based on information about the site of origin of the convulsion. Diphenylhydantoin (and, even more clearly, phenobarbital) acts on many levels of the CNS, and not all actions are necessarily related to the anticonvulsant effect. The action of diphenylhydantoin on the brain stem or cerebellum, for example, is relevant only if convulsions originate at these levels. Unfortunately, the site of origin and mechanism of action of most convulsions are not clear. Jacksonian or focal convulsions clearly originate in the cortex, and an experimental analogue can be produced by an irritative lesion in the cortex. But most convulsions begin with a loss of consciousness, and the abnormality is diffuse rather than focal. They are subcortical in origin, but the site cannot be more exactly defined. Many experimentally induced convulsions, including the pentylenetetrazol convulsions used to screen potential anticonvulsant drugs, appear even after precollicular section of the neuraxis.

2. Possible mechanisms—It is customary to assume that—whatever the level of origin—convulsions are due to the spread of activity from a focus of abnormal function into normal neural tissue. Anticonvulsant drugs could then act by suppressing the seizure focus or by preventing the spread of the impulse through normal tissue.

Diphenylhydantoin does not suppress the discharge from an experimentally produced focus, nor does it necessarily alter the EEG evidence of focal discharge in humans. Diffuse EEG abnormalities may be decreased. The best explanation for the action of diphenylhydantoin is, therefore, that it prevents the spread of abnormal electrical activity. Various explanations have been offered for the stabilization of neurons: reduction of post-tetanic potentiation, prolonged refractory period, elevation of synaptic threshold, and augmentation of some chemical inhibitory influence. The action may be on all neurons rather than on a precise area of the CNS, since one diffuse process—hypocalcemic tetany—may also be suppressed by diphenylhydantoin.

B. Effects: Effects of these drugs other than their anticonvulsant action are listed under Adverse Reactions, below.

Absorption, Metabolism, & Excretion

The maximum blood level is not reached until 8 hours after oral administration of diphenylhydantoin. The drug is metabolized by hydroxylation of the phenyl ring, a reaction governed by hepatic microsomal enzymes, and is then conjugated and excreted as a glucuronide. Metabolism is slow; the half-life of diphenylhydantoin in the plasma following discontinuance of chronic medication averages 22 hours. When the drug is given chronically a stable level is reached

TABLE 29–1. Anticonvulsant drugs: Structures, dosages, and preparations available.

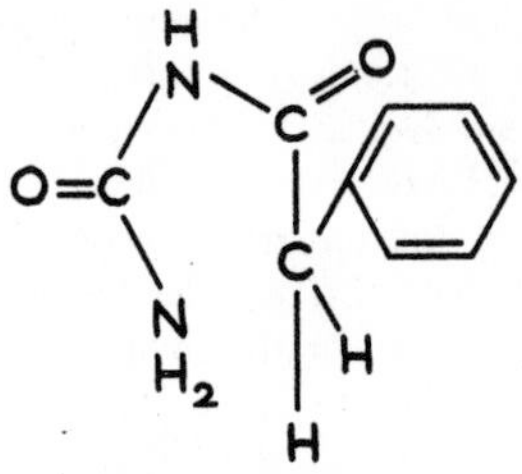

Phenylacetylurea

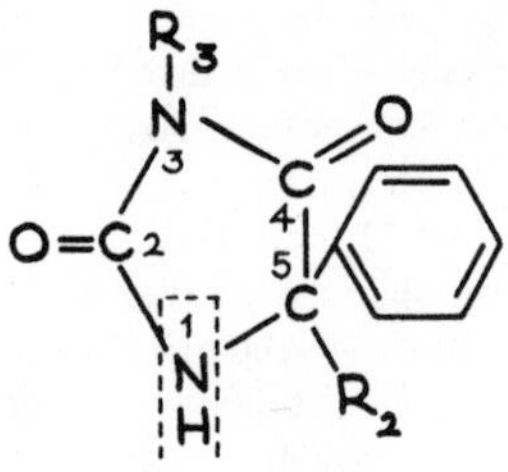

Hydantoin derivatives

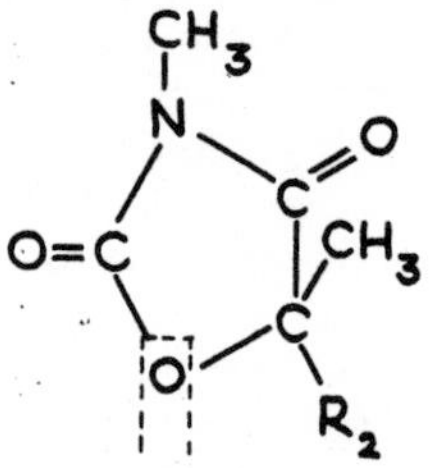

Oxazolidinediones

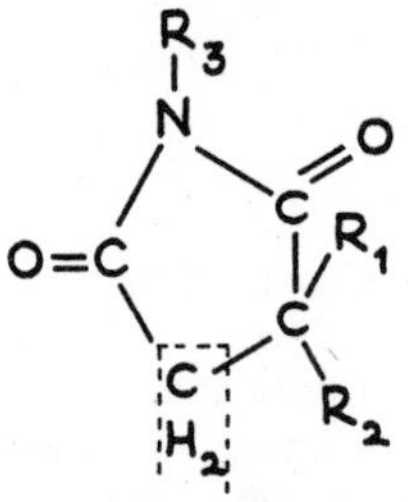

Succinimides

	R_1	R_2	R_3	Usual Adult Dose (Oral)	Preparations Available
Phenylacetylurea					
Phenacemide (Phenurone)*				1 gm 2–3 times/ day	Tablets, 500 mg
Hydantoin derivatives					
Diphenylhydantoin (Dilantin) (Phenytoin, Brit.)		–phenyl	–H	100–300 mg 1–2 times/day	Tablets, 50 and 100 mg Capsules, 30 and 100 mg Suspension, 30 and 125 mg/5 ml Suppositories, 100 and 200 mg Injectable (IM or IV), 100 and 250 mg powder in vials with diluent in separate vials
Mephenytoin (Mesantoin)		$-C_2H_5$	$-CH_3$	100–300 mg 2 times/day	Tablets, 100 mg
Ethotoin (Peganone)		–H	$-C_2H_5$	0.5–1 gm 2–3 times/day	Tablets, 250 and 500 mg
Oxazolidinediones					
Trimethadione (Tridione)		$-CH_3$		300 mg 1–4 times/day	Tablets, 150 mg Capsules, 300 mg Solution, 200 mg/5 ml
Paramethadione (Paradione)		$-C_2H_5$		300 mg 1–4 times/day	Capsules, 150 and 300 mg Solution, 300 mg/ml
Succinimides					
Ethosuximide (Zarontin)	$-C_2H_5$	$-CH_3$	–H	250–500 mg 2 times/day	Capsules, 250 mg
Methsuximide (Celontin)	–phenyl	$-CH_3$	$-CH_3$	0.3–0.6 gm 2 times/day	Capsules, 150 and 300 mg
Phensuximide (Milontin)	–phenyl	–H	$-CH_3$	0.5–1 gm 2 times/day	Capsules, 250 and 500 mg Suspension, 300 mg/5 ml

*Trade names included only for identification. These drugs are available from many suppliers under their generic names.

only after administration of a fixed dose for a week, at which time excretion matches absorption.

Administration once daily is sufficient to maintain constant blood levels. However, large doses of the alkaline drug may be divided between the morning and evening mealtimes to minimize gastrointestinal irritation.

Absorption from intramuscular injection sites is also slow, and the drug must be given intravenously when a rapid effect is needed.

Clinical Uses

A. As Anticonvulsant: Diphenylhydantoin (alone or in combination with phenobarbital) is used in the treatment of grand mal epilepsy, symptomatic convulsions, and psychomotor epilepsy. It may intensify the petit mal attacks in mixed epilepsy.

B. Trigeminal Neuralgia and Atypical Facial Pain: See carbamazepine (Tegretol) below under Other Anticonvulsant Drugs.

C. Cardiac Arrhythmias: Diphenylhydantoin has ECG and other effects comparable to those of quinidine. It has been used as an investigative drug to treat cardiac arrhythmias.

Adverse Reactions

A. Diphenylhydantoin:

1. Side-effects—

a. CNS—CNS effects are the most common dose-limiting side-effects. These include ataxia (most frequent), slurred speech, and nystagmus, accompanied in some patients by tremors and nervousness and in others by drowsiness and fatigue.

b. Gingival hypertrophy—Hypertrophy of the gums is a frequent (20%) side-effect. It may be cosmetically displeasing but causes no other difficulty beyond minor bleeding. It is both more common and more severe in younger patients.

The mechanism underlying the proliferation of the gingival stroma is not known. It has been noted that hypertrophy does not occur in edentulous patients and that diphenylhydantoin appears in the saliva whether the drug is given by mouth or parenterally.

Brushing the teeth regularly and vigorously may be of some value in minimizing gingival hypertrophy, but excision of the hypertrophied gingivas by a dental surgeon may be necessary. Neither antihistamines nor ascorbic acid is helpful in spite of isolated claims to the contrary.

c. Folate deficiency—Prolonged administration of diphenylhydantoin may lead to macrocytosis or megaloblastic anemia due to folic acid deficiency. Dietary folic acid occurs in the form of polyglutamates which must be hydrolyzed to folate monoglutamate before absorption can occur (see Chapter 44 for chemical structure). Diphenylhydantoin and, to a lesser extent, phenobarbital and primidone inhibit the deconjugation in the ileum and reduce absorption. The changes in the red cells can be prevented or treated by small oral doses of folic acid or by vitamin B_{12}.

It has also been established that youthful epileptics who are treated for extended periods may undergo progressive deterioration of their mental state that is independent of any preexisting brain damage. Combined treatment with diphenylhydantoin and primidone or phenobarbital is most likely to cause the state which is associated with decreased levels of folate in serum and CSF. Treatment with folic acid alone causes more convulsions, but combined treatment with folic acid and B_{12} is effective. Prevention requires oral doses of folic acid weekly and of vitamin B_{12} monthly.

d. Others—Diphenylhydantoin is dispensed as the sodium salt and as such is very alkaline. The resultant nausea and epigastric pain can be minimized by giving the drug with or after meals.

Low PBI values are found since this diphenylmethane compound, like others, displaces thyroxine from protein-binding sites. Thyroid function, however, is not altered.

Hirsutism of the extremities occurs in girls with no demonstrable endocrinopathy.

Rare toxic effects include toxic psychosis, hepatitis, and systemic lupus erythematosus.

2. Overdosage toxicity—The ingestion of large doses of diphenylhydantoin results in intensification of the cerebellar signs listed above and in excitement and confusion followed by depression. The acute toxicity is very low.

3. Allergic reactions—A morbilliform rash occurs in 2–10% (reports vary) of patients receiving diphenylhydantoin. In some cases the rash may be accompanied by pyrexia, eosinophilia, and lymphadenopathy. The reaction has been mistaken for measles, infectious mononucleosis, and, in at least one case, for lymphosarcoma even after biopsy. A few cases of agranulocytosis, thrombocytopenia, and exfoliative dermatitis have been reported.

B. Mephenytoin (Mesantoin): This drug has anticonvulsant properties similar to those of diphenylhydantoin but has sedative rather than excitant effects. It is metabolized by demethylation to phenylethylhydantoin, a sedative which (as Nirvanol) was abandoned in 1920 because of its bone marrow toxicity. Perhaps predictably, mephenytoin is also very toxic. Rash and neutropenia occur frequently and pancytopenia, aplastic anemia, and hepatic damage rarely (but more often than with diphenylhydantoin). Mephenytoin causes much less gingival hyperplasia and other side-effects but more drowsiness than does diphenylhydantoin.

C. Ethotoin (Peganone): This hydantoin also causes less gingival hyperplasia and hirsutism than diphenylhydantoin, but it is less effective.

Preparations & Dosages

See Table 29–1.

TRIMETHADIONE

Trimethadione (Tridione) is probably still the drug most widely used in the treatment of petit mal epilepsy, although alternative treatments are gaining in popularity. Paramethadione (Paradione) is a related oxazolidinedione compound that is both less toxic and less effective (Table 29–1).

Pharmacologic Effects

A. Mechanisms of Action: Trimethadione is useful in reducing the number of petit mal attacks whether they are of the typical pattern or one of the variants with associated motor signs. Patients subject to these attacks have characteristic abnormal EEG patterns more or less continuously rather than only during the clinical episode, as is usually the case in grand mal epilepsy. The abnormal pattern of petit mal is diffuse and symmetric and usually characterized by a 3/second spike-and-dome pattern. Trimethadione restores the EEG toward normal. In patients who respond well, the 3/second pattern no longer appears even after hyperventilation. Since the EEG abnormality is diffuse, it does not follow that trimethadione is suppressing an irritable focus.

B. Effects: Large doses of trimethadione given to animals cause sedation and respiratory depression. The drug has only a minor sedative effect in humans even when given in large doses. Its analgesic property is now clinically unimportant but led to the original trials of the drug.

Absorption, Metabolism, & Excretion

Trimethadione is rapidly and completely absorbed. The N-demethylated derivative is only slowly excreted and accumulates in the body during therapy. It may be an active metabolite.

Clinical Uses

An oxazolidinedione is used in the treatment of petit mal epilepsy and variants showing the spike-and-dome or other bilaterally synchronous or symmetric EEG pattern. It may be combined with phenobarbital. Trimethadione may increase the number of major seizures in patients with seizures of mixed types by suppressing the minor seizures, and should in these cases be combined with diphenylhydantoin. There may be a transitory increase in the number of petit mal episodes at the beginning of treatment.

Adverse Reactions

A. Trimethadione:

1. Side-effects—Sedation is uncommon and usually decreases with continued administration. A daily dose of amphetamine can be given to minimize sedation. Amphetamine so used will not antagonize and may even intensify the anticonvulsant effect.

A common side-effect, especially in adults, is a glary, blurred, or snowy appearance of objects in bright light (hemeralopia). The effect is due to an action on the retina but is reversible and controlled by reduced dosage or by wearing dark glasses. As described by the patient, it is different from photophobia, or general intolerance to light.

Most patients (80%) receiving trimethadione show a reduction in the number of neutrophils. This graded or controlled neutropenia can be followed by blood counts at intervals of 3 months. It is not dangerous but is mentioned to distinguish it from agranulocytosis.

Exacerbation of grand mal epilepsy is mentioned above. Reversible nephrosis has occurred. Hepatitis and acneiform dermatitis are apparently rare side-effects.

2. Overdosage toxicity—The acute (large or deliberate overdosage) toxicity of trimethadione is very low.

3. Allergic reactions—In contrast to the controlled neutropenia described above, agranulocytosis or pancytopenia may appear suddenly. If a morbilliform rash appears, the drug should be at least temporarily discontinued since cases of exfoliative dermatitis have been reported.

B. Paramethadione: The toxicity of paramethadione is similar to that of trimethadione, but reports of serious toxic reactions are fewer. Paramethadione may be substituted for trimethadione in an effort to reduce adverse reactions. However, if an allergic reaction to trimethadione has occurred, paramethadione should be used cautiously since cross-sensitivity may exist.

Contraindications & Cautions

When any of the anticonvulsant drugs are used, a responsible member of the patient's family should be asked to record the number of attacks and report signs of serious toxicity—bleeding or bruising, sore throat (accompanying agranulocytosis), fever, rash, pallor, behavioral changes, etc. Urinalysis and blood counts should be done monthly at first and then at intervals of about 3 months.

Because of the remote possibility of causing or aggravating hepatic or renal damage, trimethadione should be avoided or used with particular care in the presence of disease of these organs.

Trimethadione in combination with mephenytoin (Mesantoin) has been associated with aplastic anemia in several instances, and this combination should therefore not be given.

Preparations & Dosages

See Table 29–1.

SUCCINIMIDES

Many neurologists now characterize trimethadione as obsolescent and regard ethosuximide (Zarontin) as the drug of first choice in the treatment of petit mal epilepsy. They argue that it is at least as effective as trimethadione and that toxic reactions are no more frequent and are of less serious types.

Ethosuximide has recently been implicated in isolated cases of agranulocytosis and pancytopenia, and evaluation of its toxicity is difficult. Side-effects during its use are certainly no greater than those of trimethadione, especially if, as is true for all anticonvulsants, the dose is slowly increased. Side-effects include signs of gastrointestinal irritation, drowsiness or depression, ataxia, hiccup, and insomnia or agitation after larger doses.

Experience with methsuximide (Celontin) is too limited to permit confident recommendations for its use. Phensuximide (Milontin) is less effective.

PHENACEMIDE
(Phenurone)

Phenacemide is a monoureide and is thus chemically related to one class of sedative-hypnotic drugs. It is the most effective (and most toxic) of the anticonvulsants, and reference to Table 29–1 suggests that the other anticonvulsants can be regarded as closed chain derivatives of phenacemide.

Phenacemide is effective in the treatment of all types of epilepsy, but because of its toxicity it is used only in rare cases of psychomotor epilepsy which cannot be controlled with other drugs. It causes only mild sedation, but personality changes are frequent (20%). Hepatitis accounted for 4 deaths among the first 1500 patients treated. Proteinuria, exfoliative dermatitis, and aplastic anemia are also reported.

OTHER ANTICONVULSANT DRUGS

A number of drugs not primarily classified as anticonvulsants may be used in the control of some convulsive states.

Amphetamine

Dextroamphetamine or one of the related sympathomimetic stimulants (see Chapter 28) may be used to counteract the sedation induced by some anticonvulsant drugs. In addition, amphetamine probably has a minor anticonvulsant action. It modifies experimental convulsions in animals. Its awakening effect may perhaps also prevent seizures that occur during deep sleep or during drowsiness.

Sedatives & Tranquilizers

Sedatives other than the long-acting barbiturates have been used in the treatment of epilepsy. At least 2 of these—meprobamate (Equanil, Miltown) and chlordiazepoxide (Librium)—are often referred to as tranquilizers. Therefore, it must be emphasized again that the antipsychotic tranquilizers—the phenothiazines and reserpine—are convulsant agents and should not be given to patients with epilepsy. Psychomotor epilepsy

with an accompanying psychosis may be an unavoidable exception requiring the use of antipsychotic tranquilizers.

The use of chlordiazepoxide (Librium) as an anticonvulsant is still investigational. The parenteral use of diazepam (Valium), 2–10 mg IM or IV, in the control of status epilepticus or the use of oral diazepam in combination with other agents is established rather than investigational—ie, the FDA has approved marketing and advertising for this purpose.

Acetazolamide, Other Diuretics

The carbonic anhydrase inhibitors are diuretics (see Chapter 17) that produce a mild acidosis as well as a loss of sodium and potassium. The clinical efficacy of acetazolamide (Diamox) is difficult to evaluate, but it is used in the treatment of petit mal states. The same drug or a thiazide type of diuretic may be used in patients who tend to have grand mal seizures at the time of their menstrual period.

Quinacrine

Quinacrine (Atabrine) is an antimalarial drug (see Chapter 62) that may be tried in patients with petit mal who do not respond to other drugs. The mechanism of its anticonvulsant effect is not known.

Corticosteroids & Corticotropin

Hydrocortisone has been used intravenously to terminate the rarely seen continuous petit mal state. Corticosteroids and corticotropin are used in the treatment of hypsarrhythmia or myoclonic spasms of infancy.

Salicylates

In children susceptible to febrile convulsions, prompt lowering of an elevated temperature by aspirin or other antipyretic analgesics may prevent the seizures.

Carbamazepine (Tegretol)

Carbamazepine is generally equivalent to diphenylhydantoin in its pharmacologic effects but chemically is superficially similar to imipramine (Table 28–1).

Carbamazepine is not approved for marketing in the USA as an anticonvulsant but only for use in the treatment of trigeminal neuralgia. Patients with classical tic douloureux or variants should receive a trial of therapy with carbamazepine or diphenylhydantoin. Relief may be complete or partial—or may be good initially but followed by a recurrence of pain that may require the use of both drugs or of surgery.

Carbamazepine is superior to diphenylhydantoin in the treatment of trigeminal neuralgia, and side-effects are usually limited to dizziness, the tranquilizer type of sedation, ataxia, and nausea. A few cases of aplastic anemia following its use have been reported, and the package insert should be consulted if its use is contemplated because the instructions place a considerable and probably unreasonable responsibility on the prescriber.

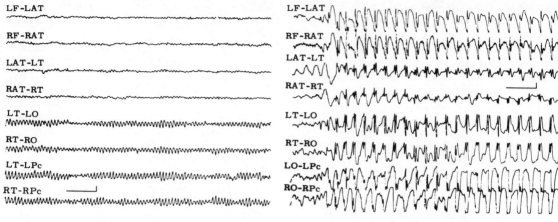

Petit mal epilepsy. This 6-year-old boy had one of his "blank spells," in which he was transiently unaware of surroundings and blinked his eyelids, during the recording.

LF-LAT
RF-RAT
LAT-LT
RAT-RT
LT-LO
RT-RO
LT-LPc
RT-RPc

Normal Adult

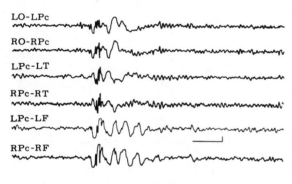

Epilepsy. Tracing of a 24-year-old man with generalized tonic-clonic convulsions and aura of nausea.

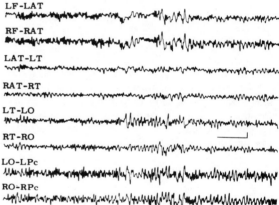

Barbiturate intoxication and withdrawal. Tracing of a 32-year-old woman, a barbiturate abuser, during a period in which she suffered intermittent confusion, amnesia, and generalized motor seizures.

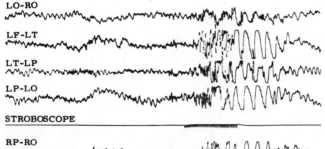

Epilepsy. This 13-year-old girl had brief episodes characterized by blinking of the eyes and absences over the past 3 years. Activation of an electric seizure was produced by photic stimulation at 20 cycles/sec frequency.

LF	= Left frontal
RF	= Right frontal
LAT	= Left anterior temporal
RAT	= Right anterior temporal
LT	= Left temporal
RT	= Right temporal
LO	= Left occipital
RO	= Right occipital
LPc	= Left precentral
RPc	= Right precentral
LP	= Left parietal
RP	= Right parietal

FIG 29–1. Representative electroencephalograms. *Calibration:* 50 μv (vertical) and 1 second (horizontal). (Reproduced, with permission, from Chusid: *Correlative Neuroanatomy and Functional Neurology,* 14th ed. Lange, 1970.)

SUMMARY OF USES OF ANTICONVULSANTS BY SEIZURE TYPES

Problems in Clinical Evaluation

There is no question that the treatment of epilepsy with the standard drugs is effective. However, the comparison of drugs within the general classes—and the evaluation of new agents—is extremely difficult. The imprecise and sometimes unsatisfactory statements often made about the usefulness of alternative drugs reflect the difficulty.

A satisfactory regimen for a patient with seizures must be highly individualized and may involve multiple drugs, especially for the one-third of patients who experience seizures of more than one type. Modification of a regimen of proved value may not only give less satisfactory results but may precipitate great difficulty. New drugs are often tried, therefore, in patients who are poorly controlled with older drugs. This technic appears to be a stringent test of the newer agent, but only if the old drug was optimally used. The interest in the new drug often results in greater care with dosage and other factors in treatment. It may be that some sort of double-blind substitution test is needed.

Another problem is statistical. If the standard drug has already reduced the incidence of seizures to a low level, the difference between old and new drugs cannot be great, and a large number of patients and a long period of observation would be necessary to establish a significant difference between groups of patients.

Laboratory Evaluation

Perhaps because clinical evaluation is so difficult, the laboratory evaluation of potential anticonvulsant drugs has attracted great interest. The influence of and interest in laboratory evaluation seem disproportionately great when one considers that intensive study has not led to the introduction of drugs of a new or unexpected chemical type.

Convulsions can be induced in experimental animals by electrical or chemical stimulation.

A. Electroshock: In this method an alternating current passes diffusely through the brain from surface electrodes. The threshold—ie, the minimum current that produces a convulsion—can be determined before and after the administration of a drug. This method does not predict the clinical usefulness of anticonvulsant drugs other than the sedatives, which do elevate the threshold.

A preferable technic is to produce a convulsion of predictable pattern by a maximal electroshock. Such convulsions are modified by the hydantoins, phenacemide, and the sedatives—ie, by drugs that are of established usefulness in the treatment of major or grand mal convulsions. In humans, these drugs prevent rather than modify the convulsions.

B. Chemoshock or Pentylenetetrazol Convulsions: The convulsions caused by pentylenetetrazol (Cardi-azol, Metrazol) are prevented or modified by trimethadione and other agents useful in the treatment of petit mal epilepsy.

Seizure Types

No single formal classification of the types of convulsions is uniformly satisfactory or accepted by all neurologists. The following common grouping permits some generalizations about treatment. The first important distinction is between symptomatic convulsions, which may have a reversible underlying organic cause, and idiopathic epilepsy.

A. Epilepsy:

1. Grand mal—A major motor seizure begins in a majority of patients with some premonitory sensory or motor change (aura) if they are awake. Following the aura, consciousness is lost and the patient falls, as all muscles are tonically contracted. As the intensity of the attack wanes, clonic movements occur, consciousness slowly returns, and a period of confusion and depression follows. These attacks may occur during sleep and may be evidenced only by incontinence or injury occurring during the clonic phase.

Phenobarbital and diphenylhydantoin are the standard drugs used in the treatment of grand mal epilepsy and are generally effective, but there is some variation in the order of their use. Some physicians argue that treatment should begin with and, if possible, be restricted to phenobarbital, the least toxic drug especially in children. Others believe that diphenylhydantoin alone should be used in order to avoid the sedative effect of the barbiturate drug. It is probable that most patients ultimately receive both drugs, either because the combination is thought to cause fewer side-effects or because both drugs are required for optimal control.

2. Petit mal group—Petit mal epilepsy, in contrast to grand mal, is associated with a distinctive EEG abnormality which is present or easily induced by hyperventilation or photic stimulation between attacks. The EEG changes (Fig 29–1) are diffuse and symmetric and are reduced by trimethadione. Brief lapses of consciousness—apparent as gaps in speech or as immobility for a few seconds—may occur scores of times each day or less frequently. There are 2 variants of petit mal epilepsy that respond similarly to treatment. The fugue may be accompanied by a complete loss of muscle tone (akinetic variant) or by isolated muscle jerks (myoclonic variant) comparable to those experienced by normal persons as sleep begins. These minor motor variants may appear without interruption of consciousness.

Phenobarbital is often tried initially in the treatment of petit mal, but the more toxic trimethadione or ethosuximide must almost always be added. If major motor attacks also occur in the same patient, diphenylhydantoin is also used. A mixed pattern is common, and petit mal attacks in children may be completely replaced by grand mal episodes after puberty.

3. Psychomotor epilepsy—The definition and diagnosis of psychomotor attacks is a matter of controversy. The usual description is of amnesic periods during which automatisms—ie, senseless or antisocial motor acts—are carried out. The EEG shows spiking activity in the anterior temporal areas even between attacks; the abnormality spreads during an attack; and the EEG changes may be activated by light sleep.

The usual treatment is with diphenylhydantoin with or without phenobarbital. The results of treatment are inconsistent, and many drugs have been tried. As is true whenever a diffuse synchronous EEG abnormality is present, trimethadione may be tried. The difficulties in management often justify the use of phenacemide (Phenurone) in spite of its toxicity.

B. Symptomatic Convulsions: The treatment of symptomatic convulsions obviously depends upon the cause. The term is most often used to include the con-

vulsions associated with intracranial tumor, scar, or vascular change. These seizures may be grand mal or focal in type, and the treatment is as discussed for grand mal epilepsy.

Convulsions due to many causes require treatment other than the anticonvulsant drugs. The treatment of hypoglycemia, hypocalcemia, isoniazid toxicity, lead poisoning, etc is discussed in other sections of this book. Convulsions caused by therapeutic agents—eg, phenothiazine tranquilizers (Chapter 25) or local anesthetics (Chapter 22)—are often less dangerous than the additional depression caused by improperly used anticonvulsant medication. Strychnine and tetanus toxin (Chapter 23) act predominantly on the spinal cord and are antagonized by barbiturates or phenothiazine tranquilizers.

● ● ●

General References

Arnold, K., & N. Gerber: The rate of decline of diphenylhydantoin in human plasma. Clin Pharmacol Therap 11:121–134, 1970.

Bogan, J., & H. Smith: Relation between primidone and phenobarbital blood levels. J Pharm Pharmacol 20:64–67, 1968.

Gunn, C.G., Gogerty, J., & S. Wolf: Clinical pharmacology of anticonvulsant compounds. Clin Pharmacol Therap 2:733–749, 1961.

Kutt, H., & F. McDowell: Management of epilepsy with diphenylhydantoin sodium. Dosage regulation for problem patients. JAMA 203:969–972, 1968.

Kutt, H., & others: Diphenylhydantoin metabolism, blood levels, and toxicity. Arch Neurol 11:642–648, 1964.

Neubauer, C.: Mental deterioration in epilepsy due to folate deficiency. Brit MJ 2:759–761, 1970.

Paddison, R.M., & others: Role of antihistamine therapy in diphenylhydantoin induced gingival hyperplasia. Clin Pharmacol Therap 1:316–318, 1960.

Rockliff, B.W., & E.H. Davis: Controlled sequential trials of carbamazepine [Tegretol] in trigeminal neuralgia. Arch Neurol 15:129–136, 1966.

Sawyer, G.T., Webster, D.D., & L.J. Schut: Treatment of uncontrolled seizure activity with diazepam. JAMA 203:913–918, 1968.

Sparberg, M.: Diagnostically confusing complications of diphenylhydantoin therapy: A review. Ann Int Med 59:914–930, 1963.

Wapner, I., Thurston, D.L., & J. Holowach: Phenobarbital: Its effect on learning in epileptic children. JAMA 182:937, 1962.

30 . . .

Drug Treatment of Parkinsonism

Parkinsonism or paralysis agitans is associated with lesions in the substantia nigra and globus pallidus which result in increased but improper modulation of motor activity by the extrapyramidal system. The manifestations of parkinsonism can be placed in 3 groups for purposes of evaluating drug therapy: (1) Akinesia: A paucity of or difficulty in initiating movement beyond that enforced by rigidity. (2) Rigidity: A rigidity that is mild and plastic ("waxy")—ie, it is easily overcome, and the limb stays in the new position forced on it. (3) Tremor: A fine, repetitive tremor may be present at rest.

Levodopa (L-dopa) through its metabolite dopamine, acts on the biochemical defect of parkinsonism and is the most effective drug available for treatment of this disease. Atropine-like drugs and other investigational drugs are less effective but can be given in combination with levodopa.

Chemistry

Dopa is a precursor of dopamine and of norepinephrine (Fig 30–1). Its biotransformation is further discussed below.

Pharmacologic Effects

A. **Mechanisms of Action:** The distribution of dopamine within the CNS parallels that of its metabolite norepinephrine. In addition, the dopamine content of the caudate nuclei and putamen is also high even though these areas contain no norepinephrine.

The idea that supplementary dopamine might be therapeutically useful was first suggested by the study of reserpine. Reserpine depletes the CNS of dopamine and causes a state of extrapyramidal rigidity that is relieved by the use of dopa but not by the administration of hydroxytryptophan, the corresponding precursor of serotonin.

Studies using fluorescence microscopy and differential centrifugation show that the dopamine is concentrated in nerve endings in the caudate nucleus and adjacent striatal areas. These fibers appear to arise from cell bodies in the substantia nigra and are assumed to be dopaminergic—ie, to act by releasing dopamine as a mediator.

In autopsy material from patients with parkinsonism, the dopamine content of the caudate nucleus and putamen is low. The primary histopathologic change in parkinsonism is a decrease in the number of pigmented neurons in the substantia nigra. These observations also suggested that restoring dopamine levels toward normal might ameliorate the signs of parkinsonism.

The first trials of levodopa gave equivocal results, but its usefulness became apparent when chronic treatment with large oral dosages was tried.

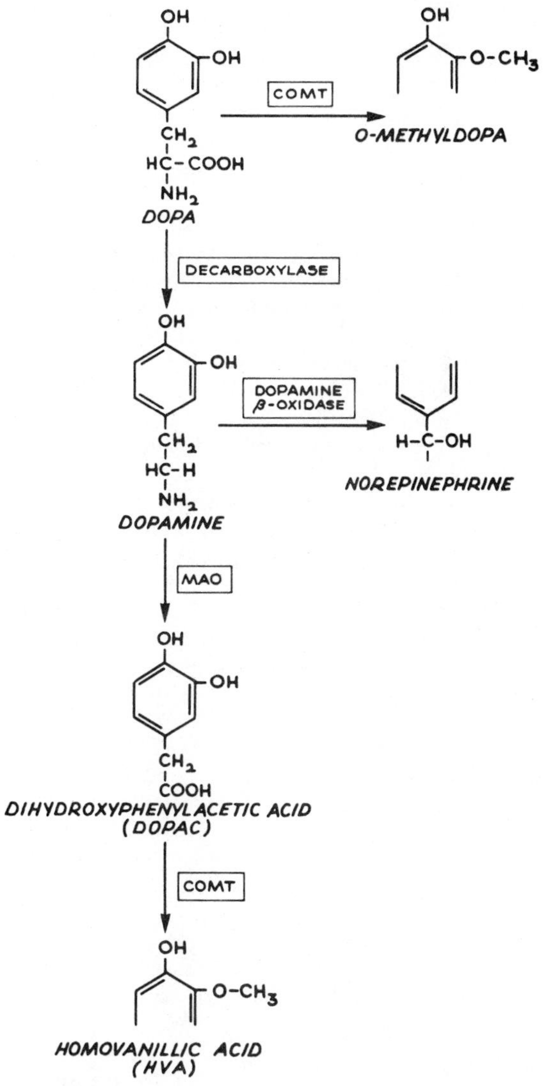

FIG 30–1. Metabolism of dopa and dopamine.

The mechanism of action as currently formulated is that levodopa administration leads to a repair of the dopamine deficiency responsible for parkinsonism. The nigrostriatal fibers that undergo degeneration are assumed to be dopaminergic and to be inhibitory on the next neuron. Symptoms then would be due to uninhibited activity of striatofugal fibers beyond the lesion. If dopamine acts on receptors in cells beyond the nigrostriatal lesion, it is difficult to explain the slow onset of action in the face of the rapid conversion of dopa to dopamine. It is also difficult to reconcile the above formulation with the observation that dopa is still effective after the postulated pathways have been interrupted by previous destructive lesions in the ventrolateral thalamus.

B. Effects:

1. On CNS—The metabolites of levodopa reduce the intensity of parkinsonism. Other CNS effects reflect a stimulant action comparable to that of the sympathomimetic stimulants.

2. Peripheral—The administration of levodopa or of dopamine itself causes some sympathomimetic changes in autonomic tissues. The pupils are dilated, the force of cardiac contraction is increased, and cardiac arrhythmias may be produced. Pupillary dilatation is prevented by the use of guanethidine, suggesting that that sympathomimetic effect at least is not due to a direct action of dopamine on receptors but to a release of norepinephrine. Large doses of dopamine may cause an elevation of blood pressure, but levodopa is more likely to cause postural hypotension through a mechanism as yet unclarified.

Absorption, Metabolism, & Excretion

Levodopa is rapidly and completely absorbed after oral administration, and, even though its effect is slow in onset and prolonged in duration, it is rapidly metabolized, with two-thirds of an oral dose appearing in the urine as metabolites within 8 hours.

The metabolism of levodopa is predominantly by decarboxylation to dopamine. The extent to which this reaction occurs after levodopa has entered the CNS and, therefore, contributes to its therapeutic effect cannot be determined since decarboxylation also occurs in the lumen of the intestine and in the liver and other organs. In addition, a significant fraction of ingested levodopa is inactivated by conversion to O-methyldopa before decarboxylation.

Dopamine is oxidatively deaminated to phenylacetic acid derivatives and O-methylated. Of the 25–30 urinary metabolites, homovanillic acid (Fig 30–1) is predominant, accounting for 40% of a single dose. Only a minute amount of the extra dopamine is converted to norepinephrine.

Levodopa must be given in large amounts to exert its beneficial effects on the CNS because most of it is wasted by metabolism in the periphery. Decarboxylase inhibitors have been used successfully to increase the amount available for entry into the CNS. MAO inhibitors might also be expected to intensify the levodopa effect by decreasing the metabolism of dopa-

mine, but they must not be used since their administration results in hypertensive episodes.

Clinical Use

The effectiveness of levodopa in the treatment of idiopathic parkinsonism has been established by double-blind studies and by studies using objective evaluations of motor function. Levodopa is clearly superior to the parasympatholytic type of drug and to amantadine, but it can be combined with those drugs for added benefit.

Akinesia is most improved—ie, the patient is more active even if rigidity and tremor persist. Rigidity usually is relieved. Tremor may subside only after a long period of treatment, or be uninfluenced. Only about one out of 4 patients fails to benefit significantly or cannot tolerate levodopa.

Improvement may not be maximal until treatment has been continued for 2–6 months. The beneficial effect persists for more than 3 weeks after the administration of levodopa is discontinued.

Patients with postencephalitic parkinsonism—a small group now since the epidemic peaked in 1917—tolerate only small doses of levodopa and experience more side-effects, especially choreiform movements. Parkinsonism that results from damage due to manganese, hypoxia, or trauma also responds.

An interesting result of the availability of effective therapy is that drug sales became an indication of the incidence of the disease, which now appears to be much lower than previously estimated.

Adverse Reactions

As levodopa is used—in gradually increasing doses—side-effects invariably occur, and the distinction between side-effects and overdosage toxicity disappears. Adverse reactions force discontinuance of therapy in only about 5% of cases, although they limit dosage in a much larger percentage of patients.

A. Gastrointestinal: Nausea and anorexia (often with vomiting) occur in virtually all patients. The symptoms are partially local in origin and to that extent can be controlled by dividing the dose and giving the drug with food or antacids. However, vomiting also occurs after the injection of levodopa.

Those antiemetics that are phenothiazines and major tranquilizers are said by some investigators to be contraindicated because they will counteract the levodopa effect; others report that they are useful.

B. Cardiovascular:

1. Cardiac arrhythmias—The sympathomimetic effect of the dopamine generated outside of the CNS can cause tachycardia, ventricular extrasystoles, and, rarely, atrial fibrillation.

2. Hypotension—The hypertension that would be predicted as a dopamine effect does occur, but only after huge doses of levodopa or in the presence of MAO inhibitors or other sympathomimetics. However, postural hypotension is always demonstrable and may cause faintness. The hypotension tends to become less severe with continued treatment.

C. Neurologic:

1. Behavioral—Levodopa has some effects comparable to those of a sympathomimetic stimulant such as amphetamine. These result in euphoria, anxiety, and insomnia and may progress to a toxic psychosis or acute brain syndrome with delusions and hallucinations and paranoid behavior.

On the other hand, depression and somnolence may also appear.

2. Dyskinetic—Patients with parkinsonism may develop abnormal, involuntary movements during treatment with levodopa—ie, in large doses the drug may precipitate some extrapyramidal signs as it is relieving others. The choreiform movements may involve the head and limbs but are often faciolingual. The grimacing and chewing movements, together with uncontrolled movement of the tongue, can be socially disabling and force a reduction in dosage even if this also reduces the therapeutic effect.

A fine tremor that is not extrapyramidal in origin may also appear.

D. Allergic: The Coombs test may become positive during treatment with levodopa but without hemolytic episodes such as are seen during methyldopa administration.

Contraindications & Cautions

Levodopa should not be given to patients with recent myocardial infarction, to those with a cardiac dysrhythmia, or to excited or paranoid psychotics.

Levodopa should be used only with caution and careful observation of the patient in the presence of depression.

Interaction With Other Drugs

Levodopa should be combined with the anticholinergic type of antiparkinson drugs and has been combined with amantadine and amphetamine without difficulty. The efforts to increase the effects of levodopa by giving it in combination with an inhibitor of decarboxylase are mentioned above.

A. Pyridoxine: The administration of pyridoxine even in the form of the ordinary vitamin preparations is equivalent to a reduction in the dosage of levodopa. The antagonism is presumably due to an increase in the activity of decarboxylases outside of the CNS for which pyridoxine is a cofactor.

B. MAO Inhibitors: MAO inhibition augments the peripheral effects of dopamine and may cause hypertension and tachycardia.

C. Major Tranquilizers: Reserpine, which depletes the basal ganglia of dopamine, should not be given with levodopa. The phenothiazine type of antipsychotic tranquilizer may also cause a parkinsonism-like state in toxic dosage, but there is no evidence—although this has often been suggested—that smaller (antiemetic) doses interfere with this action of dopa. Antidepressants of the imipramine type are pharmacologically indistinguishable from the phenothiazines but are actually recommended for use. Methyldopa, an antihypertensive drug with side-effects similar to the

tranquilizers, has been described as both useful and deleterious when combined with dopa.

Preparations & Dosages

Levodopa is given in gradually increasing dosage until the maximal therapeutic response is achieved, until side-effects severe enough to limit the dosage appear, or until a dosage of 8 gm/day is reached. The usual requirement is 4–6 gm/day.

The initial dosage is usually 0.5–1 gm/day divided into 2 doses with food. The daily amount is increased by 150–500 mg/day every 2–3 days. Extending the interval over which the final dosage is reached does not decrease the incidence of side-effects or change the maximal tolerated dose. By the time maximal dosage is reached, the drug should be given 3–4 times daily with food.

Levodopa (Bendopa, Dopar, Levopa, Larodopa) is available as capsules of 100, 250, and 500 mg or tablets of 250 and 500 mg.

ATROPINE-LIKE DRUGS

Chemistry & Classification

The central anticholinergic drugs used in the treatment of parkinsonism are selected from or related to drug classes already discussed.

A. Parasympatholytic or Cholinolytic: The belladonna alkaloids were the first drugs used to relieve the rigidity of extrapyramidal states. Scopolamine (hyoscine) is still used infrequently, but the natural alkaloids have been largely replaced by synthetic drugs related to the synthetic substitutes for atropine. (See Fig 30–2 and Table 30–1.)

B. Antihistamines: The structure and pharmacology of diphenhydramine (Benadryl) is given in Chapter 19. Orphenadrine and chlorphenoxamine (Table 30–1) are methyl- and chloro- derivatives.

C. Phenothiazine Tranquilizer: Ethopropazine is a phenothiazine derivative, the diethyl analogue of the antipsychotic tranquilizer promethazine (Table 25–1).

Pharmacologic Effects

A. Mechanisms of Action: The central anticholinergic action of these drugs is established by the observation that physostigmine (a cholinesterase inhibitor that enters the CNS) exacerbates the signs of parkinsonism and the action is blocked by tertiary amine but not by quaternary amine atropine-like drugs.

The most common suggestion is that the site of action is a cholinergic neuron immediately distal to the dopaminergic fiber that courses from the substantia nigra to the caudate nucleus. In parkinsonism, the cholinergic system is relieved of the constant inhibitory effect of dopamine following degeneration of the fibers from the substantia nigra. It is assumed that the resulting signs of parkinsonism are due to

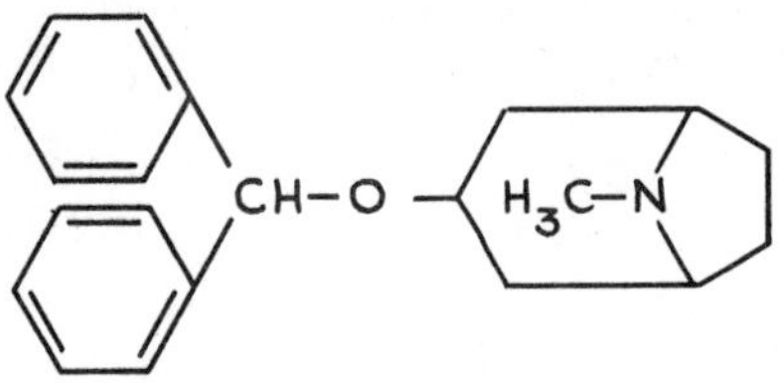

Benztropine
(Cogentin)

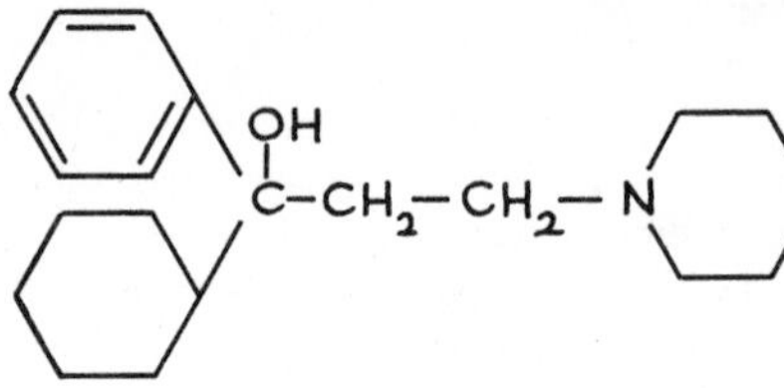

Trihexyphenidyl
(Artane)

FIG 30—2. Chemical structure of representative drugs that resemble the synthetic substitutes for atropine and the antihistamines and are used in the treatment of parkinsonism.

increased activity of the cholinergic system and are blocked by acetylcholine antagonists. The primary pathologic change is undoubtedly in the basal ganglia, but drugs may act at any of several levels to modify the resulting process. The rigidity of parkinsonism is due to persistent activity in both the agonist and antagonist muscles of a functional pair, and is associated with increased gamma-efferent outflow and a heightened sensitivity of the monosynaptic (tendon) reflexes.

A property demonstrated for some of the drugs used in the treatment of parkinsonism is the ability to suppress gamma-efferent activity. This effect, discussed in Chapter 23 in the treatment of tetanus, is most clearly demonstrated for chlorpromazine. Chlorpromazine and related tranquilizers relieve parkinsonism when given in small doses and precipitate

it in larger doses. The effect on cord reactivity is probably secondary to an action on a suprasegmental site.

B. Effects: The effects of these drugs are the same as those of the parasympatholytic agents and antipsychotic tranquilizers already described. They are less potent in their atropine-like and chlorpromazine-like effects.

Use in Parkinsonism

The effectiveness of these drugs by themselves is usually not very great. Some amelioration of the rigidity is the expected response. However, combined with levodopa, the atropine-like drugs help control hypersalivation and other symptoms.

**TABLE 30—1. Atropine-like drugs used in the treatment of parkinsonism:
Dosages and preparations available.**

	Usual Adult Dosage (3—4 Times Daily)	Preparations Available
Parasympatholytics		
Trihexyphenidyl (Artane, Pipanol, Tremin)	1—5 mg	Tablets, 2 and 5 mg Sustained release capsules, 5 mg Elixir, 2 mg/5 ml, in pints
Procyclidine (Kemadrin)	2.5—5 mg	Tablets, 5 mg
Cycrimine (Pagitane)	1.25—5 mg	Tablets, 1.25 and 2.5 mg
Biperiden (Akineton)	1—2 mg	Tablets, 2 mg Injectable lactate (IM or IV), 5 mg/ml, 1 ml ampules
Benztropine (Cogentin)	0.5—2.5 mg (twice daily)	Tablets, 0.5, 1, and 2 mg Injectable (IM or IV), 1 mg/ml, 2 ml ampules
Caramiphen (Panparnit)*	. . .	. . .
Antihistamines		
Diphenhydramine (Benadryl)	50 mg	Capsules, 25 and 50 mg Elixir, 10 mg/4 ml, 4 oz, pints, and gallons Injectable (IM or IV), 10 mg/ml, 10 and 30 ml vials; 50 mg/ml, 1 ml ampules
Orphenadrine (Disipal, Norflex)	50 mg	Tablets, 50 and 100 mg Injectable (IM or IV), 30 mg/ml, 2 ml ampules
Chlorphenoxamine (Phenoxene)	50 mg	Tablets, 50 mg
Phenothiazine		
Ethopropazine (Parsidol)	25—50 mg	Tablets, 10, 50, and 100 mg

*No longer marketed in USA except as constituent of proprietary cough mixtures.

Adverse Reactions

All of these drugs cause atropine-like effects—eg, blurred vision, dry mouth, constipation—as well as drowsiness, dizziness, and a subjectively unpleasant feeling of sedation.

Contraindications & Cautions

These atropine-like drugs can be used in the presence of glaucoma if glaucoma treatment is continued and the intraocular pressure is determined periodically.

Preparations & Dosages (See Table 30–1.)

There are no sound clinical studies to permit accurate comparison of agents or to suggest one regimen or another.

Treatment should be started with small doses and the amount slowly increased to tolerance or the maximum recommended dose. Abrupt changes in drug or dosage should not be made since it may intensify the symptoms.

OTHER DRUGS USED IN THE TREATMENT OF PARKINSONISM

In the past, dextroamphetamine was often used to minimize the tranquilizing effect of the anticholinergics. It also was said to increase mobility and prevent the oculogyric crises of postencephalitic parkinsonism.

Amantadine (Symmetrel) is another amine used investigationally in the treatment of parkinsonism. Its chemical structure is shown in Chapter 57, where amantadine is discussed as an antiviral drug. Amantadine has limited efficacy when used alone, but it can be combined with levodopa. In large doses, it has central stimulant and hallucinatory effects.

• • •

General References

Friedman, A.H., & G.M. Everett: Pharmacological aspects of parkinsonism. Advances Pharmacol 3:83–127, 1964.

Godwin-Austen, R.B., Frears, C.C., & S. Bergman: Incidence of side-effects from levodopa during the introduction of treatment. Brit MJ 1:267–268, 1971.

Hughes, R.C., & others: Levodopa in parkinsonism: The effects of withdrawal of anticholinergic drugs. Brit MJ 2:487–491, 1971.

Rushworth,.G.: Some aspects of the pathophysiology of spasticity and rigidity. Clin Pharmacol Therap 5:828–836, 1964.

Schwab, R.S., & A.C. England: Parkinson's disease. J Chronic Dis 8:488–509, 1958.

Symposium on levodopa. JAMA 218:1903–1927, 1971.

Symposium on levodopa in Parkinson's disease. Clin Pharmacol Therap 12:317–416, 1971.

Walker, J.E., & others: Amantadine and levodopa in the treatment of Parkinson's disease. Clin Pharmacol Therap 13:28–36, 1972.

Part IV. Systemic Drugs

31 . . .

Gastrointestinal Drugs

Some of the drugs that act on the gastrointestinal tract have already been discussed. The parasympatholytic drugs and narcotic analgesics decrease intestinal motility, and the parasympathomimetic drugs augment motility. The present chapter considers 2 widely used drug classes, antacids and laxatives, and defines a number of less important drug actions.

ANTACIDS

Gastric antacids are weak bases that partially neutralize the acid gastric secretion. If they elevate the pH above 4.0–4.5, they also inhibit the activity of pepsin.

Antacids are divided into 2 classes. **Systemic antacids,** of which sodium bicarbonate is the only common example, can be absorbed and cause systemic alkalosis. The more commonly used **nonsystemic antacids** either form insoluble products in the small intestine or contain a nonabsorbable cation.

Pharmacologic Effects

A. **Systemic Antacids:** Sodium bicarbonate (baking soda) is the only systemic antacid that need be considered. A fraction of the sodium bicarbonate reacts with hydrochloric acid to liberate carbon dioxide:

$$HCO_3^- + H^+ \longrightarrow H_2O + CO_2 \uparrow$$

The rapid action, the apparently beneficial effect of the gaseous distention, the subjective relief afforded by the belching induced, and its availability in most households probably account for the popularity of "soda."

Ingesting sodium bicarbonate is equivalent to ingesting additional sodium without additional chloride. Bicarbonate in the intestine is increased either (1) by that ingested and not neutralized in the stomach, or (2) by the sparing of the bicarbonate of intestinal secretions that would otherwise be used to neutralize the acid mixture reaching the small intestine. Since it is easily absorbed, the sodium bicarbonate is, in effect, added to extracellular fluid. An alkaline urine is excreted until the excess sodium is disposed of.

In addition to causing systemic alkalosis upon repeated ingestion, sodium bicarbonate—or the eleva-

tion in pH that it produces—greatly increases gastric secretion shortly after its administration, and the hypersecretion may outlast the presence of bicarbonate in the gastric contents. Rebound secretion or rebound hyperacidity is thus an additional objection to the use of soda except on infrequent occasions.

B. **Nonsystemic Antacids:**

1. **Action as antacids**—Nonsystemic antacids react to remove hydrogen ions from solution at the acid pH of the gastric contents. However, in the alkaline medium of the small intestine, hydrogen ion is again released, and the antacid is either restored to its original insoluble state or, as in the case of magnesium compounds, the products of the reaction are not absorbed even if they are slightly soluble.

For example, aluminum (or magnesium) hydroxide reacts as follows:

$$Al(OH)_3 + 3HCl \underset{\text{IN INTESTINE}}{\overset{\text{IN STOMACH}}{\rightleftarrows}}$$

$$AlCl_3 + 3H_2O$$

Magnesium trisilicate ($2MgO \cdot 3SiO_2 \cdot xH_2O$) reacts thus:

$$Mg_2Si_3O_8 + 4H^+ \longrightarrow$$

$$2Mg^{++} + 3SiO_2 + 2H_2O$$

The trisilicate is not regenerated, but the reaction is, in effect, reversible since at the alkaline pH of the intestine magnesium carbonate is formed and chloride made available for reabsorption.

Another nonsystemic antacid and perhaps the best single agent in use is calcium carbonate, which reacts in the stomach as does sodium bicarbonate:

$$CaCO_3 + 2H^+ \longrightarrow$$

$$Ca^{++} + H_2O + CO_2$$

but which at pH 8.0 in the intestine is precipitated again as $CaCO_3$.

A final example is magnesium oxide, a powder, which in suspension is hydrated to magnesium hydroxide or milk of magnesia.

2. Other properties—The insoluble nonsystemic antacids such as aluminum hydroxide or calcium carbonate are constipating. The nonabsorbable but slightly soluble magnesium salts have a slight laxative effect.

The colloidal suspensions formed by the aluminum preparations or by magnesium hydroxide or magnesium trisilicate are adsorbent, but there is no reason to relate this property to their effectiveness as antacids.

Clinical Uses

A. Treatment of Peptic Ulcer: The treatment of peptic ulcer provides a good example of the need for controlled clinical trials in all areas of therapy, whether by means of drugs or other modalities. It is impossible to present more than an intuitive evaluation of many of the diverse and strongly held opinions about treatment of this very common problem. Therapeutic trials of the drugs used in the treatment of peptic ulcer must separately evaluate the rate of healing of an ulcer, the number of recurrences and the intervals between recurrences, and the relief of pain during acute episodes. It is apparently true that treatment does relieve the pain of peptic ulcer, but it has not been established that highly restricted diets, parasympatholytic drugs, or antacids have a favorable effect on healing or recurrence of ulcers. Perhaps the only advance in this area of treatment during the past few years has been the development of skepticism and acceptance of the above conclusion as the consensus.

Even so, few would doubt that most patients are helped by consulting a physician about a peptic ulcer regimen. Relief of pain and longer-term benefits accrue from the following:

1. Nonspecific treatment—Explanation and reassurance, often in the form of hospitalization, and assistance with the problem of learning to live with stressful factors in the environment are not the least of the treatment resources the physician can offer his ulcer patients. Sedatives may be given for daytime anxiety and hypnotics for sleep.

2. Antacids—When antacids are used, the suggestions listed below (see Selection of Antacid) should be followed. Gastric emptying usually limits the duration of antacid effect to 30–60 minutes. Antacids should be given at hourly intervals or an antacid tablet kept constantly in the mouth.

3. Diet—Food, in the context of this discussion, is both an antacid and a stimulus to acid secretion. Food containing protein may neutralize acid for a few minutes and reduce motility, but will then increase gastric secretion and perhaps pain.

Frequent small feedings are equivalent to the use of antacids, and the presence of food in the stomach will slow the passage of an antacid into the intestine and prolong the buffering effect of the antacid. Certain common sense dietary restrictions, eg, all caffeine-containing foods and foods known by the patient to cause distress, are an important part of management.

4. Parasympatholytics—In the discussion of the use of atropine and its congeners, it was emphasized that the acute effects of large single doses cannot be extrapolated to predict the effects of doses that are tolerated when the drugs are chronically administered. Many explanations have been offered for the possible beneficial effects of atropine—eg, that by decreasing motility it holds the antacid in the stomach for a longer period—but the beneficial effect in the chronic rather than the acute situation has yet to be demonstrated.

Acutely, the parasympatholytic drugs do appear to reduce that fraction of discomfort associated with hypermotility or pylorospasm.

5. Other drugs—The deleterious effect of caffeine, alcohol, tobacco, phenylbutazone, and corticosteroids on the course of some patients with a peptic ulcer has been mentioned in other chapters. These drugs should be avoided in the ulcer patient, but if avoidance is not possible their ill effects can be minimized in some cases by the simultaneous administration of an antacid or atropine.

6. Investigative drugs—Carbenoxolone (Biogastrone) is an anti-inflammatory agent related to glycyrrhizinic acid and isolated from licorice. It has a demonstrated beneficial effect on gastric but not duodenal ulcers.

B. Other Uses: Many functional gastroduodenal upsets (heartburn, pylorospasm, etc) are treated with antacids with good symptomatic relief. Antacids in these as in other situations are often self-prescribed and purchased without a prescription.

Hiatal hernias are treated with drugs as are peptic ulcers.

Aluminum hydroxide gel is sometimes used in large doses to reduce phosphate absorption in uremia.

Adverse Reactions

Considering the frequency with which large amounts of antacids are chronically used, they must be regarded as almost innocuous agents.

A. Change in Bowel Habits: Some patients do not find the continuous use of a single antacid acceptable since all of them have disadvantages. Calcium carbonate is constipating; the hydrated aluminum salts are partially dried in the large intestine and result in powdery and difficult stools; and the magnesium salts by themselves may cause frequent or liquid movements. As a result, preparations that are mixtures of several antacids are more satisfactory.

B. Alkalosis: Sodium bicarbonate used chronically will cause alkalosis.

C. Milk-Alkali Syndrome: A few cases have been reported in which systemic alkalosis from soluble antacids and a high calcium intake from milk also used in the treatment of ulcers has led to hypercalcemia and metastatic calcification, especially in the kidneys, and stone formation.

TABLE 31−1. Some representative antacids.

	Usual Adult Dose	Preparations Available
Aluminum hydroxide gel or tablets (Amphojel and other proprietary preparations)	1−2 tsp in ½ glass water or 1−2 tablets chewed and swallowed with ½ glass water	Gel supplied as such, 320 mg/5 ml Tablets, 300, 320, 500, 600, and 650 mg
Aluminum hydroxide with magnesium trisilicate Gelusil	2 tablets or 1−2 tsp	Tablets containing 250 mg aluminum hydroxide and 500 mg magnesium trisilicate Liquid containing those amounts per 4 ml, in 6 oz and 12 oz
Aluminum and magnesium hydroxide Maalox	1−2 tablets or 5−10 ml	Tablets, 400 and 800 mg Liquid, 400 mg/5 ml, in 12 oz
Calcium carbonate	1−4 gm of powder suspended in water or tablets chewed and swallowed	Tablets, 600 mg
Dihydroxyaluminum aminoacetate (Alzinox, Robalate)	1−2 tablets or 5−10 ml	Tablets, 500 mg Liquid, 500 mg/5 ml, in 8 and 12 oz

Selection of Antacid

A. Time and Frequency of Administration: The ability of an antacid to neutralize gastric acid and the duration of its effect—ie, its duration in the stomach—have been studied by gastroscopic examination and by aspirating a series of samples through a gastric tube. Most studies show a duration of action of no more than 1 hour, although it is probable that, if the antacid is given within 1 hour after a meal, it may be slowly carried out of the stomach and the effect will persist for as long as 3 hours. When the treatment problem is acute, antacids are usually given hourly until the response allows a lengthening of the interval between doses.

B. Potency: No antacid exceeds calcium carbonate in its acid-neutralizing ability, but differences in potency are not great if adequate doses of the various preparations are used. The usual doses of the common antacids (2 tablets or 2 tsp) are minimal doses.

C. Patient Acceptance: Patient preference then becomes a major factor in the choice of an antacid. Antacids are available without prescription, and most patients try several and soon develop a preference for liquid or tablet or for a preparation with a particular texture or flavor. More important, they react to the changes in bowel habits. The physician and pharmacist should cooperate in finding a preparation that does not cause an intolerable change in consistency or frequency of bowel movements or should teach the patient to use more than one preparation.

Preparations Available

Antacids and mixtures of antacids are available under many brand names. The various products may differ somewhat in composition and flavor, and brand names are listed for each general group in Table 31−1 only to provide an example of composition and available preparations. The mixture of aluminum and magnesium hydroxides, for example, is available as Maalox, Mylanta, Aludrox, Bidrox, Creamalin, and Wingel—to select only a few of the more widely distributed products.

LAXATIVES

Purgation was at one time just as popular and probably just as dangerous a form of treatment as bleeding. Physicians have stopped prescribing or advising the use of purgatives, but the laity are only slowly and reluctantly giving up the idea that laxatives and enemas are an important part of general treatment for virtually all illnesses. These drugs were classified during the older period according to the intensity of their effect, and several terms persist—laxative, aperient, cathartic, purgative, "drastic"—depending upon whether the agent is mild in its action or is able to cause more frequent and liquid movements. It is probably better to avoid the old terms and to classify laxatives according to their mechanism of action. The mechanism may be simply to stimulate motility and cause defecation. However, drugs may also be given to increase the bulk of the stool or to soften it.

Pharmacologic Effects

A. Irritant or Stimulant Laxatives:

1. Castor oil—Castor oil has a distinctive and unpleasant taste. When it is hydrolyzed like other fats in the upper small intestine, irritating ricinoleic acid is liberated and acts locally to increase intestinal motility. The action of castor oil is thus prompt and is eventually exerted along the entire length of the gastrointestinal tract. By stimulating motility, it hastens its own excretion with the feces, but until this occurs it is a vigorous laxative, causing repeated movements, often with cramping.

A number of other powerful irritants such as croton oil or calomel were once used as "drastics" but are now obsolete.

2. Anthraquinone or emodin alkaloids—Cascara, senna, rhubarb, and aloes contain emodin alkaloids in the inactive form of glycosides. The active alkaloid is liberated from the glycoside after absorption, and it is then excreted into the colon. After a period of 6–8 hours (required for absorption and excretion), these drugs act locally on the colon to stimulate peristalsis.

3. Phenolphthalein is also a powerful stimulant of the large bowel. Some of it is absorbed, excreted through the bile, and absorbed again, and this enterohepatic cycle prolongs its activity. It is present in proprietaries and can cause a fixed drug eruption.

Bisacodyl (Dulcolax) is a synthetic compound that is chemically similar to phenolphthalein and is similarly absorbed and excreted.

B. Bulk Laxatives: Distention is a powerful stimulus to intestinal activity, and bulk and bulk-producing substances or solutions may therefore be used to augment intestinal activity. Furthermore, what some patients refer to as constipation is actually a subjective feeling of dissatisfaction with their bowel habits which may be relieved by increasing the bulk of the movements rather than their frequency.

1. Hydrophilic colloids—The indigestible parts of fruits and vegetables are the obvious natural source of this material, and a diet that contains adequate amounts of these items serves the same purpose as the prepared products. Bran, agar, psyllium seed, and methylcellulose are examples of substances that form gels within the large intestine and accomplish the dual purpose of distending the colon and satisfying a need of the patient.

2. Saline cathartics or nonabsorbable salts—The volume of the intestinal contents can be kept large by the ingestion of a nonabsorbable salt. The salt will hold water in the intestine in amounts sufficient to maintain its concentration isotonic, and soft or liquid bowel movements will follow when the saline solution is carried to the terminal part of the colon. Examples of this class are magnesium sulfate (Epsom salts), magnesium citrate, and magnesium hydroxide (milk of magnesia).

C. Fecal Softeners: Here again, factors other than the number of bowel movements are involved. During illness, with immobilization and dietary change, the contents of the distal colon may become desiccated, hard, or even impacted. It may be desirable to maintain a soft stool to minimize the discomfort or actual work involved in defecation. For this purpose, agents that mix with the fecal material or act as emulsifying agents are used.

Mineral oil is a commonly used example of this class. It is often referred to as a lubricant, but it softens the fecal material by becoming emulsified with it

rather than acting as a lubricant in the mechanical sense. If a slight excess of mineral oil is given, some may pass the anal sphincter and soil the skin or clothing. The concern that the chronic administration of mineral oil might dissolve significant amounts of fat-soluble vitamins and prevent their absorption is entirely theoretical.

Other examples of this class are glycerin suppositories, soapy or mineral oil enemas, and detergents such as dioctyl sodium sulfosuccinate, an anionic surface active agent marketed under many names.

Clinical Uses

A. Treatment of Constipation: These drugs may be ordered by the physician to treat constipation in specific situations of brief duration—eg, they may be used to relieve the constipation that follows the use of opiate drugs or to keep the feces soft during the period following hemorrhoidectomy.

However, most of the huge amount of these drugs consumed is self-prescribed for the treatment of what the individual considers to be constipation. Some people feel that there is a normal frequency of bowel movements that must be maintained; others still feel, perhaps as a carry-over of the concept of autointoxication, that they must clean themselves out at intervals to maintain good health; and many people have a neurotic preoccupation with their bowel habits that is not concerned solely with the number of movements.

Constipation is more common among older people, in part because of restricted activity and dietary factors, or failure to drink enough water. However, they also tend to use more laxatives because their attitudes were formed during a period when "regular bowel habits" were felt to be important to general well-being. If insufficient water is being taken, the patient should be advised to drink at least 1 (preferably 2) quarts of fluid a day. Two glasses of warm water before breakfast is of help in some situations. If the pattern of the patient's complaint justifies it, one of the above agents, particularly the hydrophilic colloids or a detergent such as dioctyl sodium sulfosuccinate, may be used even on a chronic basis. Explanation is undoubtedly preferable, but it is rarely accepted and laxatives are freely available without prescription.

The objection to the use of laxatives is that they may reinforce a neurotic preoccupation with bowel habits. Furthermore, the use of laxatives may become habitual since there must be an interval following an evacuation induced by a laxative before the next movement (while the content of the colon is replenished from above). If this interval seems to the individual to be too long, he may repeat the laxative rather than wait for an unstimulated movement. This again defers the unstimulated movement and again suggests the use of a laxative, and the cycle can be repeated indefinitely.

B. Other Uses: Castor oil and cleansing enemas are frequently used in preparation for x-ray studies. The colon must be emptied prior to outlining it with a contrast medium. Gas and fecal material that might

TABLE 31–2. Some representative laxatives: Dosages and preparations available.

	Usual Adult Dose	Preparations Available
Irritant or stimulant		
Castor oil	15 ml	As such
Emulsified castor oil (Neoloid)	2–4 tbsp	Emulsion, aqueous, 36%, 120 ml
Cascara sagrada, aromatic fluidextract	2 ml	As such
Cascara tablets	300 mg	Tablets, 120, 200, and 300 mg
Senna extract (Senokot)	275–825 mg/day	Tablets, 275 mg Granules, 450 mg packs Suppositories
Rhubarb and soda mixture	4 ml at bedtime	As such
Bisacodyl (Dulcolax)	10–15 mg at bedtime	Enteric-coated tablets, 5 mg Suppositories, 10 mg
Bulk producers		
Milk of magnesia	15–30 ml at bedtime with water	As such
Sodium phosphate	4–8 gm before breakfast with water	As such
Psyllium (plantago) seed (Metamucil, Konsyl)	1–3 rounded tsp/day in water	Granules and powder
Methylcellulose (Cellothyl, Hydrolose)	1–4 gm/day	Tablets, 500 mg Capsules, 500 mg Syrup, 5.91 gm/30 ml Solution, 9 gm/100 ml
Sodium carboxymethylcellulose (C.M.C.)	3–6 gm/day	Tablets, 500 mg and 1 gm Capsules, 650 mg
Fecal softeners		
Mineral oil	15–30 ml daily	As such
Mineral oil with agar	15–30 ml daily	As such
Dioctyl sodium sulfosuccinate Colace	50–200 mg/day	Capsules and tablets, 50, 60, 100, 150, 200, and 250 mg Liquid, 10 mg/ml Syrup, 20 mg/5 ml, 240 ml
Doxinate	50–280 mg/day	Capsules, 60 and 240 mg Pediatric solution, 50 mg/ml, 60 ml
Poloxalkol Magcyl	100–250 mg 1–3 times daily	Capsules, 250 mg Solution, 250 mg/5 ml
Polykol	100–250 mg 1–3 times daily	Capsules, 250 mg Drops, 200 mg/ml, 30 ml

otherwise cast interfering shadows are also removed by castor oil or other laxatives prior to gallbladder studies, intravenous and retrograde urograms, and other diagnostic procedures.

Adverse Reactions

The possibility that the use of laxatives may reinforce the patient's concept of constipation as a health hazard or of establishing the laxative habit has been mentioned. Cramping pain is the only other common side-effect of these drugs. The continued use of cathartics has on very rare occasions led to reversible hypokalemia or to a persistent diarrhea and hypokalemia due to damage to the colon.

Ingestion of laxatives containing oxyphenisatin, an irritant laxative related to phenolphthalein, has been associated with hepatocellular damage (chronic active hepatitis) as a hypersensitivity reaction. Oxyphenisatin has been removed from the market in the USA.

Contraindications & Cautions

Laxatives should not be used in the presence of undiagnosed abdominal pain or when the constipation is due to obstruction, including fecal impaction. Magnesium salts should not be used if renal insufficiency is present, and all but the mildest agents should be avoided during the later stages of pregnancy. The emodin alkaloids are transmitted by the nursing mother to the child.

Dosages & Preparations Available
See Table 31—2.

A FEW ADDITIONAL DEFINITIONS

Demulcents are substances with physical properties that allow them to coat and protect and soothe a surface. Antipruritic preparations applied to the skin and cough syrups are examples. Among the gastrointestinal drugs, bismuth carbonate, bismuth subacetate, and bismuth subgallate were at one time used to coat the irritated or ulcerated gastric mucosa. They are now rarely used.

Adsorbents are colloidal substances (charcoal, clays such as kaolin, and gels such as pectin) which are able to adsorb undesired constituents from solution. They are used in proprietary antidiarrheal mixtures because of their presumed ability to adsorb preformed toxins responsible for some types of food poisoning.

Bitters are preparations of alkaloids or other plant products given before meals to increase appetite.

Hydrochloric acid was formerly used as replacement therapy in a few patients with achlorhydria and symptoms thought to be related thereto. The consensus now is that there is no real indication for the use of acid.

Glutamic acid hydrochloride, which releases hydrochloric acid in the stomach, was also used in the past, but it has been withdrawn from the market.

A **carminative** is a volatile oil (in drug, liqueur, or candy) which is able to relieve the feeling of discomfort and distention after eating by aiding in the eructation or movement of gas from the stomach. Some patients with serious diseases do have their food intake limited by discomfort of this kind, and some physicians still prescribe a few drops of oil of peppermint in a small glass of warm water. Studies on the response of the gastroesophageal sphincter provide some objective basis for the practice.

A **cholagogue** is a drug or procedure that causes the gallbladder to contract and empty. The fatty meal used after the gallbladder is filled with a contrast medium to demonstrate that it empties or "functions" is an example—as is, of course, the average meal, which causes the release of 8 gm of bile salts into the intestine. Magnesium sulfate was instilled into the duodenum in the past and the duodenal contents subsequently aspirated for study.

Choleretics are drugs that increase the total flow of bile with a decrease in viscosity of the bile. Salts of bile acids (hog and ox bile extracts) do have this effect, but indications for their use have not been established. When they are used, **dehydrocholic acid** is preferred. It has a bitter taste and does have established use in measuring arm-to-tongue circulation time. In this application, 5 ml of a 20% solution of **sodium dehydrocholate (Decholin Sodium** and other names) are rapidly injected into an antecubital vein. Normally, the subject will report a bitter taste within 10—16 seconds. **Florantyrone (Zanchol)** is a synthetic drug structurally unrelated to the bile salts but which is also a choleretic.

Cholesterol is held in suspension in the bile by micelles of bile acids and lecithin. In patients with cholesterol cholelithiasis, the amounts of bile salts which appear in the bile each day are reduced. **Chenodeoxycholic acid** is one of the 3 common bile acids in humans and is an investigative drug which has dissolved or reduced the size of cholesterol gallstones in the few cases so far studied. (The structure of cholic acid is shown in Fig 15—2. Chenodeoxycholic acid lacks the hydroxyl on C12.)

PANCREATIN

Lipolytic and proteolytic enzymes must be given as replacement therapy to patients with pancreatic (exocrine) insufficiency.

Pancreatin is an alcoholic extract of hog pancreas standardized for amylase and trypsin activity. No assay for lipase is established, and the activity of the official preparation is variable.

Pancrelipase (Cotazym), a lipase-enriched pancreatin, and Viokase, which consists of desiccated gland rather than an extract, are more active than the official preparation. Problems of standardization, size and frequency of dose, and gastric inactivation persist, but some limited improvement in lipid and nitrogen absorption is usually possible.

●   ●   ●

General References

Antacids

Cameron, A.J., & M.P. Spence: Chronic milk-alkali syndrome after prolonged excessive intake of antacid tablets. Brit MJ 3:656–657, 1967.

Fordtran, J.S., & J.A.H. Collyns: Antacid pharmacology in duodenal ulcer. Effect of antacids on postcibal gastric acidity and peptic activity. New England J Med 274:921–927, 1966.

Kirsner, J.B.: Symposium: Clinical drug evaluation. Part XIII. Problems in the evaluation of gastrointestinal drugs. Clin Pharmacol Therap 3:510–518, 1962.

McMillan, D.E., & R.B. Freeman: The milk alkali syndrome: A study of the acute disorder with comments on the development of the chronic condition. Medicine 44:485–502, 1965.

Morrissey, J.F., & others: Gastric mucosal coating and gastric emptying time of antacids. A gastrocamera study. Arch Int Med 119:510–517, 1967.

Laxatives

Davidson, M., Kugler, M.M., & C.H. Bauer: Diagnosis and management in children with severe and protracted constipation and obstipation. J Pediat 62:261–275, 1963.

Rawson, M.D.: Cathartic colon. Lancet 1:1121–1124, 1966.

Reynolds, T.B., Peters, R.L., & S. Yamada: Chronic active and lupoid hepatitis caused by a laxative, oxyphenisatin. New England J Med 285:813–820, 1971.

Smith, B.: Effect of irritant purgatives on the myenteric plexus in man and the mouse. Gut 9:139–143, 1968.

Steigmann, F.: Are laxatives necessary? Am J Nursing 62:90–93, Oct, 1962.

Others

Danziger, R.G., & others: Dissolution of cholesterol gallstones by chenodeoxycholic acid. New England J Med 286:1–8, 1972.

Littman, A., & D.H. Hanscom: Pancreatic extracts. New England J Med 281:201–204, 1969.

Sigmund, C.J., & E.F. McNally: The action of a carminative on the lower esophageal sphincter. Gastroenterology 56:13–18, 1969.

Sollmann, T.: *A Manual of Pharmacology,* 8th ed. Saunders, 1957.

32...

Respiratory Drugs

Many drugs that act either primarily or incidentally on the respiratory tract or on tissue respiration are discussed in other chapters where their inclusion is determined by their mechanism of action (eg, the bronchodilators are discussed with the sympathomimetic agents). A few therapeutic agents which escape other classification are included in this chapter—ie, oxygen, expectorants, and nonnarcotic cough remedies.

OXYGEN THERAPY & ASSISTED VENTILATION

In practice, the consideration of oxygen as a therapeutic agent should not be dissociated from methods for maintaining adequate ventilation. Ventilatory assistance is needed when neural drive, muscle power, or thoracic mechanics are inadequate. Many of these situations will require the simultaneous application of mechanical assistance and oxygen administration—eg, central respiratory depression due to drugs, severe shock, and acute and chronic pulmonary disease. The use of oxygen requires an adequate airway—maintained, if necessary, by tracheal intubation or tracheostomy—and a positive pressure device that can send pulses of oxygen to the tube or mask if necessary.

Technic of Administration

The method of administering oxygen is selected from among the following depending upon the concentration desired and the need for ventilatory assistance.

Oxygen should always be administered by bubbling through water before it is delivered to the patient's airway.

A. Tent: Concentrations of 25–50% oxygen can be reached, depending upon the rate of inflow of oxygen and the permeability of the material of the tent.

B. Head Tents or Hoods: (50–80% oxygen concentration.) These are smaller than tents and can be made of less permeable material.

C. Nasal Catheter: (40–60% oxygen concentration.) This technic is adequate for most purposes and is more readily accepted by the patient than the tent or mask.

D. Mask: (80–100% oxygen concentration.) Orofacial or oronasal masks can be used with a positive pressure device.

E. Endotracheal Tube: 80–100% concentrations can be delivered by this method.

F. Hyperbaric Oxygen: When the necessary equipment is available, oxygen can be given under pressures greater than 1 atmosphere. This special technic is discussed separately below.

Mechanism of Action

The question is not how does oxygen act but how can concentrations greater than that in air exert a beneficial effect. Room air contains 20.9% oxygen, which exerts a partial pressure of 159 mm Hg in inspired air. The P_{O_2} in the alveoli is about 100 mm Hg, and there is a small (6 mm Hg) gradient across the alveolar membrane so that the P_{O_2} in arterial blood is about 90 mm Hg. Under this usual condition, hemoglobin is almost completely (96%) saturated with oxygen. How oxygen can exert a beneficial effect will depend upon the cause of the hypoxia. When hemoglobin is already nearly saturated—ie, except in anoxic anoxia—it can act only through the increase of dissolved oxygen from 0.3–2 ml/100 ml.

Clinical Uses

A. Anoxic Anoxia:

1. Inadequate ventilation—When respiratory mechanics are inadequate and arterial blood is not completely saturated during its course through the pulmonary circulation, increasing the concentration of oxygen in the ambient air can increase the P_{O_2} in the alveoli and increase the hemoglobin saturation in arterial blood. The use of oxygen will not reduce the P_{CO_2}; in fact, the respiratory depressant effect of oxygen may increase it slightly. Thus, ventilatory assistance, even if with room air, may be much more rational.

2. Interference with diffusion—States such as pulmonary edema or fibrosis, which interfere with the transfer of oxygen across the alveolar membrane, result in incomplete saturation of arterial blood. Increasing the concentration of oxygen in the inspired air will increase the alveolar P_{O_2} and increase the gradient across the alveolar membrane. Changing from room air to 100% oxygen, for example, will change the P_{O_2} in the alveoli from the 100 mm Hg mentioned above to 670 mm Hg.

3. Right to left shunts—When desaturated blood is shunted into the arterial side of the circulation, respiration is maintained or stimulated. Because that fraction of the blood flow that goes through the lungs is already well oxygenated, little is gained by the use of oxygen. However, the small increase in oxygen in solution may be useful.

B. Anemic Anoxia: Anoxia due to a decrease in the amount of hemoglobin available to transport oxygen is not often treated with oxygen. An exception is intoxication with carbon monoxide, which forms carboxyhemoglobin that cannot transport oxygen. The benefits of oxygen are due to the increase in the amount of dissolved oxygen and to the dissociation of carboxyhemoglobin brought about by the increased oxygen tension.

C. Stagnant Anoxia: Local circulatory changes can lead to a decrease in the absolute amount of oxygen available to an area. High concentrations of oxygen (but not those achieved in tents) have a demonstrable effect on the pain of myocardial infarction. Severe shock is probably also benefited.

D. Histotoxic Anoxia: Theoretically, increasing the partial pressure of oxygen in the blood—and presumably at the cristae of the mitochondria, where oxygen reduction takes place—should have no effect on the poisoned cellular functions. Actually, oxygen is clearly useful in the treatment of poisoning by cyanide, which exerts its lethal effect by the inactivation of cytochrome oxidase it causes.

Adverse Reactions

A. Respiratory Depression: After a long period of respiratory insufficiency with chronic hypercarbia and hypoxia, respiration may be maintained by the stimulus of hypoxia on peripheral chemoreceptors rather than by the effect of CO_2. Unless ventilation is assisted, administration of oxygen to a patient in this situation could lead to respiratory depression with further accumulation of CO_2.

When respiratory failure is being treated with oxygen, sedatives and narcotics should not be used unless a means of ventilating the patient is available.

B. Respiratory Tract Irritation: The use of oxygen can lead to irritation of the nose, pharynx, and trachea with a slight cough and substernal soreness. Occurrence of the symptoms depends upon the concentration of oxygen and the time of exposure. For example, 100% oxygen at a pressure of 1 atmosphere will produce symptoms in less than a day. If the concentration is kept below 60%, the reaction does not occur.

With the above respiratory tract irritation, a decrease in vital capacity may be seen, but no other signs of pulmonary damage have been established.

C. Retrolental Fibroplasia: An epidemic of retrolental fibroplasia occurred between 1946 and 1954 coincident with the increased use in nurseries of oxygen in high concentrations. This condition of bilateral, destructive retinal proliferation affects premature infants. During this period, 77% of the cases of blindness in preschool children in California were due to retrolental fibroplasia.

To avoid all but sporadic cases, oxygen should be used only if needed and the concentration should not exceed 40% except for brief periods as necessary. In premature nurseries, the concentration should actually be determined rather than calculated from flow rates.

Preparations

Medical or USP oxygen is available in cylinders which by convention are painted green. Commercial or welding oxygen is equally pure and may be used if necessary.

Hyperbaric Oxygen

Oxygen can be provided under pressures as high as 3 atmospheres if an appropriate chamber is available. The patient (and preferably the physician or attendant also) is placed in a chamber which can be pressurized with oxygen itself or can be pressurized with air and the subject given oxygen at high pressure by mask.

At 3 atmospheres pressure and 100% oxygen, enough oxygen is dissolved in the blood (6 ml/100 ml) to meet the needs of the tissues without any desaturating of hemoglobin.

Oxygen toxicity is, of course, increased at the higher pressures, and exposure times must be limited to protect the lungs, retinas, and CNS. Exposed to oxygen at 2 atmospheres pressure, 50% of subjects will show a decrease in vital capacity after 4 hours. Continued exposure can lead to pulmonary consolidation. Vasoconstriction is marked, and the oxygen supply to many tissues is reduced. At pressures above 3 atmospheres, convulsions occur.

Oxygen at high pressure is effective in the treatment of carbon monoxide poisoning and of gas gangrene if it is of a diffuse type with spreading muscle necroses uncontrollable by penicillin. Other suggested applications are still being evaluated.

ANTITUSSIVE DRUGS

Coughing is a reflex that may be initiated by irritation occurring from the pharynx to the deepest level of the respiratory tract. It may be initiated by increased secretion or irritation due to trivial or serious disease. Coughing is useful to the extent that it clears the respiratory tract of accumulated secretions or protects it from a noxious environment. In most cases, however, it can be suppressed without danger to the patient, and cough suppressant drugs are widely used to decrease discomfort and provide rest.

Treatment designed to provide symptomatic relief does not utilize only cough suppressants but also expectorants—ie, drugs that increase and liquefy bronchial secretions—and bronchodilators, usually dispensed in a demulcent vehicle which is itself active.

The antitussive drugs or cough suppressants act, with one possible exception, on the central connections in the brain stem of the cough reflex. These agents can be divided into the narcotic drugs and some nonnarcotic agents of lesser potency.

Problems of Clinical Evaluation

It is not possible to present an evaluation of the clinical efficacy of antitussive drugs that will be accepted as a consensus even by the few investigators who have worked in the area.

The drugs have been evaluated in animals on cough generated by mechanical or electrical stimulation or by chemical irritation achieved by adding ammonia or acid to inhaled air. The drugs listed below are active in this form of testing; however, in the absence of correlation with clinical effectiveness, the results are of doubtful significance.

The same conclusion applies to testing on experimental cough in humans. The significance of drug effects on cough stimulated by inhalation of aerosols containing citric acid or ammonia is vitiated by the results of trials in humans with cough due to some disease process.

Such trials have in some cases objectified the effect of antitussive drugs by recording the number and intensity of the coughs and have also collected patient evaluations for comparison with objective measurements or the records of observers.

The results of clinical trials are conflicting. It appears, however, that cough, like pain and many other symptoms, has a subjective component. Patient evaluation of an antitussive drug may be more favorable than would be predicted by the objective effects. The narcotic drugs are probably effective both in reducing cough and in altering the patient's reaction to it. The effectiveness of the nonnarcotic drugs is debatable but at best limited.

Narcotics as Cough Suppressants

The effectiveness of the narcotics as cough suppressants generally parallels their potency as analgesics and their potential for misuse. Codeine, in doses of 7.5 or 15 mg, is usually adequate, and the danger of abuse is minimal. Side-effects, especially constipation, do occur. Dextromethorphan (see Chapter 26) is a very weak analgesic which is not subject to the prescription regulations governing narcotics and, in fact, is sold without a prescription as an ingredient of many cough medicines. It is probably active but much less so than codeine.

Nonnarcotic Antitussives

The nonnarcotic cough suppressants are a diverse group pharmacologically. The following list ignores a few drugs that have practically, if not legally, disappeared from the market.

A. Peripherally Acting: Benzonatate (Tessalon, Ventussin) is a local anesthetic of the amide type related to tetracaine (see Chapter 22). In animals given the drug parenterally, it has been shown to reduce

activity from pulmonary stretch receptors, and its antitussive activity is therefore assumed to be due to a peripheral rather than a central action. The clinical studies available do not permit an evaluation of its usefulness. The usual dosage is 100 mg as often as 6 times daily. It is supplied as soft capsules or pearls containing 100 mg or as 50 mg tabs.

B. Centrally Acting: It is claimed that the following drugs are active by themselves, and they are available as such. Their wide use, however, is due to their incorporation into a number of popular prescription and nonprescription proprietary mixtures.

1. Caramiphen is the ethanedisulfonate salt of the drug also dispensed as an antiparkinson agent as the hydrochloride (Panparnit). Atropine-like side-effects may occur.

2. Carbetapentane is also anticholinergic. Like other synthetic substitutes for atropine, it is a potent local anesthetic.

3. Noscapine or narcotine is a benzylisoquinoline alkaloid isolated from opium and comparable to papaverine (Fig 26–2). It is not a narcotic in any sense. When used by itself, the usual dose is 15–30 mg.

EXPECTORANTS

Expectorants are drugs (or procedures) that increase the amount of and liquefy bronchial secretions. They thus make it easier for the patient to move secretions toward the mouth and dispose of them. In asthma or other obstructive pulmonary disease, they are useful to the extent that obstruction is due to secretions rather than to bronchiolar constriction.

In the past, a complex classification of expectorants was used. Cough suppressants were included, and some of the terminology was confusing. These terms can now be ignored.

Water, in the form of moisture in a closed room or in the form of inhaled steam or aerosol, dilutes and liquefies respiratory tract secretions. It has the great advantage of acting rapidly. Adequate hydration—ie, adequate intake—is also useful.

The common drugs used as expectorants all act reflexly by acting as gastric irritants.

Potassium Iodide

The actions of iodide related to thyroid function are discussed in Chapter 34.

In animal and human studies, potassium iodide is active in increasing the volume and decreasing the viscosity not only of the secretion of the bronchial glands but also salivary, nasal, and lacrimal secretions. The action is due at least in part to reflex secretion generated by gastric irritation. Such irritation can be effective even though frank nausea does not occur.

Even though iodides have been shown to act through the gastric reflex, they either have an additional effect or act after absorption since they do not lose their effectiveness when given as enteric-coated tablets.

The use of potassium iodide can lead to an unpleasant awareness of hypersecretion in the eyes, nose, and mouth. Sneezing and conjunctival irritation may lead to a condition closely resembling the common cold. A brassy taste may be noted. Parotid swelling may occur, and an acneiform skin rash may appear. These actions are dose-related rather than allergic. Treatment consists of discontinuing use of the drug. Potassium iodide, unlike the bromides, is rapidly excreted.

Potassium iodide is available as plain or enteric-coated tablets containing 0.3 gm. The dosage is 0.3 gm 3–4 times daily. It may also be made up as saturated solutions (SSKI) and dispensed in a dosage of 10 drops 3 times daily.

Ammonium Chloride

Ammonium chloride and other ammonium salts are demonstrably active as expectorants, but less so than potassium iodide. Ammonium chloride, like potassium iodide, acts by causing gastric irritation. Unlike potassium iodide, however, when it is used as an expectorant it must not be given as an enteric-coated tablet. (Such a preparation is available and was used in conjunction with diuretics.)

An ammonium chloride syrup is available, but the drug is most often used in mixtures.

Syrup of Ipecac

Ipecac is undoubtedly effective as an expectorant, but nausea is a common side-effect. It is included in some cough mixtures. If it is used—eg, by an asthmatic who cannot tolerate potassium iodide—the dose of the syrup is 0.5 ml 4 times daily.

Glyceryl Guaiacolate

Glyceryl guaiacolate is not used by itself but is incorporated into many cough syrups. It is much less effective than any of the above.

● ● ●

General References

Oxygen

   Campbell, E.J.M.: The management of acute respiratory failure in chronic bronchitis and emphysema. Am Rev Resp Dis 95:626–639, 1967.

   Comroe, J.H., Jr.: *Physiology of Respiration.* Year Book, 1965.

   Hugh-Jones, P., & E.J.M. Campbell (editors): Respiratory physiology. Brit M Bull 19:1–96, 1963.

   Hyperbaric oxygen therapy. Med Lett Drugs Ther 13:29–32, 1971.

Antitussive Agents

   Beecher, H.K.: *Measurement of Subjective Responses.* Oxford, 1959.

   Bickerman, H.A.: Clinical pharmacology of antitussive agents. Clin Pharmacol Therap 3:353–368, 1962.

Expectorants

   Beckman, H.: Expectorants. JAMA 167:1638–1639, 1958.

Part V. Endocrine Drugs

33...

The Hormones

This section of the book deals with a chemically, physiologically, and therapeutically diverse group of compounds called hormones. They are the biologically active agents of a single organ system, the natural products of the glands of internal secretion released directly into the circulation to act at distant sites. Along with the nervous system, they are responsible for the integration of the many different processes which allow a complicated organism to function as a unit. They are similar to catalysts in that they are not destroyed in the process of affecting cellular function and serve to control the rate at which functions occur. Furthermore, their presence in proper amounts is required for normal function.

Hormones are used to replace a deficiency of those produced endogenously or to otherwise modify endocrine and metabolic abnormalities. They are also employed in tests of endocrine function or to evaluate the response to hormones. Therefore, a somewhat more detailed description of the normal (physiologic) role of hormones as well as of the disease states produced by a deficiency or excess of hormones is required for an understanding of hormonal therapy.

The greatest use of these agents, however, is as therapeutic agents in the treatment of nonendocrine disorders by taking advantage of special physiologic or pharmacologic effects.

A large number of compounds which have properties identical or similar to the native hormones have been synthesized. In many instances these compounds differ sufficiently from the human product to provide special advantage in any given patient if the differences are appreciated.

Excessive amounts of a hormone may lead to serious disturbances. Such disorders may be the result of the therapeutic use of the hormone or may result from endogenous overproduction due to glandular hypertrophy or hyperplasia. The naturally occurring states are often treated surgically by excision of glandular tissue or tumors producing the hormones. However, an increasing number of medicinal compounds are becoming available for the treatment of such disturbances. Some are competitive inhibitors of the hormones and interfere with their action at the target cell; others interfere with their synthesis or release.

MECHANISMS OF ACTION

The means by which hormones exert their effects are the subject of intensive research. Several important kinds of effects have been found at the cellular and subcellular level. Some of these effects or actions are common to several hormones, and some hormones, if not all, act through more than one of the known mechanisms. In many instances the specificity of hormone action depends upon where rather than how the hormone acts.

Transport Effects

Several hormones have been shown to affect their target cells in such a way as to increase the transfer of substrates into the cell. In some instances, this appears to be a membrane effect and active transport does not seem to be involved. An example of this kind of effect is that of insulin on the rate of glucose and amino acid entry into muscle or fat cells. In the case of the enhancement of iodide uptake by thyrotropin, a gradient must be overcome, and alterations of membrane permeability alone could not explain the effect.

Formation of Cyclic 3',5'-Adenosine Monophosphate (Cyclic AMP)

Many hormones have been shown to effect changes in their target cells by altering levels of cyclic AMP in the cell. In most cases this is accomplished by the stimulation of the activity of adenyl cyclase, an enzyme system located in the membrane of the target cell (Fig 33-1). Adenyl cyclase stimulates the conversion of ATP to cyclic AMP, which acts upon intracellular processes to produce the effects characteristic of the hormone. Cyclic AMP is degraded by the action of the enzyme phosphodiesterase and some of the hormones may function by inhibiting its activity. This enzyme is also inhibited by theophylline derivatives, and the action of hormones which increase cyclic AMP can be enhanced by these compounds.

The high specificity of hormone action at this site depends both on the ability of the hormone to interact with the adenyl cyclase system only in its target cells and the differences which characterize the intracellular

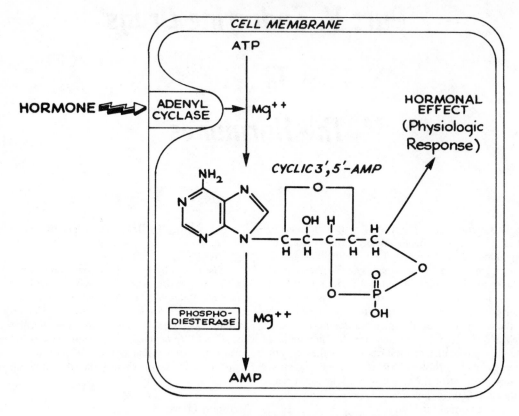

FIG 33–1. The role of adenyl cyclase in the conversion of ATP to cyclic AMP.

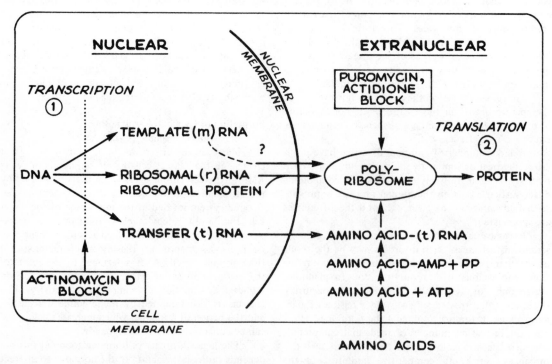

FIG 33–2. Mechanisms of protein biosynthesis and loci of action of commonly used inhibitors. (Redrawn from *Metabolic and Endocrine Physiology,* 2nd ed, by Jay Tepperman. Copyright © 1968, Year Book Medical Publishers, Inc. Used by permission.)

TABLE 33–1. Some hormonal influences on cyclic AMP levels in various tissues
and the consequence of the alteration.*

Hormone	Tissue	cAMP Level	Result
ACTH	Adrenal cortex	Increased	Increased steroidogenesis (glucocorticoids).
	Adipose tissue	Increased	Increased lipolysis.
Growth hormone	Lymphocytes	Increased	Increased mitotic activity.
LH	Ovary	Increased	Increased steroidogenesis (estrogens and progesterones).
	Corpus luteum	Increased	Increased steroidogenesis (progesterone).
	Testis	Increased	Increased steroidogenesis (androgens).
	Adipose tissue	Increased	Increased lipolysis.
MSH	Melanocytes (frog, lizard skin)	Increased	Increased melanophore dispersion.
TSH	Thyroid	Increased	Increased glucose oxidation and iodine organification; increased thyroxine and triiodothyronine synthesis and release.
	Adipose tissue	Increased	Increased lipolysis.
Parathyroid hormone	Bone, kidney	Increased	Increased serum calcium.
Vasopressin	Kidney, toad bladder	Increased	Increased water and ion movement.
Glucagon	Pancreas	Increased	Increased insulin secretion.
	Adipose tissue	Increased	Increased lipolysis.
	Heart	Increased	Positive inotropic effect.
	Liver	Increased	Increased gluconeogenesis, urea formation, and potassium release.
Insulin	Adipose tissue	Decreased	Decreased lipolysis.
	Liver	Decreased	Decreased gluconeogenesis, urea formation, and potassium release.
Catecholamines	Adipose tissue	Increased	Increased lipolysis.
	Heart	Increased	Positive inotropic effect.
	Uterus	Increased	Relaxation.
	Parotid gland	Increased	Increased amylase secretion.
	Muscle	Increased	Increased glycogenolysis.
	Liver	Increased	Increased gluconeogenesis, urea formation, and potassium release.
	Pancreas	Decreased	Decreased insulin secretion.
	Frog skin	Decreased	Decreased melanophore dispersion.
Prostaglandins	Adipose tissue	Decreased	Decreased lipolysis.
	Kidney	Decreased	Decreased water and ion movement.
	Thyroid	Increased	Increased thyroglobulin.

*From *Metabolic and Endocrine Physiology,* 2nd ed, by Jay Tepperman. Copyright © 1968, Year Book Medical Publishers, Inc. Used by permission.

enzyme activities and responses within the target cell. Some of the hormones thought to act by influencing cyclic AMP levels are listed in Table 33–1.

Induction of Protein Synthesis

In contrast to the above action of hormones (on the rate of synthesis of cyclic AMP), which seems to be a relatively direct effect on enzyme activity, it has been demonstrated that hormones can increase the amount of enzyme present. Most hormones regulate RNA and protein synthesis. Current studies suggest that the steroid hormones bind to specific receptor proteins in the cytoplasm of their target cells to form a complex. This complex is transported into the nucleus, where it binds to a specific effector site on the genome and stimulates RNA transcription (Fig 33–2). This hypothesis is supported by the demonstration of increased nuclear RNA synthesis following the addition

of hormone as well as the interference with hormone action by an inhibitor of RNA synthesis such as dactinomycin (actinomycin D).

Hormones may also affect the rate of protein synthesis at the ribosomal level. This process does not require synthesis of new RNA. Most of the evidence relating to this action of hormones is based on the finding that some hormone effects can be curtailed by treatment with inhibitors of protein synthesis (eg, puromycin) but are unaffected by the addition of dactinomycin. It has been possible to show that ribosomes obtained from hormone-treated animals have an altered capacity to synthesize protein.

The effects on membranes and enzyme activity are usually rapid. The effect of hormones on protein synthesis is slow and may not become apparent for hours or days.

TABLE 33–2. Some examples of hormonal effects on protein synthesis in target organ(s).*

Hormone	Tissue	Effect	Step Stimulated in Protein Synthesis
Cortisol	Liver	Induction of many enzymes, including those involved in gluconeogenesis.	Increased RNA synthesis, increased amino acid incorporation.
Aldosterone	Kidney	Increased sodium transport.	
Estrogen	Uterus	Increased growth.	Increased RNA synthesis.
Testosterone	Seminal vesicles, prostate, kidneys	Increased growth.	Increased amino acid incorporation.
Erythropoietin	Bone marrow	Hemoglobin synthesis.	Increased RNA synthesis.
Growth hormone	Liver, kidney, heart, spleen, adrenal	Increased protein content.	Increased RNA synthesis, increased amino acid incorporation.
Thyroxine	Whole animal	Increased BMR, increased growth rate.	Increased RNA synthesis.
Insulin (in the presence of insulin deficiency)	Muscle, liver		Increased RNA synthesis, increased amino acid incorporation.

*From *Metabolic and Endocrine Physiology,* 2nd ed, by Jay Tepperman. Copyright © 1968, Year Book Medical Publishers, Inc. Used by permission.

Although the regulatory effects of many hormones on metabolic processes are mediated by cyclic AMP, others, such as aldosterone and its effects on ion transport, require synthesis of new protein. In general, the hormonal control of growth and differentiation involves stimulation of one or more of the processes leading to increased protein synthesis (Table 33–2).

●   ●   ●

General References

Butcher, R.W.: Role of cyclic AMP in hormone actions. New England J Med 279:1378, 1968.

Williams, R.H. (editor): *Textbook of Endocrinology,* 4th ed. Saunders, 1968.

34...
Thyroid & Antithyroid Drugs

THYROID

The normal thyroid gland is responsible for the synthesis and release of 2 hormones: thyroxine (T_4) and triiodothyronine (T_3) (Fig 34—1). Both are iodine-containing amino acids that regulate the rate of cellular oxidative processes.

Metabolism of Thyroid Hormones

The major steps in the complex pathways of biosynthesis, secretion, and degradation of the active thyroid hormones are summarized in Fig 34—2.

Dietary iodine is absorbed and circulates as iodide in the blood in low concentration (0.2—0.4 μg/100 ml). It is actively removed from the blood by the cells of the thyroid gland, where it is concentrated 10—200 times or more depending upon the degree of stimulation of the concentrating mechanism by thyrotropin (TSH). The details of the iodine "trapping mechanism" in the thyroid are not completely understood, but the mechanism is known to require intact, actively respiring thyroid cells, and may be coupled to potassium transport into these cells. This reaction is of interest also because it is the site of action of a number of ions, such as perchlorate and thiocyanate, which inhibit the production of T_4 and T_3 by interfering with thyroidal iodide transport.

Inborn errors of metabolism involving this mechanism also result in goiters.

The activity of the concentrating mechanism is stimulated by TSH or by depletion of iodine stores within the gland. Iodine-concentrating mechanisms similar to that in the thyroid gland are found in the salivary and mammary glands, gastric mucosa, placenta, and skin. These differ in that they are not significantly influenced by changes in thyrotropin concentration.

Once in the gland, thyroidal iodide is oxidized to iodine. This conversion, thought to be due to the action of a peroxidase, leaves the iodine in a highly activated form.

T_3 & T_4 Synthesis

The activated iodine rapidly combines with tyrosine groups of thyroglobulin (a protein made up of approximately 5000 amino acid residues and having a molecular weight of about 650,000) to form monoiodotyrosine (MIT) and diiodotyrosine (DIT). The MIT and DIT thus formed undergo aerobic condensation to form 2 hormones: T_4 (2 DIT) and T_3 (1 MIT + DIT)

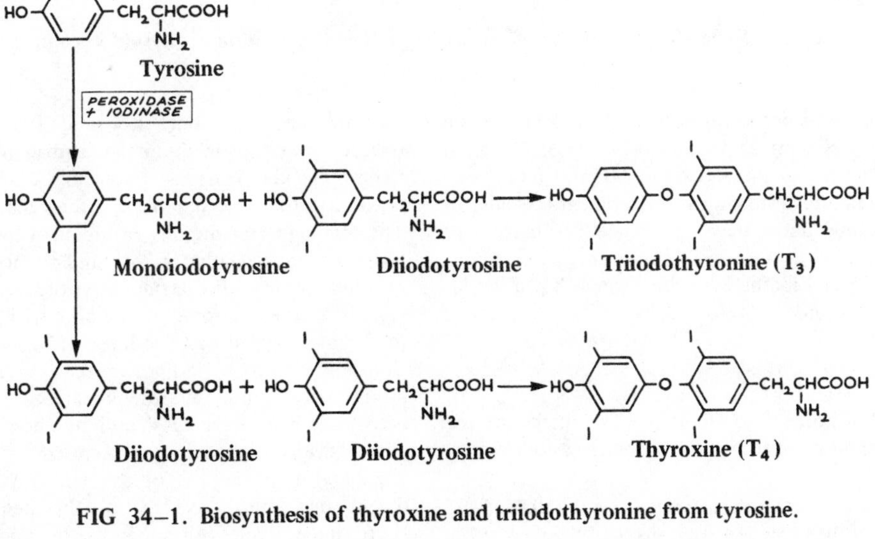

FIG 34—1. Biosynthesis of thyroxine and triiodothyronine from tyrosine.

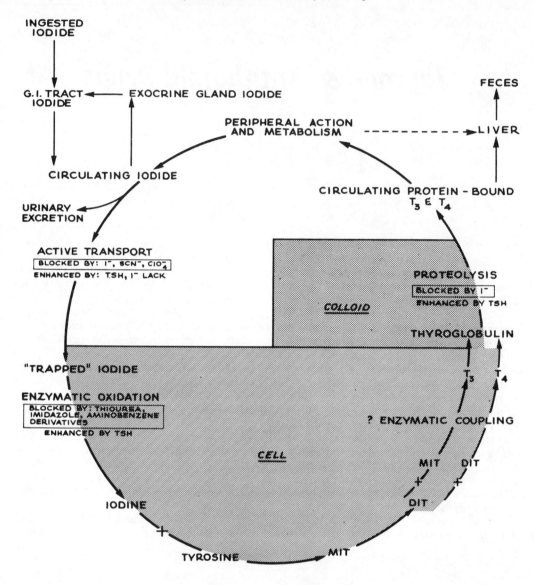

FIG 34—2. Pathways of biosynthesis, secretion, and degradation of thyroid hormones.

(Fig 34—1). A higher proportion of MIT occurs when the diet is deficient in iodine or when oxidation is blocked. The higher proportion of MIT favors the formation of T_3; however, if DIT is deficient (because of extreme iodine deficiency), the rate of formation of both thyronines is impaired. In most species about 25% of thyroidal iodine is in the form of T_4; a similar amount is present in MIT; and 30—50% is present as DIT.*

Secretion & Transport

The hormones are stored in the follicles of the thyroid gland bound to thyroglobulin as colloid. Secre-

tion of these hormones (T_3 and T_4) follows their release from thyroglobulin by a proteolytic enzyme. Each molecule yields 2—5 molecules of T_4, which are released into the capillaries by the cells of the gland. The MIT and DIT are also products of the proteolysis, but they are degraded in situ and the iodide released becomes available for hormone synthesis.

It has been estimated that about 75 μg of thyroxine (containing 50 μg of iodine) and 25 μg of triiodothyronine (15 μg of iodine) are released into the circulation daily. These figures indicate that the biologic activity is rather evenly shared by these compounds. Although the thyroxine is secreted by the thyroid gland, as much as 1/2 of the triiodothyronine produced may be derived from the deiodination of thyroxine in tissues other than the thyroid.

*It is not known whether the combination of the MIT and DIT is the result of the action of a "coupling enzyme" or a function of the structure of thyroglobulin.

Control of Secretion

The activity of the thyroid gland is normally controlled by thyrotropin (TSH) released by the anterior pituitary. In the absence of TSH (eg, after hypophysectomy), thyroid function is depressed and the gland becomes atrophic. Under the influence of TSH, the cells hypertrophy, iodine uptake increases, thyroxine synthesis is stimulated, blood flow through the gland increases, and more hormone is released into the circulation. Under stable environmental conditions in the normal individual, the rate of secretion is self-regulating since thyroid hormones act on the anterior pituitary to decrease TSH release. Disturbances of this feedback mechanism are present in several clinical disorders of thyroid function. TSH secretion is also influenced by hypothalamic neurohumor secretion. The median eminence of the hypothalamus produces a thyrotropin releasing factor (TRF) which is carried to the anterior pituitary, where it stimulates the release of TSH. A tripeptide with this activity has been isolated from hypothalamic extracts and has the structure shown in Fig 39–7. Alterations of the environmental temperature affect thyroid function through the hypothalamic centers. The depression of glandular activity observed in a variety of stressful situations and illnesses and during food deprivation is also thought to be mediated via the hypothalamic pathway.

Normal plasma levels of thyroxine are 5–12 μg/100 ml. Circulating thyroxine is bound to plasma proteins. Thyroxine-binding globulin, an acid glycoprotein with a molecular weight of about 50,000, has the highest affinity for thyroxine and binds about 85% of that present in normal plasma. Most of the remainder is bound to thyroxine-binding prealbumin, and only a fraction of 1% (0.004 μg/100 ml plasma) is free. If the more avid carriers are saturated, thyroxine will also bind to albumin. The capacity of the various carriers to bind thyroxine is inversely related to their affinity for the hormone. (See Table 34–1.)

In normal individuals plasma levels of triiodothyronine are about 0.1–0.2 μg/ml. However, the affinity of thyroxine-binding globulin for this hormone is only 10% as great as its affinity for thyroxine.

High levels of circulating estrogen, such as are seen during pregnancy and in women taking oral contraceptives, increase the thyroxine-binding globulin levels, and this in turn increases the binding of thyroxine, ie, its blood level. The binding can be competitively inhibited by related compounds and by a variety of unrelated chemicals such as diphenylhydantoin, aspirin, and dinitrophenol. Triiodothyronine levels do not appear to increase with estrogens.

Peripheral Metabolism & Excretion

Tracer studies with labeled thyroxine indicate that about 30% of the secreted hormone is in the circulation, 30% in the liver, 30% in the ECF, and 10% in the cells of the body. It is removed from the body slowly (half-life 6–7 days). The rate of removal is decreased when the metabolic rate is reduced, as in hypothyroidism (when production is decreased), or when there is increased binding to plasma proteins, as

TABLE 34–1. Thyroxine-binding proteins.

Protein	Binding Characteristic	Capacity
Thyroxine-binding α_2 globulin	Strong	Small
Prealbumin	Moderate	Moderate
Albumin	Weak	Large

in pregnancy. Thyroxine turnover is increased in hyperthyroidism, in the presence of hypoproteinemia (eg, nephrotic syndrome, cirrhosis), and when binding is inhibited by drugs (see above).

In man, 20–40% of thyroxine is eliminated in the feces. Many tissues deiodinate or deaminate thyroxine and triiodothyronine to thyroacetic and thyropropionic acid derivatives (Table 34–2). Liver, however, is the most active of these tissues; it also conjugates the hormones and their metabolites to glucuronic and sulfuric acid through the phenolic hydroxyl group.

Triiodothyronine is cleared from the circulation 5 times as rapidly as thyroxine and normally constitutes little more than 5% of hormonal iodide. Its intracellular distribution differs from thyroxine in that much less is found in liver and more in the kidneys, muscle, and skin.

Effects of Thyroid Hormones

The thyroid hormones are general metabolic stimulants affecting almost all tissues of the body.

Heat production and oxygen consumption of body tissues are increased in the intact animal under the influence of thyroxine, although in vitro studies have shown that the oxygen consumption of the pituitary is suppressed and that of some tissues (including testes, spleen, lymph nodes, and brain) is unaffected. The signs and symptoms observed when abnormally small or abnormally large amounts of thyroid hormone are present (hypo- and hyperthyroidism) are described below. Experimental work indicates that the actions of the thyroid hormones and the catecholamines epinephrine and norepinephrine may be interrelated. It has been found that the metabolic and cardiovascular effects of these amines are diminished or absent in thyroidectomized animals, whereas they are enhanced in the hyperthyroid state. On the other hand, depression of sympathetic outflow can reduce the effects of thyroxine.

Thyroid hormones are essential for normal growth and development in many species, including man. The sensitivity of this response is illustrated by the observation in thyroidectomized rats that growth can be restored to normal by one-tenth the amount of thyroxine required to restore the normal rate of metabolism.

Mechanisms of Action of Thyroid Hormones

Thyroxine has been shown to alter the activity of more than 30 enzymes in vitro and twice as many in vivo. The means by which it brings about physiologic changes has not been established. Thyroid hormones uncouple oxidative phosphorylation in mitochondria and thus interfere with the storage of metabolic energy in a usable form (high-energy phosphates). This effect could account for the increased calorigenesis and muscular weakness in hyperthyroidism, but it does not explain other actions of the hormone. Thyroxine in large amounts causes swelling of the mitochondria which could alter their permeability and function. However, many unrelated chemicals can produce this same swelling without reproducing the hormonal effects. Thyroid hormones have been shown to increase the incorporation of amino acids into proteins in the tissues in which metabolism is stimulated, suggesting an important role for protein synthesis in the metabolic action of the hormone. The observation that puromycin, an inhibitor of protein synthesis, reduces the effect of thyroxine on oxygen consumption supports this possibility.

The growth-promoting activity affects a variety of cells, and studies of tadpole metamorphosis suggest that these changes are mediated by the activation of intracellular mechanisms since they can be prevented by interference with nucleic acid metabolism.

Structure-Activity Relationships

Several metabolites of thyroxine and triiodothyronine have been found in tissues and possess hormonal activity. These include the thyroacetic, thyropropionic, and thyrolactic acid products of deamination. In addition, the activity of many other iodinated synthetic derivatives of thyronine have been investigated. Studies of these compounds indicate that 2 aromatic rings joined by an ether or thioether linkage and having a side chain containing a carboxyl group on the first ring and a phenolic hydroxyl group in the para position of the second ring are required for biologic activity. Although the specific steric arrangement of the 2 rings (perpendicular to each other) appears to be more important than the nature of the substituent groups, maximal activity requires the presence of iodine at the 3 and 5 positions. Iodine is less critical on the phenolic ring. It has been suggested that the phenylalanine ring with the 2 iodines is concerned with binding to the receptor site. An understanding of structure-function relationships has led to the development of competitive inhibitors such as 2',6'-diiodothyronine, 3,5-diiodo-4-hydroxybenzoic acid, and 3,3'5'-triiodothyronine.

It is of interest that the biologic activities of the analogues of thyroxine and triiodothyronine are not always parallel in their effects on oxygen consumption, pituitary secretion of TSH, cholesterol metabolism, and the induction of growth and metamorphosis in the tadpole (see Table 34–2).

CLINICAL DISORDERS OF THYROID FUNCTION

The clinical disorders of thyroid function in man result from a deficient or excessive production of thyroid hormones, mechanical disturbances produced by enlargement of the gland, neoplastic changes, or combinations of these factors.

Hypothyroidism

Hypothyroidism may result from a variety of congenital disorders such as athyrotic cretinism (failure of the gland to develop) and defects in hormone metabolism, eg, synthesis and release. Acquired hypothyroidism may be secondary to the failure of thyrotropin secretion by the pituitary or may be the sequel to thyroidectomy, thyroiditis, antithyroid drugs, or autoimmune disease.

When thyroid deficiency is present at birth, it produces cretinism. Although not usually recognized at birth, a characteristic syndrome may develop consisting of a puffy, expressionless face with large tongue and thick lips, yellowish skin, short extremities, poor appetite, umbilical hernia, and a reduction of body temperature and pulse rate. Replacement therapy, to be fully effective, must be started before these advanced changes occur. When the deficiency occurs later in childhood, it is associated with a reduction in the rate of growth and development.

In the adult, severe thyroid deficiency produces myxedema, characterized by marked retardation of mental and physical activity, hoarseness, dry, pale, coarse skin, dry sparse hair, thickening of the skin and subcutaneous tissues (myxedema), constipation, cold intolerance, anemia, and other changes. However, hypothyroidism is usually recognized before it has progressed to this point.

Hyperthyroidism

This disorder results from the excessive production of thyroid hormone. Although occasionally due to a neoplastic process, the disorder most commonly seen is thyrotoxic goiter (Graves' disease). The cause of Graves' disease is not established, but hyperfunction of the gland is often associated with (and may be due to) the presence of a long-acting thyroid stimulating substance (LATS). LATS is a gamma globulin found in the blood even after hypophysectomy and may be an antibody to a constituent of the cells of the thyroid gland.

Hereditary factors seem to be involved, as evidenced by the high incidence of the disorder in the families of patients. It has also been observed that some members of the patient's family who do not manifest the disorder fail to show suppression of thyroid hormone synthesis and release when given thyroid hormone, as do normal individuals.

The clinical manifestations of hyperthyroidism include the signs and symptoms of hypermetabolism such as weight loss, increased appetite, heat intolerance, perspiration, and flushing. There is overactivity of the heart, with tachycardia and bounding pulses, and neuromuscular irritability. Anxiety is a prominent complaint. Muscle wasting and weakness are sometimes striking.

TABLE 34–2. Relative potencies of thyroxine derivatives.* All of these compounds except D-thyroxine are probably formed in the body. Note that in each column the potency of the derivatives is stated relative to an arbitrary value of 100 for thyroxine.

Chemical Structure	Name	Synonyms	Relative Potency			
			[131]I†	Goiter Prev.‡	BMR§	Cholesterol Lowering
HO–⟨ ⟩–O–⟨ ⟩–$CH_2CHCOOH$ (NH_2), 4 I	L-3,5,3′,5′-Tetraiodothyronine	L-Thyroxine; T_4	100	100	100	100
HO–⟨ ⟩–O–⟨ ⟩–$CH_2CHCOOH$ (NH_2), 4 I	D-3,5,3′,5′-Tetraiodothyronine	D-Thyroxine; $D-T_4$	30	. . .	. . .	500
HO–⟨ ⟩–O–⟨ ⟩–$CH_2CHCOOH$ (NH_2), 3 I	L-3,5,3′-Triiodothyronine	Triiodothyronine; TIT; T_3	300	800	800	. . .
HO–⟨ ⟩–O–⟨ ⟩–$CH_2CHCOOH$ (NH_2), 3 I	3,3′,5′-Triiodothyronine (D, L tested)	Reverse T_3	75	< 1	< 1	. . .
HO–⟨ ⟩–O–⟨ ⟩–CH_2CH_2COOH, 4 I	3,5,3′,5′-Tetraiodothyropropionic acid	T_4 PROP	60	14	6	. . .
HO–⟨ ⟩–O–⟨ ⟩–CH_2CH_2COOH, 3 I	3,5,3′-Triiodothyropropionic acid	T_3 PROP	60	28	10	. . .
HO–⟨ ⟩–O–⟨ ⟩–CH_2COOH, 4 I	3,5,3′,5′-Tetraiodothyroacetic acid	TETRAC	75	63	9	250
HO–⟨ ⟩–O–⟨ ⟩–CH_2COOH, 3 I	3,5,3′-Triiodothyroacetic acid	TRIAC	75	51	21	. . .

*Data mostly from Money & others: Comparative effects of thyroxine analogues in experimental animals. Ann New York Acad Sc 86:512, 1960.

†Inhibition of radioactive iodine uptake.

‡Prevention of goiter in propylthiouracil-treated animals (pituitary-inhibiting effect).

§Calorigenic effect.

THYROID HORMONE PREPARATIONS
(See Table 34–3.)

Thyroid USP (Desiccated Thyroid; Thyroid Extract)

The USP thyroid preparation is powdered, acetone dried, and defatted thyroid tissue obtained from hogs, cattle, or sheep in the slaughterhouse. It is normally assayed by its iodine content, which must be between 0.17 and 0.23%. Tablets are made from the compressed powder and are not always assayed for their content of thyroxine or triiodothyronine. The variations in preparations of these substances contribute to a lack of uniformity from one product to another and probably explain why the porcine product is more calorigenic than that derived from beef or sheep. Different proportions of T_3 and T_4 will also result in different protein-bound iodine (PBI) levels for a given therapeutic effect. In spite of these variations,

TABLE 34–3. Thyroid hormone preparations.

| | $T_4:T_3$ Ratio (weight) | Onset of Activity | Values of Some Tests in Patients on Replacement Therapy Compared to Normals | | Equivalent Dosage | Preparations Available |
			PBI or Serum T_4	Resin T_3		
Thyroid USP (many preparations)	Beef, 4:1 Hog, 2–3:1	Intermediate	Normal or slightly lower	Normal or low	60 mg	Tablets, plain or enteric coated, 15, 30, 60, 120, 200, 250, and 300 mg Capsules, 60, 120, 200, 300, and 400 mg
Thyroglobulin (Endothyrin, Proloid)	2:1	Intermediate	Normal or slightly lower	Normal or low	60 mg	Tablets, 15, 30, 60, 90, 200, and 300 mg
Sodium levothyroxine (Cothroid, Letter, Levoid, Synthroid, Titroid)	Pure T_4	Slow	Slightly higher	High	0.1 mg	Tablets, 0.025, 0.05, 0.1, 0.15, 0.2, 0.3, and 0.5 mg Injectable (IV), 0.1 and 0.5 mg/ml
Sodium liothyronine (L-triiodothyronine, Cytomel)	Pure T_3	Rapid	Low	Normal	25 µg	Tablets, 5, 25, and 50 µg
Liotrix (sodium levothyroxine with sodium liothyronine, Euthroid, Thyrolar)	4:1	Intermediate	Normal	Normal	T_4: 0.06 mg T_3: 15 µg	Tablets; sizes not standardized among manufacturers

the official preparation is well absorbed and, in general, a highly satisfactory preparation for clinical use.

Synthetic iodinated proteins are quite active and have been used primarily in animal experimentation.

Thyroglobulin

Thyroglobulin, extracted from animal thyroid glands, is also available in tablet form. This preparation contains thyroxine and triiodothyronine and is standardized both by iodine content and bioassay.

Thyroxine

This preparation is widely used since it contains only one substance. The sodium salt of the natural isomer of thyroxine is employed because it is more reliably absorbed, although as much as 50% can sometimes be found in the stool. It is dispensed in the form of tablets.

Triiodothyronine

This hormone produces effects that are qualitatively similar to thyroxine. However, it has special properties that make it useful under certain circumstances. It is effective in approximately 1/5 the dose, and has a maximal effect within a few days that disappears with a half-life of about 8 days. This is in contrast to thyroxine, which requires 9 days to reach its peak effect and whose effects may require about twice as long to disappear. Triiodothyronine is generally preferred when a rapid onset of action is vital, such as in myxedema coma; but its brief effect makes it less useful for prolonged maintenance therapy in hypothyroidism. When used chronically, it is equiv-

alent to 3 times the amount of thyroxine and should be given in divided doses.

Liotrix

Liotrix is a combination of thyroxine and triiodothyronine in a 4:1 ratio. It is designed to mimic the natural secretion of the thyroid gland. Although the ratio of the 2 hormones in liotrix is higher than that in endogenously secreted thyroid hormones, the onset and duration of action and the levels of circulating hormonal iodine produced by its administration are similar. This may reflect the fact that triiodothyronine is more completely absorbed than thyroxine when given by mouth.

Its use is similar to that of thyroid USP, which also contains a mixture of T_3 and T_4. However, it is likely that the ratio will be more constant in liotrix.

THERAPEUTIC USES OF THYROID HORMONES

The 2 specific indications for the use of thyroid hormones are replacement therapy in thyroid deficiency and therapeutic or diagnostic suppression of pituitary TSH production.

Although it is usually safe to give full replacement therapy in starting doses to children and young adults, in the presence of any type of heart disease it can be quite dangerous. Gradual and cautious replacement is preferable in older individuals and in children with myxedema heart disease. Acute adrenal insufficiency may be produced by the administration of thyroid hormone to patients with hypothyroidism secondary to hypopituitarism; therefore, it is important to provide such patients with adrenal steroid replacement therapy prior to treatment with thyroid hormone.

In infants with hypothyroidism, treatment can be started with doses of 15 mg of thyroid extract and increased at intervals of 2 weeks until a euthyroid state is reached. About 45–60 mg daily are required during the first 1½ years, with doses up to 120 mg between 1½ and 3 years. Doses of 120–180 mg may be used thereafter to obtain optimal growth. The success of therapy in the infant depends upon whether it is started early enough to prevent permanent mental retardation.

Adults usually require 120–180 mg for full replacement therapy. Overtreatment with thyroid hormones is characterized by nervousness, tremor, tachycardia or arrhythmias, hypermetabolism, and hypertension. In patients with heart disease, congestive heart failure or coronary insufficiency may be provoked by the injudicious use of these hormones.

In myxedema coma it is necessary to obtain as rapid a response as possible. It may be necessary to give large doses of triiodothyronine parenterally. The desired dose can be dissolved in 0.1N NaOH and diluted with saline to bring the NaOH to one-tenth of its initial concentration. Large doses of hydrocortisone (300 mg/24 hours or more) are also administered intravenously to these patients.

Thyroid hormones, by suppressing TSH production, will cause a reduction in the size of a simple goiter such as is present when defective hormone synthesis occurs. In endemic or iodine deficiency goiter, a prompt response is usually observed unless the gland has become nodular. The maximal response may require many months of treatment.

These hormones have also been used for the treatment of functioning single nodules of thyroid tissue. If these do not regress with full replacement therapy, surgical removal is advocated.

A variety of analogues of thyroxine, particularly D-thyroxine, have been studied for use in the treatment of hypercholesterolemia since they increase the degradation of this sterol more than its synthesis, leading to a reduction in serum cholesterol levels (see p 419).

Nonspecific Therapy

Thyroid hormones are extensively used in the treatment of gynecologic conditions, including amenorrhea, anovulatory cycles, hypermenorrhea, habitual abortion, and infertility with no discernible cause. Oligospermia in the male, obesity, and metabolic insufficiency have also been reported to respond favorably to thyroxine or triiodothyronine. Although many physicians have had successful experiences with thyroid treatment of the above symptoms in the absence of diagnosable hypothyroidism, there is no evidence that the success rate is greater than that achieved by the use of placebos.

DINITROPHENOL

Dinitrophenol in a dose of 3–5 mg/kg increases the metabolic rate more than 20% for 24–48 hours. If given chronically, a 50% elevation can be maintained. Dinitrophenol has none of the hormonal effects of thyroxine. It increases the rate of oxidation by uncoupling oxidation from the formation of high-energy phosphates and leads to the generation of heat.

Dinitrophenol is a yellow dye which is rapidly absorbed from the intestine and is secreted both unchanged and in a reduced form (2-amino-4-nitrophenol). In the past it was used for the treatment of obesity; but serious side-effects, including cataracts, neuritis, anemia, agranulocytosis, purpura, and liver and kidney damage led to its withdrawal from use.

ANTITHYROID AGENTS

Reduction of thyroid activity or the effects of thyroid hormones can be accomplished by the use of drugs that interfere with the production of the thyroid hormones; by drugs that modify the actions of the hormone in the tissues; and by the destruction of part or all of the gland, either surgically or by the use of ionizing radiation.

INHIBITORS OF HORMONE BIOSYNTHESIS

The commonly used antithyroid drugs in this group are the thiocarbamides such as propylthiouracil and methimazole (Fig 34–3). These compounds interfere with the binding, into organic form, of the iodide accumulated by the thyroid gland. They are thought to act by inhibiting the oxidation of iodide to iodine. They also appear to interfere with the coupling of iodotyrosines (Fig 34–2).

The metabolism of these compounds has not been completely studied. Propylthiouracil is rapidly absorbed into the circulation. Peak plasma concentrations are reached in 2 hours. It is distributed in a space which is somewhat less than total body water. It is concentrated in the thyroid to the same degree as iodide. The thyroid can be blocked by iodide or perchlorate ion. It is rapidly removed from the body through the kidneys, and its rapid turnover makes frequent administration advisable: A dose of propylthiouracil as large as 500 mg will completely inhibit the thyroid gland for 6–8 hours. Methimazole is more slowly absorbed, reaching a peak in the plasma at about 8 hours. It has a more prolonged effect, and a

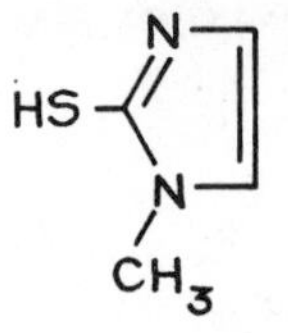

Methimazole
(1-methylimidazole-2-thiol)
(Tapazole)

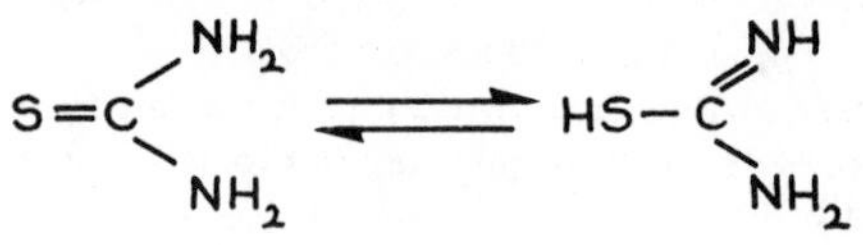

Thiourea

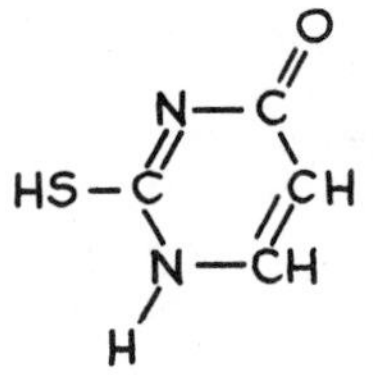

Thiouracil

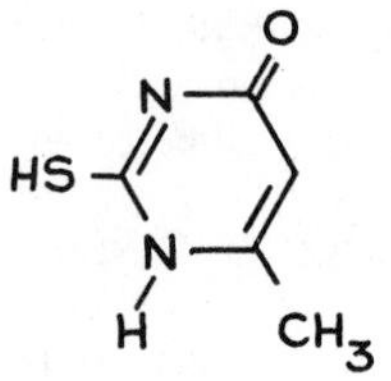

Methylthiouracil
(Methiacil)

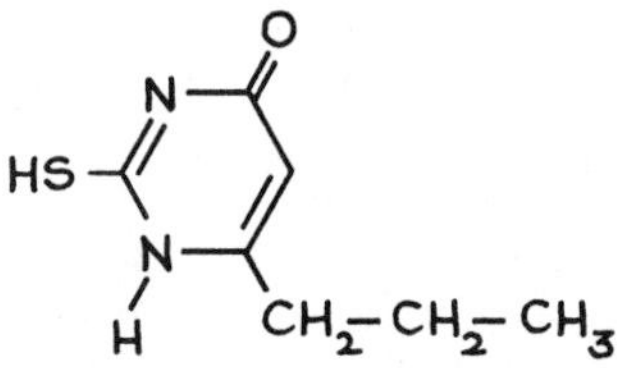

Propylthiouracil

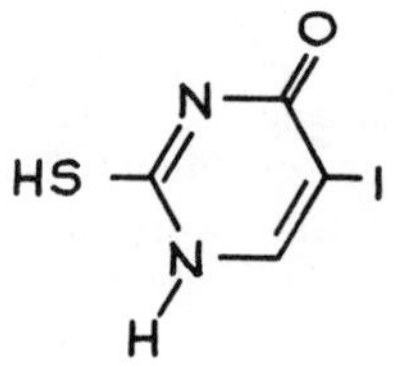

Iothiouracil sodium
(Itrumil Sodium)

FIG 34—3. Antithyroid drugs.

single dose of 30 mg continues to exert an inhibitory effect after 24 hours.

The thiocarbamides readily cross the placenta of pregnant women, and, when large doses are administered, a goiter may be produced in the fetus. Doses of propylthiouracil less than 150 mg/day (or equivalent) seldom have this effect. These drugs are also secreted into the milk in lactating women and may produce goiters in nursing infants.

These 2 drugs appear to have fewer toxic effects than some of the others used. The most common of them are a pruritic papular rash and joint pain and stiffness which may disappear with continued use; however, the arthritic manifestations may require discontinuation of the drug. These or mild gastrointestinal symptoms occur in 3% of patients receiving propylthiouracil and 7% of those taking methimazole. The incidence of agranulocytosis is less than 0.5%, and jaundice rarely occurs. When one of the drugs causes adverse effects, another may be tried.

The thiocarbamides interfere with the feedback inhibition of pituitary TSH secretion by reducing the amount of circulating thyroxine and triiodothyronine. The increase in TSH stimulates the thyroid and leads to enlargement of the gland, or goiter. Such compounds are referred to as goitrogens. This property is shared by a large number of chemically unrelated substances.

Vegetables of the Brassicaceae family such as turnips and rutabagas have been known to produce thyroid enlargement. This has been found to be due to their content of a substance (progoitrin) which can be converted to goitrin (Fig 34—4) by a heat-labile activator found in the plants, or by substances in the gastrointestinal tract. Goitrin has a potency similar to that of propylthiouracil. In addition to this naturally occurring inhibitor, a variety of useful drugs and chemicals have been shown to have low degrees of goitrogenic activity by virtue of their interference with thyroid

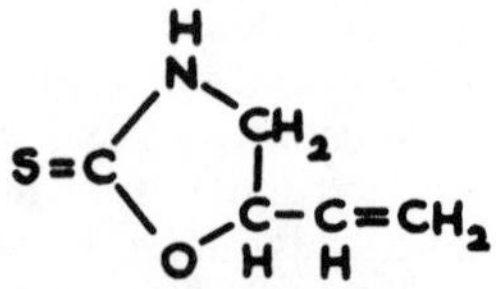

Goitrin
(L-vinyl-2-thiooxazolidone)

FIG 34—4. The naturally occurring goitrogen in vegetables of the family Brassicaceae.

hormone synthesis. This group includes sulfanilamide, phenylbutazone, para-aminobenzoic acid, cyanocobalamin, amphenone B, barbiturates, phentolamine, metahexamide, and carbutamide.

IONIC INHIBITORS

A group of monovalent hydrated anions, including thiocyanate (SCN⁻), perchlorate (ClO₄⁻), and nitrate (NO₃⁻), inhibit thyroid function and produce goiters. Their mechanism of action differs from that of the compounds discussed above and appears to result from competitive inhibition of the iodine-concentrating mechanism of the gland. They are all capable of abolishing the gradient of iodide between plasma and thyroid cells. Their goitrogenic effects can be overcome by thyroxine or iodide.

Thiocyanate is not concentrated in the thyroid gland, as is perchlorate, and is one-tenth as active. It is widely distributed in food and is normally present to a small extent in plasma. Sodium or potassium perchlorate is effective in the control of hyperthyroidism. Although the incidence of toxic effects such as fever, rash, enteric irritation, and agranulocytosis can be minimized by administering less than 1 gm daily, the usefulness of perchlorate has been limited by the occurrence of a few cases of aplastic anemia.

IODIDE

Although small amounts of iodide are required for hormone synthesis by the thyroid gland, large amounts may produce goiter and hypothyroidism when given to normal individuals for prolonged periods. Iodide can be rapidly effective in ameliorating hyperthyroidism. Maximal effects are seen in about 2 weeks, and include improvement in signs and symptoms and reduction in the size and vascularity of the gland. Unfortunately, it is not often possible to achieve a complete remission or to maintain the degree of control achieved for more than a few weeks.

Iodide administration seems to inhibit many aspects of thyroid function, including the organic binding of iodine and, in the toxic gland, the degradation of thyroglobulin. Its use in hyperthyroidism is at present limited to the preparation for thyroid surgery, although in some instances the disease has been treated with iodide alone.

Iodobrassid (Lipoiodine) is available in tablets containing 293 mg (equivalent to 150 mg of potassium iodide or 1 ml Lugol's solution). Lugol's solution is 5% iodine and 10% potassium iodide. Saturated solution of potassium iodide is available as such. In areas of endemic goiter, iodized poppyseed oil has been useful when iodized salt could not be used.

RADIOACTIVE IODINE

¹³¹Iodine (half-life 8 days) is the most commonly employed isotope of iodine. ¹³⁰I (half-life 12.3 hours) and ¹²⁵I (half-life 60 days) have also been used for experimental purposes.

¹³¹I, like stable iodine, is trapped by the thyroid gland, incorporated into thyroxine and triiodothyronine, and stored in the colloid. It emits beta rays to a mean depth of 0.5 mm (maximum 2 mm), administering radiation to the parenchyma of the gland and little else. This isotope also emits gamma rays. They account for only a small percentage of the therapeutic effect, but they do permit the study of the isotope by external counting technics.

¹³¹I is obtained essentially carrier-free from the products of uranium fission. It is supplied in low concentrations for diagnostic use and in higher concentrations for therapeutic use. It is assayed before delivery and labeled to show time of assay and activity as well as other pertinent information. The USP solution is prepared for oral or intravenous use. ¹³¹I is also available in single dose capsules.

THERAPEUTIC USES OF ANTITHYROID DRUGS & PROCEDURES

Antithyroid therapy is indicated in the treatment of hyperthyroidism and occasionally in euthyroid individuals with intractable angina pectoris.

Hyperthyroidism may be treated in several ways, depending in part upon the specific problem the patient presents and in part upon the experience and preferences of the physician.

Radioiodine Therapy

In general, radioiodine therapy is reserved for individuals over 40 years of age, and is specifically contraindicated in pregnancy. The average dose is 4–5 mc, and can be calculated on the basis of the estimated gland weight and iodine uptake to provide 7–10 thousand rads/gm of tissue. The symptoms subside gradually over a period of months, and several doses may be required. Radioiodine may be used in conjunction with other drugs to obtain more rapid control of symptoms. It has become apparent with time that an increasing number of patients treated with radioiodine become hypothyroid. The incidence of this complication is estimated to be 70% after 10 years. A similar phenomenon is observed following subtotal thyroidectomy, although the incidence is less than 50%. Since hypothyroidism can be insidious in its appearance and very disabling, the institution of thyroid hormone replacement shortly after radioiodine or surgical treatment may be advisable.

When large doses (25–75 mc) are used to destroy normal tissue in patients with intractable angina pectoris, thyroiditis may occur, and acute hyperthyroidism secondary to the loss of stored hormone from the damaged gland has been observed. Studies in patients receiving ^{131}I indicate that this treatment can produce abnormal chromosomes.

Antithyroid Drug Therapy

Antithyroid drugs may be used to control hyperthyroidism until a remission is achieved by radiotherapy (as noted above), in preparation for subtotal thyroidectomy, or as definitive treatment. Treatment is started with large doses of the drug (eg, 100–150 mg of propylthiouracil every 6 hours) in order to achieve maximal inhibition of hormone synthesis. Improvement begins rapidly, although its onset is slower after pretreatment with iodine or in the presence of a large gland with much stored hormone. When a euthyroid state is achieved, the dose can be reduced to a maintenance level of 5–10 mg of methimazole or 100–150 mg of propylthiouracil in divided doses. When continued for a year, about 50% of patients will be in a lasting remission. In 25% of cases, symptoms return upon cessation of therapy. The recurrence can be predicted if the normal suppressibility of thyroid function does not return in the post-treatment period. Patients in whom the thyroid gland is not greatly enlarged and whose disease is of short duration are more likely to respond favorably. Reduction in the size of the gland during therapy and return of normal suppressibility of thyroid function are favorable prognostic signs. This treatment is frequently used in children and young adults and in others in whom surgery and ^{131}I are contraindicated. The disadvantages of this treatment are the prolonged period of active therapy required, the toxic effects of the drugs, and the uncertainty of a lasting remission. Its advantages are the avoidance of surgery and anesthesia and the attendant risks of hypoparathyroidism and recurrent laryngeal nerve injury. Antithyroid drug therapy also avoids the risk of hypoparathyroidism associated with ^{131}I therapy.

When antithyroid drugs are used in preparation for surgery, they are administered in the same fashion. When the patient is euthyroid, iodides are given for 10 days in order to reduce the vascularity of the gland. Such treatment has reduced the surgical risk to negligible levels in the hands of an experienced thyroid surgeon.

The observation that many signs and symptoms of hyperthyroidism resemble the effects of catecholamines suggested the use of drugs such as reserpine, guanethidine, and propranolol to control the manifestations. The first 2 drugs have been disappointing in this application, and simple sedation with agents such as phenobarbital is just as effective. Propranolol will control many of the symptoms of thyrotoxicosis, but its usefulness in this disorder has not been established.

Preparations Available

Propylthiouracil: Tablets, 50 mg

Methimazole (Tapazole): Tablets, 5 and 10 mg

Iothiouracil sodium (Itrumil): Tablets, 50 mg

• • •

General References

Astwood, E.B., Cassidy, C.E., & G.D. Aurbach: Treatment of goiter and thyroid nodules with thyroid. JAMA 174:459–464, 1960.

Catz, B., & S. Russell: Myxedema, shock and coma. Arch Int Med 108:407–417, 1961.

DeGroot, L.J.: Current views on formation of thyroid hormones. New England J Med 272:243–249, 297–303, 355–361, 1965.

Greer, M.A.: The natural occurrence of goitrogenic agents. Recent Progr Hormone Res 18:187, 1962.

Greer, M.A., Meihoff, W.C., & H. Studer: Treatment of hyperthyroidism with a single daily dose of propylthiouracil. New England J Med 271:888, 1965.

Harrison, M.T.: The prevention and treatment of thyroid storm. Pharmacol Physicians 2:1–5, 1968.

Ingbar, S.H.: Management of emergencies. 9. Thyroid storm. New England J Med 274:1252–1254, 1966.

Nofal, M.M., Beierwaltes, W.H., & M.E. Patno: Treatment of hyperthyroidism with sodium iodide I131. JAMA 197:605–610, 1966.

Selenkow, H.A., & M.S. Wool: A new synthetic thyroid hormone combination for clinical therapy. Ann Int Med 67:90–99, 1967.

Stanbury, J.B., & L.J. DeGroot: The clinical chemistry and pathologic physiology of thyroid tissue. Clin Chem 13:542–553, 1967.

Symposium on the thyroid gland. J Clin Path (Suppl) 20:308, 1967.

Symposium on the Diagnosis and Treatment of Common Thyroid Diseases. Excerpta Medica International Congress Series No. 227, 1971.

Werner, S.C. (editor): *The Thyroid: A Fundamental and Clinical Text,* 3rd ed. Hoeber, 1971.

35 . . .

The Adrenocortical Steroids & Their Antagonists

The adrenocortical hormones are steroid molecules produced and released by the adrenal cortex. The secretory process is controlled by the pituitary release of corticotropin (ACTH). Secretion of the salt-retaining hormone aldosterone is also under the influence of angiotensin. Corticotropin has some actions which do not depend upon its effect on adrenocortical secretion. However, its pharmacologic value as an anti-inflammatory agent and its use in testing adrenal function depend on its trophic action. Therefore, its pharmacology will be discussed with the adrenocortical hormones.

This group of hormones has been employed in the diagnosis and treatment of a variety of disorders of adrenal function and as anti-inflammatory agents. For this reason it will be useful to outline some of the more important disturbances in adrenocortical function. Much of what is currently known about the physiology and biochemistry of this group of hormones has evolved from the careful study of these disorders.

ENDOGENOUS ADRENOCORTICOSTEROIDS

The adrenal cortex releases a large number of steroids into the circulation. Some have minimal biologic activity and function primarily as precursors, and there are some for which no function has been established. The hormonal steroids may be classified as those having important effects on intermediary metabolism (glucocorticoids), those having principally salt retaining activity (mineralocorticoids), and those having androgenic or estrogenic activity. In man, the major glucocorticoid is cortisol and the most important mineralocorticoid is aldosterone. Quantitatively, dehydroepiandrosterone (DHEA) is the major androgen since about 20 mg are secreted daily, partly as the sulfate. However, both DHEA and androstenedione are very weak androgens. A small amount of testosterone is secreted by the adrenal and may be of greater importance as an androgen. Little is known about the estrogens secreted by the adrenal. However, it has been shown that the adrenal androgens such as testosterone

and androstenedione can be converted to estrone in small amounts by nonendocrine tissues.

GLUCOCORTICOIDS
(Cortisol, Hydrocortisone, Compound F)

The major glucocorticoid in man is cortisol, a colorless, crystalline steroid with a molecular weight of 362.5 and a melting point of 217–220° C. It is slightly soluble in water (0.28 mg/ml). It is synthesized from cholesterol (as shown in Fig 35–1) by the cells of the zona fasciculata and zona reticularis and released into the circulation under the influence of ACTH. The mechanisms controlling its secretion are discussed in Chapter 39.

In the normal adult in the absence of stress, about 20 mg of cortisol are secreted daily. In plasma, cortisol is bound to plasma proteins. Corticosteroid-binding globulin, an alpha$_2$ globulin synthesized by the liver, binds 95% of the circulating hormone under normal circumstances. The remaining 5% is the metabolically active fraction. When plasma cortisol levels exceed 20–30 μg/100 ml, most of the excess is loosely bound to albumin.

The half-life of cortisol in the circulation is normally about 90–110 minutes; it may be increased when large amounts are present or in hypothyroidism. Cortisol is removed from the circulation in the liver, where it is reduced and conjugated to form water-soluble compounds which can be excreted into the urine (Fig 35–2). The side chain (C20 and 21) is removed from about 5–10% of the cortisol, and the resulting compounds are further metabolized and excreted into the urine as 11-oxy 17-ketosteroids.

In some species (eg, the rat), corticosterone is the major glucocorticoid. It is less firmly bound to protein and therefore metabolized more rapidly. The pathways of its degradation are similar to those of cortisol.

Physiologic Considerations

The glucocorticoids have widespread effects because they influence the function of most cells in the body. Although many of the effects are dose-related and become magnified when large amounts are administered for therapeutic purposes, there are also "permissive effects." In other words, many normal

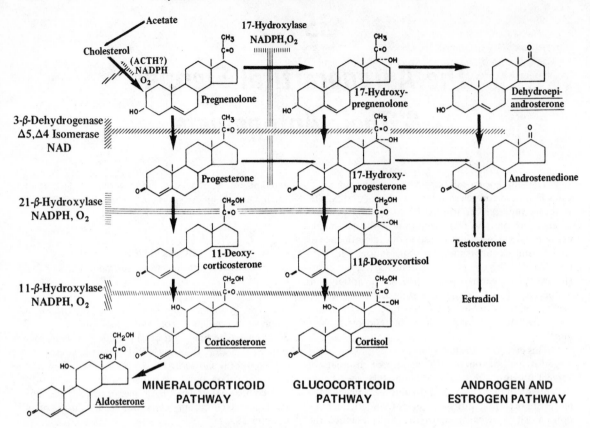

FIG 35–1. Outline of major pathways in adrenocortical hormone biosynthesis. The major secretory products are underlined. Pregnenolone is the major precursor of corticosterone and aldosterone, and 17-hydroxypregnenolone is the major precursor of cortisol. The enzymes and cofactors for the reactions progressing down each column are shown on the left and from the first to the second column at the top of the figure. When a particular enzyme is deficient, hormone production is blocked at the points indicated by the shaded bars. (Modified after Welikey, Mulrow, & others: Reproduced, with permission, from Ganong: *Review of Medical Physiology,* 5th ed. Lange, 1971.)

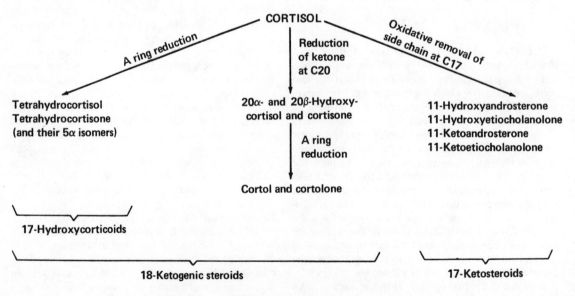

FIG 35–2. Primary excretion products of cortisol.

reactions which take place at a significant rate only in the presence of corticoids are not further stimulated in the presence of large amounts of corticoids.

These hormones have important effects on intermediary metabolism. They stimulate the production of glucose (gluconeogenesis) from proteins. The increase in circulating glucose stimulates the production of insulin and leads to the deposition of fat, particularly in the trunk, face, and mesentery. Cortisol has an anti-insulin effect and also decreases the utilization of amino acids in muscle and adipose tissue.

Cortisol or another glucocorticoid is required for maintenance of the normal alpha rhythm in the EEG. Experimentally, glucocorticoids lower the threshold to electrically induced convulsions. These compounds also inhibit the secretion of ACTH (see Chapter 39). Their presence is required for the normal function of both smooth and striated muscle. Large doses of glucocorticoids stimulate excessive production of acid and pepsin in the stomach and stimulate the formation of peptic ulcer. They facilitate fat absorption and appear to antagonize the effect of vitamin D on calcium absorption. The glucocorticoids also have important effects on the hematopoietic system, decreasing the number of lymphocytes, eosinophils, and basophils while increasing the number of neutrophils, platelets, and red blood cells.

In the absence of physiologic amounts of cortisol, renal function (particularly glomerular filtration) is impaired and there is an inability to excrete a water load.

Natural and synthetic glucocorticoids and anti-inflammatory steroids have been found to bind to specific intracellular receptors upon entering target tissues. The macromolecular complex thus formed is transported into the nucleus where it interacts with chromosomal constituents to alter gene expression. These hormones alter the regulation of many cellular processes, including enzyme synthesis and activity, membrane permeability, transport processes, and structure.

MINERALOCORTICOIDS
(Aldosterone, Deoxycorticosterone)

The most important mineralocorticoid in man is aldosterone. However, small amounts of deoxycorticosterone (DOC) are also formed and released. Although the amounts are normally insignificant, DOC is of some importance therapeutically. Its actions, effects, and metabolism are similar to those described below for aldosterone.

Aldosterone is synthesized mainly in the zona glomerulosa of the adrenal cortex (Fig 35–1).

The rate of aldosterone secretion is subject to several influences. ACTH produces a moderate stimulation of its release, but this effect is not sustained for more than a few days in the normal individual. Although aldosterone is no less than one-third as effective as cortisol in suppressing ACTH, the minute quantities of aldosterone produced by the adrenal cortex prevent it from participating in any feedback relationship in the control of ACTH secretion.

After hypophysectomy, aldosterone secretion gradually falls to about half the normal rate, which means that other factors are able to maintain and perhaps regulate its secretion. Independent variations between cortisol and aldosterone secretion can also be demonstrated by means of lesions in the nervous system such as decerebration, which decreases the secretion of hydrocortisone while increasing the secretion of aldosterone.

One of the important stimuli of aldosterone secretion is a reduction in blood volume, whether due to hemorrhage, dietary sodium restriction, or sodium loss following administration of diuretics (Fig 35–3).

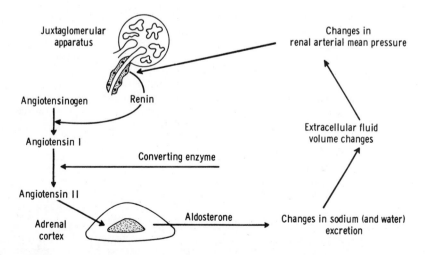

FIG 35–3. A postulated feedback mechanism regulating aldosterone secretion. (Reproduced, with permission, from Ganong: *Review of Medical Physiology,* 5th ed. Lange, 1971.)

These stimuli lead to a decrease in mean renal arterial pressure which is associated with an increase in the release of renin by the cells of the juxtaglomerular apparatus. The enzyme renin then acts upon a circulating alpha$_2$ globulin (renin substrate), releasing angiotensin I, which is then converted to angiotensin II. Angiotensin is a powerful stimulant of aldosterone production, only a few micrograms being required to show an effect in man (see p 125).

Physiologic Considerations

Aldosterone and other steroids with mineralocorticoid properties induce the reabsorption of sodium from urine by the renal tubules in exchange for potassium and hydrogen ion. Sodium reabsorption in the sweat and salivary glands, gastrointestinal mucosa, and across cell membranes in general is also increased. Excessive levels of aldosterone produced by tumors or overdosage with other mineralocorticoids lead to hypernatremia, hypokalemia, metabolic alkalosis, increased plasma volume, and hypertension.

Aldosterone has a delayed action on sodium transport. Recent experiments indicate that its action is dependent upon the synthesis of an enzyme required by the transport mechanism. The hormone appears to stimulate the formation of nuclear RNA, which in turn serves the induction of enzyme synthesis.

Metabolism

Aldosterone is secreted at the rate of 100–200 μg/day in normal individuals with a moderate dietary salt intake. The plasma level in males (resting supine) is about 0.007 μg/100 ml. The half-life of aldosterone injected in tracer quantities is 15–20 minutes, and it does not appear to be firmly bound to serum proteins.

The metabolism of aldosterone is similar to that of cortisol, about 50 μg appearing in the urine as conjugated tetrahydroaldosterone. Approximately 5–15 μg/24 hours are excreted free or as the 3-oxo glucuronide.

DOC is normally secreted in amounts of about 200 μg/day. Its half-life when injected into the human circulation is about 70 minutes. Preliminary estimates of its concentration in plasma are approximately 30 ng/100 ml. The control of its secretion differs from that of aldosterone in that the secretion of DOC is primarily under the control of ACTH. Although the response to ACTH is enhanced by dietary sodium restriction, a low-salt diet does not increase DOC secretion.

SYNTHETIC ADRENOCORTICOSTEROIDS

ACTH and steroids having glucocorticoid activity have become important agents for use in the treatment of many inflammatory and allergic disorders. This has stimulated the search for and development of many steroids with anti-inflammatory activity.

TABLE 35–1. Structure-activity relationships of commonly used glucocorticoids.

	Activity				Structure			
	Glucocorticoid and Anti-inflammatory Potency (Cortisol = 1)	Equivalent Oral Dose (mg)	Topical Activity*	Salt Retention Activity	Double Bond at Carbon 1–2(Δ^1)	Substituents at Carbons		
						R(11)	6	9	16
Cortisol	1	20	1	++		–OH			
Cortisone	0.8	25	0.8	++		=O			
Prednisolone	4	5	1–2	+	+	–OH			
Prednisone	3.5	5	1–2	+	+	=O			
Methylprednisolone	5	4	5		+	–OH	α-methyl		
Triamcinolone	5	4	1–40		+	–OH		α-fluoro	α-OH
Paramethasone	10	2			+	–OH	α-fluoro		α-methyl
Fludrocortisone	10	2	5–40	++++		–OH		α-fluoro	
Dexamethasone	30	0.75	10		+	–OH		α-fluoro	α-methyl
Betamethasone	35	0.6	5–150		+	–OH		α-fluoro	β-methyl

*Various esters of these compounds are also used for topical administration (Table 35–2).

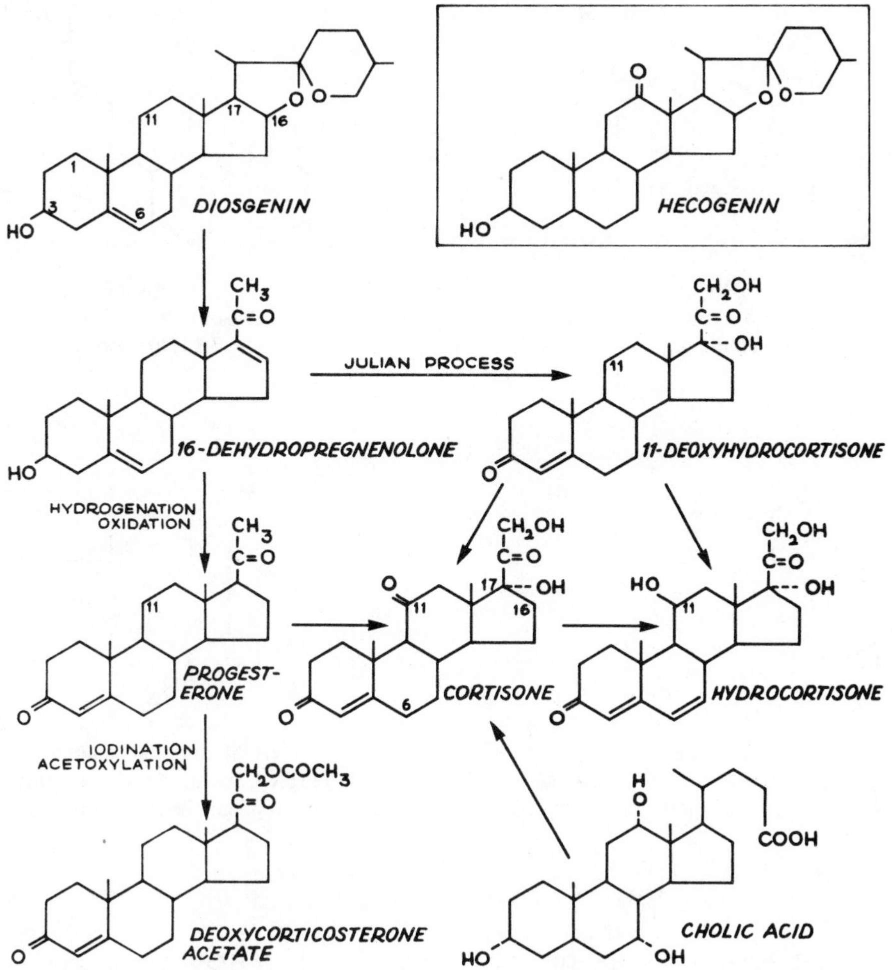

FIG 35—4. Synthesis of corticosteroids from diosgenin, hecogenin, and cholic acid. (From *Drill's Pharmacology in Medicine,* 3rd ed, 1965. J.R. DiPalma, editor. Used with permission of McGraw-Hill Book Co.)

Source & Chemistry

Although the natural corticosteroids can be obtained from animal adrenals, they are usually synthesized from cholic acid (obtained from cattle) or steroid sapogenins, diosgenin in particular, found in plants of the Liliaceae and Dioscoreaceae families (Fig 35—4). Further modifications of these steroids at the 1, 2, 6, 9, 16, and other positions have led to the marketing of a large group of synthetic steroids with special characteristics which are pharmacologically and therapeutically important (Table 35—2).

Metabolism

The metabolism of the naturally occurring adrenal steroids has been discussed above. The synthetic corticosteroids for oral use (Table 35—1) are in most cases rapidly and completely absorbed when given by mouth. Although they are transported and metabolized in a fashion similar to the endogenous steroids, important differences exist.

Alterations in the molecule influence the degree of protein binding, side chain stability, rate of reduc-

tion, and end products. Halogenation at the 9 position, unsaturation of the Δ1-2 bond of the A ring, and methylation at the 2 or 16 position will prolong the half-life by more than 50%. The 11-hydroxyl group also appears to inhibit destruction since the half-life of compound S (11-deoxycortisol) is half that of cortisol. The Δ1 compounds are excreted in the free form.

Pharmacologic Effects

The mechanism of action of the synthetic steroids is similar to that of cortisol (see above). They have been found to bind to the specific intracellular receptor protein. The specific effects leading to the suppression of inflammatory and allergic responses are not fully known. Inhibition of synthesis of specific proteins involved in chemotaxis and immunologic reactions as well as other alterations in leukocyte and macrophage function appear to be involved.

Clinical Uses

A. Diagnosis and Treatment of Disturbed Adrenal Function:

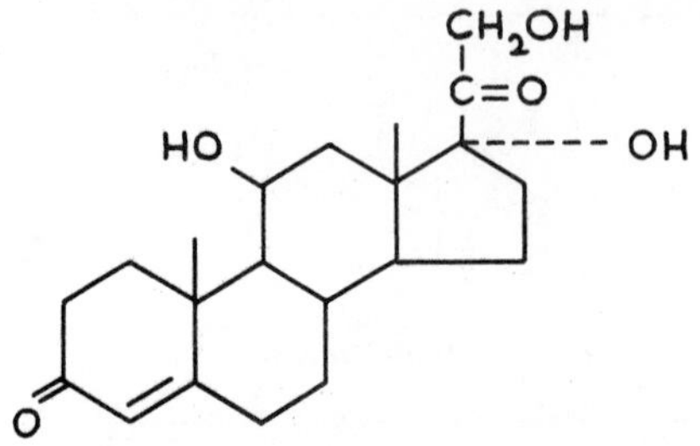

Hydrocortisone (Cortisol)
(11β,17,21-trihydroxy-4-pregnene-
3,20-dione)

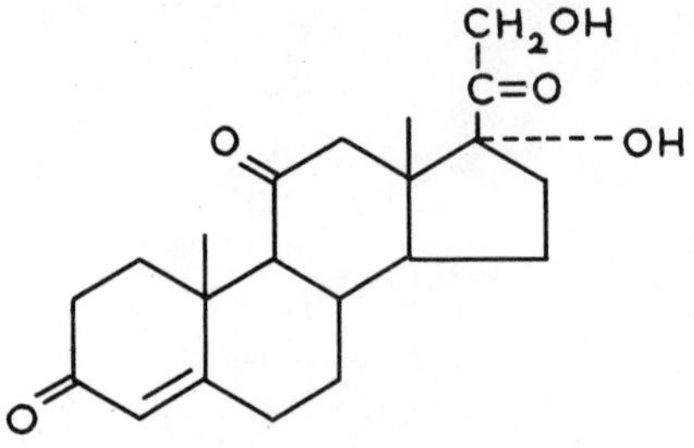

Cortisone
(17,21-dihydroxy-4-pregnene-
3,11,20-trione)

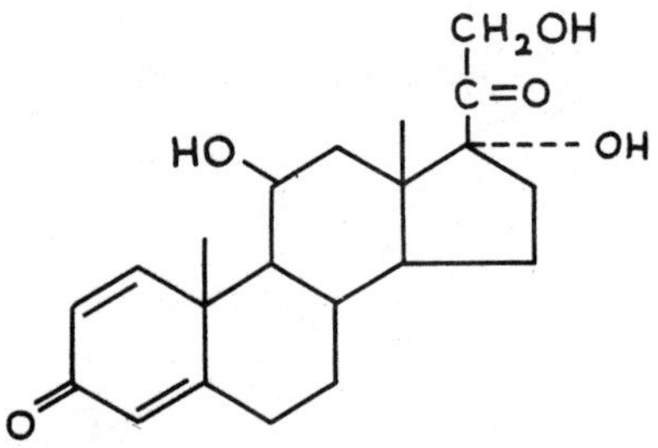

Prednisolone
(11β,17,21-trihydroxy-1,4-pregnadiene-
3,20-dione)

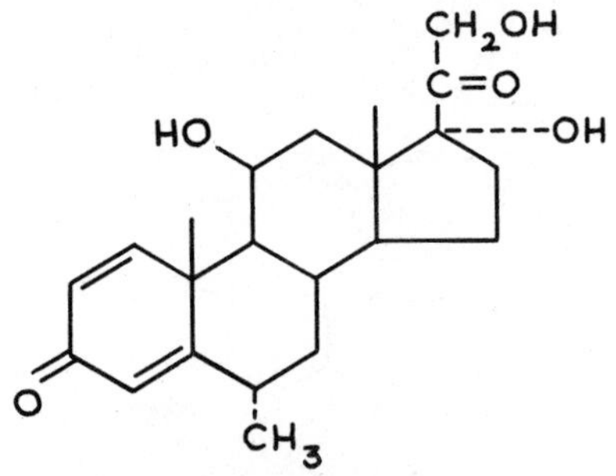

Methylprednisolone
(11β,17,21-trihydroxy-6α-methyl-1,4-
pregnadiene-3,20-dione)

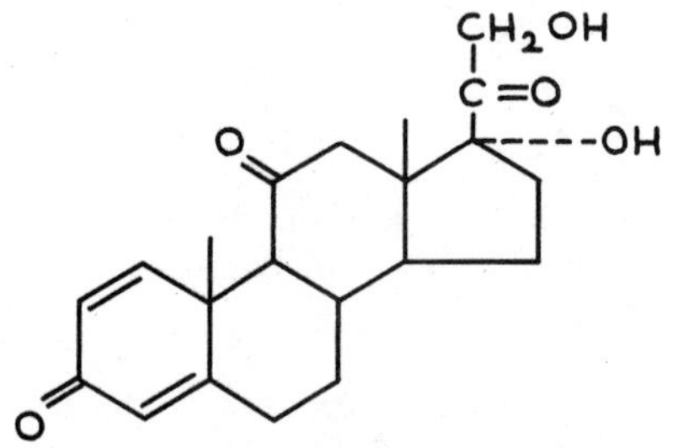

Prednisone
(17,21-dihydroxy-1,4-pregnadiene-
3,11,20-trione)

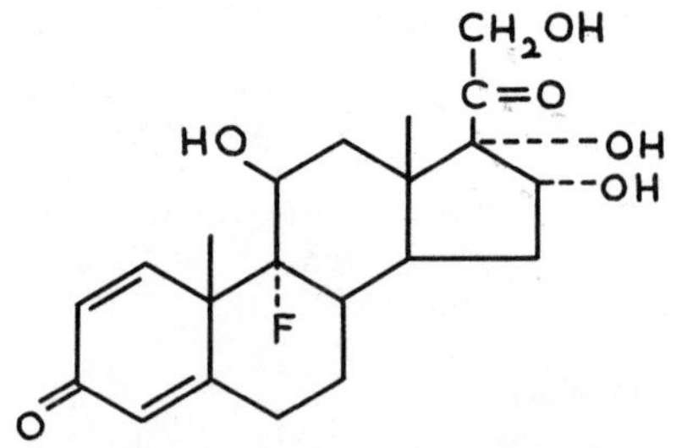

Triamcinolone
(9α-fluoro-16α-hydroxyprednisolone)

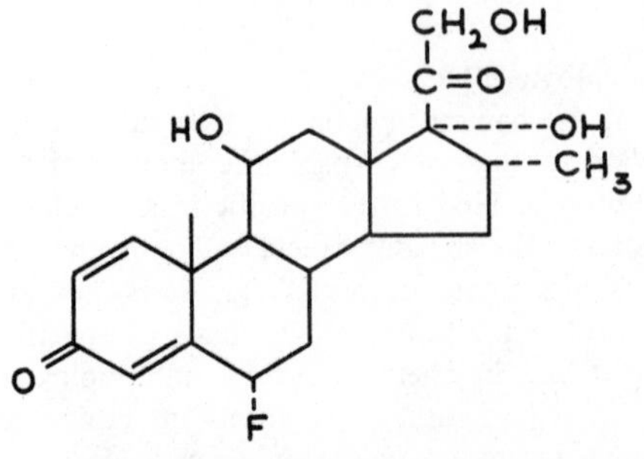

Paramethasone
(6α-fluoro-16α-methylprednisolone)

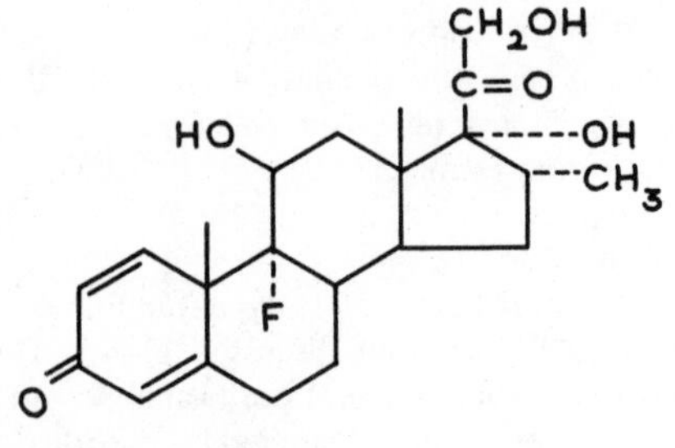

Dexamethasone
(9α-fluoro-16α-methylprednisolone)

FIG 35–5. Chemical structures of adrenocorticosteroids and derivatives.

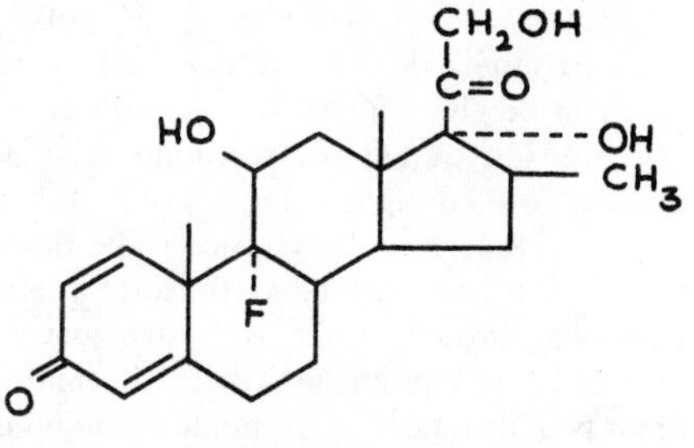

Betamethasone
(9α-fluoro-16β-methylprednisolone)

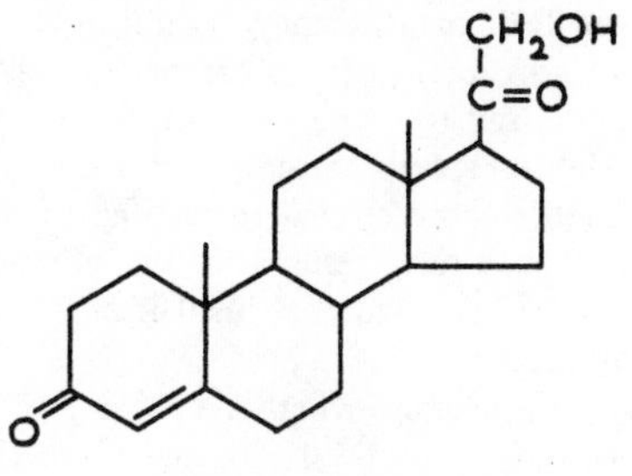

Deoxycorticosterone
(11-deoxycorticosterone)

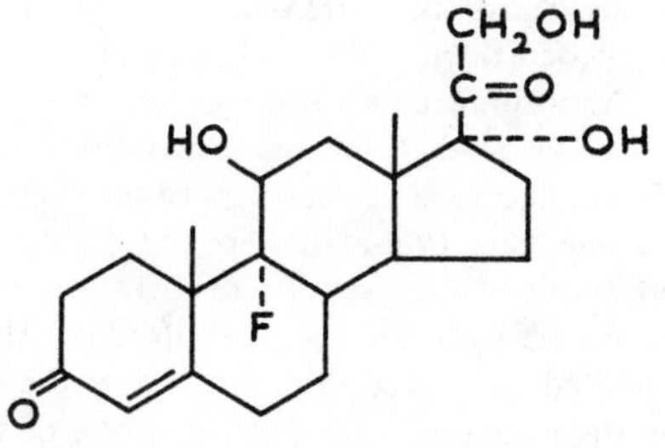

Fludrocortisone
(9α-fluoro-11β,17,21-trihydroxy-4-pregnene-
3,20-dione)

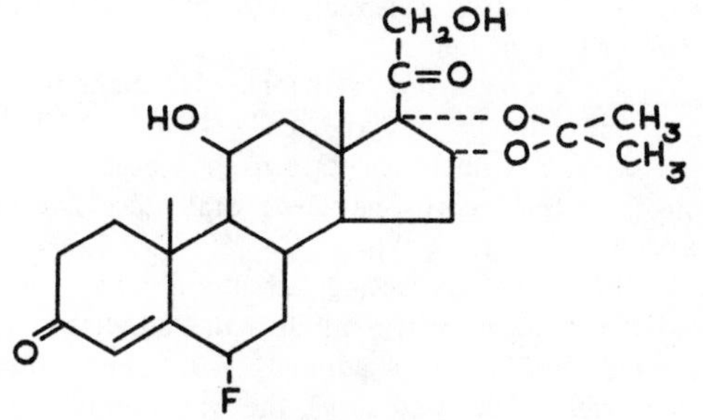

Flurandrenolone
(6α-fluoro-16α-hydroxyhydrocortisone-
16,17-acetonide)

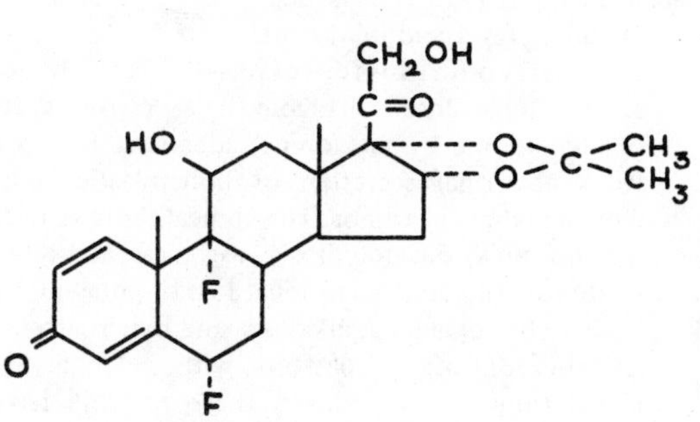

Fluocinolone
(6α,9α-difluoro-16α-hydroxyprednisolone-
16,17-acetonide)

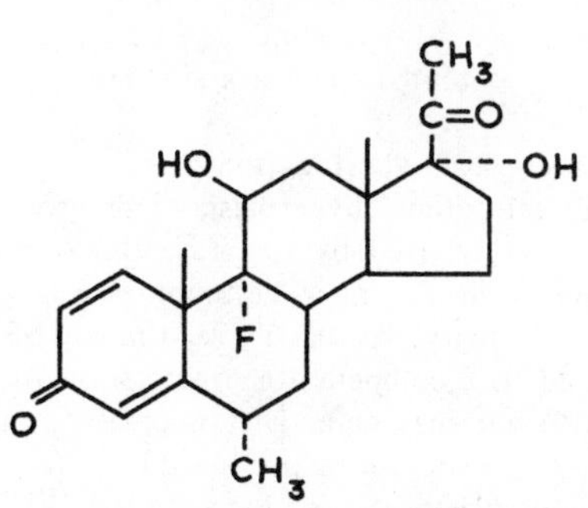

Fluorometholone
(6α-methyl-9α-fluoro-21-deoxyprednisolone)

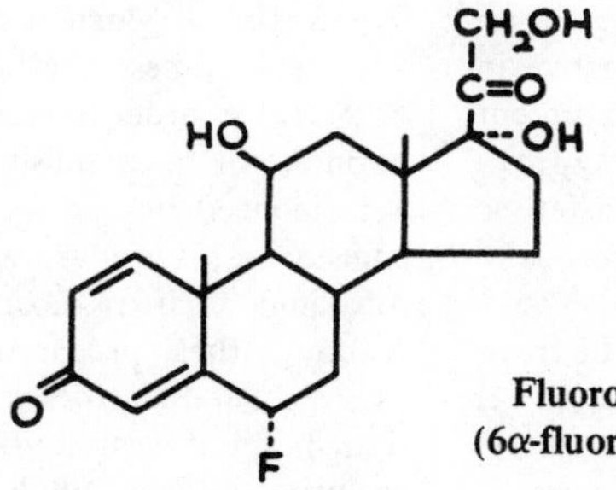

Fluoroprednisolone
(6α-fluoroprednisolone)

FIG 35–5 (cont'd). Chemical structures of adrenocorticosteroids and derivatives.

1. Adrenocortical insufficiency (Addison's disease)—Chronic adrenocortical insufficiency (addisonism) is characterized by hyperpigmentation, weakness, fatigue, weight loss, hypotension, and inability to maintain the blood glucose level with fasting. In such individuals, minor noxious, traumatic, or infectious stimuli may produce acute adrenal insufficiency with shock and finally death.

In adrenal insufficiency, whether primary or following adrenalectomy, about 20–30 mg of cortisol must be given daily, with increased amounts during periods of stress. This must be supplemented by an appropriate amount of a salt-retaining hormone such as DOC or fludrocortisone. It is for this reason that glucocorticoids devoid of salt-retaining activity are not indicated for these patients.

Aldosterone is not used for replacement therapy since the supply is too small. However, deoxycorticosterone trimethylacetate given in monthly injections and fludrocortisone given orally are excellent preparations for this purpose.

When a rapidly acting parenteral preparation is needed for the management of acute adrenal insufficiency (or to prevent adrenal insufficiency during major stress such as surgery), the water-soluble hemisuccinate of cortisol is ideal. Intramuscular administration of cortisol or cortisone or their acetates is not satisfactory because the rate of absorption is unpredictable and the onset of effect is too slow for emergency use. The availability of a good preparation of cortisol for intravenous use eliminates the need for costly and less potent aqueous and lipid adrenal extracts.

2. Adrenocortical hyperfunction—

a. Congenital adrenal hyperplasia—This group of disorders are characterized by specific defects in the synthesis of cortisol. The most common is a lack of 21-hydroxylase activity. As can be seen in Fig 35–1, this would lead to a compensatory increase in ACTH release. If sufficient enzyme activity is present, a normal amount of cortisol will be produced but the gland will become hyperplastic and produce abnormally large amounts of precursors such as 17-hydroxyprogesterone which can be diverted to the androgen pathway leading to virilization. Metabolism of this compound in the liver leads to pregnanetriol, which is characteristically excreted into the urine in large amounts in this disorder.

If the defect is in 11-hydroxylation, hypertension is prominent. When 17-hydroxylation is defective in the adrenals and gonads, hypogonadism will be present in contrast to the 11-hydroxylation deficiency. However, increased amounts of 11-deoxycorticosterone (DOC) are formed and the signs and symptoms associated with mineralocorticoid excess are found.

Cortisol and cortisone have been used in the treatment of congenital adrenal hyperplasia. Since ACTH suppression is an important objective of therapy, slowly absorbed parenteral preparations can be given in smaller amounts than the oral preparations, which are rapidly absorbed and metabolized and must be given in divided doses. When treating these patients, larger doses of cortisone (25–100 mg daily IM, depending upon age) can be given for 5–10 days to achieve adequate suppression of adrenal secretion. The dose is then reduced to 4–6 mg/day and adjusted to maintain a low urinary ketosteroid excretion. The dose must also be adjusted over the long course of therapy to permit normal growth since excessive amounts of glucocorticoids inhibit linear growth in children. In some infants, salt-retaining hormone therapy is also required.

b. Cushing's syndrome—Cushing's syndrome is usually the result of bilateral adrenal hyperplasia but occasionally is due to tumors of the gland. The manifestations are those associated with the presence of excessive glucocorticoids. When changes are marked, a rounded, plethoric face and trunk obesity are striking in appearance. In general, the manifestations of protein loss are severe and include muscle wasting, thinning of the skin, striae, easy bruisability, poor wound healing, and osteoporosis. Other serious disturbances include mental disorders, hypertension, and diabetes. This disorder is treated by the surgical removal of the tumor producing the hormone, or by the resection of hyperplastic adrenals. These patients must receive large doses of cortisol during and following the surgical procedure. Doses of 300 mg of soluble hydrocortisone intravenously are used on the day of surgery. The dose must be reduced slowly to normal replacement levels since rapid reduction in dose may produce symptoms including fever and joint pain.

c. Hyperaldosteronism—Primary hyperaldosteronism usually results from the excessive production of aldosterone by an adrenal adenoma. It may result from abnormal secretion of hyperplastic glands or from a malignant tumor. The clinical findings of hypertension, polyuria, polydipsia, weakness, and tetany are related to the continued renal loss of potassium which leads to hypokalemia, alkalosis, and hypernatremia.

In contrast to patients with secondary hyperaldosteronism (see below), these patients have low (suppressed) levels of plasma renin activity and angiotension II. When treated with deoxycorticosterone acetate (20 mg IM daily for 3 days), they fail to retain sodium and their secretion of aldosterone is not significantly reduced. They are generally improved when treated with spironolactone, and their response to this agent is of diagnostic value (see p 339).

3. Use of glucocorticoids for diagnostic purposes—It is sometimes necessary to suppress the production of ACTH in order to identify the source of a particular hormone or to establish whether or not its production is influenced by the secretion of ACTH. In these circumstances, it is advantageous to employ a very potent substance such as dexamethasone or betamethasone. Although these preparations are no more effective, the use of small quantities reduces the possibility of confusion in the interpretation of hormone assays in blood or urine. For example, if complete suppression is achieved by the use of 50 mg of cortisol, the urinary 17-hydroxycorticoids will be 15–18 mg/24 hours. If

1.5 mg of dexamethasone are employed, the excretion will be only 0.5 mg/24 hours.

In an individual with normal adrenal function, 2 mg/day of dexamethasone or betamethasone are adequate to achieve suppression in the absence of stress. In patients with Cushing's syndrome, 8 mg/day are usually effective if the excessive cortisol is produced by hyperplastic adrenals but will not suppress hormones arising from a carcinoma of the adrenal.

Suppression of the adrenal with glucocorticoids and of the ovary with estrogens can be useful in locating the source of androgen production in a hirsute woman if the effect on testosterone levels in blood or urine can be measured before and during hormone administration.

B. Adrenocorticosteroids and Nonadrenal Disorders: Cortisol and its synthetic analogues have been found to be useful in the treatment of a diverse group of diseases unrelated to any known disturbance of adrenal function.

1. Some indications for glucocorticoid therapy in therapy of nonadrenal disease—
Rheumatic fever
Rheumatoid arthritis
Systemic lupus erythematosus
Polyarteritis nodosa
Uveitis
Nephrotic syndrome
Ulcerative colitis
Sarcoidosis
Acute gout
Thrombocytopenic purpura
Hemolytic anemias
Pemphigus vulgaris
Subacute thyroiditis
Asthma
Pruritus ani and vulvae
Atopic dermatitis
Bursitis
Acute leukemia (see Chapter 45)
Immunosuppression in conjunction with tissue transplantation (see Chapter 46)
Shock due to gram-negative septicemia

When used in the therapy of these disorders, the corticosteroids are not usually curative. They may, in fact, suppress the clinical manifestations without altering the progress of the pathologic process.

2. Adverse reactions—The benefits obtained from the use of these compounds vary considerably. They must be carefully weighed in each patient against the widespread effects on every part of the organism. The major undesirable effects of the glucocorticoids are not toxic effects but exaggerations of their hormonal actions (see above) and lead to the clinical picture of iatrogenic Cushing's syndrome.

When the glucocorticoids are used for short periods (less than 1 week), it is unusual to see serious side-effects even with moderately large doses. Behavioral changes and acute peptic ulcers are occasionally observed.

a. Adrenal suppression—When physiologic amounts of corticosteroids are administered for long periods of time, adrenal suppression occurs and the patient should be given supplementary therapy at times of severe stress such as accidental trauma or surgery. The degree of adrenal unresponsiveness is a function of the length of time the patient has been treated. The dose is not an important variable when the threshold for suppression has been exceeded. With very rare exceptions, recovery occurs when the drug is withdrawn; however, a state of relative insufficiency may exist for several days, weeks, or even months after prolonged suppression.

b. Iatrogenic Cushing's syndrome—Most patients who are given daily doses of 100 mg of cortisol or more (or the equivalent amount of synthetic steroid) for longer than 2 weeks undergo a series of changes which have been termed iatrogenic Cushing's syndrome. The rate of development is a function of the dose. The appearance of the face is altered by rounding, puffiness, and plethora. Fat tends to be redistributed from the extremities to the trunk and face. There is an increased growth of fine hair over the thighs and trunk, and sometimes the face. Acne may increase or appear, and insomnia and increased appetite are noted. In the treatment of dangerous or disabling disorders, these changes may not require cessation of therapy. However, the underlying metabolic changes which accompany them can be very serious by the time they become obvious. The continuing breakdown of protein and diversion of amino acids to glucose increases the need for insulin and over a period of time results in weight gain, fat deposition, muscle wasting, thinning of the skin with striae and bruising, hyperglycemia, growth suppression (in children), and eventually the development of steroid diabetes and osteoporosis.

Other serious complications include the development of peptic ulcers and their complications. The clinical findings associated with other disorders, particularly bacterial and mycotic infections, may be masked by the corticosteroids, and patients must be carefully watched to avoid serious mishap when large doses are used. Some patients develop a myopathy, the nature of which is unknown. The frequency of myopathy is greater in patients treated with triamcinolone. The administration of this drug as well as of methylprednisolone has been associated with nausea, dizziness, and weight loss in some patients. It is treated by changing drugs, reducing dosage, and increasing the potassium and protein intake. When diabetes occurs, it is treated by diet and insulin, although these patients rarely develop ketoacidosis. In general, patients treated with corticosteroids should be on high-protein diets, and increased potassium and anabolic steroids should be used when required.

When given in greater than physiologic amounts, the use of steroids such as cortisone and hydrocortisone, which have mineralocorticoid effects, cause, in addition to glucocorticoid effects, some sodium and fluid retention and loss of potassium. In patients with normal cardiovascular and renal function, this leads to

TABLE 35–2. Adrenal corticosteroids: Preparations available.

	Oral	Parenteral*	Topical
Hydrocortisone (cortisol; many trade names)	Tablets, 5, 10, and 20 mg Suspension, 2 mg/ml	Solution, 50 and 125 mg/ml Suspension, 50 mg/ml Aqueous suspension, 5, 25, 50, and 125 mg/ml	Cream, 0.2, 0.25, 0.5, 1, 1.5, 2, and 2.5% Ointment, 0.25, 0.5, 1, 1.5, 2, and 2.5% Lotion, 0.125, 0.25, 0.5, and 1% Drops, 0.2% Suppositories, 25 and 50 mg
Cortisone acetate (Cortone)	Tablets, 5, 10, and 25 mg	Suspension, 25 and 50 mg/ml	Ointment, 1.5% Solution, 0.5 and 2% Ophthalmic solution, 2%
Prednisolone (many trade names)	Tablets, 1, 2.5, and 5 mg Timed capsules, 5 mg	Aqueous suspension, 10, 25, and 50 mg/ml Powder, 50 mg/vial	Ointment, 0.25 and 0.5% Cream, 0.5% Ophthalmic solution, 0.1, 0.25, and 0.8% Aerosol, 50 mg/150 gm container
Methylprednisolone (Depo-Medrol, Medrol, Solu-Medrol)	Tablets, 2, 4, and 16 mg Sustained-action capsules, 2 and 4 mg	Suspension, 20, 40, and 80 mg/ml Solution, 40 and 62.5 mg/ml	Ophthalmic ointment, 0.1% "Cream-ointment," 0.25 and 1%
Prednisone (many trade names)	Tablets, 1, 2.5, and 5 mg	. . .	. . .
Triamcinolone (Aristocort, Aristo-span, Kenacort, Kena-log)	Tablets, 1, 2, 4, 8, and 16 mg Syrup, 2 and 4 mg/5 ml	Suspension, 10, 20, 25, and 40 mg/ml	Cream, ointment, or lotion, 0.025, 0.1, 0.25, and 0.5% Spray, 0.0066% Foam, 0.1%
Paramethasone (Haldrone, Stemex)	Tablets, 1 and 2 mg	. . .	. . .
Dexamethasone (Decadron, Deronil, Dexameth, Gamma-corten, Hexadrol)	Tablets, 0.25, 0.5, 0.75, and 1.5 mg Elixir, 0.5 mg/5 ml	Solution, 4 mg/ml	Ophthalmic ointment, 0.05% Ophthalmic solution, 0.1% Cream, 0.04% Metered aerosol spray, 0.084 mg/spray
Betamethasone (Celestone, Valisone)	Tablets, 0.6 mg Syrup, 0.6 mg/5 ml	Suspension, 6 mg/ml	Cream, ointment, 0.1%
Desoxycorticosterone (Cortate, Cortinaq, Doca, Percorten)	Linguets, 2 and 5 mg	In oil, 5 mg/ml Aqueous suspension, 5 mg/ml Pellets, 75 and 125 mg	. . .
Fludrocortisone (F-Cortef, Florinef)	Tablets, 0.1 and 1 mg	. . .	Ophthalmic ointment, 0.1% Ophthalmic suspension, 0.1%
Flurandrenolone (Cordran)	. . .	. . .	Cream, ointment, 0.025 and 0.05% Tape, 4 μg/sq cm
Fluocinolone (Fluonid, Synalar, Lidex)	. . .	. . .	Ointment, 0.025% Cream, 0.01, 0.025, and 0.2% Solution, 0.01 and 0.05%
Fluorometholone (Oxylone)	. . .	. . .	Cream, ointment, 0.025%
Fluoroprednisolone (Alphadrol)	Tablets, 0.75 and 1.5 mg	. . .	. . .

*Solutions usually as sodium succinate or 21-phosphate for intramuscular or intravenous injection.

a hypokalemic, hypochloremic alkalosis and eventually a rise in blood pressure. In patients with hypoproteinemia, renal disease, or liver disease, edema may also occur. In patients with heart disease, even small degrees of sodium retention may lead to congestive heart failure. These effects can be minimized by sodium restriction and judicious potassium supplements. Many of the synthetic steroids have so little mineralocorticoid effect that these problems can be avoided. However, for the same reason, such compounds are not indicated for replacement therapy in adrenal insufficiency.

Contraindications & Cautions

A. Special Precautions: Patients receiving these drugs must be observed carefully for the development of hyperglycemia, glycosuria, sodium retention with edema or hypertension, hypokalemia, peptic ulcer, osteoporosis, and hidden infections. In order to minimize undesirable effects, periodic clinical examination with determinations of urine glucose and serum potassium are useful. A high-protein diet and adequate calcium intake are necessary. In patients with limited cardiac reserve, sodium restriction may be required. Sudden cessation of therapy should be avoided when more than physiologic amounts of steroids have been used in order to prevent an acute exacerbation of the disease process or symptoms of adrenal insufficiency.

The dosage should be kept as low as possible and intermittent dosage (eg, alternate-day) employed when satisfactory therapeutic results can be obtained on this schedule. In patients being maintained on relatively low doses of corticosteroids, supplementary therapy may be required at times of stress such as when surgical procedures are performed or accidents occur.

B. Contraindications: These agents must be used with the greatest of caution in patients with the following disorders.

1. Peptic ulcer—In the presence of active peptic ulcer disease, these steroids may cause hemorrhage or perforation. In patients with previous ulceration, activation is likely. Careful dietary control and antacids should be used when corticosteroid must be given to these patients.

2. Heart disease or hypertension with congestive heart failure—Measures to avoid the accumulation of extracellular fluid should be utilized. The concomitant use of potassium-wasting diuretics may create serious problems in patients receiving digitalis.

3. Infections—Since natural indicators of and defenses against infection are attenuated, great care is required even when antibiotics are used. Antituberculosis therapy may be required even in patients with inactive tuberculosis. Ophthalmic herpes simplex is particularly dangerous in the presence of corticosteroids.

4. Psychoses—Serious behavioral disturbances may occur in patients on steroid therapy, and prior disturbances are thought to predispose patients to acute psychoses.

5. Diabetes—Since these agents increase glucose production, more insulin may be required. However,

the corticosteroids do not cause acidosis or coma unless complications (such as an infection) occur.

Selection of Drug & Dosage Schedule

Since these preparations differ with respect to relative anti-inflammatory and mineralocorticoid effect (Table 35–1), duration of action, cost, and dosage forms available, these factors are taken into account in selecting the drug to be used.

A. ACTH Vs Adrenocortical Steroids: In patients with normal adrenals, ACTH has been used to induce the endogenous production of cortisol to obtain similar effects. However, when exogenous ACTH is given, the total amount of cortisol released by the adrenal can only be measured in retrospect. Furthermore, following ACTH administration the adrenal also increases its output of other hormones, including the androgens, which may not be desirable. Therefore, with rare exceptions, the use of ACTH as a therapeutic agent is probably unjustified. The instances in which ACTH has been claimed to be more effective than the glucocorticoids can probably be explained as being due to comparison of ACTH with the effect of smaller amounts of corticosteroids than are being produced by the administration of ACTH.

B. Dosage: In determining the dose to be used, the physician must consider the seriousness of the disease, the amount of drug likely to be required to obtain the desired effect, and the duration of therapy. In some diseases, the amount required for maintenance of the desired therapeutic effect is less than the dose needed to obtain the initial effect, and the lowest possible dose for the needed effect should be determined by gradually lowering the dose until an increase in signs or symptoms is noted.

Many types of dosage schedules have been used in administering glucocorticoids. When it is necessary to maintain continuously elevated plasma corticosteroid levels in order to suppress ACTH, a slowly absorbed parenteral preparation or small doses at frequent intervals are required. In order to maintain the same level throughout the day, a much larger dose would be required and very high plasma levels would be present for a short period of time. The opposite situation exists with respect to the use of corticosteroids in the treatment of inflammatory and allergic disorders. The same total quantity given in a few doses may be more effective than when given in many smaller doses or in a slowly absorbed parenteral form. In addition, the other less desirable effects of the hormone may be less marked because there is a recovery period between each dose. The intermittent use of large doses of corticosteroids has been very helpful in the chronic treatment of disorders such as asthma and the nephrotic syndrome. When used in this manner, very large amounts (eg, 100 mg prednisone daily) can sometimes be administered with only minimal side-effects.

When selecting a drug for use in large doses, a synthetic steroid with little mineralocorticoid effect is advisable.

C. Special Dosage Forms: The use of local therapy such as topical preparations for skin disease, ophthalmic forms for eye disease, intra-articular injections for joint disease, and hydrocortisone enemas for ulcerative colitis provides a means of delivering large amounts of steroid to the diseased tissue without serious systemic effects.

ADRENAL ANTAGONISTS

It has been possible to partially separate the mineralocorticoid and glucocorticoid effects by structural modifications of corticosteroids. However, it has not been possible to develop a compound that strongly inhibits ACTH production without having glucocorticoid activity.

o,p′DDD

Attempts to suppress adrenal steroidogenesis using derivatives of DDT have met with limited success. One compound, 2,2-bis(o-chlorophenyl-p-chlorophenyl)-1,1,dichloroethane—o,p′DDD—will produce adrenal atrophy in dogs and will interfere with biosynthetic pathways. Doses of up to 10 gm daily have been administered to patients with carcinoma of the adrenal. The production of corticosteroids was reduced, and in a few patients some reduction in tumor size was noted. However, severe toxic effects, including CNS depression, tremors, and skin and gastrointestinal disturbances limit the effective use of this experimental compound.

Amphenone B

Amphenone B is a more potent inhibitor of synthesis, blocking hydroxylation at the 11, 17, and 21 positions. It does not have a destructive effect on

the tissue, and the synthetic block leads to increased production of ACTH and hyperplasia of the gland. Amphenone also causes CNS depression, gastrointestinal tract and skin disorders, and impairs liver and thyroid function.

Metyrapone

Metyrapone (Metopirone) has a more selective effect at low doses. It inhibits 11-hydroxylation, interfering with cortisol and corticosterone synthesis and leading to the secretion of 11-deoxycorticosterone (compound S). In the presence of a normal pituitary gland, there is a compensatory increase in compound S production. This response is a measure of the capacity of the anterior pituitary to produce ACTH and has been adapted for clinical use. Although the toxicity of metyrapone is much lower than that of the above agents, it does produce transient dizziness and gastrointestinal disturbances. It is of no value in the treatment of adrenal hyperfunction due to adrenal hyperplasia because increased ACTH production can overcome the partial synthetic block.

Metyrapone is most commonly used in tests of adrenal function. The blood levels of compound S and the urinary excretion of 17-hydroxycorticoids are measured before and after administration of the compound. Normally, there is a 2-fold or greater increase in the urinary 17-hydroxycorticoid excretion. A dose of 300–500 mg every 4 hours for 6 doses is commonly used, and urine collections made on the day before and the day after treatment. In patients with Cushing's syndrome, a normal response to metyrapone indicates that the cortisol excess is not the result of adrenal carcinoma.

Adrenal function may also be tested by administering metyrapone, 2–3 gm orally at midnight, and measuring the level of ACTH or 11-deoxycortisol in blood drawn at 8:00 a.m., or by comparing the excretion of 17-hydroxycorticosteroids in the urine during

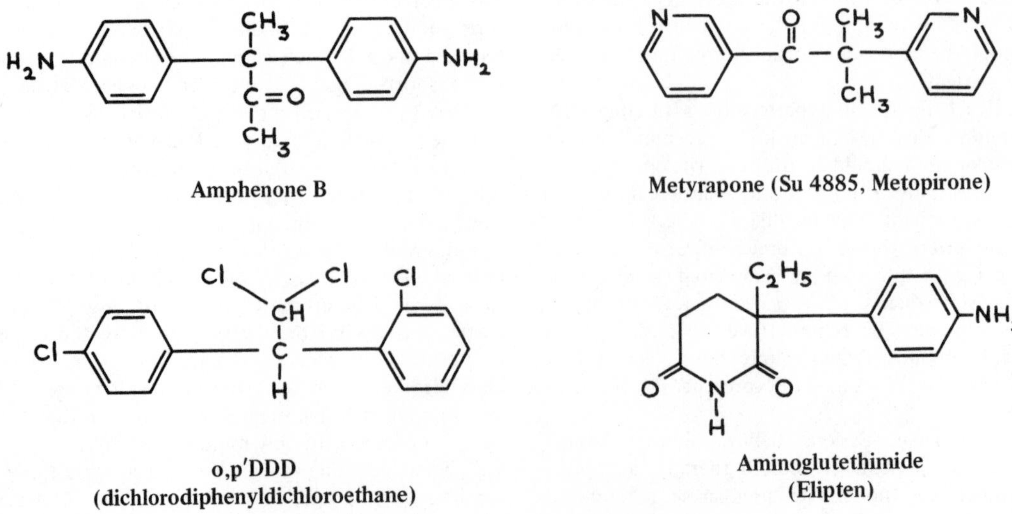

Amphenone B

Metyrapone (Su 4885, Metopirone)

o,p′DDD
(dichlorodiphenyldichloroethane)

Aminoglutethimide
(Elipten)

FIG 35–6. Adrenal antagonists.

the 24-hour periods preceding and following administration of the drug.

In patients with suspected or known lesions of the pituitary, this procedure is a means of estimating the ability of the gland to produce ACTH.

Other Adrenocortical Antagonists

A number of other agents have been used in experimental work, including Su 9055, which inhibits 17-hydroxylation. Studies of the toxicity of these compounds have been sufficient to discourage extensive trials in man although a recently studied drug, **aminoglutethimide,** which blocks conversion of cholesterol to pregnenolone, may prove useful in reducing mineralocorticoid and glucocorticoid excess in adrenocortical malignancy.

Spironolactone
(Aldactone; 3-[3-oxo-7α-acetylthio-17β-
hydroxy-4-androsten-17α-yl] propionic
acid γ-lactone)

ALDOSTERONE INHIBITORS

In addition to agents which interfere with aldosterone synthesis such as amphenone B, there are steroids which compete with aldosterone for binding sites and decrease its effect peripherally. Progesterone is mildly active in this respect. However, it has been found that substitution of a 17-spironolactone group for the C20-21 side chain of deoxycorticosterone results in a compound capable of blocking the sodium-retaining effect of aldosterone.

Spironolactone (Aldactone) is a 7α-acetylthio-spironolactone. Little is known about its metabolism. The onset of activity is slow, and the effects last for 2–3 days after the drug is discontinued. It is used in the treatment of primary hyperaldosteronism in doses

of 50–100 mg/day in divided doses. When used diagnostically for the detection of hyperaldosteronism in hypokalemic patients with hypertension, doses of 400–500 mg/day for 4–8 days—with an adequate intake of sodium and potassium—will restore potassium levels to or toward normal.

Spironolactone finds limited use as a diuretic in patients with secondary hyperaldosteronism who are resistant to other diuretics (see Chapter 17). This agent will reverse many of the findings of hyperaldosteronism. It has been useful in establishing the diagnosis in some patients and in ameliorating the signs and symptoms when surgical removal of an adenoma is delayed.

Occasional sedative effects, headache, gastrointestinal symptoms, and skin rashes are the only reported adverse reactions.

Spironolactone (Aldactone) is available as 25 mg scored tablets.

● ● ●

General References

Bartter, F.C. (editor): *The Clinical Use of Aldosterone Antagonists.* Thomas, 1960.

Bongiovanni, A.M., & A.W. Root: The adrenogenital syndrome. New England J Med 268:1283–1289, 1342–1351, 1391–1399, 1963.

Brown, J., & C.M. Pearson (editors): *Clinical Uses of Adrenal Steroids.* McGraw-Hill, 1962.

Burdick, K.H., Poulsen, B., & V.A. Place: Extemporaneous formulation of corticosteroids for topical usage. JAMA 211:462–466, 1970.

Davis, J.O.: The control of aldosterone secretion. Physiologist 5:65, 1962.

Edelman, I.S., & G.M. Fimognari: On the biochemical mechanism of action of aldosterone. Recent Progr Hormone Res 24:1–34, 1968.

Hutter, A.M., Jr., & D.E. Kayhoe: Adrenal cortical carcinoma. Results of treatment with o,p'DDD in 138 patients. Am J Med 41:581–592, 1966.

Jubiz, W., & others: Plasma metyrapone, adrenocorticotropic hormone, cortisol, and deoxycortisol levels: Sequential changes during oral and intravenous metyrapone administration. Arch Int Med 125:468–471, 1970.

Kaplan, N.M.: Assessment of pituitary ACTH secretory capacity with Metopirone [metyrapone]. J Clin Endocrinol 23:945–952, 1963.

Makman, M.H., Nakagawa, S., & A. White: Studies on the mode of action of adrenal steroids on lymphocytes. Recent Progr Hormone Res 23:195–219, 1967.

Mills, L.G., & J.H. Moyer (editors): *Inflammation and Diseases of Connective Tissue.* Saunders, 1961.

Miner, R.W. (editor): Hydrocortisone, its newer analogs, and aldosterone as therapeutic agents. Ann New York Acad Sc 61:281–636, 1955.

Nelson, D.H. (editor): Treatment of adrenal disorders. Mod Treat 3:135–434, 1966.

Schedl, H.P.: Absorption of steroid hormones from the human small intestine. J Clin Endocrinol 25:1309–1316, 1965.

Scoggins, R.B., & B. Kliman: Percutaneous absorption of corticosteroids: Systemic effects. New England J Med 273:831–839, 1965.

Slaunwhite, W., Jr., & A. Sandberg: Transcortin: A corticosteroid-binding protein of plasma. J Clin Invest 38:384–391, 1959.

Thorn, G.W.: Clinical considerations in the use of corticosteroids. New England J Med 274:775–781, 1966.

36...

Parathyroid Hormones, Calcium, & Vitamin D

CALCIUM METABOLISM

Calcium is the fifth most abundant element in the body. More than 90% of it is found in bone, largely as hydroxyapatite, but the small amounts found in the extracellular fluid and in the soft tissues have vitally important functions.

Plasma calcium exists in several forms. The normal distribution of the element in normal plasma is shown in Fig 36–1. However, the amount bound to protein is a function of the protein concentration and may vary accordingly in the presence of a normal level of ionized calcium. Since it is the ionized calcium that

is physiologically active in plasma, none of the pathologic changes associated with hypo- or hypercalcemia are found in pathologic states of plasma protein concentrations.

The calcium in bone exchanges with extracellular fluid. The concentration of calcium ion in plasma and extracellular fluid is the resultant of several factors, including the relative rates of bone formation and dissolution, absorption from the bowel, and excretion into the bowel and by the kidney. Physiologic concentrations of the ion are normally maintained by the interplay of parathyroid hormone, calcitonin, and vitamin D and their effects on the above processes.

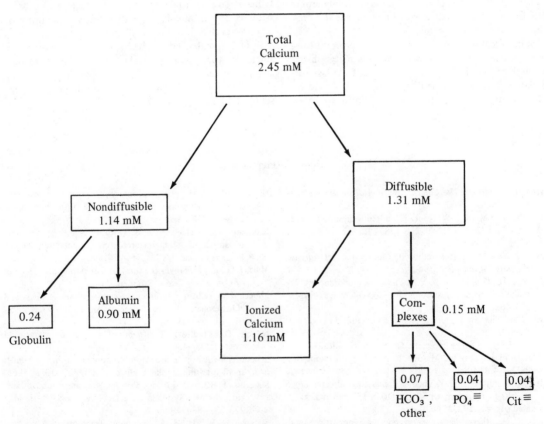

FIG 36–1. **Distribution of the calcium in 1 liter of plasma.** (Reproduced, with permission, from Neuman & Neuman: *The Chemical Dynamics of Bone Mineral.* University of Chicago Press, 1958. Copyright by the University of Chicago.)

Calcium absorption is an active transport process that takes place in the proximal part of the small bowel. It is increased by parathyroid hormone and vitamin D and possibly by lactose and amino acids. Calcium absorption is decreased in the presence of phytate, oxalate, and phosphate, which form insoluble salts or complexes with it. In the presence of steatorrhea, a severe loss of calcium may take place; the amount may be in excess of that in the diet. Not only is calcium lost in the form of calcium soaps, but less vitamin D is absorbed, which increases the loss of calcium normally secreted into the intestinal lumen.

Calcium is also excreted in the urine. It is present in the glomerular filtrate, and about 70% is reabsorbed in the proximal tubule, about 20% in the loop of Henle, and about 10% in the distal tubule. Calcium is not secreted by the tubules. The urinary excretion of calcium is relatively constant on a given diet, but can be enhanced by loading the body with sodium salts. Calcium excretion may also be increased by renal tubular dysfunction and depressed by kidney disorders associated with reduced glomerular filtration.

The rate at which calcium leaves and enters the circulation from the readily exchangeable portion of the bone pool is controlled largely by parathyroid hormone and calcitonin (see below).

Physiologic Role of Calcium

In addition to its role in bone formation, calcium ion is necessary for the normal coagulation of blood; substances which combine with it to form soluble complexes or precipitates (such as oxalate, citrate, or EDTA) can be used as anticoagulants in vitro. In conjunction with potassium and magnesium ion, calcium regulates cardiac and skeletal muscle and nerve excitability. The effect is inversely proportionate to the ionized calcium concentration in these tissues. (For example, reduction of serum calcium concentration increases excitability.) The opposite relationship exists at the myoneural junction. Calcium is also a constituent of the intercellular cement substance.

For a more detailed discussion of calcium, see Chapter 43.

PARATHYROID HORMONE

Parathyroid hormone is secreted by 4 small glands located bilaterally at the upper and lower poles of the thyroid gland. (The number and positions may vary at times.) Although all of the details of its structure have not been elucidated, several highly purified preparations of parathyroid hormone are available for study. The structure of human parathyroid hormone has not been defined. However, it appears to circulate in more than one form and may differ slightly from the form in which it is extracted from glandular tissue.

The structure of bovine parathyroid hormone has been determined (Fig 36–2). Its amino acid composition is similar to that reported for the porcine hormone. A peptide composed of the first 34 amino acids has been synthesized and studied. Although less active when injected into animals, it is qualitatively identical with the larger polypeptide.

Polypeptides with parathyroid hormone activity are also formed by malignant tumors of other tissues, including the ovaries, kidneys, and lungs.

Metabolism

Very little is known about the fate of this hormone following its release from the gland. Studies with labeled hormones indicate a half-life of 16–21 minutes. Indirect evidence obtained from a study of its effects indicates that its onset of action is rapid and that it is cleared from the circulation quickly. A detectable lowering of plasma calcium occurs within 1 hour after parathyroidectomy. The hormone is partly excreted by the kidney.

A radio-immunoassay for parathyroid hormone has been developed. Preliminary studies indicate that the blood level in normal subjects is under 1 ng/ml. The level falls when calcium is infused and rises when calcium levels fall.

Physiologic Considerations

A. Effects of Deficiency or Excess: Serious disturbances occur when the plasma ionized calcium level deviates from normal (see Disorders of Parathyroid Function, below). When the parathyroid glands are removed, the plasma calcium falls from its normal level of about 4.5–5.5 mEq/liter to 3.5 mEq/liter or less, resulting in tetany. This fall occurs within hours in the rat, but it may take several days in man. Fall in plasma calcium is associated with an increase in serum inorganic phosphate. When parathyroid hormone is injected, the reverse occurs.

The above changes are mediated largely via the effect of the hormone on bone metabolism and renal function. Bone is the major reservoir of calcium in the body, and parathyroid hormone acts directly on bone to release calcium into the extracellular fluid by stimulating osteoclastic resorption of bone. Although the evidence is somewhat contradictory, it is possible that parathyroid hormone increases the intestinal absorption of calcium. Crude parathyroid extracts have been shown to increase the proximal renal tubular reabsorption of calcium, but studies with highly purified preparations do not seem to have this property consistently.

In addition to the effects on calcium, parathyroid hormone inhibits the renal reabsorption of phosphate at the proximal convoluted tubule.

B. Mechanisms of Action: Parathyroid hormone activates adenyl cyclase in renal and bone cells. It has been postulated that this leads to increased formation of cyclic AMP, which promotes the synthesis and release of specific lysosomal enzymes which break down the organic matrix of bone and release calcium. The calcium release may be aided by the increase in plasma citrate concentration, which is also produced by parathyroid hormone. It has been shown that large

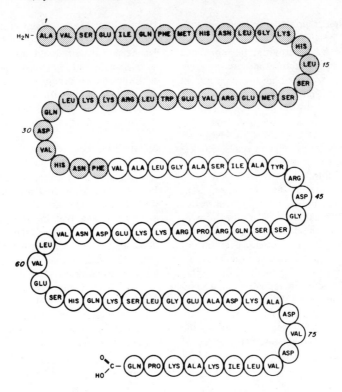

FIG 36-2. Amino acid sequence of bovine PTH. Amino acids 1—34 represent the fragment produced by solid phase peptide synthesis and found to be biologically active, in vivo and in vitro, on both bone and kidney receptors. (Reproduced with permission, from Potts, J.T., Jr., & others: Parathyroid hormone: Sequence, synthesis, immunoassay studies. Am J Med 50:639—649, 1971.)

amounts of purified parathyroid hormone will stimulate the oxidation and phosphate uptake of actinomycin-inhibited mitochondria. The physiologic significance of this action, if any, is not known. Parathyroid hormone in the presence of vitamin D will also stimulate the release of calcium from mitochondria under certain conditions. The response to this hormone is also diminished in vitamin D-deficient animals.

C. Regulation of Secretion: Parathyroid hormone secretion appears to be under the control of a negative feedback mechanism mediated by the direct effect of the plasma calcium level perfusing the parathyroid gland. Hypertrophy of the gland can be induced by hypocalcemia, and involution by hypercalcemia.

Disorders of Parathyroid Function

A. Hypoparathyroidism: A deficiency of parathyroid hormone most often follows accidental damage to or removal of the glands during thyroid surgery. The glands are also removed at times in the course of radical neck surgery for various malignancies or in the treatment of hyperparathyroidism (see below).

Idiopathic hypoparathyroidism also follows atrophy of these glands. This disorder, particularly when associated with adrenal atrophy, is associated with the presence of autoantibodies which may play a role in the genesis of the disorder.

Apparent deficiency of the hormone occurs in "pseudohypoparathyroidism," a congenital disorder characterized by a lack of response to the hormone rather than by a lack of the hormone itself. Pseudohypoparathyroidism is associated with short stature, subcutaneous calcification, mental deficiency, and dental and skeletal abnormalities. This constellation of congenital abnormalities also occurs with normal tissue responsiveness to parathyroid hormone (pseudopseudohypoparathyroidism).

These disorders (except for pseudopseudohypoparathyroidism) produce the symptoms of hypocalcemia (see p 347).

B. Hyperparathyroidism: Excessive production of parathyroid hormone may result from its overproduction by tissues not responsive to feedback control, such as is seen with adenomas, carcinoma, or hyperplasia of the parathyroid glands. The symptoms are due to hypercalcemia, renal calculi produced by the hypercalciuria, and skeletal lesions, including osteoclastic tumor and bone dissolution. The symptoms of hypercalcemia are discussed below.

Excessive production of parathyroid hormone also occurs as a compensatory mechanism when chronic hypocalcemia is present, such as with intestinal malabsorption, vitamin D lack, and with renal insufficiency. Under these circumstances, hypercalcemia is not present and bone lesions may be prominent.

Clinical Uses

The usefulness of parathyroid extract is quite limited. Although it has been given as replacement therapy to maintain plasma calcium in hypoparathyroidism for prolonged periods of time, a combination of vitamin D preparations and calcium is much more useful.

Parathyroid extract has been used most extensively for the control of hypocalcemic manifestations of parathyroid deficiency while vitamin D and calcium are being started. It is given in doses of 50—150 units, and the initial dose may be given intravenously to obtain a more rapid effect. In any case, it is usual to give calcium intravenously for immediate relief (see below).

Preparations Available

Parathyroid injection USP (parathyroid solution, parathyroid extract), the official preparation, is an aqueous extract of parathyroid glands with a pH of 2.5–3.0 and containing 100 units/ml. One unit is defined as 1/100 of the amount required to raise the blood calcium of an intact dog 1 mg/100 ml 15–18 hours after subcutaneous injection.

Since it is protein in nature, parathyroid extract is destroyed in the intestines and must be given parenterally. Its effects are delayed and prolonged in comparison with the highly purified preparations. When given subcutaneously in large doses, the peak effect occurs within 18 hours and may last for 38 hours. Some effect may be seen in 4 hours.

Paroidin (Parke, Davis) and parathyroid injectable (Lilly) are aqueous extracts of beef parathyroids containing 100 USP units/ml for subcutaneous or intramuscular injection. The recommended dose is 20–40 USP units/12 hours for 5–6 days as required to maintain serum calcium levels.

CALCITONIN
(Thyrocalcitonin)

It was found that under some circumstances the plasma calcium level may fall more rapidly than could be accounted for by cessation of parathyroid secretion. A substance capable of lowering plasma calcium levels was postulated and named calcitonin.

Calcitonin has now been isolated and purified and its structure determined. Porcine calcitonin differs considerably from parathyroid hormone, having only 32 amino acid residues and a molecular weight of 3585. Its structure is shown in Fig 36–3. There is a disulfide loop at the N terminus. The first 25 amino acids appear to be necessary for activity. Calcitonin has been isolated from the thyroid glands of man and many other mammals and from the ultimobranchial glands of lower vertebrates. These preparations are all small peptides containing 32 amino acids. Although their biologic activity is similar, there are important differences in amino acid sequence and potency (Fig 36–4).

Metabolism

Calcitonin is secreted by the cells of the ultimobranchial glands in lower vertebrates. In man and other mammals, the ultimobranchial cells, which are derived from the sixth branchial pouch, invade the thyroid gland and other nearby tissues. The parafollicular cells of the thyroid (light cells, C cells) appear to be the source of calcitonin in man and other mammals. Since the hormone is antigenic, it has been possible to develop a radio-immunoassay to measure it. Few studies have been published concerning the details of its metabolism. Its secretion is controlled by the concentration of calcium in the blood perfusing the secretory tissue. A rise in serum calcium causes a prompt increase in the release of the hormone into the circulation. In rabbits, the blood concentration is about 0.1–0.15 ng/ml, and 10- to 15-fold rises occur when hypercalcemia is induced. The estimated half-life is 5–15 minutes. It is estimated that in man the secretion

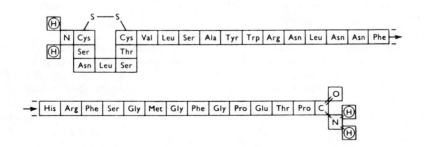

FIG 36–3. Chemical structure of porcine calcitonin.

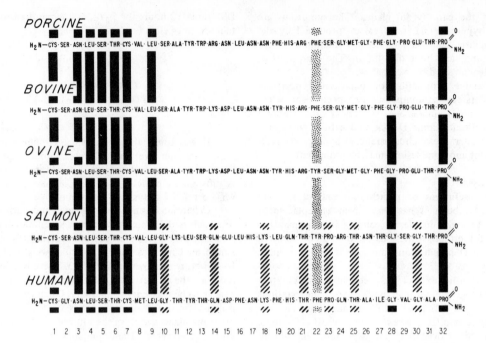

FIG 36–4. Amino acid sequences of the calcitonins.

of calcitonin may be as high as 0.4 mg/day. In contrast to parathyroid hormone, the reserve of calcitonin is large.

Physiologic Considerations

Calcitonin appears to act by inhibiting bone resorption. It has been shown to inhibit or antagonize the bone resorption induced by parathyroid hormone or vitamin D. In the rat, human calcitonin lowers serum phosphate and magnesium. Chronic administration of active extracts leads to increased bone mass, which can be accounted for entirely by the inhibition of bone resorption.

The mechanism of action has not been established. Calcitonin has been shown to reduce the release of citrate into the medium when bone is cultured in vitro. Inhibitors of phosphodiesterase such as theophylline block the hypocalcemic effect of calcitonin. This observation has led to the hypothesis that calcitonin may inhibit bone resorption by increasing the rate of destruction of cyclic AMP.

Although the physiologic role of calcitonin has not been established, studies in young animals suggest that it may function to decrease the mobilization of calcium from bone when calcium is ingested.

Disorders of Calcitonin Secretion

Since calcitonin inhibits the resorption of bone, it would not be expected to alter calcium levels when bone turnover is slow. When calcitonin is injected into normal adults, little change is observed. However, more marked changes are observed in the presence of a hypercalcemic state. When bone turnover is elevated,

as in Paget's disease, the reduction of calcium levels is marked even though serum calcium levels are normal. Increased circulating levels of calcitonin have been detected in patients with medullary carcinoma of the thyroid, a tumor arising from the parafollicular cells.

Preparations

Several preparations of calcitonin are now under study for use in man. The most potent of these is salmon ultimobranchial calcitonin, which has detectable effects in doses as low as 0.3 µg (1/10 the dose of synthetic human calcitonin and 1/100 the amount of porcine calcitonin required for comparable effects).

Preliminary studies indicate that calcitonin can produce remissions in patients with Paget's disease. It will also lower serum calcium levels in some hypercalcemic patients.

The appearance of antibodies to salmon calcitonin has been reported in some patients under treatment with this preparation.

VITAMIN D

The vitamins D are natural sterols derived from precursors (provitamins) which have been subjected to irradiation with ultraviolet light. In man this occurs in the skin and the vitamin D formed is stored in the liver. About 400 IU are required daily for children and for women during pregnancy and lactation. The daily allowances for adults have not been established.

Metabolism

Vitamin D is well absorbed following parenteral administration and it can be absorbed through the skin. It is usually administered by mouth and absorbed without difficulty in the absence of hepatic, biliary, or intestinal disorders. However, in the presence of steatorrhea or continuous mineral oil administration, the absorption of the vitamin is poor.

The metabolism of vitamin D is very slow. When absorbed into the circulation, it binds to alpha globulins and albumin. Significant amounts are found in the liver, kidney, intestine, bone, and adrenal gland. The normal plasma level is 1–3 units/ml. Although the details of its degradation and disposal are not known, in animals about 50% of a dose of radioactive vitamin D appears in the feces.

When radioactive vitamin D_3 is given to normal individuals, about 80% is absorbed. Most of the remainder can be recovered from the feces unchanged. When analyzed several hours later, the plasma radioactivity is found in the chylomicron fraction. This indicates that it is absorbed via the lymphatics.

When given intravenously, vitamin D_3 disappears slowly, with an initial half-life of approximately 12 hours. Much of it appears to be converted to 25-hydroxycholecalciferol, an important biologically active metabolite. This sterol has a half-life of about 20 days. Vitamin D_3 and 25-hydroxycholecalciferol bind to a specific transport protein in the circulation. Physiologic effects are not usually observed within 4–6 hours of administration. Less than 3% of an oral or intravenous dose is recovered in the urine in the first 48–72 hours, and most of this material is in the form of biologically inactive water-soluble conjugates (glucuronides).

Studies of the metabolism of vitamin D are complicated by the presence of circulating metabolites, some of which are inactive. Sufficiently sensitive chemical methods for the measurement of these sterols are not available.

Physiologic Considerations

Vitamin D is one of several factors required for normal calcium and phosphorus metabolism. As noted above, it may be required for the normal activity of parathyroid hormone. The D vitamins and related sterols increase the gastrointestinal absorption of ingested calcium and phosphorus. Administration of this vitamin causes an increase in the citrate content of bone, heart, kidneys, and blood of experimental animals.

The mechanism of action of vitamin D on bone is not well understood. However, its effects on the gastrointestinal absorption of calcium have been extensively studied. Vitamin D enhances the transfer of calcium across the intestine in both directions. It increases the uptake and release of this ion. It has been shown to induce the formation of a calcium-binding protein responsible for the transfer. The normal lack of permeability of the intestine to calcium is an active process requiring energy to be maintained.

A. Vitamin D Deficiency: A deficiency in vitamin D leads to inadequate absorption of calcium and phosphorus. In order to maintain plasma calcium levels, parathyroid hormone is secreted, leading to the mobilization of calcium and phosphorus from bone. In children, the resulting demineralization produces rickets; in adults, osteomalacia.

Recent studies indicate that patients with vitamin D-resistant rickets have abnormal vitamin D metabolism. These individuals have been found to have a decreased rate of conversion of vitamin D to its active metabolites. Patients with renal osteodystrophy also show defective conversion.

B. Vitamin D Excess: Hypervitaminosis D results from the chronic ingestion of large doses (150,000 units/day) of the vitamin. This is a serious disorder in which hypercalcemia is produced by mobilization of the ion from bone. This would indicate either that there is a simultaneous lack of ingested calcium or that vitamin D acts mainly as a calcium mobilizing agent. In addition to the usual signs, symptoms, and sequelae of hypercalcemia (see below), metastatic calcification of soft tissues is common.

Clinical Uses

Vitamin D is most commonly used (with calcium) to supplement the diet of infants in order to prevent rickets. With rare exceptions, an intake of about 400 units/day is sufficient to provide optimal concentrations of vitamin D.

When a deficiency has become established, large doses may shorten the recovery time. Doses of 3000–4000 units daily may be administered for several weeks. In vitamin D-resistant rickets, as much as 500,000 units may be required daily.

Vitamin D and dihydrotachysterol are useful in the treatment of hypocalcemia due to hypoparathyroidism. Ergocalciferol in doses of 50–250 thousand units/day is frequently given with supplemental calcium salts, the dose being determined by the effects on the serum calcium level.

Vitamin D in large doses has been used in the treatment of other diseases such as rheumatoid arthritis and psoriasis. There is no convincing evidence that it is effective in controlling these disorders, and the incidence of serious toxicity makes its use inadvisable.

Preparations Available

Previously utilized bioassay procedures have been abandoned now that chemical procedures for the measurement of the sterols are available. One IU is the biologic activity contained in 0.025 μg of calciferol.

Vitamin D can be taken with foods to which it has been added such as milk and various formula diets. It is also available in multivitamin preparations and in combination with vitamin A. Fish liver oils and concentrates are also marketed. A common dosage form contains 4000 units of vitamin A and 400 units of vitamin D per capsule or teaspoon.

Ergocalciferol USP (vitamin D_2, calciferol) is a white crystalline substance dispensed in capsules containing 10,000, 25,000, and 50,000 units in vegetable oil and in tablets containing 10,000 units. It is also dispensed in solution containing 10,000 units/ml in

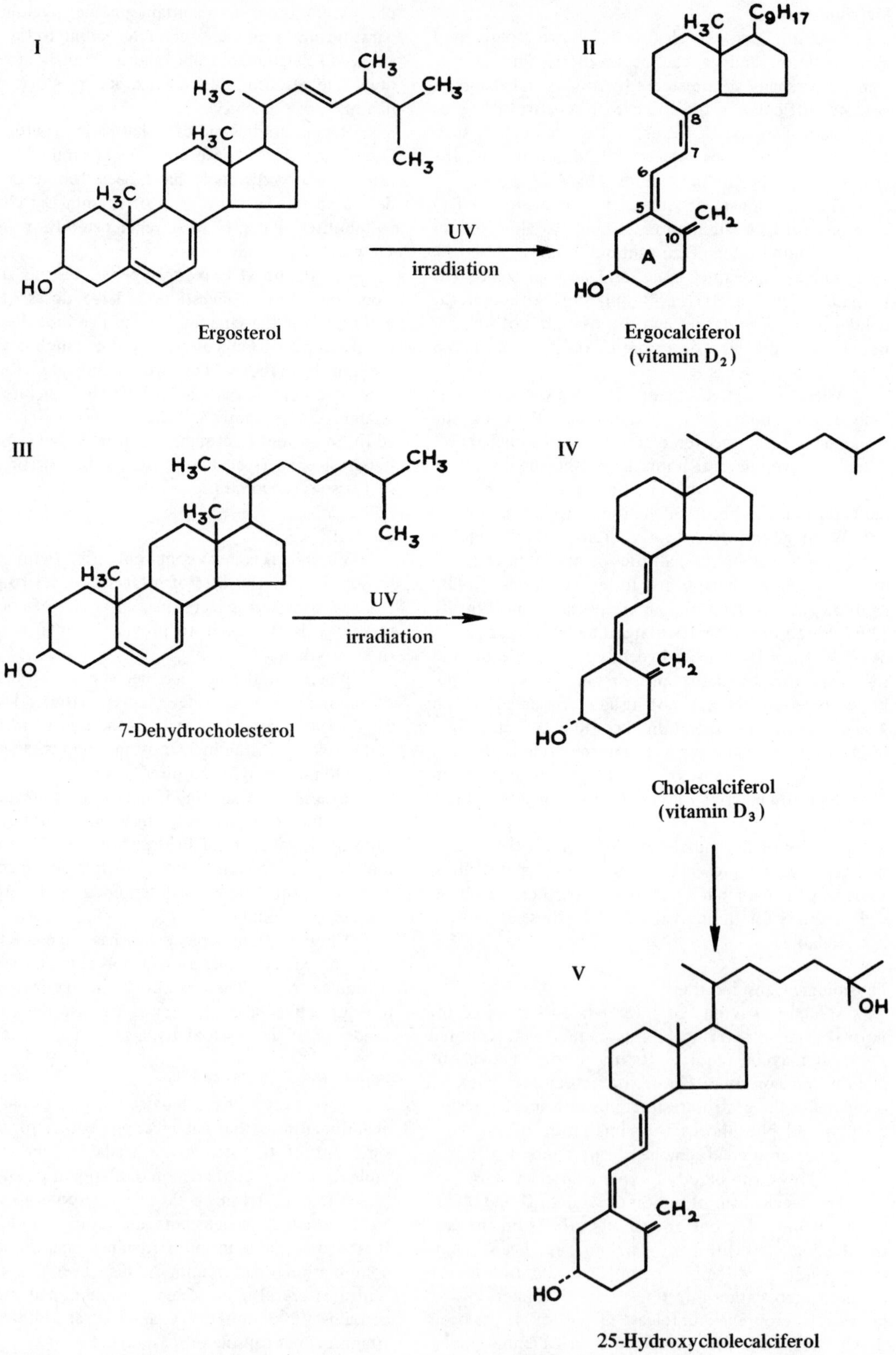

FIG 36−5. Compounds II and IV, ergocalciferol (vitamin D_2) and cholecalciferol (vitamin D_3), are produced by
irradiation of compounds I and III, ergosterol and 7-dehydrocholesterol. Cholecalciferol is converted to the
active metabolite 25-hydroxycholecalciferol after ingestion.

vegetable oil, propylene glycol, or polysorbate 80. Injectable preparations are available containing 50,000, 100,000, and 500,000 units/ml.

Cholecalciferol USP (activated 7-dehydrocholesterol) and decavitamin capsules and tablets USP are preparations containing at least 400 units of some form of vitamin D.

Dihydrotachysterol USP is a colorless, odorless, crystalline material. It is dispensed in tablets containing 0.2 mg of the active sterol. On the basis of weight, it is 3 times as effective as calciferol (vitamin D_2). Its effect also dissipates more rapidly, and it is especially useful in patients who require large doses of calciferol.

Dihydrotachysterol (AT 10, Hytakerol) is available in capsules containing 0.125 mg in solution, and as solution (in oil) containing 0.25 mg/ml. Even though this preparation is assayed for dihydrotachysterol content, it does not appear to be as potent or reliable as the USP material.

New forms of vitamin D such as 25-hydroxycholecalciferol are under study for clinical use.

Dihydrotachysterol$_2$

TREATMENT OF HYPOCALCEMIA

Hypocalcemia is characterized by neuromuscular excitability, tetanic muscular contractions, and positive Chvostek's and Trousseau's signs. When chronic, it is commonly associated with cataracts, papilledema, skin disorders, and calcification of the basal ganglia. It is most often seen following removal of the parathyroid glands, in malabsorption syndromes, and in chronic renal failure.

When manifestations of hypocalcemia are severe, they are relieved by the slow intravenous administration of 5–20 ml of 5% calcium chloride or 10% calcium gluconate. The oral preparations, in doses suggested in Table 36–1, can be used when symptoms are mild. In the treatment of hypoparathyroidism, these preparations are given with vitamin D, the dose being adjusted to maintain serum calcium at normal concentrations.

TREATMENT OF HYPERCALCEMIA

Hypercalcemia is seen in a variety of circumstances including malignant tumors of the breast and other tissues, hyperparathyroidism, vitamin D intoxication, milk-alkali syndrome, hyperthyroidism, idiopathic hypercalcemia of infants, and others. Regardless of the cause, serious complications may follow if there is calcium deposition in the kidney or if the serum calcium is markedly elevated.

The immediate treatment of hypercalcemia is directed at a reduction of serum calcium levels and prevention of renal stones and calcification by maintaining a dilute urine. The cause of the disorder should be treated promptly when possible.

Fluids should be administered in large quantities (parenterally if necessary) in order to correct dehydration, improve glomerular filtration, and increase urine volume. These changes will dilute serum calcium and increase its loss in the urine. In more severe disturbances, sodium sulfate orally (5–10 gm/day) or IV (200 mEq/liter) will enhance the loss of calcium.

Phosphate is also used (investigationally at present) in the treatment of hypercalcemia. Although a fall in serum calcium is produced by phosphate, much of the calcium is deposited in the body rather than excreted in the urine, and is thought to lead to metastatic calcification as well as being deposited in bone. This form of therapy may be more useful when phosphate depletion and hypophosphatemia accompany hypercalcemia, as is the case in patients with renal transplants or primary hyperparathyroidism.

Potent diuretics such as furosemide may be of value in selected patients such as those with decreased cardiac reserve. In such a patient, the careful measurement and replacement of other substances lost (water, potassium, magnesium, etc) may be required.

Sodium phytate (Rencal), a drug currently being studied, administered in doses of 3 gm 3 times daily by mouth, will reduce calcium absorption. Disodium ethylenediaminetetraacetate (EDTA) has been used to chelate calcium ion, but the rapid reduction of calcium levels which may occur is dangerous and this form of therapy is rarely used.

When renal failure is present, hemodialysis may be useful. In patients with heart failure, the enhancement of digitalis toxicity should be kept in mind.

Glucocorticoids such as prednisone (30–50 mg/day) will usually reduce hypercalcemia in patients with sarcoidosis and malignancies, but this rarely happens in patients with hyperparathyroidism. Once the level is lowered, the improvement can usually be maintained by lower doses of the steroid and the elimination of milk and dairy products from the diet.

TABLE 36−1. Calcium: Dosages and preparations available.

	Usual Adult Dose	Preparations Available
Oral preparations		
Calcium gluconate	1−5 gm	Tablets, 300, 500, 600, and 1000 mg Capsules, 325 mg
Calcium gluconogalactogluconate	15 ml 2−3 times/day (children, 5 ml 3 times/day)	Syrup, containing equivalent of 1.3 gm calcium gluconate/5 ml
Calcium lactate	1−5 gm 3 times/day with meals	Tablets, 300, 325, 500, 600, and 650 mg
Dicalcium phosphate	1 gm 3 times/day	Tablets, 500 and 1000 mg Capsules, 1000 mg Powder, 0.4 dicalcium phosphate per gm powder
Dicalcium phosphate with calcium gluconate	6−12 capsules or tablets/day 3−6 wafers/day	Capsules and tablets, 290 mg dicalcium phosphate and 190 mg calcium gluconate Wafers, 580 mg dicalcium phosphate and 380 mg calcium gluconate
Parenteral preparations		
Calcium chloride	5−20 ml IV	Ampules, 5 and 10% solution
Calcium gluconate	5−10 ml IV or IM	Ampules, 10% solution
Calcium gluconogalactogluconate	10−20 ml IV or IM	Ampules, 10 and 20% solution
Calcium gluceptate (glucoheptonate)	5−20 ml IV, 2−5 ml IM	Ampules, 5 ml equivalent to 90 mg calcium
Calcium gluconate-glucoheptonate	10 ml IV or IM	Ampules, 10 ml containing 500 mg calcium gluconate and 620 mg calcium glucoheptonate
Calcium levulinate	5−10 ml IV or IM	Ampules, 10% solution
Calcium lactate and calcium glycerophosphate	10−20 ml IV, IM, or subcut	Ampules and vials, 5 mg of each/ml

• • •

General References

Anast, C., & others: Thyrocalcitonin and the response to parathyroid hormone. J Clin Invest 46:57−64, 1967.

Aurbach, G.D., & others: Polypeptide hormones and calcium metabolism. Ann Int Med 70:1243−1265, 1969.

Avioli, L.V.: Absorption and metabolism of vitamin D_3 in man. Am J Clin Nutr 22:437−446, 1969.

Chakmakjian, Z.H., & J.E. Bethune: Sodium sulfate treatment of hypercalcemia. New England J Med 275:862−869, 1966.

Copp, D.H.: Endocrine control of calcium homeostasis. J Endocrinol 43:137−161, 1969.

F. Raymond Keating Jr. Memorial Symposium: Hyperparathyroidism, 1970. Am J Med 50:557−700, 1971.

Gaillard, P.J., & others (editors): *The Parathyroid Glands*. Univ of Chicago Press, 1965.

Graham, G.G.: Johns Hopkins conjoint clinic on vitamins. J Chronic Dis 19:1067−1081, 1966.

Harrison, H.E.: Parathyroid hormone and vitamin D. Yale J Biol Med 38:393−409, 1966.

Harrison, H.E., Lifshitz, F., & R.M. Blizzard: Comparison between crystalline dihydrotachysterol and calciferol in patients requiring pharmacologic vitamin D therapy. New England J Med 276:894−900, 1967.

Hirsch, P.F., & P.L. Munson: Thyrocalcitonin. Physiol Rev 49:548−622, 1969.

Howard, J.E., & W.C. Thomas: Clinical disorders of calcium homeostasis. Medicine 42:25−45, 1963.

International Symposium on Calcitonin. (London, 1969.) Springer-Verlag (New York), 1970.

Potts, J.T., Jr., Aurbach, G.D., & L.M. Sherwood: Parathyroid hormone: Chemical properties and structural requirements for biological and immunological activity. Recent Progr Hormone Res 22:101−143, 1966.

37 . . .

Insulin, Glucagon, Oral Antidiabetic Drugs, & Hyperglycemic Agents

INSULIN

Insulin and glucagon, the known hormones of the pancreatic islets, are intimately involved in various phases of intermediary metabolism. The marked effects of these hormones on the blood levels and metabolism of glucose are of pharmacologic importance in the treatment of disorders of carbohydrate metabolism. Other agents, though chemically unrelated, are also important in this respect and will be discussed in this chapter.

Chemistry

Insulin is a small protein with a molecular weight of approximately 6000. It contains 51 amino acids arranged in 2 chains (A and B) linked by disulfide bridges, and there are species differences in the amino acids of both chains (Fig 37–1). Insulin is synthesized in the pancreas by the beta cells of the islets of Langerhans, from which it can be extracted for pharmaceutical purposes. It is usually obtained from beef or pork pancreas. When purified it crystallizes in the presence of

zinc as an odorless white powder which is insoluble at neutral pH but soluble in dilute mineral acids or alkali.

Structural modifications which have been found to destroy biologic activity include esterification of the carboxyl groups; oxidation or reduction of the disulfide groups; degradation by chymotrypsin, pepsin, or papain and removal of the C-terminal group of the A chain; modification of the free amino groups or aliphatic hydroxyl groups; and reduction with thioglycolate and removal of the C-terminal alanine from the B chain. Although limited proteolysis with carboxypeptidase or trypsin will not destroy the biologic activity of the insulin molecule, destruction by the proteolytic activity in the digestive tract prevents its oral use.

Physiologic Considerations

A. Secretion: Insulin is synthesized by the beta cells and is stored in intracellular granules. During the process of secretion, the granules move to the cell membrane. The membranes appear to rupture, releasing the granules into the extracellular space. In man, the pancreas stores about 10 mg of insulin. It is estimated that approximately 2 mg (50 units) are released into the portal vein daily.

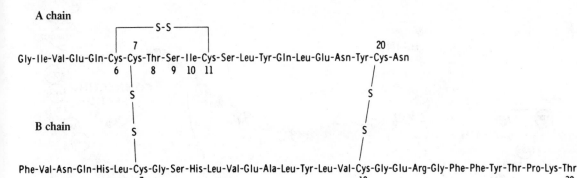

	A Chain		B Chain
	8	10	30
Man	Thr	Ile	Thr
Pig	Thr	Ile	Ala
Rabbit	Thr	Ile	Ser
Beef	Ala	Val	Ala

FIG 37–1. Structure of human insulin. The differences in the structure of insulin in different animal species are shown in the table.

Normally, the release of insulin is controlled by the concentration of glucose in the plasma perfusing the gland. A fall in glucose inhibits—and a rise increases—its release. Mannose—and fructose to a lesser extent—will also stimulate insulin release, whereas nonmetabolizable sugars (eg, galactose, ribose, and xylose) will not.

Other stimuli are known to affect the rate of secretion. It is increased by vagal stimulation, by amino acids such as leucine and arginine, by glucagon, by secretory products of the gastrointestinal tract such as secretin, gastrin, pancreozymin, and a glucagon-like factor, and by some of the oral hypoglycemic agents (see below). It is inhibited by epinephrine and related compounds with alpha-adrenergic activity.

B. Metabolism: Insulin is synthesized by the beta cells of the pancreas as part of a larger single chain molecule which is called proinsulin (Fig 37–2). During the biosynthetic process, proinsulin is converted to insulin by cleavage of the polypeptide connecting the amino terminal of the A chain to the carboxy terminal of the B chain. There are species differences in the amino acid sequence of the connecting peptide. This conversion normally takes place in the beta cell, presumably as a result of proteolytic enzyme activity. However, small amounts of proinsulin gain entrance into the circulation and are converted to an active moiety in peripheral tissues. Considerable evidence suggests that the circulating proinsulin and partially fragmented intermediates make up the large molecules detected by immunoassay procedures and called "big" insulin.

When secreted, insulin may be bound in part to the serum globulins, but the specificity of this binding in persons not treated with insulin has not been established. Once insulin has entered the circulation, it is taken up by the tissues or metabolized rapidly, as indicated by a half-life of about 10 minutes. A large proportion of the secreted hormone is taken up by the liver. In spite of the rapid rate of clearance from the circulation, its effects may be manifest for hours. In the fasting or postabsorptive state, the concentration of insulin is about 25 μU/ml plasma by immunoassay, and the concentration may rise to as much as 5 times that level after a glucose load. Plasma concentrations of insulin-like activity (ILA), when determined by in vitro bioassay utilizing changes in glucose uptake by rat diaphragm or epididymal fat pad, appear to be much higher.

The breakdown of insulin is the result of the action of peptidases on the A and B chains which have been separated by reductive cleavage of the disulfide linkages. These changes occur mainly in the liver. However, kidney, placenta, muscle, and, to a lesser extent, plasma exhibit the ability to degrade insulin.

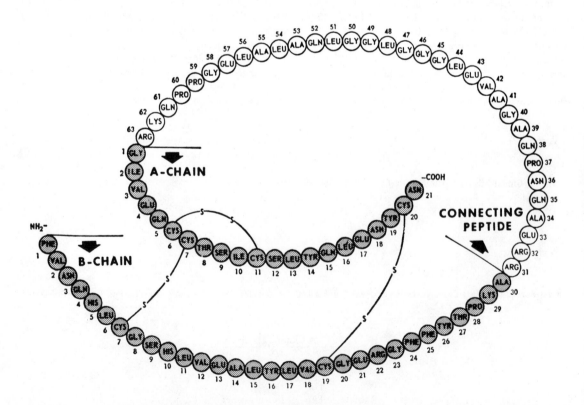

FIG 37–2. Structure of porcine proinsulin. (Reproduced, with permission, from Chance & others: Porcine proinsulin: Characterization and amino acid sequence. Science 161:165–166, 1968. Copyright 1968 by the American Association for the Advancement of Science.)

The uptake by tissue and rate of destruction may be inhibited by the binding of insulin to antibodies and other proteins under abnormal circumstances (eg, diabetes mellitus).

C. Effects of Insulin: Insulin influences the metabolism of a wide variety of tissues. It plays a key role in the intermediary metabolism of muscle and adipose tissue and has important effects in the liver.

In muscle and adipose tissue, insulin increases the cellular uptake of amino acids, glucose, and other monosaccharides along with potassium and phosphate ions. (Similar effects occur in connective tissue and leukocytes but not in brain, kidney, or red blood cells.) Insulin is adsorbed to tissues in vitro and can be dissociated by agents which split disulfide bonds but not by mechanical washing. This suggests that insulin may affect transport processes across cell membranes by forming disulfide links with them.

In muscle and adipose tissue, the uptake of glucose is a rate-limiting step in the subsequent metabolism of this sugar. The uptake of nonmetabolizable sugars is also increased, indicating that the further metabolism of glucose is not required for this action of insulin. The transport effects of insulin occur in minutes and are not inhibited by actinomycin, suggesting that the synthesis of new proteins is not required. Insulin appears to activate glycogen synthetase and hexokinase, although the effect has not been proved to be directly on the enzyme.

Insulin has important effects on fatty acid synthesis and release in adipose tissue. This results in part from the inhibition of the lipase, which breaks down triglycerides to glycerol and fatty acids, and in part by promoting the production of glycerophosphate from glucose, leading to the resynthesis of triglycerides from fatty acids.

In the liver the intracellular glucose concentration is dependent upon the concentration of glucose in the perfusing plasma and is not directly altered by insulin. However, insulin decreases the output of glucose and urea by the liver and increases the uptake of potassium and phosphate by this organ. Insulin stimulates glycolysis and inhibits gluconeogenesis by inducing the formation of enzymes controlling the former and repressing those promoting the latter process. These changes may also be secondary to other metabolic alterations rather than direct effects of insulin.

D. Insulin Deficiency: Insulin deficiency occurs most commonly in diabetes mellitus but may follow pancreatectomy or destruction of the organ by pancreatitis or a tumor. It can be induced experimentally by drugs such as alloxan and can be seen with excessive production of glucose (eg, glucocorticoid therapy or Cushing's syndrome), in which case the deficiency is relative to the need rather than absolute.

Clinical Uses

A. Diabetes Mellitus: Diabetes mellitus is a complex disorder which appears to be the result of one or more inherited defects. Two important aspects of the disorder are the deficiency in insulin effect and the basement membrane thickening found in small blood vessels. These are the earliest detectable findings, and their relationship to each other is not known. The characteristic symptoms of the disorder are the consequence of the relative or complete lack of insulin on intermediary metabolism, whereas many of the complications result from disease of the blood vessels. Unfortunately, even properly treated and well controlled diabetes (from the metabolic standpoint) may progress to serious vascular complications. The symptoms of diabetes result from decreased utilization of glucose in peripheral tissues such as muscle and adipose tissue and increased release of glucose (gluconeogenesis) into the circulation by the liver.

The clinical disorder is not detectable in its earliest stages. As the severity increases, the above-mentioned defect in insulin action can be identified. This is followed by an alteration in carbohydrate metabolism characterized by a reduction in the rate at which glucose is removed from the circulation (impaired glucose tolerance). The disorder progresses until blood glucose levels are sufficiently high to permit the loss of this sugar in the urine. When insulin deficiency is marked, as in early onset or "juvenile" diabetes, large amounts of glucose appear in the urine, and the ensuing osmotic diuresis and loss of carbohydrate leads to the full-blown syndrome of polyphagia; polydipsia, polyuria, and weight loss.

The increased utilization of fat from adipose tissue stores as a source of energy and the conversion of protein to glucose—much of which is lost in the urine—leads to weight loss in spite of increased food intake.

Fat which is mobilized as free fatty acids is partly converted to triglyceride in the liver and partly oxidized in the liver and other tissues. An excess of acetyl-coenzyme A is formed in the liver and converted to ketones, some of which are organic acids. When ketone production exceeds the rate of utilization, organic acids accumulate in the body and cause metabolic acidosis. This in turn leads to the loss of fixed base (sodium and potassium). These changes can be prevented or corrected by the administration of insulin and a proper diet. However, if not checked by the institution of an appropriate therapeutic program, the loss of water and electrolytes and the accumulation of hydrogen ion lead to diabetic acidosis and coma, which may be fatal in severe diabetes.

The dose and type of insulin must be determined for each patient by clinical trial. In a given patient the amount required will depend upon the amount of endogenous insulin available, the diet, and exercise (which tends to decrease the need for insulin). Insulin requirements rise with increased metabolic activity due to fever, thyrotoxicosis, pregnancy, and also during periods of stress such as surgery, traumatic injuries, infections, and diabetic acidosis. Increased insulin requirements may be associated with the presence of high titers of insulin-binding antibodies.

B. Insulin Tolerance Test: The insulin tolerance test consists of the administration of crystalline insulin in a dose of 0.1 unit/kg body weight and the measurement of blood glucose at frequent intervals thereafter (eg, 0, 15, 30, 45, and 60 minutes; or 0, 20, 30, 40, and 60 minutes). A normal individual, after an overnight fast, will have a fall in blood glucose of about 50–70% in 20–40 minutes and a return to normal in 60–90 minutes. A decrease in the hypoglycemic effect of insulin is found in acromegaly (excessive growth hormone production), Cushing's syndrome, and diabetes mellitus. Patients with pituitary or adrenocortical insufficiency are highly sensitive to insulin, and the test should not be administered to such patients.

Insulin-induced hypoglycemia also increases the plasma levels of growth hormone as measured by immunoassay and is used to test the reserve of this hormone. Arginine infusions will provoke a similar rise in growth hormone levels; in patients suspected of having a deficiency of growth hormone, arginine is safer than insulin for this purpose.

C. Insulin Coma Therapy: Insulin is still occasionally used in the treatment of serious psychiatric disorders. Increasing doses of regular insulin are injected until coma is produced. The induction of hypoglycemic coma is repeated daily except on weekends for periods of many weeks in the hope of improving the mental state.

Adverse Reactions

A. Hyperinsulinism: The toxicity of insulin is essentially confined to the effects of overdosage (hyperinsulinism), usually the result of unanticipated changes in the insulin requirements of diabetic patients.* This often occurs because of the omission of meals or increased exercise. It may also occur as a result of errors in filling syringes and failure to understand the physician's directions, particularly when more than one preparation of insulin is employed.

The predominant symptoms vary with the type of insulin–probably a reflection of the rate at which the blood glucose falls. Although symptoms do not usually occur unless the blood glucose falls to levels below 50 mg/100 ml, a rapid fall from very high to slightly elevated or normal levels will sometimes provoke characteristic symptoms. The signs and symptoms stem primarily from alterations in the nervous system, which under these circumstances is deprived of its major substrate. The changes affect first the cerebral cortex and then the lower centers.

Hypoglycemic reactions following the administration of regular insulin usually start with a feeling of hunger and weakness followed by light-headedness, sweating, tachycardia, anxiety, numbness, a tingling sensation, and tremor. These symptoms are largely due to sympatho-adrenal activation. When produced by a long-acting insulin, headache and mental, motor, and emotional disturbances are more characteristic. The intermediate-acting preparations produce a mixture of

*Excessive insulin leading to hypoglycemia may be due to islet cell tumors of the pancreas and perhaps to malignancies of other organs. Functional hyperinsulinism also occurs, and is common in prediabetic individuals.

these symptoms. If severe, all reactions may lead to convulsions, coma, and death.

A variety of mechanisms designed to restore the blood glucose to normal come into play during a hypoglycemic reaction. These include the release of epinephrine and glucagon, which mobilize glucose from glycogen stores in the liver, and glucocorticoids, which increase gluconeogenesis. Sympathetic nerve fibers to adipose tissue and growth hormone released by the pituitary increase the amount of free fatty acids available to meet energy requirements of many tissues.

Treatment consists of giving 50% glucose solution, by vein if necessary, to restore consciousness. Glucagon has also been used to increase blood glucose (see below).

B. Allergic Reactions: About 25% of diabetics under treatment with insulin will, at some time, show an allergy to insulin. The reactions are usually mild and transient and consist of localized itching, swelling, and erythema at the site of injection. A few patients develop generalized urticaria, particularly after the intermittent use of insulin. Demonstrable IgE antibodies are present in these patients. Patients sensitive to beef and pork insulin can be managed with insulin derived from another species (sheep, fish) if necessary. Antihistamines are also useful in the treatment of mild allergies. When the allergy is more severe, treatment with corticosteroids, desensitization to insulin, or, in certain maturity onset cases, treatment with an oral hypoglycemic agent may be required.

Preliminary studies suggest that highly purified (monocomponent, single component) insulin may be used in sensitized individuals without causing allergic reactions.

Preparations Available

The types of insulin currently used in the USA are listed in Table 37–1. They are dispensed in 10 ml multiple injection vials. All of the preparations are available in 2 concentrations. U40 insulin is labeled in red and contains 40 units/ml. U80 insulin is labeled in green and contains 80 units/ml. Regular insulin is also packaged in concentrations of 100 units/ml (orange label) and 500 units/ml (brown and white stripes) which are useful when very large doses of insulin are required for the treatment of insulin-resistant diabetes.

The international unit of insulin is defined as the amount required to lower the blood glucose of a fasting, 2 kg rabbit from 120 to 45 mg/100 ml. The international reference material has an activity of 22 units/mg. However, crystalline insulin contains about 25 units/mg.

Although the above assay is used for pharmaceutical purposes, exquisitely sensitive methods are needed and have been developed for studies of insulin secretion and metabolism in intact animals. These include immunochemical assays and in vitro bioassays involving changes in the metabolism of rat diaphragm (muscle) or epididymal fat pad (adipose tissue).

A. Crystalline Zinc Insulin (Regular Insulin): This preparation is used for a brief effect with rapid onset,

TABLE 37–1. Insulin: Sources and activity.

Type of Preparations	Animal Source*	Activity (Hours)		Manufacturer
		Peak	Duration†	
Rapid-acting				
Insulin injection USP (regular, crystalline zinc)	Beef, pork, or mixture	½–1	5–7	Lilly, Squibb
Insulin zinc suspension USP (prompt, semi-lente)	Beef, pork, or mixture	1–2	12–16	Lilly, Squibb
Intermediate-acting				
Globin zinc insulin USP	Beef	2–4	18–24	Burroughs Wellcome
Isophane insulin suspension USP (NPH insulin)	Beef, pork, or mixture	2–8	24–28	Lilly, Squibb
Insulin zinc suspension USP (lente)	Beef, pork, or mixture	2–8	24–28	Lilly, Squibb
Long-acting				
Protamine zinc insulin suspension USP (PZI)	Beef, pork, or mixture	8–12	36+	Lilly, Squibb
Insulin zinc suspension extended USP (ultra-lente)	Beef, pork, or mixture	8–14	36+	Lilly, Squibb

*Fish insulin is available commercially in Japan but not in the USA; sheep insulin is an investigational drug in the USA.
†The duration of action is increased with increasing doses.

often in combination with long-acting preparations. It is the only preparation that can be given intravenously and is so used in the treatment of diabetic acidosis. It is also used for testing purposes (see above) and in insulin coma therapy for psychiatric disorders. It is a clear solution with a pH of approximately 3.0 containing 0.02–0.04 mg of zinc per 100 units.

B. Globin Insulin: Globin insulin is a clear solution with a pH of 3.7 containing 3.8 mg of erythrocyte globin and 0.3 mg of zinc per 100 units of crystalline insulin. When injected, the solution is neutralized in the tissues and the insulin-protein complex precipitates. The action of insulin in this form is not sufficiently prolonged to be generally useful for single dose administration of the 24-hour requirement.

C. Protamine Zinc Insulin (PZI): PZI is a preparation in which crystalline insulin is combined with an excess of protamine in phosphate buffer at pH 7.2 to form a fine precipitate containing 1.25 mg of protamine per 100 units insulin. The preparation is stabilized by the addition of 0.2 mg of zinc per 100 units. The insulin is released from the protein by proteolytic enzymes, resulting in a steady prolonged effect. Since there is an excess of protamine, this preparation is given in a separate syringe when used in conjunction with regular insulin in order to prevent binding of the regular insulin. Free protamine also combines with prothrombin and may cause local plugging of the lymphatics and irregular absorption.

D. Isophane (Neutral-Protamine-Hagedorn, NPH) Insulin: NPH insulin is a suspension of crystals of protamine zinc insulin (0.4 mg protamine per 100 units insulin) in neutral phosphate buffer (pH 7.2) containing just enough protamine to bind the insulin. Its

action is intermediate between that of PZI and regular insulin. It may be mixed with regular insulin without altering either preparation. It is frequently useful in a single dose per 24 hours, alone or in combination with regular insulin. When insulin requirements are very high, it can be administered in divided doses (2/3 in the morning and 1/3 in the late afternoon).

E. Insulin Zinc Suspensions: These preparations are made by substituting acetate for phosphate buffer, making the insulin insoluble at pH 7.2. This process may result in the formation of small amorphous particles or larger crystals. The amorphous preparation is called prompt insulin zinc suspension USP (semi-lente) and has an action similar to that of regular insulin. The crystalline form is more slowly absorbed, having an action slightly more prolonged than PZI, and is called extended insulin zinc suspension USP (ultra-lente). An intermediate preparation, insulin zinc suspension USP (lente), is a mixture consisting of 30% semi-lente and 70% ultra-lente.

F. Dalanated Insulin: Desalaninated (dalanated) pork insulin is an investigational preparation being used experimentally in the management of insulin-resistant diabetes. It is apparently less antigenic than the other preparations, or at least does not bind as readily with the antibodies that reduce the effectiveness of insulin. It is not commercially available.

ORAL HYPOGLYCEMIC AGENTS

A wide variety of compounds are capable of causing a reduction in blood glucose. These include sulfonamides, salicylates, and a variety of plant substances as well as the compounds discussed more fully below. Although insulin is a practical and satisfactory agent for the treatment of diabetes, it has the disadvantage of requiring parenteral administration one or more times daily. The search continues for a means of controlling hyperglycemia in diabetes by the use of oral preparations of insulin or therapeutic agents other than insulin. Early attempts to treat patients with guanidine derivatives (synthalin) and hypoglycin (a West Indian plant derivative) met with failure because of the toxicity of these agents. At present, 2 classes of compounds, the sulfonylureas and the biguanides, have provided clinically useful preparations. There is evidence that these compounds, when used early in the course of the disease, may ameliorate the disorder.

Synthalin A
(decamethylene diguanidine)

Hypoglycin A
(α-amino-β-[2-methylenecyclopropyl] propionic acid)

SULFONYLUREAS

Several members of this class of compounds are in current use (Fig 37–3). Their mechanism of action is thought to be the same, but they differ in their metabolism sufficiently to produce important and possibly useful differences in potency and duration of action.

Metabolism

The sulfonylureas are promptly and completely absorbed from the intestine after oral administration. They are distributed throughout the extracellular fluid compartment. In the plasma they are partially bound to serum protein. The rate and means of degradation of these drugs vary.

Tolbutamide, the shortest acting drug, is readily converted in the liver to hydroxy- and carboxytolbutamide, which is rapidly excreted by the kidney. Its half-life in the body is 4–6 hours. Carbutamide is acetylated in the liver and excreted in the urine. Almost all of it is removed from the body in 36 hours. The peak hypoglycemic effect occurs in about 5 hours.

Acetohexamide has a very short half-life in the circulation (½–2 hours). However, it is metabolized to 1-hydroxyhexamide, which is even more potent than its precursor. The half-life of the reduced compound is 4–5 hours, so that the action of the drug has a time course slower than that of tolbutamide. It also differs from tolbutamide in that about 10% of the metabolites are excreted in the bile and appear in the stool.

Tolazamide is more slowly absorbed than the other sulfonylureas, and its effects on blood glucose are not apparent for several hours. Its half-life is about 7 hours. It is metabolized to p-carboxytolazamide, 4-hydroxymethyltolazamide, and other compounds, some of which have potent hypoglycemic effects.

The half-life of chlorpropamide in the circulation is 36 hours, so that its effects last for several days. Most of this drug is slowly excreted by the kidney without significant alteration. It is bound to plasma albumin, and a maximum blood level is not reached until after 4 days of therapy. Several weeks may be required for elimination of this drug from the body. The peak of its hypoglycemic effect is reached 10 hours after ingestion.

Glyburide (Glibenclamide), a recently introduced oral sulfonylurea derivative, appears to be suitable for use in the treatment of patients with diabetes. It is a very active compound, and patients can be maintained on as little as 2.5 mg daily. When administered orally, peak concentrations occur in 4 hours. More than 95% is removed from the circulation in 24 hours. After a single oral dose of 5 mg, the plasma glucose levels remain lower than control levels for more than 15 hours. Experience has not been sufficient to evaluate toxicity with prolonged use.

Although the rate of metabolism of these drugs tends to increase as treatment progresses, in the presence of hepatic dysfunction and, particularly, with impaired renal function, marked reduction in the clearance of these drugs leading to serious reactions has been observed.

Glymidine (sodium glymidine, glycodiazine) although not a sulfonylurea derivative, is closely related to this group of compounds. It is a sulfapyrimidine without antibacterial activity, and its mechanism of action is similar to that of the sulfonylureas. It is marketed in Europe under the following trade names: Lycanol, Gondafon, Redul, and Glyconormal. It is

Glymidine

Tolbutamide
 Artosin
 Orinase
 Rastinon

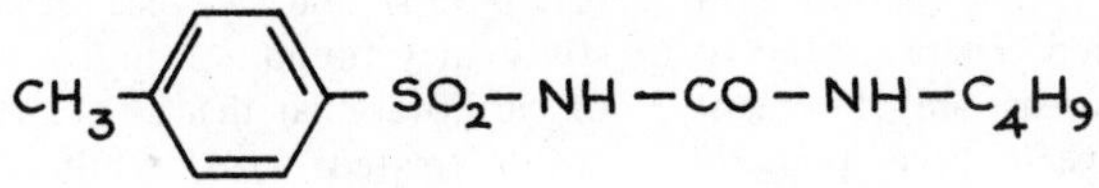

$$CH_3 - \text{⟨benzene⟩} - SO_2 - NH - CO - NH - C_4H_9$$

Tolazamide
 Tolinase

$$CH_3 - \text{⟨benzene⟩} - SO_2 - NH - \overset{O}{\overset{\|}{C}} - NH - N\text{⟨azepane⟩}$$

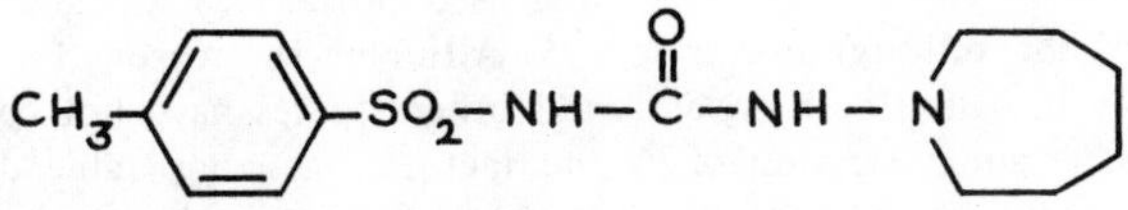

Acetohexamide
 Dymelor

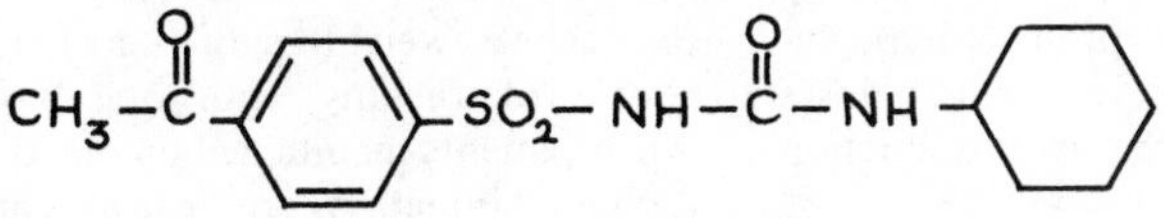

$$CH_3 - \overset{O}{\overset{\|}{C}} - \text{⟨benzene⟩} - SO_2 - NH - \overset{O}{\overset{\|}{C}} - NH - \text{⟨cyclohexane⟩}$$

Chlorpropamide
 Diabinese

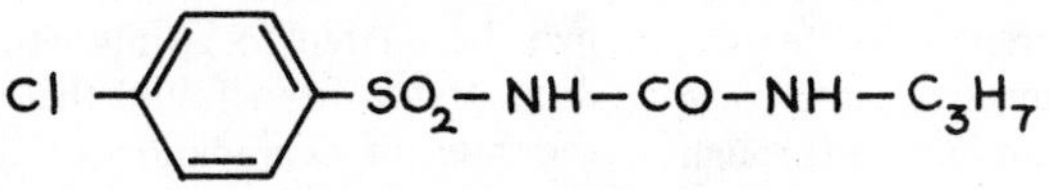

$$Cl - \text{⟨benzene⟩} - SO_2 - NH - CO - NH - C_3H_7$$

Carbutamide*
 Invenol
 Nadisan

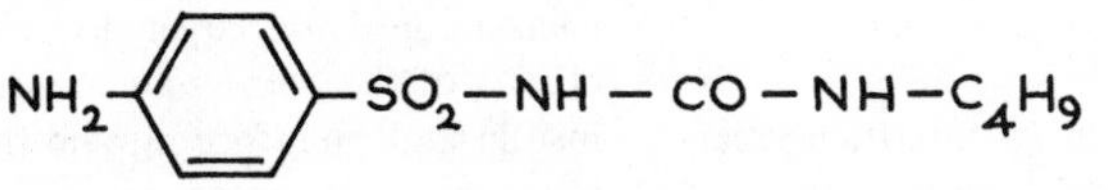

$$NH_2 - \text{⟨benzene⟩} - SO_2 - NH - CO - NH - C_4H_9$$

Tolcylamide
 (glycyclamide)*
 Diaboral
 Tolhexamide

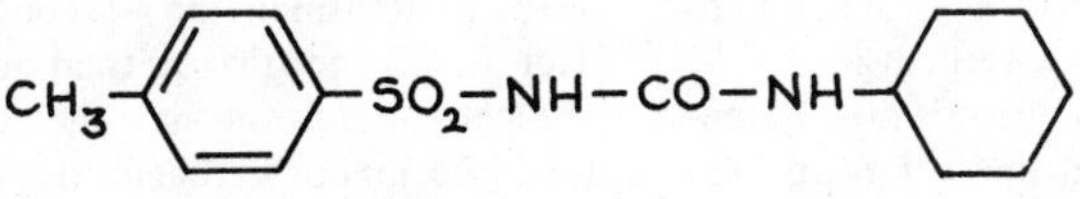

$$CH_3 - \text{⟨benzene⟩} - SO_2 - NH - CO - NH - \text{⟨cyclohexane⟩}$$

Glyburide
 (glybenclamid)*
 Daonil*
 Euglucon*

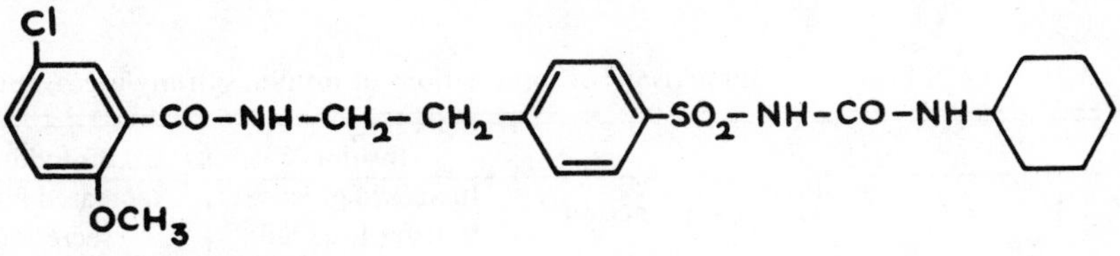

$$\text{⟨benzene, Cl and OCH}_3\text{⟩} - CO - NH - CH_2 - CH_2 - \text{⟨benzene⟩} - SO_2 - NH - CO - NH - \text{⟨cyclohexane⟩}$$

*In clinical use outside the USA, principally in Europe.

FIG 37–3. Chemical structures of sulfonylureas. Examples of trade names and code designations are given. Some of the preparations have many trade names.

used in doses of 0.5–2 gm/day. It has a half-life of 4 hours and is generally well tolerated. There appears to be no cross-allergy with sulfonylureas, and this agent may be useful in patients sensitive to other preparations.

Pharmacologic Effects

The hypoglycemic effect of the sulfonylureas is thought to be due to their ability to cause the release of insulin from the pancreas. The administration of one of these agents is attended by an increase in plasma insulin level and by a decrease in the insulin content of the pancreas. In the dosages usually employed, these compounds do not produce hypoglycemia in the absence of the pancreas; larger doses appear to have a direct effect on the liver production of glucose.

The peripheral metabolic events following the administration of this class of compounds are similar to but not exactly the same as the effects of parenterally administered insulin. These differences are thought to be due to the fact that the insulin is released for a prolonged period in small amounts and passes through the liver before entering the general circulation. A comparison of the effects of the sulfonylureas to insulin and biguanide is shown in Table 37–2.

Clinical Uses

A. Diabetes Mellitus: These drugs find their greatest use in the treatment of maturity onset diabetes in the patient whose pancreas still has the capacity to produce insulin. They are usually ineffective even in this group when more than 25–35 units of insulin are required for maintenance. The long-term use of oral hypoglycemic agents in diabetes mellitus is now extensive. In one large study (The University Group Diabetes Program [UGDP]) in which 12 clinics participated, the effects of insulin, tolbutamide, phenformin

(see p 358), and a lactose placebo were studied. In this study they found a significant increase in the number of cardiovascular deaths (12.7%) after 8 years in the group treated with tolbutamide as compared with placebo-treated controls (4.9%). The use of phenformin in this study was also discontinued because of increased mortality.

Although the reasons for the deaths are not clear and other studies have not confirmed these findings, the fact that a comparable degree of restoration of glucose tolerance and control of hyperglycemia can be achieved by weight reduction alone must not be overlooked by the physician. Every attempt must be made to achieve weight reduction before or during the course of therapy with oral hypoglycemic agents. When patients maintained on oral hypoglycemic agents develop infections or other complications which increase insulin requirements, they often require treatment with parenteral insulin.

The failure of therapy after a period of treatment may be related to an alteration in metabolism of the drug. It has been found that some patients, in whom the rate of degradation of tolbutamide may be increased, will respond to chlorpropamide. If therapy cannot be maintained with 0.5 gm chlorpropamide, 2 gm tolbutamide, 1.25 gm acetohexamide, or 0.75 gm tolazamide daily, larger doses should not be used. The effects of these drugs are additive when combined with insulin and phenformin, and they may be used in combination.

The effectiveness of these drugs varies with time. There may be an increased effect during the first 4–6 weeks of treatment or a secondary failure of the drug after 6–12 months of treatment. Lack of continued medical supervision may therefore lead to death from hypoglycemia or ketoacidosis.

Another important factor altering the effectiveness of these drugs is the enhancement of activity,

TABLE 37–2. Comparisons of some actions of insulin, sulfonylureas, and phenethylbiguanide.*

	Insulin	Sulfonylureas	Phenethylbiguanide
Major action:	Increased glucose transfer into cells	Increased insulin secretion	Increased anaerobiosis
Some subsidiary effects			
Insulin secretion	Decreased	Increased†	Decreased
Glucose uptake by peripheral tissues	Increased	Increased	Increased
Hepatic glucogenesis	Decreased	Decreased	Decreased
Gluconeogenesis	Decreased	Decreased	Decreased
Liver glycogen	Increased	Increased	Decreased
Oxidative phosphorylation	Increased	Increased	Decreased
Blood sugar-lowering effect			
Normal subjects	Marked	Moderate	None
Depancreatized subjects	Marked	None	Slight
Marked hypoglycemia	Common	Rare	None
Lactate utilization	Increased	Increased	Decreased
Irreversible side-effects	Present	Rare	None

*Reproduced, with permission, from Williams: *Textbook of Endocrinology,* 4th ed. Saunders, 1968.

†Plasma ILA is lowered after 2 weeks of therapy with chlorpropamide.

observed in patients simultaneously treated with other drugs. Phenylbutazone, phenyramidol, bishydroxy-coumarin, and sulfaphenazole have been shown to increase the half-life of one or more of the sulfonyl-ureas. Salicylates, probenecid, and monoamine oxidase inhibitors also potentiate the hypoglycemic effects of the sulfonylureas.

B. Diagnostic Tests: The response to tolbutamide is also used for testing purposes. In most patients with insulinomas (insulin-producing tumors of the pancreas), 1 gm of sodium tolbutamide in 20 ml saline, given IV in 2 minutes, will produce a profound and prolonged hypoglycemia. A similar test has been used to determine whether or not a diabetic patient would be a suitable candidate for sulfonylurea therapy. However, therapeutic trial is more reliable.

Tolbutamide is also useful for testing patients with borderline abnormalities in the glucose tolerance test or postprandial blood glucose levels. The oral administration of 2 gm of tolbutamide with 2 gm of sodium bicarbonate produces a fall in blood glucose levels to 78% of the control value or less in more than 90% of normal subjects even in the presence of obesity, liver disease, hyperthyroidism, and other abnormalities affecting carbohydrate tolerance.

C. Chlorpropamide in Diabetes Insipidus: Chlorpropamide has been found to have an antidiuretic effect in patients with diabetes insipidus. This effect appears to be similar to that produced by vasopressin. It causes a reduction of free water clearance without reducing glomerular filtration or osmolal clearance. This property is not shared by other sulfonylureas. It has been used in doses of 0.25–0.5 gm/day or more in the treatment of patients with diabetes insipidus. It may act by enhancing the effects of low concentrations of vasopressin on the kidney.

Adverse Reactions

The undesirable side-effects of these drugs are due to their toxicity; allergic reactions are rare. All of the sulfonylureas cause similar toxic reactions, but the frequency of untoward reactions does vary. It is usually possible to reduce the dose or substitute another drug when toxic reactions occur.

The incidence of undesirable effects is estimated to be about 5% for this group of drugs—somewhat lower for tolbutamide than for carbutamide and the longer-acting agents. The increased gastric secretion produced by these drugs may lead to heartburn, nausea, abdominal pain, and diarrhea. These effects are

TABLE 37–3. Sulfonylureas and biguanides: Dosages and preparations available.

	Daily Dose	Duration of Action	Preparations Available
Sulfonylureas			
Tolbutamide (Orinase, Artosin, Rastinon)	0.5–3 gm in divided doses	6–12 hours	Tablets, 500 mg (Rastinon also available as 1 gm tablets)
Tolazamide (Tolinase)	0.1–0.5 gm as single dose or in divided doses	10–14 hours	Tablets, 100 and 250 mg
Acetohexamide (Dymelor, Dymelin, Ordimel)	0.25–1.5 gm as single dose or in divided doses	12–24 hours	Tablets, 250 and 500 mg
Chlorpropamide (Diabinese, Mellinase, Diabetil, Dialane)	0.1–0.5 gm as single dose	Up to 60 hours	Tablets, 100 and 250 mg
Carbutamide* (Alentin, Invenol, Inbuton, Glucidoral, Nadisan, Oranil, Talanton)	0.5–3 gm	Up to 60 hours	Tablets, 500 mg
Glycyclamide* (tolhexa-mide, Diaboral, Subose)	0.2–1.2 gm	. . .	Tablets, 200 mg
1-Butyl-3-metanilylurea* (Sucrida Berna)	0.5–1 gm	. . .	Tablets, 500 mg
Biguanides			
Phenformin (DBI, Meltrol)	0.025–0.15 gm as single dose or in divided doses	4–6 hours / 8–12 hours	Tablets, 25 mg / Timed-disintegration capsules, 50 and 100 mg
Buformin* (Silubin)	0.05–0.3 gm in divided doses	. . .	Tablets, 50 mg / Sustained-action tablets, 100 mg
Metformin* (Diabex, Glucophage, Glecofago, Modulan, Haurymellin)	1–3 gm in divided doses	. . .	Tablets, 500 mg

*In clinical use outside the USA.

dose-related and are treated by reduction of dose, administration of antacids, and use of a bland diet. CNS effects such as confusion, vertigo, ataxia, and weakness have been observed with the use of large doses of chlorpropamide. Flushing reactions to alcohol, also dose-related, occur most frequently with carbutamide and chlorpropamide. The sulfonylureas have also been reported to produce hypothyroidism.

The more serious toxic effects, granulocytopenia and cholestatic jaundice, are frequently preceded by fever, malaise, and skin eruptions or photosensitivity. These tend to occur in the first 1–2 months of therapy. They are more frequent with large doses of chlorpropamide. Exacerbation of hemolytic anemia has been reported in the presence of red blood cell enzyme deficiency.

The most serious acute problems connected with the use of these agents are profound hypoglycemia and diabetic acidosis. The long-term problems have been mentioned above (see p 356).

Preparations Available

See Table 37–3.

BIGUANIDES

Although guanidine and many of its derivatives can produce hypoglycemia, only phenethylbiguanide (phenformin) is in use at the present time in the USA. It is a white crystalline powder with the structure shown in Fig 37–4. Although it has been found to have the effects noted in Table 37–2 in various experi-

mental studies, its hypoglycemic effect in patients with diabetes is not well understood. It is of interest that the compound does not cause a reduction in blood glucose in normal human subjects. It has been shown to potentiate the effects of insulin in vivo and in vitro and may antagonize anti-insulin factors. It has also been shown to decrease glucose absorption from the gut.

Phenformin (DBI) is dispensed as rapidly disintegrating 25 mg tablets or as slow-release 50 mg capsules (DBI-TD) designed to release one-third of the drug during the first hour, two-thirds by the fourth hour, and the remainder within 8 hours. The slow-release capsules are easier to use in most patients. Half to two-thirds of the dose can be given in the morning and the rest with the evening meal.

The average dose is slightly less than 1 mg/lb body weight. The symptoms of an excessive dose include nausea, anorexia, foul breath, vomiting, diarrhea, and abdominal cramps. A metallic taste may be noted, as well as malaise. These symptoms are less common with doses of 100 mg/day or less and can be controlled by reduction of the dose or cessation of therapy. Lactic acidosis has been noted, particularly in patients with severe hepatic, renal, or cardiac disease and when other symptoms of toxicity have been present for several days.

Phenformin has been reported by some investigators to lead to a slow but consistent weight loss. This observation has not been confirmed by carefully controlled studies. However, this agent lowers blood sugar without promoting insulin release. Therefore, in addition to reducing the postprandial need for insulin from the pancreas, it might reduce the deposition of fat.

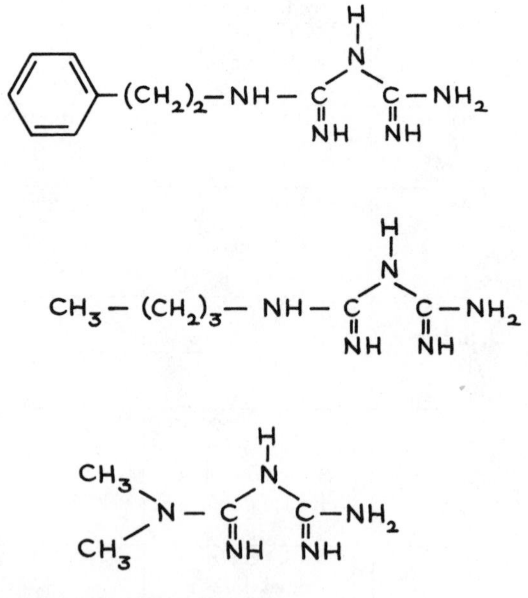

*In clinical use outside the USA, principally in Europe.

FIG 37–4. Chemical structures of biguanides. Examples of trade names and code designations are given. Some of the preparations have many trade names.

Phenformin is often used in combination with sulfonylureas or insulin. About half of patients on sulfonylureas alone will become unresponsive to therapy within 4 years, and the majority of these can be controlled for a variable period by the addition of phenformin. In patients in whom diabetes is difficult to control, even with large doses of insulin, the addition of phenformin to the therapeutic regimen has improved blood sugar control.

HYPERGLYCEMIC AGENTS

Blood glucose levels can be increased by several means. Therapeutically, the usual method is to give glucose orally or, in unconscious patients, intravenously in concentrated solutions. Glucagon or epinephrine is occasionally used to achieve a rapid rise in blood glucose concentrations from glycogen stores. More prolonged effects (for experimental or therapeutic purposes) can be achieved by pancreatectomy, by destruction of the islets with drugs such as alloxan and streptozotocin; and, under certain circumstances, by hormones such as the glucocorticoids and growth hormone or drugs such as diazoxide.

GLUCAGON

Chemistry

Glucagon is produced by the alpha cells of the islets of Langerhans and a "glucagon-like" hormone is produced by cells in the gastric and duodenal mucosa. Glucagon is a polypeptide composed of a single chain of 29 amino acids (Fig 37-5) and has a molecular weight of 3485. When isolated, it is a white crystalline material which is soluble in acid and alkali but relatively insoluble in the range of pH 4.0-9.0.

Glucagon has been measured by immunoassay procedures and found to be present in serum in the range of 1-3 mμg/ml. In the circulation it does not appear to be bound to a specific protein.

Pharmacologic Effects

When glucose is given orally, a "glucagon-like" substance is released from the gastrointestinal tract. When glucose is given intravenously, this release does not occur. There is a decline in plasma glucagon levels. The glucagon-like material that is released following

the ingestion of glucose stimulates the release of insulin by the pancreas. This may be one of the reasons that plasma insulin concentrations rise more rapidly and remain higher after oral than after intravenous administration of glucose when comparable plasma glucose levels are achieved. Glucagon release is also stimulated by prolonged fasting and by intravenous administration of arginine and oral administration of amino acids.

Glucagon has been shown to increase gluconeogenesis from amino acids and lactic acid in the perfused liver. However, the rise in blood glucose produced by this hormone is primarily the result of glycogenolysis. Glucagon stimulates the formation of cyclic AMP from ADP in the liver. This leads to the activation of phosphorylase, the rate-limiting enzyme in the conversion of glycogen to glucose. Although glucagon is active in adipose tissue, it does not activate muscle phosphorylase.

Little is known about the metabolism of glucagon in vivo. Beef liver has been found to contain an enzyme which hydrolyzes the glucagon at the peptide bond between serine and glutamine, removing the first 2 amino acids.

Although no clinical syndrome due to a deficiency of glucagon has been established, glucagon-secreting tumors have been found. A patient with a glucagon-producing alpha cell carcinoma of the pancreas has been described. He was found to be diabetic.

Clinical Uses

Glucagon is used as an adjunct to glucose for the treatment of acute hypoglycemic reactions. It is particularly useful when oral and intravenous administration of glucose is not possible. It is effective in doses of 0.5-1 mg subcut, IM, or IV. In managing a labile diabetic, the family of the patient, when instructed by the physician, can administer glucagon to a person with a severe hypoglycemic reaction while awaiting the arrival of the physician.

The response may occur as early as 5 minutes after administration of glucagon, but more commonly it takes 10-25 minutes. If no response occurs in 25 minutes, a second dose may be administered. Glucagon and glucose may be administered concomitantly, and glucose should be used if there is no response to glucagon.

Recent studies indicate that glucagon has an important inotropic effect on the heart which resembles that produced by the catecholamines. It is not prevented by propranolol. The observation that it does not seem to increase the tendency toward arrhythmias in the failing or damaged heart indicates that it may be of therapeutic value clinically. Under some circumstances, it has been useful in the treatment of cardiogenic shock and congestive heart failure.

His-Ser-Gln-Gly-Thr-Phe-Thr-Ser-Asp-Tyr-Ser-Lys-Tyr-Leu-Asp-Ser-Arg-Arg-Ala-Gln-Asp-Phe-Val-Gln-Trp-Leu-Met-Asn-Thr

FIG 37-5. Amino acid sequence of glucagon polypeptide.

Glucagon is useful as a diagnostic agent. The intravenous injection of 0.5–1 mg of glucagon will usually provoke a paroxysm in patients with pheochromocytomas. It appears to be as reliable as histamine, and its injection is not accompanied by the unpleasant flush and headache produced by the injection of histamine.

Glucagon in 1 mg doses will also increase the pituitary release of growth hormone and ACTH by the pituitary and can be used to test pituitary function. It has also been used to provoke insulin release by the pancreatic beta cells for testing purposes.

Adverse Reactions

Except for occasional episodes of nausea and vomiting, particularly with large doses, the administration of glucagon has not caused serious side-effects. Hypotensive reactions due to glucagon sensitivity have been reported following intravenous administration.

Contraindications & Cautions

There are no established contraindications to the use of glucagon. The greatest danger in its use is the possibility of overlooking coma due to other causes in the mistaken belief that the unconscious patient is having an insulin reaction.

Preparations Available

Glucagon USP is supplied in 1 ml ampules containing 1 mg and 10 ml vials containing 10 mg of dry crystalline glucagon hydrochloride mixed with lactose (49 and 140 mg, respectively). It is supplied with an appropriate diluent that contains phenol as a preservative. When reconstituted, the solution can be kept for 3 months under refrigeration.

DIAZOXIDE
(Hyperstat)

Diazoxide is chemically related to the thiazide diuretics. It was first studied because of its antihypertensive properties but has proved to be more useful in the treatment of hypoglycemia. Although it has not been marketed, it has been used investigatively in the treatment of several disorders associated with hypoglycemia.

Diazoxide (Hyperstat)

Diazoxide can increase blood glucose by several mechanisms. In large doses it leads to the adrenal medullary release of epinephrine. It also inhibits the release of insulin. However, in the presence of adequate glycogen stores it can produce an increase in plasma glucose and free fatty acid (FFA) levels in pancreatectomized and adrenalectomized animals. In the intact animal, diazoxide increases hepatic release of glucose, inhibits glucose utilization in the periphery, and increases the rate of mobilization of FFA. Little is known about its metabolism.

Diazoxide (Hyperstat) has been used experimentally in several hypoglycemic states, including idiopathic hypoglycemia and Von Gierke's disease. Its most important potential use at present is in the management of insulin-producing tumors which are not amenable to or have not responded to surgery or irradiation. Doses as high as 200 mg every 6 hours have been used in patients with islet cell tumors. However, at doses this high and at even lower doses, persistent nausea and vomiting, edema, and excessive hair growth occur. Hypogammaglobulinemia has also been reported in patients under treatment with this drug. In order to minimize its undesirable effects, diazoxide has been used in combination with other agents such as growth hormone, glucocorticoids, and benzothiadiazines.

Diazoxide (Hyperstat) is dispensed as compressed tablets containing 100 mg/tablet and in ampules containing 300 mg in 20 ml of diluent for intravenous use.

OTHER HYPERGLYCEMIC AGENTS

Many compounds such as uric acid, dehydroascorbic acid, quinolones, and alloxan have been reported to selectively destroy the insulin-secreting cells of the pancreas. Alloxan has been used extensively. It has proved to be a convenient means of producing insulin deficiency in laboratory animals. Attempts to use this compound in the treatment of insulin-secreting tumors have not been successful.

Alloxan

Streptozotocin, an antibiotic derived from *Streptomyces achromogenes,* causes a highly specific and irreversible destruction of the activity of pancreatic beta cells when given in doses of 50–100 mg/kg to rats. At doses of 65 mg/kg, there is a prompt initial rise in plasma glucose, reaching a peak in 2 hours. This is followed in 2 hours by marked hypoglycemia. In 24 hours, a marked and permanent hyperglycemia is present. This agent has been used to treat insulin-producing islet cell tumors with some success. However, its usefulness is limited by severe renal and hepatic toxicity.

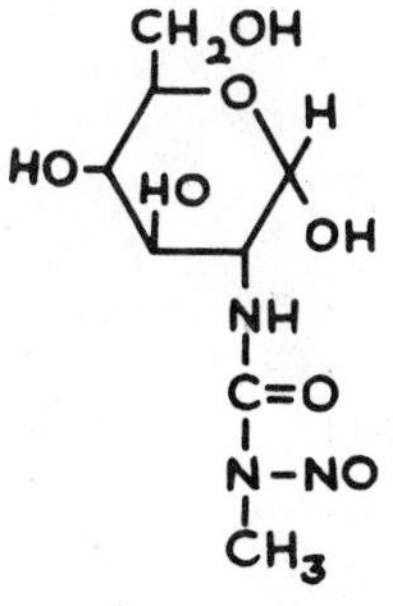

Streptozotocin

• • •

General References

Balodimos, M.C., Camerini-Dávalos, R.A., & A. Marble: Nine years' experience with tolbutamide in the treatment of diabetes. Metabolism 15:957–970, 1966.

Bond, V.P. (moderator): Symposium on insulin. Am J Med 40:651–772, 1966.

Bressler, R., Corredor, C., & K. Brendel: Hypoglycin and hypoglycin-like compounds. Pharmacol Rev 21:105–130, 1969.

Campbell, G.D. (editor): *Oral Hypoglycaemic Agents.* Academic Press, 1969.

Foa, P.P., & G. Galansino: *Glucagon: Chemistry and Function in Health and Disease.* Thomas, 1962.

Frawley, T.F. (editor): Symposium on treatment of diabetes mellitus. Mod Treat 2:597–696, 1965.

Goldschlager, N., & others: The effect of glucagon on the coronary circulation in man. Circulation 40:829–837, 1969.

Goodman, J.I.: Role of phenformin (DBI) as an adjuvant in oral antidiabetic therapy. Metabolism 14:1153–1157, 1965.

Graber, A.L., Porte, D., Jr., & R.H. Williams: Clinical use of diazoxide [Hyperstat] and mechanism for its hyperglycemic effects. Diabetes 15:143–148, 1966.

Grodsky, G.M., & P.H. Forsham: Pancreas: Endocrine function. Ann Rev Physiol 28:347–380, 1966.

Junod, A., & others: Diabetogenic action of streptozotocin: Relationship of dose to metabolic response. J Clin Invest 48:2129–2139, 1969.

Levine, R.: Insulin: The biography of a small protein. New England J Med 277:1059–1064, 1967.

Lukens, F.D.: The rediscovery of regular insulin. New England J Med 272:130–136, 1965.

Martin, H.E., Smith, K., & M.L. Wilson: The fluid and electrolyte therapy of severe diabetic acidosis and ketosis. A study of 29 episodes (26 patients). Am J Med 24:376–389, 1958.

Mayhew, D.A., Wright, P.H., & J. Ashmore: Regulation of insulin secretion. Pharmacol Rev 21:183–212, 1969.

Mereu, T.R., Kassoff, A., & A.D. Goodman: Diazoxide in the treatment of infantile hypoglycemia. New England J Med 275:1455–1460, 1966.

Romanoff, N.E.: Factors controlling release of insulin from the beta cell in relation to diabetes mellitus. New York J Med 68:385–391, 1968.

Rosenbloom, A.L., Smith, D.W., & R.C. Cohan: Zinc glucagon in idiopathic hypoglycemia of infancy. Am J Dis Child 112:107–111, 1966.

Roth, H., & others: Zinc glucagon in the management of refractionary hypoglycemia due to insulin-producing tumors. New England J Med 274:493–497, 1966.

Rubenstein, A.H., & I. Spitz: Role of the kidney in insulin metabolism and excretion. Diabetes 17:161–169, 1968.

Symposium on diabetes mellitus. Arch Int Med 123:219–322, 1969.

The University Group Diabetes Program: A study of the effects of hypoglycemic agents on vascular complications in patients with adult-onset diabetes. Diabetes 19 (Suppl 2):747–830, 1970.

Williams, R.H.: Recent advances relative to diabetes mellitus. Ann Int Med 63:512–529, 1965.

38 . . .

The Gonadal Hormones & Inhibitors

THE OVARY
(Estrogens, Progestins, Other Ovarian Hormones,
Oral Contraceptives, Other Uses of Estrogens
& Progestins, & Ovulation-Inducing Agents)

The ovary has important gametogenic functions which are integrated with its complex hormonal activity. Our present understanding of these functions, their interrelationships, and the differences from one species to another is incomplete. In the human female, the gonad is relatively quiescent during the period of rapid growth and maturation. At puberty the ovary begins a 30–40 year period of cyclic function called the menstrual cycle because of the regular episodes of bleeding that are its most obvious manifestation. It then fails to respond to gonadotropins secreted by the anterior pituitary gland, and the cessation of cyclic bleeding which occurs is called the menopause.

The nature of the mechanism responsible for the onset of ovarian function at the time of puberty is unknown. It is thought that the maturation of centers in the brain such as the amygdala releases an inhibition

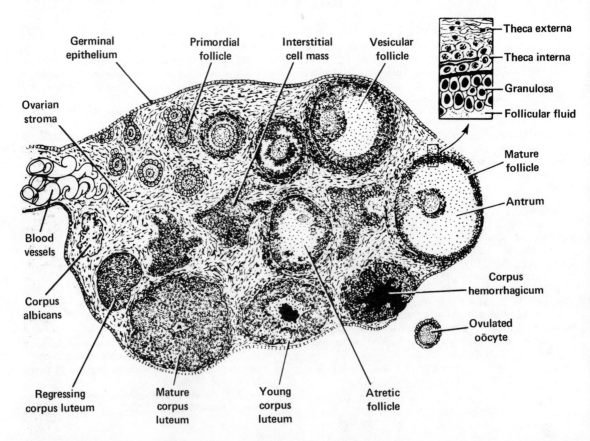

FIG 38–1. Diagram of a mammalian ovary, showing the sequential development of a follicle, formation of a corpus luteum, and, in the center, follicular atresia. A section of the wall of a mature follicle is enlarged at the upper right. The interstitial cell mass is not prominent in primates. (After Patten & Eakin. Reproduced, with permission, from Gorbman & Bern: *Textbook of Comparative Endocrinology*. Wiley, 1962.)

of the cells in the median eminence of the hypothalamus, allowing them to produce releasing factors for follicle-stimulating hormone (FSH) and luteinizing hormone (LH) (see Chapter 39), which are carried to the anterior pituitary, where they stimulate the secretion of FSH and LH. At first, small amounts of these hormones are released and the limited quantities of estrogens secreted cause breast development, alterations in fat distribution, and a growth spurt associated with epiphyseal closure in the long bones. The small amounts of androgens produced by the ovary and adrenal contribute to the appearance of axillary and pubic hair at this time.

After a year or two, sufficient amounts of estrogen are produced to induce endometrial changes and periodic bleeding. After the first few cycles, which may be anovulatory, normal cyclic function is established.

At the beginning of each cycle a variable number of follicles, each containing an ovum, begin to enlarge in response to FSH. After 5 or 6 days, one of the follicles begins to develop more rapidly. The granulosa cells of this follicle multiply and, under the influence of LH, synthesize estrogens and release them at an increasing rate. The estrogens appear to inhibit FSH release, which may lead to the regression of the smaller, less mature follicles. The ovum undergoes meiotic reduction division at this time. This structure is called the graafian follicle and consists of an ovum surrounded by a fluid-filled antrum lined by granulosa and theca cells (Fig 38–1). The estrogen secretion reaches a peak just before midcycle and may be responsible for the brief surge in LH and FSH release which immediately precedes (and may cause) ovulation. At the time of ovulation, the granulosa cells are beginning to secrete progesterone. When the follicle ruptures, the ovum is released into the abdominal cavity.

Following the above events, the cavity of the ruptured follicle fills with blood and the luteinized theca and granulosa cells proliferate and replace the blood to form the corpus luteum. The cells of this structure produce estrogens and progesterone for the remainder of the cycle unless pregnancy occurs. The maintenance of a functioning corpus luteum requires the elaboration of prolactin in the rodent. However, in the human female the structure is able to persist for a period of time independently. Its life can be prolonged by chorionic gonadotropin and, when the ovum is fertilized and implants in the endometrium, it produces sufficient amounts of gonadotropin to maintain the corpus luteum for a prolonged period of time.

If pregnancy does not occur, the corpus luteum begins to degenerate and ceases hormone production. The endometrium, which proliferated during the follicular phase and developed its glandular structure during the luteal phase, is shed in the process of menstruation. These hormonal events are summarized in Fig 38–2.

Disturbances in Ovarian Function

The control of ovarian function is complex. It involves several parts of the brain, including the hypothalamus and the limbic system. Chemical transmitters produced by the ventral hypothalamus appear to regulate the production of the gonadotropic hormones by the pituitary; these hormones in turn control follicular development, ovulation, and hormone production in the ovary. Disturbances of cyclic function are common even during the peak years of reproduction. A minority of these result from inflammatory or neoplastic processes which destroy the uterus, ovaries, or pituitary, but the causes of most menstrual problems are poorly understood. Many of the minor disturbances leading to periods of amenorrhea or anovulatory cycles are functional in nature and self-limited. They are often associated with emotional or environmental changes and are thought to represent temporary disorders in the centers in the brain which control the secretion of the hypothalamic releasing factors. Amenorrhea is at times associated with inappropriate lactation, indicating a loss of the inhibitory influence of the hypothalamus on the pituitary secretion of prolactin. In some instances, the biosynthesis of estrogens is deranged in a fashion which allows increased amounts of androgens, including testosterone, to be secreted by the ovary. This produces hirsutism in association with menstrual disturbances. Normal ovarian function can be modified by androgens produced by the adrenal cortex or tumors arising from it. The ovary also gives rise to androgen-producing neoplasms such as arrhenoblastomas and Leydig cell tumors.

THE ESTROGENS

Estrogenic activity is shared by a large number of chemical substances. In addition to the variety of steroidal estrogens derived from animal sources, nonsteroidal estrogens have been synthesized. Many phenols are estrogenic, and estrogenic activity has been identified in such diverse forms of life as those found in the sediments of the seas and certain species of clover.

The Natural Estrogens

The major estrogens produced by women are estradiol, estrone, and estriol (Fig 38–3). Estradiol appears to be the major secretory product of the ovary. Although some estrone is produced in the ovary, most of it (and estriol) is formed in the liver from estradiol or converted in peripheral tissues from androstenedione and other androgens. As noted above, during the first part of the menstrual cycle estrogens are produced in the graafian follicle by the theca cells. After ovulation, the estrogens as well as progesterone are synthesized by the granulosa cells of the corpus luteum, and the pathways of biosynthesis are slightly different. The biosynthetic pathways during both of these phases are illustrated in Fig 38–4.

During pregnancy, a large amount of estrogen is synthesized by the fetal-placental unit. Neither the pla-

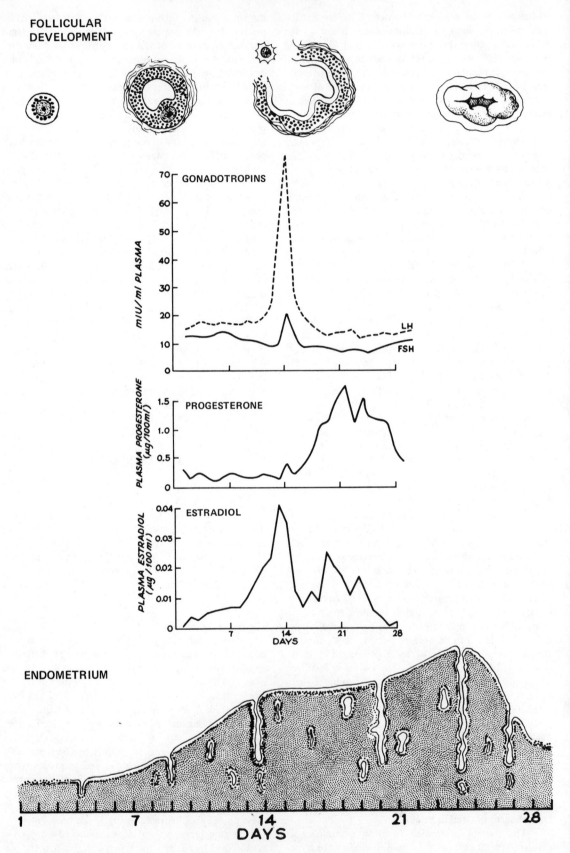

FIG 38–2. The menstrual cycle, showing pituitary and ovarian hormones and histologic changes.

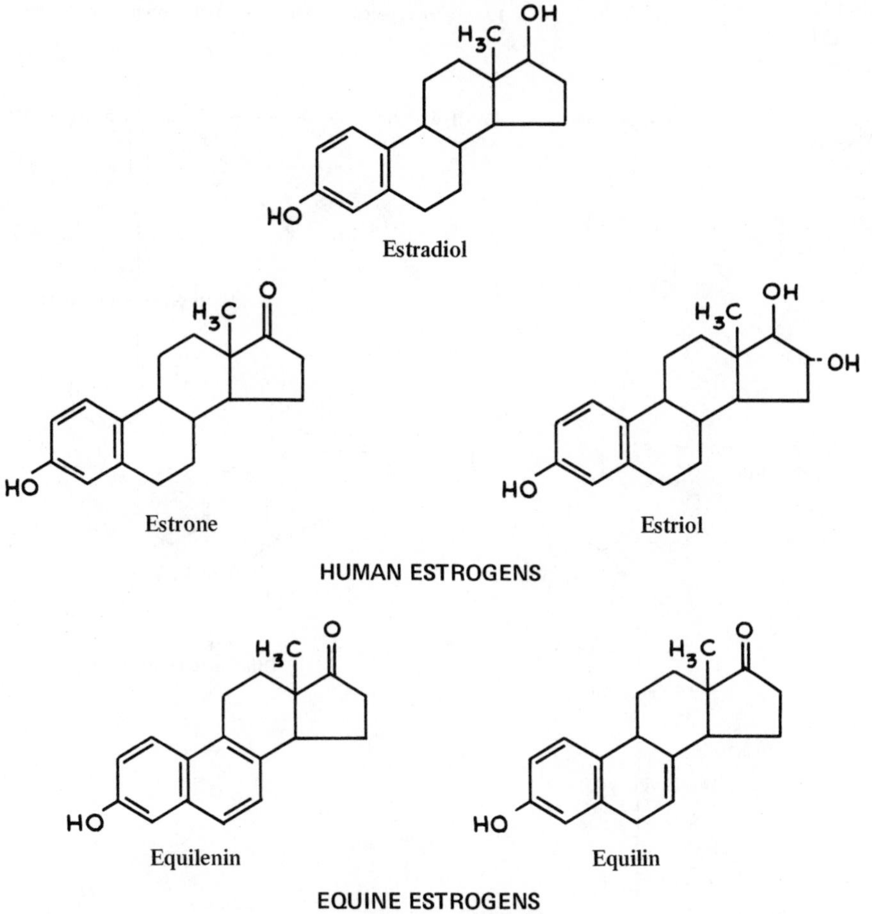

Estradiol

HUMAN ESTROGENS

Estrone

Estriol

EQUINE ESTROGENS

Equilenin

Equilin

FIG 38—3. The estrogens.

centa nor the fetal adrenal contain all the enzymes necessary for this synthesis, and there is a remarkable coordination of activity leading to the production of this hormone. The pathways involved and the locations of the enzymes are shown in Fig 38—5.

One of the most prolific natural sources of estrogenic substances is the stallion, which liberates more of this hormone than the pregnant mare or pregnant human women. The equine estrogens—equilenin and equilin—and their congeners are unsaturated in the B as well as the A ring and excreted in large quantities in the uring, from which they are recovered and used for medicinal purposes (Fig 38—3).

As noted above, the control of estrogen secretion is poorly understood. Estradiol is produced at a rate which varies from 50—350 μg/day during the cycle, in the pattern illustrated in Fig 38—2. According to the few preliminary estimates available, the blood level is of the order of 1—25 ng/100 ml (Fig 38—2). There is very little precise information about the binding of natural estrogens to plasma proteins and what role this might play in their function and metabolism. However, the initial half-life of tracer amounts of estradiol infused into the circulation is approximately 50 minutes. Estradiol is converted by the liver and other tis-

sues to estrone and estriol (and many other metabolites) which are found in the urine as the water-soluble sulfates and glucuronides (Fig 38—4).

Synthetic Estrogens

A variety of chemical alterations have been produced in the natural estrogens. The most important effect of these alterations has been to increase their effectiveness by mouth. Those which have found pharmaceutical use are listed in Table 38—1.

In addition to the steroidal estrogens, a variety of nonsteroidal compounds with estrogenic activity have been synthesized and used clinically (Fig 38—6). The most potent and widely used compound in this country is diethylstilbestrol. It is effective by mouth, but very little is known about its metabolism. Its rate of degradation in the body appears to be slower than that of the natural estrogens because it has a longer duration of action.

Physiologic Effects

The estrogens are required for the normal maturation of the female. They stimulate the development of the vagina, uterus, and fallopian tubes as well as the secondary sex characteristics. They stimulate

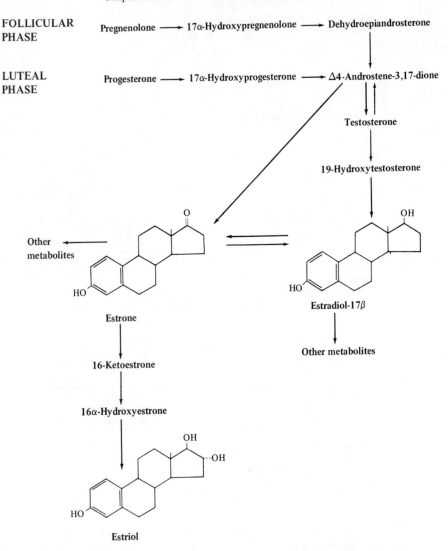

FOLLICULAR PHASE

Pregnenolone ⟶ 17α-Hydroxypregnenolone ⟶ Dehydroepiandrosterone

LUTEAL PHASE

Progesterone ⟶ 17α-Hydroxyprogesterone ⟶ Δ4-Androstene-3,17-dione

Testosterone

19-Hydroxytestosterone

Other metabolites

O

Estrone

Estradiol-17β

Other metabolites

16-Ketoestrone

16α-Hydroxyestrone

OH

OH

Estriol

FIG 38–4. Biosynthesis and metabolism of estrogens.

stromal development and ductal growth in the breast and are responsible for the accelerated growth phase and the closing of the epiphyses of the long bones which occurs at puberty. They contribute to the growth of the axillary and pubic hair and alter the distribution of body fat so as to produce typical female body contours, including some accumulation of body fat around the hips and breasts. Larger quantities also stimulate development of pigmentation in the skin which is most prominent in the region of the nipples and areola and in the genital region.

In addition to the growth effects on the uterine muscle, estrogen also plays an important role in the development of the endometrial lining. Continuous exposure to estrogens for prolonged periods leads to an abnormal hyperplasia of the endometrium which is usually associated with abnormal bleeding patterns. When the estrogen production is properly coordinated with the production of progesterone during the normal

human menstrual cycle, periodic bleeding and shedding of the endometrial lining occur.

Estrogens have a number of important metabolic effects. They seem to be partially responsible for the maintenance of the normal structure of the skin and blood vessels in women. Estrogens decrease the rate of resorption of bone in hypogonadal females but do not stimulate bone formation. Estrogens may have important effects on intestinal absorption because they reduce the motility of the bowel. In addition to stimulating the synthesis of enzymes leading to uterine growth, they alter the production and activity of many other enzymes in the body. In the liver, metabolism of a_2 globulin is altered, so that there is a higher circulating level of this group of proteins (Table 38–2.) This results in an increase in proteins which bind the glucocorticoids produced by the adrenal, the copper-containing oxidative enzymes, and other important substances.

TABLE 38–1. Commonly used estrogens.*

	Average Replacement Dose	Route of Administration	Preparations Available
Ethinyl estradiol (Estinyl, Lynoral, Menolyn, Roldiol, Ylestrol, Spanestrin)	0.02–0.06 mg/day	Oral	Tablets, 0.02, 0.05, 0.1, and 0.5 mg Capsules, 0.06 mg
Estradiol (Almediol, Altrad, Aquagen, Microdiol, Progynon, Propagone)	0.2–0.5 mg/day	IM or subcut	Aqueous suspension, 0.2, 0.25, 0.5 and 1 mg/ml Pellets, 25 mg
Estradiol benzoate (Progynon-B and others)	0.33–1.66 mg 2 times/week	IM	In oil, 1 and 3.33 mg/ml
Estradiol dipropionate (Ovocyclin and others)	0.5–1.25 mg/ week	IM	In oil, 1 and 5 mg/ml
Estradiol valerate (Atladiol, Deladiol, Delestrogen, Dura-Estradiol, Estate, Lastrogen, Valergen)	2–20 mg every other week	IM	In oil, 10, 20, and 40 mg/ml
Estradiol cypionate (Depo-Estradiol)	2–5 mg every 3–4 weeks	IM	In oil, 1 and 5 mg/ml
Piperazine estrone sulfate (Ogen)	1.5–4.5 mg/day	Oral	Tablets, 0.625, 1.25, and 2.5 mg
Conjugated estrogenic substances			
Oral: (Amnestrogen, Conestron, Estratab, Estrosan, Evex, Femogen, Menest, Premarin)	0.2–3.75 mg/day	Oral	Tablets, 0.1, 0.3, 0.625, 1.25, and 2.5 mg
Parenteral: (Aquest, Neo-Amniotin, Premarin)	0.2–20 mg	IV, IM, subcut	Injectable, 1, 2, 4, and 5 mg/ml
Topical: (Premarin)		Topical	Lotion, 1 mg/ml Cream, 0.625 mg/gm
Diethylstilbestrol (Des, Stilbetin, Vagestrol, and others)	0.1–0.5 mg/day	Oral, topical (vaginal suppository)	Tablets, 0.1, 0.25, 0.5, 1, 2, 5, 10, 25, 50, and 100 mg Enseals, 0.1, 0.25, 0.5, 1, 5, 25, and 100 mg Liquid, 25 mg/tsp Vaginal suppositories, 0.1, 0.25, and 0.5 mg
Diethylstilbestrol dipropionate (various manufacturers)	0.1–0.5 mg/day	Oral, IM	Tablets, 0.5, 1, and 5 mg In oil, 0.5, 1, and 5 mg/ml
Dienestrol (Synestrol)	Oral, 0.1–1.5 mg/day	Oral, topical	Tablets, 0.1, 0.5, and 10 mg Cream, 0.01%
Chlorotrianisene (Tace)	12–25 mg/day	Oral	Capsules, 12 and 25 mg
Methallenestril (Vallestril)	3–6 mg/day	Oral	Tablets, 3 and 20 mg

*Mestranol is not used as such. It is widely used in combination with progestins (Table 38–5). Its potency is equivalent to that of ethinyl estradiol.

Alterations in the composition of the plasma lipids caused by estrogens are characterized by an increase in the alpha lipoproteins, a slight reduction in the beta lipoproteins, and a reduction in plasma cholesterol levels. Plasma triglyceride levels are increased (Table 38–3).

Estrogens may also produce alterations in carbohydrate metabolism. The reduction of gastrointestinal motility can reduce the rate of sugar absorption. Estrogens appear to antagonize the hypoglycemic action of insulin, leading to increased levels of circulating insulin, and glucose tolerance may be measurably impaired. It is this change, in conjunction with a decrease in post-heparin lipolytic activity, which leads to the elevation of plasma triglycerides. Effects on the clotting factors and clotting mechanisms are discussed below in the section on oral contraceptives.

Caution: A number of papers have appeared reporting the occurrence of adenocarcinoma of the vagina in young women whose mothers were treated with large doses of diethylstilbestrol early in pregnancy. There is no good indication for its use at that time, and it should be avoided.

Preparations & Dosages

The commonly used natural and synthetic preparations, equivalent dosages, and routes of administration are given in Table 38–1.

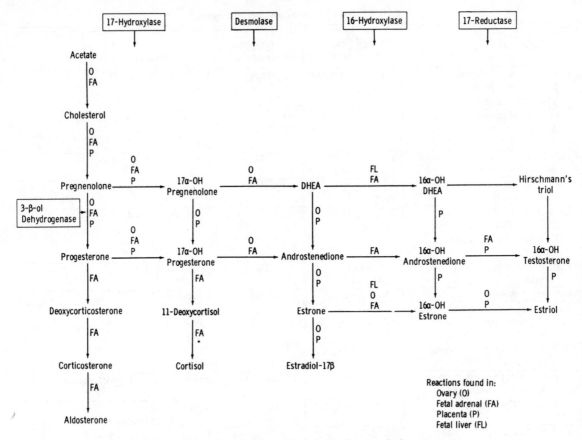

FIG 38—5. Steroid biosynthesis in the fetus and placenta.

THE PROGESTINS

1. PROGESTERONE

Progesterone is the most important progestin in man. In addition to having important hormonal effects, it serves as a precursor to the estrogens, androgens, and adrenocortical steroids. It is synthesized in the ovary, testes, and adrenal from acetate, cholesterol, and pregnenolone as shown in Fig 38—7. Large amounts are also synthesized and released by the placenta during pregnancy (Fig 38—5).

In the ovary, progesterone is produced primarily by the corpus luteum and secreted in amounts of 20—30 mg/day during the luteal phase. Normal males appear to secrete 1—5 mg of progesterone daily, resulting in plasma levels of about 0.03 μg/100 ml. The level is only slightly higher in the female during the follicular phase of the cycle, when only a few milligrams per day of progesterone are secreted. During the luteal phase, 20—30 mg/day are released into the circulation and the plasma levels range from 0.5 to more than 2 μg/100 ml (Fig 38—2).

Progesterone is rapidly absorbed following administration by any route. Its half-life in the plasma is approximately 5 minutes, and small amounts are stored temporarily in body fat. It is almost completely metabolized in one passage through the liver, and for that reason it is quite ineffective when administered by mouth.

In the liver, progesterone is metabolized to pregnanediol and conjugated to glucuronic acid. It is excreted into the urine as pregnanediol glucuronide (Fig 38—7). The urinary content of pregnanediol has been used as an index of progesterone secretion. It has been very useful in spite of the fact that the proportion of secreted progesterone converted to this compound varies from day to day and from individual to individual. Although a variety of biologic assays have been used for the measurement of the progesterone in the past, several excellent methods including double-isotope derivative technics, gas chromatographic technics, and ligand-binding assays are now available.

In addition to progesterone, 20α- and 20β-hydroxyprogesterone (20α- or 20β-hydroxy-4-pregnene-3-one) are also found. These compounds have about 1/5 the progestational activity of progesterone in man and other species. Little is known of the role of these compounds, but 20α-hydroxyprogesterone is produced in large amounts in some species and may be of some importance biologically.

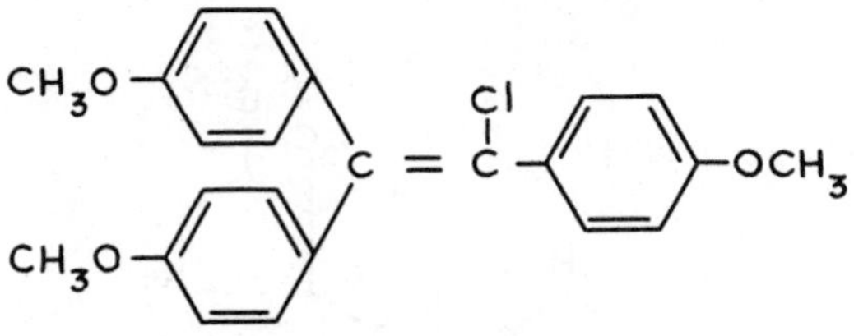

CH_3O— ... —C=C— ... —OCH_3 (Cl)

Chlorotrianisene (Tace;
tri-*p*-anisylchloroethylene)

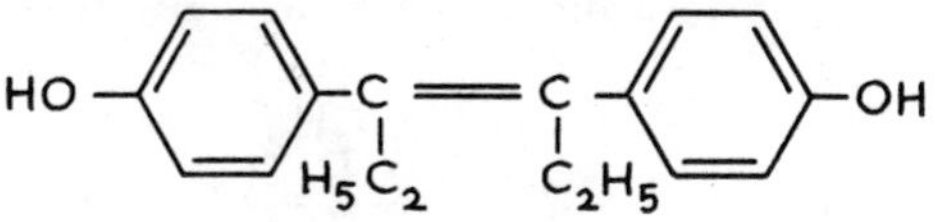

HO— ... —C=C— ... —OH
H_5C_2 C_2H_5

Diethylstilbestrol

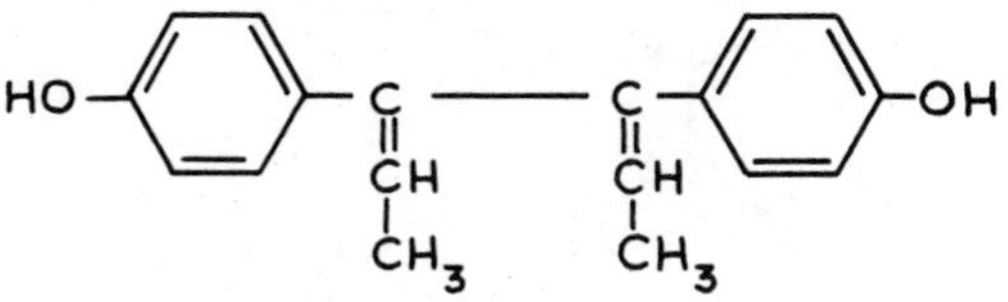

HO— ... —C — C— ...—OH
CH   CH
CH_3 CH_3

Dienestrol

CH_3O— ... —C—C—COOH
H CH_3
C_2H_5 CH_3

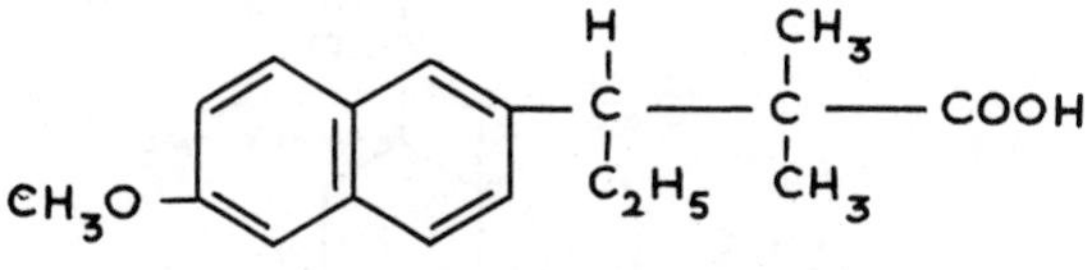

Methallenestril
(Vallestril)

FIG 38—6. Synthetic nonsteroidal compounds with estrogenic activity.

Acetate
↓
Cholesterol
↓

CH_3
C=O

Pregnenolone
HO

CH_3
C=O

Progesterone
O

CH_3
CHOH

Pregnanediol
HO

↓

Sodium-pregnanediol-20-glucuronide

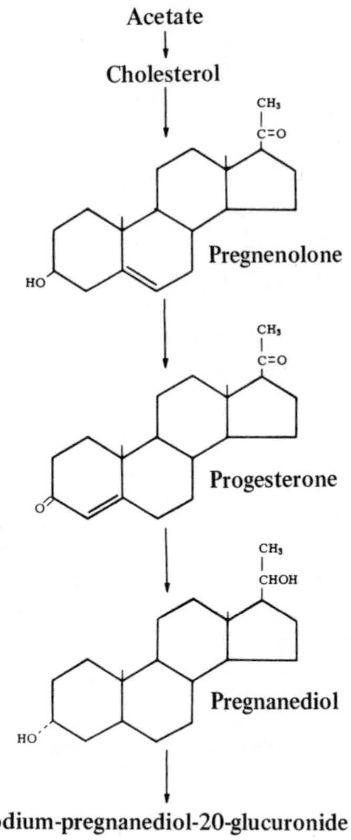

FIG 38—7. Biosynthesis of progesterone and major pathway for its metabolism. Other metabolites are also formed. (Reproduced, with permission, from Ganong: *Review of Medical Physiology,* 5th ed. Lange, 1971.)

The effects of progesterone on lipid and protein metabolism are summarized in Tables 38—2 and 38—3. It is not known to have important effects on carbohydrate metabolism. Preliminary studies suggest that some progestins may antagonize or otherwise modify the effects of estrogens on carbohydrate metabolism.

Progesterone can compete with aldosterone at the renal tubule, causing a decrease in Na^+ reabsorption. This leads to an increased secretion of aldosterone by the adrenal cortex. Progesterone increases the body temperature in man. The mechanism of this effect is not known, but an alteration of the temperature regulating centers in the hypothalamus has been suggested. Progesterone also alters the function of the respiratory centers. The ventilatory response to CO_2 is increased (synthetic progestins with an ethinyl group do not have respiratory effects). This leads to a measurable reduction in arterial and alveolar CO_2 during pregnancy and in the luteal phase of the menstrual cycle. Progesterone and related steroids also have hypnotic effects on the brain.

Progesterone is responsible for the alveolobular development of the secretory apparatus in the breast. It also causes the maturation and secretory changes in the endometrium which are seen following ovulation (Fig 38—2).

Progesterone decreases the plasma levels of many amino acids and leads to increased urinary nitrogen excretion. It has been found to induce changes in the smooth endoplasmic reticulum and its functions in experimental animals.

2. SYNTHETIC PROGESTATIONAL AGENTS

A variety of progestational compounds have now been synthesized. Some of these are active when given by mouth. They are not a uniform group of compounds, and all of them differ from progesterone in one or more respects. Table 38—4 shows some of the important pharmacologic effects and dosage forms of many of these compounds. The chemical structures are shown in Fig 38—8.

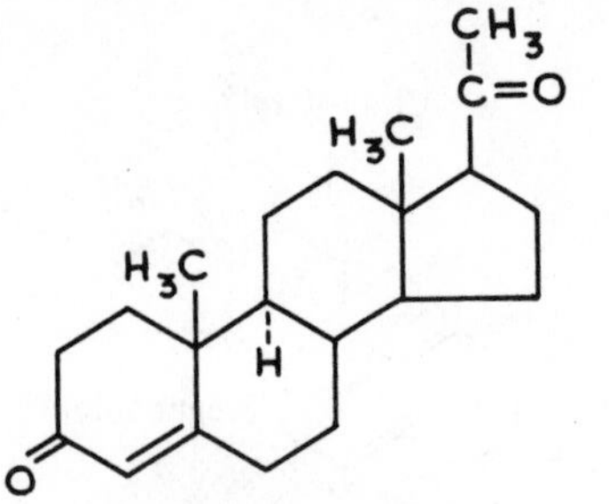

FIG 38–8. Chemical structures of progesterone and progesterone derivatives.

Progesterone
(Δ^4-pregnene-3,20-dione)

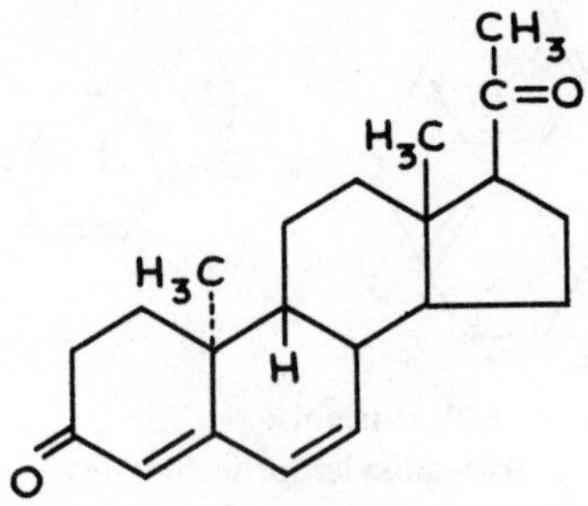

Dydrogesterone
(6-dehydro-retroprogesterone)

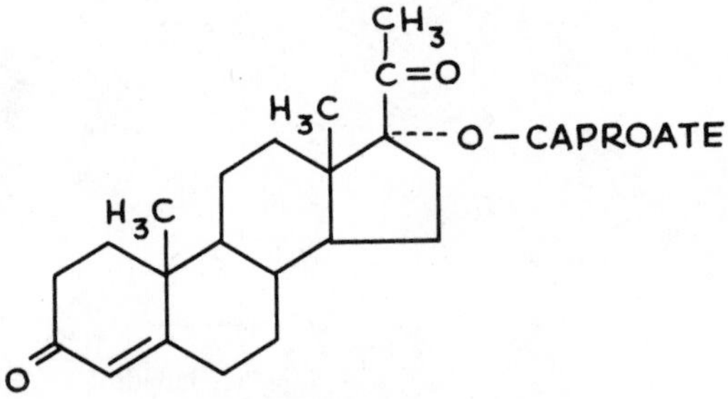

17α-Hydroxyprogesterone caproate

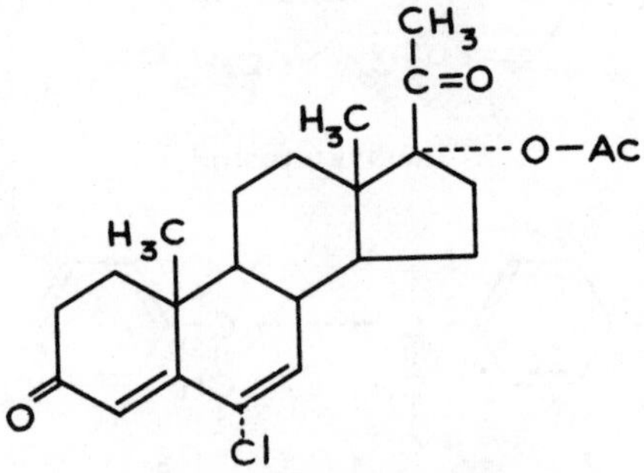

Chlormadinone acetate
(6α-chloro-Δ^6-17α-acetoxyprogesterone)

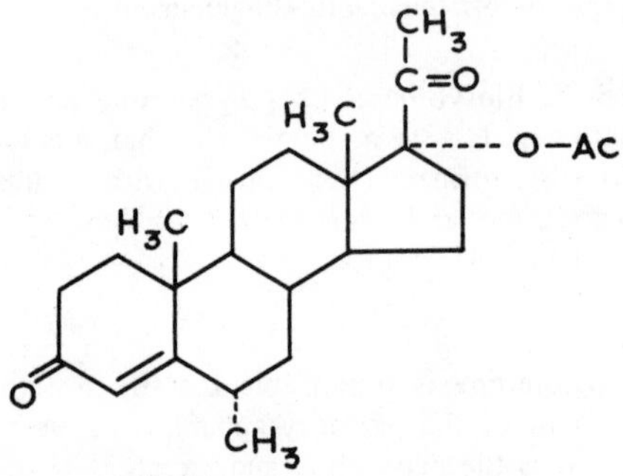

Medroxyprogesterone acetate
(6α-methyl-17α-acetoxyprogesterone)

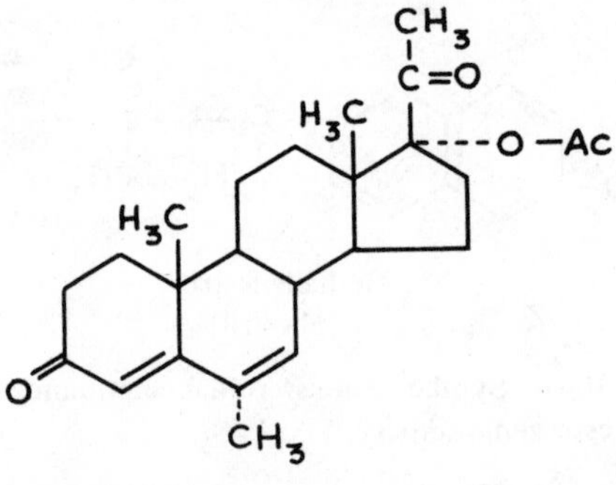

Megestrol acetate
(6α-methyl-Δ^6-17α-acetoxyprogesterone)

3. COMBINATIONS OF ESTROGENS

Since estrogens and progestins are often used in combination with one another, a variety of combined preparations are available. Most of them have been designed for use as oral contraceptives, and their properties as a class of drugs will be discussed below.

OTHER OVARIAN HORMONES

The normal ovary produces small amounts of androgens, including testosterone, androstenedione, and dehydroepiandrosterone. Only testosterone has a significant amount of biologic activity, although androstenedione can be converted to estrone in peripheral tissues. The normal woman produces a total of less than 200 μg of testosterone in 24 hours, and about 1/3 of this is probably formed in the ovary directly. The physiologic significance of these small amounts of androgens is not established, but they may be partly responsible for normal hair growth at puberty and may have other important metabolic effects. The androgen production by the ovary may be markedly increased in some abnormal states, usually in association with amenorrhea as noted above.

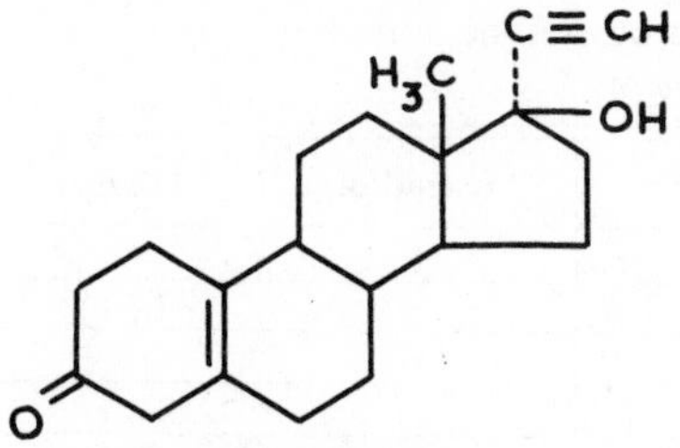

Norethynodrel
(17α-ethinyl-Δ⁵[¹⁰]-19-nortestosterone)

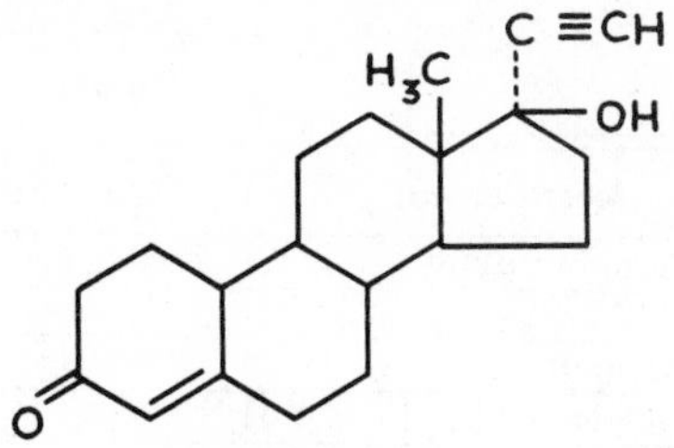

Norethindrone
(17α-ethinyl-19-nortestosterone)

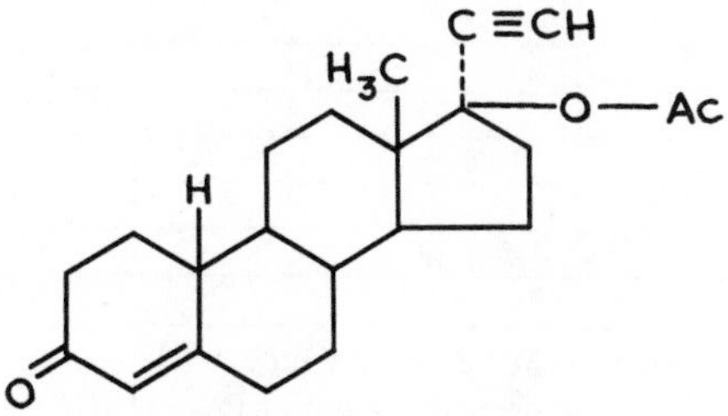

Norethindrone acetate
(17α-ethinyl-19-nortestosterone acetate)

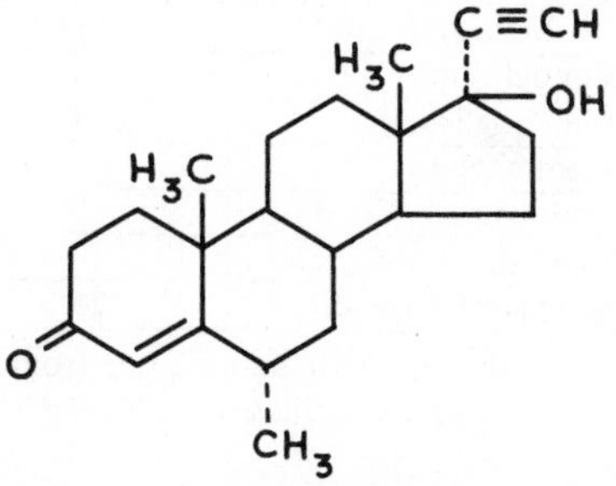

Dimethisterone
(6α-methyl-17α[1-propynyl] testosterone)

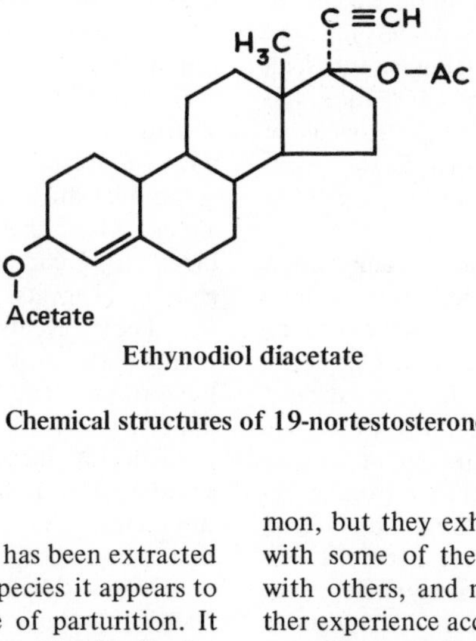

Ethynodiol diacetate

FIG 38-9. Chemical structures of 19-nortestosterone derivatives.

Relaxin

Relaxin is a polypeptide which has been extracted from the ovary. In certain animal species it appears to play an important role at the time of parturition. It causes relaxation of the pelvic ligaments and softening of the uterine cervix. In man, clinical trials with relaxin have been carried out in patients with dysmenorrhea. Relaxin has also been administered to patients in premature labor and during prolonged labors. The therapeutic value of this hormone has not been established.

ORAL CONTRACEPTIVES

A large number of oral contraceptives containing estrogens or progestins (or both) are now available for clinical use. These preparations vary chemically, and, as might be expected, have many properties in com-

mon, but they exhibit definite differences. Experience with some of the drugs has been much greater than with others, and more differences may emerge as further experience accumulates.

Three types of preparations have been used for oral contraception: (1) combinations of estrogens and progestins; (2) the sequential use of estrogens followed by combined estrogens and progestins; and (3) continuous progestin therapy without concomitant administration of estrogens.

The preparations for oral use are all well absorbed, and the metabolism of the drugs is not known to be profoundly altered by simultaneous administration. Little information is available concerning the turnover time and excretion of these compounds.

Pharmacologic Effects

A. Mechanism of Contraceptive Action: The combinations of estrogens and progestins and the sequential agents appear to exert their effect largely through

TABLE 38–2. The effects of testosterone, progesterone, estradiol, and pregnancy on plasma proteins.*

Measurement	Testosterone	Progesterone	Estradiol	Pregnancy
Serum proteins	0	0	−	−
TBPA	+	0	−	−
Albumin	0	0	−	−
Orosomucoid		0	−	−
TBG	−	0	+	+
Trypsin inhibitor	0	0	+	+
CBG	−	0	+	+
Transferrin	−	0	0	+
Ceruloplasmin	0	0	+	+
Haptoglobin	0	0	−	0
Immunoglobulins	0	0	0	0
Plasminogen	0	0	+	+
Fibrinogen	−	0	+	+
Renin substrate		0	↑	↑
Plasma amino acids	↑	↓	↑	

*Reproduced, with permission, from Salhanick, H.A., Kipnis, D.M., & R.L. Vande Wiele (editors): *Metabolic Effects of Gonadal Hormones and Contraceptive Steroids.* Plenum Press, 1969.

inhibition of ovulation. The combination agents containing estrogens and progestins also produce a change in the cervical mucus, in the uterine endometrium, and in the motility and secretion in the fallopian tubes, all of which decrease the likelihood of conception and implantation. The continuous use of progestins alone does not inhibit ovulation. The other factors mentioned, therefore, play a major role in the prevention of pregnancy when these agents are used.

B. General Effects: Chronic use of combination or sequential agents appears to depress ovarian function. The gross appearance of the ovary is that of relative inactivity; there is a minimum of follicular development, and corpora lutea, larger follicles, stromal edema, and other morphologic features which are normally seen in ovulating women are absent. In general, the amounts of the endogenous estrogens excreted in the urine are less than those observed in normal menstruating women, and pregnanediol excretion is not usually increased in the latter phase of the cycle. It is not known whether the few instances in which pregnanediol excretion is elevated are due to escape ovulation in these patients or whether corpora lutea have been formed without ovulation. Although cystic follicles have been described in patients being treated with oral contraceptives, the ovaries usually become smaller even when enlarged before therapy.

The great majority of patients return to normal menstrual patterns when therapy is terminated. About 75% will ovulate in the first post-treatment cycle, and 98% by the third post-treatment cycle. Patients who have a history of irregular cycles seem more liable to the development of amenorrhea following cessation of therapy.

A very few patients remain amenorrheic for periods of up to several years after therapy has been concluded. It is not possible at present to know whether the amenorrhea occurred as a result of the therapy or was in any way influenced by it.

These preparations have important effects on the genital tract. The cytologic findings on vaginal smears vary depending on the preparation used. For example, with the use of sequential regimens a high maturation index—ie, cornified epithelium—is noted until the progestational drug is added during the last 5 days. With almost all of the combined drugs, a low maturation index is found because of the presence of progestational agents.

These agents have important effects on the uterus. After prolonged use, the cervix may show some hypertrophy and polyp formation. There are also important effects on the cervical mucus. Normally, through the menstrual cycle, there is an increasing amount of clear liquefied mucus which is altered by the secretion of progesterone following ovulation. At that time it becomes thick and less copious and contains much cellular debris. This sequence is not much altered by the sequential preparations; however, the combined products as well as continuous progesterone therapy produce the expected changes in the mucus.

Initially there is some stimulation of the uterine muscle, resulting in some softening and increase in size. This effect is neither common nor marked and is due to the estrogens. The endometrial changes vary markedly with the preparation. With sequential agents the sequence of changes does not vary greatly from normal. During the last 5 days, progressive progestational effects on the glandular tissues are observed. In contrast to this, agents containing both estrogens and progestins produce a stromal deciduation toward the end of the cycle. The agents containing the 19-nor compounds—particularly those with the smaller amounts of estrogen—tend to produce more glandular atrophy and usually less bleeding, whereas combina-

TABLE 38-3. Some effects of oral contraceptives on plasma lipids (Dec. 1968).*

	Estrogen	Progestin	Cholesterol	Phospholipid	Triglyceride
	All	. . .	↓	↑	↑
	. . .	All	0	0	0
Provest	Ethinyl estradiol	Medroxyprogesterone	0	↑	↑
Volidan	Ethinyl estradiol	Megestrol	0	↑	↑
Anovlar	Ethinyl estradiol	Norethisterone	↓	sl↓	?↑
Enovid	Mestranol	Norethynodrel	0	. . .	↑
Ovulen	Mestranol	Ethynodiol	0	↑	↑

*Reproduced, with permission, from Salhanick, H.A., Kipnis, D.M., & R.L. Vande Wiele (editors): *Metabolic Effects of Gonadal Hormones and Contraceptive Steroids.* Plenum Press, 1969.

tion agents containing progestins which produce more physiologic changes in the endometrium (eg, medroxyprogesterone) are associated with spotting between periods and more bleeding at the time of menses. The flow during menses tends to be slightly heavier than or similar to that prior to therapy when sequential regimens are used.

Although studies in rodents suggest that the development of the blastocyst and the endometrium must be very precisely matched for implantation to occur, pregnancies occur in some patients who omit a few tablets or when the medication was begun too late in a given cycle to prevent ovulation.

Although studies in man are not available, animal experiments indicate that alterations in the transport of the gamete through the oviduct are produced by estrogens and progestins. The effect on germ cell transport is thought by some to be an important mechanism for the impairment of fertility, particularly with the use of low-dosage continuous progestin therapy as noted above.

Stimulation of the breasts occurs in most patients receiving estrogen-containing agents. Some enlargement is generally noted. The administration of estrogens and combinations of estrogens and progestins tends to suppress lactation. When the doses are small, the effects on breast feeding are not appreciable. However, when postpartum mothers are examined, milk is found in the breasts of fewer patients taking oral contraceptives than in untreated mothers. Preliminary studies of the transport of the oral contraceptives into the breast milk suggest that only small amounts of these compounds are found, and they have not been considered to be of importance.

C. Extragenital Effects of the Oral Contraceptives: The state of knowledge about these effects is incomplete at present, even though they reflect effects of either estrogens or progestins which have been used for many years. The possible consequences of these compounds have been brought to our attention more forcefully because of the large and growing number of normal individuals using them. In some cases the effects are known to be secondary to the estrogens and

in other cases to the progestins. However, in many instances the agent responsible for the effects is not known. Various effects may be more pronounced with one of the preparations than with others.

1. CNS effects—The CNS effects of the oral contraceptives have not been well studied in man. A variety of effects of estrogen and progesterone have been noted in animals. Estrogens tend to lower the threshold of excitability in the brain, whereas progesterone tends to increase it. The thermogenic action of progesterone and some of the synthetic progestins is also thought to be in the CNS. The suppression of ovarian function which results from inhibition of gonadotropin secretion is also thought to be due to an influence on the hypothalamus or other parts of the nervous system.

It is very difficult to evaluate any behavioral or emotional effects of these compounds. Although the incidence of pronounced changes in mood, affect, and behavior reported in most studies is low, milder changes are common. These changes are variable and therefore difficult to evaluate in relation to the pharmacologic effects of the drug. They may be psychologically induced by the act of using contraception or the circumstances surrounding it. However, it is possible that the changes in neuronal activity and thresholds produced by these drugs may lead to changes conditioned by other factors.

2. Effects on endocrine function—The effects on the endocrine system are not well understood at present. The inhibition of pituitary gonadotropin secretion has been mentioned. Estrogens are known to alter adrenal structure and function. In man, a few changes are of note. Estrogens increase the plasma concentration of the α_2 globulin which binds hydrocortisone (cortisol-binding protein). This does not appear to lead to any chronic alteration in the rate of secretion of cortisol, but plasma concentrations may be more than double the levels found in untreated individuals. It has also been observed that the ACTH response to the administration of metyrapone (see Chapter 39) is attenuated by estrogens and the oral contraceptives.

The estrogen-containing preparations cause alteration in the angiotensin-aldosterone system. Plasma

TABLE 38–4. Progesterone, progesterone derivatives, and 19-nortestosterone derivatives: Pharmacologic actions and preparations available. (After E.W. Overstreet, MD.)

	Duration of Action	Amount Required to Produce Secretory Endometrium	Amount Required to Delay Menses	Gonado-tropin Inhibition	Pregnancy Maintained (Castrate Animals)	BBT Rise	Estro-genic Activity	Androgenic Activity in Man	Nitrogen Metabolism	Sodium Metabolism	Preparations Available
Progesterone	1–3 days	100 mg for 5 days		+	Yes	Yes	0	0	Slightly catabolic	Slight Na loss	25, 50, and 100 mg in oil or aqueous suspension
Progesterone derivatives											
Dydrogesterone	1–3 days	10 mg for 15 days	25 mg*	0	Yes	No	0	0	Slightly catabolic	Slight Na loss	Tablets, 5 and 10 mg
Hydroxyproges-erone caproate	8–14 days	250 mg IM once		+	Rabbits, yes; rats and mice, no	Yes	0	0	Slightly catabolic	0	In oil, 125 and 250 mg/ml
Chlormadinone	1–3 days	2 mg for 12 days	4 mg		Yes	No	0	0	0	Slight diuresis	(Not available)
Medroxyproges-erone acetate	Oral: 1–3 days IM (50 mg): 4–6 weeks	50 mg for 10 days	30 mg		Yes	Yes	0	0	Slightly catabolic	0	Tablets, 2.5 and 10 mg Depot, 50 mg/ml
Megestrol	1–3 days	5 mg for 10 days	10 mg		Yes	Yes	0	0	Slightly catabolic	Slight diuresis	
19-Nortestosterone derivatives											
Norethynodrel	1–3 days		15 mg	+	No	Yes	Some	Slight	Slightly anabolic	Slight retention	(See Enovid, Table 38–5.)
Norethindrone	1–3 days		15 mg	++	No	Yes	Some	Slight	Anabolic	Slight retention	Tablets, 5 mg
Norethindrone acetate	1–3 days		7.5 mg	+++ to ++++	No	Yes	Some	Slight	Anabolic	Slight retention	Tablets, 5 mg
Dimethisterone	1–3 days		30 mg	+ to ++	Poor	Yes	0	0	0	0	(See Oracon, Table 38–5.)
Ethynodiol	1–3 days		3 mg	++	?	No	Some	0	Anabolic	0	(See Ovulen, Table 38–5.)

*With mestranol, 100–200 mg.

renin activity has been found to increase, and there is an increase in aldosterone secretion. Preliminary studies indicate that the increase in plasma renin activity is due mainly to increased levels of circulatory renin substrate, since renin levels may be decreased. The relationship between these alterations and the hypertension which occurs in patients taking oral contraceptives is not clear.

Thyroxine-binding globulin is increased. As a result, the plasma PBI and BEI levels are increased to those commonly seen during pregnancy. Since more of the thyroxine is bound, red cell T_3 uptake is also decreased. However, there are no alterations in thyroid function clinically, and the thyroid uptake of radioactive iodine is not altered. The free thyroxine level in these patients is also normal.

3. Hematologic effects—Serious thromboembolic phenomena occurring in women taking oral contraceptives have stimulated a great many studies of the effects of these compounds on blood coagulation. A clear picture of such effects has not yet emerged. The oral contraceptives do not consistently alter bleeding or clotting time. Many studies have been reported of the effects of this group of agents on the clotting factors. A great deal of conflicting information has arisen from these studies. Preliminary indications are that the changes observed are similar to those reported in pregnancy. There is an increase in factors VII, VIII, IX, and X. Increased amounts of coumarin derivatives are required to produce a reduction in prothrombin time in patients on oral contraceptives. Vitamin K-dependent clotting activity is increased in vitro only after the storage of blood for 16 hours in plastic tubes.

In addition to the changes in clotting factors, there are important changes in serum proteins. There is an increase in the α_2 globulins which affects the concentrations of hormones and other serum constituents which are protein-bound (Table 38-2). There is an increase in serum iron and total iron-binding capacity similar to that reported in patients with hepatitis.

Significant alterations in the cellular components of blood (including platelets) have not been reported with any consistency. A number of patients, however, have been reported to develop folic acid deficiency anemias. Preliminary studies indicate that the oral contraceptives inhibit the conversion of polyglutamic folate (found in food) to the monoglutamic folate which can be absorbed in the gastrointestinal tract. This can be reversed by supplementary folic acid or cessation of oral contraceptives.

4. Hepatic effects—The liver plays an important role in the inactivation and conversion to water-soluble conjugates of the estrogens and progestins used in oral contraceptives. These hormones have profound effects on the function of the liver in other respects. Some of these effects are deleterious and will be considered below under Adverse Reactions.

The effects on serum proteins noted above result from the effects of the estrogens on the synthesis of the various α_2 globulins and fibrinogen. Serum haptoglobins which also arise from the liver are depressed rather than increased by estrogen.

Some of the effects on carbohydrate and lipid metabolism are probably influenced by changes in liver metabolism. However, detailed studies of these changes have not been reported.

Important alterations in drug excretion and metabolism are also found in the liver. Estrogens in the amounts seen during pregnancy or used in oral contraceptive agents delay the clearance of BSP and reduce bile flow. These alterations result from impairment of the transfer of cholephilic substances from hepatic cells into the bile. Some of these effects of estrogens and progestins may be indirectly induced or due to metabolites of the hormones rather than the hormones themselves.

5. Effects on lipid metabolism—(Table 38-3.) The effects on lipid metabolism are potentially of great importance in evaluating the long-term use of these compounds. Estrogens are known to increase the alpha lipoproteins, decrease beta lipoproteins (the major cholesterol-carrying faction), decrease serum cholesterol, and increase phospholipids. There are conflicting reports about the effects of the oral contraceptive drugs containing mixtures of estrogens and progestins. At present it appears that some of the progestins, particularly the 19-nortestosterone derivatives, antagonize the effects of estrogens. However, each of the compounds will have to be thoroughly studied since the net effect depends in part on the type of progestin and in part on the relative amounts of estrogen and progestin.

6. Effects on carbohydrate metabolism—The administration of oral contraceptives produces alterations in carbohydrate metabolism similar to those observed in pregnancy. There is a reduction in the rate of absorption of carbohydrates from the gastrointestinal tract. Many individuals exhibit decreases in glucose tolerance; others, although their glucose tolerance has not been altered, have been shown to secrete increased amounts of insulin following the ingestion or injection of glucose. In general, these changes have been more marked in patients with a family history of diabetes. Since estrogens are known to enhance the secretion of growth hormone by the pituitary, it has been suggested that this may be responsible for some of the observed effects. Studies in experimental animals indicate that estrogens stimulate islet cell function and increase the ability of the pancreas to secrete insulin. Progesterone, on the other hand, clearly interferes with insulin action. Preliminary observations indicate that both effects occur in women. Although the changes in glucose tolerance are reversible on discontinuing medication, the implications of long-term treatment in patients who inherit the trait for diabetes is not known.

7. Cardiovascular effects—Increases in blood pressure have been reported in a small number of patients. This may be related to the enhancement of plasma renin activity as a result of oral contraceptive drugs. (See Effects on Endocrine Function, above.) The pressure slowly returns to normal when treatment is terminated. Although the magnitude of the pressure change is small in many patients, it is marked in others. It is

TABLE 38–5. Steroid contraceptive agents in common use.

1. Oral Combination Single Tablets

	Composition				Total Steroid/ One Treatment Cycle	
	Estrogen		Progesterone Derivative		Estrogen	Progestin
Demulen	Ethinyl estradiol	0.05 mg	Ethynodiol diacetate	1 mg	1 mg	20 mg
Enovid E	Mestranol	0.1 mg	Norethynodrel	2.5 mg	2 mg	50 mg
Enovid 5 mg*		0.075 mg		5 mg	1.5 mg	100 mg
Enovid 10 mg*		0.15 mg		9.85 mg	3 mg	197 mg
Norinyl–1	Mestranol	0.05 mg	Norethindrone	1 mg	1 mg	20 mg
Norinyl 1+80		0.08 mg		1 mg	1.6 mg	20 mg
Norinyl 2 mg		0.1 mg		2 mg	2 mg	40 mg
Norlestrin 1 mg	Ethinyl estradiol	0.05 mg	Norethindrone	1 mg	1 mg	20 mg
Norlestrin 2.5 mg		0.05 mg		2.5 mg	1 mg	50 mg
Ortho-Novum 1/50	Mestranol	0.05 mg	Norethindrone	1 mg	1 mg	20 mg
Ortho-Novum 1/80		0.08 mg		1 mg	1.6 mg	20 mg
Ortho-Novum 2 mg		0.1 mg		2 mg	2 mg	40 mg
Ortho-Novum 10 mg*		0.06 mg		10 mg	1.2 mg	200 mg
Ovral	Ethinyl estradiol	0.05 mg	Norgestrel	0.5 mg	1 mg	10 mg
Ovulen	Mestranol	0.1 mg	Ethynodiol diacetate	1 mg	2 mg	20 mg

2. Oral Sequential Agents

	Tablet 1		Tablet 2		Total Steroid/ One Treatment Cycle	
	Estrogen	Days Taken	Progesterone Derivative Plus Estrogen	Days Taken	Estrogen	Progestin
Norquen	Mestranol 0.08 mg	14	Norethindrone, 2 mg plus mestranol, 0.08 mg	6	1.6 mg	12 mg
Oracon	Ethinyl estradiol 0.1 mg	16	Dimethisterone, 25 mg plus ethinyl estradiol, 0.1 mg	5	2.1 mg	125 mg
Ortho-Novum SQ	Mestranol 0.08 mg	14	Norethindrone, 2 mg plus mestranol, 0.08 mg	6	1.6 mg	12 mg

*These agents are more commonly used to suppress ovulatory function in patients with endometriosis (see p 364).

important that blood pressure be followed in each patient. An increase in blood pressure has been reported to occur in postmenopausal women treated with estrogens alone.

Although not found consistently, venous engorgement has been reported in some patients. Changes in the connective tissue in the arteries of rodents have been reported, but the significance of these changes is not known.

8. Effects on the skin—The oral contraceptives have been noted to increase pigmentation of the skin of patients (chloasma). This effect seems to be enhanced in women who have dark complexions and by exposure to ultraviolet light. Some of the androgen-like progestins may increase the production of sebum. The sequential oral contraceptive preparations as well as estrogens often decrease sebum production. This may be due to suppression of the ovarian production of androgens.

Clinical Uses

The most important use of the estrogens and progestins is for oral contraception. A large number of preparations are available for this specific purpose. They are specially packaged to provide for ease of administration. In general, they are very effective; when these agents are taken according to directions, the risk of conception is extremely small. The pregnancy rate is estimated to be about 0.5–1/100 women years at risk with combination agents and slightly higher for the sequential preparations.

The preparations are listed in Table 38–5.

When these agents are not taken as directed and one or more doses are missed, there appears to be a significantly higher pregnancy rate in patients on the sequential agents than when the combinations are employed. It would seem, therefore, that when the slightest possibility of conception must be avoided, a combination rather than a sequential preparation should be selected for use.

As is true with most hormonal preparations, many of the side-effects are physiologic or pharmacologic effects of the drugs which are objectionable only because they are not pertinent to the situation for which they are being used. Therefore, the product containing the smallest amounts of hormones should be selected for use.

The differences between preparations can be used to advantage in selecting a preparation for an individual patient when special needs arise. These differences reflect differences in the amounts of estrogen, the amounts of progestin, and the type of progestin. Preparations containing larger amounts of estrogen tend to produce more withdrawal bleeding, nausea, and mastalgia. Preparations containing 19-nortestosterone derivatives tend to reduce the amount of withdrawal bleeding and have more anabolic or androgenic effects.

Adverse Reactions

The incidence of serious known side-effects associated with the use of these drugs is low. There are a number of reversible changes in intermediary metabolism. However, the long-term effects of such changes as an increase in plasma triglycerides or decrease in glucose tolerance cannot be assessed as yet. Minor side-effects are frequent, but most are mild and many are transient. Although it is not often necessary to discontinue medication for these, as many as 1/3 of all patients started on oral contraception, with combined or sequential agents, discontinue therapy.

It is difficult to evaluate the significance of some of the complaints. The great variability of side-effects in different patients taking the same preparation suggests that they are not directly or entirely due to the hormones. This does not mean that they can be ignored in the context of the oral contraceptive administration, however, and each case must be evaluated individually.

A. Mild Side-Effects:

1. Nausea, mastalgia, breakthrough bleeding, and edema are related to the amount of estrogen in the preparation. They are more common with the sequential preparations because of the larger amounts of estrogen present, and can often be alleviated by a shift to a combination agent or to a preparation containing smaller amounts of estrogen or to agents containing progestational compounds with androgen-like effects.

2. Changes in serum proteins and other effects on endocrine function (see above) must be taken into account when thyroid, adrenal, or pituitary function is being evaluated. Increases in sedimentation rate are thought to be due to increased levels of fibrinogen.

3. Psychologic changes are often transient and are not predictable with any of the preparations. In general, most patients "feel better" because they are relieved of anxiety about becoming pregnant. Some patients experience premenstrual-like symptoms of irritability and depression throughout the cycle.

4. Headache is mild and often transient. Migraine is often made worse and has been reported to be associated with an increased frequency of cerebrovascular accidents. When this occurs, or when migraine has its onset during therapy with these agents, treatment should be discontinued.

5. Libido is increased or decreased in a few patients and unchanged in the majority. Similar changes have been observed with placebo therapy.

6. Withdrawal bleeding sometimes fails to occur—most often with combination preparations—and may cause confusion with regard to pregnancy. If this is disturbing to the patient, sequential preparations may be tried or other methods of contraception used.

B. More Annoying Side-Effects: Any of the following may require discontinuation of oral contraceptives:

1. Breakthrough bleeding is more common with sequential agents and with Provest. Excessive bleeding can sometimes be reduced by changing to a combination agent—particularly one containing an androgen-like progestin.

2. Weight gain is more common with the combination agents containing androgen-like progestins. It can usually be controlled by shifting to sequential agents or by dieting.

3. Increased skin pigmentation may be distressing in dark-skinned women. It tends to increase with time, the incidence being about 5% at the end of the first year and about 40% after 8 years. It is thought to be exacerbated by vitamin B deficiency. It is often reversible upon discontinuance of medication, but in occasional cases the pigmentation disappears very slowly.

4. Acne may be exacerbated by agents containing androgen-like progestins, whereas agents containing large amounts of estrogen frequently cause marked improvement in acne.

5. Hirsutism may also be aggravated by the 19-nortestosterone derivatives, and the combination containing nonandrogenic progestins or the sequential agents is preferred.

6. Ureteral dilatation similar to that observed in pregnancy has been reported, but no increase in the incidence of urinary tract infections.

7. Vaginal infections are more common and more difficult to treat in patients who are receiving oral contraceptives.

8. Amenorrhea after discontinuation—Following cessation of administration of oral contraceptives, 95% of patients with normal menstrual histories resume normal periods and all but a few resume normal cycles during the next few months. However, some patients remain amenorrheic for several years. Many of these patients also have galactorrhea. Patients who have had menstrual irregularities before taking oral contraceptives are particularly susceptible to prolonged amenorrhea when the agents are discontinued.

C. Severe Side-Effects:

1. **Jaundice**—Many cases of cholestatic jaundice have been reported in patients taking these drugs. The differences in incidence of these disorders from one population to another suggest that genetic factors may be involved.

The jaundice caused by these agents is similar to that produced by other 17-alkyl substituted steroids. It is most often observed in the first 3 cycles and is particularly common in women with a history of cholestatic jaundice during pregnancy. Liver biopsies taken from such women show bile thrombi along the canaliculi and occasional focal necrosis. Serum alkaline phosphatase and SGPT are increased. The BSP retention, serum enzyme changes, and increases in thymol turbidity observed in some patients may indicate structural liver damage.

Jaundice and pruritus disappear 1–8 weeks after the drug is discontinued.

2. Vascular disorders—The most serious disorders observed in association with the use of oral contraceptives are thrombophlebitis, pulmonary embolization, and cerebrovascular thrombosis. The results of most studies indicate a 5- to 10-fold increase in the incidence of thromboembolic disorders in women taking oral contraceptives. The underlying changes leading to thrombophlebitis in these patients have not been identified. Although the risk is small, the seriousness of the consequences is so great that many clinicians are of the opinion that women who can satisfactorily and successfully use other forms of contraception should be advised to do so. There appear to be fewer untoward vascular complications in patients with blood group O as compared with A, B, or AB.

3. Depression of sufficient degree to require cessation of therapy occurs in about 6% of patients treated with some preparations.

4. Some patients show an increased blood pressure during oral contraceptive therapy.

In addition to the above effects, a number of other adverse reactions have been reported for which a causal relationship has not been established. These include alopecia, erythema multiforme, erythema nodosum, and other skin disorders.

Contraindications & Cautions

These drugs are contraindicated in patients with thrombophlebitis, thromboembolic phenomena, and cerebrovascular disorders or a past history of these conditions. They should not be used to treat vaginal bleeding when the cause is unknown. They should be avoided in patients known or suspected to have a tumor of the breast or other estrogen-dependent neoplasm.

Since these preparations have caused aggravation of preexisting disorders, they should be avoided or used with caution in patients with liver disease, asthma, migraine, diabetes, hypertension, or convulsive disorders.

Since these compounds may produce edema, they should be used with great caution in patients in congestive failure or in whom edema is otherwise undesirable or dangerous.

Estrogens may increase the rate of growth of fibroids. Therefore, for women with these tumors, agents with the smallest amounts of estrogen and the most androgenic progestins should be selected and sequential agents avoided. The use of progestational agents alone for contraception has been investigated. Effective contraception has been achieved by the administration of small oral doses daily, by the injection of long-acting esters, and by periodic implantation of pellets. These methods have not come into wide use because they produce erratic bleeding in many patients. Such agents, however, might be especially useful in the occasional patient in whom estrogen therapy is inadvisable.

In some patients, aggravation of preexisting liver disease, asthma, eczema, migraine, epilepsy, diabetes, hypertension, and optic or retrobulbar neuritis have been reported.

At present these agents are contraindicated in adolescents in whom epiphyseal closure has not yet been completed.

Since the long-term consequences of the changes in lipid and carbohydrate metabolism are unknown, and since estrogens are such potent carcinogens in some mammals, the precise risks involved in the prolonged use of these doses of estrogenic and progestational agents cannot be accurately assessed. This fact (and the known risks) should be explained to all patients for whom these drugs are prescribed.

Studies in progress indicate that either estrogens or progestins alone can be effectively used for contraception. Chlormadinone or norgestrel given in small doses daily by mouth, medroxyprogesterone or norethisterone enanthate injected at intervals up to 3 months, or subcutaneous implantation of silastic capsules containing megestrol acetate are capable of preventing pregnancy. They do not appear to be quite as reliable as the oral contraceptives in current use and are associated with a high incidence of abnormal bleeding.

Estrogens in large doses given for several days immediately following intercourse at the time of ovulation can prevent pregnancy. The safety and effectiveness of this regimen are under study.

Preparations Available

Table 38–5 shows the contraceptive agents and the amounts of estrogen and progestin they contain.

OTHER USES OF ESTROGENS & PROGESTINS

Therapeutic Uses

Estrogens have been used extensively for replacement therapy in estrogen-deficient patients. The estrogen deficiency may be due to primary failure of development of the ovaries, castration, or menopause. When used for this purpose, small doses are usually adequate, eg, diethylstilbestrol, 0.5–2 mg. When doses of less than 2 mg are used, withdrawal bleeding may not occur. Since prolonged unopposed estrogen therapy usually leads to endometrial hyperplasia, estrogens are administered cyclically unless the uterus has been removed. A typical regimen consists of giving the medication daily for 3 or 4 weeks, followed by 1 week without therapy. A more regular cycle can usually be obtained by the addition of a progestational agent for the last 5 days of each cycle. Although sequential contraceptive agents are a convenient form of medication for estrogen replacement, the amounts of estrogen contained are frequently in excess of the amount indicated.

Large doses of estrogens or contraceptive agents can be used to suppress ovulation in patients with intractable dysmenorrhea or when suppression of ovarian function is used in the treatment of hirsutism and amenorrhea due to excessive secretion of androgens by the ovary.

Estrogens are widely used in the menopause. The need for and response to estrogen are quite variable, and many symptoms and disorders in menopausal women are probably unrelated to estrogen deficiency. Hot flushes, sweating, and atrophic vaginitis are generally relieved by estrogens. However, they have often been prescribed with the hope of preventing atherosclerosis of the coronary and cerebral vessels and promoting repair of osteoporosis. Most studies in patients with atherosclerosis indicate that estrogens do not protect men or postmenopausal women from myocardial infarction or cerebrovascular accidents. In fact, it is possible that in some patients estrogens may increase the risk of these disorders. Estrogens decrease the rate of bone resorption but do not increase the rate of bone formation, and their usefulness in the prevention or treatment of osteoporosis is not established.

Estrogen therapy has now become the major cause of postmenopausal bleeding. Unfortunately, vaginal bleeding at this time in life may be due to carcinoma of the endometrium, and a large number of women have been and will be subject to dilatation and curettage of the uterus unnecessarily. In order to avoid this complication, patients should be treated with the smallest amount of estrogen possible. When moderate doses are necessary, they should be given cyclically so that bleeding, when it occurs, will be more likely to occur during the withdrawal period. Endometrial hyperplasia which leads to this bleeding can be prevented by administration of a progestational agent for several days with the last doses of estrogen in each cycle. For example, the patient may take 0.1–0.5 mg stilbestrol for the first 20 days of each month and 10 mg of medroxyprogesterone can be added on days 18, 19, and 20. This will usually produce regular and predictable withdrawal bleeding. Endometrial hyperplasia and consequent bleeding can also be minimized by combining the estrogen with an androgen such as methyltestosterone in doses of 5 mg daily. The long-term metabolic effects of androgens in postmenopausal women have not been adequately assessed.

Estrogens have been used to stop excessive vaginal bleeding due to endometrial hyperplasia. Repeated doses of 10 mg of diethylstilbestrol every few hours or the administration of 20 mg of Premarin intravenously have been useful in arresting blood loss temporarily.

Progestins and estrogens are useful in the treatment of endometriosis. When severe dysmenorrhea is the major symptom, the suppression of ovulation with estrogen may be followed by painless periods. However, in most patients this approach to therapy is inadequate. The long-term administration of large doses of progestins or combinations of progestins and estrogens prevents the periodic breakdown of the endometrial tissue and in some cases will lead to endometrial fibrosis and prevent the reactivation of implants for prolonged periods. Parenteral injection of agents such as Depo-Provera (medroxyprogesterone) can induce prolonged amenorrhea, although normal menstrual function generally reappears in time.

Progestins do not appear to have any place in the therapy of threatened or habitual abortion. Early reports of the usefulness of these agents resulted from the unwarranted assumption that after several abortions the likelihood of repeated abortions was over 90%. When progestational agents were administered to patients with previous abortions, a salvage rate of 80% was obtained. It has since been recognized that similar patients abort only 20% of the time even when untreated.

In some patients with "threatened" abortion it has been noted that progesterone production is decreased. It is likely that the decrease in progesterone reflects damage to the placenta or fetus and is another result of the events leading to abortion rather than the cause of the abortion. The administration of progesterone in these circumstances does not appear to be useful and may result in delaying recognition of an abortion which has occurred. In addition, progesterone and progestational agents administered early in pregnancy have been incriminated in the masculinization of the external genitalia in the female fetus. Prolonged postpartum bleeding has been reported in some patients treated with repository medroxyprogesterone or hydroxyprogesterone caproate, and delay in the spontaneous expulsion of the dead fetus occurs.

Progesterone and medroxyprogesterone have been used in the treatment of women who have difficulty in conceiving and who demonstrate a slow rise in basal body temperature. Some investigators believe that these patients suffer from a relative luteal insufficiency, and progesterone or related compounds are given to replace the deficiency. There is no convincing evidence that this is an effective means of treatment. The successes reported are impossible to evaluate in the absence of satisfactory controls.

Diagnostic Uses

Progesterone can also be used as a test of estrogen secretion. The administration of progesterone, 150 mg/day, or hydroxyprogesterone, 10 mg/day for 5–7 days, is followed by withdrawal bleeding in amenorrheic patients only when the endometrium has been stimulated by estrogens. Administration of a combination of estrogen and progestin can be used to test the responsiveness of the endometrium in patients with amenorrhea.

The absence of withdrawal bleeding following the administration of these agents in women with amenorrhea of recent onset is indicative of pregnancy.

OVULATION-INDUCING AGENTS

1. CLOMIPHENE CITRATE
(Clomid)

Interest in the discovery of antiestrogenic compounds has been stimulated by the increasing need for antifertility compounds. Several of the synthetic estrogens have been shown to have significant antiestrogen properties. They are able to successfully compete for binding sites, yet have weaker hormonal properties. Clomiphene citrate is one such compound. It is closely related to other pharmacologically active compounds such as the estrogen chlorotrianisene (Fig 38–6) and the cholesterol inhibitor triparanol.

This compound is active when taken by mouth since it is readily absorbed. Very little is known about its metabolism, but available studies indicate that about half of the compound is excreted into the stools within 5 days after administration. Studies of the metabolism of clomiphene have been more extensive in animals. In monkeys the half-life of clomiphene citrate, when given intravenously, is approximately 48 hours. When 90% of the dose has been eliminated from the body, the liver, gallbladder, and bile have the highest concentrations of the remaining compound. It has been suggested that clomiphene is slowly excreted from an enterohepatic pool.

Pharmacologic Effects
A. Mechanisms of Action: Clomiphene citrate is a weak estrogen. The estrogenic effects are best demonstrated in animals with marked gonadal deficiency. Clomiphene has also been shown to effectively inhibit the action of stronger estrogens. In humans it leads to an increase in the secretion of gonadotropins and estrogens.

B. Effects: The pharmacologic importance of this compound rests on its ability to stimulate ovulation in women with amenorrhea and other ovulatory disorders. The mechanism by which ovulation is produced

is not known. It has been suggested that it blocks an inhibitory influence of estrogens on the hypothalamus and increases the production of gonadotropins. Clomiphene will not work in the absence of a pituitary gland which is capable of producing gonadotropins. It has been shown in the rat that crystals of this compound implanted in the pituitary have no effect, whereas those implanted in parts of the median eminence are able to induce ovulation. The observation that this compound can induce ovulation in patients with very low estrogen levels does not support the hypothesis that it works by breaking a feedback inhibition. However, it does stimulate gonadotropin production by the pituitary by an action on the hypothalamus.

Clinical Uses
Clomiphene citrate is used for the treatment of disorders of ovulation in patients wishing to become pregnant. In general, a single ovulation is induced by a single course of therapy, and the patient must be treated repeatedly until pregnancy is achieved since normal ovulatory function does not usually resume. The compound is of no use in patients with ovarian or pituitary failure. However, the latter diagnoses cannot be made solely on the basis of low or high values of total urinary gonadotropins.

Standardized procedures for the use of clomiphene as a testing substance have not been established. This substance can serve as a useful test of the ability of the pituitary gland to secrete gonadotropins.

When clomiphene is administered in doses of 100 mg daily for 5 days, a rise in plasma LH and FSH is observed several days after starting. In patients who ovulate, the initial rise is followed by a second rise of gonadotropin levels just prior to ovulation.

Adverse Reactions
The most common side-effect in patients treated with this drug are hot flushes, which resemble those experienced by menopausal patients. They tend to be mild, and disappear when the drug is discontinued. There have been occasional reports of eye symptoms due to intensification and prolongation of after-images. These are generally of short duration. Headache, constipation, allergic skin reactions, and reversible hair loss have been reported occasionally.

The effective use of clomiphene is associated with some stimulation of the ovaries and usually with ovarian enlargement. The degree of enlargement tends to be greater and its incidence higher in patients who have enlarged ovaries at the beginning of therapy.

$$(C_2H_5)_2 NCH_2 CH_2 O - \bigcirc - \overset{\underset{\displaystyle |}{}}{C} = \overset{\overset{\displaystyle Cl}{|}}{C} - \bigcirc \cdot C_6H_8O_7$$

Clomiphene citrate (Clomid)

A variety of other symptoms such as nausea, vomiting, increased nervous tension, depression, fatigue, breast soreness, weight gain, urinary frequency, and heavy menses have also been reported. However, these appear to be due to the hormonal changes associated with an ovulatory menstrual cycle rather than a result of the medication. The incidence of multiple pregnancy is approximately 10%.

Clomiphene has not been shown to have an adverse effect in human pregnancy. However, since the only current indication for clomiphene therapy is to achieve pregnancy, existing pregnancy is a contraindication to its use.

Contraindications & Cautions

Special precautions should be observed in patients with enlarged ovaries. These women are thought to be more sensitive to this drug and should receive small doses. Any patient who complains of abdominal symptoms should be carefully examined. The maximum ovarian enlargement occurs after the 5-day course has been completed, and many patients can be shown to have a palpable increase in ovarian size by the seventh to tenth days.

Special precautions must also be taken in patients who have visual symptoms associated with clomiphene therapy since these symptoms may make activities such as driving more hazardous.

Preparations & Dosages

Clomiphene citrate (Clomid) is available as 50 mg scored tablets. The recommended dose at the beginning of therapy is 50 mg/day for 5 days. If ovulation occurs, this same course may be repeated until pregnancy is achieved. If ovulation does not occur, the dose is doubled to 100 mg/day for 5 days. If ovulation and menses occur, the next course can be started on the fifth day of the cycle. Experience to date suggests that patients who do not ovulate after 3 courses of 100 mg/day of clomiphene are not likely to respond to continued therapy.

About 80% of patients with anovulatory disorders or amenorrhea can be expected to respond by having ovulatory cycles. Approximately half of these patients will become pregnant. In the patients in whom pregnancy is achieved, the incidence of early abortion seems to be slightly increased. Although a variety of congenital defects have been described in the children resulting from these pregnancies, the incidence does not appear to be greater than occurs spontaneously.

2. HUMAN MENOPAUSAL GONADOTROPIN (HMG, Menotropins)

Because of antibody formation and species differences in response, animal preparations of FSH have not been very useful in man. Studies are currently in progress utilizing partially purified extracts of human pituitary glands or pooled urine obtained from postmenopausal women which contains both FSH and LH activity. The LH content is estimated by observing changes in the weight of the ventral prostate in hypophysectomized immature rats or depletion of ascorbic acid from the ovaries of immature rats. An ovarian augmentation assay is available for measuring FSH content. The pituitary extracts are available in only a few laboratories, but HMG has been more widely distributed for investigational purposes in the USA.

Clinical Uses

HMG—in conjunction with human chorionic gonadotropin (HCG); see p 398—is used to stimulate ovulation in patients who do not ovulate but have potentially functional ovarian tissue. It has been successful in the induction of ovulation in patients with hypopituitarism and other defects in gonadotropin secretion. It has also been used in patients with amenorrhea or anovulatory cycles and in patients in whom ovulatory disturbances are associated with galactorrhea or hirsutism. Ovarian failure should be excluded in patients considered for therapy. Since therapy is difficult and expensive, it is useful to look for the existence of other factors such as obstruction of the fallopian tubes or abnormalities in sperm production by the husband. The acceptability of multiple birth by the patient must be considered.

Preparations of human menopausal gonadotropin can stimulate spermatogenesis in males with isolated gonadotropin deficiency. In conjunction with HCG (see Chapter 39), endocrine and gametogenic function has been restored in a few of these patients.

Contraindications & Cautions

HMG is a potentially dangerous agent and should be administered only after thorough acquaintance with its use and by physicians experienced in dealing with endocrine disturbances and problems of reproductive function. Careful selection of patients is required.

This preparation should not be used in early pregnancy (which may be difficult to diagnose in patients with irregular cycles), nor in patients with ovarian failure except as a diagnostic procedure. In patients with pituitary and other intracranial tumors, the primary disease process should be treated before undertaking therapy with HMG. HMG should not be used in patients with other causes of infertility than lack of ovulation.

Adverse Reactions

The most common problem encountered is excessive ovarian stimulation. Ovarian enlargement is common. When marked (hyperstimulation syndrome), it may be accompanied by pain, ascites, and pleural effusion. Arterial thromboembolism has been reported in 2 patients. Occasional patients experience swelling and fever along with discomfort at the injection site. Undesirable results of therapy include the high incidence of multiple pregnancy and abortion (Table 38–6). The frequency of birth defects has not been

TABLE 38–6. Results of treatment with HMG.

Pregnancy Achieved	Multiple Pregnancy		Aborting	Hyper-stimulation Syndrome
	Twins	Triplets, Etc		
25–40%	10–20%	5–10%	20–30%	0.5–1.5%

elevated in the offspring of patients who have succeeded in carrying their pregnancy to term.

The typical outcome of therapy in suitably selected patients treated by experienced physicians is shown in Table 38–6.

It is clear that this mode of therapy is complicated, time-consuming, and expensive. It should not be undertaken lightly but can be very helpful to the proper patient.

Preparations & Dosages

Human menopausal gonadotropins (menotropins, Pergonal) are supplied in lyophilized form in ampules containing 75 IU each of FSH and LH and 10 mg of lactose. The usual dosage is 1 or more ampules IM daily until estrogen production is optimal (as indicated by estrogen assay or cervical mucus examination). HCG (see Chapter 39) in doses of 5000–10,000 IU IM is then administered on one or more occasions; if estrogen production becomes excessive, HCG should be withheld. Patients must be examined frequently for 2 weeks following the last injection (daily or on alternate days) to detect signs of overstimulation. Frequent intercourse near the time of expected ovulation is advisable.

THE TESTIS
(Androgens & Anabolic Steroids)

The testis, like the ovary, has both gametogenic and endocrine functions. The gametogenic function of the testes is controlled largely by the secretion of FSH by the pituitary. Androgens are also required for sperm production in the seminiferous tubules. The Sertoli cells in the seminiferous tubules may be the source of the estrogens produced in the testes. The androgens are produced in the interstitial or Leydig cells which are found in the spaces between the seminiferous tubules.

In man the most important androgen appears to be testosterone. The pathways of synthesis of testosterone in the testes are similar to those previously described in the ovary and the adrenal except that the hormone and its precursors are the primary secretory products of the gland (Fig 38–10).

In the male, about 8 mg of testosterone, almost all of which is derived from the testes, are secreted daily. Plasma levels of testosterone in males are about 0.6 μg/100 ml after puberty and do not appear to vary significantly with age. Testosterone is also present in the plasma of women in concentrations of approximately 0.03 μg/100 ml and is derived in approximately equal parts from the ovaries, the adrenals, and by the peripheral conversion of other hormones. .

About 65% of circulating testosterone is bound to protein. This protein has been shown to be specific, and, as is the case with many other hormone-binding proteins, its concentration can be increased with estrogens and is elevated during pregnancy.

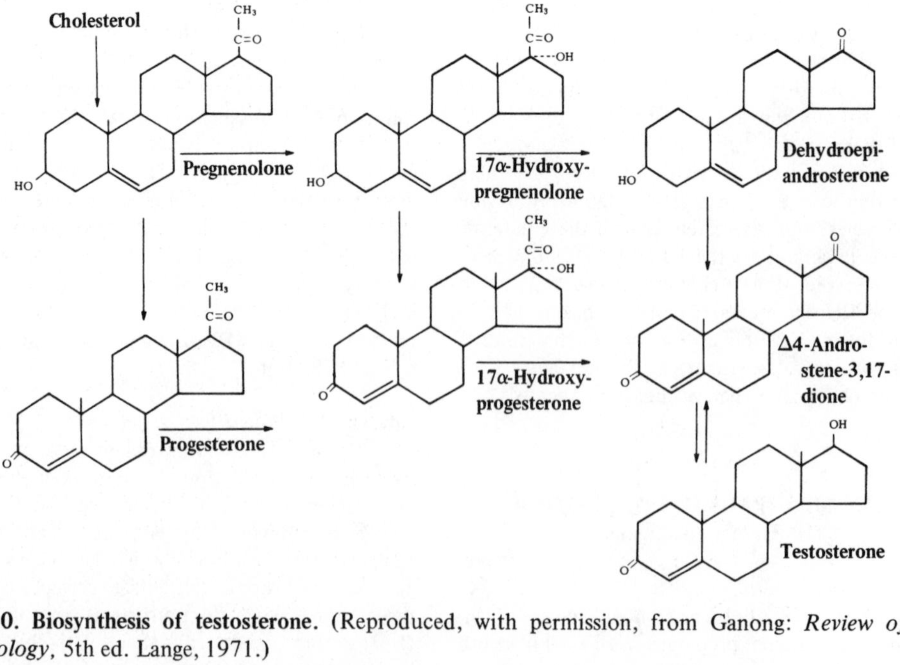

FIG 38–10. Biosynthesis of testosterone. (Reproduced, with permission, from Ganong: *Review of Medical Physiology,* 5th ed. Lange, 1971.)

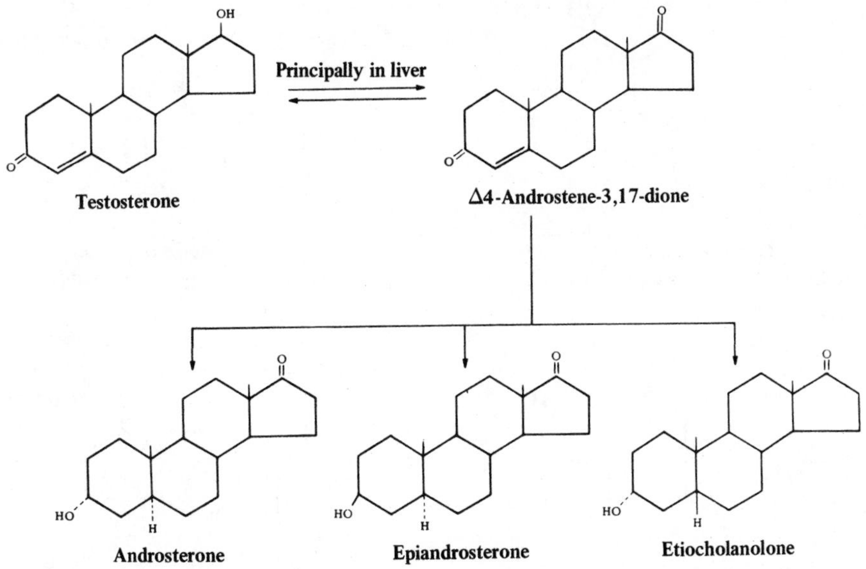

FIG 38–11. Metabolism of testosterone. (Reproduced, with permission, from Ganong: *Review of Medical Physiology,* 5th ed. Lange, 1971.)

Metabolism

The major pathway of metabolism of testosterone in man is illustrated in Fig 38–11. In the liver, the reduction of the double bond and ketone in the A ring, as is seen in other steroids with a Δ4-ketone configuration in the A ring, leads to the production of inactive substances such as androsterone and etiocholanolone which are then conjugated and secreted into the urine.

Androstenedione and dehydroepiandrosterone (Fig 38–10) are also produced in significant amounts in man, although largely in the adrenal rather than in the testes. These compounds do not have significant biologic activity, but they are to a large extent metabolized in the same fashion as testosterone. Both compounds—but particularly androstenedione—can be converted by peripheral tissues to estrone in very small amounts.

Dihydrotestosterone is another highly active natural androgen. In the rat it appears to be the major androgen, and recent studies indicate that testosterone exerts its hormonal activity in this species by conversion to dihydrotestosterone. The enzyme responsible for conversion of testosterone to dihydrotestosterone is also found in man. Its importance in the mediation of the androgenic effects of testosterone has not been determined. Preliminary findings suggest that its activity is secondarily reduced in hypoandrogenic states. When administered to man, it is less active than testosterone—in contrast to the rat, in which it is more potent.

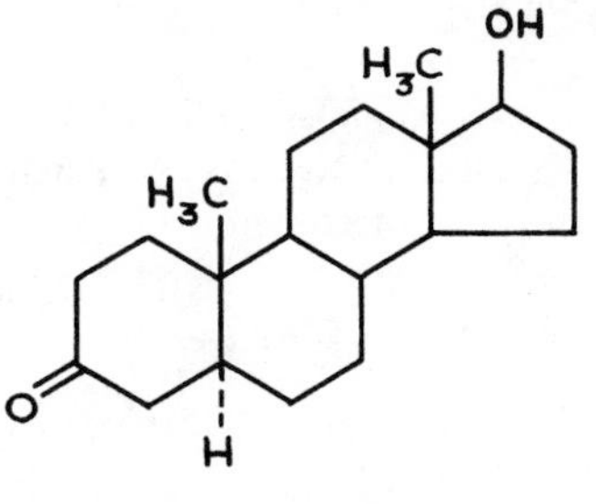

Control of Secretion

The production of testosterone by the testes is controlled by the pituitary release of LH, which in turn is controlled by luteinizing hormone-releasing factor (LHRF) produced in the median eminence of the hypothalamus. The administration of testosterone not only suppresses LH but in large doses can reduce the secretion of FSH by the pituitary. It is not known whether the physiologic control of FSH secretion is a negative feedback effect of testosterone or whether it is influenced by estrogens or other substances produced in the testes.

Physiologic Effects

In the normal male, testosterone is responsible for the many changes that occur in puberty. In addition to the general growth-promoting properties of androgens on the body tissues, these hormones are responsible for penile and scrotal growth. Changes in the skin include the appearance of pubic hair, axillary hair, and beard hair. The sebaceous glands become more active, and the skin tends to become thicker and oilier. The larynx grows and the vocal cords become thicker, leading to a lower pitched voice. Skeletal growth is stimulated and epiphyseal closure accelerated. Other effects include growth of the prostate and seminal vesicles, darkening

Dihydrotestosterone

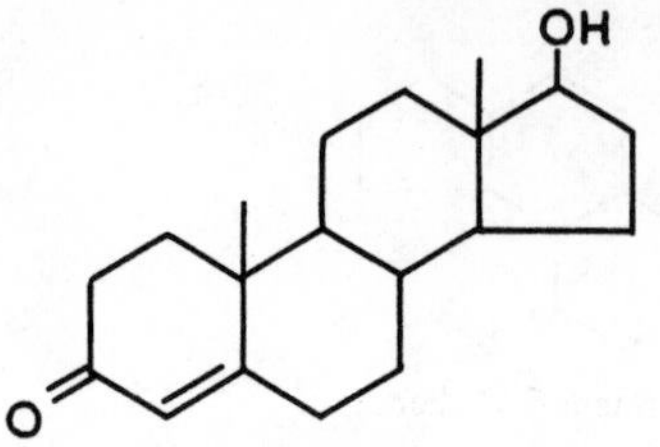

Testosterone
(17β-hydroxy-4-androsten-3-one)

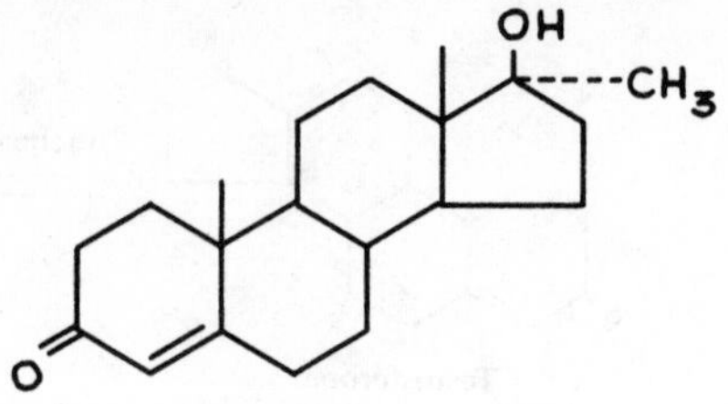

17α-Methyltestosterone
(17β-hydroxy-17α-methyl-4-androsten-3-one)

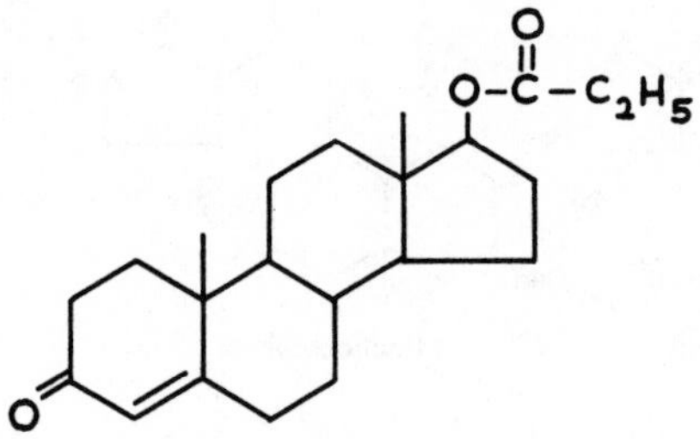

Testosterone propionate
(17β-hydroxy-4-androsten-3-one
propionate)

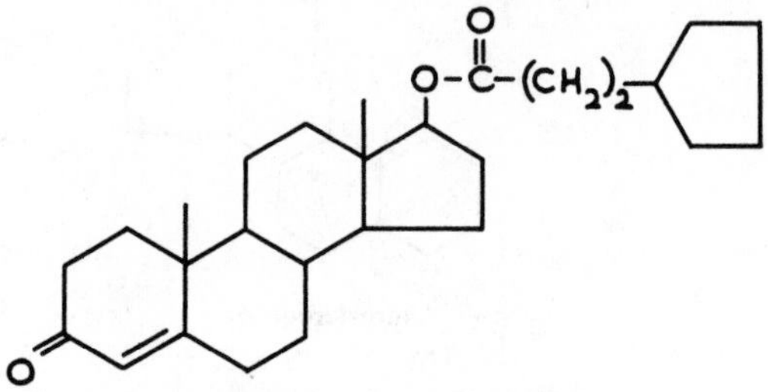

Testosterone cyclopentylpropionate
(testosterone 17β-cyclopentanepropionate)

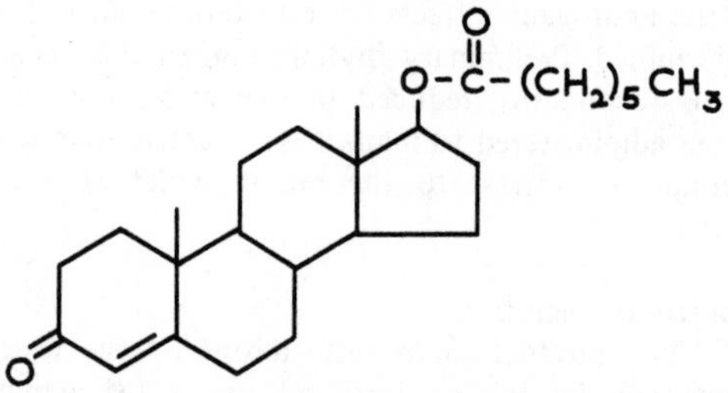

Testosterone enanthate
(4-androstene-17β-heptanoate-3-one)

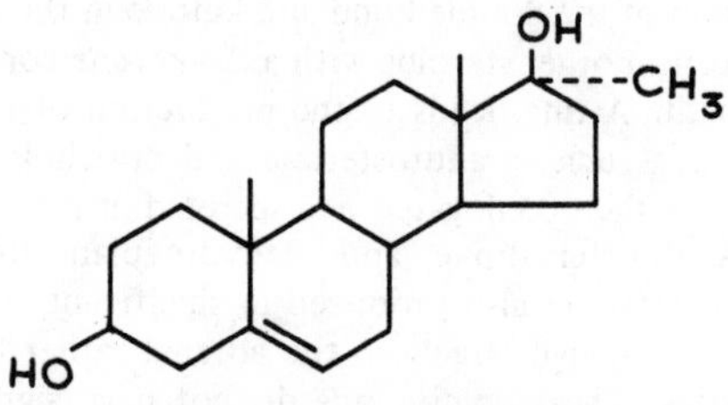

Methylandrostenediol
(methandriol; 17α-methyl-5-androstene-
3β,17β-diol)

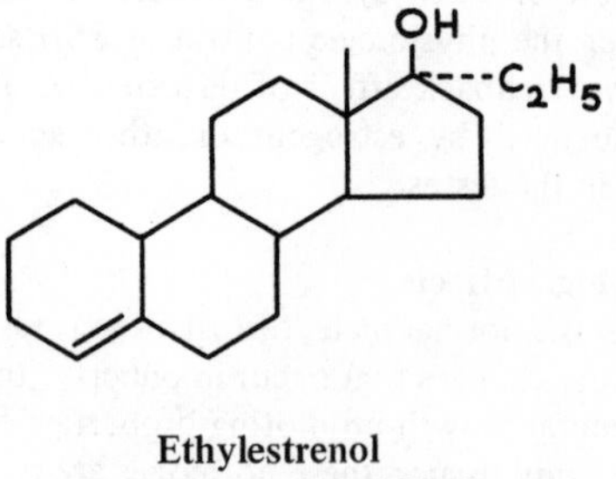

Ethylestrenol
(17α-ethylestr-4-en-17β-ol)

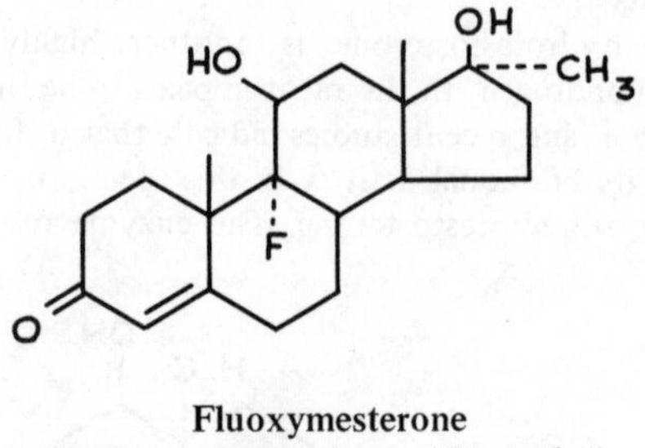

Fluoxymesterone
(9α-fluoro-11β-hydroxy-17α-methyl-
testosterone)

FIG 38–12. Chemical structures of androgenic steroids and derivatives.

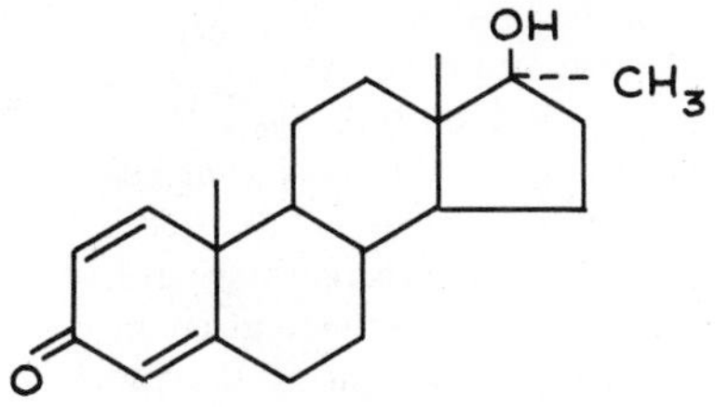

Methandrostenolone
(17α-methyl-1-testosterone)

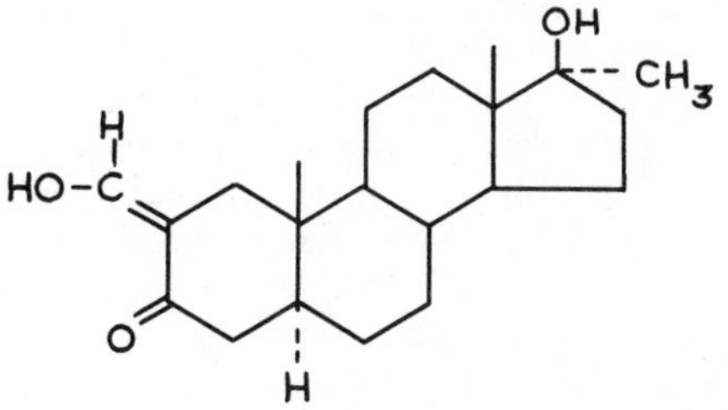

Oxymetholone
(17β-hydroxy-2-[hydroxymethylene]-17α-
methyl-5α-androstan-3-one)

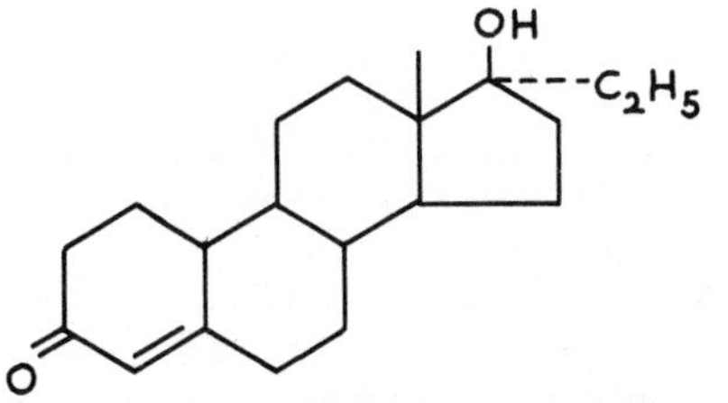

Norethandrolone
(17α-ethyl-17β-hydroxy-4-norandrosten-
3-one)

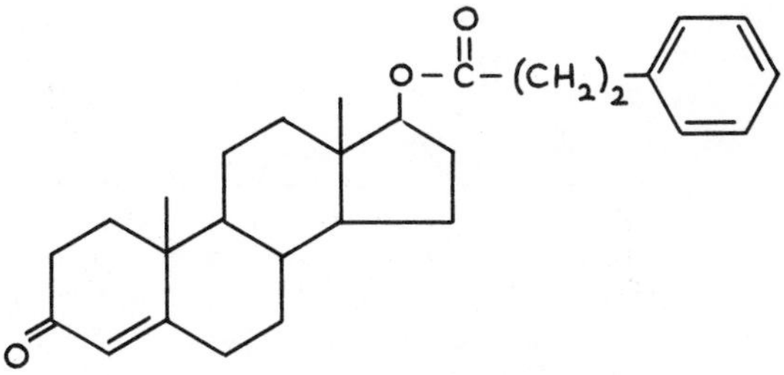

Nandrolone phenpropionate
(17β-hydroxyestr-4-en-3-one
phenylpropionate)

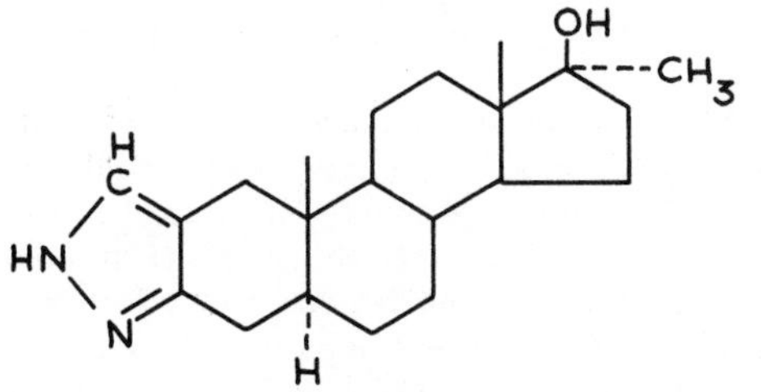

Stanozolol
(androstanozole; 17β-hydroxy-17α-methyl-
androstano-[3,2-c]-pyrazole)

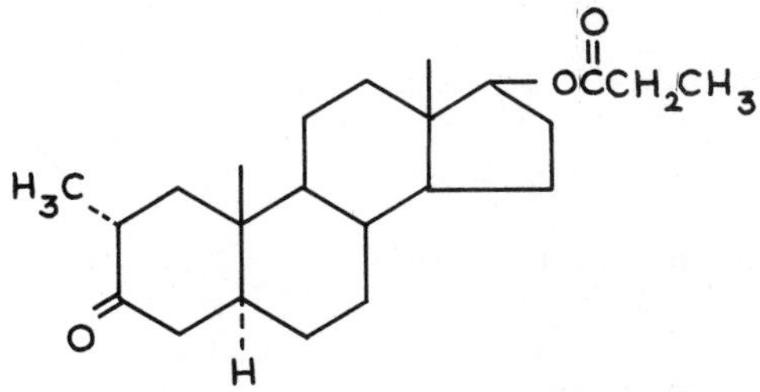

Dromostanolone propionate
(17β-hydroxy-2α-methyl-androstan-
3-one propionate)

FIG 38—12 (cont'd). Chemical structures of androgenic steroids and derivatives.

of the skin, and increased skin circulation. Psychologic and behavioral changes also occur.

Synthetic Steroids With Androgenic & Anabolic Action

Testosterone, when administered by mouth, is rapidly absorbed. However, it is largely converted to inactive metabolites, and only about 1/6 of the hormone is available in active form. Testosterone can be administered parenterally, but it has a more prolonged absorption time and greater activity when esterified. Methyltestosterone and fluoxymesterone are active when given by mouth.

Testosterone and its derivatives have been used for their anabolic effects as well as for the replacement of testosterone deficiency. Although testosterone and other known active steroids can be isolated in pure form and measured by weight, biologic assays are still used in the investigation of new compounds. In some of these studies in animals, the anabolic effects of the compound—as measured by trophic effects on muscles or the reduction of nitrogen excretion—may be dissociated from the other androgenic effects. This has led to the marketing of a substantial group of compounds which are supposed to have marked anabolic activity associated with only weak androgenic effects. This dissociation does not appear to be complete, and in man it is less marked than in the animals used for testing. Though they may be less virilizing than equivalent doses of testosterone, doses of these drugs large enough to promote nitrogen retention can also produce unwanted androgenic effects.

Pharmacologic Effects

A. Mechanisms of Action: Little is known about the mechanisms of action of androgens. In target cells, testosterone appears to bind to a protein associated with the genetic material in the nucleus. It stimulates the production of RNA and protein. A variety of enzymes, particularly in the liver, are known to be influenced by androgens. In the rat, testosterone is converted to dihydrotestosterone in the nucleus; the latter compound appears to be more firmly bound to the receptor protein than testosterone itself and is probably the active form of the hormone.

B. Effects: In the male at puberty, androgens cause development of the secondary sex characteristics (see above). In the adult male, large doses of testosterone or its derivatives suppress the secretion of gonadotropins and result in some atrophy of the interstitial tissue and the tubules of the testes. Since fairly large doses of androgens are required to suppress gonadotropic secretion, it has been postulated that estrogens produced in the testis—rather than androgens—are responsible for the feedback control of secretion. In the adult woman, androgens are capable of producing changes similar to those observed in the prepubertal male. These include growth of facial hair and body hair, deepening of the voice, enlargement of the clitoris, frontal baldness, and prominent musculature. The natural androgens stimulate red cell production.

The administration of androgens reduces the excretion of nitrogen into the urine, indicating an increase in protein synthesis or decrease in protein breakdown within the body. This effect is much more pronounced in women and children than in normal men.

Clinical Uses

A. Androgen Replacement Therapy in Men: The most important indication for androgen therapy is for replacement of androgen deficiency in men with hypogonadism or hypopituitarism. When therapy is begun in patients with hypogonadism which occurs after maturation, 1–2 injections of 50 mg of testosterone propionate weekly are usually sufficient. It is often more convenient to use a long-acting preparation in doses of 200–300 mg/month. Oral preparations, eg, methyltestosterone or fluoxymesterone, may also be used. When treating patients in whom deficiency occurred before maturation, larger doses of testosterone must be used, and even then full masculinization may not be achieved. In younger people one can start with smaller doses to allow the gradual development of the changes as they naturally occur in puberty. However, for a period of 2–3 years, therapy must be pursued with relatively large doses of androgen. In patients with hypopituitarism, androgens are not added to the treatment regimen until puberty, at which time they are instituted in gradually increasing doses to achieve the growth spurt and the development of secondary sex characteristics.

B. Gynecologic Disorders: Androgens are used occasionally in the treatment of certain gynecologic disorders, but the undesirable effects in women are such that they must be used with great caution. Andro-gens have been used to reduce breast engorgement during the postpartum period, usually in conjunction with estrogens. For example, 4 ml of a preparation containing 90 mg/ml of testosterone enanthate and 4 mg/ml of estradiol are useful for this purpose when given at the onset of the second stage of labor.

Androgens are sometimes given in combination with estrogens for replacement therapy in the postmenopausal period in an attempt to eliminate the endometrial bleeding which may occur when only estrogens are used. They are also used for the chemotherapy of breast tumors in premenopausal women.

C. Use as Protein Anabolic Agents: Androgens and anabolic steroids have been used in conjunction with dietary measures and exercises in an attempt to reverse protein loss after trauma, surgery, or prolonged immobilization, and in patients with debilitating diseases.

D. Anemia: Large doses of androgens have been employed in the treatment of refractory anemias and have resulted in some increase in reticulocytosis and hemoglobin levels. The large amounts required prevent this from being a useful method of therapy in women.

E. Osteoporosis: Androgens and anabolic agents have been used in the treatment of osteoporosis, either alone or in conjunction with estrogens. The benefits of androgens in these patients have not been substantiated by careful studies and their use should be limited to very small amounts which will not cause undesirable effects.

F. Use as Metabolic Stimulators: These agents have been used to stimulate growth in prepubertal boys. If the drugs are used carefully, these children will probably achieve their expected adult height (and sooner). If treatment is too vigorous, the patient may grow rapidly at first but will not achieve full stature because of the accelerated epiphyseal closure that occurs. It is difficult to control this type of therapy adequately even with frequent x-ray examination of the epiphyses since the action of the hormones on epiphysial centers may continue for many months after therapy is discontinued.

Adverse Reactions

The adverse effects of these compounds are due largely to their masculinizing actions and are most noticeable in women and prepubertal children. In women, the administration of more than 200–300 mg of testosterone per month is usually associated with hirsutism, acne, depression of menses, clitoral enlargement, and deepening of the voice. These effects may occur on even smaller doses in some women. Some of the androgenic steroids exert progestational activity leading to endometrial bleeding. These hormones also alter serum lipids and could conceivably increase susceptibility to atherosclerotic disease of the vessels in women. Except under the most unusual circumstances, androgens should not be used in infants. Recent studies in animals suggest that in early life administration of androgens may have profound effects on maturation of CNS centers governing sexual development, particularly in the female. Administration of these drugs to pregnant females may lead to masculinization of the external genitalia in the infant. Although the above-mentioned effects may be less marked with the anabolic agents, they do occur.

Sodium retention and edema are not common but must be carefully watched for in patients with heart and kidney disease.

Most of the synthetic androgens and anabolic agents are 17-alkyl substituted steroids. Administration of drugs with this structure is associated with increase in BSP retention and SGOT levels. Alkaline phosphatase values are also elevated. These changes usually occur early in the course of treatment, and the degree is proportionate to the dose. Bilirubin levels occasionally increase until clinical jaundice is apparent. The cholestatic jaundice is reversible upon cessation of therapy, and permanent changes do not occur.

Contraindications & Cautions

The use of androgenic steroids is contraindicated in pregnant women or women who may become pregnant during the course of therapy.

Androgens should not be administered to male patients with carcinoma of the prostate or breast.

Until more is known about the effects of these hormones on the CNS in developing children, they should be avoided in infants and young children.

Special caution is required in giving these drugs to children to produce a growth spurt.

Care should be exercised in the administration of these drugs to patients with renal or cardiac disease predisposed to edema. If sodium and water retention occur, they will respond to diuretic therapy.

Methyltestosterone therapy is associated with creatinuria, but the significance of this finding is not known.

TABLE 38–7. Androgens: Preparations available and relative androgen/anabolic activity.

	Preparations Available	Androgenic/ Anabolic Activity
Testosterone (Andronaq, Glutest, Homogene-S, Malestrone, Malotrone, Neo-Hombreol [F], Oreton, Sterotate, Tesamone, Testadenos)	Aqueous suspension, 25, 50, and 100 mg/ml Pellets, 75 mg (for subcutaneous implantation)	1:1
Methyltestosterone (Glutest, Metandren, Oreton [M], Neo-Hombreol [M], Steronyl)	Tablets, 2, 5, 10, and 25 mg Linguets, 5 and 10 mg Buccal tablets, 10 mg	1:1
Testosterone propionate (Androlan, Homogene-P, Malotrone-P, Neo-Hombreol, Oreton [P], Perandren [P], Testadenos, Testonate, Testeplex)	In oil, 25, 50, and 100 mg/ml Buccal tablets, 5 and 10 mg	1:1
Testosterone cyclopentylpropionate (Depo-Testosterone Cypionate)	In oil, 50, 100, and 200 mg/ml	1:1
Testosterone enanthate (Atlatest, Delatest, Delatestryl, Dura-Testosterone)	In oil, 100 and 200 mg/ml	1:1
Methandriol (Stenediol)	Aqueous suspension, 25 and 50 mg/ml Tablets, 10 and 25 mg Linguets, 10 and 25 mg	1:2
Methandriol dipropionate (Anabol, Crestabolic)	In oil, 50 mg/ml	1:2
Ethylestrenol (Maxibolin)	Tablets, 2 mg Elixir, 2 mg/5 ml	1:3*
Fluoxymesterone (Halotestin, Ora-Testryl, Ultandren)	Tablets, 2, 5, and 10 mg	1:1
Methandrostenelone (Dianabol)	Tablets, 2.5 and 5 mg	1:1
Oxymetholone (Adroyd)	Tablets, 2.5, 5, and 10 mg	1:2.5
Norethandrolone (Nilevar)	Tablets, 10 mg Drops, 0.25 mg/drop (8.3 mg/ml) In oil, 25 mg/ml	1:3
Nandrolone phenpropionate (Durabolin, Durabolin-50)	In oil, 25 and 50 mg/ml	1:2.5
Nandrolone decanoate (Deca-Durabolin)	In oil, 50 mg/ml	1:2.5
Stanozolol (Winstrol)	Tablets, 2 mg	1:3
Dromostanolone propionate (Drolban)	In oil, 50 mg/ml	1:3

*Not definitely established; may be higher.

Preparations & Dosages

Table 38–7 lists the dosage forms available, equivalent dosages, and special properties of the androgens in common use as well as the anabolic steroids. Their structural formulas are shown in Fig 38–12.

ANTIANDROGENS

The potential usefulness of antiandrogens for the treatment of patients producing excessive amounts of testosterone has led to the search for effective drugs that can be used for this purpose. Two approaches to the problem have met with limited success experimentally.

Several compounds have been developed which inhibit the 17-hydroxylation of progesterone or pregnenolone, therefore preventing the action of the side chain-splitting enzyme and the further transformation of these steroid precursors to active androgens. A few of these compounds have been tested clinically but have been too toxic for prolonged use.

Another approach has been the development of steroids which are chemically similar and act as competitive inhibitors. A few of these have been tried in patients on a limited basis, but useful compounds are not available for therapeutic purposes.

• • •

General References

Advisory Committee on Obstetrics and Gynecology: *Second Report on the Oral Contraceptives.* Food and Drug Administration, 1969.

Cohen, H.: Relaxin: Studies dealing with the isolation, purification, and characterization. Tr New York Acad Sc 25:313, 1963.

Drill, V.A.: *Oral Contraceptives.* McGraw-Hill, 1966.

Gallagher, T.F., Jr., Mueller, M.N., & A. Kappas: Estrogen pharmacology. IV. Studies on the structural basis for estrogen-induced impairment of liver function. Medicine 45:471–479, 1966.

Glick, I.D.: Mood and behavioral changes associated with the use of the oral contraceptive agents. Psychopharmacologia 10:363–374, 1967.

Gold, J.J. (editor): Symposium on treatment of menstrual disorders. Mod Treat 2:117–212, 1965.

Hahn, H.B., Jr., Hayles, A.B., & A. Albert: Medroxyprogesterone [Provera] and constitutional precocious puberty. Mayo Clin Proc 39:182–190, 1964.

Hertz, R.: Physiologic effects of androgens and estrogens in man. Am J Med 21:671–678, 1956.

Howard, R.P., & others: Testicular deficiency: A clinical and pathologic study. J Clin Endocrinol 10:121–186, 1950.

Kappas, A.: Studies in endocrine pharmacology: Biologic actions of some natural steroids on the liver. New England J Med 278:378, 1968.

Salhanick, H.A., Kipnis, D.M., & R.L. Vande Wiele (editors): *Metabolic Effects of Gonadal Hormones and Contraceptive Steroids.* Plenum Press, 1969.

Taft, P., & others: The clinical uses of human gonadotrophins. Australasian Ann Med 17:96–101, 1968.

Vande Wiele, R.L., & R.N. Turksoy: Treatment of amenorrhea and of anovulation with human menopausal and chorionic gonadotropins. J Clin Endocrinol 25:369–384, 1965.

Wolstenholme, G.E.W., & M. O'Connor (editors): Endocrinology of the testis. Ciba Found Colloq Endocrinol 16:1–331, 1967.

39 . . .

Hypothalamic & Pituitary Hormones

The pituitary gland is a remarkable structure consisting of an anterior lobe (adenohypophysis), intermediate lobe, and posterior lobe (neurohypophysis). This organ is known to produce or release 10 hormones and may produce others (Table 39–1). Since the secretion of these hormones is regulated by chemical mediators or hormones released by the hypothalamus, the 2 organs are considered together.

THE ANTERIOR PITUITARY & ITS HORMONES

The anterior lobe of the pituitary gland constitutes 2/3 of the organ and is derived from the ventral portion of Rathke's pouch (an outpocketing of oral ectoderm). It is made up of several types of cells which have been classified in several ways on the basis of morphologic and staining characteristics. In man, about half of the cells appear agranular and are called chromophobes. It is thought that these cells differentiate into cells with granules which readily accept acidic or basic dyes. Approximately 2/3 of the chromophilic cells are acidophils and the rest basophils. In man, luteinizing hormone (LH), follicle-stimulating hormone (FSH), and thyroid-stimulating hormone (TSH)—all glycoproteins—are produced by basophils. The acidophils secrete growth hormone and prolactin. Corticotropin (ACTH) was once thought to be synthesized in the basophils, but it is probably formed in the chromophobes.

The secretion of the known hormones of the anterior lobe is regulated by chemical mediators formed in the median eminence of the hypothalamus (Fig 39–1) and carried to the adenohypophysis by a portal system of blood vessels which traverse the pituitary stalk and form sinusoids in the anterior pituitary.

GROWTH HORMONE
(GH, Somatotropin, STH)

Growth hormone is synthesized in the anterior pituitary gland. It has been prepared in highly purified

TABLE 39–1. Pituitary hormones.*

Name and Source	Principal Actions
Anterior lobe	
Thyroid stimulating hormone (TSH, thyrotropin)	Stimulates thyroid secretion and growth
Adrenocorticotropic hormone (ACTH, corticotropin)	Stimulates adrenocortical secretion and growth
Growth hormone (GH, somatotropin, STH)	Accelerates body growth
Follicle stimulating hormone (FSH)	Stimulates ovarian follicle growth in female and spermatogenesis in male
Luteinizing hormone (LH, interstitial cell stimulating hormone, ICSH)	Stimulates ovulation and luteinization of ovarian follicles in female and testosterone secretion in male
Prolactin (luteotropic hormone, LTH, luteotropin, lactogenic hormone, mammotropin)	Stimulates secretion of milk and maternal behavior. Maintains corpus luteum in female rodents but apparently not in other species.
Intermediate lobe	
α-and β-Melanocyte stimulating hormones (α- and β-MSH; referred to collectively as melanotropin or intermedin)	Expand melanophores
Posterior lobe	
Vasopressin (antidiuretic hormone, ADH)	Promotes water retention
Oxytocin	Causes milk ejection

*Reproduced, with permission, from Ganong, W.F.: *Review of Medical Physiology,* 5th ed. Lange, 1971.

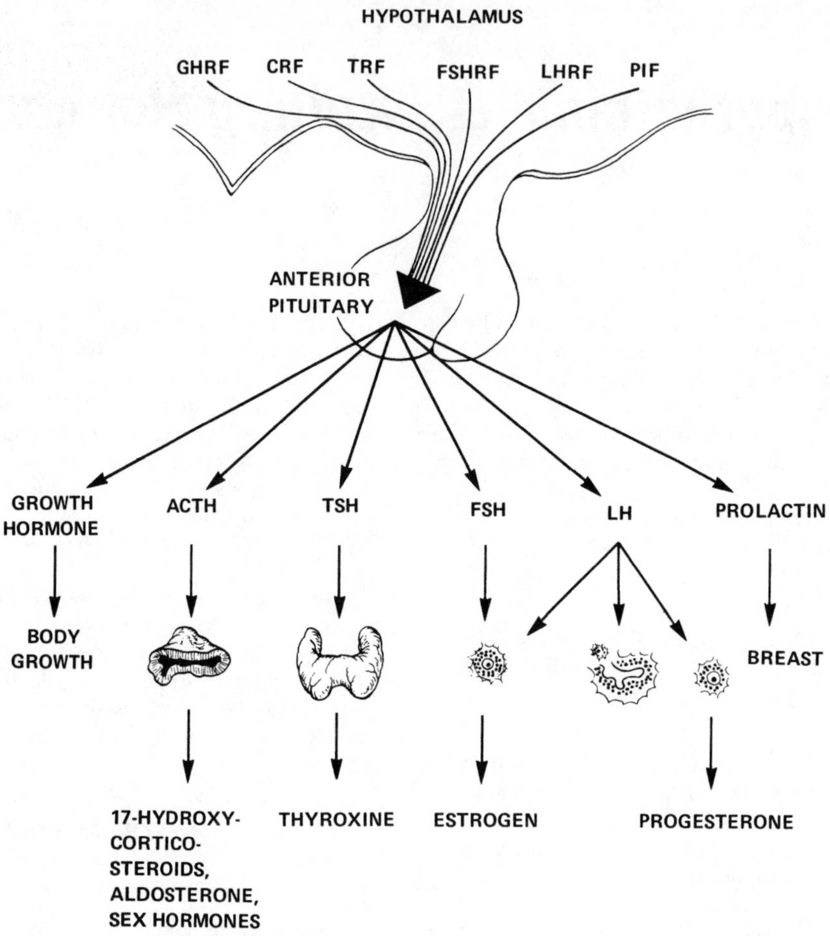

HYPOTHALAMUS

GHRF   CRF   TRF   FSHRF   LHRF   PIF

ANTERIOR
PITUITARY

GROWTH   ACTH   TSH   FSH   LH   PROLACTIN
HORMONE

BODY
GROWTH

17-HYDROXY-   THYROXINE   ESTROGEN   PROGESTERONE
CORTICO-
STEROIDS,
ALDOSTERONE,
SEX HORMONES

BREAST

FIG 39–1. Hypothalamic releasing factors and actions of anterior pituitary hormones. GHRF, growth hormone-releasing factor; CRF, corticotropin-releasing factor; TRF, thyrotropin-releasing factor; FSHRF, follicle-stimulating hormone-releasing factor; LHRF, luteinizing hormone-releasing factor; PIF, prolactin-inhibiting factor.

form from a variety of animal sources including man and monkeys. The structure varies considerably from one species to another. Human growth hormone (Fig 39–2) contains 188 amino acids in a chain and has 2 disulfide bridges. The molecular weight is 21,500. Growth hormone prepared from the rhesus monkey has a molecular weight of 25,400 and 4 disulfide bridges. In contrast to this, the cattle hormone contains about 400 amino acids with a molecular weight of 46,000 and has a branched Y-type structure. The relationships between structure and activity have not been clearly established. Preliminary studies indicate that the entire molecule is not required for activity. The smallest active fragment of human growth hormone has not been identified, but preparations smaller than the natural hormone have been found to be active.

The marked structural variation may account for the fact that growth hormone from one species may not be active in another (Table 39–2). This phenom-

enon, called species specificity, was first well characterized in the study of this substance.

This hormone comprises about 10% of the weight of the anterior pituitary, and its activity is relatively stable with chemical manipulation. Even the most highly purified preparations can be separated into several active components by various technics such as starch gel electrophoresis and gel filtration with Sephedex or other forms of chromatography. Relatively simple procedures are successful in extracting almost half of the material in the gland in clinically useful form.

Growth hormone is destroyed in the gastrointestinal tract and must be administered parenterally. Very little is known about its transport, metabolism, and excretion in man.

Growth hormone has many important effects in the body. It stimulates protein synthesis and growth in almost all tissues of the body including bone, skin, muscle, collagen, and visceral organs. Although the

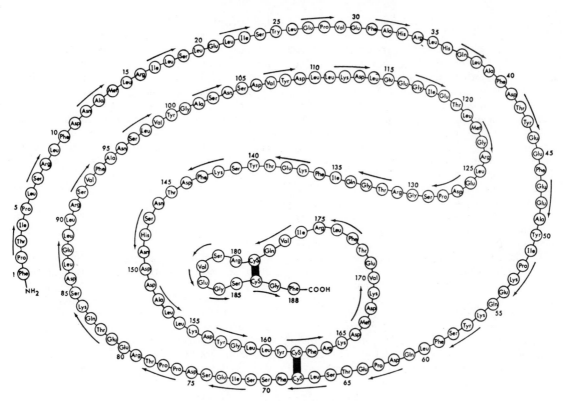

FIG 39–2. Human growth hormone.

mechanism by which growth hormone exerts these effects is not known in detail, it has been shown to increase the transport of amino acids into cells and to stimulate the synthesis of ribonucleic acids.

Growth hormone also has important effects on fat metabolism. In vitro, it appears to stimulate the hormone-sensitive lipase in adipose tissue. When

TABLE 39–2. Activity of growth hormones in other species.* (+), active; (–), inactive.

Growth Hormone From	Stimulates Growth In				
	Fish	Birds	Rat	Monkey	Man
Fish			–		
Reptiles			+		
Amphibia			+		
Birds			+		
Cows	+	–†	+	–	–‡
Sheep	+		+		–
Pigs	+	–†	+	–	–‡
Whales			+		–
Monkeys	+		+		+
Humans	+		+	+	

*Reproduced, with permission, from Ganong: *Review of Medical Physiology,* 5th ed. Lange, 1971.
†Probable diabetogenic effect.
‡Slight diabetogenic effect.

administered to the intact animal or man, the available preparations of growth hormone produce a brief fall in blood glucose and fatty acids followed by a slow rise over a period of several hours in the free fatty acids in plasma.

Growth hormone also has important effects on carbohydrate metabolism. When injected over a prolonged period, it can lead to the development of diabetes mellitus in animals and impairment of glucose tolerance in man. In muscle, growth hormone influences several steps in the metabolism of glucose which impairs glycolysis and glucose transport. It is not known whether these are direct effects of growth hormone or secondary to the mobilization of free fatty acids from adipose tissue. Hyperglycemia, which can be produced by growth hormone, results from a combination of the above effects associated with increased hepatic gluconeogenesis.

The growth effects of this hormone are associated with the retention of mineral substances such as calcium, sodium, potassium, and phosphate in proportion to the amount of tissue added to the body.

Metabolism

In man, growth hormone is secreted at the rate of about 4 mg/day. Little is known about its transport or degradation. However, it is rapidly removed from the circulation. The half-life is estimated to be 20–30 minutes. The circulating levels of growth hormone in man have been measured by an immunoassay. Under basal conditions, the levels are low—usually less than 5 ng/ml. In adult women with normal ovarian function or under treatment with estrogen, the circulating levels may reach 15 ng/ml even with normal activity. The levels are somewhat higher in very young children. They gradually decrease until age 4–5.

Growth hormone can be measured by bioassay as well as immunologically. The bioassay involving the growth in width of the tibial epiphysis is an excellent measure of the growth-promoting activities of this hormone. The immunoassay is a more rapid, sensitive, and simple technic that has markedly increased our understanding of growth hormone secretion. However, it is not entirely clear whether all of the activities associated with preparations extracted from the pituitary are represented by the immunologically active hormone under all circumstances. In men, plasma levels of growth hormone range from 0–5 ng/ml of plasma.

Growth hormone is at least in part regulated by a substance produced in the median eminence of the hypothalamus (Fig 39–1). It has a molecular weight of approximately 2000 and is called growth hormone releasing factor (GHRF). Levels of growth hormone are increased rapidly by a wide variety of stresses, including exercise; by hypoglycemia; and by amino acids such as arginine. The release of this hormone can be inhibited by glucose and by hydrocortisone-like compounds.

Disorders of Growth Hormone Production

Excessive production of growth hormone occurs in the presence of adenomas of the pituitary (eosinophilic) which produce this substance. When this occurs before puberty, excessive growth (gigantism) occurs. After fusion of epiphyseal plates of the long bones, acromegaly is produced. This disorder is accompanied by an overgrowth of the soft tissues, mandible, sinuses, and visceral organs, leading to an easily recognizable characteristic appearance.

Growth hormone may be congenitally absent or defective, leading to dwarfism. Deficiency may also result from partial or complete destruction of the anterior pituitary gland. Such patients fail to grow and may have episodes of hypoglycemia. They often have symptoms due to the deficiency of other tropic hormones.

The ability of the pituitary to produce growth hormone can be tested in several ways. The basal levels can be measured as well as the responses to several stimuli. Among those for which standardized procedures have been developed are the responses to insulin-induced hypoglycemia, intravenous infusions of arginine monochloride, and the injection of glucagon. The injection of vasopressin or production of fever with pyrogen have also been used to test growth hormone reserve.

Clinical Uses

No preparations of human growth hormone are commercially available for clinical use. However, small amounts have been made available to investigators for the treatment of patients with growth hormone deficiency. A small number of patients have been treated for growth failures secondary to hypopituitarism. The majority have shown a significant improvement in growth rate, although a few have failed to respond. Antibiodies have been found in some of these patients after prolonged treatment but as a rule have not been associated with diminished response. Growth failures for reasons other than growth hormone deficiency have not responded well to treatment with this substance. The undesirable side-effects associated with treatment have been discomfort, pain, and swelling associated with frequent injections and occasional allergic reactions. It has not been possible to assess the long-term effects on carbohydrate metabolism, although the hormone has been observed to make diabetes mellitus worse.

Growth hormone is conceivably useful in a variety of other circumstances because of its fat mobilizing and protein anabolic effects. It is not likely that these will be thoroughly investigated until a more abundant supply of active material is available. Although larger amounts of growth hormone derived from nonhuman sources have been available (Table 39–2), these preparations are not fully active in man. There is a specificity of action that is probably related to the structural differences of hormones from various species.

The placenta produces a substance that has chemical and biologic properties similar to those exhibited by human growth hormone. It has been named human chorionic somatomammotropin (HCS). Although this is a very low specific activity protein, it is produced by the placenta in very large amounts. Preliminary studies also suggest that this substance has growth hormone-like activity when given to individuals with hypopituitarism. Its structure is closely related to that of human growth hormone.

PROLACTIN
(Luteotropic Hormone, LTH; Luteotropin, Lactogenic Hormone, Mammotropin)

Although preparations of highly purified prolactin have been obtained from ovine sources (Fig 39–3), the most active substances promoting lactation in the human pituitary thus far are found in preparations of growth hormone. The inability to separate these activities completely suggests that the 2 substances are chemically and structurally similar. The comparative effects of prolactin are remarkably diverse and include the stimulation of milk production in mammals, the maintenance of corpus luteum function (luteotropic action) in some rodents, and important behavioral effects in lower vertebrates. The advent of sensitive bio- and immunoassay technics for the estimation of prolactin is providing some understanding of the control of its secretion in man. Its secretion can be stimulated by estrogens, phenothiazines, and other tran-

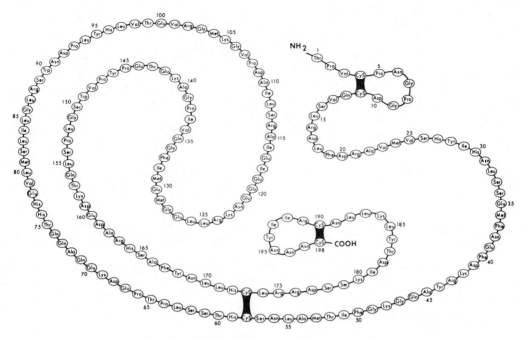

FIG 39–3. Ovine prolactin. (Courtesy of C.H. Li.)

quilizers and dopamine, and the secretion can be inhibited by ergot derivatives. Until a purified preparation of the human material is available, very little will be learned of its functions in man. Preparations of growth hormone with high prolactin activity have been administered successfully in an attempt to improve milk production in lactating women.

The human placenta also produces a protein hormone with growth hormone-like and prolactin-like activities. This material is produced in large amounts throughout pregnancy and has a specific activity which is much lower than that of the pituitary hormones (see above).

CORTICOTROPIN
(Adrenocorticotropic Hormone, ACTH)

Corticotropin is a polypeptide that in man contains 39 amino acids in the sequence illustrated in Fig 39–4. In other species, the isolated polypeptide shows minor variations in amino acids 25–33. The molecular weights of these preparations are between 4500 and 4600.

Corticotropin is assayed biologically by its ability to cause an increase in adrenocortical steroid production or ascorbic acid depletion—or sometimes by its ability to maintain adrenal weight in the hypophysectomized animal. It is now possible to measure small amounts of corticotropin in the circulation by means of an immunoassay.

Pure corticotropin has a biologic activity of 150–200 units/ml. (One USP unit is the activity contained in 1 mg of the international standard.) It is a white powder, soluble in water and 70% alcohol or acetone, and has an iso-electric point of about 4.7. It is stable in neutral or slightly acidic solutions, but labile in alkaline solutions.

Studies with fragments of this polypeptide and with synthetic polypeptides indicate that the entire molecule is not required for biologic activity. Synthetic polypeptides having as few as 19 and 23 amino acids have essentially complete activity.

It has been found that structural changes can independently alter the biologic and immunologic properties of this hormone. Modification of the N-terminal amino acid can reduce or eliminate biologic activity without materially altering its immunologic activity. The reverse is true when alterations are confined to the C-terminal amino acid.

Effects of Corticotropin

Corticotropin stimulates the growth of the adrenal gland and the production and release of hormonal steroids by the adrenal cortex; to some extent, it also increases the flow of blood through the gland.

In addition to controlling adrenocortical secretion, corticotropin has some direct effects. It has a melanocyte-stimulating activity which is probably related to the fact that it is structurally related to melanocyte-stimulating hormone (MSH). α-MSH of beef origin has a sequence of 13 amino acids in common with corticotropin (Fig 39–4). Corticotropin mobilizes lipids from adipose tissue in the form of free

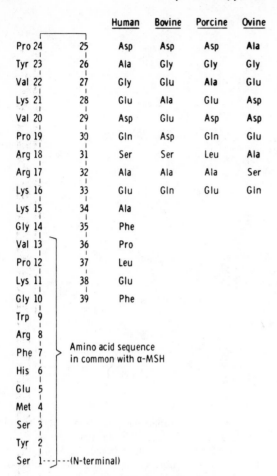

		Human	Bovine	Porcine	Ovine
Pro 24	25	Asp	Asp	Asp	Ala
Tyr 23	26	Ala	Gly	Gly	Gly
Val 22	27	Gly	Glu	Ala	Glu
Lys 21	28	Glu	Ala	Glu	Asp
Val 20	29	Asp	Glu	Asp	Asp
Pro 19	30	Gln	Asp	Gln	Glu
Arg 18	31	Ser	Ser	Leu	Ala
Arg 17	32	Ala	Ala	Ala	Ser
Lys 16	33	Glu	Gln	Glu	Gln
Lys 15	34	Ala			
Gly 14	35	Phe			
Val 13	36	Pro			
Pro 12	37	Leu			
Lys 11	38	Glu			
Gly 10	39	Phe			
Trp 9					
Arg 8					
Phe 7		Amino acid sequence			
His 6		in common with α-MSH			
Glu 5					
Met 4					
Ser 3					
Tyr 2					
Ser 1	----(N-terminal)				

FIG 39—4. Amino acid sequences of human, bovine, porcine, and ovine corticotropin.

fatty acids (FFA). The FFA are in part converted to neutral lipids and ketones by the liver. The remaining FFA are oxidized or reesterified into triglycerides in muscle and other tissues. The effect on adipose tissue is probably mediated by stimulation of a hormone-sensitive lipase. Corticotropin has been shown to have additional effects in adrenalectomized animals. It causes a reduction of the rate of disappearance of plasma glucose and a reduction in the level of glucose and amino acids, and it inhibits the degradation of the corticosteroids. It also has a minor positive inotropic effect on the heart. It is doubtful that any of these effects are of more than minor importance physiologically.

Corticotropin also decreases the further release of corticotropin by inhibiting the secretion of corticotropin-releasing factor (CRF; Fig 39—1)—an example of "short loop" feedback inhibition of pituitary hormones.

Action of Corticotropin on Adrenal Steroidogenesis

Corticotropin increases the production of cortisol and its precursors primarily in the zona fasciculata and

zona reticularis and of aldosterone in the zona glomerulosa of the adrenal cortex (see Chapter 35). Many of the precursors are common to both pathways; however, the enzymes involved may be specific for each pathway (Fig 35—1).

The rate-limiting step in synthesis which is stimulated by corticotropin appears to be the conversion of cholesterol to pregnenolone. The precise mechanism of action involved in the stimulation of the adrenal cortex is not known, but a number of associated molecular events have been described. These include an increase in the cellular uptake of glucose and amino acids and production of cyclic AMP (cyclic 3',5'-adenosine monophosphate). The latter substance activates dephosphorylase kinase, which produces an increase in active phosphorylase in the zona fasciculata. It has been shown that cyclic AMP is capable of markedly stimulating steroidogenesis, probably as the result of increased production of energy substrate and dihydronicotinamide adenine dinucleotide phosphate (NADPH), which can increase corticosteroid production in vitro. A number of structural changes in the adrenal involving the mitochondria are observed to follow corticotropin stimulation.

Metabolism

Corticotropin has a half-life of less than 20 minutes. At rest, the plasma level is 0.3—0.88 mU/100 ml (21—63 pg/ml); with activity or stress, the level may increase to as high as 2.8 mU/100 ml (200 pg/ml). The human anterior pituitary contains 5—10 mg of corticotropin per gram of tissue and releases a fraction of a milligram per day at rest. In the circulation it is associated with plasma proteins (Cohn fractions II and III) and is concentrated in several tissues, including the adrenal cortex, kidneys, and placenta. Some appears in the urine.

Regulation of Secretion

The control of corticotropin secretion is dual in nature and appears to be mediated by the hypothalamic secretion of a substance which has been named corticotropin-releasing factor (CRF; Fig 39—1). Increased circulating cortisol levels depress corticotropin release; decreased cortisol levels increase the rate of its secretion. This phenomenon is referred to as negative feedback control.

A second mechanism, activated by stress, involves other parts of the brain. Stimulation of portions of the anterior median eminence of the hypothalamus, the limbic system, and the amygdaloid complex and removal of the cerebral cortex also increase corticotropin secretion. Lesions in the anterior median eminence and transection of the midbrain interfere with the normal increase observed in response to stress.

In the absence of stress and in the presence of intact feedback regulation, the rate of corticotropin secretion varies throughout the day, reaching its maximum in the morning hours and being low during the evening. This variation can be blocked by morphine and does not occur in patients with diseases of the nervous system associated with widespread destruction of tissues. It therefore appears that the level at which feedback regulation occurs is determined by a center in the brain. It is not known whether this center is related to or identical with those controlling circadian rhythms of other bodily processes such as temperature and renal function.

Noxious stimuli can overcome feedback inhibition unless there is severe atrophy of the biochemical mechanism involved in the formation and release of corticotropin and adrenocortical steroids. Atrophy of this degree is seen after prolonged administration of corticotropin or one of the glucocorticoids or following the removal of a cortisol-producing tumor.

The pituitary reserve can be tested by utilizing both pathways. The feedback response can be provoked by the 11-hydroxylase inhibitor metyrapone (see Chapter 35). Increased ACTH release can also be provoked by hypoglycemia, lysine vasopressin, or pyrogen.

Clinical Uses

A. Therapeutic Uses: The most obvious use for corticotropin is in the replacement of a deficiency of endogenous corticotropin such as might be found when the anterior pituitary is destroyed by a tumor, thrombosis of its vascular supply, or other injury. However, it has been found to be more convenient, comfortable, and accurate (as well as less expensive) to replace the adrenocortical hormones whose production is stimulated by corticotropin directly since corticotropin must be given parenterally (see Chapter 35).

Corticotropin is occasionally used in the treatment of allergic and inflammatory disorders which are favorably influenced by glucocorticoids. It has been proposed that the tropic effect on the adrenal cortex might prevent or minimize the occurrence of iatrogenic adrenal insufficiency (produced by prolonged suppression of endogenous adrenocortical secretion). However, careful studies of pituitary and adrenal function following prolonged treatment with large doses of glucocorticoids or corticotropin indicate that the response to stress is inhibited to a similar degree in patients receiving both preparations.

B. Diagnostic Uses: Corticotropin is widely used in the study of adrenocortical function. In the patient suffering from adrenocortical insufficiency, the increase in production of cortisol and other corticosteroids following administration of corticotropin will be absent if the disorder resides in the adrenal. When the deficiency is due to a reduction in corticotropin, the adrenal response will be present—albeit sluggish if the deficiency is severe and of long duration.

The patient who is able to produce a normal amount of corticosteroid at rest but is unable to increase the rate of secretion during periods of stress can be identified by a failure to respond to corticotropin even though the resting levels of secretion are normal.

The infusion of corticotropin may be helpful as an adjunct to suppression tests in the differential diagnosis of Cushing's syndrome. In patients with bilateral adrenal hyperplasia, the steroidogenic response to corticotropin is marked. When the source of the excessive hormone production is carcinoma of the adrenal, this hyperactive response is usually absent. Benign adenomas producing adrenocortical steroids vary in their response to corticotropin.

Corticotropin tests can be performed in several ways. When possible, the intravenous infusion of synthetic corticotropin is preferred because the responses are more reproducible and because the source of material can be immediately removed if an allergic reaction occurs.

When synthetic corticotropin (0.25 mg) is injected intravenously in a few ml of saline, peak plasma cortisol levels are reached in 45–60 minutes. The levels are sufficiently elevated in 30 minutes to yield reliable results in most patients. When the same amount is infused over 8 hours in saline or glucose, the increase in plasma cortisol or urinary 17-hydroxycorticoid excretion can be measured as an index of adrenal response.

Contraindications & Cautions

The major contraindication to the administration of corticotropin is a history of a previous hypersensitivity reaction. Most patients exhibiting such responses will tolerate synthetic corticotropin. However, a few reactions have occurred, and an intradermal test should be done even with this preparation.

Preparations Available

Corticotropin is available in preparations suitable for intravenous or intramuscular use (Table 39–3). The latter consist of corticotropin in gelatin solution or adsorbed to zinc hydroxide to prolong the action of the drug.

The corticotropin in these preparations is derived from animal pituitary glands since synthetic materials have not been made available for commercial use until recently. The potency is determined by bioassay. The USP unit is equivalent to the activity contained in 1/5 of an ampule (1 mg) of the Third International Standard for Corticotropin using the adrenal ascorbic acid depletion assay.

A synthetic preparation of corticotropin (cosyntropin) is now available for clinical use. It contains the first 24 amino acids of β-corticotropin. A dose of 0.25 mg is equivalent to 25 IU. This preparation appears to be free of allergic reactions and, in contrast to others, can be given as reliably by the intramuscular as by the intravenous route. It will cause a significant elevation of plasma corticosteroids in 60–70 minutes in normal subjects.

Clinical preparations of corticotropin are derived largely from bovine, porcine, and ovine pituitary glands. Since it is rapidly destroyed by proteolytic enzymes, corticotropin cannot be administered orally. However, it is readily absorbed when given by intramuscular injection or as an intravenous infusion.

Since the half-life is less than 20 minutes, the effects of intravenously administered corticotropin do

TABLE 39–3. Corticotropin: Preparations available.

	Route of Administration	Preparations Available
Corticotropin Injection USP	Subcut or IM; IV only if specifically so indicated on the label of the particular product.	10 units/ml, 1 and 10 ml vials 20 units/ml, 2 and 10 ml vials 40 units/ml, 1 and 5 ml vials 80 units/ml, 5 ml vials Powder, 25 and 40 units/vial
Repository corticotropin injection USP	Subcut or IM; IV only if specifically so indicated on the label of the particular product.	20 units/ml, 5 ml vials 40 units/ml, 1 and 5 ml vials 80 units/ml, 5 ml vials
Sterile corticotropin zinc hydroxide suspension USP	IM only	20 units/ml, 5 ml vials 40 units/ml, 5 ml vials 40 units/1 ml syringe
Cosyntropin (synthetic a1-24 corticotropin)	IV	Powder, 0.25 mg (25 units/vial)

not persist for a long period following injection; when larger doses are given (eg, more than 10 mg), the steroidogenic effect is directly related to the duration of the infusion. When corticotropin is given by the intramuscular route, the effects are not greatly prolonged unless gelatin is added or the drug is adsorbed to zinc hydroxide.

GONADOTROPINS

The pituitary hormones regulating ovarian and testicular function are known as gonadotropins. The control of ovarian function varies from one species to another. Three hormones are known to have gonadotropic activity in some species. They are luteinizing hormone (LH), follicle-stimulating hormone (FSH), and prolactin (see above). The function of the latter is well established in the rodent, but its activity in controlling ovarian function in the human female has not been established. FSH and LH appear to be important in all species studied. In addition to these hormones produced by the anterior pituitary, human placenta produces chorionic gonadotropin (HCG) which is related and will be considered below.

Preparations of LH and HCG have been used experimentally to stimulate the production of androgens by the testes or by the ovary for the purpose of testing endocrine function. They are also used in conjunction with FSH, human menopausal urine gonadotropin preparations, and clomiphene (Clomid) to produce ovulation in women with abnormal menstrual function (see Chapter 38).

The gonadotropins—LH, FSH, and HCG—and thyrotropin are glycoproteins. They have each been shown to consist of 2 chains designated a and β. The a chains are quite similar to each other and can be interchanged without altering biologic activity (Table 39–4). The β chains confer biologic specificity.

The regulation of FSH and LH secretion from the pituitary is complex. It involves feedback regulation by

the gonadal hormones at the hypothalamus and pituitary level and direct feedback effects of the gonadotropins on the secretion of hypothalamic releasing factors or hormones. A polypeptide with FSH and LH releasing activity has been isolated and its structure determined, and it has been synthesized (Fig 39–5). This material (FSH-RH/LH-RH) can increase LH levels in 15 minutes when 1 μg is injected intravenously. About 3 μg will induce a comparable increase in serum FSH. This agent can be used to distinguish hypothalamic from pituitary deficiency as the cause of hypogonadism in patients with responsive ovaries and low levels of circulating gonadotropins. Its potential uses for inducing ovulation and otherwise altering the menstrual cycle or spermatogenesis and fertility are being explored.

TABLE 39–4. Properties of the pituitary glycoprotein subunits.*

	ICSH-a	TSH-a	FSH-a
Hexose (%)	8.3	7.3	2.8
Hexosamine (%)	8.6	13.3	2.3
Sialic acid (%)	. . .	. . .	0.8
N-terminal	Phe	Phe	Phe
C-terminal	Ser	Ser	Ser
Partial amino acid content†			
Lysine	10	10	10.5
Arginine	3	3	4.5
Proline	7	7	5.6
Half-cystine	10	10	4.9
Methionine	4	4	0.3
Leucine	2	2	9.0
Tyrosine	5	5	2.7

*Reproduced, with permission, from Papkoff, H.: Gen Comp Endocr. In press.

†Values for ICSH-a and TSH-a are residues per molecule determined by structure analysis; values for FSH-a are expressed as residues/100 residues determined by amino acid analysis.

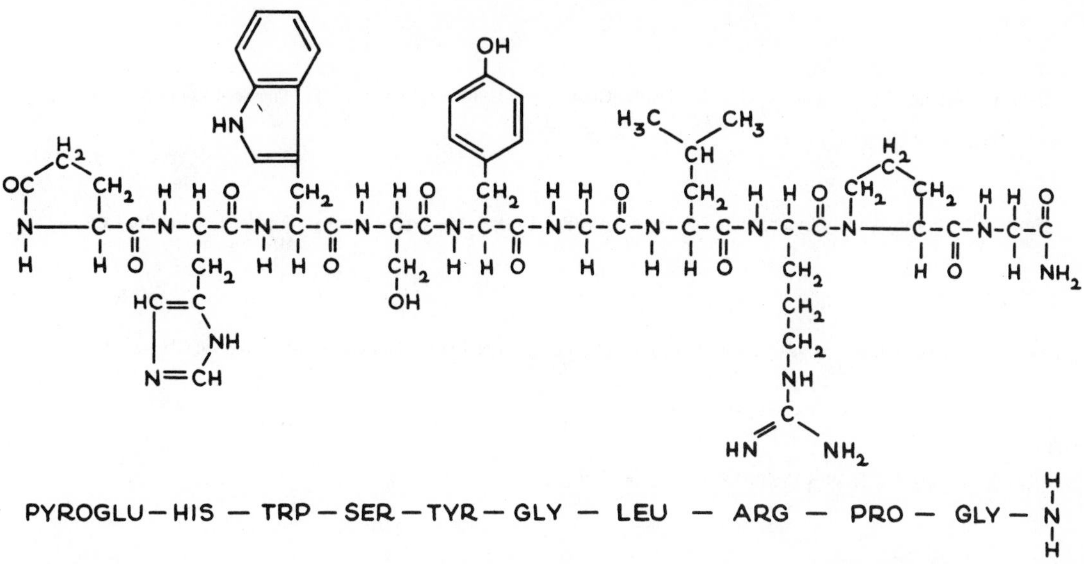

PYROGLU—HIS — TRP — SER —TYR— GLY — LEU — ARG — PRO — GLY — N⟨H,H⟩

FIG 39—5. The molecular structure of porcine LH and FSH-releasing hormone (LH-RH/FSH-RH). (Reproduced, with permission, from Schally, A.V., Kastin, A.J., & A. Arimura: Hypothalamic follicle-stimulating hormone [FSH] and luteinizing hormone [LH]-regulating hormone: Structure, physiology, and clinical studies. Fertil Steril 22:703—721, 1971.)

1. FOLLICLE-STIMULATING HORMONE (FSH)

FSH is a glycoprotein composed of 2 polypeptide chains. The *a* chain, as noted above, is similar to that of LH (Fig 39—6). It has a molecular weight of approximately 32,000 and a carbohydrate content of 18%. Its high solubility, acidity, and resistance to inactivation by proteolytic enzymes have served to facilitate its separation. It is inactivated by neuraminidase with the release of sialic acid.

FSH appears to be responsible for the stimulation of the growth and possibly the secretion of estrogen by the graafian follicle. In the male, this hormone stimulates the development of the germinal elements leading to the production of sperm cells.

Very few studies of the metabolism of FSH have been reported. Preliminary studies indicate that the premenopausal production rate in women is in the range of 200—300 IU/day and that it may be 10—15 times as high in postmenopausal women. The initial half-life is approximately 10 minutes. Studies of the blood level of this hormone throughout the menstrual cycle in women have been performed by several methods utilizing both immunoassay and bioassay procedures. Recent studies utilizing immunoassay procedures indicate that there is an increase in plasma FSH concentration early in the cycle as well as a peak coincident with the peak in LH secretion at midcycle (Fig 38—2). These peaks appear to precede ovulation by about 16 hours.

The release of FSH is controlled by FSH releasing factor, which is produced by the median eminence of the hypothalamus. The secretion of this material is complex. It is influenced by levels of estrogen and progesterone and by neural stimuli from other neural centers in the brain.

Little is known about the metabolism of FSH except that an estimated 10—20% of the amount secreted can be identified in the urine by immunoassay or bioassay.

Preparations & Dosages
See Human Menopausal Gonadotropin, Chapter 38.

2. LUTEINIZING HORMONE
(LH; Interstitial Cell-Stimulating Hormone, ICSH; Ovulating Hormone)

The structure of LH is shown in Fig 39—6. It is similar to those of FSH and thyrotropin.

Good preparations have been obtained from the pituitary glands of several species, including man. However, only small amounts of the latter preparation have been available.

LH is produced at about 2—4 times the rate of FSH in normal menstruating women. However, it is not secreted at a constant rate. The rate of secretion is somewhat higher in the first half of the cycle than in the second, but there is a high peak which seems to be associated with (and may be the cause of) ovulation in man and other species. Its half-life in man appears to be about 20—25 minutes. Plasma levels of LH during the menstrual cycle are plotted in Fig 38—2.

Little is known about the metabolism of LH except that a portion is excreted into the urine in a biologically active form detectable by immunoassay.

Alpha chain:

H-Phe-Pro-Asp-Gly-Glx-Phe-Thr-Met-Glx-Gly-Cys-Pro-Glx-Cys-Lys-Leu-Lys-Glu-Asn-Lys-Tyr-Phe-Ser-Lys-Pro-Asx-Ala-
                              10   20

Pro-Ile-Tyr-Gln-Cys-Met-Gly-Cys-Cys-Phe-Ser-Arg-Ala-Tyr-Pro-Thr-Pro-Ala-Arg-Ser-Lys-Lys-Thr-Met-Leu-Val-Pro-Lys-
                    30   40   50

CHO   CHO
| |
Asn-Ile-Thr-Ser-Glu-Ala-Thr-Cys-Cys-Val-Ala-Lys-Ala-Phe-Thr-Lys-Ala-Thr-Val-Met-Gly-Asn-Val-Arg-Val-Glx-Asn-His-
                    60   70   80

Thr-Glx-Cys-His-Ser-Cys-Thr-Cys-Tyr-Tyr-His-Lys-Ser-OH
                    90

Beta chain:

                                        CHO
                                        |
H-Ser-Arg-Gly-Pro-Leu-Arg-Pro-Leu-Cys-Glu-Pro-Ile-Asn-Ala-Thr-Leu-Ala-Ala-Glu-Lys-Glu-Ala-Cys-Pro-Val-Cys-Ile-Thr-
                            10   20

Phe-Thr-Thr-Ser-Ile-Gly-Ala-Tyr-Cys-Cys-Pro-Ser-Met-Lys-Arg-Val-Leu-Pro-Val-Pro-Pro-Leu-Ile-Pro-Met-Pro-Gln-Arg-Val-
            30   40   50

Cys-Thr-Tyr-His-Gln-Leu-Arg-Phe-Ala-Ser-Val-Arg-Leu-Pro-Gly-Pro-Cys-Pro-Val-Asp-Pro-Gly-Met-Val-Ser-Phe-Pro-Val-
            60   70   80

Ala-Leu-Ser-Cys-His-Gly-Pro-Cys-Cys-Arg-Leu-Ser-Ser-Thr-Asp-Cys-Gly-Pro-Gly-Arg-Thr-Glu-Pro-Leu-Ala-Cys-Asp-His-
            90   100   110

Pro-Pro-Leu-Pro-Asp-Ile-Leu-OH
            120

FIG 39—6. Amino acid sequence of ovine ICSH.

LH is responsible for the stimulation of the Leydig cells in the testes, leading to the production of testosterone. In the female it is thought also to stimulate the interstitial cells in the ovary, leading to the production of some androgens; and it has also been shown to stimulate the production of progesterone by the cells of the corpus luteum obtained from the human ovary. Although the actual site of LH action in the production of progesterone in the corpus luteum is unknown, experimental evidence suggests that it accelerates the conversion of acetate to squalene and of cholesterol to 20α-hydroxycholesterol. LH has been shown to increase the production of cyclic AMP, leading to an increase in the activation of phosphorylase. This enzyme, by its effects on carbohydrate metabo-lism, provides NADPH, which is required for the conversion of cholesterol to progesterone in the corpus luteum.

Although no preparations of LH are available for clinical use, HCG is commonly used to obtain this activity.

3. CHORIONIC GONADOTROPIN
(Human Chorionic Gonadotropin, HCG)

Human chorionic gonadotropin is a water-soluble glycoprotein resembling the above compounds except that it is more highly acidic. The study of highly purified preparations indicate that the hormone may be composed of 2 polypeptide chains. Amino acid analyses of these preparations suggest a molecular weight of about 27,000. However, other technics have suggested a larger molecule. The nature of the carbohydrate chains indicate that the structure is highly complex. The specific activity of the hormone is about 12,000 IU/mg. It sufficiently resembles LH so that an antiserum prepared from HCG will cross-react with LH extracted from human pituitary glands. Its biologic activities are similar to those of LH, but little is known of its metabolism. HCG is produced in detectable amounts by trophoblast of the placenta shortly after implantation of the blastocyst. Its production is greatest 6–8 weeks later, and levels remain high until parturition. It disappears from the circulation slowly (over a period of days) at the termination of pregnancy. It is obtained for clinical use by extraction from the urine of pregnant women.

Clinical Uses

HCG is used in conjunction with FSH for the induction of ovulation (Chapter 38). It is also used for diagnostic purposes in order to determine the ability of the gonads to produce gonadal steroids. Doses of 5000–10,000 IU daily for several days are required to produce a marked effect. HCG has also been used in conjunction with a 600-calorie diet to produce weight loss. It is said to reduce the appetite and aid in adherence to the stringent diet. Although the regimen can be effective, there is no evidence that the HCG contributes by a pharmacologic or metabolic action. A combination of the expense and the biweekly visit to the physician may be an important incentive for the patient to remain on the diet.

Preparations Available

Antuitrin-S (for IM injection only), vials of 5000 IU powder plus 10 ml sterile aqueous diluent

A.P.L. (for IM injection only), Secules containing 5000, 10,000, or 20,000 IU in dry form plus 10 ml ampule sterile aqueous diluent (1 of each per package)

Follutein (IM rather than IV injections recommended), vials of 10,000 IU powder plus 10 ml sterile aqueous diluent

Stemutrolin: (For IM injection only. Male treatment is the only use listed.) Vials of 5000 IU powder plus 10 ml sterile aqueous diluent

THYROID-STIMULATING HORMONE
(TSH, Thyrotropin)

TSH, the pituitary hormone responsible for the regulation of thyroid gland activity, is a glycoprotein.

Chemistry

TSH has not been completely purified and characterized although some aspects of its structure are known. It appears to be a single chain polypeptide with several disulfide bonds. It contains glucosamine and galactosamine and has a molecular weight of approximately 25,000. The structural differences in TSH derived from different species are thought to be small since the preparations are active in species other than the one from which it is derived. It has been shown, however, that antibodies may form under these circumstances, limiting the time during which the hormone will be effective in other species. These observations indicate that the determinants of biologic and immunologic activity differ as was noted with corticotropin.

Assay

TSH can be assayed by its effects on the thyroid gland. Thyroid weight, hormone synthesis, iodine or phosphorus uptake, and morphologic changes (follicular cell height) have been employed. More recently, radio-immunoassay and fluorescent staining procedures have been used.

Effects

TSH has an important effect in the regulation of most processes leading to the synthesis and release of thyroxine and triiodothyronine. Its administration is followed by the biologic effects of these hormones. TSH stimulates the accumulation of iodine, glucose, and amino acids by the cells of the thyroid and increases oxidative metabolism, proteolysis of colloid, and release of hormone.

The molecular mechanisms involved in these actions have not been defined. TSH enhances the metabolism of glucose via the hexose monophosphate shunt pathway. This leads to an increase in available NADPH. TSH has been reported to increase cyclic AMP, but its known actions do not appear to be dependent upon protein synthesis.

Control of Secretion

The release of TSH by the pituitary is regulated in part by negative feedback control which involves the inhibition of release by thyroxine acting both at the pituitary and at hypothalamic centers which secrete a thyrotropin-releasing factor or hormone (TRF, TRH). TRH has recently been isolated, purified, and characterized. It appears to be a tripeptide with the structure illustrated in Fig 39–7. Its release is controlled by thyroxine, as mentioned above, and directly by higher centers in the nervous system in response to environmental changes.

TRH has been synthesized and is being tested clinically for use as a diagnostic agent in the assessment of thyroid function. Doses of 1 mg IV elicit a significant elevation of plasma TSH levels. As little as 10 μg can produce an increase of TSH levels in hypothyroid patients. Thus far, only minimal side-effects such as transient nausea have been observed. The hormone is

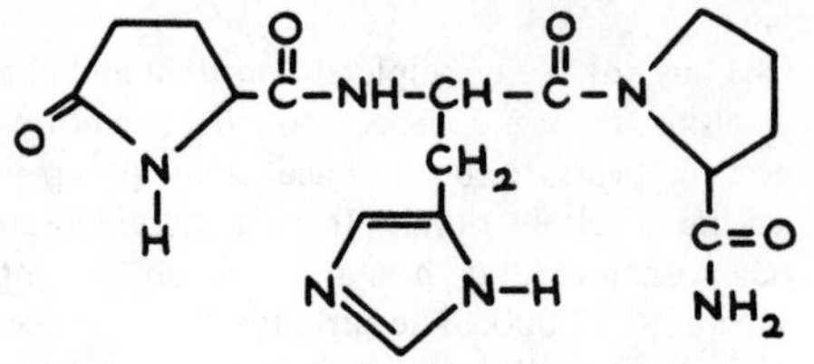

FIG 39–7. Thyrotropin-releasing factor.

orally active, but larger doses are required. Potential therapeutic uses of the agent are being explored. Possible applications include the stimulation of ^{131}I uptake for increased efficacy of ^{131}I therapy of thyrotoxicosis and thyroid carcinoma. TSH release is increased by cold and reduced by heat.

Metabolism

When released into the circulation, TSH is rapidly cleared by the kidney. Its half-life is about 35 minutes in the normal individual but is increased in patients with hypothyroidism and decreased in patients with hyperthyroidism.

Plasma levels, as determined by the most sensitive assay available, have been found to range from less than 1 to 50 ng/ml in normal subjects (0.01–0.05 mU/ml). Plasma TSH can be suppressed by the administration of thyroid hormone and may be 50 times normal in the presence of thyroid deficiency.

Disorders of Thyrotropin Secretion

A deficiency of thyrotropin production is caused by destructive lesions of the anterior pituitary gland. Hyperfunction of the thyroid is not produced by TSH, but is thought to be caused by long-acting thyroid stimulator (LATS). This protein is a gamma globulin and is thought to be an antibody to microsomal proteins derived from the thyroid.

Clinical Uses

A. Therapeutic Uses: TSH (as thyrotropin; Thytropar) is not used for the replacement of endogenous deficiencies of the hormone because it is less satisfactory than administering thyroid hormone orally. In addition, bovine TSH is active for only a short time in man because of antibody formation.

TSH has been successfully used to stimulate the iodine uptake of toxic adenomatous goiters and in the treatment of metastatic thyroid disease in patients with thyroid cancer to enhance the effectiveness of therapy with radioactive iodine (^{131}I). It can be given in 3 or more daily doses of 10 units IM for several days until an adequate response is obtained.

B. Diagnostic Uses: TSH has also been used for diagnostic purposes. Hypothyroidism due to disturbances of the thyroid gland can be distinguished from that secondary to pituitary deficiency of TSH production. In addition, it is possible to distinguish primary hypothyroidism from iatrogenic suppression of thyroid

function in patients who have been treated with thyroid hormone for prolonged periods. When used for these purposes, 10 units of TSH given for 1–3 days will cause an increase in the serum thyroxine and an increase in the ^{131}I uptake by the thyroid gland in the presence of normal thyroid tissue.

Contraindications & Cautions

TSH should not be given to patients in whom an increase in thyroid function might be harmful. This would include patients with angina pectoris, recent myocardial infarction, or congestive heart failure. It should be used with caution in patients with hypopituitarism or adrenal insufficiency.

TSH may produce temporary swelling of the thyroid; arrhythmias, including atrial fibrillation and tachycardias; fever; and nausea and vomiting.

In addition to the problems caused by the hormonal effects, anaphylactic reactions have occurred. Other allergic reactions including urticaria, fever, and transient hypotension have been reported and can usually be prevented by prior administration of antihistamines.

Preparations Available

Thyrotropin (Thytropar), derived from beef pituitaries, is available for intramuscular administration in ampules (10 units) as a partially lyophilized powder which is devoid of significant amounts of corticotropin, gonadotropin, somatotropin, oxytocin, and vasopressin. It is stable at room temperature and is dissolved in normal saline prior to injection. The solution is stable for several weeks if refrigerated.

INTERMEDIATE LOBE OF THE PITUITARY

The intermediate lobe of the pituitary is formed from the dorsal part of Rathke's pouch and is separated from the anterior lobe by the residual of the pocket formed by that structure. This part of the gland is less well developed in man than in other species. Two polypeptides have been isolated from the cells of this lobe which disperse melanin granules in pigment cells. They have been named α- and β-melanocyte-stimulating hormone (MSH). Their structures have a number of amino acids in a sequence found in corticotropin (Fig 39–4). Corticotropin has "MSH-like" activity but is much less potent than α- or β-MSH. Preliminary studies of changes in plasma MSH levels, as measured by immunoassay, indicate that, in man, the secretion of this hormone follows that of corticotropin and is not related to alterations in pigmentation other than those produced by changes in adrenocortical function.

TABLE 39–5. The relationship between the structure of the MSH's and amino acids 1–19 of the 39 amino acids in ACTH.*

		Ser-1	Tyr-2	Ser-3	Met-4	Glu-5	His-6	Phe-7	Arg-8	Trp-9	Gly-10	Lys-11	Pro-12	Val-13	Gly-14 Lys-15 Lys-16 Arg-17 Arg-18 Pro-19
ACTH (pig, sheep, beef)		Ser-1	Tyr-2	Ser-3	Met-4 Glu-5 His-6 Phe-7 Arg-8 Trp-9 Gly-10							Lys-11	Pro-12	Val-13	Gly-14 Lys-15 Lys-16 Arg-17 Arg-18 Pro-19
α MSH (pig, beef, horse)	CH₃CO-	Ser-1	Tyr-2	Ser-3	Met-4 Glu-5 His-6 Phe-7 Arg-8 Trp-9 Gly-10							Lys-11	Pro-12	Val-13	NH₂
β MSH (pig)	Asp-1 Glu-2 Gly-3 Pro-4		Tyr-5	Lys-6	Met-7 Glu-8 His-9 Phe-10 Arg-11 Trp-12 Gly-13							Ser-14	Pro-15	Pro-16	Lys-17 Asp-18
β MSH (beef)	Asp-1 Ser-2 Gly-3 Pro-4		Tyr-5	Lys-6	Met-7 Glu-8 His-9 Phe-10 Arg-11 Trp-12 Gly-13							Ser-14	Pro-15	Pro-16	Lys-17 Asp-18
β MSH (horse)	Asp-1 Glu-2 Gly-3 Pro-4		Tyr-5	Lys-6	Met-7 Glu-8 His-9 Phe-10 Arg-11 Trp-12 Gly-13							Ser-14	Pro-15	Arg-16	Lys-17 Asp-18
β MSH (human)	Ala-1 Glu-2 Lys-3 Lys-4 Asp-5 Glu-6 Gly-7 Pro-8		Tyr-9	Arg-10	Met-11 Glu-12 His-13 Phe-14 Arg-15 Trp-16 Gly-17							Ser-18	Pro-19	Pro-20	Lys-21 Asp-22

*Reproduced, with permission, from Li: Some aspects of the relation of peptide structure to activity in pituitary hormones. Vitamins & Hormones 19:313, 1961.

In fish, amphibia, and reptiles, MSH appears to play a role in the control of skin coloration. MSH secretion causes darkening of the skin in these species, and its secretion is under the control of neural centers and regulated by photoreceptors. Its function in man is not known.

THE POSTERIOR PITUITARY (NEUROHYPOPHYSIS)

The posterior lobe of the pituitary is an extension of the nervous system derived from the floor of the thalamic portion of the brain. It contains neuroglial cells, pituicytes, and the axons of neurons in the supraoptic and paraventricular nuclei of the hypothalamus.

Although vasopressin and oxytocin have been extracted from the posterior pituitary, it is now known that they are neurosecretory products of neurons of the supraoptic and paraventricular nuclei. The structures of these hormones in man are illustrated in Fig 39–8, and some of the species differences which have been documented are noted.

VASOPRESSIN (Antidiuretic Hormone, ADH)

Although methods are available for the measurement of vasopressin, the lack of agreement in results from different laboratories leaves us with little information about the rates of secretion, plasma levels, and metabolism of this substance. When vasopressin is injected intravenously or secreted into the blood stream, it behaves as though it were cleared by a single passage through the liver and kidney. When relatively large amounts are injected, the half-life is less than 20 minutes. When it is given intramuscularly or subcutaneously, its effects may persist for several hours, and its activity can be further prolonged by injecting it as vasopressin tannate in oil.

Vasopressin has now been synthesized and is available for use in a highly purified form.

The mechanism of action of vasopressin in the kidneys is under study. It binds firmly to renal tissue, and its action can be inhibited by agents which block the sulfhydryl group. It is known that vasopressin activates the enzyme increasing concentrations of cyclic AMP in the kidney; and cyclic AMP is able to duplicate many of the actions of vasopressin in this tissue.

Control of Secretion

Vasopressin is produced by the nerve cells in the supraoptic and paraventricular nuclei of the hypothalamus. It appears to then be transported along the nerve fibers to the pituicytes of the posterior lobe of the pituitary. In the pituitary gland, it is bound to a specific group of proteins called neurophysin, which contains 3 polypeptide binding sites per molecule. It can be discharged from this area by electrical stimulation or acetylcholine. The control of vasopressin release is mediated in part through osmoreceptors, and an increase in plasma osmolality resulting from water withdrawal or dehydration leads to increased rates of release of the hormone. Hydration, on the other hand, reduces the secretion to a level that cannot be detected in the plasma or urine. In addition to the osmoreceptors, which are thought to be located in the region of the hypothalamic nuclei, the secretion of vasopressin can be modified by changes in volume. In addition to these homeostatic mechanisms, the secretion of vasopressin can be increased by emotional and physical stress as well as by drugs such as nicotine and mor-

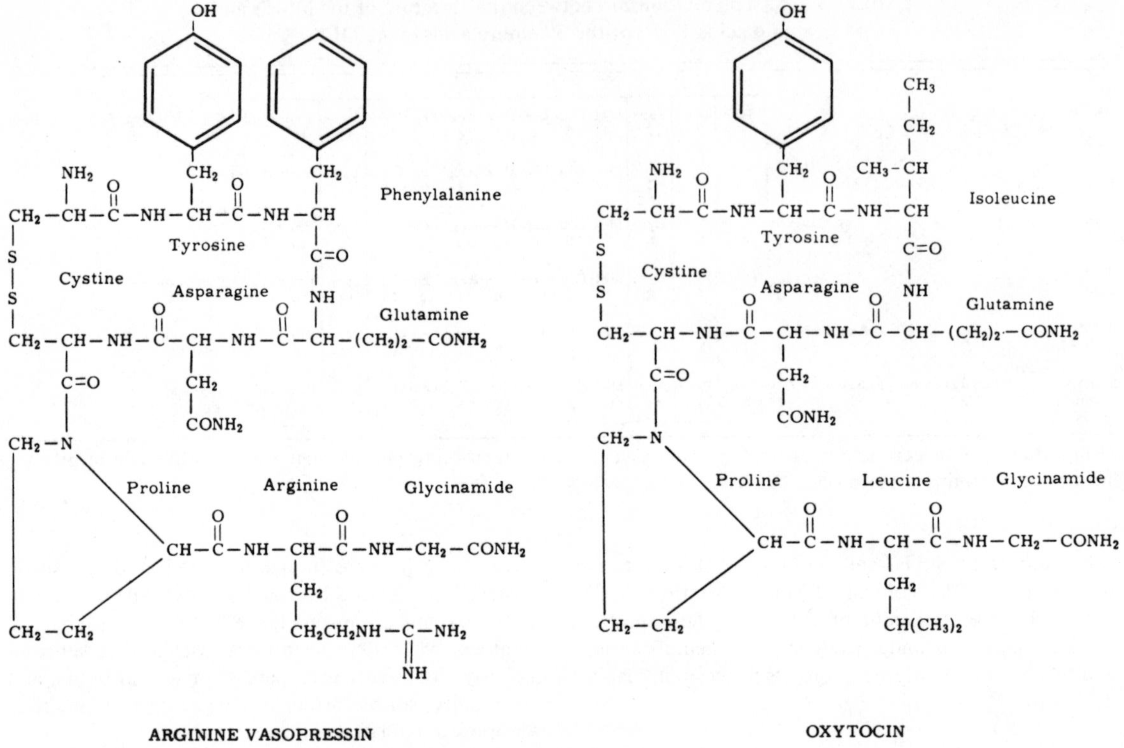

FIG 39—8. Formulas of arginine vasopressin and oxytocin. In the pig and hippopotamus, lysine is substituted for arginine in the vasopressin side chain. (Reproduced, with permission, from Ganong: *Review of Medical Physiology,* 5th ed. Lange, 1971.)

phine. Vasopressin secretion can be inhibited by alcohol.

Effects of Deficiency or Excess

The absence of vasopressin causes diabetes insipidus, a disorder characterized by severe polyuria.

An excess of vasopressin results in water retention and dilutional hyponatremia. This disorder occurs under a variety of circumstances, particularly in the presence of pulmonary disease. Tumors have also been reported which appear to produce vasopressin or a similar substance.

Clinical Uses

The major therapeutic use of vasopressin is in the treatment of diabetes insipidus due to a deficiency of this hormone. Since the half-life of vasopressin is short, aqueous solutions are not convenient for chronic control and vasopressin tannate in oil is used instead. A dose of 0.25—1 unit/day or more may be required, and a few patients can be maintained on injections at greater intervals.

Vasopressin deficiency may not be the only cause of diabetes insipidus since some individuals with renal tubular defects fail to respond to the hormone. Although vasopressin is not useful in treatment of these patients, it can be used as a diagnostic test—keeping in mind that after prolonged polyuria even the normal renal tubule will not immediately respond to vasopressin.

In addition to the intramuscular preparations, vasopressin can be given as nasal snuff, 30—60 mg 2—3 times a day; this is the least expensive form of treatment, but it may be quite irritating and absorption is uncertain.

For patients who are allergic to animal vasopressin, a synthetic substitute, lysine-8 vasopressin, is available as a nasal spray. This preparation is free of local side-effects, and water intoxication, which is not unusual with vasopressin tannate in oil, does not occur.

Large doses of vasopressin produce a reduction in portal blood pressure and blood flow and have been used along with other measures in the treatment of esophageal bleeding. With the large doses used (10—20 units), a moderate rise in arterial blood pressure is observed.

Lysine vasopressin given in doses of 5 units IV has been used to stimulate growth hormone and ACTH secretion in order to test pituitary function. Atropine can be given to minimize gastrointestinal disturbances without affecting the test. Since normal individuals may fail to respond, it has been used in conjunction with other stimuli such as insulin and pyrogen.

Adverse Reactions

When large doses of vasopressin are injected, vasoconstriction occurs, leading to some increase in blood pressure and pallor of the skin. There is also an increase in intestinal activity which may result in nausea and cramping. Women occasionally experience uterine cramps. Coronary vessels may also constrict, resulting in anginal attacks in patients with coronary atherosclerosis. These attacks may be precipitated by very small amounts, and vasopressin must be used with the greatest of care and only if absolutely necessary in such individuals.

Preparations Available

Vasopressin (Pitressin) injection, 20 units/ml, 0.5 and 1 ml ampules, for subcut or IM injection

Vasopressin (Pitressin) tannate (in peanut oil), 5 units/ml, 1 ml ampules, for IM injection

Posterior pituitary powder for nasal insufflation, 1/8 oz (3.54 gm) bottles

Lypressin (Syntopressin Spray; lysine-8 vasopressin), nasal spray, 50 units/ml, providing a dose of 5 units with each squeeze of the plastic bottle

OXYTOCIN

Oxytocin was the first polypeptide hormone to be synthesized. As shown in Fig 39–8, it is a cyclic polypeptide containing 8 amino acids and having a molecular weight of about 1000. This hormone also contains a disulfide bond and in other respects is quite similar to vasopressin. Analogues of these hormones have been produced by substitution of various groups. Desamino oxytocin, which lacks a free primary amino group in the terminal cystine residue, has 5 times the antidiuretic activity of oxytocin. Other modifications of biologic activity have been produced by changes in structure.

Oxytocin stimulates uterine smooth muscle, resulting in contraction of the uterus; it also stimulates smooth muscle of the mammary gland, causing the letdown of milk. The action of oxytocin on the uterus is conditioned by the levels of estrogens and progesterone present as well as by concentrations of ions such as calcium, magnesium, and potassium. The sensitivity of the human uterus to oxytocin increases gradually during pregnancy. It is not known whether oxytocin plays a physiologic role in stimulating the onset of labor. However, stimulation of the nipple by suckling leads to the reflex release of oxytocin which causes contraction of the smooth muscle of the mammary gland and leading to the reflex ejection of milk. If large amounts are administered, oxytocin appears to have a transient relaxing effect on the smooth muscle, resulting in a decrease in systolic and diastolic blood pressure, flushing, and increased brain blood flow. Reflex tachycardia may also occur. The chicken, a species in which this response is particularly marked, has been used to assay oxytocin.

Oxytocin has also been observed to have an insulin-like effect when incubated with the epididymal fat pad of the rat. Nothing is known of its metabolic actions in man. As is true of vasopressin also, oxytocin is destroyed when given by mouth. Vasopressin is destroyed by trypsin, whereas oxytocin is resistant to trypsin but is inactivated by chymotrypsin. It can be given by any parenteral route, including intranasal application. Once in the body, it is rapidly removed, having a half-life of less than 15 minutes. It is thought to be removed primarily by the kidney. During pregnancy, an enzyme (aminopeptidase) appears which is capable of rapidly destroying this hormone. The concentration of this enzyme increases throughout pregnancy, reaching a maximum at the time of parturition.

Clinical Uses

Oxytocin is employed in the induction of labor in pregnant women. In general, larger amounts are required earlier in pregnancy. The administration of small amounts of oxytocin is capable of stimulating apparently normal labor; however, when large amounts are given, tetanic contractions of the uterus occur.

Oxytocin is most safely administered in the form of a dilute intravenous solution containing about 10 units/liter of 5% dextrose. The solution is administered at a very slow rate which can be gradually increased until effective contractions occur. This procedure should be carried out under the supervision of a physician, with careful attention to the frequency and intensity of contractions and the effects of these contractions on the fetal heart tones. When oxytocin is used in combination with amniotomy, it is possible to induce labor in almost any patient at or near the end of pregnancy.

Oxytocin is also used after delivery to facilitate recovery of the placenta. It may also be given to enhance uterine contractions for the purpose of reducing the amount of bleeding. However, it is not usually employed in this way since the ergot derivatives (see Chapter 14) produce a rapid and long-lasting response with low toxicity.

Contraindications & Cautions

The major adverse reaction is related to the production of tetanic contractions of the uterus. However, lack of care and control of infusions occasionally leads to the administration of large amounts of water and the production of hyponatremia.

Labor should not be induced by oxytocin if there are any abnormalities of the uterus or if the patient has had previous uterine surgery, nor if the pelvic structures are too small to allow passage of the baby through the birth canal.

Preparations Available

Buccal tablets (Pitocin), 200 units/tablet

Nasal spray (Pitocin), 40 units/ml in plastic squeeze bottles, 2 and 5 ml

Injectable (subcut, IM, or IV):
  Pituitary oxytocin (Pitocin) ampules, 5 units/0.5 ml ampule and 10 units/1 ml ampule

Synthetic oxytocin (Syntocinon), 5 units/0.5 ml ampule and 10 units/1 ml ampule

• • •

General References

Bahl, O.P.: Human chorionic gonadotropin. I. Purification and physicochemical properties. J Biol Chem 244:567–574, 1969.

Bahl, O.P.: Human chorionic gonadotropin. II. Nature of the carbohydrate units. J Biol Chem 244:575–583, 1969.

Carroll, B.J., Pearson, M.J., & F.I.R. Martin: Evaluation of three acute tests of hypothalamic-pituitary-adrenal function. Metabolism 18:476–483, 1969.

Deutsch, S., & H. Mescon: Melanin pigmentation and its endocrine control. New England J Med 257:222–226, 268–272, 1957.

Douglas, R.G., Kramer, E.E., & R. Bonsnes: Oxytocin, newer knowledge and present clinical usage. Am J Obst Gynec 73:1206–1217, 1957.

Eik-Nes, K.B.: Effects of gonadotrophins on secretion of steroids by the testis and ovary. Physiol Rev 44:609–630, 1964.

Ganong, W.F., & L. Martini (editors): *Frontiers in Neuroendocrinology, 1969.* Oxford University Press, 1969.

Gemzell, C.A., Roos, P., & E.E. Loeffler: The clinical use of pituitary gonadotrophins in women. J Reprod Fertil 12:49–64, 1966.

Growth Hormone. Excerpta Medica, International Congress Series No. 158, Excerpta Medica Foundation, 1968.

Harris, G.W., & B.T. Donovan: *The Pituitary Gland.* 3 vols. *I. Anterior Pituitary. II. Anterior Pituitary. III. Pars Intermedia and Neurohypophysis.* Univ of California Press, 1966.

Hollenberg, M.D., & D.B. Hope: The isolation of the native hormone-binding proteins from bovine pituitary posterior lobes. Crystallization of neurophysin-I and -II as complexes with (8-arginine)-vasopressin. Biochem J 106:557–564, 1968.

Kleeman, C.R., & M.P. Fichman: The clinical physiology of water metabolism. New England J Med 277:1300, 1967.

Knobil, E., & J. Hotchkiss: Growth hormone. Ann Rev Physiol 26:47, 1964.

Lerner, A.A., & J.D. Case: Melatonin. Fed Proc 19:590, 1960.

Li, C.H.: Some aspects of the relation of peptide structure to activity in pituitary hormones. Vitamins & Hormones 19:313, 1961.

Li, C.H.: Current concepts on the chemical biology of pituitary hormones. Perspectives Biol Med 11:498–521, 1968.

Martini, L., & W.F. Ganong (editors): *Neuroendocrinology.* 2 vols. Academic Press, 1967.

Peake, G.T., & others: Ultrastructural, histologic and hormonal characterization of a prolactin-rich human pituitary tumor. J Clin Endocrinol 29:1383–1393, 1969.

Prader, A., & others: The metabolic effect of a small uniform dose of human growth hormone in hypopituitary dwarfs and in control children. I. Nitrogen, α-amino-N, creatine-creatinine and calcium excretion and serum urea-N, α-amino-N, inorganic phosphorus and alkaline phosphatase. Acta endocrinol 57:115–128, 1968.

Prader, A., & others: The metabolic effect of a small uniform dose of human growth hormone in hypopituitary dwarfs and control children. II. Blood glucose response to insulin-induced hypoglycaemia. Acta endocrinol 57:129–135, 1968.

Raben, M.S.: Growth hormone. 1. Physiologic aspects. 2. Clinical use of human growth hormone. New England J Med 266:31–35, 82–86, 1962.

Reichlin, S.: Neuroendocrinology. New England J Med 269:1182–1190, 1246–1250, 1296–1303, 1963.

Saffran, M.: Hypothalamic regulation of ACTH secretion. A Res Nerv Ment Dis Proc 43:36–46, 1966.

Treatment of abnormal height in children. Med Lett Drugs Ther 11(No. 4):13–14, February 21, 1969.

Part VI. Agents Used in the Treatment of Nutritional & Metabolic Derangements

40...

Drugs Used in the Treatment of Gout

Unlike most other mammals, man is unable to convert poorly soluble uric acid to allantoin because he does not possess the enzyme uricase. Since uric acid is a major metabolic end-product of amino acid metabolism (and, to a much less important extent, of purine metabolism), normal plasma and urinary uric acid levels are near the saturation point. A moderate increase in uric acid production can lead to the deposition of sodium urate microcrystals in and around the joints and in the kidneys and other tissues, and uric acid stones may form in the lumen of the urinary tract —ie, gout occurs.

The treatment of gout may be aimed at (1) relieving an acute attack of gouty arthritis or (2) reducing the serum urate concentration in order to prevent recurrent attacks of inflammatory arthritis or to lead to resorption of urate deposits. In this chapter we will discuss, correspondingly, (1) colchicine, phenylbutazone, and other drugs used in treating an acute attack of gout; (2) urate diuretics such as probenecid and sulfinpyrazone; and (3) allopurinol, an inhibitor of uric acid synthesis.

COLCHICINE

Chemistry

Colchicine is an alkaloid isolated from the meadow saffron (autumn crocus, *Colchicum autumnale*).

Colchicine

Pharmacologic Effects

Colchicine can dramatically relieve pain and bring about a decrease in the inflammatory changes of gout in 12–24 hours. Yet it does not alter the metabolism or excretion of urates and has no analgesic or anti-inflammatory action in any clinical situation other than gouty and sarcoid arthritis.

Colchicine reduces the inflammatory response to experimentally deposited microcrystals of sodium urate and alters some metabolic activities of granulocytes that are associated with phagocytosis. It is presumed to act by interfering with phagocytosis of urate crystals. Studies with derivatives of colchicine have established that the effect on mitosis, mentioned next, is not essential to its action in gout.

Colchicine is able, in the intact organism and in cultures, to arrest mitosis at metaphase. It is thus used to facilitate studies on the morphology of chromosomes and the rate of mitotic activity. It has been superseded by newer agents in cancer chemotherapy.

Clinical Uses

Colchicine is probably still the drug most often used to reduce the pain and inflammation of an attack of acute gouty arthritis, and it may also be given on a long-term basis to prevent or reduce the frequency of attacks. The specificity of the response to colchicine provides diagnostic information, but diarrhea is a common and disturbing side-effect. Phenylbutazone and indomethacin are at least as satisfactory as colchicine for the brief treatment of an acute attack, but colchicine is preferable for prolonged prophylactic use because of the greater toxicity of the nonspecific analgesics.

With the availability of drugs effective in lowering serum urate concentrations, the prolonged use of colchicine is now uncommon. Colchicine should be given concurrently with the hypouricemic agents early in treatment since the patient is vulnerable to acute attacks when the urate deposits are mobilized.

Adverse Reactions

A. Side-Effects: The important toxic effect which limits dosage is diarrhea accompanied by nausea, vomiting, and abdominal pain. These effects are systemic rather than local in origin and also follow parenteral administration.

The effect of colchicine in inhibiting mitosis is not a source of toxicity in this application.

B. Overdosage Toxicity: Acute intoxication following ingestion of large (nontherapeutic) doses of the alkaloid or its plant source is characterized by burning throat pain, bloody diarrhea, shock, hematuria and oliguria, and ascending CNS depression.

Preparations & Dosages

Tablets containing 0.5 mg are available, but 0.6 mg tablets (a carry-over of the 1/100 gr dosage of the apothecary system) are often more easily available.

For terminating an attack, the dosage is usually 1 or 1.2 mg orally initially followed by 0.5 or 0.6 mg every hour until the pain is relieved or nausea and diarrhea appear. When the need or tolerance of the patient has been previously established (usually 4–8 mg), the initial dose should be 1 mg less.

The prophylactic dose of colchicine is 0.5 mg 3 times daily.

OTHER DRUGS USED FOR ACUTE ATTACKS OF GOUT

Phenylbutazone (Butazolidin)

Phenylbutazone may be used either as initial treatment or when treatment with colchicine is unsuccessful. The toxic effects mentioned in Chapter 27 are not a problem if treatment is limited to 3 days and to an initial dose of 400 mg followed by 200 mg every 6 hours. Phenylbutazone has a slight uricosuric effect in addition to its anti-inflammatory action.

Indomethacin (Indocin)

Indomethacin is also effective but is appreciably more toxic (see Chapter 27).

Corticotropin or Corticosteroids

Prednisone or other anti-inflammatory steroid or ACTH will terminate an acute attack of gout. However, the effect is a nonspecific suppression of the inflammatory reaction which reappears when the drug is discontinued. Since colchicine or phenylbutazone will probably have to be used ultimately, treatment should be started with one of these drugs and the steroid added only if necessary.

URICOSURIC AGENTS
(Sulfinpyrazone & Probenecid)

Two drug effects can be used to control serum urate concentrations for indefinite periods in order to prevent arthritis and renal damage. The first is the increase of urinary excretion of uric acid by interference with renal tubular reabsorption. The second is the decrease of uric acid synthesis by allopurinol.

Chemistry

Uricosuric agents or urate diuretics compete with uric acid at the anionic transport sites of the renal tubule. To do this they must be organic acids. The structures of the 2 most commonly used uricosuric drugs, sulfinpyrazone and probenecid, are shown below together with that of uric acid. Sulfinpyrazone is a metabolite of an analogue of phenylbutazone (Table 27–3).

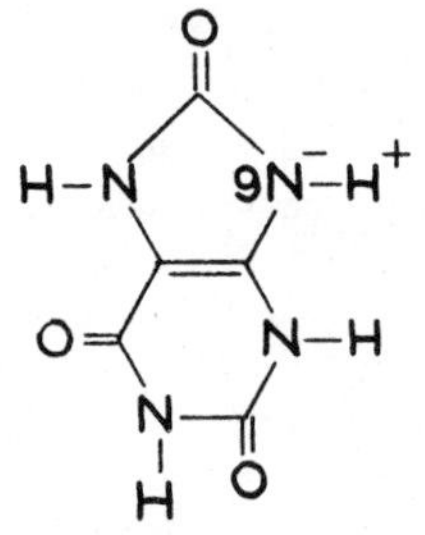

Uric Acid

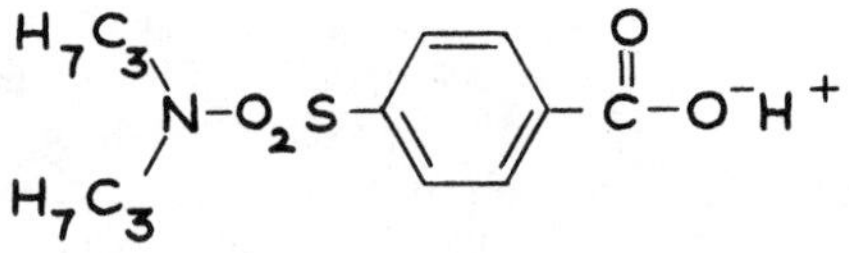

Probenecid
(Benemid)

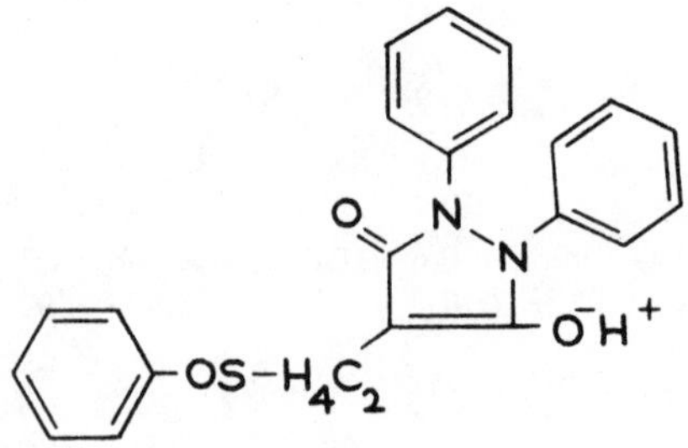

Sulfinpyrazone
(Anturane)
(enol form)

Absorption, Metabolism, & Excretion

Probenecid is completely reabsorbed by the renal tubules and very slowly metabolized. Sulfinpyrazone or its active hydroxylated derivative is rapidly excreted by the kidneys. Yet, after oral administration, the duration of its effect is almost as long as that of probenecid.

Pharmacologic Effects

A. **Mechanisms of Action**: Uric acid, like many other anions of weak acids, appears in the glomerular filtrate in a significant fraction of its concentration in plasma. It is completely reabsorbed in the proximal convolution and then secreted by another system for the transport of organic acids in the distal tubule. Another anion with a greater affinity for the carrier presumed to be involved in the tubular transport mechanism could preempt the capacity (tubular maximum) at either the reabsorbing or the secreting sites.

Small doses of uricosuric agents may preferentially reduce secretion and have a uric acid retaining effect, but therapeutic doses block reabsorption and greatly increase the urinary output of uric acid. (The salicylates are unsatisfactory agents because of the large doses required to reach a uricosuric effect; smaller doses cause a net retention of uric acid. They should not be used even as analgesics in patients with gout.)

The secretion of other organic acids—eg, PSP and penicillin—is reduced by uricosuric agents. Probenecid was developed as an agent to prolong penicillin blood levels.

The reabsorption of phosphate anion is also reduced.

B. **Effects**: As the urinary excretion of uric acid increases, the plasma level may not be greatly reduced but the size of the urate pool decreases. In patients who respond favorably, tophaceous deposits of urate will be resorbed, with relief of arthritis and remineralization of bone. With the ensuing increase in uric acid excretion, the predisposition to the formation of renal stones is augmented rather than decreased; therefore, the urine volume should be maintained at a high level and, at least early in treatment, the urine pH kept above 6.0 by the administration of alkali.

Clinical Uses

The effectiveness of probenecid and sulfinpyrazone is established not only by increased urinary excretion and somewhat lower plasma levels of uric acid but also by decreased frequency of acute arthritic attacks and by x-ray and gross observations of the depletion of urate deposits in the tissues.

Therapy should be initiated when acute attacks have occurred, when physical or x-ray evidence of tophi appear, or when plasma levels of uric acid are so high (> 8 mg/100 ml) that tissue damage is almost inevitable. Therapy should not be started until 2–3 weeks after an acute attack.

Probenecid was used in the past to block the renal tubular secretion of penicillin and reduce penicillin excretion to that amount provided by glomerular filtration. It is now more practical to merely increase the dosage of penicillin.

Adverse Reactions

Side-effects do not provide a basis for preferring one or the other of the uricosuric agents. Both of these organic acids cause gastrointestinal irritation, but sulfinpyrazone is more active in this regard and should be administered with food. Probenecid is more likely to cause allergic dermatitis, but a rash may appear after the use of either compound.

Contraindications & Cautions

The essential caution is to maintain a large urine volume to minimize the possibility of stone formation. The urine of patients with gout tends to be acid— perhaps, as one hypothesis suggests, because the synthesis of ammonia from glutamine is reduced. If urine volume can be maintained at 2 liters or more per day, the addition of alkali is not essential but is advisable early in treatment.

Initiation of treatment with the urate diuretics is believed by some physicians to be associated with an increased risk of acute arthritic attacks. This impression may be carried over from experience with the salicylates. Some physicians give colchicine (0.5 mg 3 times a day) for some weeks when beginning therapy with probenecid or sulfinpyrazone. Salicylates should not be used in combination with these drugs, since some of the uricosuric effect will be lost.

Preparations & Dosages

Probenecid (Benemid) is available as 0.5 gm scored tablets. Give 0.25 gm twice daily for 1 week and 0.5 gm twice daily thereafter. If necessary (and tolerated), the dosage may be increased in 0.5 gm increments to 2 gm/day.

Sulfinpyrazone (Anturane) is available as scored 100 mg tablets. Begin with 50 mg 4 times daily with meals and at bedtime with milk, increasing to 400 mg/day (divided as above) within 1 week. If necessary (and tolerated), dosage may be increased to 800 mg/day.

Urinary output should be maintained at 2 liters or more to prevent precipitation of uric acid in the urinary tract. In early treatment, maintain urine pH above 6.0 by administration of alkalinizing agents.

ALLOPURINOL
(Inhibitor of Uric Acid Synthesis)

An alternative to increasing uric acid excretion in the treatment of gout is to reduce its synthesis by inhibiting xanthine oxidase with allopurinol.

Chemistry

The structure of allopurinol, an isomer of hypoxanthine, is shown in Fig 40–1.

Metabolism

Allopurinol is itself acted upon by xanthine oxidase, and the resulting compound retains the ability to inhibit xanthine oxidase.

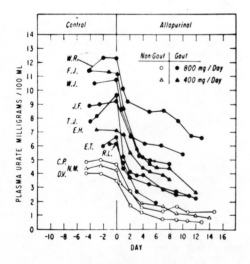

FIG 40–1. Inhibition of uric acid synthesis by allopurinol. Hypoxanthine (from inosine) or xanthine (from guanine) is converted to uric acid by aerobic oxidation. Xanthine oxidase is inhibited by allopurinol and its metabolite alloxanthine.

Pharmacologic Effects

A. Mechanisms of Action: Dietary purines are a comparatively unimportant source of uric acid. The quantitatively important fractions of purines are formed from amino acids, formate, and CO_2 in the body. Those purine ribonucleotides not incorporated into nucleic acids and those derived from the degradation of nucleic acids are converted to xanthine or hypoxanthine and oxidized to uric acid. When this last step is inhibited by allopurinol, there is a fall in the plasma urate level and a decrease in the size of the urate pool (Fig 40–2).

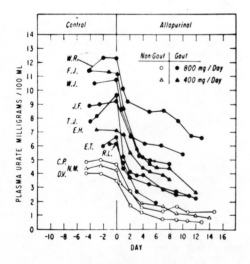

FIG 40–2. The effect of allopurinol on the concentration of urate in plasma of gouty and normal subjects. (Reproduced, with permission, from Klinenberg & others: The effectiveness of the xanthine oxidase inhibitor allopurinol in the treatment of gout. Ann Int Med 62:643, 1965.)

B. Effects: The only pharmacologic effects of allopurinol are those that result from inhibition of uric acid synthesis. Serum uric acid levels begin to fall immediately, and normal or subnormal levels are reached in 7–10 days. Resorption of tophaceous deposits is gradual, but is usually impressive within 6–12 months.

Clinical Uses

Treatment with allopurinol, as with the uricosuric agents, is begun with the expectation that it will be continued for many years if not for life. One of the indications or predictors of damage listed above should be present before treatment is initiated.

Whether allopurinol or one of the uricosuric agents is selected is a matter of individual preference. Both are effective and relatively safe. Allopurinol is a newer agent, and some investigators continue to express concern about the possible toxicity of an agent that causes such interesting biochemical changes.

Allopurinol clearly would be preferable (1) when probenecid or sulfinpyrazone cannot be used because of side-effects or allergic reactions; (2) when the uricosuric agents are providing a less than optimal therapeutic effect; (3) in patients whose renal function is sufficiently impaired so that urate excretion is limited; (4) in patients with gouty nephropathy or attacks of renal colic during uricosuric treatment; and (5) when plasma uric acid levels are or threaten to become greatly elevated. This elevation may occur with severe primary gout, or the hyperuricemia may follow the use of cytotoxic drugs or radiation therapy in the treatment of leukemias (secondary gout).

Adverse Reactions

After effective doses of allopurinol, the patient becomes equivalent to a subject with xanthinuria. Urinary xanthine levels are elevated, but xanthine stones or crystals have not yet been reported. No decrease in alcohol tolerance or changes in iron metabolism have been reported, although these could conceivably have followed xanthine oxidase inhibition.

A. Side-Effects: Acute attacks of gouty arthritis occur early in treatment with allopurinol when urate crystals are being withdrawn from the tissues and plasma levels are below normal. To prevent acute attacks, colchicine should be given during the initial period of therapy with allopurinol unless allopurinol is being used in combination with probenecid or sulfinpyrazone.

B. Allergic Reactions: As many as 3% of patients develop a pruritic maculopapular rash. A type of allergic reaction similar to drug fever occurs less commonly. Isolated cases of exfoliative dermatitis have been reported.

Preparations & Dosages

Allopurinol (Zyloprim) is available as scored 100 mg tablets. The initial dose is 50 mg 2−3 times daily. Increase the dose over a period of 2−3 weeks to 200−400 mg/day in 2 or 3 divided doses.

Colchicine, 0.5 mg twice daily, should be given also during the first few weeks of therapy.

●　　●　　●

General References

Goldfinger SE: Drug therapy: Treatment of gout. New England J Med 285:1303−1306, 1971.

Gutman, A.B., & T.F. Yü: Uric acid metabolism in normal man and in primary gout. New England J Med 273:252−258, 313−320, 1965.

Krakoff, I.H.: Clinical pharmacology of drugs which influence uric acid production and excretion. Clin Pharmacol Therap 8:124−138, 1967.

Muggia, F.M., Ball, T.J., Jr., & J.E. Ultmann: Allopurinol in the treatment of neoplastic disease complicated by hyperuricemia. Arch Int Med 120:12−18, 1967.

Rundles, R.W., Metz, E.N., & H.R. Silberman: Allopurinol in the treatment of gout. Ann Int Med 64:229−258, 1966.

Scott, J.T.: Symposium on allopurinol. Ann Rheumat Dis 25:599−718, 1966.

Velayos, E.E., & C.J. Smyth: Urate diuretic therapy in chronic gout. A comparative study of probenecid and sulfinpyrazone. Arch Int Med 116:212−219, 1965.

Wilson, G.M., Jr., Huffman, E.R., & C.J. Smyth: Oral phenylbutazone in the treatment of acute gouty arthritis. Am J Med 21:232−236, 1956.

Yü T.F., & A.B. Gutman: Efficacy of colchicine prophylaxis in gout: Prevention of recurrent gouty arthritis over a mean period of five years in 208 gouty subjects. Ann Int Med 55:179−192, 1961.

41 . . .

Vitamins & Other Therapeutic Nutritional Agents

This chapter will discuss vitamins as therapeutic agents and the reduction of atherosclerosis, a metabolic disease treated by diet as well as by hypolipidemic drugs.

THE VITAMINS

The skeptical and negative attitude with which many people now approach the discussion of vitamins as therapeutic agents suggests to others either that they do not appreciate the importance of vitamins or they are callously forgetting that not all populations are overfed. Let us begin, therefore, by acknowledging the biochemical importance of the vitamins and the great contribution to human welfare that has been made by those who have elucidated the role of vitamins in nutrition.

However, the function of this section is not to review the biochemistry of vitamins but to discuss vitamins as drugs used in humans. Several vitamins with specific, well understood therapeutic functions are discussed elsewhere in this book. Cyanocobalamin (vitamin B_{12}), folic acid, the K vitamins, and vitamin D have already been discussed. The problem with the therapeutic applications of the remaining vitamins is that the need is mostly to argue against their use except in the form of natural foodstuffs. The important exceptions of infants, some pregnant women, and those rare individuals suffering from vitamin deficiencies will not be ignored, but the burden of this discussion is to evaluate the promiscuous and unestablished uses of vitamins. The intention is not to deprecate nutritional studies. On the contrary, preoccupation with the vitamins has probably delayed our understanding of other areas of nutritional therapy—eg, the treatment of atherosclerosis.

For each vitamin, certain information is needed to judge the advisability or necessity of its supplementation in the diet. The most important of these factors is the daily requirement. The data on a representative water-soluble vitamin and a representative fat-soluble vitamin will be examined in detail in order to provide information against which certain suggested minimum daily requirements can be measured.

VITAMIN A

The fat-soluble vitamins, of which vitamin A is a convenient example, have several characteristics in common. They may occur in plant tissues either as the vitamin or as a provitamin, but in animals they are concentrated in a few tissues. Their absorption parallels that of other fats, and deficiencies may occur during interference with fat absorption—eg, the deficiency of vitamin K with hypoprothrombinemia that occurs during obstructive jaundice. Fat-soluble vitamins are stored in the liver and to a lesser extent in other fatty tissues. The stores are large, and utilization or excretion extremely slow.

Source & Chemistry

Vitamin A is provided by butterfat, eggs, liver, and, to a lesser extent, by other meats. Precursors of vitamin A, the carotenoid pigments, are present in large amounts in colored vegetables and fruits and are converted, although inefficiently, to vitamin A in the intestinal mucosa.

Human Requirement

Early in World War II, the governments of the USA and Great Britain became concerned with possible nutritional deficiency in the civilian population and attempted to establish minimum daily requirements. In the USA the effort was made by a committee of the National Research Council (NRC). Although the report of the committee was labeled as conjectural, the high allowances it reported provided an authoritative basis for the exploitation of fears of undernutrition. In 1955, presumably because of misuse of the recommendations, the Food & Nutrition Board decided to withhold further printing of the report. However, a revised report with essentially the same allowances was recently published.

The British effort involved the collection of new data, and this experience will be discussed here and in the section on vitamin C to show that the theoretical allowances are unreasonably high. Twenty-three conscientious objectors were isolated and placed on a diet lacking butter, whole milk, liver, fat, fish, and all colored vegetables. The trial was continued for 14 months, at which time only 3 of the volunteers showed changes in dark adaptation greater than the seasonal variation seen in control subjects on a diet adequate in vitamin A. This minor change was effectively treated with 1300 units of vitamin A per day—ie, the therapeutic dose appears to be 1300 units or less per day even though the NRC maintenance allowance has been placed at 5000 units/day. Plasma carotenoids disappeared within a few weeks on the above diet, but the mean plasma vitamin A content fell less than 30% during the 14 months. Thus, vitamin A stores in the body are adequate to meet the needs of humans for extended periods without supplementary vitamins.

Vitamin A deficiency does occur in malnourished children in tropical countries of Southeast Asia, Latin America, Africa, and the Middle East. In very young children, the corneal epithelium may be irreversibly damaged (xerophthalmia), and an associated susceptibility to infection leads to many deaths.

Toxicity

The indiscriminate use of vitamin A, unlike the use of most vitamins, cannot be justified on the basis that it at least does no harm. Toxic reactions have occurred in children given large amounts of high-potency oils by their mothers and in adults who have taken unusually large amounts because of the alleged anti-infective action of an excess of the vitamin or some other faddist concept. In studies of possible pharmacologic actions of vitamin A, toxicity has been therapeutically induced. In children, the important toxicity consists of cortical (subperiosteal) hyperostosis and interference with bone growth. In adults, changes include dry, itching, scaling skin, hyperkeratosis, and altered liver function, but no bone changes or alterations in calcium dynamics.

VITAMIN E

A variety of heavy oils, the tocopherols, possess vitamin E activity. α-Tocopherol, the synthetic form used as a dietary supplement, is given in the form of the stable acetate which is converted in the body to the free alcohol that is the active form of the vitamin. The richest sources of tocopherols are vegetable oils, especially wheat germ oil, but they are so widely distributed in common foods that a dietary deficiency is probably impossible except transiently in the newborn. However, defects in absorption are possible.

Deficiency State in Humans

The effect of vitamin E deficiency in animals varies widely with the species studied. In humans, vitamin E deficiency has been associated in a few cases with anemia which is presumed to be due either to hemolysis or to interference with heme synthesis.

Administration of vitamin E prevents an experimental porphyria in rats and, according to one report, is effective in the treatment of porphyria cutanea tarda. Abnormal amounts of precursors of heme (ALA, porphobilinogen, porphyrins) are excreted in these conditions, suggesting that the anemia of vitamin E deficiency is due to a block in heme synthesis.

Vitamin E is also able to protect the erythrocyte against peroxide-induced hemolysis. If erythrocytes from deficient animals or humans are exposed to hydrogen peroxide, the cell membrane is altered and hemolysis occurs in a larger fraction of the cells than in a sample from a normal subject. Vitamin E, either fed or added in vitro, protects against the hemolysis. In the presence of steatorrhea, depletion of tocopherol can be demonstrated and the red cells of a fraction of these patients will be unusually susceptible to peroxide hemolysis. In a few premature infants, vitamin E deficiency with edema and hemolytic anemia has occurred in association with the use of a formula containing large amounts of polyunsaturated fats, which increases the requirement of vitamin E, and added iron, which interferes with its absorption.

Human Requirement

The nominal human requirements are based on the amounts of vitamin E found in an adequate diet and not on any dietary or careful therapeutic trials. In the presence of impaired fat absorption, the requirement appears to be more than 15 IU/day of α-tocopherol. (An international unit is the activity of 1 mg of DL-α-tocopherol acetate.)

ASCORBIC ACID
(Vitamin C)

Ascorbic acid and the B vitamins are water-soluble. Interference with the absorption of the water-soluble vitamins is not a problem, but rediffusion into the intestinal lumen (as may occur during diarrhea) and excretion by the kidney can remove significant amounts. The water-soluble vitamins are distributed more uniformly throughout the tissues, and there are no large depots such as that of vitamin A in the liver. The water-soluble vitamins are therefore more rapidly depleted than the fat-soluble vitamins. The rapidity of the process and the amount of supplementation required are probably less than is generally stated.

Source & Chemistry

Vitamin C is present in significant amounts in all fruits and vegetables. Foods of animal origin, with the exception of milk, are not important sources of vitamin C. Ascorbic acid is stable only when in acid solution and protected from air; it is destroyed by heating in contact with oxygen. Fruits maintain their vitamin C content. Vegetables lose their vitamin C content during storage unless they are "living foods" such as potatoes or bananas—ie, plants whose cells continue metabolic activity during storage. Frozen and canned

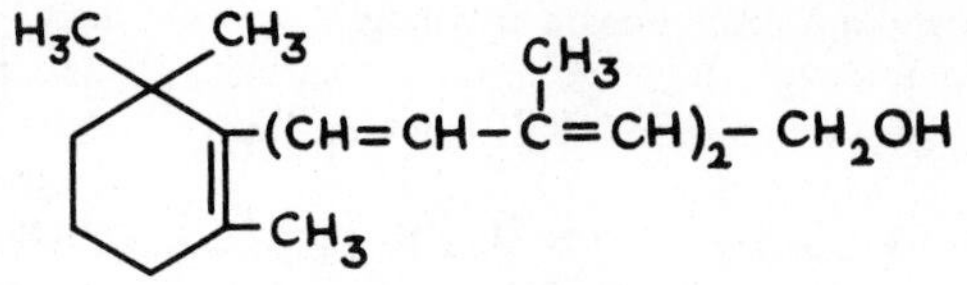

Vitamin A₁
(alcohol)

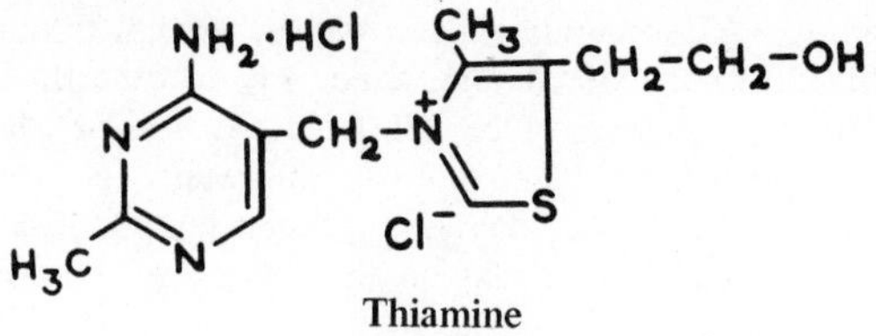

Thiamine
(vitamin B₁)

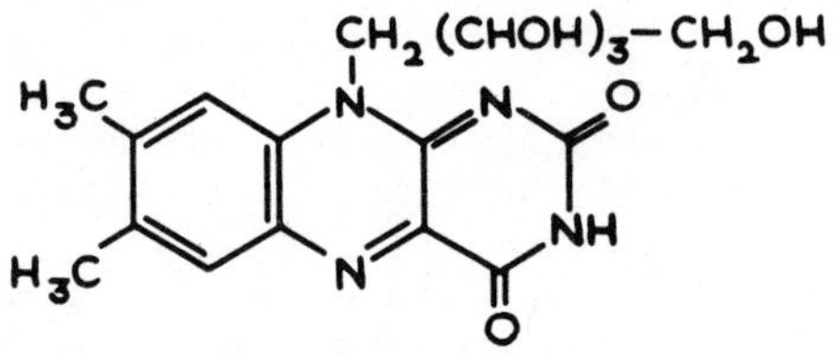

Riboflavin
(vitamin B₂)

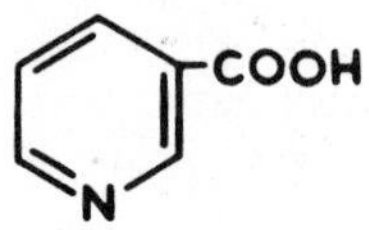

Niacin
(nicotinic acid)

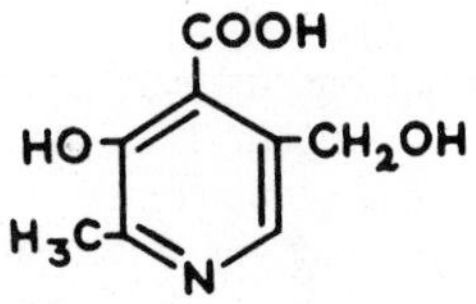

Pyridoxine
(vitamin B₆)

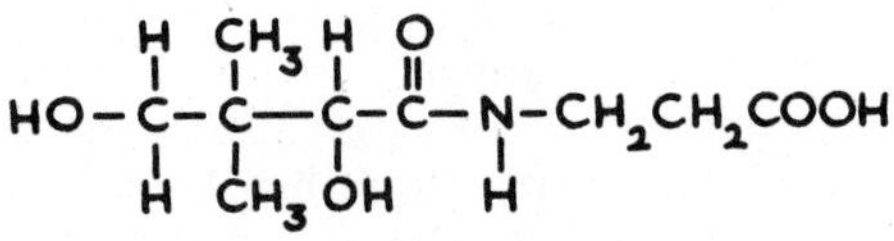

Pantothenic
acid

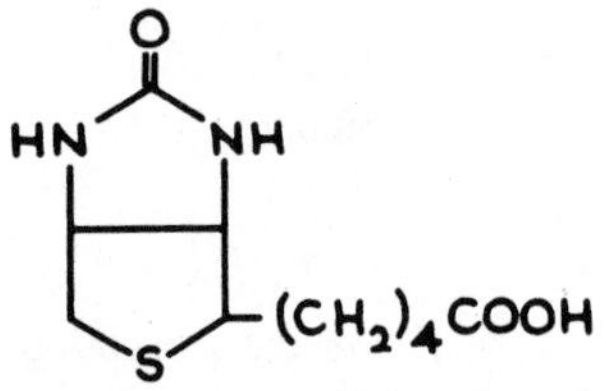

Biotin

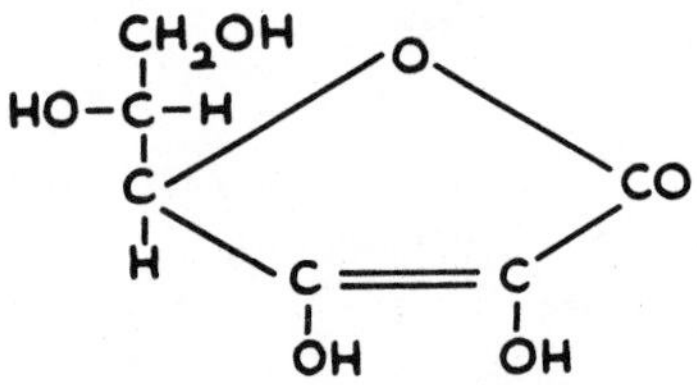

Ascorbic acid (vitamin C)—
Synthesized by all mammals
except guinea pigs and primates

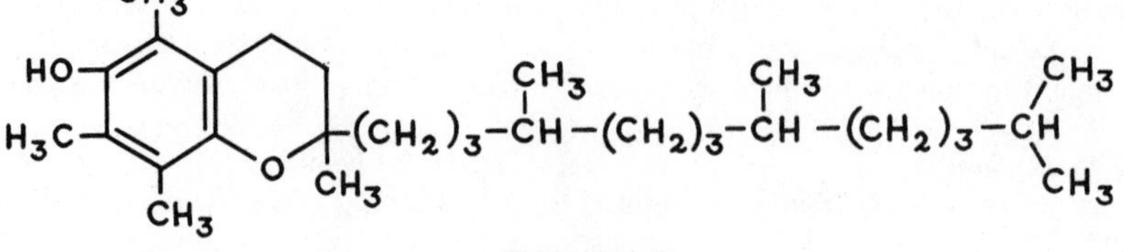

α-Tocopherol
(β- and γ-tocopherols
are also active)

FIG 41–1. Vitamins essential to or probably essential to human nutrition.

TABLE 41-1. Vitamins essential or probably essential to human nutrition.

Vitamin*	Action	Deficiency Symptoms	Sources	RDA†
Vitamin A (A$_1$ and A$_2$)	Constituents of visual pigments; maintain epithelia.	Night blindness, hyperkeratosis	Colored vegetables and fruit	5000 IU
B complex Thiamine (B$_1$)	Coenzyme for pyruvate decarboxylation and in hexose monophosphate shunt	Beriberi, neuritis	Liver, unrefined cereal grains	1.4 mg
Riboflavin (B$_2$)	Constituent of riboflavin adenine dinucleotide (FAD)	Glossitis	Liver, milk	1.7 mg
Niacin	Constituent of NAD	Pellagra	Yeast, lean meat, liver	18 mg
Pyridoxine (B$_6$)	Forms prosthetic group of decarboxylases and transaminases. Converted in body to pyridoxal phosphate and pyridoxamine phosphate.	Convulsions, hyperirritability	Yeast, wheat, corn, liver	2 mg
Pantothenic acid	Constituent of Co A	Burning feet syndrome in man (?)		None established
Biotin	Catalyzes CO_2 "fixation" (in fatty acid synthesis, etc)	Dermatitis, enteritis in animals	Egg yolk, liver, tomatoes	None established
Vitamin C	Role in collagen synthesis and other unknown actions	Scurvy	Fruits and vegetables	60 mg
Vitamin E		Hemolytic anemia in man	Milk, eggs, meat, leafy vegetables, wheat germ	30 IU

*Cyanocobalamin (vitamin B$_{12}$) and folic acid are discussed in Chapter 44; vitamin K in Chapter 18; and the D vitamins in Chapter 36.
†Recommended Daily Allowances for adult men, Food and Nutrition Board, NAS-NRC, revised 1968.

vegetables vary in their content of ascorbic acid but usually contain useful amounts.

Human Requirement

A. In Infants: Scurvy can occur at any age, but the needs of the very young will be considered separately since there is no disagreement about the need for vitamin C supplementation. The extremely rare cases of scurvy seen today occur most often between the ages of 7 months and 2 years.

Breast milk contains vitamin C in adequate amounts. Commercial (powdered) formulas contain added vitamin C, but the amount preserved or destroyed depends upon the extent of heating during preparation. It is, therefore, standard practice to add supplementary ascorbate to the diet until the infant is eating fresh or commercially canned or frozen fruits or vegetables and "living foods" such as bananas. A solution of ascorbic acid or a preparation containing several other vitamins may be added drop-wise to the formula *after* sterilization, or multivitamin drops may be given orally.

B. In Adults: Scurvy does occur in adult primates, but the decision about when supplementation is indicated should be based on information on how long a period of deprivation is required to produce scurvy and what the minimum daily requirement is. The NRC allowance of 60 mg may be compared with the figure derived from a human experiment. Under double-blind conditions, volunteers (conscientious objectors) were

placed in several groups. All received a diet that contained no more than 1 mg/day of ascorbic acid.

One group of 7 subjects received a supplement of 10 mg/day of vitamin C and showed no abnormalities after 160 days, and 4 of these were continued on the trial for 14 months without the appearance of abnormal signs.

A group of 10 subjects received no vitamin C supplementation. The subjects in this group developed hyperkeratosis and enlargement of the hair follicles after 17–21 weeks of deprivation. After 26–34 weeks, perifollicular hemorrhages were seen; after 30–38 weeks, swelling and bleeding from the gums occurred. The effect on wound healing was assayed by observing the healing of standardized incisions made on the thigh down to the fascia lata. Only after 7 months on the experimental diet did old scars become livid and new scars heal poorly. The other expected or classical signs of scurvy were not demonstrated. It should be noted that 100 days elapsed between the disappearance of vitamin C from the plasma and the appearance of symptoms—ie, biochemical and clinical criteria of deficiency are not the same. All of the changes regressed in 1–2 weeks in response to 10 mg/day of ascorbic acid with the exception of the gum changes, which required 10–14 weeks.

Both the maintenance and the therapeutic dose of ascorbic acid appear to be less than 10 mg/day rather than the much larger amounts suggested by the NRC.

The usefulness of supplementary ascorbic acid has not been established. Vitamin C, alone or in combination with the flavonoids, does not reduce the incidence or duration of colds or provide any other measurable benefit when tested in controlled studies involving groups as diverse as young athletes and aged patients Two qualifications must be added pending further information: (1) It is possible that supplementary ascorbic acid may favorably influence bacterial pharyngitis and tonsillitis, and (2) the requirement for ascorbate is increased postoperatively, especially if inflammation is prominent, and amounts as large as 300 mg/day may be necessary to establish biochemical repair. However, no relationship between the biochemical defect—ie, decreased levels of ascorbate—and defective wound healing has been established, although the adverse effect of true ascorbic acid deficiency on wound healing is well established. The role of vitamin C in wound healing is presumably related to the importance of the vitamin in collagen formation; vitamin C is essential for the conversion of proline to hydroxyproline in a protein precursor of collagen.

OTHER WATER-SOLUBLE VITAMINS

1. THIAMINE
(Vitamin B$_1$)

Thiamine deficiency occurs in 2 widely different situations. It may occur in populations subjected to real nutritional deficiency, or in groups that still use polished rice as a staple food—ie, discard all but the starch-containing portion—to the exclusion of other foods. (The daily requirement of thiamine is proportionate to the amount of carbohydrate metabolized.)

It may also occur in an occasional chronic alcoholic patient who derives most of his caloric need from alcohol and the sugar in fortified wine. These patients may develop cardiac (wet) beriberi with high output congestive failure, Wernicke's encephalopathy (cerebral beriberi), or Korsakoff's psychosis due to thiamine deficiency. The peripheral neuropathy also seen (dry beriberi) is less clearly related to thiamine deficiency.

Vitamin deficiencies are often multiple in the above situations, and treatment should provide supplements of more than just thiamine.

2. NIACIN
(Nicotinic Acid)

Nicotinic acid is converted to nicotinic acid amide in the body or may be ingested as the amide. Nicotinic acid amide is incorporated into nicotinamide adenine dinucleotide (NAD, DPN). Niacin and niacinamide are the official names in the USA.

The deficiency state associated with niacin is pellagra. Niacin can be synthesized in the body from tryptophan. Epidemic pellagra, now controlled, therefore occurred only in the southern USA and a few other areas (Egypt, South Africa) where corn, which is virtually free of tryptophan, was a staple in the diet. Sporadic pellagra is extremely rare; dietary sources of tryptophan or niacin are abundant; in fact, in many countries several times the minimum daily requirement is present in the beans and coffee consumed.

Secondary pellagra, with dermatitis (but not necessarily the expected triad including diarrhea and dementia), has been reported rarely in association with isoniazid therapy, carcinoid syndrome, and Hartnup's disease.

Niacin and niacinamide have been used for nonnutritional or pharmacologic effects in 3 situations without demonstrated efficacy in any of them:

(1) Nicotinic acid (but not the amide) is a vasodilator. Except when large doses are given intravenously, its action is limited to the skin, causing a flush and an intense feeling of warmth. No beneficial action on the cerebral or peripheral circulation has been shown.

(2) The action of nicotinic acid in lowering blood lipid levels is discussed below.

(3) Niacinamide or NAD has been used in the treatment of schizophrenia and drug-induced hallucinatory states, and nicotinic acid is used in the treatment of alcoholism. The effectiveness claimed initially has not been verified by controlled studies.

3. PYRIDOXINE
(Vitamin B$_6$)

Dietary Deficiency

The pyridoxine deficiency state cannot ordinarily be produced by dietary restriction, its demonstration requiring the use of a competitive antagonist, deoxypyridoxine, or depletion with an amine as described below. In one incident or brief epidemic, infants maintained on a proprietary formula lacking pyridoxine (and perhaps because of the particular fat added) exhibited irritability and even convulsions relieved by supplemental pyridoxine.

Pyridoxine Depletion by Isoniazid

When this vitamin is used as a drug, it is administered in the form of pyridoxine, an alcohol (Table 41–1). It is converted in the body to pyridoxal and functions as a coenzyme in the form of pyridoxal phosphate. Aldehydes such as pyridoxal can react with compounds that are amines to form Schiff bases which may be stable. (See reaction below.)

Isoniazid (isonicotinic acid hydrazide) given chronically can deplete the organism of pyridoxal by increasing its excretion, presumably by the reaction shown below. Peripheral or even optic neuritis can

$$R_1-\overset{\overset{\displaystyle H}{|}}{C}=O \ + \ H_2N-R_2 \rightleftharpoons R_1-\overset{\overset{\displaystyle H}{|}}{C}=N-R_2 \ + \ H_2O$$

result. If more than 5 mg/kg/day of isoniazid is administered, pyridoxine, 50 or 100 mg daily, should be given.

Pyridoxine-Responsive Anemias

These rare anemias are hypochromic microcytic anemias accompanied by hyperferremia and hemosiderosis. Large doses of pyridoxine (50–200 mg IM daily) elevate hemoglobin to normal, but the cells remain hypochromic and small. No other signs of pyridoxine deficiency appear.

4. FLAVONOIDS

The flavonoids or vitamin P are of interest in relation to the question of how drug efficacy is evaluated rather than because of any nutritional effect. These compounds are yellow plant pigments with a distribution similar to that of vitamin C. From animal experiments it was concluded that in scurvy they are able to correct capillary fragility more effectively than vitamin C alone. This tentative conclusion was extended to provide indications for their use in many forms of vascular disease and bleeding and in the prevention of colds. When the reevaluation of the efficacy of drugs first marketed in the USA between 1938 and 1962 was begun by the Food & Drug Administration and its outside advisors, these were the first drugs to be ordered withdrawn from the market. At the time, more than 200 prescription and over-the-counter preparations were in use.

GENERAL CONSIDERATIONS IN THE USE OF VITAMINS

"Subclinical Deficiencies"

Recognizable vitamin deficiencies are extremely rare. However, it is conceivable that persistent slight deficiencies might impair bodily functions before the overt signs of deficiency appear, and the claim is constantly made that routine vitamin supplementation is beneficial to health. If these claims are justified, it should be possible to support them by objective evidence under controlled experimental conditions—ie, the criteria of effectiveness should be the same as for any other drug. The fact is that no beneficial effects from multivitamin supplementation have been shown in trials that include placebo control groups. Groups of

senile patients in a rest home and groups of steel workers, to select very diverse examples, have been used in trials of this kind. In the latter case, the work records, absenteeism, subjective reports, and slit-lamp examination of the eyes did not show any difference between vitamin-supplemented and placebo control groups.

Trials with groups of older patients show that the usual "stigmas" of vitamin deficiency cannot be accepted as evidence of deficiency unless control groups receiving adequate nutrition are shown not to develop the same signs as a result of aging or other causes. Thickening of the bulbar conjunctivas, cheilosis, corneal vascularization, sublingual purpura, and glossodynia are examples of signs that occur independently of the nutritional status and are not altered by treatment with vitamins.

A Biochemical Fallacy

Chemical determinations and nutritional surveys can contribute to the impression that subclinical vitamin deficiencies are a widespread health problem if clinical defects are not used as one criterion of deficiency. If plasma levels of a vitamin, values for excretion products, or even calculated dietary intakes are tabulated for a specific group, the values will be normally distributed and reflect the normal dietary pattern established by cultural and economic factors acting on the group; however, they do not establish minimal or optimal standards. Subjects falling outside of the usual range of variation may be labeled as vitamin deficient, but this does not establish that a deficiency important to the individual exists unless verified by clinical data.

Effects of Real Dietary Deprivation

From the foregoing it may be inferred that most of the vitamins prescribed in our overfed culture are wasted. This conclusion is reinforced by the observation that vitamin deficiency accounts for very little of the difficulty even when dietary restriction is extreme. Consider, for example, an incident in western Holland at the end of World War II. This population, conditioned by wartime restrictions, was isolated for 6–10 months between the German withdrawal and the Allied occupation. The diet was 1000 calories/day (500 if the individual was unable to forage). Five percent of the population developed serious malnutrition, as evidenced by the fact that 10% of the patients admitted to hospitals died. These emaciated, exhausted people showed no signs of vitamin deficiency except, occasionally, redness and tenderness of the top of the tongue, possibly due to nicotinic acid deficiency.

Prisoners of war repatriated from the Far East did show signs of vitamin deficiency after their long imprisonment, but even in these cases much of the "beriberi" was unresponsive to thiamine and represented protein deficiency.

The results of dietary deprivation in the very young also emphasize the greater importance of protein and total calories rather than vitamins. Undernutrition—ie, deficiency of total calories—in an infant leads to marasmus. The child shows terrible atrophy of muscular and subcutaneous tissues, and growth stops; but organ structure and function and even behavior are less affected.

Protein deficiency in the growing child, usually with some caloric restriction, is seen in many tropical countries beset by poverty and ignorance of nutrition. It is most often called kwashiorkor. Growth and nutrition are arrested; the child is apathetic and anorexic; decreased plasma protein and edema are present; the skin is atrophic and shows hyperkeratosis and pigmentation not distributed in such a way as to suggest pellagra; and the liver is fatty. Vitamin A deficiency may coexist, but no vitamin deficiency is of importance compared to the deficiency of essential amino acids.

When Are Vitamins Indicated?

The ordinary diet in our western culture is more than adequate in quality and amount, and supplementary vitamins have already been added to many staple foods—especially milk, bread, and cereals. Deficiency states will occur only in the presence of a specific disease, during the use of some specific drug, or when alcoholism or other aberrant behavior has led, as it sometimes does, to a deficient diet. Vitamins should be used as other drugs are used—when specific indications are present—and should not be used as tonics or placebos. The danger of indiscriminate use of vitamins does not lie in the extremely rare toxic effect nor even the expense involved, but in the manner in which they may delay or prevent the understanding and treatment of the complaint of the patient. For example, in the treatment of fatigability or other symptoms of neurotic anxiety, the use of vitamins as a "tonic" or simply to provide some positive action may reinforce the patient's conviction that some organic problem is present.

Vitamin Supplementation in Pregnant & Lactating Women

Vitamin supplements have been almost routinely provided as part of prenatal care, but no evidence has accumulated to suggest that they have a favorable effect on the health of the mother or the newborn. For reasons discussed below, the only routine dietary supplements required are iron, calcium, and perhaps, in some communities, folic acid.

Staple foods and infant foods are now enriched with iodine (a most important nutritional factor during pregnancy), vitamins, and even iron. It is customary to justify supplementary vitamins by reasoning that they at least do no harm. However, there is evidence that hypercalcemia and permanent damage may be induced in a few infants by the amounts of vitamin D provided in fortified foods, and less substantial evidence connects excessive intake of vitamin D during pregnancy with congenital heart defects. The British government has acted to reduce the potency of vitamin D supplements. Drastic vitamin deficiencies, often induced with antimetabolites rather than by dietary means, can cause congenital defects in laboratory animals, but there is no epidemiologic evidence associating any diet pattern with the incidence of congenital defects in humans.

The definition of "quality" in the diets of pregnant women is incomplete, but protein content is probably more important than vitamins.

Preparations Available

Preparations of single vitamins are available, and there are indications for the use of a few of them—eg, ascorbic acid in infants, pyridoxine during isoniazid therapy, and perhaps thiamine early in the treatment of malnutrition associated with chronic alcoholism. Usually, however, a preparation containing many vitamins is preferable. Official preparations based on the recommended maintenance and therapeutic allowances are established, and there are many equivalent preparations. Specific preparations or retailers may be suggested, but there is no need to prescribe in the usual way since even the preparations of single vitamins are available without prescription and are less expensive when so ordered.

Vitamin A is not given by itself. Vitamin D is discussed in Chapter 36.

Ascorbic acid:
    Tablets, 25, 30, 50, 100, 250, and 500 mg
    Chewable tablets, 30, 50, 100, 250, and 500 mg
    Capsules, 250 and 500 mg
    Wafers, lozenges, troches, 100 mg
    Solution (drops), 50 mg/0.6 ml, 50 ml; and 100 mg/ml (2.5 mg/drop), 10 and 50 ml
    Injectable (IM, IV, or subcut):
        50 mg/ml, 2 ml
        100 mg/ml, 1, 2, 5, and 10 ml
        200 mg/ml, 5 and 10 ml
        250 mg/ml, 2 and 30 ml
        500 mg/ml, 1 and 2 ml

Pyridoxine:
    Tablets, 5, 10, 25, 50, and 100 mg
    Injectable (IM or IV), 50 mg/ml, 1, 5, 10, and 30 ml; 100 mg/ml, 1, 5, 10, and 30 ml

Thiamine:
    Tablets, 5, 10, 25, 50, 100, and 250 mg
    Elixir, 0.25 mg/5 ml and 2.25 mg/5 ml
    Injectable (IM or IV), 50 mg/ml, 10 ml; 100 mg/ml, 1, 2, 5, 10, and 30 ml; and 200 mg/ml, 30 ml

Nicotinic Acid: See p 419.

TREATMENT OF HYPERLIPIDEMIA & ATHEROSCLEROSIS

The intense interest in hyperlipidemia and in methods for lowering the concentration of lipids in the plasma is due to the overwhelming importance of atherosclerotic arterial disease as a cause of mortality and morbidity.

Atherosclerosis is a disease of arteries rather than of arterioles (as in hypertension) and can lead to occlusion of coronary, cerebral, and other peripheral arteries. Atherosclerotic lesions develop from the intimal and subintimal deposition of lipid material. Initially the composition of the lipids deposited resembles that of plasma lipids, and it is generally held that lipids are deposited in atherosclerotic plaques by filtration from plasma.

The distribution of the lesions is patchy rather than uniform, and the process shows a predilection for areas of tortuosity and turbulent flow—eg, the sharply branching coronary arteries. The mechanical factors are mentioned as a reminder that hypertension accelerates the progression of atherosclerosis. Restoration of a normal blood pressure in a hypertensive patient (Chapter 12) is an important factor in controlling atherosclerosis.

As the atherosclerotic plaque ages, the composition of the included lipids changes and fibrosis and calcification occur. However, the process is more or less reversible even late in its course—ie, there is a hopeful basis for treatment.

THE PREDICTIVE VALUE OF HYPERLIPIDEMIA

Many large-scale prospective studies, some lasting for as long as 20 years, have shown a strong positive correlation between the plasma level of cholesterol and excess mortality and morbidity due to coronary artery disease. The relationship is graded—ie, as levels rise progressively from 200 mg/100 ml, the risk doubles at 250 mg/100 ml and is fourfold at 280 mg/100 ml.

If serum cholesterol is lowered by caloric restriction and a diet high in unsaturated fats, a small lowering results in a substantial gain—eg, a 15% decrement in cholesterol level decreases the risk 35%.

To be successful, the dietary regimen requires a degree of patient cooperation that is rarely possible or achieved, and a drug with effects equivalent to the diet would have great practical advantages.

The Hyperlipidemias

Serum cholesterol and triglyceride determinations are inexpensive and suitable for following the results of treatment, especially in large studies such as those mentioned above. These water-insoluble substances are transported in the plasma as components of different lipoproteins. These lipoproteins may be described on the basis of their behavior in the ultracentrifuge or their electrophoretic mobility, or they may be chemically analyzed.

This discussion will refer to (1) VLDL—very low density lipoproteins, pre-β-lipoproteins, rich in triglycerides; and (2) LDL—low density lipoproteins, β-lipoproteins, cholesterol-rich lipoproteins.

The hyperlipidemias may be a primary entity or may occur secondary to some other pathologic state.

Plasma lipids may be elevated secondary to the altered lipid metabolism of diabetic ketosis, hypothyroidism, the nephrotic syndrome, biliary obstruction, or acute alcoholism. Treatment of these secondary hyperlipidemias is aimed at the underlying disease, but drugs may be used—eg, cholestyramine in biliary obstruction.

The major clinical features of the primary hyperlipidemias are summarized in Table 41–2.

The balance of this discussion (except as otherwise noted) refers to type IV, the common endogenous hyperlipemia.

DIETARY TREATMENT

The hazards of untreated hypertension and of cigarette smoking have already been mentioned. Dietary therapy should also precede the use of hypocholesterolemic drugs.

Weight Reduction

Treatment should begin with caloric restriction, a procedure of established efficacy.

Diet Low in Cholesterol & Saturated Fats

To achieve gains beyond those of caloric restriction, dietary restriction must be rigid and is usually so burdensome that patient cooperation becomes a problem. Initially at least, 40% of the calories should be derived from fat, and as much as 75% of these should be from unsaturated fats—ie, a diet low in saturated fats cannot be achieved by increasing carbohydrate intake. Such a diet requires avoidance of meat, eggs, and dairy products.

DRUG TREATMENT

1. CLOFIBRATE
(Atromid-S)

Drugs may be used to supplement the effects of dietary treatment. The long-term benefits of the chemical changes induced by hypocholesterolemic drugs

TABLE 41-2. Major clinical features of primary hyperlipidemias.

Hyper-lipemia Pheno-type	Elevated Plasma Compo-nent	Incidence	Plasma Choles-terol	Plasma Triglyc-erides	Accel-erate Athero-sclerosis	Treatment
I	Chylo-microns	Rare	N/↑	↑	No	Diet: Low-fat.
II	LDL VLDL (less)	Common	↑	N/↑	Yes	Diet: Low in saturated fats and choles-terol. Increased unsaturated fats. Cholestyramine Clofibrate Nicotinic acid
III	Abnormal VLDL	Uncom-mon	↑	↑	Yes	Weight reduction Diet: Low in saturated fats and carbo-hydrate. Clofibrate
IV	VLDL	Common	N/↑	↑	Yes	Weight reduction Diet: Increased unsaturated fats, decreased carbohydrates. Clofibrate
V	Chylo-microns	Uncom-mon	↑	↑	Not known	Weight reduction Diet: Low-fat, low-carbohydrate. Clofibrate(?)

↑　　= Elevated
N/↑　= Elevated or normal but not diagnostic
LDL　= Low density lipoprotein (β)
VLDL = Very low density lipoprotein (pre-β)

have not yet been determined, but many physicians believe that their use is justified pending evaluation. The most widely used drug is clofibrate, selected as the most promising agent some years ago on the mistaken premise that it is an inhibitor of cholesterol synthesis.

Chemistry

Clofibrate (ethylchlorophenoxyisobutyrate) is the only one of a large number of comparable compounds yet available for use.

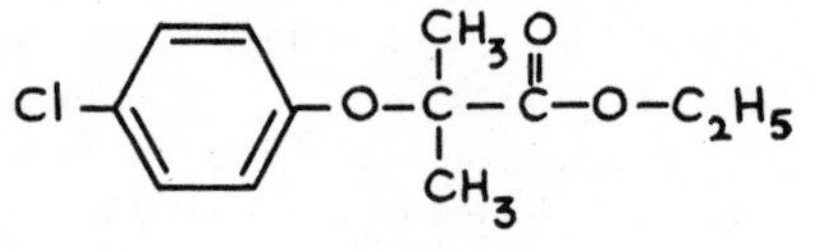

**Clofibrate
(Atromid-S)**

Absorption & Metabolism

Clofibrate is well absorbed after oral administration. After absorption it is rapidly hydrolyzed to the free acid, bound to plasma albumin, and distributed to extracellular sites. Excreted in the urine as the glucuronide, it is comparatively long-acting, with a chemical half-life of 12 hours, but is nevertheless given 4 times daily.

Pharmacologic Effects

A. Mechanisms of Action: The mechanism by which clofibrate reduces the plasma levels of triglyceride-rich VLDL and, to a lesser extent, the level of cholesterol-rich LDL is not known. Perhaps the most likely of the 5 hypotheses based on observed effects is that it inhibits lipoprotein release from the liver by reducing plasma free fatty acid (FFA).

Clofibrate was originally held to be an inhibitor of cholesterol synthesis on the basis of its effects in isolated tissues. It appears unlikely that such inhibition is of importance in the intact organism.

B. Effects: In a population with some initial elevation of plasma lipid levels, clofibrate will reduce the levels of VLDL (pre-β, triglyceride-rich); of LDL (β-lipoprotein, cholesterol-rich) to a lesser extent; and of free fatty acids. As a result, triglyceride levels decrease 30 or 40% and cholesterol levels 15-20%. The higher the initial levels, the greater the decrease. The effect has been maintained for more than 6 years in individual patients and in groups of patients.

Clofibrate also corrects abnormal platelet adhesiveness, decreases fibrinogen levels, and increases fibrinolysis. Since the therapeutic effects discussed below do not correlate with the lipid lowering action of clofibrate, these other less completely studied mechanisms may be very important.

Clinical Uses

There are 2 indications for the use of clofibrate as a supplement to other treatment. The first (and less controversial use) is in the treatment of a hyper-lipidemia which is symptomatic—eg, with xanthomas or abdominal pain—and which cannot be treated with diet alone. Clofibrate may even be used in a patient with secondary hyperlipemia—eg, a diabetic with lipemic retinopathy.

The other use, still unestablished, is in asymptomatic patients with the common endogenous hyperlipemia to defer or prevent coronary occlusions and, presumably, other atherosclerotic disease.

Clofibrate can decrease the level of cholesterol and β-lipoproteins, the best predictors of coronary artery disease, although it is more active in lowering triglyceride levels. Whether such lowering will decrease morbidity must be established by clinical trial. At this time, 2 studies are available which bear on this question.

The first is a collaborative study in hospitals of Scotland and England using patients with preexisting atherosclerotic heart disease. This more vulnerable group of 1214 patients was given clofibrate or a placebo under careful double-blind conditions for as long as 6 years. Fatal myocardial infarctions occurred in 13% of the controls and 10% of the treated subjects. If patients with angina are excluded, there was little difference in total infarctions in the 2 groups. Surprisingly, patients with angina, who would seem to have less reversible lesions, benefited more than those without angina, and the overall effect did not correlate well with the lipid-lowering effect.

A trial in this country, not double-blind, used a younger group for only 2 or 3 years and found a great difference between the incidence of nonfatal infarcts in the 2 groups—again unrelated to lowering or persistence of the hyperlipidemia.

These results are in contrast with the effect of dietary treatment, which has no demonstrable benefit when coronary artery disease is already manifest.

Adverse Effects

Adverse reactions to clofibrate have been surprisingly infrequent for a drug that must be given continuously for years. Nausea is common (5%) but usually disappears with continued treatment. Liver function tests (SGOT) are depressed early in treatment. Brittle hair is noted by some women patients, and isolated cases of alopecia have been reported.

Contraindications & Cautions

In many (but not all) patients, administration of clofibrate leads to intensification of the effect of anticoagulants of the warfarin type. When clofibrate is added to the regimen of a patient receiving an inhibitor of prothrombin synthesis, the dosage may have to be reduced by 30–50%. The mechanism of this interaction has not been established. Like other drugs that are acids, clofibrate displaces warfarin from the albumin to which it is bound in the plasma. However, plasma levels of warfarin rise rather than fall as they would if displacement were the only mechanism acting; this suggests that clofibrate interferes with the metabolism of warfarin.

Preparations & Dosages

Clofibrate (Atromid-S) is supplied as 500 mg capsules. The dosage is 500 mg 4 times a day.

2. OTHER DRUGS

Nicotinic Acid

Given in the large doses required, nicotinic acid or niacin (but not the related nicotinic acid amide or niacinamide) causes a reduction in VLDL and LDL. Fat is stored in adipose tissue as triglycerides but is released from fat cells for transport as free fatty acids. It is assumed that the demonstrated ability of nicotinic acid to partially block the release of free fatty acids explains its effect on blood lipids. As with other drugs of this class, an effect on the clinical course of atherosclerotic disease has not been established. Furthermore, its use is attended by frequent adverse reactions.

In the dosage necessary, nicotinic acid almost invariably causes side-effects. These can be reduced by slowly increasing the dosage to the desired level, and the side-effects often ameliorate as treatment is continued. Nicotinic acid is a vasodilator of cutaneous vessels and causes a cutaneous flush with itching and feelings of warmth. Gastrointestinal irritation is apparent as nausea, heartburn, and diarrhea. The skin may become dry, and brown pigmentation may appear.

Tests of liver function are depressed. Jaundice may occur.

Nicotinic acid (niacin) is available in tablets containing 20, 25, 50, 100, 250, 500, and 1000 mg, in buffered tablets containing 500 mg, and in sustained release capsules containing 125 and 250 mg. Treatment should begin with low dosage—eg, 250 mg 4 times daily—which is increased over a period of 2–3 weeks to 3 gm/day.

Dextrothyroxine (Choloxin)

Endogenous or exogenously induced hyperthyroidism leads to a decrease in cholesterol levels by increasing the rate of excretion and metabolism of cholesterol more than it increases its rate of synthesis. Laboratory studies suggest that some thyroxine analogues can achieve the effect on cholesterol catabolism without increasing the metabolic rate and perhaps precipitating anginal pain in susceptible individuals. The margin between the effective and toxic doses of the one compound used, dextrothyroxine, is narrow.

Dextrothyroxine (Choloxin) is supplied as 2 and 4 mg tablets. A daily dose of less than 4 mg is not likely to be effective; 8 mg or more per day often causes angina or signs of hypermetabolism as may doses in between.

Estrogens

Premenopausal women are much less susceptible to atherosclerosis than men of the same age. The administration of estrogens to men produces a female pattern of plasma lipids—eg, total cholesterol is not decreased but occurs more as α-lipoproteins and less as the β-lipoproteins presumed to be associated with the development of atherosclerosis. Feminizing effects occur with the dosage necessary, and an effect on survival is not demonstrable in trials of synthetic estrogens. Additional clinical trials of naturally occurring estrogens are in progress, but this use of the estrogens must, for the time being, be regarded as investigational.

Triparanol

Cholesterol present in the organism is derived in part from dietary sources, but synthesis in the liver is more important because it can increase to compensate for changes in the diet. Inhibition of hepatic synthesis would lower plasma cholesterol.

Triparanol (MER/29), a drug no longer marketed, blocked the synthesis of cholesterol at the last step in the series of reactions. The immediate precursor of cholesterol, desmosterol or 24-dehydrocholesterol, accumulated in the organism. After the drug had been marketed for 18 months, an association with the development of cataracts and other less serious adverse reactions was established. It was also established that the manufacturer and 3 scientists had withheld data from animal toxicity testing that anticipated the human toxicity.

Cholesterol is synthesized from acetate. One of the first reactions in the complex sequence is the production of mevalonic acid, and it is this early reaction that is blocked in isolated tissues by clofibrate. Thus, even if the inhibition of cholesterol synthesis should be a property of clofibrate, the triparanol type of toxicity would not be anticipated.

Sitosterols

The sitosterols are plant sterols that are chemically very similar to cholesterol. They are not absorbed following oral administration and decrease the absorption of dietary cholesterol and the enterohepatic cycling of endogenous cholesterol and bile acids. The resulting reduction in plasma cholesterol and LDL is small even when very large doses of this expensive drug

are given. Sitosterols (Cytellin) are available as a suspension containing 3 gm/15 ml.

Cholestyramine (Cuemid, Questran)

Cholestyramine may lower plasma cholesterol, but it is still an investigational drug for that purpose. It also increases the excretion in the feces of bile acids and is used to reduce itching associated with partial biliary obstruction.

Cholestyramine is a basic anion exchange resin, a quaternary ammonium chloride able to exchange the chloride for the cholate ion. It is not absorbed after oral administration but appears in the feces together with the bile salt bound to it.

Bile acids—eg, cholic acid or, in the alkaline medium of the small intestine, the bile salt, cholate—are metabolites of cholesterol. They are usually reabsorbed from the intestine and undergo repeated enterohepatic cycling. If they are bound by cholestyramine, their daily excretion is greatly increased, with 2 consequences: (1) In the presence of partial biliary obstruction and jaundice, itching due to the accumulation of bile salts may be relieved; and (2) cholesterol may be depleted as cholic acid synthesis is stimulated.

Adverse Reactions

Cholestyramine causes gastrointestinal irritation (nausea, heartburn, and diarrhea) and irritation of the tongue or perianal region. It may cause depletion of vitamins A and D, and there have been rare reports of depletion of vitamin K. The drug may also combine with other drugs and interfere with their absorption.

Contraindications & Cautions

Consider the need for supplementary vitamins A, D, and K when cholestyramine is used. Give other drugs 1 hour before giving the resin. It should be given suspended in an adequate volume of fluid.

Preparations & Dosages

Cholestyramine resin is supplied in packets containing 4 gm (Questran) and in bottles of 216 gm (Cuemid). The dosage is 4 gm (1 tsp) of the granules 3 times each day with meals, mixed with water or juice.

●   ●   ●

General References

Vitamins

Cox, E.V., & others: The anemia of scurvy. Am J Med 42:220–227, 1967.

Crandon, J.H., & others: Ascorbic acid economy in surgical patients as indicated by blood ascorbic acid levels. New England J Med 258:105–113, 1958.

Goldsmith, G.A.: Niacin: Antipellagra factor, hypocholesterolemic agent. JAMA 194:167–173, 1965.

Hume, E.M., & H.A. Krebs: Vitamin A requirements in human adults. An experimental study of vitamin A deprivation in man. Special Report Series, No. 264, Medical Research Council, London, 1949 or Brit MJ 2:932, 1950.

Lane, M., & C.P. Alfrey, Jr.: The anemia of human riboflavin deficiency. Blood 25:432–442, 1965.

Muenter, M.D., & others: Chronic vitamin A intoxication in adults. Am J Med 50:129–136, 1971.

Nair, P.P., & others: The effect of vitamin E on porphyrin metabolism in man. Arch Int Med 128:411–415, 1971.

Ritchie, J.H., & others: Edema and hemolytic anemia in premature infants. A vitamin E deficiency syndrome. New England J Med 279:1185–1190, 1968.

Scriver, C.R.: Pyridoxine deficiency and dependency. Am J Dis Child 113:109–114, 1967.

Silverman, S., Jr., Eisenberg, E., & G. Renstrup: A study of the effects of high doses of vitamin A on oral leukoplakia, including toxicity, liver function and skeletal metabolism. J Oral Therap Pharmacol 2:9–23, 1965.

Vitamin-C requirement of human adults. Experimental study of vitamin-C deprivation in man. Medical Research Council. Lancet 1:853–858, 1948.

Walker, G.H., Bynoe, M.L., & D.A.J. Tyrrell: Trial of ascorbic acid in prevention of colds. Brit MJ 1:603–606, 1967.

Undernutrition

György, P.: Protein-calorie and vitamin A malnutrition in Southeast Asia. Fed Proc 27:949–953, 1968.

Keys, A., & H. Sinclair: Real nutritional deficiency. Brit M Bull 8:262–264, 1952.

Scrimshaw, N.S., & M. Béhar: Malnutrition in underdeveloped countries. New England J Med 272:137–144, 193–198, 1965.

Hypolipidemic Agents

Council on Foods and Nutrition: The regulation of dietary fat. JAMA 181:411–429, 1962.

Fallon, H.J., & J.W. Woods: Response of hyperlipoproteinemia to cholestyramine resin. JAMA. 204:1161–1164, 1968.

Keys, A., & R.W. Parlin: Serum cholesterol response to changes in dietary lipids. Am J Clin Nutr 19:175–181, 1966.

Krasno, L.R., & G.J. Kidera: Clofibrate in coronary heart disease. JAMA 219:845–851, 1972.

Lees, R.S., & D.E. Wilson: The treatment of hyperlipidemia. New England J Med 284:186–194, 1971.

Orgain, E.S., Bogdonoff, M.D., & C. Cain: Clofibrate and androsterone effect on serum lipids. Arch Int Med 119:80–85, 1967.

Owen, W.R.: Efficacy of drugs in lowering blood cholesterol. M Clin North America 48:347–353, 1964.

Parsons, W.B.: Treatment of hypercholesteremia by nicotinic acid. Arch Int Med 107:639–652, 653–667, 1961.

Stamler, J., & others: Effectiveness of estrogens for therapy of myocardial infarction in middle-aged men. JAMA 183:632–638, 1963.

Various authors: Clofibrate in ischemic heart disease. Brit MJ 4:765, 1971.

42...

Specific Ions: Iron, Fluoride

Ions with osmotic as well as specific chemical effects are discussed as components of parenteral fluids in Chapter 43. Many metals are discussed as toxic agents (Chapter 65), and other ions—eg, calcium, lithium, iodide, or ammonium—are discussed in appropriate places elsewhere in this book.

IRON

Absorption

There are 2 mechanisms for the absorption of ferrous ion. The physiologically important mechanism involves active transport and is able to alter the absorption of iron as need changes. The second mechanism, diffusion across the mucosal barrier, is important after administration of large doses.

The first or physiologic process occurs in the duodenum and adjacent jejunum. Of the ferrous iron that enters the mucosal cell, a fraction is transported to the blood but some is converted to ferric iron and, after combination with the protein apoferritin, is stored in the mucosal cells as ferritin. The iron in ferritin is lost into the feces when the mucosal cells are shed. When an excess of iron is available and stores of ferritin are large, absorption of iron is limited—ie, a "mucosal block" is established.

The large amounts of iron administered therapeutically can partially bypass the above mechanism. However, the control mechanisms must still operate since administration of an initial dose of ferrous sulfate decreases the amount absorbed from a second dose given 6 hours later, and chronic toxic effects from the prolonged administration of iron are extremely rare.

The presence or absence of gastric acid has little effect on the absorption of iron in the ferrous form. The absorption of dietary iron or ferric salts is greatly enhanced by gastric acid, which favors conversion of iron to the ferrous form and perhaps also favors the formation of chelates with ascorbate and other dietary components. Such chelates remain soluble in the alkaline intestinal contents. The absorption of iron is decreased by gastrectomy (subtotal). The concurrent administration of antacids decreases absorption, as does the combination of iron with phosphate and other components of food also.

Supplemental iron is best absorbed when given in the fasting state but is nevertheless given with meals to reduce local irritation.

Metabolism & Pharmacologic Effects

Following absorption, iron (as ferrous ion), combines with CO_2 and a globulin, transferrin, and is carried to several sites. A small fraction (3 mg) functions in metallo-enzymes; about 200 mg are incorporated into myoglobin; and the largest fraction (2500 mg) is incorporated into hemoglobin within red blood cells. About 1 gm of iron is stored in marrow, liver, and spleen and is available for the synthesis of hemoglobin should blood be lost from the body. Ordinarily, of course, erythrocytes are destroyed and replaced without the loss of any component.

The daily loss of iron in desquamated cells is as low as 1 mg/day. Women may lose an additional 20–30 mg/month, and pregnancy requires replacement of about 500 mg. With the exception of the toxic effect of large doses of iron on the gastrointestinal tract, its pharmacologic action is comparable to its action as a dietary factor—ie, to maintain iron stores and hemoglobin synthesis.

Clinical Uses

The only use of systemically administered iron salts is to correct or prevent iron deficiency anemias. Only about half of the iron in food is available for absorption, and the dietary supply is not much above the need. Iron is added to white bread, but there is no evidence that it is significantly absorbed when the bread is part of an ordinary meal rather than a simple test meal. Consequently, a slight increase in blood loss rapidly leads to depletion of the iron stores. Anemia—ie, depletion of hemoglobin iron—follows, and with severe deficiencies tissue iron is also depleted. Until the last stage, the symptoms of iron deficiency are entirely those of anemia.

In addition to blood loss (including that of menstruation), there are other situations that may precipitate iron deficiency and anemia.

Pregnancy places an additional demand on iron stores that are often marginal at the beginning of pregnancy. Supplementary iron during the later months of pregnancy can maintain hemoglobin to some extent and hasten its resynthesis after the blood loss of deliv-

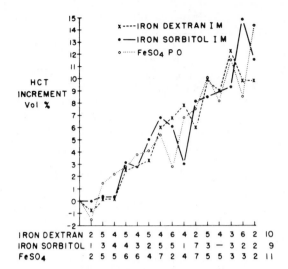

IRON DEXTRAN	2	5	4	5	4	5	4	6	4	2	5	4	3	6	2	10
IRON SORBITOL	1	3	4	4	3	2	5	5	1	7	3	—	3	2	2	9
FeSO₄		2	5	5	6	6	4	7	2	4	7	5	5	3	3	2	11

FIG 42–1. **Comparison of the similar rates at which 2 parenteral iron preparations and oral ferrous sulfate correct an iron deficiency anemia.** The figures at the bottom are the number of patients included at each point on the graph. (Reproduced, with permission, from McCurdy: Oral and parenteral iron therapy. JAMA 191:861, 1965.)

ery. However, most of the anemia of pregnancy is dilutional, and the increase in plasma volume is accompanied by a smaller increase in red cell mass.

Iron deficiency anemia is also common in infants during their first year, and supplementary iron may be needed. The iron stores of full-term infants (but not prematures) are large enough for the needs of the first few months even if the mother was deficient in iron. Rapid growth takes place at a time when dietary iron may be scant since cow's milk, including the evaporated milk from which the most economical formula is made, contains very little iron. Some prepared formulas and the cereals prepared for infant feeding contain added iron, but these are least likely to be used in the families where they are most needed. In all prematures and in the children of economically marginal families, supplementary iron (as drops providing 1–2 mg/kg in each daily dose) should be supplied during the first year.

Following subtotal gastrectomy, iron absorption is reduced and the need for supplementary iron should be anticipated.

Adverse Reactions

A. Side-Effects: Gastrointestinal side-effects—eg, gastric discomfort, cramps, and diarrhea—are very common (20% or more of patients) but are usually mild. The patient should be warned to expect black stools.

Side-effects are minimized by taking iron after meals.

B. Overdosage Toxicity: Acute toxicity in young children who accidentally ingest iron tablets is a common occurrence because iron is frequently prescribed

for the mother and left about the house in some easily accessible place. As few as 10–30 tablets have been fatal in very young children.

The large amounts of iron involved cause a necrotizing gastroenteritis with bleeding and transudation into the lumen. Shock occurs either because of the loss of fluid or because of some more subtle change—eg, the vasodilating effect of large amounts of ferritin or the action of bacterial toxins that can cross the damaged intestinal wall. Metabolic acidosis and liver damage occur late in the course.

The course of the intoxication is conveniently but only approximately divided into 4 phases. For the first 1–6 hours, the manifestations are those of gastroenteritis and shock—eg, vomiting and diarrhea of bloody material, shock, dyspnea, lethargy. Thereafter, the patient may recover or, after a transient period (6–24 hours) of improvement, develop a metabolic acidosis followed by coma and the appearance of liver damage.

Treatment: If the victim is not vomiting, he should be given eggs, milk, or water and emesis induced. If the history justifies it, gastric lavage should then be carried out using a lavage solution that contains phosphate ion to combine with dissolved iron.

Specific treatment depends upon the use of chelating agents (see Chapter 65), which complex with metal ions, removing them from solution and incorporating them into a less toxic chelate.

Deferoxamine (Desferal; see Fig 65–2) forms a nontoxic complex with iron with such avidity that it is able to extract iron from transferrin and ferritin. If signs of systemic iron toxicity appear, deferoxamine should be given either intramuscularly or by slow intravenous infusion.

Deferoxamine can cause a precipitous hypotension and should not be used unless an accurate history, the appearance of systemic signs of iron toxicity (shock), or the demonstration of an excess of serum iron over iron-binding capacity is present. It should not be used in the presence of anuria or severe renal disease. Deferoxamine (Desferal) is supplied as ampules containing 500 mg of the lyophilized deferoxamine mesylate.

Calcium disodium edathamil (Calcium Disodium Versenate) should be used if deferoxamine is not available. Following lavage or emesis, 35–45 mg/kg should be placed in the stomach. Intravenous infusions of the same dose can be given daily if needed.

C. Chronic Toxicity: Hemochromatosis—ie, the deposition of hemosiderin in the parenchyma of the liver and other organs—has occurred in a few patients given iron for many years. Hemochromatosis also occurs idiopathically and following multiple transfusions. Deferoxamine is still an investigational and probably toxic drug when used chronically in such cases. Moreover, it is less efficient than venesection.

Preparations & Dosages

The iron salts and chelates suggested for use can differ in their acute toxicity and in the incidence of

TABLE 42–1. Iron for oral administration: Dosages and preparations available.

	Iron Content	Usual Adult Dose (3–4 Times Daily)	Iron/ Dose	Preparations Available
Ferrous sulfate	20%	300 mg	60 mg	Tablets (plain, coated, or enteric-coated), 200, 300, and 325 mg Controlled release tablets, 525 mg Syrup or elixir, 125 mg/1 ml, 150 mg/5 ml, and 220 mg/5 ml Drops, 75 mg/0.6 ml
Ferrous sulfate, exsiccated (eg, Feosol)*	30%	200 mg	60 mg	Tablets and capsules, 200 mg Sustained release capsules, 150 mg
Ferrous gluconate (eg, Fergon)*	12%	300 mg	36 mg	Tablets (plain, coated, or enteric-coated), 325 mg Elixir, 300 mg/5 ml
Ferrous fumarate (eg, Toleron, Ircon)*	33%	200 mg	66 mg	Tablets (plain, coated, or chewable), 200, 225, 250, and 325 mg Suspension, 100 mg/5 ml
Ferroglycine sulfate (eg, Ferronord)†	16%	250 mg	40 mg	Tablets (coated), 250 mg
Ferrocholinate (iron choline citrate; eg, Ferrolip, Chel-Iron)†	12%	330 mg	40 mg	Tablets (coated), 330 and 360 mg Syrup, 280 mg/1 ml and 417 mg/5 ml
Polysaccharide-iron complex (eg, Niferex)†	...	...	50 mg	Tablets (coated), 50 mg elemental iron Elixir, 100 mg elemental iron per 5 ml

*Available as generic preparations. Protected names shown only for identification.
†Not recommended for use. See text.

side-effects that accompany their use. Both of these properties, like the therapeutic effect, depend upon the amount of iron contained in a dose, and in comparing available preparations equivalent amounts of iron rather than equal doses of the salt must be compared. If this caution is accepted and if the studies are controlled as in other clinical trials, no superiority over ferrous sulfate can be demonstrated for any of the available preparations.

Ferrous sulfate is the standard drug. If side-effects interfere when it is used, the dose can be decreased or less iron given by substituting ferrous gluconate.

Several preparations are inferior to the sulfate. Ferroglycine sulfate is a chelate that is decomposed by stomach acid and is, therefore, merely an expensive way to administer ferrous sulfate. A polysaccharide-iron complex can be made into a palatable pediatric preparation, but little if any of the iron can be absorbed.

Some sustained release preparations have been shown to provide less iron for absorption than ordinary tablets; another delivers exactly the same amount of iron as the inexpensive tablet.

The rapidity of the response to ferrous sulfate increases as the dose is increased up to 2 gm/day. Such dosage almost always causes side-effects. Dosage should be started at a low level and increased slowly if necessary. Treatment should be continued for several months after restoration of normal levels of hemoglobin to replenish iron stores.

A. Oral Preparations: See Table 42–1.

B. Injectable Iron Preparations: Injectable iron preparations are available when the parenteral route is indicated. It is generally thought that such indications are uncommon—eg, intolerance or failure of response to orally administered iron. Parenteral iron should not be used in patients with anemias other than iron deficiency—eg, hemolytic anemias—since iron overload will result. The response to intramuscularly administered iron is no more rapid than that after oral administration.

1. Iron-dextran injection (Imferon)—The iron-dextran complex contains 5% iron—ie, 50 mg of iron per ml of solution. Give 1 ml (50 mg iron) IM on the first day and then 2–5 ml daily or at longer intervals until the calculated dose has been given. Give 250 mg for each gram of hemoglobin below normal. Follow the directions for deep intramuscular injection to avoid discoloring the skin. Anaphylactic reactions have been reported.

2. Iron sorbitex (Jectofer) is an iron-sorbitol complex comparable to iron-dextran complex (Imferon). It also contains 50 mg of iron per ml and is supplied as 2 ml ampules.

3. Dextriferron (Astrafer) is an iron-dextrin complex that is given intravenously. Additional precautions are necessary in its use, and the package literature should be consulted.

FLUORIDE

This discussion relates to fluoride ion—ie, to compounds that release fluoride ion upon ionization or decomposition but not to fluorine contained in organic compounds. The incidence of dental caries is much reduced by the ingestion of adequate amounts of fluoride.

Absorption, Metabolism, & Excretion

Soluble fluorides—eg, sodium fluoride—are rapidly absorbed following oral ingestion. Less soluble salts are only slowly absorbed. Thus the formation of calcium fluoride by the administration of calcium ions in the antidotal treatment of fluoride toxicity delays but does not prevent absorption of fluoride.

Once absorbed, fluoride is initially distributed much as chloride is—ie, it remains extracellular to a large extent. It is slightly less well reabsorbed by the renal tubules than is chloride and is consequently rapidly excreted into the urine. Unlike chloride, however, it is also concentrated in bone. Because of the prompt excretion and deposition, fluoride levels in plasma are only transiently elevated following an oral dose.

At a given dietary level of fluoride, the deposition and release of fluoride from bone are equal. If an increased amount of fluoride is given, half of each dose will be deposited in bone until a new state of equilibrium is reached. It is this increased amount of fluoride in bone and teeth that is important in the action of supplementary fluoride.

Mechanism of Action

A. In Tooth Enamel: The surface layer of enamel contains a higher concentration of fluoride than deeper layers of enamel or dentine, suggesting that enamel takes up fluoride from the surrounding fluid. Enamel with a higher fluoride content is more resistant to erosion by acid—ie, to dental decay. Enamel (and bone) is composed of apatite, a form of crystalline calcium phosphate that contains hydroxyl groups in its crystal lattice. The most probable explanation for the effect of fluoride on the teeth is that the fluoride exchanges for hydroxyl in the crystal structure.

B. In Bone: In bone, hydroxyapatite is similarly converted to fluorapatite. However, to explain the osteosclerosis that larger doses of fluoride causes, some as yet unclarified additional mechanisms must be present—eg, stimulation of osteoblastic activity.

Clinical Uses

A. Prevention of Dental Caries: Dental decay, which is probably the most widespread of all diseases, follows localized erosion of the enamel of a tooth. Progressively deeper destruction leads to pain, abscess formation, and loss of the tooth. The process is due to the growth of acid-producing bacteria that require carbohydrate for their growth. Control of decay can in part be accomplished by brushing the teeth or rinsing the mouth to remove bacteria and their substrate and by some restriction of sugars in the diet. The most effective prophylactic measure that is applicable to whole populations is to increase the resistance of the enamel by providing fluoride for incorporation into apatite.

1. Fluoridation of water supplies—Studies of communities in which there was a high incidence of mottling of the teeth showed an association with a high level of fluoride in the communal water supply and also a low incidence of dental decay. Further epidemiologic studies established that protection against caries could be provided by adding fluoride to drinking water in amounts that did not cause mottling or dental fluorosis.

The addition of fluoride to the water supplies of communities receiving less than optimal amounts of fluoride began on a trial basis in 1945. Large-scale evaluations of the effect of added fluoride for periods of 10 and 15 years are now available, and there is no question that fluoridation is effective. Benefit is most striking in the younger age groups who have received the supplement before eruption of their teeth. In general, the numbers of decayed, missing, or filled teeth are reduced 50–60% in children at age 14–16.

Fluoride, usually as sodium silicofluoride, is added to the water supply to a final fluoride concentration of about 1 ppm or 1 mg/liter, although the concentration is varied with the climate—ie, with the predicted intake of water. This amount of fluoride has no toxic effects; does not affect the taste or odor of water; and usually costs 5–15 cents a year per individual, a negligible cost compared to the savings in the cost of restorative dentistry.

Nevertheless, objections to fluoridation persist and voters in a number of cities have rejected proposals to fluoridate. Some of the objections are unjustified since the possibility of toxic effects has been carefully studied. The one basis for argument is the philosophic one that the individual is being medicated against his will. However, it is no more difficult for an individual to remove fluoride from his water supply than for the majority of householders to add it on an individual basis.

About half of the population of the USA is now supplied with water that contains supplemental or natural fluoride in protective amounts. If the communal water supply is not fluoridated, each child should receive fluoride supplements up to age 12. The amount of supplement depends upon the fluoride content of the available water, but the total intake should not exceed 1 mg/day.

2. Topical application of fluorides—Topical application of a fluoride salt will supplement the effect of systemic fluoride in producing acid-resistant tooth structures. If caries is a clinical problem, topical application by a dentist is indicated.

When solutions of sodium fluoride or stannous fluoride are painted on the dry tooth, fluoride is not immediately incorporated into apatite. A depot of calcium fluoride is first formed on the surface of the tooth from which fluoride is released.

Toothpastes containing stannous fluoride are a less effective way of applying fluoride topically. Their regular and frequent use adds a modest gain to the benefits of regular frequent brushing with any tooth cleanser.

No claim can be made that fluoride is effective against any dental disease other than decay. There are hints from epidemiologic studies that periodontal disease is influenced by added fluoride, but no completed studies are available.

B. Investigative Use in Osteoporosis: The progressive loss of bone in osteoporosis has for many years been treated with estrogens or other anabolic steroids on the assumption that the basic process is a loss of protein matrix with secondary loss of calcium. Use of the steroids has not resulted in demonstrable recalcification, and there is current interest in developing other methods of treatment such as giving supplementary calcium salts by mouth. In the present context, the possible role of fluoride in maintaining normal bone density should be mentioned. In the epidemiologic studies of communities with varying fluoride levels in the drinking water, it was reported that 10−15% of the inhabitants receiving enough fluoride to develop mottled enamel also had coarsened trabeculae and increased density of bone. Even more striking was the higher incidence of osteoporosis in the residents of one city with very little fluoride in the water.

Additional field studies and evaluation of the use of large dosages of sodium fluoride in the treatment of osteoporosis are now in progress. Evaluation of changes may require many years. Osteoporosis is the result of a very small daily negative calcium balance continued for decades.

Other investigative studies of large amounts of sodium fluoride on otosclerosis, multiple myeloma, and Paget's disease appear to establish that recalcification can be accomplished.

Because fluoride is concentrated at areas of rapid remolding of bone, a scan done after the administration of $Na^{18}F$ can be used to identify early bony metastases.

Adverse Reactions

Fluoride in large doses is, as opponents of fluoridation emphasize, dangerously toxic. In the range of milligrams per day it causes only dental fluorosis. The adverse effects of high fluoride intake from natural sources and the possible adverse effects of supplementary fluoride have been investigated on larger samples and with far more care than is expended on other therapeutic agents. No cause for concern has been found.

It must be emphasized that, in areas where fluoridation of water is public policy, the daily intake is about 1 mg/day. The acute ingestion of 250 mg leads only to nausea and vomiting.

A. Dental Fluorosis: Excess fluoride during the first 8 years of life leads to areas of irregular and hypo-plastic enamel formation. These may be apparent as chalky or paper-white areas. In more advanced form they may appear as yellowish-brown pits and ridges. These areas are resistant to the development of caries. If they are cosmetically disturbing, the brownish color can be bleached with 30% hydrogen peroxide.

Significant mottling is rare when less than 2 mg/day of fluoride are ingested. It is detectable but cosmetically negligible in almost half of children who received 1.7 ppm of fluoride in drinking water. With 4−6 ppm of fluoride—ie, 4−6 mg/day—mottling is invariable and may be disfiguring.

In communities suffering from endemic mottling, fluoride is removed from the water.

B. Skeletal Fluorosis: Ingestion of fluoride in amounts of 8−20 mg/day for years can lead to increased osteoblastic activity and increased density of bone. Signs include osteosclerosis or thickened, more dense trabeculae, periosteal hyperostoses, and calcification of soft tissues attached to bone.

With large doses (20−80 mg/day for 10−20 years), the changes may become crippling. Osteoporosis may replace osteosclerosis after a long period.

A more acute form of osteosclerosis can follow industrial exposure to larger amounts of fluoride.

C. Acute Toxicity: Acute fluoride intoxication does not result from exposure to therapeutic fluoride. An entire tube of fluoride toothpaste does not contain a dangerous amount of fluoride. Sodium fluoride is prescribed so that no more than 200 mg are in the home at any time.

Acute fluoride toxicity usually results from ingestion of an insecticide. Fluoride in these large amounts reacts with calcium and depresses the activity of many enzymes. Initial symptoms are due to gastrointestinal irritation—ie, nausea, vomiting, cramping pain, and diarrhea. Convulsions can occur, and blood pressure and respiration are progressively depressed. Hypoglycemia and hypocalcemia may be prominent findings.

Treatment consists of the following: (1) Lavage with a calcium salt—eg, lime water or calcium chloride—or the induction of emesis following ingestion of the same solution. After lavage or emesis, give calcium salts by mouth. (2) Begin an intravenous infusion of glucose in water or saline, in part to treat hypoglycemia but also so that a calcium salt can be injected intravenously if needed.

The fluoride salts used as agricultural chemicals are rapidly absorbed, and treatment must be prompt. Reported lethal doses are as small as 0.5 gm in a child, but doses many times that size have not been fatal.

Preparations Available

Bottled water containing added fluoride and sodium fluoride tablets and solutions are available for use in communities without fluoridation of the water supply. The amount of fluoride in the untreated water supply is variable, and information about dosage should be solicited from local public health officials. In the following preparations of sodium fluoride, the amounts given represent fluoride content:

Tablets, 0.5 and 1 ml

Drops, 0.1 mg/0.04 ml, 0.5 mg/ml, 1 mg/0.5 ml, and 1 mg/4 drops

Gel drops, 0.5%, 24 ml

Solution, 1 mg/5 ml

Topical, 1.23%, solution and gel, 250 ml

●　　●　　●

General References

Iron

Barr, D.G.D., & D.K.B. Fraser: Acute iron poisoning in children: Role of chelating agents. Brit MJ 1:737–741, 1968.

Beutler, E., & S.E. Larsh: Relative effectiveness of ferroglycine sulfate and ferrous sulfate. New England J Med 267:538–540, 1962.

Callender, S.T.: Quick- and slow-release iron: A double-blind trial with a single daily dose regimen. Brit MJ 4:531–534, 1969.

Committee on Nutrition of the American Academy of Pediatrics: Iron-fortified formulas. Pediatrics 47:786, 1971.

Fairbanks, V.F., Fahey, J.L., & E. Beutler: *Clinical Disorders of Iron Metabolism,* 2nd ed. Grune & Stratton, 1971.

Fischer, D.S., Parkman, R., & S.C. Finch: Acute iron poisoning in children: The problem of appropriate therapy. JAMA 218:1179–1184, 1971.

Jacobs, J., Greene, H., & B.R. Gendel: Acute iron intoxication. New England J Med 273:1124–1127, 1965.

Marchasin, S., & R.O. Wallerstein: The treatment of iron-deficiency anemia with intravenous iron dextran. Blood 23:354–358, 1964.

Middleton, E.J., Nagy, E., & A.B. Morrison: Studies on the absorption of orally administered iron from sustained-release preparations. New England J Med 274:136–139, 1966.

Pritchard, J.A.: Hemoglobin regeneration in iron-deficiency anemia. JAMA 195:717–720, 1966.

Ross, J.D.: Failure of iron-deficient infants to respond to an orally administered iron-carbohydrate complex. New England J Med 269:399–401, 1963.

Fluorides

Bernstein, D.S., & P. Cohen: Use of sodium fluoride in the treatment of osteoporosis. J Clin Endocrinol 27:197–210, 1967.

Dunning, J.M.: Current status of fluoridation. New England J Med 272:30–34, 84–88, 1965.

Fluoridation. Symposium. J Am Dent A 65:578–717, 1962.

Hodge, H.C., & F.A. Smith: Fluorides and man. Ann Rev Pharmacol 8:395–408, 1968.

Sapolsky, H.M.: Science, voters, and the fluoridation controversy. Science 162:427–432, 1968.

Shambaugh, G.E., & A. Petrovic: Effects of sodium fluoride on bone. Application to otosclerosis and other decalcifying bone diseases. JAMA 204:969–980, 1968.

43...

Fluids & Electrolytes

Marcus A. Krupp, MD

Water and solute made up of electrolyte and non-ionized organic molecules constitute the body fluids which vary somewhat in composition in individual organs and compartments.

The body fluids support homeostasis by virtue of 3 closely related factors: volume, concentration, and pharmacologic activity.

Water Volume

(1) Extracellular (plasma, interstitial fluid) and transcellular (CSF, intraluminal intestinal fluid, ocular fluid).

(2) Intracellular.

Concentration

(1) Osmolality (total solute concentration).

(2) Concentration of individual electrolytes.

Pharmacologic Activity

(1) Concentration of hydrogen ion (pH).

(2) Concentration of electrolytes which exert pharmacologic actions.

WATER VOLUME

"Volume" and "water" are substantially interchangeable in the context of this discussion. Volume of body water is maintained by a balance between intake and excretion. Water as such, in foods and as a product of combustion, is excreted by the kidneys, skin, and lungs. Electrolytes important in maintaining volume and distribution include the cations sodium for extracellular fluid and potassium and magnesium for intracellular fluid, and the anions chloride and bicarbonate for extracellular fluid and phosphate and protein for intracellular fluid.

Loss of water or excess of water results in corresponding change in volume in both extra- and intracellular compartments. Loss of sodium (with accompanying anion) or excess of sodium results in decrease or increase, respectively, of the volume of extracellular fluid, with water moving out of the extracellular compartment with sodium loss and into the extracellular compartment with sodium retention.

In response to changes in volume, appropriate servo or feedback mechanisms come into play. The principal elements in regulation are antidiuretic hormone for water, aldosterone and other steroids for sodium (and potassium), and vascular responses affecting glomerular filtration rate for water and sodium.

The average adult requires at least 800–1300 ml of water per day to cover obligatory water needs. A normal adult on an ordinary diet requires 500 ml of water for renal excretion of solute in a maximally concentrated urine plus an additional amount of water to replace that lost via the skin and respiratory tract.

Fluid losses most often include electrolyte as well as water. Sweat, gastrointestinal fluids, urine, and fluid escaping from wounds contain significant quantities of electrolyte. In order to ascertain deficits of water and electrolytes, one must consider the history, change in body weight, clinical state, and appropriate determinations in plasma of concentration of each of the electrolytes, osmolality, protein, and pH. Assessment of renal function is required before repair and maintenance requirements can be determined and prescribed.

TABLE 43–1. Body water distribution in an average normal young adult male.*

	ml/kg† Body Weight	% of Total· Body Water
Total extracellular fluid	270	45
Plasma	45	7.5
Interstitial fluid	120	20
Connective tissue and bone	90	15
Transcellular fluid	15	2.5
Total intracellular fluid	330	55
Total body water	600	100

*Modified from Edelman & Liebman: Anatomy of water and electrolytes. J Med 27:256, 1959.

$†\dfrac{ml/kg}{10}$ = %, eg, 45 ml/kg = 4.5%

Dr. Krupp is Clinical Professor of Medicine, Stanford University School of Medicine, Palo Alto, California; Director, Palo Alto Medical Research Foundation, Palo Alto, California.

WATER DEFICIT

Water deficit results in a decrease in volume of both extracellular and intracellular fluids with a corresponding increase in concentration of both extracellular and intracellular solute in these fluids. In the blood, the loss of body water is reflected in an increased plasma osmolality as concentrations of plasma electrolyte and protein rise. With decreased blood volume, renal blood flow is reduced and excretion of urea falls, resulting in an elevation of urea in body fluids. Antidiuretic hormone secretion is stimulated, providing some protection from water loss by the kidney.

Water deficit results from reduced intake or unusual losses. Reduced intake is likely when the patient is unconscious, disabled, unable to ingest water because of esophageal or pyloric obstruction, or receives inadequate fluids to meet maintenance and replacement needs. Fever or a hot environment increases loss from the lungs and skin. The kidney fails to conserve water when there is inadequate ADH (diabetes insipidus) or insensitivity to ADH (nephrogenic diabetes insipidus), osmotic diuresis in diabetes mellitus, inadequate tubule function due to renal disease, and impaired capacity to reabsorb water secondary to potassium depletion, hypercalcemia, correction of obstructive uropathy, or from intensive diuretic therapy.

Water deficit is characterized by thirst, flushed skin, "dehydrated" appearance, dry mucous membranes, tachycardia, and oliguria. As dehydration increases, hallucinations and delirium, hyperpnea, and coma ensue.

Treatment

Water may be provided with or without electrolyte. If water alone is needed, 2.5–5% dextrose solution may be given intravenously; even the dextrose is oxidized to yield water.

In the presence of normal renal function, 2000–3000 ml of water per day (1500 ml/sq M of body surface) will provide a liberal maintenance ration. If dehydration is present with increased serum sodium concentration and osmolality, extra water replacement can be estimated on the basis of restoring normal osmolality for the total body fluid volume. The need for intracellular water is reflected in the extracellular fluid with which it is in osmotic equilibrium; therefore, any correction of deviation in osmolality must be considered on the basis of the total volume of body water.

WATER EXCESS

Water excess (overhydration, dilution syndrome) results in expansion of volume of body fluid and decreased concentration (dilution) of plasma electrolyte and protein, a reduced osmolality of plasma. Similar dilutions occur intracellularly. Normally, ADH secretion is inhibited, enabling the kidneys to excrete the excess water. Water excess results from intake in excess of capacity for excretion, usually from too large a water ration during parenteral administration; or from impaired excretory capacity resulting from acute or chronic renal insufficiency, renal functional changes (lowered glomerular filtration and increased water reabsorption) accompanying heart failure, liver disease with ascites, or administration of ADH or inappropriate secretion of ADH by neoplasms or in complex endocrine disturbances.

Water excess, particularly if severe or if it develops acutely, produces the syndrome of water intoxication, characterized by headache, nausea, vomiting, abdominal cramps, weakness, stupor, coma, and convulsions.

Treatment

The basic treatment consists of water restriction. If a real deficit of sodium exists as well, saline solutions should be employed. In the presence of severe water intoxication, administration of hypertonic saline solution may be useful to promote movement of excess intracellular water to the extracellular space, ie, to increase osmolality and diminish intracellular water volume.

CONCENTRATION

The total concentration of solute (osmolality) is apparently the same in intracellular and extracellular water. In the intracellular compartment, protein concentration plays a more important osmolal role than in the plasma. The protein content of interstitial fluid is small, and osmolal effects are therefore negligible. The most accessible and best index of osmolality is the measurement of the solute concentration in the plasma by ascertaining the depression of the freezing point. An indirect and useful measurement is that of plasma sodium concentration, provided due attention is paid to hyperglycemia and high urea concentrations, which cause a significant increase in osmolality; and lipemia and hyperproteinemia, which provide a nonaqueous addition to plasma volume. In the latter situations, sodium concentration determinations yield low values which must be interpreted with consideration of the concentration of the other constituents, ie, in terms of plasma or serum water rather than of the plasma specimen per se.

HYPERNATREMIA

Increased concentration of sodium in extracellular fluid and hyperosmolality may result from water loss without equivalent sodium loss (pure water volume deficit) or from excessive sodium administration with inadequate water replacement. Hypernatremia may be due to inappropriate regulation of osmolality, occasionally present with intracranial tumors.

Hypernatremia is not an index of total body content of sodium. Increased total body sodium is usually due to retention of sodium with heart failure, cirrhosis of the liver, and nephrosis. In these states, sodium concentration in extracellular fluid is usually normal or low as a result of expansion of the total volume of body fluid.

Treatment

Treatment must be based on accurate appraisal of the significance of the alteration of the plasma sodium concentration. The clinical history and examination and corroborating laboratory data provide a guide for therapy. Hypernatremia due to water deficit is treated by replenishing water deficit (see above). If treatment with excessive quantities of sodium salts produces hypernatremia, withholding sodium may suffice. Natriuretic drugs (diuretics) may be employed to hasten excretion of the excess sodium; attention must be paid to replacement of water when diuretics are so employed.

HYPONATREMIA

A decreased concentration of sodium in extracellular fluid may result from loss of sodium or from dilution by retention of water. Sodium loss occurs with adrenocortical insufficiency, vigorous diuretic therapy, unusual losses of gastrointestinal secretions, renal insufficiency, and unusual sweating. When the deficit of water is replaced with inadequate sodium replacement, hyponatremia ensues. Retention of water occurs with the therapeutic use of ADH or with the secretion of excess antidiuretic substances by some types of carcinoma of the lung, with chronic severe heart failure, cirrhosis of the liver with ascites, and nephrotic syndrome. These states produce dilution syndromes characterized by hyponatremia (dilutional hyponatremia).

TABLE 43–2. Relationship of serum sodium to total body sodium in various clinical states.*

Serum Sodium	Total Body Sodium	Clinical States	Fluid and Electrolyte Therapy
Low (hyponatremia) < 130 mEq/liter	High	Edematous states (eg, nephrosis, cirrhosis, cardiac disease). May also occur after severe burns and in the immediate postoperative period.	Not indicated to raise serum sodium.
	Normal	Patients on low sodium intake retaining water as a metabolic response to trauma or surgery, particularly if given excess water (dilution syndrome; water intoxication). May also occur in cirrhotic patients after paracentesis.	Mild: Restrict fluids. Severe: Hypertonic (3–6%) sodium chloride solution may be needed.
	Low	Addison's disease; salt-wasting nephritis; gastrointestinal fluid and electrolyte losses; prolonged sweating with free access to water; perhaps in prolonged use of diuretic agents and on salt-free diets.	Isotonic sodium chloride solution.
Normal 135–145 mEq/ liter	High	Renal, cardiac, or hepatic disease; also carcinoma involving pleural or peritoneal cavities. Caused by renal retention of water and salt in the same osmotic ratio.	
	Low	In the early stages of rapid salt depletion from gastrointestinal losses, renal excretion of a dilute urine preserves osmolarity of body fluids. A similar situation prevails in diabetic acidosis.	
High (hypernatremia) > 150 mEq/liter	High	Excess administration of sodium salts.	Water by mouth or dextrose and water intravenously. Withhold electrolytes.
	Normal	Simple dehydration due to deprivation of water; diabetes insipidus (congenital, or acquired, as in the diuretic phase of acute renal insufficiency or after cerebral trauma).	
	Low	Prolonged sweating without access to water.	Hypotonic sodium chloride solution.

*Reproduced, with permission, from Wilson: *Handbook of Surgery,* 4th ed. Lange, 1969.

Treatment

If there is a deficit of sodium, sodium chloride with or without sodium bicarbonate may be used for replacement. For replacement of moderate deficits, 0.9% sodium chloride (155 mEq of Na^+ and Cl^-/liter), or Ringer's solution with or without lactate, may be employed. For severe sodium deficit, 3% sodium chloride (513 mEq/liter) or 5% sodium chloride (855 mEq/liter) may be used with caution. More comprehensive texts on water and electrolyte metabolism must be consulted for specific information on treatment.

Hyponatremia due to dilution of electrolyte because of water retention should be treated by restriction of intake of water. In states associated with dilutional hyponatremia, total body sodium is elevated or normal and, therefore, sodium should not be administered.

The concentrations of other electrolytes in extracellular fluids have insignificant osmolar effects.

PHARMACOLOGIC ACTIVITY OF FLUIDS & ELECTROLYTES

HYDROGEN ION CONCENTRATION

The hydrogen ion concentration (H^+) of body fluids is closely regulated with intracellular concentrations of 10^{-7} molar (pH 7.0) and extracellular fluid concentrations of 4×10^{-8} molar (pH 7.4). In spite of accumulation or loss of H^+, these concentrations are maintained at nearly normal by buffer substances which remove or release H^+. The capacity of buffers is limited, however, and regulation is accomplished principally by the lungs and kidneys. The principal buffer substances include proteins, the oxyhemoglobin-reduced hemoglobin system, primary and secondary phosphate ions, some intracellular phosphate esters, and the carbonic acid-sodium bicarbonate systems.

Most of the food used for energy is completely utilized, with production of water, CO_2 and urea. Sulfate and, to a limited extent, phosphate end-products are strong acid anions which must be "neutralized" by cation such as sodium. In the utilization of fat and carbohydrate, intermediate products include the strong acids acetoacetic acid and lactic acid. Buffers provide cation and remove H^+, which is ultimately excreted by the kidney as acid or as ammonium ion and by the lung as CO_2 and H_2O, equivalent to carbonic acid. The anions of strong acids with cation such as sodium and ammonium are eliminated by the kidney.

The role of the lung and kidney in removal of H^+ and in regulation of H^+ concentration can be viewed as,

$$\frac{[H^+] \ [HCO_3^-] \ \rightleftarrows \ P_{CO_2} \ \text{lung}}{[HCO_3^-] \ \text{kidney}}$$

Respiratory control of the partial pressure of CO_2 (P_{CO_2}) in the pulmonary alveoli and therefore in the arterial plasma determines the H_2CO_3 concentration in body fluids:

$$CO_2 + H_2O \rightleftarrows H_2CO_3$$

The elimination of CO_2 via the lung in effect removes carbonic acid. The kidney is responsible for $BHCO_3$ concentration in body fluids, which, with H_2CO_3, constitutes one of the buffer systems for regulation of pH.

The kidney produces carbonic acid from metabolic CO_2 and water by the following reaction:

$$CO_2 + H_2O \xrightarrow{\boxed{\text{Carbonic anhydrase}}} H_2CO_3$$

The carbonic acid serves as a source of H^+ which can be exchanged for Na^+ in the tubular urine so that H^+ is excreted and Na^+ reabsorbed. The exchange affects anions of weak acids:

$$Na^+ + HCO_3^- + H^+ \rightarrow H_2CO_3 \rightarrow CO_2 + H_2O$$

with Na^+ reabsorbed. Although the pH of urine cannot be lowered below pH 4.5, additional H^+ ion can be excreted by combination with NH_3, generated principally from glutamine within the tubule cell. NH_3 diffuses from the tubule cell into the urine within the tubule where it combines with $H^+ \rightarrow NH_4^+$, providing cation for excretion with anions of strong acids with no increase in H^+ concentration (no lowering of pH). These exchanges in the renal tubule involve active transport systems capable of maintaining a gradient in concentration of extracellular fluid H^+ of 4×10^{-8} molar (pH 7.4) against a tubular urine H^+ of 32×10^{-6} molar (pH 4.5), an 800-fold increase in H^+ concentration.

The clinical term **acidosis** signifies a decrease in pH (increase in H^+) of extracellular fluid; the term **alkalosis** signifies an increase in pH (decrease in H^+) of extracellular fluid. The change in H^+ concentration may be the result of metabolic or respiratory abnormalities.

1. RESPIRATORY ACIDOSIS

Respiratory acidosis follows ventilatory abnormalities resulting in CO_2 retention and elevation of P_{CO_2} in alveoli and arterial blood (hypercapnia). Inadequate ventilation during anesthesia, following suppression of the respiratory center by CNS disease or drugs or resulting from respiratory muscle weakness or paralysis, produces CO_2 retention. Anatomic changes in structure of the lung (emphysema) or pulmonary circulation and abnormal thoracic structure (kyphoscoliosis) may alter alveolar-capillary blood exchange or diminish effective ventilation to prevent CO_2 excretion. Associated with impaired CO_2 excretion there may be impaired O_2 exchange with low alveolar and arterial P_{O_2} (hypoxia). In the presence of CO_2 retention and the resultant increase in H_2CO_3 concentration, compensatory reabsorption of HCO_3^- by the kidney provides buffer to reduce H^+ concentration, but this protection cannot be accomplished rapidly and is effectively available only in chronic situations that develop slowly.

Treatment

Treatment is directed toward improving ventilation with mechanical aids, bronchodilators, correction of heart failure, and antidotes for anesthetics or drugs suppressing the respiratory center. Close monitoring of P_{CO_2}, P_{O_2}, and pH of arterial blood is essential. The respiratory center is readily rendered unresponsive by high P_{CO_2} (hypercapnia), and recovery may be very slow. In the presence of hypercapnia, relief of hypoxia with oxygen therapy may deprive the patient of the only remaining stimulus to the respiratory center and produce more severe hypoventilation with resultant CO_2 narcosis and death. Assistance with respiration is required until the respiratory center becomes normally responsive to normal CO_2 concentrations.

2. RESPIRATORY ALKALOSIS

Respiratory alkalosis is a result of hyperventilation which produces lowered P_{CO_2} and elevated pH of extracellular fluid. Anxiety is the usual cause. Hyperventilation during anesthesia or from incorrectly used mechanical respiratory aids occurs more commonly than is generally appreciated. Renal compensation by excretion of HCO_3^- (with Na^+ predominantly) is too slow a response to be effective, and elevation of pH may reach a point at which asterixis, tetany, and increased neuromuscular irritability appear.

Treatment

Treatment of spontaneous hyperventilation consists of reducing anxiety by drugs or psychotherapy. Tetany may be alleviated by rebreathing exhaled air, which will increase P_{CO_2} and lower blood pH. Regulation of devices used in assisting with respiration should be determined by measurement of the P_{CO_2} and pH of arterial blood.

3. METABOLIC ACIDOSIS

Metabolic acidosis occurs with starvation, uncontrolled diabetes mellitus with ketosis, electrolyte (including bicarbonate) and water loss with diarrhea or enteric fistulas, and renal insufficiency or tubular defect producing inadequate H^+ excretion. Cation loss (Na^+, K^+, Ca^{++}) and organic acid anion retention occur with starvation and uncontrolled diabetes mellitus. In the presence of renal insufficiency, phosphate and sulfate are retained and cation (especially Na^+) is lost because of limited H^+ secretion for exchange with cation in the renal tubule. Respiratory compensation for metabolic acidosis by hyperventilation provides reduction of P_{CO_2} and thereby reduction of H_2CO_3 in extracellular fluid.

Treatment

Treatment is directed toward correcting the metabolic defect (eg, insulin for control of diabetes) and replenishment of water and of deficits of Na^+, K^+, HCO_3^-, and other electrolytes. Renal insufficiency requires careful replacement of water and electrolyte deficit and closely controlled rations of water, sodium, potassium, calcium, chloride, and bicarbonate to maintain normal extracellular fluid concentrations; the elevated serum phosphate may be lowered by interfering with phosphate absorption from the gut by oral administration of aluminum hydroxide preparations. In the presence of renal insufficiency, elevated extracellular K^+ concentrations may be reduced by either oral administration of ion exchange resins which bind K^+, either ingested or secreted, and prevent absorption in the intestine (see Hyperkalemia, below), or by hemodialysis or peritoneal dialysis.

4. METABOLIC ALKALOSIS

Metabolic alkalosis results from loss of gastric juice rich in HCl or from excessive sodium bicarbonate ingestion, and occurs also in association with K^+ deficit which is characteristically accompanied by increased urinary excretion of H^+. All of these result in renal retention of HCO_3^-, producing elevated extracellular fluid bicarbonate. Respiratory compensation by hypoventilation produces an elevation in P_{CO_2}, increasing the H_2CO_3 fraction of the bicarbonate buffer system.

Treatment

Treatment consists of replacing Cl^- and K^+ as well as any deficit of water and other electrolyte.

POTASSIUM

Potassium is one of the major intracellular cations, occupying a role that is parallel to that of sodium in extracellular fluid. Physiologic actions of potassium are related primarily to concentration of the cation in extracellular fluid, although the intracellular concentration may have some influence. Potassium plays an important part in muscular contraction, conduction of nerve impulses, enzyme action, and cell membrane function.

Cardiac muscle excitability, conduction, and rhythm are markedly affected by changes in concentration of K^+ in extracellular fluid. Both an increase and a decrease of extracellular K^+ concentration diminish excitability and conduction rate. Higher than normal concentrations produce a marked depression of conductivity with cardiac arrest in diastole; in the presence of very low concentrations, cardiac arrest occurs in systole. The effects of abnormal K^+ concentrations in extracellular fluid upon cell membrane potential of cardiac muscle and upon depolarization and repolarization are manifested in the ECG.

Membrane potential and excitability of skeletal and smooth muscle are profoundly affected by the concentrations of K^+, Ca^{++}, and Mg^{++}, with H^+ and Na^+ also involved. Conduction across the myoneural junction is under the influence of these cations as well. At both extremes of abnormal concentration of K^+ in extracellular fluid, muscle contractility is impaired and flaccid paralysis ensues.

Potassium concentration of extracellular fluid is closely regulated between 3.5–5 mEq/liter. Excretion of the 35–100 mEq of potassium contained in the daily diet of the average adult is predominantly via the kidney. There is good evidence that the potassium in glomerular filtrate is reabsorbed in the proximal tubule and that active secretion of potassium into the tubular fluid occurs in the distal portion of the tubule.

1. HYPERKALEMIA

Causes of increased extracellular K^+ concentration include failure of the kidney to excrete ingested potassium (acute and chronic renal failure, severe oliguria due to severe dehydration or trauma); unusual release of intracellular potassium in burns, crush injuries, or severe infections; and overtreatment with potassium salts. In metabolic acidosis, extracellular K^+ concentration is increased, as K^+ shifts from cells.

The elevated K^+ concentration interferes with normal neuromuscular function to produce weakness and paralysis; abdominal distention and diarrhea may occur. As extracellular concentration of K^+ increases, the ECG reflects impaired conduction by peaked T waves of increased amplitude, atrial arrest, spread in the QRS, biphasic QRS–T complexes, and finally ventricular fibrillation and cardiac arrest.

Treatment

Treatment consists of withholding potassium and employing cation exchange resins by mouth or enema.

Kayexalate, a sodium cycle sulfonic polystyrene exchange resin, 40–80 gm/day in divided doses, is usually effective. In an emergency, insulin may be employed to deposit K^+ with glycogen in the liver, and Ca^{++} may be given intravenously as an antagonist ion. Sodium bicarbonate can be given intravenously as an emergency measure in severe hyperkalemia; the increase in pH so induced results in a shift of K^+ into cells. Hemodialysis or peritoneal dialysis may be required to remove K^+ in the presence of protracted renal insufficiency.

2. HYPOKALEMIA

Potassium deficit may or may not be accompanied by lowered extracellular fluid K^+ concentration; however, when hypokalemia is present, total potassium deficit is usually profound. Exceptions to this common circumstance include the hypokalemia of alkalosis and that following administration of insulin. Causes of potassium deficit include reduced intake due to starvation or upper gastrointestinal obstruction; poor absorption in steatorrhea, short bowel syndrome, and regional enteritis; loss via the gastrointestinal tract due to emesis, diarrhea, and suction; loss via the kidney due to congenital tubule malfunction, diuresis resulting from diabetes or diuretics, accompanying metabolic alkalosis, and following excessive treatment with saline solutions containing little or no potassium; loss of interstitial fluid with burns or freezing; loss of K^+ due to adrenocortical hormone (cortisol or aldosterone) excess; and intracellular shift in bouts of familial periodic paralysis. A low concentration of K^+ in extracellular fluid results in impaired neuromuscular function with profound weakness of skeletal muscle, leading to impaired ventilation, and of smooth muscle, producing ileus. The ECG shows decreased amplitude and broadening of T waves, prominent U waves, sagging S–T segments, atrioventricular block, and, finally, cardiac arrest. Metabolic alkalosis with elevated plasma pH and bicarbonate concentration develops as a result of potassium deficit which is accompanied by renal excretion of H^+ and reabsorption of bicarbonate and by movement of Na^+ and H^+ from extracellular fluid into cells as K^+ is lost. A defect of water reabsorption by the renal tubule also occurs, producing polyuria and hyposthenuria; this is only slowly ameliorated following treatment.

Treatment

Treatment requires replacement of potassium orally or parenterally. Because of the toxicity of potassium, it must be administered cautiously to prevent hyperkalemia. Furthermore, confirmation of adequate renal function is important when potassium is administered since the principal route of excretion is via the kidney. KCl in a total dose of 1–3 mEq/kg/24 hours may be given parenterally in glucose or saline solutions (or both) at a rate that will not produce hyperkalemia. Cl^- is almost always needed to relieve the hypochloremia that is associated with the accompanying metabolic alkalosis.

CALCIUM

Calcium constitutes about 2% of body weight, but only about 1% of the total body calcium is in solution in body fluid. In the plasma, calcium is present as a nondiffusible complex with protein (33%); as a diffusible but undissociated complex with anions such as citrate, bicarbonate, and phosphate (12%); and as Ca^{++} (55%). The normal total plasma (or serum) calcium concentration is 4.5–5.5 mEq/liter (9–11 mg/100 ml). Bone serves as a reservoir of calcium available to body fluids. Excretion of Ca^{++} is via the kidney.

Calcium functions as an essential ion for many enzymes. It is an important constituent of mucoproteins and mucopolysaccharides, and is essential in blood coagulation.

Calcium along with other cations exerts an important effect on cell membrane potential and permeability manifested prominently in neuromuscular function. It plays a central role in muscle contraction as it is released from the sarcolemma to enter into the ATP-ADP reaction. During muscle relaxation, the calcium is actively transferred back to the sarcolemma and sarcoplasmic reticulum.

Neural function is sensitive to Ca^{++} concentration of interstitial fluid. Excitability is diminished by high Ca^{++} concentration and increased by low concentration. Signs of elevated Ca^{++} concentration include dulling of consciousness and stupor and muscular flaccidity and weakness. Low Ca^{++} concentration increases excitability to produce hyperirritability of muscle, tetany, and convulsions.

Cardiac muscle responds to elevated Ca^{++} concentration with increased contractility, ventricular extrasystoles, and idioventricular rhythm. These responses are accentuated in the presence of digitalis. With severe calcium toxicity, cardiac arrest in systole may occur. Low concentration of Ca^{++} produces diminished contractility of the heart and a lengthening of the Q–T interval of the ECG by prolonging the S–T segment.

1. HYPERCALCEMIA

Hypercalcemia results from hyperparathyroidism, invasion of bone by neoplasm (lung, breast, kidney, thyroid), production of a parathyroid-like hormone by isolated neoplasms (ovary, kidney, lung), sarcoidosis, multiple myeloma, and vitamin D intoxication.

Hypercalcemia per se affects neuromuscular function to produce weakness, and produces polyuria, thirst, anorexia, vomiting, and constipation.

Treatment

Treatment consists of control of the primary disease. In the presence of increase of Ca^{++} concentration in extracellular fluid producing symptoms and signs of intoxication, inorganic phosphate may be administered intravenously or orally; sodium sulfate may be given intravenously; or disodium edetate (disodium ethylenediaminetetraacetate) may be given intravenously. Changes in Ca^{++} concentration may be evanescent. When elevated Ca^{++} concentrations result from sarcoid or neoplasm, corticosteroids such as prednisone may be very effective.

2. HYPOCALCEMIA

Hypocalcemia results from hypoparathyroidism (idiopathic or postoperative), chronic renal insufficiency, rickets and osteomalacia, and malabsorption syndromes.

Hypocalcemia affects neuromuscular function to produce muscle cramps and tetany, convulsions, stridor and dyspnea, diplopia, abdominal cramps, and urinary frequency. Personality changes may occur. In chronic hypoparathyroidism and pseudohypoparathyroidism, cataracts may appear and calcification of basal ganglia of the brain may occur. Mental retardation and stunted growth are common in childhood.

Treatment

Treatment depends on the primary disease. Treatment of hypoparathyroidism with vitamin D and calcium is discussed in Chapter 36. For tetany due to hypocalcemia, calcium gluconate, 1–2 gm, may be given IV. A continuous infusion to sustain plasma calcium concentration may be required. Oral medication with the chloride, gluconate, levulinate, lactate, or carbonate salts of calcium will usually control milder symptoms or latent tetany.

MAGNESIUM

About 50% of total body magnesium exists in the insoluble state in bone. Only 5% is present as extracellular cation; the remaining 45% is contained in cells as intracellular cation. The normal plasma concentration is 1.5–2.5 mEq/liter, with about 1/3 bound to protein and 2/3 as free cation. Excretion of magnesium ion is via the kidney, with no evidence of active tubule secretion.

Magnesium is an important prosthetic or activator ion participating in the function of many enzymes involved in phosphate transfer reactions, including those requiring ATP or other nucleotide triphosphate as coenzymes.

Magnesium exerts physiologic effects on the nervous system resembling those of calcium. Elevated

Mg^{++} concentration of interstitial fluid produces sedation and central and peripheral nervous system depression. Low concentrations produce increased irritability, disorientation, and convulsions.

Magnesium acts directly upon the myoneural junction. Elevated levels produce blockade by decreasing acetylcholine release, reducing the effect of acetylcholine on depolarization, and diminishing excitability of the muscle cell. Calcium ion exerts an antagonistic action. Low levels of magnesium increase neuromuscular irritability and contractility, partly by increasing acetylcholine release. Tetany and convulsions may occur.

Cardiac muscle is affected by large increases in magnesium concentration in the range of 10–15 mEq/liter. Conduction time is increased, with lengthened duration of P–R and QRS components of the ECG. As the concentration of Mg^{++} increases further, cardiac arrest in diastole occurs.

Elevated magnesium concentrations produce vasodilation and a drop in blood pressure by blockade of sympathetic ganglia as well as a direct effect on smooth muscle.

1. HYPERMAGNESEMIA

Magnesium excess is almost always the result of renal insufficiency and inability to excrete what has been absorbed from food or infused. Occasionally, with the use of magnesium sulfate as a cathartic, enough magnesium is absorbed to produce toxicity, particularly in the presence of impaired renal function. Manifestations of hypermagnesemia include muscle weakness, fall in blood pressure, and sedation and confusion. The ECG shows increased P–R interval, broadened QRS complexes, and elevated T waves. Death usually results from respiratory muscle paralysis.

Treatment

Treatment is directed toward alleviating renal insufficiency. Calcium acts as an antagonist to Mg^{++} and may be employed parenterally for temporary benefit. Extracorporeal or peritoneal dialysis may be indicated.

2. HYPOMAGNESEMIA

Magnesium deficit may be encountered in chronic alcoholism in association with delirium tremens, starvation, diarrhea, malabsorption, prolonged gastrointestinal suction, vigorous diuresis, primary aldosteronism, and hypoparathyroidism.

Magnesium deficit is characterized by neuromuscular and CNS hyperirritability with athetoid movements; jerking, coarse, and flapping tremor; positive Babinski response, nystagmus, tachycardia, hypertension, and vasomotor changes.

Treatment

Treatment consists of the use of parenteral fluids containing magnesium as chloride or sulfate, 10–40 mEq/day during the period of severe deficit followed by 10 mEq/day for maintenance. Magnesium sulfate may also be given IM, 4–8 gm (66–133 mEq) daily in 4 divided doses.

MAINTENANCE & REPLACEMENT THERAPY

The range of tolerance for water and electrolytes (homeostatic limits) permits reasonable latitude in therapy provided normal renal function exists to accomplish the final regulation of volume and concentration.

Deficits should be restored within 24–48 hours, during which time maintenance requirements must also be met. Continuing unusual losses from the gastrointestinal tract, kidney, burns, etc must also be replaced as they are incurred.

In administering fluids parenterally to those who cannot take fluids orally, the total daily ration should be administered continuously over the 24-hour period in order to assure the best utilization by the patient. This is particularly true when losses are large and the total daily infusion is large. With modern technics for continuous intravenous infusions, around-the-clock administration produces little discomfort or hardship.

TABLE 43–3. Daily maintenance rations for patients requiring parenteral fluids.

	Per sq M Body Surface	Average Adult (60–100 kg)
Glucose	60–75 gm	100–200 gm
Na⁺	50–70 mEq	80–120 mEq
K⁺	50–70 mEq	80–120 mEq
Water	1500 ml	2500 ml

TABLE 43–4. Composition of solutions for parenteral infusion.*

	Ionic Concentration in mEq/liter							
	Na⁺	K⁺	Ca⁺⁺	Mg⁺⁺	NH₄⁺	Cl⁻	HCO₃⁻ Equiv	PO₄≡
Isotonic saline (0.9%)	155					155		
Sodium chloride (5%)	855					855		
Ringer's solution	147	4	4			155		
Ringer's lactate (Hartmann's)	130	4	3			109	28	
M/6 sodium lactate	167						167	
Darrow's solution (KNL)	121	35				103	53	
Potassium chloride								
0.2% in dextrose 5%		27				27		
0.3% in dextrose 5%		40				40		
"Modified duodenal solution" with dextrose, 10%	80	36	5	3		64	60	
"Gastric solution" with dextrose, 10%	63	17			70	150		
Ammonium chloride, 0.9%					170	170		
Examples of "maintenance solutions":								
Pediatric electrolyte "No. 48" with dextrose 5%	25	20		3		22	23	3
Maintenance electrolyte "No. 75" with dextrose 5%	40	35				40	20	15
Levulose and dextrose with electrolyte (Butler's II)	57	25		5		49	25	13
Dextrose in 0.2% saline	34					34		
Dextrose in 0.45% saline	77					77		

Ampules (note directions with ampule). Contents per ampule.†

	Na⁺	K⁺	Ca⁺⁺	Mg⁺⁺	NH₄⁺	Cl⁻	HCO₃⁻ Equiv	PO₄≡
Potassium phosphate‡, 20 ml		40						40
Potassium chloride‡, 40 mEq		40				40		
KMC‡		25	10	10		45		
Calcium gluconate, 10%, 10 ml			4.5				4.5	
Sodium bicarbonate§, 7.5%, 50 ml	45						45	
Sodium lactate§, molar, 40 ml	40						40	
Ammonium chloride, 100 mEq					100	100		

*Modified and reproduced, with permission, from Krupp, Sweet, Jawetz, & Biglieri: *Physician's Handbook,* 16th ed. Lange, 1970.

†Many other types of solutions are commercially available and may be used.

‡Dilute to 1 liter.

§Dilute as indicated by manufacturer.

TABLE 43–5. Oral electrolyte preparations.*

Preparation	Supplied as	Electrolyte Content†					
		Na⁺	K⁺	NH₄⁺	Ca⁺⁺	Cl⁻	HCO₃⁻ (or equivalent)
NaCl	Salt	17				17	
NaHCO₃	Salt	12					12
KCl	Salt		14			14	
K-triplex	Elixir		15 mEq/ 5 ml				15
K gluconate (Kaon)	Elixir		7 mEq/ 5 ml				7
Ca gluconate	Salt				4.5		
Ca lactate	Salt				10		
NH₄ Cl (acidifying salt)	Salt			19‡		19	
Kayexalate (ion-exchange resins)	Salt	3§	§				

*Reproduced, with permission, from Krupp & Chatton: *Current Diagnosis & Treatment 1972.* Lange, 1972.

†mEq/gm unless otherwise specified.

‡NH₄⁺ is converted to H⁺ in the body, mEq for mEq.

§1 gm resin removes 1 mEq K⁺ and contributes 3 mEq Na⁺ to patient.

TABLE 43–6. Equivalent values of salts
used for therapy.*

Salt	gm	mEq of Cation per Amount Stated
IV or Oral		
NaCl	9	155
NaCl	5.8	100
NaCl	1	17
NaHCO$_3$	8.4	100
Na lactate	11.2	100
KCl	1.8	25
K acetate	2.5	25
{ K$_2$HPO$_4$	1.84	25
{ KH$_2$PO$_4$	0.4	
CaCl$_2$	0.5	10
Ca gluconate	2	10
MgCl$_2$	0.5	10
Oral		
K citrate	3	25
K tartrate	5	27

*Reproduced, with permission, from Krupp, Sweet, Jawetz, & Biglieri: *Physician's Handbook,* 16th ed. Lange, 1970.

●　　●　　●

General References

General

Black, D.A.K.: Symptoms and signs in disorders of body fluid. J Chronic Dis 11:340–347, 1960.

Bland, J.H.: *Clinical Metabolism of Body Water and Electrolytes.* Saunders, 1963.

Jenkins, M.T., & others: Clinical questions related to fluids. Clin Anesth 3:212–225, 1968.

Pitts, R.F.: *Physiology of the Kidney and Body Fluids,* 2nd ed. Year Book, 1968.

Robinson, J.R.: Metabolism of intracellular water. Physiol Rev 40:112–149, 1960.

Sunderman, F.W., & F.W. Sunderman, Jr.: *Clinical Pathology of the Serum Electrolytes.* Thomas, 1966.

Fluid Volume–Sodium

Clift, G.V., & others: Syndrome of inappropriate vasopressin secretion. Arch Int Med 118:453–460, 1966.

Dodge, P.R., & others: Studies in experimental water intoxication. Arch Neurol 3:513–529, 1960.

Earley, L.E.: Sodium metabolism. New England J Med 281:72–86, 1969.

Finberg, L.: Hypernatremic dehydration. Advances Pediat 16:325–344, 1969.

Gauer, O.H., & J.P. Henry: Circulatory basis of fluid volume control. Physiol Rev 43:423–481, 1963.

Githers, J.H.: Hypernatremic dehydration. Clin Pediat 2:453–462, 1963.

Goldberg, M.: Hyponatremia and the inappropriate secretion of antidiuretic hormone. Am J Med 35:293–298, 1963.

Leaf, A.: The clinical and physiologic significance of the serum sodium concentration. New England J Med 267:24–30, 77–83, 1962.

Maffly, R.H., & I.S. Edelman: The role of sodium potassium and water in the hypoosmotic states of heart failure. Progr Cardiovas Dis 4:88–104, 1961.

Warhol, R.M., Eichenholz, A., & R.O. Mulhausen: Osmolality. Arch Int Med 116:743–749, 1965.

Welt, L.G.: Hypo- and hypernatremia. Ann Int Med 56:161–164, 1962.

Hydrogen Ion

Albert, M.S., Dell, R.B., & R.W. Winters: Quantitative displacement of acid-base equilibrium in metabolic acidosis. Ann Int Med 66:312–322, 1967.

Blumentals, A.S. (editor): Symposium on acid-base balance. Arch Int Med 116:647–742, 1965.

Diarrhea and acid-base disturbances. Leading article. Lancet 1:1305–1306, 1966.

Elkinton, J.R.: Hydrogen ion turnover in health and disease. Ann Int Med 57:660–684, 1962.

Kassirer, J.P., & W.B. Schwartz: The response of normal man to selective depletion of hydrochloric acid. Correction of metabolic alkalosis in man without repair of potassium deficiency. Am J Med 40:10–26, 1966.

Manfredi, F.: Effects of hypocapnia and hypercapnia on intracellular acid-base equilibrium in man. J Lab Clin Med 69:304–312, 1967.

Schwartz, W.B., & W.C. Waters: Lactate versus bicarbonate. Am J Med 32:831–834, 1962.

Statement of acid-base terminology. Ann Int Med 63:885–890, 1965; Anesthesiology 27:7–12, 1966; Ann New York Acad Sc 133:251–258, 1966.

Tranquada, R.E., Grant, W.J., & C.R. Peterson: Lactic acidosis. Arch Int Med 117:192–202, 1966.

Van Ypersele de Strihou, C., Brasseur, L., & J. DeConinck: The "carbon-dioxide response curve" for chronic hypercapnia in man. New England J Med 275:117–122, 1966.

Waddell, W.J., & others: Intracellular pH. Physiol Rev 49:285–329, 1969.

Potassium

Bellet, S.: The cardiotoxic effects of hyperpotassemia and its treatment. Postgrad Med 25:602–609, 1959.

Berlyne, G.M., Janabi, K., & A.B. Shaw: Dangers of resonium A (Kayexalate) in the treatment of hyperkalemia in renal failure. Lancet 1:167–169, 1966.

Black, D.A.K.: Current concepts of potassium metabolism. J Pediat 56:814–825, 1960.

Christy, N.P., & J.H. Laragh: Pathogenesis of hypokalemic alkalosis in Cushing's syndrome. New England J Med 265:1083–1088, 1961.

Kassirer, J.P., & others: The critical role of chloride in the correction of hypokalemic alkalosis in man. Am J Med 38:172–189, 1965.

Leaf, A., & R.F. Santos: Physiologic mechanisms in potassium deficiency. New England J Med 264:335–341, 1961.

Papper, S., & R. Whang: *Hyperkalemia and Hypokalemia.* Disease-A-Month. Year Book, June 1964.

Surawicz, B.: Electrolytes and the electrocardiogram. Am J Cardiol 12:656–662, 1963.

Weatherall, M.: Ions and the actions of digitalis. Brit Heart J 28:497–504, 1966.

Calcium

Chakmakjian, Z.H., & J.E. Bethune: Sodium sulfate treatment of hypercalcemia. New England J Med 275:862–869, 1966.

Copp, D.H.: Endocrine control of calcium homeostasis. J Endocr 43:137–161, 1969.

Goldsmith, R.S., & S.H. Ingbar: Inorganic phosphate treatment of hypercalcemia of diverse etiologies. New England J Med 274:1–7, 284, 1966.

Hebert, L.A., & others: Studies of the mechanism by which phosphate infusion lowers serum calcium concentration. J Clin Invest 45:1886–1894, 1966.

Howard, J.E., & W.C. Thomas: Clinical disorders of calcium homeostasis. Medicine 42:25–45, 1963.

Krane, S.M.: Selected features of the clinical course of hypoparathyroidism. JAMA 178:472–475, 1961.

Mannheimer, I.H.: Hypercalcemia of breast cancer: Management with corticosteroids. Cancer 18:679–691, 1965.

Parathyroid insufficiency. Leading article. Lancet 2:1441–1442, 1961.

Magnesium

Aikawa, J.K.: *The Role of Magnesium in Biologic Processes.* Thomas, 1963.

Dunn, M.J., & M. Walser: Magnesium depletion in normal man. Metabolism 15:884–895, 1966.

MacIntyre, I.: Magnesium metabolism. Advances Int Med 13:143–154, 1967.

Wacker, W.E.C., & A.F. Parisi: Magnesium metabolism. New England J Med 278:772–776, 1968.

44...

Cyanocobalamin & Folic Acid

Folic acid and vitamin B_{12} (cyanocobalamin) are chemically unrelated essential food factors that can be conveniently considered together because a deficiency of either produces a morphologically similar arrest of bone marrow maturation and megaloblastic anemia. This is not surprising since both compounds are essential for the normal synthesis of deoxyribonucleic acid (DNA), and a deficiency of either interferes with normal mitosis. Other systems characterized by rapid cell division—eg, the gastrointestinal epithelium and the myeloid cells—are also affected by a deficiency state.

Folic acid and vitamin B_{12} are involved in widely differing metabolic reactions, but the pathways are linked at some points and a deficiency of either factor can be at least partially corrected by administration of the other factor. However, the neurologic lesions resulting from cobalamin deficiency are not corrected by folic acid administration.

FOLIC ACID

Source & Chemistry

Folic acid (pteroylmonoglutamic acid, folacin) consists of a pteridine nucleus, para-aminobenzoic acid, and glutamic acid. Sources of folic acid are widespread in foods of both animal and vegetable origin, the highest contents occurring in yeast, liver, and green vegetables such as spinach, asparagus, lettuce, and endive. The term "folate content" is often used to include folic acid (folate monoglutamate) and also conjugates that contain more than one glutamic acid residue. The degree of absorption and utilization of folate may vary depending on the degree of liberation of folic acid by conjugase enzymes present in the jejunum. Folic acid is destroyed only by prolonged boiling, and the presence of reducing agents such as ascorbic acid reduce the loss.

Absorption, Distribution, & Excretion

Folic acid is readily and completely absorbed by the proximal third of the small intestine. Low concentrations probably utilize an active transport mechanism, but at high concentrations folic acid is probably also absorbed by diffusion. Absorption of orally administered supplemental folic acid is usually satisfac-

tory even in the presence of disorders of the small bowel which have produced a deficiency state. Conjugated folate in food is less readily absorbed, and dietary correction of the deficiency is usually impractical in the presence of intestinal disease. Folic acid is widely distributed to all tissues and concentrated in the CSF. Only small amounts of folic acid appear in the urine of subjects on normal diets, but excretion by this route is high following large doses.

Requirements & Stores of Folic Acid

The dietary intake of folate in the USA varies widely between $50-2000$ µg. The availability of the vitamin probably also varies with the type of glutamate conjugate. Stores of folic acid are low compared with stores of vitamin B_{12}, being exhausted in $1-3$ months depending upon the previous nutritional status and the rate of utilization.

The minimum daily intake required by a healthy adult is probably about 50 µg daily. Experimental folate deficiency, manifested by slight anemia and megaloblastic changes in the bone marrow, has been produced in man by administration of a diet containing only 5 µg folate daily for 4½ months. Dietary requirements of an individual subject vary with both physiologic and disease states. Pregnancy can precipitate clinical deficiency in women receiving inadequate diets.

Folate deficiency can be diagnosed on clinical grounds—ie, the appearance of macrocytosis or an overt megaloblastic anemia—or by one of several laboratory procedures. Serum folate levels can be measured by a microbiologic assay or the urinary excretion of formiminoglutamic acid (FIGLU) measured following the administration of histidine. Histidine is enzymatically converted to FIGLU and reacts with tetrahydrofolic acid to form formiminotetrahydrofolic acid and glutamic acid. In folic acid deficiency this reaction cannot occur, and excess FIGLU accumulates and is excreted in the urine. Both the FIGLU test and serum folate levels have proved to be unreliable in some cases of undisputed folic acid deficiency occurring in pregnancy.

Mechanisms of Action

Folic acid is the inactive precursor of several coenzymes, and the main step in their formation is reduction to tetrahydrofolic acid by the enzyme folate

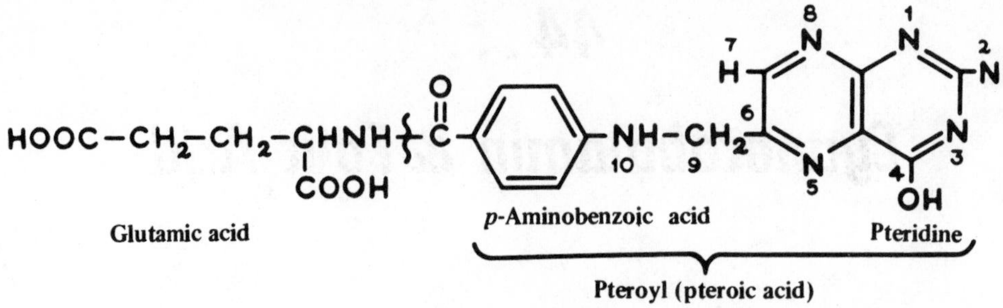

$$HOOC-CH_2-CH_2-CHNH \{ \quad C \quad \} \quad NH-CH_2$$

Glutamic acid   p-Aminobenzoic acid   Pteridine

Pteroyl (pteroic acid)

Folic acid

reductase. Several derivatives of tetrahydrofolic acid accept and donate single carbon atom units. Formyl, formate, or hydroxymethyl derivatives are formed at the N_{10} (or N_5 and N_{10}) positions. Folinic acid (5-formyltetrahydrofolic acid) is widely regarded as an active form of the coenzyme. This is not strictly true, because conversion to the 10-formyl or 5,10-formyl derivative is required before the compound can be utilized, and this is accomplished by the enzyme tetrahydrofolic acid isomerase. Deficiency of folic acid is not uncommonly associated with deficiency of ascorbic acid, and it has been suggested that ascorbic acid is required for the reduction of folic acid to the tetrahydro derivative. Recent work suggests that this is unlikely, and dietary deficiency of both vitamins appears to be a more reasonable explanation.

Single carbon units are utilized in several reactions, of which the most important are the following:

(1) Purine synthesis entirely from single carbon units via inosinic acid.

(2) Pyrimidine nucleotide synthesis with the methylation of deoxyuridylic acid to thymidylic acid. It is suggested that deficiency of folic acid coenzymes limits DNA production at this stage.

(3) Amino acid interconversions, including conversion of homocysteine to methionine, a reaction also requiring vitamin B_{12}.

The biologic aspects of the disordered metabolism resulting from folic acid deficiency are related chiefly to disordered growth secondary to defective synthesis of purine and pyrimidine nucleotides. Failure to produce new DNA impairs mitosis, and the biologic effects of this are readily seen in all tissues that contain rapidly dividing cells. Erythropoiesis changes from a normoblastic to megaloblastic appearance. The megaloblast is a large cell with an increased ratio of cytoplasmic to nuclear material. The chromatin is fine-grained, suggesting relative immaturity of the nucleus. The DNA content of the cell is normal or slightly increased, whereas the ribonucleic acid (RNA) is markedly increased. The cytoplasmic development continues largely unimpaired, later resulting in hemoglobin production, whereas nuclear changes lag behind. Thymine will reverse the megaloblastic changes produced by folic acid deficiency (but not those secondary to vitamin B_{12} deficiency), suggesting that failure of thymidylate synthesis is the chief limiting factor in this case.

Clinical Uses

In the presence of a megaloblastic anemia, the differentiation between deficiency of folate and vitamin B_{12} must be made and the nature of the process causing a deficiency then clarified.

Deficiency of folic acid may be due to dietary deficiency, although this is rare unless there are increased requirements, as during pregnancy; to decreased utilization due to the use of drugs that are folic acid antagonists; or to interference with absorption.

Supplementary folic acid may, therefore, be used to correct the following states:

A. Dietary Deficiency: Dietary deficiency of folic acid, previously thought to be rare because of the ubiquitous nature of the vitamin, is now more commonly reported. In alcoholics the diet is often deficient in vegetable and animal products, and elderly people may live on restricted diets either for socioeconomic reasons or out of apathy. A recent study of regional ileitis showed that folic acid deficiency was only partly due to defective absorption. Defective intake associated with anorexia was also an important factor. The main treatment in all of these cases consists of correction of the diet, but folic acid, 100–200 μg daily orally, quickly corrects the deficiency.

B. Increased Requirement During Pregnancy: The chief condition precipitating megaloblastic anemia secondary to increased utilization of folic acid is pregnancy. A degree of dietary deficiency also plays a part. The megaloblastic anemia of pregnancy occurs predominantly in poor, multiparous women; it is now uncommon in Western society but still occurs in underdeveloped communities. The greater incidence in twin pregnancies and during the third trimester emphasizes the importance of increased fetal requirements. Folic acid in a dose of 0.5–1 mg daily orally is usually curative. Antenatal care in poor socioeconomic areas frequently includes prophylactic administration of folic acid, 100–300 μg daily orally, often in a preparation that also includes iron. This greatly reduces the incidence of macrocytosis and anemia.

C. Interference with Utilization by Other Drugs: Megaloblastic anemia occurs in many patients receiving the anticonvulsant diphenylhydantoin (Dilantin), and also in some patients receiving primidone (Mysoline), carbamazepine (Tegretol), or mephobarbital (Mebaral). Folate deficiency is a rare result of the use of oral contraceptives. These drugs act to inhibit intestinal deconjugase activity and reduce absorption of dietary folate polyglutamates. The anemia is corrected by folic acid or, where practical, by stopping the causative drug.

D. **Malabsorption Syndrome**: Folic acid deficiency occurs commonly in the malabsorption syndrome, due usually to disease of the small intestine but sometimes following partial gastrectomy. Malabsorption syndrome secondary to atrophy of the intestinal villi is seen classically in celiac disease, adult idiopathic steatorrhea, and tropical sprue. The first 2 conditions are often due to intolerance to gluten, and dramatic clinical responses often follow treatment with gluten-free diets. Folic acid supplements are often needed, however, especially in adults.

The cause of tropical sprue is less well understood, and folic acid deficiency probably results from poor intake, poor absorption, and perhaps the increased requirements caused by associated infection. The clinical manifestations often respond quickly to folic acid treatment, though broad spectrum antibiotics also are sometimes needed for several months.

Folic acid deficiency may also be produced by malabsorption syndromes secondary to gross structural disease of the small intestines—eg, regional ileitis, intestinal tuberculosis, infiltrations by reticuloses and Whipple's disease, intestinal amyloidosis, multiple diverticula, blind loops, extensive surgical resections, and irradiation damage.

For many years the therapeutic dose of folic acid has been 10–20 mg daily orally. This is unnecessarily high, and 0.5–1 mg daily is probably sufficient. Even this dose can produce a therapeutic response in anemia due to vitamin B_{12} deficiency, and evidence of vitamin B_{12} deficiency should be sought before treatment with folic acid is begun, particularly if the terminal ileum is diseased or has been surgically removed. If doubt exists regarding the ability of the intestine to absorb folic acid, intramuscular injection is practical for a short period.

Contraindications & Cautions

Because folic acid is generally held to be free of toxic effects, it is frequently given in unnecessarily large doses and sometimes in the absence of a clear indication for its use. An observation that 15 mg/day for as short a period as 1 month may cause behavioral changes has not yet been repeated, but some caution is advisable until the possible toxicity is studied.

Folic acid alone must not be administered to patients with pernicious anemia. Correction of the anemia may occur, but progression of neurologic complications frequently follows.

To treat or mask the development of an anemia due to vitamin B_{12} deficiency requires doses of folic acid that are large compared to the amounts needed for the prevention of folate deficiency. To prevent the masking of the anemia and the development of peripheral nerve and spinal cord changes from vitamin B_{12} deficiency in patients not recognized to have pernicious anemia, multivitamin preparations that may be sold without a prescription are not permitted to contain more than 0.1 mg of folate per daily dose. Vita-min preparations sold only upon prescription are not so regulated.

Preparations Available

Tablets, 0.4, 5, and 20 mg
Elixir (flavored), 5 mg/5 ml
Injectable (IM), 15 mg/ml, 1, 2, and 10 ml ampules

FOLINIC ACID
(Citrovorum Factor, Leucovorin)

A folic acid deficiency is produced during therapy with the folic acid analogues aminopterin and amethopterin (methotrexate) used as antineoplastic agents and with the chemotherapeutic agent pyrimethamine. These agents competitively inhibit the conversion of folic acid to folinic acid, but their affinity for the enzyme (folate reductase) is so much greater than that of folic acid that not even large doses of folic acid will correct the drug induced deficiency. In the event of a severe toxic reaction to the folic acid antagonist, the already reduced form, folinic acid, can be given since it can be used to form new coenzyme.

Folinic acid is supplied (as Calcium Leucovorin) for intravenous or intramuscular injection as 1 ml ampules containing 3 mg/ml.

VITAMIN B_{12}
(Cyanocobalamin)

Sources & Chemistry

Several related compounds are able to correct vitamin B_{12} deficiency. Cyanocobalamin was the first member of the group to be isolated, and it is still widely used therapeutically. Composed of 2 main groups, the planar group consists of 4 reduced pyrrole rings holding a central cobalt atom. Below the planar group and linked between the central cobalt atom and pyrrole ring IV is a "nucleotide" not found in the usual nucleic acids but composed of ribose and the base 5,6-dimethyl-benzimidazole. Above the planar group, linked to the cobalt atom, is a cyanide radical. This cyanide group can be replaced, without loss of biologic activity, by several other substituents: a hydroxyl group, giving hydroxycobalamin; and a 5-deoxyadenosyl substitution, forming coenzyme B_{12} (or cobamide) found in highest concentrations of the 3 cobamides.

The ultimate source of the vitamin is synthesis by microorganisms, and it is found only in foodstuffs of animal origin. Liver, kidney, and shellfish have the highest content; muscle, fish, and some cheeses contain moderate amounts. It does not occur in plant products except when they contain symbiotic bacteria (as is the case with legumes).

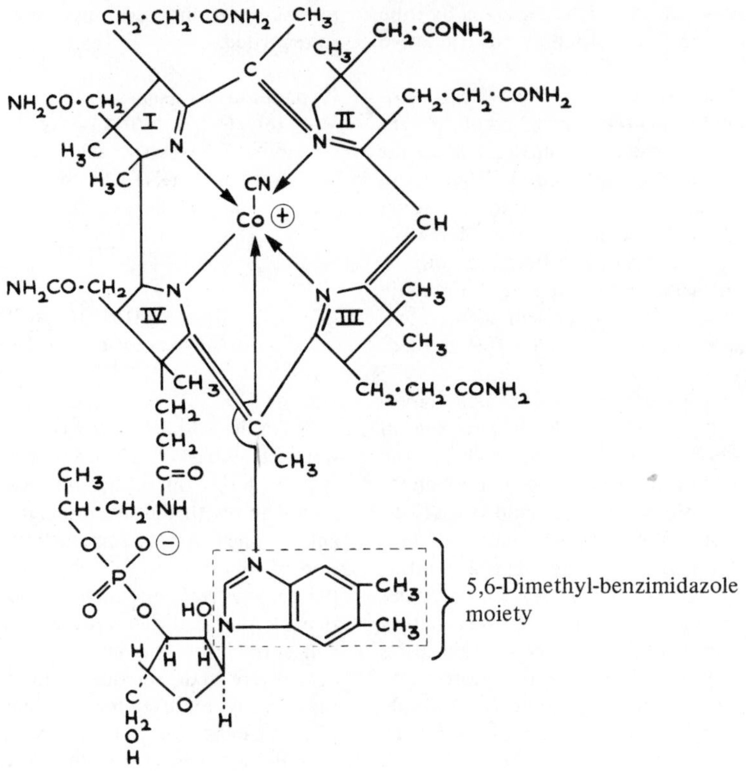

$$CH_2 \cdot CH_2 \cdot CONH_2 \quad CH_3 \quad CH_2 \cdot CONH_2$$

I, II, III, IV (pyrrole rings)

$$NH_2CO \cdot CH_2 \qquad CH_3 \qquad CH_2 \cdot CH_2 \cdot CONH_2$$

$$H_3C \qquad H_3C$$

$$CN$$
$$Co\ \oplus$$

$$CH$$

$$NH_2CO \cdot CH_2 \qquad CH_3 \qquad CH_3 \qquad CH_2 \cdot CH_2 \cdot CONH_2$$

$$CH_3$$
$$CH_2$$
$$CH_2$$
$$C=O$$
$$CH_3 \quad CH_3$$
$$CH \cdot CH_2 \cdot NH$$

$$P \qquad O\ \ominus$$

$$HO$$

5,6-Dimethyl-benzimidazole moiety (CH_3, CH_3)

$$C\ H_2\ O\ H$$

Cyanocobalamin (vitamin B_{12})

Bacteria in the human colon synthesize vitamin B_{12}, and the patients who used to die of pernicious anemia had fecal excretions of the vitamin far greater than their needs. Vitamin B_{12} in food sources is usually bound to protein and peptides which are removed before recombination of the vitamin with intrinsic factor in the gut prior to absorption.

The commercially available B_{12} is prepared by fermentation using *Streptomyces griseus*.

Absorption, Distribution, & Excretion

There are 2 mechanisms for the absorption of vitamin B_{12}. The more important of the 2 is applicable to the small amounts of the vitamin present in the diet. In the stomach, vitamin B_{12} is released from associated peptides and proteins and combines preferentially with intrinsic factor, a glycoprotein (mol wt 50,000) secreted by the parietal or chief cells of the fundus and body of the stomach. Absorption of vitamin B_{12} then takes place in the lower ileum by a highly specific transport system that requires calcium ions and a pH above 5.7. It is the loss of intrinsic factor and subsequent failure of absorption of vitamin B_{12} that is the cause of pernicious anemia. When large quantities of vitamin B_{12} are given orally, a small percentage is absorbed by diffusion, and this process is independent of the intrinsic factor mechanism. This type of absorption is of therapeutic importance only when patients with pernicious anemia refuse parenteral vitamin B_{12} therapy and are treated with 1000 μg of vitamin B_{12} daily by mouth.

In theory, pernicious anemia could be treated by the combined oral administration of cyanocobalamin and hog intrinsic factor—ie, liver-stomach preparations. However, a refractory state quickly develops.

Isotopically labeled vitamin B_{12} appears to remain in the wall of the lower ileum for several hours before entering the blood. In the plasma the vitamin is carried by 2 proteins, an α_1-globulin and a β-globulin, to its storage site in the liver. Intramuscular administration of cyanocobalamin produces a rapid rise in blood level with saturation of the binding sites on plasma proteins. A large fraction of the injected vitamin (up to 98%) may then be excreted in the urine. Hydroxocobalamin, however, is more completely bound to proteins; a lower fraction of an intramuscular dose is excreted in the urine; and plasma levels following a single injection are maintained 2–3 times as long.

In healthy subjects, excretion of vitamin B_{12} is negligible. Most of the loss occurs as a result of biliary excretion, the vitamin appearing in the feces together with that produced by colonic bacteria. Only a small proportion of vitamin B_{12} excreted in the bile appears in the feces because most is reabsorbed by the terminal ileum.

Requirements & Stores of Vitamin B_{12}

The adult human requires about 1 μg of vitamin B_{12} daily to replace the loss that occurs chiefly in the bile and feces. This amount maintains the stores and makes vitamin B_{12} the most potent known vitamin. Dietary intake varies from 1–85 μg daily. The total vitamin B_{12} store for an adult human averages 5 mg, most of this being in the liver. It follows that serious deficiency does not usually appear for 3–6 years even in the absence of dietary intake or complete failure of absorption.

Mechanisms of Action

The methylation of homocysteine to methionine requires methyl B_{12}, which receives the methyl group from N_5-methyltetrahydrofolic acid and subsequently transfers it to homocysteine. In the absence of methyl B_{12}, N_5-methyltetrahydrofolic acid cannot be utilized and is trapped, resulting in a situation similar in end result to folic acid deficiency. Experiments performed on microorganisms suggest that vitamin B_{12} may be required for the synthesis of deoxyribose; if this work also applies to mammalian cells, deficiency of the vitamin could limit production of DNA without affecting RNA synthesis. Propionic acid can be metabolized via methylmalonate to succinate, and the last reaction requires coenzyme B_{12}. This reaction, together with the regeneration of methionine, associates vitamin B_{12} with lipid metabolism, and tenuous suggestions have attempted to link these biochemical findings with the defective formation of myelin seen in the nervous system in vitamin B_{12} deficiency. The widespread disturbance of DNA production resulting in the changes seen in cells of the hematopoietic system and most epithelial cells—and which have been previously described for folic acid deficiency—are more easily understood than the lesions of the nervous tissue.

Clinical Uses

Vitamin B_{12}, because of its relative cheapness and lack of toxic effects, is widely used as a placebo and "tonic." This practice should be deplored. Administration should be confined to cases of established deficiency, and, since replacement therapy is usually required for life, a complete investigation of the case should be performed. The degree of deficiency and the underlying cause of the deficiency should then be recorded and the healthy skepticism of successive physicians allayed without the need for repeated studies.

A. Pernicious Anemia: By far the most common justified use of vitamin B_{12} is in the treatment of pernicious anemia (addisonian anemia), a conditional deficiency due to failure of absorption. The primary lesion in pernicious anemia is atrophy of the gastric mucosa with achlorhydria and failure to secrete intrinsic fac-

tor. As a result, dietary vitamin B_{12} is not absorbed by the terminal ileum and is excreted in the feces together with that produced by colonic bacteria. The initial treatment of pernicious anemia consists of parenteral cyanocobalamin or hydroxocobalamin. Doses as high as 1000 μg IM on alternate days for 10–15 days and as low as 30 μg daily IM for 5–10 days have been suggested. The tendency has been to use unnecessarily high doses, most of the vitamin appearing in the urine, but the use of hydroxocobalamin reduces the urinary loss. Higher dosages are probably advisable when neurologic changes are present. Within hours of commencing treatment with the vitamin, mental symptoms such as lassitude often improve dramatically and the mild fever that is frequently present may subside. The megaloblastic changes in the marrow disappear in 2–3 days. The reticulocyte response begins in about 3 days, reaching a peak in about 1 week. The hemoglobin and erythrocyte count return to normal in 4–6 weeks. The rate of rise of hemoglobin and the height of the reticulocyte count are greater in cases of greater severity.

The reliability of the response of pernicious anemia to vitamin B_{12} and the insidious fall of hemoglobin which allows cardiovascular compensation largely obviate the need for the transfusion of packed red cells. The response of the neurologic syndrome is slower and less certain than the anemia. Peripheral neuropathy is usually corrected. The subacute combined degeneration of the cord is arrested by vitamin B_{12}, but improvement, if it occurs, is slow. Changes of short duration carry a much better prognosis than a long-standing condition.

Maintenance therapy must be continued for life. Unless the patient understands his disease, the basis for its diagnosis, and the need for repeated treatment, he will be subject to relapses and repeated diagnostic studies. Cyanocobalamin, 100 μg IM monthly, is effec-

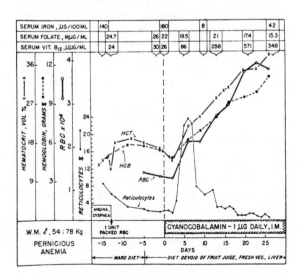

FIG 44–1. Response to 1 μg of vitamin B_{12} daily in a patient with pernicious anemia. (Reproduced, with permission, from Herbert: Megaloblastic anemia. New England J Med 268:370, 1963.)

tive. Hydroxocobalamin, which is stored in the body for a slightly longer period, may be used instead of cyanocobalamin.

Large amounts of cyanocobalamin by mouth (1000 μg/day) are effective but less reliable than parenteral vitamin B_{12}. Injectable liver preparations are now standardized in terms of their vitamin B_{12} content and there is no reason to use them. Folic acid will correct the anemia of vitamin B_{12} deficiency but allows the neurologic damage to progress.

B. Investigation of B_{12} Absorption: The cause of suspected vitamin B_{12} deficiency can be investigated by oral administration of a small amount of vitamin B_{12} labeled with radioactive cobalt (^{57}Co). Radioactivity only appears in the urine if the isotopically labeled vitamin is absorbed from the gut. An intramuscular injection of 1000 μg of nonradioactive vitamin B_{12} precedes the oral vitamin and saturates the depleted stores, increasing urinary excretion of the labeled vitamin (Schilling test). Failure of absorption can be further investigated by repeating the test but also by giving intrinsic factor in addition to isotopically labeled vitamin B_{12}. If absorption of vitamin B_{12} follows this procedure, then deficiency of intrinsic factor is the likely cause; but failure of absorption probably indicates disease of the terminal ileum. Continued and severe deficiency of vitamin B_{12} from any cause produces the classical clinical picture of macrocytic megaloblastic anemia with mild hemolytic features together with glossitis and weight loss. Varying degrees of peripheral neuropathy, subacute combined degeneration of the spinal cord, retrobulbar neuritis, and mental changes occur, and may be present when anemia is absent and megaloblastic changes are slight.

C. Other Uses: All patients who have had a total gastrectomy develop vitamin B_{12} deficiency if they live long enough to exhaust their stores of the vitamin. The deficiency in these cases should be anticipated and parenteral maintenance therapy given. Some cases of partial gastrectomy subsequently develop deficiency of vitamin B_{12}, possibly due to atrophy in the remaining stomach. The treatment is identical to that described for pernicious anemia. Following both total and subtotal gastrectomy, an iron deficiency anemia is likely to develop before the macrocytic anemia.

Dietary deficiency of vitamin B_{12} is extremely rare and has been reported only in association with strict vegetarian diets excluding all meat, eggs, and dairy products. The high intake of folic acid usually prevents any marked hematologic changes. If vitamin B_{12} deficiency is suspected, it can be adequately treated by cyanocobalamin, 5 μg daily orally. The origin of the material from *Streptomyces griseus* can be stressed to avoid any conflict.

It has been claimed that the form of retrobulbar neuritis seen in heavy smokers (tobacco amblyopia) is due to the combination of smoking and vitamin B_{12} deficiency. Correction of the deficiency with cyanocobalamin has produced improvement of vision in some cases.

Disorders of the ileum sometimes lead to defective absorption of vitamin B_{12}. Patients with regional ileitis (Crohn's disease), in which the terminal ileum is either diseased or removed, are most prone to this deficiency. All patients with surgical resections, strictures, and bypass operations involving the ileum should be observed periodically for vitamin B_{12} deficiency. Occasionally the generalized mucosal diseases—celiac disease, idiopathic steatorrhea, and tropical sprue—produce vitamin B_{12} deficiency, but this is rare in comparison with the incidence of folic acid deficiency in these cases. Vitamin B_{12} deficiency is not uncommon in association with the blind loop syndrome, possibly because of bacterial competition for the vitamin. Treatment consists of replacement of vitamin B_{12} together with antibiotic therapy and perhaps surgical correction. Another esoteric cause of deficiency is infestation with the tapeworm *Diphyllobothrium latum* which occurs predominantly in people eating uncooked fish from the Baltic Sea. Anthelmintic treatment and dietary advice are indicated.

Preparations Available

　　Cyanocobalamin: (Various mfrs.)

　　　　Tablets, 5, 10, 25, 30, 50, 100, and 1000 μg

　　　　Soluble tablets, 25, 50, 100, and 250 μg

　　　　Capsules, 25 μg

　　　　Solution, 2 μg/drop, 15, 60, and 480 ml; 30 μg/ml, 30 ml

　　　　Elixir, 5 μg/5 ml

　　　　Injectable (IM), 30, 50, 60, 100, 120, 250, 500, 1000, 2000, and 5000 μg/ml, in 1, 5, 10, and 30 ml ampules and vials

　　Cyanocobalamin ^{57}Co (Racobalamin-57) and cyanocobalamin ^{60}Co (Racobalamin-60):

　　　　Available from the manufacturer to qualified departments and individuals.

　　Hydroxocobalamin: (Various mfrs.)

　　　　Injectable (IM), 100 μg/ml, 10 ml; 1000 μg/ml, 1, 5, and 10 ml

•　　•　　•

General References

Vitamin B$_{12}$

Castle, W.B.: Treatment of pernicious anemia: Historical aspects. Clin Pharmacol Therap 7:147–161, 1966.

Herbert, V.: Megaloblastic anemia. New England J Med 268:201–203, 368–371, 1963.

Weir, D.G., & P.B.B. Gatenby: Subacute combined degeneration of the cord after partial gastrectomy. Brit MJ 2:1175–1176, 1963.

Folate

Baldwin, J.M., & D.J. Dalessio: Folic acid therapy and spinal cord degeneration in pernicious anemia. New England J Med 264:1339–1342, 1961.

Conley, C.L., & J.R. Krevans: Development of neurologic manifestations of pernicious anemia during multivitamin therapy. New England J Med 245:529–531, 1951.

Gough, K.R., Thirkettle, J.L., & A.E. Read: Folic acid deficiency in patients after gastric resection. Quart J Med 34:1–14, 1965.

Herbert, V.: Folic acid. Ann Rev Med 16:359–370, 1965.

Lawrence, C., & F.A. Klipstein: Megaloblastic anemia of pregnancy in New York City. Ann Int Med 66:25–34, 1967.

Streiff, R.R.: Folate deficiency and oral contraceptives. JAMA 214:105–108, 1970.

Willoughby, M.L.N., & F.G. Jewell: Folate status throughout pregnancy and in the postpartum period. Brit MJ 4:356–360, 1968.

Part VII. Chemotherapeutic Agents

45 . . .

Cancer Chemotherapy

Sydney E. Salmon, MD, & Martin Apple, PhD

Cancer is a group of neoplastic diseases that occur in man in all age groups and in all races, as well as in animal species. The incidence, geographical distribution, and behavior of specific types of cancer are related to multiple factors including sex, age, race, genetic predisposition, and exposure to environmental carcinogenic factors. Recent evidence suggests that certain herpes group DNA viruses and "type C" RNA virus particles which have been implicated as etiologic agents in causation of a wide variety of animal cancers might possibly be causative agents in human malignancies as well. Additionally, oncogenic RNA viruses have been found to contain a "reverse transcriptase" enzyme which may permit reading of the oncogenic message of viral RNA into the base sequence of host cell DNA. Even if a viral genome is proved to be essential for the initiation of certain human cancers, it is likely that additional hereditary and environmental factors modulate the neoplastic expression of latent virus infections.

Irrespective of etiology, cancer is basically a disease of cells characterized by a reduction or loss of effectiveness of normal cellular control and maturation mechanisms which regulate multiplication and other functions required for homeostasis in a complex multicellular organism. The 5 major features of cancer are as follows: (1) Excessive cell growth, usually in the form of a tumor. (2) Undifferentiated cells and tissues, similar to embryonic tissues. (3) Invasiveness, the ability to grow into adjacent tissue (a basic distinction from normal tissue). (4) The ability to metastasize—spread to new sites and establish new growths of cancer. (5) A type of "acquired heredity" in which the progeny of the cancer cells all retain the same cancerous properties.

The abnormal behavior of the cancer cell leads to illness in the host (1) as a result of the pressure effects due to local tumor growth; (2) by destruction of organs involved with the primary tumor or its distant metastases, and (3) by deleterious systemic effects secondary to the growths.

Next to heart disease, cancer is the major cause of death in the USA, causing over 300,000 fatalities a year. With present methods of treatment, one-third of patients are cured with initial surgery or radiation therapy. The cures are almost entirely in patients whose disease has not disseminated by the time of treatment. Earlier diagnosis might enable 50% of patients to be cured by means of therapy aimed at eradicating local tumor growth. In most of the remaining cases, relatively early metastasis appears to be one of the biologic features of tumor growth, indicating that a systemic approach, as can be attained with chemotherapy, will be required for effective cancer management.

Chemotherapy as presently used is usually curative in choriocarcinoma in women, Burkitt's lymphoma, Wilms's tumor in children, and occasionally in certain testicular tumors and perhaps insulinoma, and in occasional cases of acute leukemia of childhood and other tumors. It should be emphasized that chemotherapeutic cures are currently attained only in relatively rare tumors. Thus, in many tumors, chemotherapy is the third line of attack inasmuch as surgery or intensive x-ray therapy is usually indicated when cancer appears to be localized. Over 75% of cancer cases in the USA are of the type called carcinoma (derived from epithelium), and most of the rest are sarcomas (derived from mesothelium). The 8 commonest cancers account for over 70% of cancer incidence, and about 70% of these cases will have a fatal outcome. The commonest cancers are as follows: lung carcinoma (70,000 cases annually in the USA), colon and rectal cancer (75,000), female breast cancer (70,000), uterine carcinoma (45,000), prostatic carcinoma (35,000), bladder and kidney cancer (31,000), lymphoma (22,000), and leukemia (19,000). Although early diagnosis has reduced cancer mortality, many of the common cancers have spread by the time of diagnosis and are not susceptible to cure by current technics.

Thus, in most forms of disseminated cancer, the therapeutic emphasis cannot presently be directed aggressively toward cure but rather toward the palliation of symptoms, prevention and management of complications, psychologic support, and prolongation of useful life. Cancer chemotherapeutic agents have

Dr. Salmon is Associate Professor of Medicine and Head, Division of Hematology and Oncology, University of Arizona College of Medicine, Tucson. Dr. Apple is Assistant Professor of Pharmacology and Pharmaceutical Chemistry and Research Biochemist, Cancer Research Institute, University of California, San Francisco.

done much to make effective palliation more attainable.

In principle, drug research may provide the ultimate cure for cancer, although the agents at present available, most of which have been discovered empirically, fall far short of this goal. The concerted attempt to develop effective anticancer drugs has intensified during the past 2 decades. This effort has employed testing in well characterized animal tumor systems, tissue culture studies, and preclinical pharmacology and pharmacokinetics prior to the initiation of controlled drug trials of the most promising agents in cancer patients. Although ideal anticancer drugs would theoretically be those which only destroy cancer cells and do not harm normal tissues, this goal has not yet been reached.

New information on cell kinetics and tumor cell mass may partially explain the limited effectiveness of most anticancer agents. Patients with disseminated cancer (eg, acute leukemia) may have as many as 10^{12} (1 trillion) cancer cells distributed in various sites in the body at the time of diagnosis. If a given drug, administered optimally, is capable of killing 99.9% of cancer cells without intolerable toxicity to the patient, this effect might result in symptomatic improvement but would only reduce the number of tumor cells by 3 orders of magnitude (from 10^{12} to 10^9, or 1 billion cells). In bacterial infections, a response of this magnitude to antibiotics might be curative because of the substantial host resistance factors which can eliminate large numbers of residual microorganisms. In the cancer patient, it is not clear to what extent host factors (eg, the immune system) can potentially limit cancer growth. Because of the overlap of toxicity of most anticancer agents on normal cells, therapy with these agents is usually of limited intensity. Predictive chemotherapeutic studies in mouse leukemia have suggested that treatment with a variety of agents must be adequate to eliminate all malignant cells to attain a cure. The conclusions from such kinetic studies, as well as new information on the biochemistry of the cell's proliferative cycle, have given impetus to reassessment of existing drugs. These studies have included evaluation of the effects of combinations of agents which might have noncumulative toxicities on normal cells but additive or synergistic effects on cancer cells, leading to a greater "log-kill." Such combinations, while still investigational for most tumors, have already made possible significant therapeutic advances for several human malignancies.

Applications of these kinetic concepts to cancer chemotherapy are illustrated in Fig 45–1. A schematic diagram of the cell cycle and probable sites of action of the various cancer chemotherapeutic agents is presented in Fig 45–2. It must be emphasized that the exact "phase" of the cell cycle of cycle-specific agents is still somewhat uncertain, especially for the various drugs designated for phases other than the S-phase.

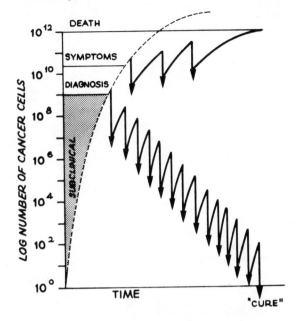

FIG 45–1. **Relationship of tumor cell number to time of diagnosis, symptoms, treatment, and survival.** Two alternative outcomes of drug treatment are shown for comparison with the course of tumor growth when no treatment is given (dotted line). In the protocol diagrammed at top, treatment (indicated by the arrows) is given infrequently. Although it induces some regression in the amount of tumor in the body, regrowth exceeds regression, and the result is manifested as prolongation of survival but with recurrence of symptoms between courses of treatment and eventual death of the patient. The treatment diagrammed in the lower section is more intensive and frequent and induces a greater magnitude of regression; tumor cell kill exceeds regrowth, and "cure" results. In the second example, treatment has been continued long after all clinical evidence of cancer has disappeared.

POLYFUNCTIONAL ALKYLATING AGENTS

History

This group of agents was developed from the sulfur mustard vesicant gas dichloroethyl sulfide which was used in World War I. During World War II, the nitrogen mustards were developed for use as chemical warfare agents. In addition to their vesicant effect upon the skin, these compounds produced atrophy of lymphoid tissue and bone marrow. Because of these latter effects, they were introduced for the treatment of malignant lymphomas and leukemias and were later found to be effective against bronchogenic carcinoma and carcinoma of the ovary as well. Since the introduc-

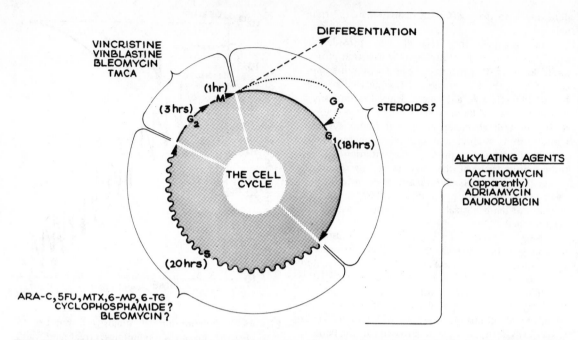

**FIG 45–2. The cell cycle and tentative points of action of cancer chemotherapeutic agents, showing the bio-
chemical steps necessary for cell proliferation by normal and cancer cells.** Many of the effective cancer
chemotherapeutic drugs appear to exert their action on cancer cells going through the cell cycle. G_1 is the
phase prior to DNA synthesis during which various enzymes, including those necessary for DNA synthesis,
are synthesized; the S phase is the actual period of commitment to division during which DNA is replicated
for the various chromosomes; G_2 is a phase of specialized protein and RNA synthesis and manufacture of the
mitotic spindle apparatus, followed by the brief M phase of mitosis with its prophase, metaphase, and
telophase steps. G_0 refers to a long resting state in which cells are not cycling and therefore are not affected
by drugs which act only on cells going through the cell cycle. The designations of phases of the cell cycle
where various drugs act must be considered tentative.

tion of the parent nitrogen mustard "HN2"—methyl-
bis(β-chloroethyl)amine, mechlorethamine, Mustargen
—new and more stable polyfunctional alkylating drugs
have been developed in the search for more effective
and less toxic agents.

(R is CH_3)

Mechlorethamine

Chemistry

Most of the useful drugs classified as alkylating
agents contain a bis(chloroethyl)amine or ethyleneimine structure:

(R is HOOC–$CH_2CH_2CH_2$–⟨⟩–)

Chlorambucil

Bis(chloroethyl)amine   **Ethyleneimine**

(R is HOOC–C–CH_2–⟨⟩–)
with NH_2 and H

Melphalan

Clinically used bis(chloroethyl)amines include
mechlorethamine, chlorambucil, melphalan, cyclophosphamide, and bis(chloroethyl)nitrosourea or BCNU:

Cyclophosphamide

$$NH-CH_2CH_2Cl$$
$$O=C$$
$$N-CH_2-CH_2Cl$$
$$O=N$$

BCNU

An ethyleneimine used clinically is triethylenethiophosphoramide (Thio-TEPA):

$$H_2C—CH_2$$
$$H_2C \quad N \quad CH_2$$
$$N-P-N$$
$$H_2C \quad S \quad CH_2$$

Thio-TEPA

A third group of alkylating agents, of which only one is currently used clinically, are the alkylsulfonates such as busulfan:

$$CH_3-\overset{O}{\underset{O}{S}}-O-CH_2CH_2CH_2CH_2-O-\overset{O}{\underset{O}{S}}-CH_3$$

Busulfan

These drugs act to alkylate, ie, to transfer their alkyl groups to biologically important cell constituents whose function is then impaired.

The polyfunctional alkylating agents have both a cytolytic and a mutagenic or radiomimetic action. They also inhibit glycolysis, respiration, protein synthesis, nucleic acid synthesis, and a number of membrane functions. This diversity of cellular effects is produced because these drugs readily react chemically with carboxyl, sulfhydryl, amino, and phosphate groups which occur in almost all cell constituents. Their general chemical mechanism of action is summarized as follows: The drug molecule ionizes, forming a carbonium or positive carbon ion which then alkylates (transfers carbonium ion) a cell constituent such as an amino, carboxyl, sulfhydryl, or phosphate group.

The DNA constituent guanine is apparently the most important cell molecule which is alkylated. Alkylation of the N^7 of guanine in DNA has 4 important consequences for DNA function: (1) alteration of the guanine so that it forms an abnormal base pair with thymine (miscoding); (2) cleavage of the imidazole ring of guanine (destroying it); (3) linking of guanine pairs, producing cross-linked DNA strands (which cannot

replicate); and (4) depurination of the DNA (causing actual breakage of the DNA strands) (Fig 45–3). Single-stranded damage can potentially be corrected by DNA repair mechanisms, but cross-linking alkylations produce chromosome fragmentation.

Most alkylating agents act primarily as cyclephase nonspecific agents and therefore can be used clinically in tumors which have a small fraction of dividing cells.

Pharmacologic Effects

The alkylating drugs are vesicants, having both local and systemic toxicity. Toxicity is primarily in tissues having a rapid rate of cellular proliferation, ie, those of the hematopoietic system, gastrointestinal tract, and gonads. In general, the aliphatic compounds produce similar toxic manifestations which are dose-related. These can be divided into (1) immediate or acute and (2) delayed. The parent drug, mechlorethamine, will be described in some detail since it serves as a prototype of the action of all the alkylating drugs.

Following the intravenous administration of mechlorethamine, the immediate effects are frequently nausea and vomiting occurring within a few minutes to half an hour. This is due to an effect on the medulla. In the event of skin contamination or subcutaneous infiltration of the drug, vesication and tissue necrosis with eventual sloughing occur, producing a slowly healing indolent ulcer.

The important delayed effects of mechlorethamine are on the hematopoietic system. Within a few hours after administration of a therapeutic dose of the drug, lymphopenia occurs. The lymphocytes fall to very low levels which persist for about 2 weeks. Cell necrosis with shrinkage of lymphopoietic centers in the lymph nodes also results. In the bone marrow, evidence of cell necrosis and disintegration appears within 12 hours and continues for 4–6 days, resulting in marked hypoplasia. Recovery begins at about 10 days, and by 3–4 weeks normal cellularity is restored. The hypoplastic period in the marrow is manifested in the peripheral blood at the fifth to sixth day after administration by a moderate leukopenia, with leukocyte counts often falling to 2500–3000/cu mm and persisting until the 10th–12th day. Regeneration of the marrow is reflected by an increase in leukocyte count until normal or slightly elevated levels are reached by the third or fourth week. The effect on megakaryocytes and platelets follows a similar course of depression and regeneration. As a result of the long life span of the erythrocyte, the effect of mechlorethamine on bone marrow depression is masked and the red cell count is usually not significantly decreased.

These effects upon the bone marrow limit the use of mechlorethamine injections to intervals of 4–6 weeks. Following hematopoietic recovery, the agent may again be administered on repeated occasions. The fact that the effect on normal tissue is only slightly different from that on tumor tissue also limits the effectiveness of this drug. Severe and prolonged mar-

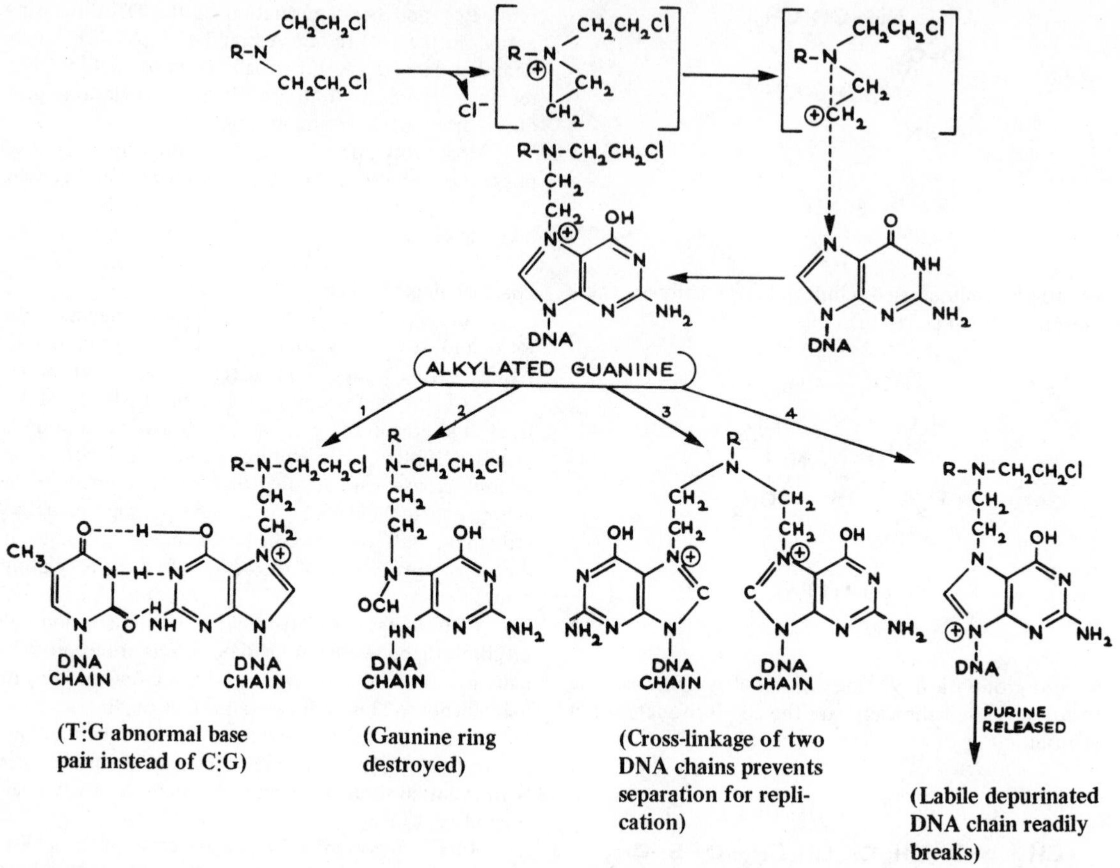

FIG 45-3. Effect of alkylating agents on DNA purines. A bis(chloroethyl)amine forms an ethyleneammonium ion which opens to form a carbonium ion. The carbonium ion reacts with a base such as N^7 of guanine in DNA, producing an alkylated purine. The alkylated purine, through one or more of the illustrated mechanisms, leads to cell death.

row depression occasionally occurs, especially in patients who have been extensively treated with systemic radiation and other chemotherapeutic drugs. Effects on the gastrointestinal tract are transient. The alkylating drugs also inhibit spermatogenesis and can, in principle, induce chromosome alterations and mutations.

The above description of the effects of mechlorethamine serves as the basis for a description of the effects of all of the alkylating agents.

The desirability of oral dosage forms of these agents led to the development of more chemically stable alkylators which are effective when given orally.

Cyclophosphamide, chlorambucil, melphalan, and triethylenethiophosphoramide can produce similar therapeutic responses in tumors sensitive to alkylating agents. If a tumor shows resistance to one alkylating agent, it is usually resistant to all others in this class except the nitrosoureas. Repeated blood counts are mandatory during administration of these drugs, and severe leukopenia or thrombocytopenia requires discontinuance of the agent.

Busulfan (Myleran), the methanesulfonate type of alkylator, has been found to have a relatively selective effect on myeloid tissue, producing granulocytopenia. As a result, it has been effectively employed in the treatment of chronic granulocytic leukemia. Busulfan is insoluble in ordinary physiologic solutions and is administered orally. It causes no nausea or vomiting and is uniformly absorbed. Increased melanin pigmentation is a frequent sequel of busulfan therapy. Occasional patients have also developed pulmonary fibrosis after prolonged treatment.

BCNU, which apparently alkylates via its nitroso and chloroethyl branches, also produces severe thrombocytopenia and leukopenia. The drug is lipid-soluble and therefore has activity in the CNS, including brain tumors. It is active in tumors resistant to alkylating agents and therefore can be used in disorders such as lymphoma in relapse on other alkylators. Important congeners under study are CCNU and methyl-CCNU.

Clinical Uses

The alkylating drugs are primarily used in the treatment of malignancies of the hematopoietic tissues, neuroblastoma, and disseminated carcinomas of the lungs, ovaries and testes, and breasts. They are curative only in Burkitt's lymphoma, but often provide significant palliation of the other neoplasms listed above. The details of their use will be discussed in a later section (see p 462).

Table 45–6 summarizes the neoplastic diseases that respond to chemotherapy with the alkylating drugs.

Adverse Reactions

Nausea and vomiting are almost universally reported with intravenously administered mechlorethamine and cyclophosphamide, and with moderate frequency with oral cyclophosphamide.

The important toxic effect of therapeutic doses of all the alkylating drugs is depression of bone marrow and subsequent leukopenia and thrombocytopenia. Severe infections and septicemia may result, with granulocytopenia below 600 PMN's/cu mm. Platelet depression below 40,000/cu mm may be accompanied by induced hemorrhagic phenomena. In excessively high doses, mechlorethamine can produce parasympathomimetic toxicity, convulsions, and eventual CNS depression and death. The oral agents do not ordinarily produce these effects. Cyclophosphamide may produce slight to severe transient alopecia in up to 30% of patients. It may also cause hemorrhagic cystitis. The cystitis can often be averted with adequate hydration.

The hematopoietic effects of toxic doses of alkylating drugs are treated by discontinuing the agent. Red cell and platelet transfusions and antibiotics to control infections are employed as needed until the marrow has regenerated.

Contraindications & Cautions

Because of their depressant action on the hematopoietic system, caution must be employed when alkylating drugs are given concurrently with antimetabolites or with radiation therapy.

Alkylating drugs may reduce the impaired host resistance to levels which permit localized chronic infection to disseminate. They should be used with caution in patients known to have active tuberculous or mycotic infections. (See also Table 45–1.)

STRUCTURAL ANALOGUES OF METABOLITES ("ANTIMETABOLITES")

The metabolite structural analogues are important for their antineoplastic effects and for their significance in rational attempts to design specific antitumor drugs. Based on the same idea as the bacterial growth-inhibiting metabolite structural analogues such as the sulfonamides, these chemicals differ greatly in structure, but each is closely related to some substances utilized by cells for metabolism and growth. Although all of these agents are structurally similar to normal metabolites, in only one case (methotrexate, which acts directly as an antifolate) is the drug itself known unequivocally to act directly as a metabolite substitute.

Biochemical Mechanisms

The analogues or their active (biotransformation) products act in one of 4 ways to block growth: (1) By

TABLE 45–1. Polyfunctional alkylating agents: Dosages and toxicity.

Alkylator	Dose	Acute Toxicity	Delayed Toxicity
Nitrogen mustard (HN2, mechlorethamine, Mustargen)	0.4 mg/kg IV in single or divided doses	Nausea and vomiting	Moderate depression of peripheral blood count.
Chlorambucil (Leukeran)	0.1–0.2 mg/kg/day orally; 6–12 mg/day	None	Excessive doses produce severe bone marrow depression with leukopenia, thrombocytopenia, and bleeding. Alopecia and hemorrhagic cystitis occasionally occur with cyclophosphamide. Cystitis can be prevented with adequate hydration.
Cyclophosphamide (Cytoxan)	3.5–5 mg/kg/day orally for 10 days; 40 mg/kg IV as single dose	Nausea and vomiting	
Melphalan (Alkeran)	0.25 mg/kg/day orally for 4 days; 2–4 mg/day as maintenance dose	None	
Triethylenethiophosphoramide (Thio-TEPA)	0.2 mg/kg IV for 5 days	None	
Busulfan (Myleran)	2–8 mg/day orally; 150–250 mg/course	None	
BCNU (bischlornitrosourea)	100 mg/sq m IV every 6 weeks	Nausea and vomiting	Leukopenia and thrombocytopenia.

substituting for the normal metabolite in a series of metabolic reactions, so that the analogue is incorporated into a key molecule instead of the normal metabolite, making the key molecule functionally abnormal. (2) By competing with a normal metabolite which acts at an enzyme regulatory site (the "allosteric" or noncatalytic site) to alter the regulated catalytic rate of a key enzyme. (3) By competing successfully with a normal metabolite for temporary occupation of the catalytic site of a key enzyme. (4) By binding so tightly to the catalytic site of a key enzyme that the enzyme is inactivated.

Among the major biochemical alterations in cancer cell metabolism is an exaggeration of nucleic

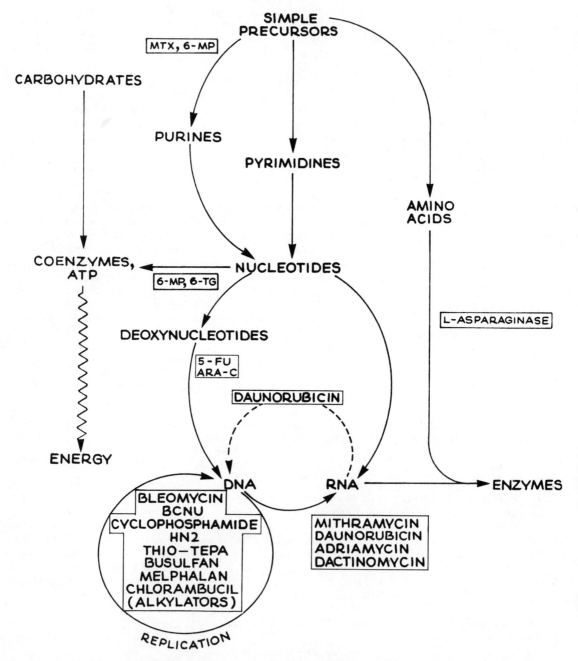

FIG 45—4. **Proposed major sites of action of anticancer drugs.** The major cellular processes for growth include energy capture and use for synthesis of DNA, RNA, and proteins such as enzymes. Cytotoxic anticancer drugs can act to block these processes as shown.

acid synthesis. A major effect of the structural analogues used clinically is that they interfere with the synthesis of nucleic acids, preventing the proliferation of many types of normal and neoplastic cells (Fig 45-4). Structural analogues all appear to act in a cycle-phase specific manner and thus are most useful clinically when tumors have a high fraction of dividing cells.

These drugs and their dosages and toxicities are shown in Table 45-2. The principal drugs are discussed below.

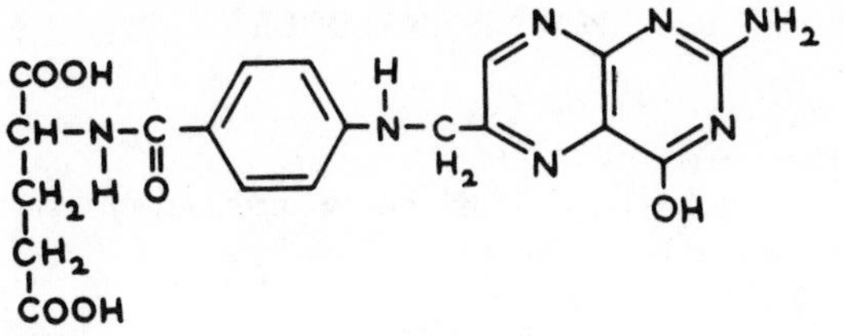

METHOTREXATE

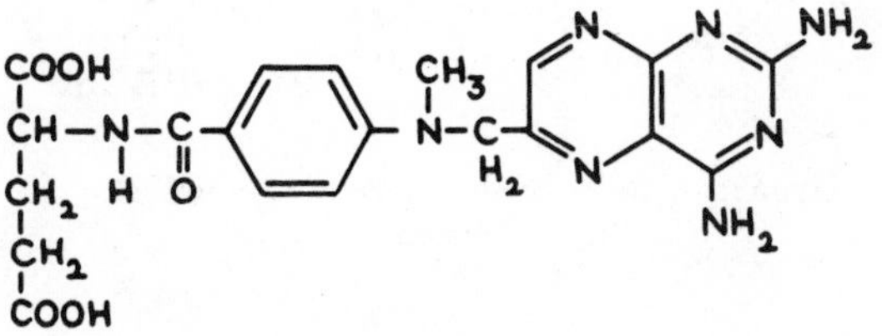

Chemistry

Methotrexate (4-amino-N^{10}-methylpteroylglutamate) is also known as MTX and amethopterin.

Mechanism of Action

Methotrexate acts by binding tightly to the catalytic site of dihydrofolate reductase, inactivating the key enzyme needed to create the active form of folic acid. Blockage of active tetrahydrofolate synthesis soon stops the formation of the purine precursors of DNA, RNA, ATP, and key coenzymes and arrests cell growth.

Folic acid

Methotrexate

Absorption, Metabolism, & Excretion

Methotrexate is rapidly absorbed from the gastrointestinal tract, and up to 90% of the oral dose can be excreted in the urine in about 12 hours. It is generally not metabolized significantly in man. In the blood it binds readily to plasma proteins and can be displaced by sulfonamides and salicylates, increasing its apparent toxicity. That fraction of it which binds in tissues is cleared very slowly. Adequate renal function is essential for rapid excretion.

TABLE 45-2. Structural analogues: Dosages and toxicity.

Chemotherapeutic Agent	Dose	Delayed Toxicity*
Methotrexate (amethopterin, MTX)	2.5-5 mg/day orally; 5 mg intrathecally 1-2 times weekly	Oral and gastrointestinal tract ulceration, bone marrow depression, leukopenia, thrombocytopenia.
6-Mercaptopurine (Purinethol, 6-MP)	2.5 mg/kg/day orally	Usually well tolerated. Larger dosages may cause bone marrow depression.
6-Thioguanine (thioguanine, 6-TG)	2 mg/kg/day orally	Usually well tolerated. Larger dosages may cause bone marrow depression.
5-Fluorouracil (5-FU)	15 mg/kg/day IV for 3-5 days or 15 mg/kg weekly for 6 weeks	Nausea, oral and gastrointestinal ulceration, bone marrow depression.
Cytarabine (1-β-D-arabinofuranosylcytosine; Ara-C, Cytosar)	1-3 mg/kg IV over 24 hours for up to 10 days	Nausea and vomiting, bone marrow depression, megaloblastosis, leukopenia, thrombocytopenia.
Supportive Agent With All Drugs	**Dose**	**Delayed Toxicity**
Allopurinol (Zyloprim)	300-800 mg/day orally for prevention or relief of hyperuricemia	Usually none. Enhances effects and toxicity of 6-MP when used in combination.

*These drugs do not cause acute toxicity.

PURINE ANALOGUES

Chemistry

The structures of the purine analogues are shown below.

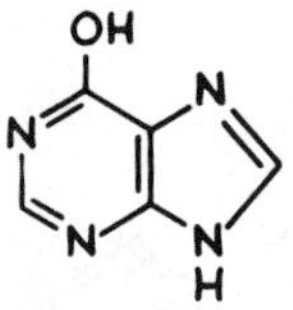

| Hypoxanthine | 6-Mercapto-purine | MMPR |

| Allopurinol | Guanine | 6-Thioguanine |

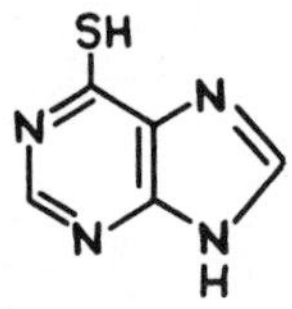

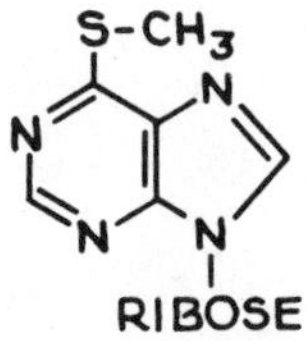

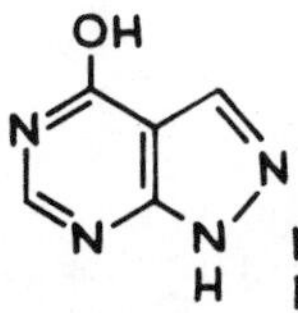

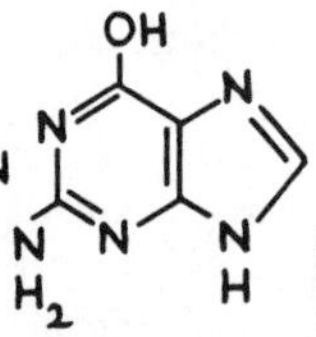

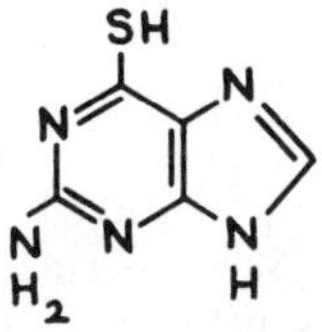

Mechanism of Action

6-Mercaptopurine (Purinethol, 6-MP) is metabolized to the nucleotide structurally corresponding to inosinic acid (hypoxanthine ribotide). It competes successfully for the catalytic site of enzymes metabolizing inosinic acid to adenine and xanthine ribotides.

An alternative, probably more important path of metabolism is conversion of 6-MP into 6-methyl-mercaptopurine ribotide (MMPR). MMPR is a potent inhibitor of de novo purine biosynthesis. It acts by competing with inosinic acid for the feedback regulatory site of the enzyme catalyzing formation of phosphoribosylamine, an essential precursor of all nucleic acid purines. The MMPR-enzyme complex fails to synthesize phosphoribosylamine and thus stops RNA and DNA synthesis.

6-Thioguanine is metabolized to the nucleotide structurally corresponding to guanine. Although it is metabolized along pathways similar to those described above in the case of 6-MP, and partially inhibits purine metabolizing enzymes, its major growth-inhibiting action seems to be substitution for guanine in nucleic acid synthesis, producing functionally altered polynucleotides.

Absorption, Metabolism, & Excretion

6-Mercaptopurine is rapidly absorbed from the gastrointestinal tract. Its half-life in blood is about 90 minutes. It is rapidly metabolized and mainly excreted in urine. Much of the therapeutic dose is converted into 6-thiouric acid, and inactive metabolite, by oxidation catalyzed by xanthine oxidase.

6-Thioguanine is also rapidly absorbed if given orally. 6-TG clears from plasma with a half-life of 1−1½ hours and is mainly excreted in urine as 6-thiourate and methylated 6-TG.

ALLOPURINOL

Allopurinol (Zyloprim) is a structural analogue of hypoxanthine which is frequently used in cancer chemotherapy but is not a cytotoxic drug. It acts by successfully competing with other purines for the catalytic site of xanthine oxidase to prevent catabolic oxidation of purines to uric acid. Xanthine oxidase normally converts hypoxanthine to xanthine and xanthine to uric acid. Although allopurinol has no direct therapeutic effect, it plays an important supportive role in the therapy of acute leukemia and other neoplasms during times of high nucleic acid turnover and uric acid formation. Potentially lethal hyperuricemia is often observed in such patients after effective cytotoxic chemotherapy and sometimes in the untreated state. Administration of allopurinol reduces formation of uric acid. Because of the greater solubility and renal clearance of hypoxanthine, acute gouty nephropathy can be prevented by prophylactic use of allopurinol.

Since most 6-mercaptopurine is detoxified by xanthine oxidase-mediated conversion to thiouric acid and since allopurinol effectively stops xanthine oxidase catalysis, simultaneous therapy with both of these agents will potentiate the effects and toxicity of 6-mercaptopurine unless the 6-MP dose is reduced to 25−30% of its usual therapeutic level. Since so much 6-thioguanine is excreted as the methylated metabolite, the dosage of 6-TG need not be correspondingly reduced.

PYRIMIDINE ANALOGUES

1. CYTARABINE

Chemistry

Cytarabine (1-β-arabinofuranosylcytosine; Ara-C; Cytosar) has the structure shown below.

Mechanism of Action

Cytarabine is metabolized to nucleotide forms which apparently successfully compete with normal metabolites at the catalytic center of enzymes converting cytidine nucleotide to deoxycytidine nucleotide and the enzymes incorporating deoxycytidine triphosphate into DNA, thus curtailing DNA synthesis.

Cytosine
deoxyriboside

Cytosine
arabinoside

Absorption, Metabolism, & Excretion

Cytarabine is not active orally. The intravenous dose is cleared from the blood in 15–30 minutes. Most of the drug is deaminated to form uracil arabinoside, an inactive metabolite which is readily excreted in urine.

2. 5-FLUOROURACIL (5-FU)

Chemistry

Uracil

5-FU

Mechanism of Action

5-Fluorouracil is converted to 5-FU nucleotide and reduced to 5-fluorouracil deoxyribotide (FdR),

the active form. The fluorodeoxyribotide successfully competes with uracil deoxyribotide for the catalytic center of the enzyme which catalyzes thymidine (TMP) synthesis. Since thymidine is absolutely essential for DNA synthesis, the 5-FU metabolite effectively blocks DNA synthesis this way (Fig 45–5).

Absorption, Metabolism, & Excretion

5-FU is readily absorbed orally but is usually given intravenously. Most of an intravenous dose is excreted as expired CO_2 within 24 hours.

5-Fluorodeoxyuridine (floxuridine, FUDR) acts similarly to 5-FU and is used for intra-arterial infusion into solid carcinomas.

PLANT ALKALOIDS

VINBLASTINE

Vinblastine (Velban) is an alkaloid derived from *Vinca rosea*, the periwinkle plant (Fig 45–6). Its mechanism of action is not completely understood, but it binds to the microtubular protein of the mitotic spindle, inactivating it, and causes arrest of mitosis at the metaphase. It produces nausea and vomiting and marrow depression as well as alopecia. It has value in the treatment of systemic Hodgkin's disease and lymphosarcoma in patients who fail to respond to the alkylating agents. See clinical section below and Table 45–6.

Vinblastine (Velban) is available in 10 mg vials for intravenous use.

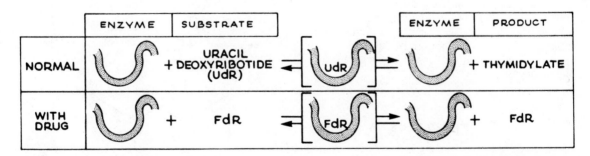

FIG 45–5. Block of DNA synthesis by 5-fluorouracil. When the enzyme is occupied with the normal metabolite UdR, it rapidly produces thymidylate. When the drug metabolite FdR is present, it occupies the enzyme catalytic site and prevents the normal metabolite from being converted to thymidylate. FdR is released from the enzyme slowly and is chemically unchanged.

Vincristine

Vinblastine

R is O=C–H

R is CH$_3$

FIG 45–6. Vincristine (Oncovin) and vinblastine (Velban).

VINCRISTINE

Vincristine (Oncovin) is also an alkaloid derivative of *Vinca rosea,* and is closely related to vinblastine. It also appears to be a "spindle poison" and causes arrest of the mitotic cycle. Despite its marked structural similarity to vinblastine, it has a strikingly different spectrum of activity and qualitatively different toxicities.

Vincristine has been used with considerable success in combination with prednisone for remission induction in childhood acute leukemia. It is also useful in certain other rapidly proliferating neoplasms. It causes a significant incidence of neurotoxicity, which limits its use to short courses. The principal serious toxic effects are areflexia, peripheral neuritis, and paralytic ileus. It occasionally produces bone marrow depression.

Vincristine (Oncovin) is available in 1 and 5 mg ampules for intravenous use.

TRIMETHYLCOLCHICINIC ACID (TMCA)

This chemical derivative of the plant alkaloid colchicine appears to have a mode of action identical to that of the vinca alkaloids (binding to microtubular proteins) despite the fact that it is structurally very different. TMCA is an investigational drug which appears to be active in chronic myelogenous leukemia and melanoma.

ANTIBIOTICS

A number of compounds produced as growth inhibitors by microorganisms, the antibiotics, have found clinical utility in cancer chemotherapy. They exert their cytotoxic effects by similar mechanisms of binding to polynucleotides and preventing new polynucleotide synthesis, particularly blocking the transcription of new DNA or RNA.

DACTINOMYCIN

Dactinomycin (actinomycin D, Cosmegen) is an antibiotic which is important for research in molecular biology and in clinical cancer therapy of Wilms's tumor, choriocarcinoma, and some other cancers. The drug consists of a 3-ring aromatic chromophore (actinocin) and 2 peptide loops.

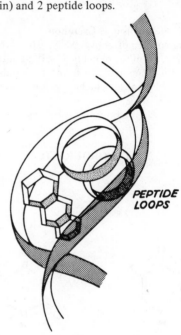

PEPTIDE LOOPS

An actinomycin anchored in DNA helix

SARCOSINE   SARCOSINE

L–PROL   N–MET-VAL   L–PROL   N–MET-VAL

D–VAL   L–THREO   D–VAL   L–THREO

Dactinomycin

Mechanism of Action

The ability of actinomycins to react with DNA appears to be the major factor in their cytotoxicity. Dactinomycin inhibits DNA-dependent RNA synthesis —particularly the synthesis of ribosomal RNA in cancer cell nucleoli. The peptide loops act as anchors to hold the actinocin ring at a purine-pyrimidine base pair, preventing DNA transcription. The actinocin ring structure is inactive as a drug.

Absorption, Metabolism, & Excretion

About half of an intravenous dose of dactinomycin is excreted unmetabolized in bile and about 10% is excreted in urine. The drug is significantly less potent when given orally. Most of an intravenous dose leaves the plasma within 2–5 minutes. The drug is irritating at the local injection site.

Adverse Reactions

Dactinomycin produces delayed bone marrow depression with severe thrombocytopenia, nausea and vomiting, diarrhea, oral ulcers, and skin eruptions. Significant skin reactions are prone to develop on sites of prior x-ray radiation therapy.

ANTHRACYCLINES
(Daunorubicin & Adriamycin)

These agents are still investigational in the USA but show definite promise of becoming major anticancer drugs.

Chemistry

The structural formulas of daunorubicin (daunomycin, daunoblastine, rubidomycin) and adriamycin are shown below.

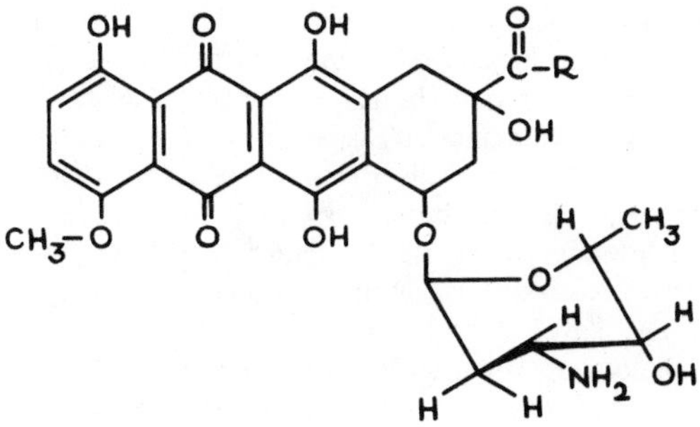

Daunorubicin R = CH$_3$
Adriamycin R = CH$_2$OH

Mechanism of Action

Physicochemical studies of the interaction between anthracycline antibiotics and DNA suggest that the ring portion intercalates between adjoining nucleotide pairs. Additionally, with the stabilizing effect of the amino sugar, the drug binds tenaciously to DNA, preventing DNA-directed RNA or DNA transcription.

Absorption, Metabolism, & Excretion

The initial half-life of daunorubicin in plasma is about 45 minutes. It goes into kidney, spleen, liver, and lung. It is mainly excreted in bile; about one-sixth is excreted in the urine. The plasma protein-bound drug has a half-life of over 40 hours, delaying clearance of part of each drug dose.

Clinical Uses

Studies in acute leukemia suggest that daunorubicin will find utility as an additional agent for combination chemotherapy. Adriamycin appears to be active in lung and bladder carcinoma, lymphomas, and a wide variety of sarcomas, and is otherwise similar to daunorubicin. Because of its slightly greater therapeutic index, its cardiotoxicity is sometimes less severe than that of daunorubicin. The broad spectrum of action of this investigational agent has prompted extensive trials by cooperating chemotherapy groups.

Adverse Reactions

An optimal dosage schedule for the anthracyclines has not been established. Bone marrow depression and cardiac toxicity are the major adverse effects. Daunorubicin-induced cardiotoxicity begins with tachycardia and other arrhythmias and is followed by cardiorespiratory symptoms.

MITHRAMYCIN

Mithramycin (Mithracin) is a cytotoxic antibiotic consisting of a polycyclic chromophore with 2 chains of sugars (see next page).

It apparently acts similarly to actinomycin (the polycyclic chromophore with 2 peptide loops) by intercalating and anchoring in DNA and specifically inhibiting DNA-directed RNA synthesis. It is active in testicular cancers and in preventing intractable hypercalcemia secondary to bone metastases.

Toxic manifestations of mithramycin are (in order of appearance) nausea, vomiting, thrombocytopenia (often lethal), hemorrhage, and hepatotoxicity.

BLEOMYCIN

Bleomycin is a preparation consisting of about a dozen different antibiotic peptides produced by a streptomycete. The bleomycin mixture inhibits cell mitosis and DNA synthesis. It is extremely active in

Mithramycin

squamous cell skin cancers, testicular tumors, and most lymphomas. Toxic effects include blistering and hyperkeratosis of the palms, anorexia, nausea, fever, fatigue, finger hyperesthesia, stomatitis, and alopecia. Pulmonary fibrosis is a somewhat uncommon but often fatal adverse effect which has been seen principally in elderly patients with a reduced pulmonary diffusion capacity for oxygen who have received a total dose of over 200 mg. Development of nonproductive cough, decreased diffusion capacity for oxygen, or pulmonary infiltrates is an indication to discontinue the drug and institute antibiotic and corticosteroid treatment.

L-ASPARAGINASE
(L-Asparagine Amidohydrolase)

This is a promising new agent which is currently undergoing clinical investigation and is not available to the practicing physician in the USA. Certain animal tumors which are dependent on the amino acid L-asparagine for growth have been found to be sensitive to the deprivation of this amino acid and respond to L-asparaginase therapy. Similar observations have now been made in certain human malignancies, especially acute lymphoblastic leukemia. The enzyme preparation used is prepared from *Escherichia coli* and is, therefore, a foreign antigenic protein. Contamina-

tion of asparaginase preparations with endotoxin and other bacterial products was initially a major problem, but this has been greatly reduced with more recent preparations of the enzyme. L-Asparaginase is administered intravenously, and 80% of the activity remains within the intravascular space with a half-life of more than 24 hours. Blood aspargine levels fall almost immediately to undetectable levels and remain so as long as therapy is continued. The drug appears to affect leukemic cells, which are incapable of converting aspartic acid to asparagine via the asparagine synthetase reaction and therefore depend on blood asparginase for growth. The intravascular asparaginase converts asparagine to aspartic acid in the blood, and the leukemic cells therefore receive insufficient asparagine to synthesize essential proteins. Prompt decrease in peripheral leukemic leukocyte counts, marrow infiltration, lymphadenopathy, and splenomegaly have been noted in sensitive patients, but remissions obtained with this single agent have been of relatively short duration. In some instances, the development of resistance has been associated with increased levels of asparagine synthetase in the malignant cells. Toxic effects of the enzyme preparations include fever, chills, nausea, liver dysfunction, mental depression, reduced levels of certain serum proteins, and occasional instances of acute pancreatitis. In some patients, immunologic response to the enzyme occurs with detectable circulating antibodies. Anaphylactic reactions have been observed with repeated use. Tech-

TABLE 45–3. Natural product cancer chemotherapy drugs: Dosages and toxicity.

Drug	Dosage and Route	Acute Toxicity	Delayed Toxocity
Vinblastine (Velban)	0.1–0.2 mg/kg IV weekly	Nausea and vomiting	Alopecia, loss of reflexes, bone marrow depression.
Vincristine (Oncovin)	0.01–0.03 mg/kg IV weekly	None	Areflexia, muscle weakness, peripheral neuritis, paralytic ileus, mild bone marrow depression, alopecia.
Dactinomycin (actinomycin D, Cosmegen)	0.04 mg/kg IV weekly	Nausea and vomiting	Stomatitis, gastrointestinal tract upset, alopecia, bone marrow depression.
Daunorubicin (daunomycin, rubidomycin)	30–60 mg/sq m daily IV for 3 days, or 30–60 mg/sq m IV weekly	Nausea, fever, red urine (not hematuria)	Cardiotoxicity, bone marrow depression, alopecia.
Adriamycin	60 mg/sq m IV every 3 weeks to a maximum total dose of 600 mg/sq m	Nausea, red urine (not hematuria)	Cardiotoxicity, alopecia, bone marrow depression, stomatitis.
Mithramycin (Mithracin)	25–50 μg/kg IV every other day for up to 8 doses	Nausea and vomiting	Thrombocytopenia, hepatotoxicity.
Bleomycin	0.1 mg/kg IV twice weekly to a total dose of 200 mg	Nausea and vomiting	Edema of hands, fever, pulmonary fibrosis, stomatitis, alopecia.
L-Asparaginase	250–1000 IU/kg/day IV	Nausea and fever	Hepatotoxicity, mental depression, pancreatitis.

nics involving plasma dialysis against the enzyme have been investigated as potentially less toxic means of using this antigenic compound. Inasmuch as the mechanism of action of L-asparaginase is independent of all other known chemotherapeutic agents, it may prove most useful in intensive combination chemotherapy for remission induction in leukemia and other sensitive malignancies.

Asparaginase also represents a theoretical advance, because its development was predicated on the demonstration of a specific metabolic deficiency of malignant cells.

STEROID HORMONES

Sex hormones and adrenocortical hormones are employed in the management of several types of neoplastic disease. The sex hormones are concerned with the stimulation and control of proliferation and function of certain tissues, including the mammary and prostate glands. Cancer arising from and retaining properties of these tissues may be inhibited or stimulated by appropriate changes in hormone balance. Cancer of the breast and cancer of the prostate have been effectually palliated with sex hormone therapy or ablation of certain endocrine organs.

The adrenal corticosteroids (particularly the glucocorticoid analogues) have been useful in the treatment of acute leukemia, lymphomas, myeloma, and other hematologic malignancies as well as in advanced breast cancer, and as supportive therapy in the management of hypercalcemia resulting from many types of cancer. These steroids produce dissolution of lymphocytes, regression of lymph nodes, and inhibition of growth of certain mesenchymal tissues.

The most useful steroid hormones are as follows:

(1) Androgens: Testosterone propionate, fluoxymesterone, testolactone

(2) Estrogens: Diethylstilbestrol, ethinyl estradiol

(3) Progestins: Hydroxyprogesterone caproate, medroxyprogesterone

(4) Adrenocortical compounds: Hydrocortisone acetate, prednisone, prednisolone, dexamethasone

Absorption, Metabolism, & Excretion

With the exception of testosterone propionate and hydroxyprogesterone caproate, the corticosteroids are administered orally and are readily absorbed. Testosterone and hydroxyprogesterone are oil-soluble and must be administered intramuscularly. The mechanisms of their metabolism and excretion are described in Chapter 38.

Pharmacologic Effects

The precise mechanism of action of the sex hormones in mammary and prostate cancer has not been determined. Recent observations indicate that steroid hormones must bind to cytoplasmic receptor proteins of tumor cells in order for their anticancer effects to be exerted on the nucleus of the tumor cell. One mechanism of resistance to the effects of steroid hormones is the loss of the specific cytoplasmic steroid-binding protein. For example, estrogen-sensitive breast cancers have cytoplasmic receptor proteins specific for estradiol, and prednisone-sensitive lymphoma cells

TABLE 45—4. Steroid hormones: Dosages and toxicity.

	Usual Adult Dose	Acute Toxicity	Delayed Toxicity
Androgens			
Testosterone propionate	100 mg IM 3 times weekly	None	Fluid retention, masculiniza-tion. Cholestatic jaundice in some patients receiving fluoxy-mesterone.
Fluoxymesterone (Halotestin)	10—20 mg/day orally	None	
Estrogens			
Diethylstilbestrol	1—5 mg 3 times a day orally	Occasional nausea and vomiting	Fluid retention, feminization, uterine bleeding.
Ethinyl estradiol (Estinyl)	3 mg/day orally		
Progestins			
Hydroxyprogesterone cap-roate (Delalutin)	1 gm IM twice weekly	None	
Medroxyprogesterone (Provera)	100—200 mg/day orally; 200—600 mg orally twice weekly	None	
Adrenocorticosteroids			
Hydrocortisone	50—200 mg/day orally	None	Fluid retention, hypertension, diabetes, increased susceptibil-ity to infection, "moon facies."
Prednisone	20—100 mg/day orally or, when effective, 50—100 mg every other day orally as single dose.	None	

bind this steroid. In contrast, steroid-resistant breast cancers and lymphomas appear to have lost these specific cytoplasmic receptors. Androgens and estrogens act, in part, by antagonizing the action of the opposing sex hormone and by inhibiting the pituitary gland.

The adrenocortical hormones act by an unknown mechanism to injure specific cell types. They interfere with lymphoid proliferation, produce dissolution of lymphocytes and regression of lymphatic tissue, and inhibit the growth of certain mesenchymal tissues. It is believed that the anti-inflammatory activity of the adrenal steroids is similar to their therapeutic effects against certain tumors.

Clinical Uses

The sex hormones are employed in cancer of the female and male breast, cancer of the prostate, and cancer of the endometrium of the uterus.

The relationship between hormones and hormone dependent tumors was initially demonstrated by Beatson in 1896 when it was shown that oophorectomy produced improvement in women with advanced breast cancer. It is now established that the therapeutic effect was the result of the unopposed action of the patient's androgenic hormones which became apparent following removal of the ovaries. Extensive studies with the androgenic, estrogenic, and progestational sex hormones have demonstrated their value in advanced inoperable mammary cancer, cancer of the prostate, and cancer of the endometrium (see pp 466—468).

Adverse Reactions

Androgens, estrogens, and adrenocortical hormones all can produce fluid retention through their

sodium-retaining effect. Prolonged use of androgens and estrogens will cause masculinization and feminization, respectively. Extended use of the adrenocortical steroids may result in hypertension, diabetes, increased susceptibility to infection, and the development of cushingoid appearance ("moon facies"). (See Chapter 35.)

<h2 style="text-align:center">MISCELLANEOUS ANTICANCER DRUGS</h2>

<h3 style="text-align:center">PROCARBAZINE</h3>

Procarbazine (N-methylhydrazine, Matulane) is a recently developed methylhydrazine derivative that has been shown to have cytotoxic (antineoplastic) activity and to have teratogenic, immunosuppressive, and carcinogenic properties.

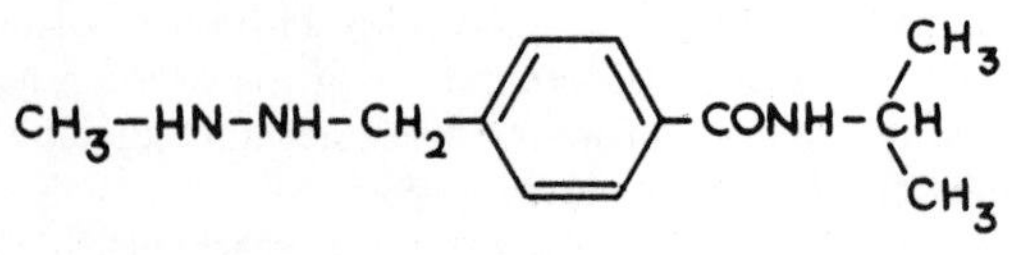

$$CH_3-HN-NH-CH_2- \bigcirc -CONH-CH\begin{smallmatrix}CH_3\\ \\CH_3\end{smallmatrix}$$

N-Isopropyl-α-(2-methylhydrazino)-
p-toluamide (procarbazine, Matulane)

The biochemical mechanism of action is unclear. During the oxidative breakdown of procarbazine in cells, H_2O_2, HCHO, azo-procarbazine, and hydroxyl radicals are generated, all of which could cause the chromosome breakage frequently observed.

Procarbazine is a monoamine oxidase inhibitor. It is rapidly absorbed from the gastrointestinal tract and has a half-life in blood of 7 minutes. About 75% of a dose is excreted in the urine in 24 hours, most of which is terephthalic N-isopropylamide.

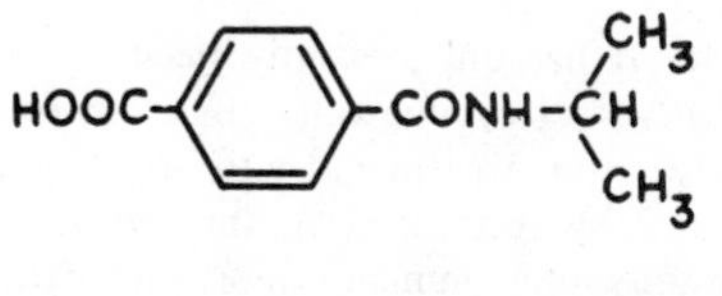

Clinical studies indicate that this drug is of value in the treatment of advanced Hodgkin's disease. There is no cross-resistance between procarbazine and either vinblastine or the alkylating agents; for this reason, it has been used in patients who are refractory to the latter agents as well as in combination therapy.

Procarbazine produces nausea, leukopenia, thrombocytopenia, and occasional gastrointestinal symptoms. Concomitant use of CNS depressants or alcohol with procarbazine is contraindicated.

IMIDAZOLE CARBOXAMIDE

Imidazole carboxamide is currently classed as an investigational agent in the USA. It is a synthetic compound with the following structure:

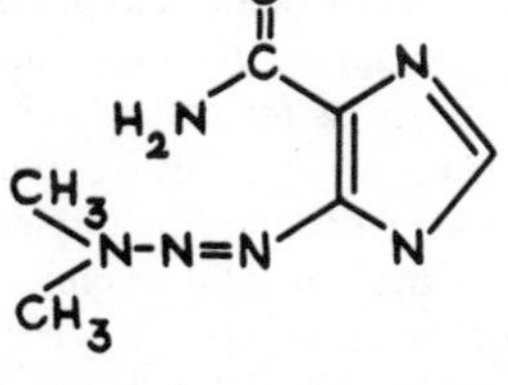

Its mechanism of action is not known. Speculation has centered around possible roles either as an alkylating agent or as an antimetabolite of a purine precursor. Only the parenteral route has proved feasible in man, and there is no apparent schedule dependency: single-dose daily treatment at a dosage of 10 mg/kg (300 mg/sq m IV) daily for 9 days appears to be optimal. The drug is active in melanoma and has a 30% response rate. It has some activity in various sarcomas, and its action in sarcomas seems to be potentiated by combination with adriamycin.

O,P'DDD

This drug (1,1-dichloro-2-[o-chlorphenyl]-2-[p-chlorophenyl]-ethane) is a DDT congener, and was first found to be adrenolytic in dogs. Subsequently, it was found to be of use in the treatment of adrenal carcinoma. The drug produces tumor regression and relief of the excessive adrenal steroid secretion which often occurs with this malignancy. Toxicities include skin eruptions, diarrhea, and mental depression.

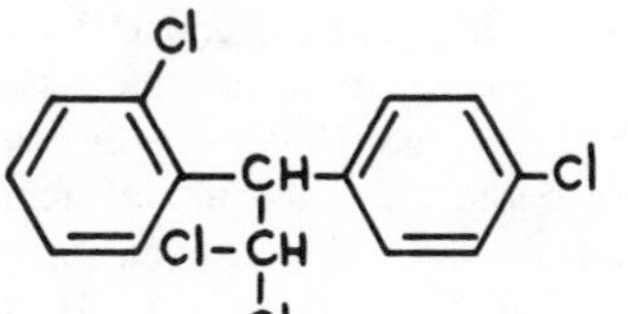

About 40% of an oral dose is absorbed, and 60% is excreted in stool. Of the amount reaching the tissues, most is stored in fat for several weeks. About 25% of an absorbed dose is excreted as a urinary metabolite. It produces anorexia, nausea, somnolence, and dermatitis.

Since this is an experimental drug, indicated only for a rare cancer, patients requiring o,p'DDD therapy are usually referred to appropriate investigational centers in the USA after inquiry through the National Cancer Institute.

QUINACRINE

This antimalarial drug has been found to be of occasional use in the control of malignant pleural, pericardial, and abdominal effusions. It is instilled directly into the fluid-containing cavity. Although its exact mechanism of action is uncertain, it is a local irritant and leads to the production of local fibrous adhesions.

INVESTIGATIONAL AGENTS

Several of the drugs mentioned in the text remain in an investigational status in the USA until their efficacy and safety for cancer chemotherapy can be established. In specific instances where treatment with one of these agents seems warranted, it usually can be arranged through a university hospital, a cancer chemotherapy center, or by contacting the Chemotherapy Branch of the National Cancer Institute, which can provide further information and identify investigators who are authorized to administer these drugs.

TABLE 45—5. Miscellaneous anticancer drugs: Dosages and toxicity.

Drug	Usual Dose	Acute Toxicity	Delayed Toxicity
Procarbazine (Matulane)	50—200 mg/day orally	Nausea and vomiting	Bone marrow depression, CNS depression.
Imidazole carboxamide	10 mg/kg (300 mg/sq m) daily IV for 9 days	Nausea and vomiting	Bone marrow depression.
o,p'DDD	6—15 gm/day orally	Nausea and vomiting	Dermatitis, diarrhea, mental depression.
Quinacrine	100—300 mg/day by intra-cavitary injection for 5 days	Local pain and fever	None.

This status applies to several antibiotics: (1) bleomycin, a Japanese antibiotic which has activity in squamous cancer and Hodgkin's disease; (2) daunorubicin (daunomycin), useful in acute leukemia; (3) adriamycin, which is active in various sarcomas, carcinomas, and lymphomas; and (4) streptozotocin, which is active in insulinoma. Chemical compounds and other natural products to which this designation also applies include bischlornitrosourea (BCNU) and its CCNU and methyl-CCNU congeners, imidazole carboxamide, o,p'DDD, and trimethylcolchicinic acid. All of these drugs have substantial toxicities. Until their pharmacology is more completely understood and their net effects have proved to be beneficial, their use will be restricted to clinical research. It appears likely that adriamycin, BCNU, and bleomycin will all have major uses in cancer chemotherapy and will be added to the practicing oncologist's list of effective anticancer drugs.

CLINICAL APPLICATIONS OF CANCER CHEMOTHERAPEUTIC DRUGS

Knowledge of the kinetics of tumor cell proliferation and total body tumor cell number (as summarized in Fig 45—1), as well as information on the pharmacology and mechanism of action of cancer chemotherapeutic agents, have become important in designing optimal therapeutic regimens for patients with advanced cancer. The strategy for developing drug regimens requires a knowledge of the particular characteristics of specific tumors—eg, Is there a high growth fraction? Is there a high spontaneous cell death rate? Are most of the cells in G_O? Are their normal counterparts under hormonal control? Similarly, knowledge of the pharmacology of specific drugs is equally important—eg, Does the drug have a particular affinity for uptake by the tumor cells (streptozotocin)? Are the tumor cells sensitive to the drug? Is the drug cycle-stage specific?

Probable sites of action of various drugs are illustrated in Fig 45—2 and are shown in reference to the

cell cycle. It has only recently been recognized that drugs that affect cycling cells can often be used most effectively after treatment with a cycle-nonspecific agent (eg, alkylating agents); this principle has been tested in only a few human tumors, but with increasing success. Similarly, recognition of true drug synergism (tumor cell kill due to the drug combination greater than the additive effects of the individual drugs) or antagonism is important in the design of combination chemotherapeutic programs. The combination of cytarabine with 6-thioguanine in the treatment of acute myelogenous leukemia is an example of true synergism, whereas the combination of L-asparaginase with methotrexate has been found to be antagonistic; in the latter instance, the results are worse than can be achieved with either drug used alone.

The application of these principles is well illustrated in the current approach to the treatment of acute leukemia, lymphomas, Wilms's tumor, and testicular neoplasms.

ACUTE LEUKEMIA

Acute leukemia is a general term for a group of malignant disorders of blood leukocytes. Age at onset of disease and certain morphologic characteristics have significant implications for patient survival and responsiveness to chemotherapy. With current agents, childhood acute leukemia is more treatable than that which occurs later in life. In all leukemic patients, major emphasis must be given to intensive support of the patient with necessary red cell and platelet transfusions, prevention of hyperuricemia, and infection.

A useful distinction can be drawn between *remission induction* and *maintenance* chemotherapy because the therapeutic agents used, dosage schedules, and objectives are somewhat different. Remission induction is in general a more intensive type of chemotherapy and often uses multiple agents administered simultaneously. The objective of induction therapy is to clear the body of all detectable leukemic leukocytes, ie, to reduce the leukemic cell number by many logs. This objective can sometimes be obtained using drugs which would have prohibitive toxicities if used on a chronic basis. The objective of maintenance therapy is to keep the population of residual leukemic cells in check so that they do not repopulate the blood and bone marrow and lead to the return of symptoms. In general, drugs used for remission maintenance are those which have relatively little delayed or cumulative toxicity and can be taken for months or years on an outpatient basis. Current schemes of chemotherapy often use courses of "reinduction" medications between remission treatments even though the patient has remained in complete remission. This is intended to further reduce the body's burden of leukemic cells. Thus, the objective today is not remission maintenance but complete cure of acute leukemia.

Acute Leukemia of Childhood

Acute lymphoblastic leukemia is the predominant form of leukemia in children, and until 1948 had a median survival of 3 months. With the advent of the folic acid antagonists, a major increase in survival was attained. Subsequently, corticosteroids, mercapto-purine, cyclophosphamide, vincristine, and L-aspara-ginase were all found to have activity in this disease. In general, current practice is to employ a combination of vincristine and prednisone for initial induction of remission. Over 85% of children undergo complete remission with this therapy, with only minimal toxic-ity. Maintenance therapy usually consists of oral methotrexate or mercaptopurine, and is continued indefinitely or until resistance and clinical relapse occur. This form of maintenance, although still fre-quently used, is being supplanted by "total therapy" regimens designed to eliminate all subclinical residues of leukemia. It is often continued for 2–3 years to provide a minimum duration of therapy considered likely to induce cure. If the disease does recur, an attempt is made at reinduction with the same inducing drugs. If resistance is observed, reinduction is attempted with a different drug, eg, cyclophos-phamide, and maintenance with mercaptopurine, methotrexate, or cyclophosphamide. Because each sub-sequent relapse appears to be more difficult to reverse, the greatest effort must be made to maintain the child in remission. Prolongation of survival is clearly related to the duration of remission. Currently, the median duration of survival in childhood acute leukemia is approaching 3 years.

Relapse is often the result of development of CNS leukemia. Many of the drugs do not cross the blood-brain barrier, and the brain and CSF thus provide a favored reservoir for leukemic cell proliferation. Intra-thecal methotrexate is used for CNS leukemia, often with great effectiveness. Prophylactic intrathecal methotrexate therapy has been strongly advocated, and its efficacy has recently been demonstrated. Cytarabine is also useful for treatment and prevention of CNS leukemia. The very small number of children who currently survive for 5 years without evidence of recurrence appear to have about a 50% chance of having a permanent remission or cure. Until recently, only about 130 documented cases of permanent remis-sion have occurred in the world. Recent efforts at com-bination chemotherapy seem to be further improving this picture.

The fact that cure can potentially be obtained in this most disturbing disorder has lent great impetus to current investigations of intensive chemotherapy employing combinations of proved agents plus L-asparaginase, daunorubicin (daunomycin), and other experimental agents.

Acute Leukemia in Adults

Acute leukemia in adults is predominantly of the myelocytic variety, although some cases of lympho-blastic leukemia are also seen. The lymphoblastic form is managed in similar fashion to that described for chil-dren but with somewhat less rewarding therapeutic results. Acute myelogenous leukemia (AML) is exceed-ingly difficult to treat, and only an occasional patient lives longer than a year after the diagnosis is estab-lished. The single most active agent for adult acute leukemia is cytarabine; however, it is best used in com-bination. It has recently been observed that a combina-tion of cytarabine and 6-thioguanine is capable of inducing remissions in up to 50% of previously un-treated patients with AML. Combinations of 4 drugs—cyclophosphamide, vincristine, cytarabine, and pred-nisone—can also induce remissions in about 40% of patients, but this therapy makes tremendous demands for supportive therapy during remission induction. Patients over the age of 50 respond less well to chemo-therapy, primarily because their host resistance is weaker. Remission maintenance is usually with 6-thio-guanine, 6-mercaptopurine, or methotrexate, but remission duration is considerably shorter with cur-rently available therapy.

CHRONIC MYELOCYTIC LEUKEMIA

Chronic myelogenous leukemia arises from a chromosomally abnormal hematopoietic stem cell. The clinical symptoms and the course are related to the leukocyte level and its rate of increase. Most patients with leukocyte counts over 20,000/cu mm should be treated. The goal of treatment is to reduce and main-tain the granulocytes at normal levels and to raise the hemoglobin concentration to normal. The most useful form of treatment is chemotherapy with busulfan (Myleran), although other oral alkylating agents can also be used. Systemic radiation therapy with ^{32}P, and local splenic x-ray radiation, are alternative treatments occasionally used. In the early stages of the disease, treatment produces a prompt decrease in spleen size and a fall in the leukocyte count which are associated with subjective well-being. Current therapy has not been proved to prolong survival, but it markedly relieves symptoms.

Busulfan is considered the treatment of choice because of its ease of administration, freedom from side-effects, and low cost.

Initial chemotherapy consists of giving busulfan, 4 mg daily orally, until the number of leukocytes falls to 12,000/cu mm. If the initial white count is higher than 100,000/cu mm, allopurinol should be used prophylactically to prevent the development of hyperuricemia. Maintenance therapy is advisable if the leukocyte count doubles within 1 month after discontinuance of the initial course of treatment. A maintenance dose of 2 mg of busulfan daily is usually sufficient, but as the disease progresses it may be necessary to increase the dose to 6 or 8 mg daily.

Resistance to busulfan eventually develops. The hemoglobin falls, the spleen enlarges, and the differential count shows increasing cellular immaturity with large numbers of myeloblasts. At this point, busulfan is discontinued and mercaptopurine is given, but only partial and temporary success can be anticipated. Late in the course of the disease (between 3½ and 5 years), "blast crisis" develops and the disease converts to an acute leukemia. Therapy at that point is still investigational, but combination chemotherapy, including vincristine and prednisone, may have some benefit. The leukocyte count falls, but there is often little or no effect on bone marrow myeloblastosis. Although there may be some subjective improvement, true remissions rarely occur in patients who have undergone blast crisis.

CHRONIC LYMPHOCYTIC LEUKEMIA

Treatment of chronic lymphocytic leukemia is markedly different than that of chronic myelogenous leukemia. Whereas chronic myelogenous leukemia is a proliferative neoplasm requiring chemotherapy for symptomatic control, chronic lymphocytic leukemia appears to result from a gradual accumulation of long-lived β-lymphocytes rather than from rapid neoplastic cell proliferation. Chronic lymphocytic leukemia is often detected accidentally long before the development of symptoms. Although the average life expectancy is only 3 years, the disease occurs frequently in elderly patients, which skews the survival data. Many patients who are asymptomatic may have prolonged survival (eg, 5–15 years) without any therapy. In patients whose disease is restricted to lymphocytosis in the peripheral blood, it is reasonable to withhold treatment because in chronic lymphocytic leukemia one does not "treat the lymphocyte count" unless it is well above 150,000/cu mm. When anemia, weight loss, fever, and generalized organ and bone marrow involvement do occur, treatment is indicated.

The therapeutic resources available for the treatment of chronic lymphocytic leukemia include localized x-ray therapy, systemic radiation with ^{32}P, and corticosteroid and alkylating agent chemotherapy. Prednisone is often quite effective, and after an initial course of 80 mg/day for several weeks the dose can be tapered to low levels or switched to an intermittent (every other day) schedule which virtually eliminates side-effects. Hemolytic anemia may respond dramatically to prednisone, although thrombocytopenia is often more refractory. Alkylating agents will also decrease the number of lymphocytes and organ enlargement in most patients, and the choice between corticosteroids and alkylating agents is frequently based on relative contraindications of one drug or the other in varying clinical circumstances.

Chlorambucil (Leukeran) is probably the most easily administered oral alkylating agent and has fewest side-effects. The dose is usually 0.1 mg/kg daily, with monitoring of the blood counts at weekly intervals. More aggressive therapy is only rarely indicated in instances of severe hemolytic anemia and rapidly progressive disease. The goal of therapy is to eliminate the systemic manifestations of the disease, and complete normalization of the lymphocyte count is not necessary. Therapy can be discontinued once the patient's condition has stabilized, but maintenance therapy should be considered if symptoms reappear quickly. Local x-ray therapy is useful for shrinking symptomatic enlarged lymph nodes but is only occasionally indicated. Systemic therapy with ^{32}P can also be used to relieve the generalized symptoms of chronic lymphocytic leukemia. It is important not to overtreat these patients and to choose therapeutic modalities carefully because of the poor host resistance present in elderly patients.

THE LYMPHOMAS

1. HODGKIN'S DISEASE

Although remarkably little is known about the cause of Hodgkin's disease, its therapy is currently undergoing revolutionary improvement. Hodgkin's disease is a lymphoma with certain unique characteristics in its natural history: its apparent tendency to progress from a single involved node to anatomically adjacent nodes in a somewhat "orderly" fashion, and its tendency to appear confined to the lymphoid system for a long period of time, with progression to involve retroperitoneal nodes and the spleen. Extranodal involvement may also occur, and involvement of the liver, bone marrow, lungs, or other sites is taken as evidence of more "malignant" behavior of the tumor. A concerted attempt at adequate staging of the extent of disease is essential to effective treatment of this disorder, and newly diagnosed cases must be adequately studied with x-rays, lymphography, and exploratory laparotomy and splenectomy (looking for occult disease) in order to prepare a rational treatment plan. Widespread involvement is manifested by symptoms such as sweats, fever, anorexia, and weight loss and symptoms of infiltration of other organs, including the lungs, liver, and bone marrow.

Intensive x-ray therapy with supervoltage equipment is curative in most cases of early Hodgkin's disease confined to one lymph node area or several adjacent areas above the diaphragm (stages I and II). Radiation therapy is also of some use in more generalized Hodgkin's disease limited to the lymphoid system above and below the diaphragm (stage III), and occasionally in stage IV for palliation of symptoms due to enlarging lymph nodes. As can be seen in Table 45–6, a variety of chemotherapeutic agents are active in Hodgkin's disease; however, as of the past few years, it is clear that optimum treatment is with combination chemotherapy.

Combination chemotherapy is now indicated in patients presenting with stage III or stage IV Hodgkin's disease. The results have been sufficiently promising to lead to present trials of combination chemotherapy along with x-ray therapy in stage I and stage II disease. The most effective form of chemotherapy at present is with a 4-drug combination known as "MOPP," consisting of mechlorethamine (HN2, Mustargen), Oncovin (vincristine), procarbazine (Matulane), and prednisone. This form of treatment, which was developed by De Vita and his associates at the National Cancer Institute, is given repeatedly for at least 6 months, and sometimes for as long as a year. Over 90% of previously untreated patients with advanced Hodgkin's disease (stages III and IV) go into complete remission, with disappearance of all symptoms and objective evidences of tumor.

A current schedule for use of MOPP includes repeated courses every 2 months with M (mechlorethamine), 6 mg/sq m IV on days 1 and 8; O (vincristine), 1.4 mg/sq m IV on days 1 and 8; P (procarbazine), 50 mg orally on day 1, 100 mg orally on day 2, and 100 mg/sq m on days 3–10; and P (prednisone), 40 mg/sq m orally on days 1–10. Complex treatment regimens such as these should be under the direction of a medical oncologist who is familiar with the individual and synergistic toxicities and contraindications for each of the drugs involved. Frequent blood counts are obtained, and treatment is modified or suspended temporarily in the event of severe depression of the white cell or platelet count. With this form of remission induction with at least 6 courses of MOPP, approximately 50% of patients will remain free of all signs of Hodgkin's disease for over 2 years.

Current trials which employ either continued MOPP or other drugs for maintenance of remission make it possible for over 75% of patients to remain in complete remission with no evidence of recurrence of Hodgkin's disease. Theoretical calculations based on the number of logs of tumor cells likely to be killed with this type of intensive therapy suggest that a cellular cure of Hodgkin's disease may be accomplished in some of these cases, but follow-ups of 5–15 years after cessation of all chemotherapy will be required for confirmation. This form of chemotherapy therefore represents a major improvement in the management of advanced Hodgkin's disease, and patients should be afforded every chance to achieve complete remission.

Some of the reasons for the success of this approach to chemotherapy were the prior demonstrations of antineoplastic activity of each of the individual drugs used in Hodgkin's disease, the differing modes of action of the alkylating agents, procarbazine, vinca alkaloids, and corticosteroids, and the lack of cross-resistance of tumors to these different drugs. There is now little question, however, that the drugs should be used in combination rather than sequentially, since in the latter instance the tumor will develop resistance to the various agents and prolonged complete and unmaintained remissions cannot be attained.

Other single agents which appear promising in Hodgkin's disease are bleomycin and adriamycin. These drugs are currently under investigation and may find a role in combination chemotherapy. Bleomycin has the advantage of being cycle-specific while not a marrow depressant, whereas adriamycin, a marrow suppressant, is cycle-nonspecific but does not have cross-resistance with alkylating agents.

2. LYMPHOSARCOMA & RETICULUM CELL SARCOMA

Unlike Hodgkin's disease, which often appears to be unicentric in origin with evidence of probable active host resistance to the disease, lymphosarcoma and reticulum cell sarcoma often appear to be multicentric or generalized at the time of diagnosis. Staging is important in these lymphomas also, since predominantly localized disease can be treated first with radiation therapy followed by treatment of systemic lymphoma, if evidence of it is detected by staging procedures. Lymphosarcoma may be variable in onset and is often indistinguishable from chronic lymphocytic leukemia except for the absence of leukocytosis. Reticulum cell sarcoma is the most aggressive tumor in the lymphoma category, and the median survival of untreated patients is little more than 8 months. Lymphosarcoma is more amenable to chemotherapy than reticulum cell sarcoma, but neither responds as favorably as Hodgkin's disease.

Alkylating agents, vincristine, and prednisone all have a place in the management of these lymphomas; as in the case of Hodgkin's disease, combination chemotherapy is now the preferred approach to treatment and offers the best chance of inducing complete remission. Attainment of complete remission is a major objective since it not only leads to relief of all symptoms but also significantly lengthens the patient's life expectancy. One useful combination approach includes cyclophosphamide, vincristine (Oncovin), and prednisone in combination ("COP"). With COP therapy, complete remissions occur in 50% of patients with lymphosarcoma and about 40% of patients with reticulum cell sarcoma. These results are clearly superior to those that can be achieved with single agent therapy.

Once complete remission is attained, in the case of lymphosarcoma, it is apparently preferable to continue the same form of chemotherapy. However, in reticulum cell sarcoma, continuation of COP therapy does not appear to prolong the period of complete remission; some other form of chemotherapy will probably have to be developed to handle the subclinical phase of this tumor (less than 10^9 tumor cells).

Bertino at Yale has recently developed a new approach to combination chemotherapy for reticulum cell sarcoma which exploits knowledge of drug action and cellular kinetics in experimental animals as developed by Skipper and Schabel. This approach uses an alkylating agent (cyclophosphamide) to induce a multilog kill of G_O as well as cycling tumor cells, followed by vincristine, cytarabine, and methotrexate therapy to kill the residual tumor cells which are predominantly cycling. Results with this approach appear to be superior to those of COP therapy in reticulum cell sarcoma, and further exploration is warranted.

MULTIPLE MYELOMA

This plasma cell malignancy is now one of the "models" of neoplastic disease in man because the tumor arises from a single tumor stem cell and the tumor cells all produce a marker protein (myeloma immunoglobulin) which allows for quantitation of the total body burden of tumor cells. The tumor grows principally in the bone marrow and the surrounding bone, causing anemia, bone pain, lytic lesions, bone fractures, and anemia as well as increased susceptibility to infection. It has been clear for about 10 years that patients do improve if treated with oral alkylating agents such as melphalan or cyclophosphamide and that intermittent high doses of prednisone also have an oncolytic effect. Relatively simple combination chemotherapy was therefore developed by combining melphalan and prednisone, administering both drugs for courses of 4 days every 4–6 weeks. About 75% of myeloma patients improve with this treatment, and those patients who have the greatest reduction in total body tumor cell number (generally only 1–2 logs) have significant relief of symptoms and prolongation of survival with this treatment, and return to a more active life. Such therapy, although beneficial, is far from optimal, because between 10^{10} and 10^{11} myeloma cells persist in a "plateau" and resistance to chemotherapy (presumably by "subcloning") usually occurs after 2–3 years of treatment in most responding cases.

It has recently become clear that vincristine is also active if given when the population has been reduced in size by one or more logs (in which case more cells are cycling), and new efforts at developing combination chemotherapy must have as their objective the maximum degree of reduction in total body tumor cell number rather than just prolongation of survival. This objective can be followed serially, and intensified treatment can be administered during the "plateau."

Treatment of complications of myeloma is another important aspect of comprehensive therapy, and this effort is most important shortly after diagnosis, when they are most likely to be present.

The anemia of myeloma often responds well to androgen therapy, eg, testosterone enanthate (Delatestryl), 600 mg IM every 6 weeks for 2 or 3 doses. Hypercalcemia should be treated with fluids, corticosteroids, and calcium restriction; if this is not sufficient, mithramycin (Mithracin), 25 µg/kg IV, should be given every second or third day for 2 or 3 doses. The initial induction course of chemotherapy with alkylating agents and prednisone will often correct the hypercalcemia, but this complication is potentially lethal and should be viewed as a medical emergency and treated promptly. Painful bone lesions should be treated with x-ray therapy (if the area is not too extensive), as this will help ready the patient for ambulation and thereby minimize the possibility of hypercalcemia. Myeloma patients are often subject to recurrent infection because of a functional hypogammaglobulinemia. Prophylactic administration of gamma globulin does not correct the susceptibility to infection, but induction of a remission with chemotherapy often does. Sodium fluoride may increase the density of osteoporotic bone in some instances; however, this approach remains investigational and unproved despite many years of effort. The degree of reduction of myeloma globulin in the serum or urine is the most useful objective measure of the effectiveness of chemotherapy.

Similar comments apply to macroglobulinemia of Waldenström, which is a related plasma cell neoplasm. The growth characteristics of this tumor are more analogous to those of chronic lymphocytic leukemia; treatment need not be quite so aggressive, because the macroglobulin-producing cells rarely attack the skeleton. In most instances, low-dosage chlorambucil therapy proves adequate, and the patients have a relatively long life expectancy.

CANCER OF THE BREAST

In both men and women, palliative therapy of metastatic breast cancer is achieved by hormone administration and, in some cases, by nonhormonal chemotherapy. These drugs produce only moderate objective tumor regression but considerable subjective improvement. Because the hormones often cause serious undesirable side-effects, their use must be carefully individualized and controlled.

The rationale of hormone therapy of breast cancer is based on the concept that some breast cancers retain the characteristics of normal breast tissue, particularly with respect to hormone control. It has been empirically established that the progress of mammary carcinoma may often be favorably (although temporarily) affected by large doses of the sex hormones or by removal of the sources of endogenous hormone production by oophorectomy (orchiectomy in the male), adrenalectomy, or hypophysectomy.

The response to hormone therapy depends upon the age and menopausal status of the patient and the extent and nature of metastatic involvement.

Treatment with hormones is indicated only in patients with disseminated disease.

Androgenic Hormones

The androgens are used as palliative agents in women at any stage of disseminated breast cancer, without relation to the menopause. They are employed in premenopausal patients with progressive metastatic disease following relapse or failure to respond to oophorectomy. Testosterone propionate, 100 gm IM 3 times weekly, results in subjective improvement characterized by euphoria and relief of pain in 20–25% of patients, and about 2/3 of patients with bone metastases experience pain relief within 1–2 weeks after beginning therapy. Soft tissue metastases are less responsive to androgens, and regression occurs slowly. Metastases in the liver and brain rarely respond.

The duration of androgen-induced remissions is usually not over 6–8 months and seldom more than a year. Treatment with androgens must be continued for 10–12 weeks before its effect can be appraised. Occasionally, a transient "flare" or exacerbation of symptoms produced by the tumor may precede the onset of a regression. Following response to therapy, the androgen is continued until a relapse occurs. Further regression often follows discontinuation of therapy, so that it is desirable to wait several weeks before employing other methods of therapy. When relapse occurs in premenopausal patients after an adequate trial with androgen, adrenocorticosteroids or surgical measures (eg, adrenalectomy or hypophysectomy) may be considered.

Unpleasant and distressing side-effects of androgen therapy include virilism, hirsutism, deepening of the voice, acne, flushing, sodium retention, and increased libido. Hypercalcemia, which occurs in about 10% of patients with extensive osteolytic metastases, is significantly increased with androgen treatment. Symptoms, which appear after several weeks or months of treatment, include drowsiness, unusual behavior, nausea and vomiting, constipation, polyuria, and ultimately coma and death.

If patients develop evidence of hypercalcemia, prompt corrective measures are instituted. These include withdrawal of the androgen, institution of a high fluid intake, ambulation when possible, removal from the diet of calcium-rich foods such as milk and cheese, and the administration of large doses of corticosteroids. Prednisone in doses of 60–100 mg/day often produces dramatic clinical improvement and a decrease in serum calcium levels. When hypercalcemia is resistant to these measures, mithramycin (Mithracin)

is usually successful. In these patients, resumption of androgen therapy is undertaken with caution. A minimally androgenic synthetic compound, testolactone (Teslac), was released by the FDA for general use in 1969. Although virtually without side-effects, it has a favorable effect in only 8–10% of women who are treated.

Estrogenic Hormones

Estrogens are employed in both men and women with widespread breast cancer. In women, they are not used until at least 5 years after the menopause. Tumor regression with this form of therapy in women is surprising in view of the stimulating effect of estrogens on these tumors in premenopausal patients. Nevertheless, the palliative value of estrogens has been established by empirical use. A standard drug is diethylstilbestrol, 1–5 mg 3 times daily orally. Large doses often produce objective regressions lasting several weeks or months in soft tissue metastases and pulmonary metastases, and ulcerated primary lesions may heal. Estrogens are less effective in the palliation of osseous metastases, and patients with liver metastases seldom respond. Subjective improvement has been reported by about half of the patients treated.

The effect of estrogen therapy is usually evident within 1–3 months. The drug should be administered for at least 3 months before concluding that treatment is without value.

The complications of estrogen therapy include sodium retention and edema, anorexia, nausea and vomiting, uterine bleeding, pigmentation of the nipples, and occasionally exacerbation of tumor growth.

Adrenocorticosteroid Hormones

Administration of the corticosteroids (cortisone, prednisone, or equivalent cortisone compounds) produces marked subjective improvement in the form of euphoria, increased appetite and vigor, and other manifestations. Unfortunately, they do not produce significant tumor regression and are best reserved for palliation of patients with far-advanced disease who have received all of the above-described methods of treatment. Dramatic relief of symptoms produced by cerebral metastases and by hypercalcemia may follow the administration of these drugs. They are also of occasional value in the treatment of hemolytic anemia accompanying breast cancer.

Nonhormonal Chemotherapy of Breast Cancer

Systemic chemotherapy is in general reserved for use in breast cancer after refractoriness to hormonal measures is manifest. 5-Fluorouracil is perhaps the simplest agent to use, and causes virtually no toxicity when given in a dosage of 15 mg/kg IV once weekly. Responses occur in about 30% of women, and can be often maintained for 4–6 months. A variety of other agents, including cyclophosphamide, vincristine, and methotrexate, also show activity, although the remissions are of short duration with the latter 2 agents.

Combination therapy for breast cancer is currently investigational. Although rather striking remissions have been observed, toxicity is sometimes considerable. The current sequence of therapy for women with disseminated breast cancer would appear to be (1) hormonal manipulation, (2) 5-fluorouracil, (3) alkylating agent therapy, and (4) other agents. Management of this type requires the skill of a competent cancer chemotherapist or medical oncologist.

CARCINOMA OF THE ENDOMETRIUM

Progesterone derivatives cause dramatic objective tumor regression and symptomatic improvement lasting for many months in about 30% of patients with metastatic endometrial carcinoma. Patients showing objective response have definite prolongation of survival; unresponsive patients have a median life expectancy of 7 months, whereas the responders have a life expectancy of 27 months. The responses observed are primarily regressions of pulmonary metastases. Hydroxyprogesterone caproate (Delalutin) and medroxyprogesterone (Provera) have been employed with minimal side-effects.

CHORIOCARCINOMA OF THE UTERUS

This is a rare tumor of women arising from fetal trophoblastic tissue. It has been found that massive doses of methotrexate—25 mg daily for 4—5 days—will produce a high percentage of cures associated with complete regression of metastatic lesions and disappearance of chorionic gonadotropic hormones in the urine. Therapy should be given repeatedly until all evidence of the disease has disappeared. In some cases, combination or sequential chemotherapy with methotrexate, chlorambucil, vincristine, dactinomycin, and mercaptopurine is required to achieve cure when methotrexate alone is not adequate. It had been believed that this tumor genetically resembles a homograft and that maternal immunologic resistance is developed against antigens present in the trophoblastic tissue. However, recent studies indicate that chemotherapy is equally effective when the tumor is HL-A identical to the mother. This evidence refutes the hypothesis that the benefit of chemotherapy is enhanced by histo-incompatibility of the tumor. That is, cures are obtained even in the absence of histo-incompatibility. The effect of the antimetabolite presumably is to produce additional toxicity on rapidly growing trophoblastic tissue. Males with choriocarcinoma of the testes do not respond as well to chemotherapy, presumably because the tumor arises from host cells and is not a homograft.

CARCINOMA OF THE PROSTATE

Carcinoma of the prostate was one of the first forms of cancer shown to be responsive to hormonal manipulation. Orchiectomy and estrogen therapy have resulted in prolonged improvement from metastatic bone lesions. Hormonal treatment produces symptomatic benefit in 70—80% of patients and a significant degree of objective tumor regression. Responsive patients are treated indefinitely until relapse occurs. Prednisone will sometimes produce brief remissions at that point.

Treatment with other agents is experimental.

CARCINOMA OF THE OVARY

This neoplasm often remains occult until it has metastasized to the peritoneal cavity and may present as malignant ascites. The origin of this adenocarcinoma can usually be identified by histologic and secretory characteristics. The tumor responds dramatically to alkylating agents in at least 30—40% of patients, with resolution of ascites, disappearance of pain, and marked shrinkage of evident tumor.

Chlorambucil, mechlorethamine, cyclophosphamide, melphalan, and triethylenethiophosphoramide (Thio-TEPA) have all been demonstrated to be effective; however, all appear to have been used with suboptimal dose scheduling. Triethylenethiophosphoramide is particularly useful for intraperitoneal administration for malignant ascites since it is relatively nonirritating and causes fewer subjective side-effects than other agents. Despite the success at remission induction that is reported with alkylating agents in ovarian carcinoma, the remissions tend to last only 6 months to 1 year. Fluorouracil and vincristine also have activity in ovarian carcinoma, and this has prompted some exploration of combination therapy. The anthracycline antibiotic adriamycin also appears promising for ovarian carcinoma which is resistant to alkylating agents; however, its optimal dose and schedule have yet to be established.

CARCINOMA OF THE GASTROINTESTINAL TRACT

For many years, no chemotherapeutic drug had been shown to affect the course of neoplasms of the alimentary tract. It has now been demonstrated that fluorouracil can produce temporary remissions in adenocarcinoma of the colon. Responses occur in 20% of patients and average 4—5 months in duration. Treatment with fluorouracil is accompanied by significant toxicity in the form of stomatitis, nausea, intestinal ulceration, and bone marrow depression. These effects can be avoided without impairment of therapeutic efficacy by giving the drug in a single weekly injection of 15 mg/kg. Responses are also seen in some gastric and biliary tract adenocarcinomas.

Hepatic artery infusion of 5-FU or 5-FUDR have both been used with some success in the management of liver metastases from colon cancer; however, the same effect may be possible with oral administration of 5-FU. This latter approach should be considered experimental; nonetheless, it is fairly simple and sometimes useful.

Islet cell carcinoma of the pancreas arising from β cells and secreting insulin has been found to be exquisitely sensitive to the diabetogenic antibiotic streptozotocin. The results have been exceedingly good in this rare tumor, and it appears likely that this therapy may be curative.

BRONCHOGENIC CARCINOMA

The management of bronchogenic carcinoma is very unsatisfactory, and prevention (primarily through avoidance of cigarette smoking) remains the most important means of control. The average life expectancy after diagnosis has been 8 months. The tumor can rarely be cured by surgery, and x-ray therapy is used primarily for palliation of pain, obstruction, or bleeding. Distant metastases (including spread to the bone marrow) have usually occurred by the time of diagnosis, and chemotherapy therefore appears to be the only feasible approach.

Although this tumor had been notoriously resistant to all conventional forms of cancer chemotherapy, several novel approaches now show promise. Tumor histology has been found to be important in identifying which patients will respond to chemotherapy. Patients with the "oat cell" variety of lung cancer (the most rapidly growing type) show the best responses to cyclophosphamide as well as to combination chemotherapy. Administration of extraordinarily high doses of methotrexate (3–30 gm IV every 6 weeks) combined with a citrovorum factor (folinic acid) rescue technic has produced tumor regressions which have lasted for over 1 year; however, this approach remains investigational.

There is little doubt, however, that citrovorum factor administration after methotrexate does "rescue" the bone marrow cells from the otherwise lethal toxicity of the folic acid antagonist, while the tumor cells do not appear to recover despite the folinic acid administration. Similar results have been obtained with combination chemotherapy, and adriamycin also shows activity. Thus, although systemic treatment is still unsatisfactory, it has shown signs of promise.

Several local complications also deserve mention, as they can be improved with chemotherapy. Mechlorethamine treatment of patients with superior vena

caval compression often relieves this acute and frequently fatal complication of bronchogenic carcinoma. Pleural effusion due to carcinomatous metastasis may be controlled by intrapleural injection of mechlorethamine or quinacrine (see below).

MALIGNANT MELANOMA & MISCELLANEOUS SARCOMAS

Metastatic melanoma is one of the most difficult neoplasms to treat. Most chemotherapeutic agents are reported to induce regressions in at least 10% of melanoma patients; however, spontaneous regressions also occur, especially in skin metastases, and regressions of cutaneous lesions thus may not necessarily imply sensitivity to chemotherapy. Immunologic reactivity to the tumor by host lymphocytes may partially explain the evanescent changes in skin lesions, but "spontaneous regression" of visceral disease is rare and metastases occur in virtually every organ in the body. Alkylating agents such as melphalan and hydroxyurea occasionally cause visceral regressions. Imidazole carboxamide, a new experimental compound, may cause regressions, and trimethylcolchicinic acid also appears to be active. Combinations of BCNU and vincristine have been tried with limited success.

The picture in various sarcomas had also been rather bleak until recently, with responses occasionally noted with dactinomycin, vinblastine, vincristine, or alkylating agents. Within the last year it has become clear that osteogenic sarcoma and Ewing's sarcoma may respond to adriamycin, and one of the cooperative chemotherapy groups has just established that a combination of adriamycin and imidazole carboxamide may induce substantial regressions in about 40% of cases of rhabdomyosarcoma, fibrosarcoma, osteogenic sarcoma, and related tumors. Although both of these agents are still investigational in the USA, it appears likely that they will gain widespread use for these formerly resistant tumors.

CONTROL OF MALIGNANT EFFUSIONS & ASCITES

The direct injection of mechlorethamine into the involved cavity will eliminate or suppress an effusion in about 2/3 of patients with ascites and effusions due to carcinoma. This method of control compares favorably with the results obtained using radioactive gold or chromium phosphate. It has the important advantage of being easily administered, readily available, inexpensive, and without radiation hazard. The method is useful irrespective of the types of primary tumor.

The procedure is as follows: Most of the pleural or ascitic fluid is withdrawn, and mechlorethamine is

TABLE 45–6. Malignancies responsive to chemotherapy.

Diagnosis	Alkylating Agents	Antimetabolites	Steroid Hormones	Miscellaneous Drugs
Acute lymphocytic leukemia	Cyclophosphamide	Mercaptopurine, thioguanine, methotrexate, Ara-C	Prednisone	Vincristine, asparaginase,* daunorubicin* (daunomycin)
Acute myelocytic leukemia		Thioguanine, Ara-C, mercaptopurine	Prednisone	Vincristine, allopurinol†
Chronic myelocytic leukemia	Busulfan	Mercaptopurine, thioguanine		Vincristine, allopurinol†
Chronic lymphocytic leukemia	Chlorambucil, cyclophosphamide, triethylenethiophosphoramide		Prednisone	Vincristine
Hodgkin's disease	Chlorambucil, mechlorethamine, cyclophosphoramide, triethylenethiophosphoramide		Prednisone	Vinblastine, vincristine, procarbazine, bleomycin,* adriamycin*
Lymphosarcoma and reticulum cell sarcoma	Chlorambucil, cyclophosphamide, mechlorethamine		Prednisone	Vincristine, adriamycin*
Multiple myeloma	Melphalan, cyclophosphamide		Prednisone	Androgens,† vincristine, procarbazine
Macroglobulinemia	Chlorambucil			
Polycythemia vera	Busulfan, chlorambucil			Allopurinol†
Carcinoma of lung	Cyclophosphamide, mechlorethamine	Methotrexate	Prednisone	Atabrine†
Carcinoma of larynx and other "head and neck" tumors		Methotrexate		Bleomycin,* adriamycin*
Carcinoma of endometrium			Progestins	
Carcinoma of ovary	Triethylenethiophosphoramide, cyclophosphamide, chlorambucil	Fluorouracil		Adriamycin*
Breast carcinoma	Cyclophosphamide, chlorambucil, mechlorethamine	Fluorouracil, methotrexate	Estrogens, androgens, Δ^1-testonolactone, prednisone	Vincristine, adriamycin*
Choriocarcinoma (trophoblastic neoplasms)		Methotrexate, mercaptopurine		Dactinomycin, vinblastine, vincristine
Carcinoma of testis	Cyclophosphamide, chlorambucil	Methotrexate		Dactinomycin, vincristine, mithramycin, bleomycin*
Carcinoma of prostate			Estrogens	Adriamycin*
Wilms's tumor (children)	Mechlorethamine, cyclophosphamide		Prednisone	Dactinomycin, vincristine
Neuroblastoma	Cyclophosphamide			Vincristine
Carcinoma of adrenal				o,p'DDD*
Carcinoma of colon		Fluorouracil		
Carcinoid	Cyclophosphamide			Dactinomycin
Insulinoma				Streptozotocin*
Miscellaneous sarcomas and carcinomas	Mechlorethamine, cyclophosphamide, chlorambucil	Fluorouracil, methotrexate	Prednisone	Dactinomycin, vincristine, adriamycin,* imidazole carboxamide*

*Investigational agent.
†Valuable supportive agent, not oncolytic.

injected into the cavity. The dose employed is 0.4 mg/kg, or a total dose of 20–30 mg in the usual patient. The solution is prepared immediately before administration so as to avoid loss of potency through hydrolysis. A free flow of fluid from the cavity must be established before the drug is injected to avoid injection into the tissues. After the drug is injected, the patient is placed in a variety of positions in order to distribute the drug throughout the pleural or abdominal cavity. On the following day, the remaining fluid is withdrawn from the body cavity.

Pain sometimes occurs following injection of mechlorethamine into the pleural cavity, but pain, nausea, vomiting, and peritoneal irritation may be experienced for several days following injection into the peritoneal cavity. Nausea and vomiting usually occur within a few hours after administration, but can be controlled with chlorpromazine, 25 mg IM given immediately before the procedure and at intervals following the injection. Bone marrow depression is mild with this method of administration, except in patients who have received extensive radiation therapy.

Quinacrine (Atabrine) has been employed in place of mechlorethamine with similar therapeutic benefit. The drug is customarily injected daily over a 5-day period. Local pain and fever are commonly noted. There is no systemic hematopoietic depression.

• • •

General References

General

Baserga, R. (editor): *The Cell Cycle and Cancer.* Dekker, 1971.

Bruce, W.R., & H. Lin: Cellular approach to cancer chemotherapy. Cancer Res 29:2308–2310, 1969.

Cline, M.J.: *Cancer Chemotherapy.* Saunders, 1971.

Krakoff, I.H. (editor): Symposium on medical aspect of cancer. M Clin North America 55:525–787, 1971.

Livingston, R.B., & S.K. Carter: *Single Agents in Cancer Chemotherapy.* Plenum, 1970.

Perry, S. (editor): *Human Tumor Cell Kinetics Lecture Series.* Nat Cancer Inst Monogr No. 30, 1969.

Ryser, H.J.-P.: Chemical carcinogenesis. New England J Med 285:721–734, 1971.

Salmon, S.E.: Malignant disorders. Chap 30, pp 891–902, in: *Current Diagnosis & Treatment.* Krupp, M.A., & M.J. Chatton (editors). Lange, 1972.

Skipper, H.E.: Biochemical, biological, pharmacologic, toxicologic, kinetic and clinical relationships. Cancer 21:600–610, 1968.

Skipper, H.E., & others: Implications of biochemical, pharmacologic and toxicologic relationships in the design of optimal therapy. Cancer Chemother Rep 54:431, 1970.

Alkylating Agents

Fairley, K.F., & J.M. Simister: *Cyclophosphamide.* Williams & Wilkins, 1965.

Karnofsky, D.A. (editor): Comparative clinical and biological effects of alkylating agents. Ann New York Acad Sc 66:657–1266, 1958.

Lawley, P., & P. Brooks: Interstrand crosslinking of DNA by difunctional alkylating agents. J Molec Biol 25:143–160, 1967.

Schmidt, L.H., & others: Comparative pharmacology of alkylating agents. Parts I–III. Cancer Chemother Rep (Suppl 2):1–1528, 1965.

Van Duuren, B.L. (editor): Biological effects of alkylating agents. Ann New York Acad Sc 163:589–1029, 1969.

Wheeler, G.P.: Studies related to the mechanisms of action of cytotoxic alkylating agents. Cancer Res 22:651–688, 1962.

Antimetabolites

Bertino, J.R., & F.M. Huennekens (editors): Folate antagonists as chemotherapeutic agents. Ann New York Acad Sc 186:1–519, 1971.

Burchenal, J.H., & R.R. Ellison: The pyrimidine and purine antagonists. Clin Pharmacol Therap 2:523–541, 1961.

Cohen, S.S.: Introduction to the biochemistry of D-arabinosylnucleosides. Progr Nucleic Acid Res Molec Biol 5:1–88, 1966.

Heidelberger, C.: Cancer chemotherapy with purine and pyrimidine analogs. Ann Rev Pharmacol 7:101–124, 1967.

Hitchings, G.H., & C.P. Rhoads (editors): 6-Mercaptopurine. Ann New York Acad Sc 60:183–508, 1954.

Krakoff, I.H., & R. Meyer: Prevention of hyperuricemia in leukemia and lymphoma: Use of allopurinol. JAMA 193:1–6, 1965.

Livingston, R.B., & S.K. Carter: Cytosine arabinoside: A clinical brochure. Part I. Cancer Chemother Rep 53:179–205, 1968.

Steroids

American Cancer Society: Hormones and chemotherapy for cancer. Cancer 18:1517–1666, 1965.

Baxter, J.D., & others: Glucocorticoid receptors in lymphoma cells in culture: Relationship to glucocorticoid killing activity. Science 171:189–191, 1971.

Krakoff, I.H.: Chemotherapy and hormonal therapy of carcinoma of the breast. Pages 77–83 in: *Cancer Chemotherapy.* Brodsky, I., & others (editors). Grune & Stratton, 1967.

Pincus, G., & E. Vollmer (editors): *Biological Activities of Steroids in Relation to Cancer.* Academic Press, 1960.

Tait, J.F., & S. Burstein: In vivo studies of steroid dynamics in man. The Hormones 5:441–557, 1964.

Antibiotics & Other Natural Products

Adamson, R.H.: Antitumor activity and other biological properties of L-asparaginase: A review. Cancer Chemother Rep 52:617–626, 1968.

Antitumor Antibiotic Bleomycin. Nippon Kayaku Ltd (Tokyo), 1969.

Apple, M.A., & C.M. Haskell: Potent inhibition of sarcoma virus RNA-directed RNA:DNA duplex synthesis and arrest of ascites murine leukemia and sarcoma in vivo by anthracyclines. Phys Chem Physics 3:307–318, 1971.

Jones, B., & others: Daunomycin in the treatment of advanced childhood lymphoblastic leukemia. Cancer Res 31:84–90, 1971.

Livingston, R.B., & S.K. Carter: Daunomycin: A chemotherapy fact sheet of the National Cancer Institute. March 1970.

Newton, B.A.: Chemotherapeutic compounds affecting DNA structure and function. Advances Pharmacol Chemother 8:149–184, 1970.

Shastri, S., & others: Clinical study with bleomycin. Cancer 28:1142–1146, 1971.

Symposium: The actinomycins and their importance in the treatment of tumors in animals and man. Ann New York Acad Sc 89:283–486, 1960.

Symposium on vincristine. Cancer Chemother Rep 52:455–535, 1968.

Miscellaneous Anticancer Drugs

Dollinger, M.R., & others: Quinacrine in the treatment of neoplastic effusions. Ann Int Med 66:249–257, 1967.

Hutter, A.M., & D.E. Kayhoe: Adrenal cortical carcinoma: Results of treatment with o,p'DDD in 138 patients. Am J Med 41:572–592, 1966.

Jell, A.M., & J. Marks (editors): *Natulan-Ibenzmethyzin.* J. Wright & Sons (Bristol), 1965.

Clinical Oncology: Acute Leukemia

Crowther, D., & others: Combination chemotherapy using L-asparaginase, daunorubicin, and cytosine arabinoside in adults with acute myelogenous leukaemia. Brit MJ 4:513–517, 1970.

Frei, E., III, & E.J. Freireich: Progress and perspectives in the chemotherapy of acute leukemia. Advances Chemother 2:269, 1965.

Frei, E., III, & others: Advances in the chemotherapy of acute leukemia: Comparative leukemia research, 1969. Bibl haemat 36:689–700, 1970.

Gee, T., Yu, K.P., & B.D. Clarkson: Treatment of adult leukemia with arabinosylcytosine and thioguanine. Cancer 23:1019–1032, 1969.

Henderson, E.S.: Treatment of acute leukemia. Seminars Hemat 6:271–319, 1969.

Hryniuk, W., & others: Treatment of leukemia with large doses of methotrexate and folinic acid: Clinical-biochemical correlates. J Nat Cancer Inst 48:2140–2155, 1969.

Shambron, E., Miller, S., & V.F. Fairbanks: Intrathecal administration of amethopterin (methotrexate) in leukemic encephalopathy of young adults. New England J Med 265:169–171, 1961.

Clinical Oncology: Chronic Leukemias, Hodgkin's Disease, Lymphosarcoma, & Multiple Myeloma

Alexanian, R., & others: Treatment of multiple myeloma: Combination chemotherapy with different melphalan dose regimens. JAMA 208:1685, 1969.

De Vita, V.T., Jr., & others: Combination chemotherapy in the treatment of advanced Hodgkin's disease. Ann Int Med 73:881–895, 1970.

Galton, D.A.G., & others: The use of chlorambucil (Leukeran) and steroids in the treatment of chronic lymphocytic leukemia. Brit J Haemat 7:73–98, 1961.

Huguley, C.M., & others: Comparison of 6-mercaptopurine (Purinethol) and busulfan (Myleran) in chronic granulocytic leukemia. Blood 21:89–101, 1963.

Luce, J.K., & others: Combined cyclophosphamide, vincristine, and prednisone therapy of malignant lymphoma. Cancer 28:306–317, 1971.

Rhomes, J.A., & others: Central nervous system therapy and combination chemotherapy of childhood lymphocytic leukemia. Blood 37:272–281, 1971.

Salmon, S.E., & others: Role of gamma globulin for immunoprophylaxis in multiple myeloma. New England J Med 277:1336–1340, 1967.

Salmon, S.E., & B.A. Smith: Immunoglobulin synthesis and total body tumor cell number in IgG multiple myeloma. J Clin Invest 49:1114–1121, 1970.

Stolinsky, D.C., & others: Clinical experience with procarbazine in Hodgkin's disease, reticulum cell sarcoma, and lymphosarcoma. Cancer 26:984–990, 1970.

Sullivan, P.W., & S.E. Salmon: Kinetics of growth and regression in IgG multiple myeloma. J Clin Invest. In press.

Young, R.C., & others: Treatment of advanced Hodgkin's disease with (1,3 bis[2-chloroethyl]-1-nitrosourea) BCNU. New England J Med 285:475–479, 1971.

Clinical Oncology: Other Neoplasms

Carbone, P.P. (moderator): Lung cancer: Perspectives and prospects. Ann Int Med 73:1003–1024, 1970.

Eisman, S.H.: The therapy of advanced female breast cancer: An appraisal of its present status and problems. M Clin North America 50:1457–1467, 1966.

James, D.H., Jr., Beckwith, J.B., & J.L. Swinn: Vincristine in children with malignant solid tumors. J Pediat 64:534–541, 1964.

Kaufman, R.J.: Management of advanced ovarian carcinoma. M Clin North America 50:845–856, 1966.

Kennedy, B.J.: Mithramycin therapy in advanced testicular neoplasms. Cancer 26:755–766, 1970.

Li, M.C., Hertz, R., & D.B. Spencer: Effect of methotrexate therapy upon choriocarcinoma. Proc Soc Exper Biol Med 93:361–366, 1956.

Reifenstein, E.: Hydroxyprogesterone caproate therapy in advanced endometrial cancer. Cancer 27:485–502, 1971.

Selawry, O.S., & J. Hananian: Vincristine treatment of cancer in children. JAMA 183:741–746, 1963.

Tilney, N.L., & S.G. Economou: Chemotherapy of gastrointestinal cancer. Geriatrics 20:265–276, 1965.

Whitmore, W.F., Jr.: Hormone therapy in prostatic cancer. Am J Med 21:697–713, 1956.

Wilson, C.B., & others: 1,3-Bis(2-chloroethyl)-1-nitrosourea (NSC-409962) in the treatment of brain tumors. Part I. Cancer Chemother Rep 54:273–281, 1970.

46...

Drugs & the Immune System

Sydney E. Salmon, MD

IMMUNOSUPPRESSIVE AGENTS

THE IMMUNE MECHANISM

With the increase in understanding of normal mechanisms of immunity and the role of immunologic abnormalities in the pathophysiology of certain disorders, agents that suppress the immune response now play an important role in tissue transplantation procedures and in certain diseases associated with disorders of immunity. Although some of the details of the overall immune mechanism are still uncertain, a general scheme of the steps involved in the genesis of specific immunity can be sketched (Fig 46–1) as a means

of placing the effects and toxicities of immunosuppressive agents in perspective.

Specific immunity appears to result from the interaction of antigens (substances the host normally recognizes as foreign) with mononuclear cells that circulate in the blood and lymph. The nature of self-recognition, or "tolerance," remains obscure, but it appears to be defined in utero, during development of the lymphoid tissues. Although lymphoid cells derived embryologically from the thymus and bone marrow play the major role in the development of specific immunity, an initial "antigen-processing" step seems to occur in the mononuclear phagocyte (the blood monocyte or the tissue macrophage), which then makes the antigen more readily recognizable or available to lymphoid cells. The ability of lymphoid cells to interact with specific antigens appears to be genetically

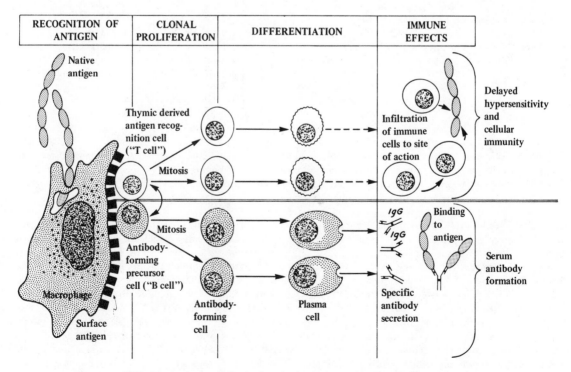

FIG 46–1. A theoretical scheme of cellular and humoral immunity.

Dr. Salmon is Associate Professor of Medicine and Head, Division of Hematology and Oncology, Department of Medicine, University of Arizona, Tucson.

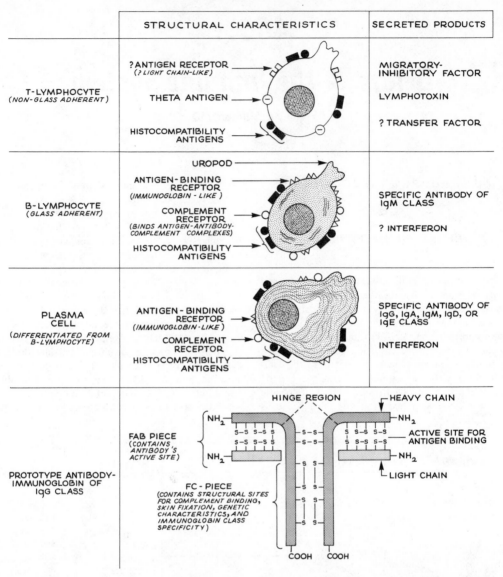

FIG 46—2. Effectors in the immune response. Specific cell types including T-lymphocytes, B-lymphocytes, and plasma cells—as well as secreted antibody-immunoglobulin—have binding sites for specific antigen as well as differential genetic and functional characteristics. Membrane features as well as secreted products can thus be seen to have important functions in the immune response.

determined, with different lymphoid clones having individual specificities for different antigenic determinants.

A basic dualism seems to govern the function of the lymphoid system. Two different types of lymphoid cells mediate—respectively—cellular immunity and serologic immunity. Long-lived clones of small lymphoid cells derived from or influenced by the thymus (T cells) appear to recognize the antigen and presumably bind to it. The proliferation of such clones of antigen recognition cells, which occurs after contact with antigen, is presumably responsible for the development of "cellular immunity," which can be demonstrated in delayed hypersensitivity reactions and

is important in tissue graft rejection. The T cells may have surface receptors which allow them to recognize a foreign antigen and react to it. T cells appear to exert their effects by direct cytotoxic interaction (eg, with tumor cells or transplants), and by release of various "lymphokines" (eg, lymphotoxin, migration-inhibitory factor). The genesis of specific antibody immunoglobulins resides in the progeny of a second type of lymphoid cell, the antibody precursor cell (B cell), derived from the bone marrow. B cells can be identified by the presence of monoclonal immunoglobulins on their surfaces which are located in "spots" on the cell membrane and appear to serve as antigen receptors. By the time of birth, lymph node and splenic architecture

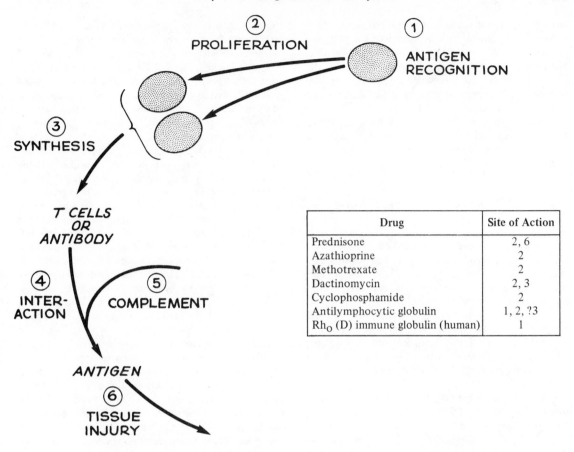

FIG 46–3. The sites of action of immunosuppressive agents on the immune response.

Drug	Site of Action
Prednisone	2, 6
Azathioprine	2
Methotrexate	2
Dactinomycin	2, 3
Cyclophosphamide	2
Antilymphocytic globulin	1, 2, ?3
Rh_O (D) immune globulin (human)	1

includes parafollicular cuffs of thymus-derived lymphocytes and follicular nests of immunoglobulin-synthesizing cells that form germinal centers. Intimate cell-cell interaction between macrophages bearing the antigen in an immunogenic form on the cell surface and complementary clones of T cells and B cells is thought to be required before the clonal proliferation of T cells can develop cellular immunity and the B cells can form antibody-forming cells (Fig 46–1). The antibody-forming cells can increase their synthetic capacity by further differentiation into plasma cells, clones of which specifically secrete large amounts of antibody of one of the immunoglobulin classes IgG, IgA, IgM, IgD, and IgE. During the course of this differentiation, individual clones may "switch" their immunoglobulin type from IgM to IgG, even though the active site of the secreted antibody retains the identical structure after this "switch." Finally, specific antibody binds to the foreign antigen, leading to its precipitation, inactivation (eg, virus), lysis (eg, red cells), or phagocytosis (eg, bacteria). In some of these circumstances, complement is bound to the antigen-antibody complex and facilitates the destruction or phagocytosis of the antigen. Once an antibody response is established, reexposure to antigen leads to an immediate chemical combination of antigen and antibody and also serves to provide a "booster" for a rapid secondary wave of cell proliferation and anti-

body synthesis. The dual nature of immunity is underscored by certain "experiments of nature," or genetic diseases. For example, the Di George syndrome, resulting from absence of the third branchial cleft, is associated with absent thymic development and impaired delayed hypersensitivity but normal antibody formation, whereas delayed hypersensitivity is usually normal in X-linked congenital agammaglobulinemia, which presents as an antibody deficiency syndrome.

The complexity of the immune system appears to provide a sufficient number of control points to render the emergence of a "forbidden clone," which is reactive against the host's own constituents, a relatively rare event. Normally, most components of the lymphoid system remain in a highly "repressed" state until they are selectively activated for a specific immune response. The numerous steps of the process also imply that immunosuppressive agents can be directed at various steps along this pathway (Fig 46–3), including the induction of specific tolerance. Because the immune system provides a major barricade against microorganisms (including oncogenic viruses), toxins, and foreign cells, generalized immunosuppression can potentially be very dangerous to the host.

With only one notable exception–Rh_O (D) immune globulin (human)–the clinically useful immunosuppressive agents which are now available may have general immunosuppressive properties and must be used with caution. Generalized immunosuppression increases the risk of infection and may also increase the risk of development of lymphoreticular malignancies or other forms of cancer. In general, it is easier to block or attenuate a primary immune response with immunosuppressive drugs than to suppress an established immune response.

Even with these limitations and cautions, immunosuppression is of proved usefulness in a number of acquired immune disorders as well as in organ transplantation.

TESTS OF IMMUNOSUPPRESSION

A wide variety of clinical and basic research technics have been used to test immunologic competence and its drug-induced suppression. The simplest tests which can be used to detect the effects of immunosuppressive agents include the following:

(1) Delayed hypersensitivity testing with skin test antigens to detect the ability to respond to mumps, trichophyton, *Candida albicans,* and other antigens to which most individuals have been exposed or to respond to sensitizing chemicals such as dinitrochlorobenzene.

(2) Measurement of serum immunoglobulins, serum complement, and specific antibodies to various natural and acquired antibodies.

(3) Serial measurements of antibody response after primary immunization or a secondary booster injection (Fig 46—2).

(4) Absolute circulating lymphocyte counts.

These relatively simple tests plus the evaluation of clinical responses in organ transplantation and autoimmune disorders have provided most of the current information on the in vivo effects of the immunosuppressive agents in man. However, evidence of immunosuppression as measured by these tests of immune response does not always correlate well with the clinical response of the disease state being treated. For example, in the case of skin testing, adequate control of such studies also requires that the patient's nonspecific inflammatory response be tested also; if this is impaired, the delayed hypersensitivity testing will be difficult to interpret. The relevance to in vivo events of cell responses in various in vitro tests of lymphoid function, such as lymphocyte transformation testing and inhibition of macrophage migration, is in most instances even more uncertain. Nonetheless, it is clear that once the in vitro tests are well standardized and made quantitative, they will take on increasing importance and may supplant some of the in vivo studies.

RELATIONSHIP OF IMMUNOSUPPRESSIVE THERAPY TO CANCER CHEMOTHERAPY

Although there is definite overlap between the drugs used for immunosuppression (Fig 46—3) and those used in cancer chemotherapy (Chapter 45), different principles govern their use in these 2 disease categories. The general pharmacologic properties and toxicities of several of these agents (corticosteroids, alkylating agents, and certain structural analogues) were described in Chapter 45. The unique applications of these and other immunosuppressive drugs will be reviewed in this chapter in relationship to the action of these agents on the immune system and their effects in specific disease states. Since many cytotoxic drugs (eg, structural analogues) act primarily on proliferating cells, there is, in a sense, a similarity between their uses against proliferating cancer cells and against proliferating immune cells. However, the character and kinetics of cancer cell proliferation (Chapter 45) are somewhat dissimilar to immune cell proliferation and allow different features to be exploited in immunosuppression. For example, whereas cancer cell proliferation appears to be uncontrolled, immune cell proliferation usually occurs in response to the presence of a specific antigen. While division of individual malignant cells within a large cancer cell population appears to occur randomly in an apparently unsynchronized way, immune cell proliferation appears to be "synchronized" in a burst of mitotic division which occurs after introduction of the antigen, with a large fraction of the responding cells going through the generation cycle in order to produce specific immunity. Thus, when cytotoxic drugs are used at the time of initial exposure to foreign antigen (eg, a kidney transplant), a very high percentage of an initially small number of precursor cells can be destroyed because the antigen stimulates selected relevant clones to proliferate rather than all clones of immune cells. Therefore, a greater degree of selective toxicity can be initially obtained against the unwanted immune clone, whereas this objective is harder to achieve in cancer chemotherapy.

The selective nature of immunosuppression in a synchronized response can result in less damage to other normal cells, and dosages of the drugs are sometimes lower than those used in cancer chemotherapy. When dealing with an established immune response, the selective advantage in immunosuppression is not so great as in the instance of the primary immune response. Lymphoid cells can still be damaged somewhat more than other host tissues, however, because they are generally more sensitive to cytotoxic drugs and radiation than are other types of normal cells. Macrophages are relatively radioresistant cells and presumably also are less affected by immunosuppressive drugs than are lymphoid cells.

CORTICOSTEROIDS

Corticosteroids were the first class of hormonal agents which were recognized to have lympholytic properties. Administration of a glucocorticoid (eg, prednisone, dexamethasone) reduces the size and lymphoid content of the lymph nodes and spleen, although it has essentially no toxic effect on proliferating myeloid or erythroid stem cells in the bone marrow. Glucocorticoids are thought to interfere with the cell cycle of activated lymphoid cells, but the exact mechanism remains obscure. Prednisone can suppress both cellular immunity and antibody synthesis. Plasma cells seem to be less sensitive to the effects of corticosteroids. However, since the precursor lymphoid cells are sensitive to this agent, the primary response can be diminished, and, with continued use, previously established antibody responses are also decreased.

Prednisone is used in a wide variety of clinical circumstances where it is thought that the immunosuppressive properties of the drug account for its beneficial effects. Indications include auto-immune disorders such as auto-immune hemolytic anemia, idiopathic thrombocytopenic purpura, and lupus erythematosus and some cases of Hashimoto's thyroiditis. Corticosteroids are also used liberally in organ transplant recipients and are of particular value during rejection crises because the dosage can be increased without fear of bone marrow toxicity. The usual dose range for prednisone as an immunosuppressive agent is 10–100 mg orally daily or on an intermittent schedule. The potential side-effects of corticosteroids, including adrenal suppression (Chapters 35 and 45), are also relevant when these agents are used chronically for immunosuppression.

AZATHIOPRINE & OTHER CYTOTOXIC AGENTS

1. AZATHIOPRINE
(Imuran)

Azathioprine is an imidazolyl derivative of mercaptopurine (6-mercaptopurine, 6-MP) and functions as a structural analogue or "antimetabolite" (Chapter 45). Although its action is presumably mediated by mercaptopurine as the active form, it has received more widespread use than mercaptopurine for immunosuppression in man. These agents may represent prototypes of the structural analogue or cytotoxic types of immunosuppressive drugs, and many other agents which kill proliferative cells seem to work at a similar level in the immune response.

Azathioprine
(Imuran)

Azathioprine is absorbed well from the gastrointestinal tract and is split in vivo, primarily into the parent compound, mercaptopurine. Xanthine oxidase splits much of the active material to 6-thiouric acid prior to excretion in the urine. After administration of azathioprine, small amounts of unchanged drug and mercaptopurine are also excreted by the kidney, and as much as a 2-fold increase in toxicity may occur in anephric or anuric patients. Since much of the drug's inactivation depends on xanthine oxidase, patients who are also receiving allopurinol (Chapter 45) for control of hyperuricemia should have the dose of azathioprine reduced to 1/4–1/3 the usual dose to prevent excessive toxicity.

As with mercaptopurine, the chief toxicity of azathioprine is bone marrow depression, usually manifest as leukopenia although anemia, thrombocytopenia, and bleeding may also occur. Skin rashes, drug fever, nausea and vomiting, and sometimes diarrhea occur, with the gastrointestinal symptoms seen mainly at higher dosages. Hepatic dysfunction, manifested by very high serum alkaline phosphatase levels and mild jaundice, occurs occasionally.

Immunosuppression with azathioprine or mercaptopurine therapy seems to result from interference with nucleic acid metabolism at steps that are required for the wave of cell proliferation that follows antigenic stimulation. The purine analogues are thus cytotoxic agents and destroy stimulated lymphoid cells. Although continued messenger RNA synthesis is necessary for sustained antibody synthesis by plasma cells, these analogues appear to have less effect on this process than on nucleic acid synthesis in proliferating cells. Cellular immunity as well as primary and secondary serum antibody responses can be blocked by these cytotoxic agents. Animal studies have shown that, if a course of mercaptopurine therapy is completed prior to exposure to a new antigen, the subsequent antibody response may actually be potentiated rather than suppressed. Although this latter phenomenon has yet to be substantiated clinically, such observations emphasize the need for precise timing of therapy relative to organ transplantation.

Azathioprine and mercaptopurine appear to be of definite benefit in maintaining renal homografts and may also be of value in transplantation of other tissues. These analogues have also been used with some success in the management of acute glomerulonephritis and in the renal component of systemic lupus erythematosus.

Although these agents are potentially toxic to bone marrow elements, including the megakaryocytes and red cell precursors, the favorable effects sometimes outweigh the toxic effects. The drugs have been of occasional use in prednisone-resistant antibody-mediated idiopathic thrombocytopenic purpura and auto-immune hemolytic anemias.

2. OTHER CYTOTOXIC AGENTS

Other cytotoxic agents, including methotrexate and cytosine arabinoside (Chapter 45), also have immunosuppressive properties. Although these agents can be used for immunosuppression, they have not received as widespread use as the purine antagonists and their indications for immunosuppression are less certain. The use of methotrexate (which can be given orally) appears reasonable in patients with idiosyncratic reactions to purine antagonists. The antibiotic dactinomycin has also been used with some success at the time of impending renal transplant rejection.

CYCLOPHOSPHAMIDE

The alkylating agent cyclophosphamide (Cytoxan) has recently been the focus of considerable interest as an immunosuppressive agent in animals and man. It is perhaps the most potent immunosuppressive drug that has been synthesized. Cyclophosphamide destroys proliferating lymphoid cells but also appears to alkylate some resting cells. It has been observed that very large doses (eg, > 120 mg/kg IV over several days) may induce an apparent specific tolerance to a new antigen if the drug is administered simultaneously with—or shortly after—the antigen. In smaller doses, it has been very effective in auto-immune disorders, including systemic lupus erythematosus, and in patients with acquired factor XIII antibodies and bleeding syndromes.

Although treatment with large doses of cyclophosphamide carries considerable risk of pancytopenia and hemorrhagic cystitis, the drug has aided in "takes" of bone marrow transplants and may have value in other types of organ transplantation also. Although cyclophosphamide appears to induce tolerance for marrow or immune cell grafting, its use does not prevent the subsequent "graft-versus-host" syndrome, which may be serious or lethal if the donor is a poor histocompatibility match. This form of therapy must be considered investigational in the USA and requires the informed consent of the recipient. Highly specialized medical care and supportive facilities are mandatory for patient survival during the period of intensive therapy.

ANTIBODIES AS IMMUNOSUPPRESSIVE AGENTS

1. HETEROLOGOUS ANTILYMPHOCYTIC GLOBULIN

Although antisera directed against lymphocytes had been prepared sporadically since Metchnikoff's first observations just before the turn of the century, detailed evaluation was not made of antilymphocytic serum until the 1960's. With the arrival of the era of human organ homotransplantation, heterologous antilymphocytic globulin (ALG) suddenly took on new importance. It has subsequently been the subject of many basic and clinical studies. ALG remains an investigational agent in the USA, but it is used in many medical centers that have organ transplantation programs.

The antiserum is usually obtained by immunization of large animals (eg, horses) with human lymphoid cells. The IgG fraction of the antiserum is prepared by cold alcohol precipitation or chromatographic fractionation. The potency of each batch of ALG is determined by lymphocyte agglutination and cytotoxicity testing in vitro. Cytotoxicity titers correspond somewhat to the clinical responses, but the activity of ALG has yet to be adequately standardized.

Antilymphocytic antibody acts primarily on the small, long-lived peripheral lymphocytes which circulate between the blood and lymph. With continued administration, the "thymus-dependent" lymphocytes from the cuffs of lymphoid follicles are also depleted, as they normally participate in the recirculating pool. Antilymphocytic antibody binds to the surface of these small "antigen recognition" cells (Fig 46–1), with the cytotoxic destruction of the cells mediated by serum complement. As a result of the destruction of the AR cells, a rather specific impairment of delayed hypersensitivity and cellular immunity occurs while humoral antibody formation remains relatively intact. The pattern of immunosuppression obtained with ALG is similar to that which occurs when circulating small lymphocytes are depleted by prolonged thoracic duct drainage. The selectivity of ALG for the cellular immune system accounts for its usefulness in preventing rejection of transplanted organs.

Since ALG has still not been adequately standardized, only generalizations about dosage and treatment can be given. After transplantation of an organ such as the kidney, ALG is often administered (by intramuscular injection) first on a daily basis and subsequently cut back in frequency. Because ALG is usually administered along with azathioprine and prednisone, it has not been possible to assess the effects of ALG alone in human kidney transplants. Investigators who treat their renal transplant recipients with ALG believe that it reduces the dosage requirements for the other immunosuppressive drugs and improves survival in patients who receive kidneys from unrelated or cadaver donors. Recently there has been some success in the use of ALG alone for recipient preparation for bone marrow transplantation. In this procedure the recipient is treated with ALG in large doses for 7–10 days, followed by transplantation of $1–3 \times 10^{10}$ bone marrow cells from the donor. Residual ALG appears to destroy the T cells in the donor marrow graft, and the severe graft-versus-host syndrome has not been observed. These limited data do indicate that ALG given alone is a potent immunosuppressive agent in man.

The side-effects of ALG are mostly those of the injection of a foreign protein obtained from horse serum. Local pain and erythema often occur at the injection site. Since the humoral antibody mechanism remains active, skin-reactive and precipitating anti-bodies can be formed against the horse IgG.

Anaphylactic and serum sickness reactions have been observed and usually require cessation of ALG therapy. In addition, complexes of host antibodies with horse ALG may precipitate and localize in the glomerulus of the transplanted kidney. Even more disturbing has been the development of reticulum cell sarcoma in the buttock at the site of ALG injection. The incidence of lymphoma as well as other forms of cancer is increased in kidney transplant patients, and may be as high as 2% in long-term survivors. It appears likely that part of the increased risk of cancer is related to the suppression of a normally potent defense system against oncogenic viruses or transformed cells. Thus, it remains to be seen whether ALG is any more carcino-genic than the other immunosuppressive agents.

Antilymphocytic antibody has great potential as an immunosuppressive agent but presents significant problems in its present form. Some investigators now hope that a more highly purified and selective anti-body can be developed which would have activity against just those clones that respond to transplanta-tion antigens rather than all antigen recognition cells.

2. RH$_O$ (D) IMMUNE GLOBULIN (HUMAN) (RhoGAM)

One of the major advances in medicine during the past decade has been the development of a technic of preventing Rh hemolytic disease of the newborn. The technic is based on the observation that a primary anti-body response to a foreign antigen can be blocked if specific antibody is administered passively at the time of exposure to antigen.

Rh$_O$ (D) immune globulin (human) (RhoGAM) is a concentrated (15%) solution of human IgG globulin containing a high titer of antibodies against the Rh$_O$ (D) antigen of the red cell. The IgG is prepared by cold alcohol fractionation of carefully selected plasma from Rh$_O$ (D)-negative, D^u-negative mothers sensitized by repeated Rh-incompatible pregnancies or from Rh-negative volunteers who have been deliberately immunized for plasma collection.

Sensitization of Rh-negative mothers to the D antigen occurs usually at the time of birth of an Rh$_O$ (D)-positive or D^u-positive infant, when fetal red cells may leak into the mother's blood stream. Sensitization might also occur occasionally with miscarriages or ectopic pregnancies. With subsequent pregnancies maternal antibody against Rh-positive cells is trans-ferred to the fetus during the third trimester, leading to the development of erythroblastosis fetalis or hemo-lytic disease of the newborn.

If an injection of Rh$_O$ (D) antibody is adminis-tered to the mother within 72 hours after the birth of an Rh-negative baby, the mother's own antibody response to the foreign Rh$_O$ (D)-positive cells is sup-pressed. When the mother has been treated in this fashion, Rh hemolytic disease of the newborn has not been observed in the subsequent pregnancy. For this prophylactic treatment to be successful, the mother must be Rh$_O$ (D)-negative and D^u-negative and must not already be immunized to the Rh$_O$ (D) factor. Treatment is also often advised for Rh-negative mothers who have had miscarriages, ectopic pregnan-cies, or abortions in which the blood type of the fetus is unknown.

Note: Rh$_O$ (D) immune globulin (human) is administered to the mother and must not be given to the infant.

The usual dose of RhoGAM is 2 ml IM. Adverse reactions are infrequent and consist of local discomfort at the injection site or, rarely, a slight temperature elevation.

The mechanism of suppression of the immune response by passive administration of specific antibody may consist of prompt elimination of the foreign anti-gen after combination with the antibody or may be a type of "feedback immunosuppression" in which a change in the antigen results from its combination with antibody, so that it is no longer recognized as foreign. If antibody produces "feedback" immunosuppression, it presumably acts either on the macrophage, the T-lymphocyte, or the B-lymphocyte (Figs 46–1 and 46–2).

CLINICAL USES OF IMMUNOSUPPRESSIVE DRUGS

Immunosuppressive agents are currently used in 3 clinical circumstances: (1) organ transplantation, (2) auto-immune disorders, and (3) iso-immune dis-orders (Rh hemolytic disease of the newborn). The agents used differ somewhat for the specific disorders treated (see specific agents and Table 46–1), as do administration schedules also. Optimal treatment schedules have yet to be established in many clinical situations in which these drugs are used, and objective evaluations of their relative efficacy are uncertain in many instances, especially with newer agents such as ALG. Other considerations related to the conditions to be treated also affect the evaluation of effectiveness of the immunosuppressive agents.

Organ Transplantation

In organ transplantation, tissue typing, based on donor and recipient histocompatibility matching with the HLA haplotype system, is of definite value. Close histocompatibility matching reduces the likelihood of graft rejection and may also reduce the requirements for intensive immunosuppressive therapy. Response to transplantation and immunosuppressive drugs in renal disease may be dependent on the nature of the primary renal lesions in patients undergoing the transplant pro-cedure.

Primary renal disease itself is frequently immuno-logic in nature. Two major types of glomerular injury are mediated by immune mechanisms. The first type results from the passive deposition of antigen-antibody complexes from the circulation as blood is filtered through the glomerulus. Deposition of antigen-antibody complexes in a "lump and bump" fashion is associated with the renal disease of systemic lupus erythematosus and with the majority of cases of acute glomerulonephritis. The second form of glomerulonephritis is associated with linear deposition of specific anti-basement membrane antibody in the renal glomerulus.

Although immunosuppressive therapy may be of benefit in both of these circumstances, the data in the literature are incomplete. Since patients with severe glomerulonephritis are often candidates for kidney transplantation, those pathogenetic factors which might persist and also damage the transplanted kidney are of great importance. It has been observed that patients with anti-basement membrane antibody may experience an acute graft rejection when they receive a kidney transplant. Patients with anti-basement membrane antibodies are likely to need management with immunosuppressive therapy for 6–8 weeks after bi-

lateral nephrectomy, being maintained on a dialysis program, before transplantation of a donor kidney can be considered. Similarly, patients with a disease such as systemic lupus erythematosus are poor candidates for renal transplant until the systemic cause of the renal injury is under control.

Even with all these considerations, the response to renal transplantation has become increasingly gratifying, including that with unmatched kidneys from cadaver donors. At present, over 80% of carefully selected but nonrelated recipients may survive beyond 2 years after the transplant, and 5-year survival is not an unrealistic hope.

Transplantation of other organs, such as liver, heart, bone marrow, pancreas, and lungs (in order of decreasing success), has also been performed. In some of these instances, technical problems account for the poorer results; in others, immunosuppression has proved to be less potent than in renal transplants.

Auto-immune Disorders

The effectiveness of immunosuppressive drugs in auto-immune disorders varies widely. Most of these disorders are of unknown cause and the rationale for immunosuppression is sometimes strained, although it is usually thought that faulty recognition mechanisms or antibody cross-reactivity account for the proliferation of unneeded lymphoid clones. In the auto-immune diseases, unlike the situation in immunosuppression for transplantation, the unwanted immune response is already established when the disease is diagnosed, and a large proliferating mass of lymphoid cells must be dealt with. Nonetheless, with immunosuppressive therapy, remissions can be obtained in most instances of auto-immune hemolytic anemia, idiopathic thrombocytopenic purpura, Hashimoto's thyroiditis, and temporal arteritis. Apparent improvement is also often seen in patients with systemic lupus erythematosus, acute glomerulonephritis, acquired factor VIII inhibitors (antibodies), and certain other auto-immune states.

In most instances it is only assumed that it is the immunosuppressive properties of drugs such as prednisone, cyclophosphamide, and mercaptopurine that produce these improvements. Once the cause of these autoreactive states is defined, therapy may become more rational.

Hemolytic Disease of the Newborn

The success of prevention of Rh hemolytic disease of the newborn currently stands as a landmark in immunosuppressive therapy. It is hoped that this example of precise suppression without side-effects will also apply to other disease states once the offending antigens can be identified.

TABLE 46–1. Clinical uses of immuno-suppressive agents.

Disease	Immunosuppressive Agents Used	Response
Auto-immune		
Idiopathic thrombocytopenic purpura	Prednisone,* occasionally mercaptopurine or azathioprine	Usually good
Auto-immune hemolytic anemia	Prednisone,* cyclophosphamide, chlorambucil, mercaptopurine, azathioprine	Usually good
Acute glomerulonephritis	Prednisone,* mercaptopurine, alkylating agents	Usually good
Acquired factor XIII antibodies	Cyclophosphamide plus factor XIII	Usually good
Iso-immune		
Hemolytic anemia of the newborn	Rh$_O$ (D) immune globulin (human)*	Excellent
Organ transplantation		
Renal	Azathioprine,	Usually good
Heart and liver	prednisone, anti-lymphocytic globulin, dactinomycin	Fair to poor
Bone marrow	Cyclophosphamide, prednisone, anti-lymphocytic globulin	Some successes; generally poor thus far

*Drug of choice.

IMMUNOLOGIC REACTIONS TO DRUGS & DRUG ALLERGY

The basic immune mechanism and the ways in which it can be suppressed by drugs are discussed in the foregoing section of this chapter. Drugs often serve also to *activate* the immune system, usually in undesirable ways that appear as adverse drug reactions. These reactions are generally lumped in a broad classification as "drug allergy." Indeed, many drug reactions such as those to penicillin, iodides, diphenylhydantoin, and sulfonamides are allergic in nature. These drug reactions are manifested as skin eruptions, edema, anaphylactoid reactions, fever, and eosinophilia. The fundamentals of the allergic sensitization to drugs have been clarified by the recent discovery of the IgE class of immunoglobulins by the Ishizakas, and a clearer understanding of the process of sensitization and activation of blood basophils and tissue mast cells.

Other drug reactions are also mediated by immune mechanisms but, as will be seen, may have different mechanisms.

Some adverse reactions to drugs may be mistakenly classified as allergic or immune when they are in reality genetic deficiency states or are idiosyncratic and not mediated by immune mechanisms (eg, hemolysis due to primaquine in G6PD deficiency, or aplastic anemia due to chloramphenicol).

MECHANISMS OF IMMEDIATE DRUG ALLERGY

The mechanisms of immune activation that are operative in drug allergy are similar to the normal humoral antibody responses to foreign macromolecules. These mechanisms can now be placed in a theoretical construct which includes an afferent limb of the immune response (Fig 46–4a) as well as an efferent limb which includes the pharmacologic mediators of allergy (Fig 46–4b). Landsteiner and his associates first demonstrated that animals could be sensitized to simple chemicals such as picric acid (a hapten) if the chemical was linked to a carrier protein. This linkage can occur in the body with a normal tissue or serum protein serving as the carrier. The subsequent immune response will be specific for the hapten even though linkage to a carrier is necessary for immune recognition. Surprisingly, carrier recognition is genetically determined even though the host does not produce antibodies against the carrier protein. When drugs serve as haptens, the antibody-forming precursor cells which respond are often the precursors of cells which produce antibodies of the IgE class. In nonallergic individuals, IgE globulin levels are the lowest of any immunoglobulin (less than 1 μg/ml), whereas in allergy they may be increased 10-fold or more. IgE antibodies have the interesting property of fixing to blood basophils and tissue mast cells, and are described as skin-sensitizing or reaginic antibodies.

The fixation of the IgE antibody to blood basophils or their tissue equivalent (mast cells) sets the stage for an acute allergic reaction. When the offending drug is reintroduced into the body, IgE antibody molecules on the surface of sensitized basophilic leukocytes bind to the antigenic form of the drug (Fig 46–4b). Sensitized tissue mast cells or blood basophils are stimulated to degranulate and produce a burst of histamine release. It appears likely that the process of degranulation depends upon the mast cell's capability to increase its intracellular levels of 3',5'-cyclic AMP. Agents that inhibit the destruction of cyclic AMP (eg, theophylline), as well as those that enhance the activity of the synthesis of cyclic AMP (eg, catecholamines), block histamine release. Other vasoactive substances such as kinins may also be generated during histamine release. These mediators initiate immediate skin and smooth muscle responses and thus initiate tissue injury and the inflammatory response. Such reactions can be devastating or lethal to the patient, especially when they produce laryngospasm, bronchospasm, or hypotension.

DRUG TREATMENT OF IMMEDIATE ALLERGY

One can test an individual for possible sensitivity to a drug by a simple scratch test, ie, by applying an extremely dilute solution of the drug to the skin. If allergy is present, an immediate wheal and flare will occur. Skin reactivity to a specific drug can also be transferred from an allergic individual to a normal recipient (human or primate) with serum which contains the reaginic IgE antibodies (the Prausnitz-Küstner reaction).

Drugs that modify allergic responses act at several links in this chain of events. Prednisone, which is often used in severe allergic reactions, is immunosuppressive and probably blocks proliferation of the IgE-producing clones. In the efferent limb of the allergic response, isoproterenol and theophylline act synergistically to block the release of histamine from the mast cell, while antihistamines and epinephrine serve to rapidly block or counteract the effects of the vasoactive mediators of allergy. Corticosteroids may also act to reduce tissue injury and edema in the inflammatory response.

DESENSITIZATION TO DRUGS

When reasonable alternatives are not available, certain drugs (eg, penicillin) must be used for life-threatening illnesses even in the presence of known allergic sensitivity. In such cases, desensitization can sometimes be accomplished by starting with minute

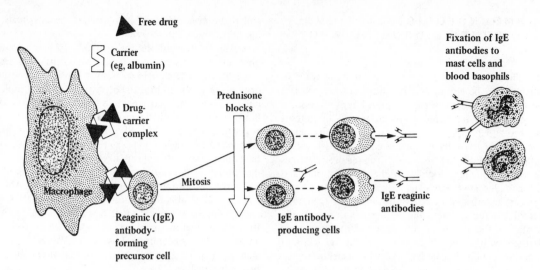

FIG 46–4a. Induction of IgE-mediated allergic sensitivity to drugs and other allergens.

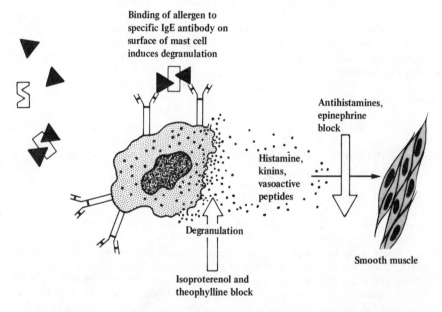

FIG 46–4b. Response of IgE-sensitized cells to subsequent exposure to allergens.

dosages of the drug and gradually increasing the dose over a period of days to the full therapeutic range. This practice can be quite hazardous, and one must always be ready to treat the patient for an episode of acute anaphylactic shock before desensitization has been achieved. This form of desensitization differs from immunosuppression in that the immune mechanism often appears to be stimulated and reactivity is only predictably diminished while the treatment is continued.

The exact mechanism of desensitization to drugs is complex. In some instances, allergic desensitization appears to be accomplished by the stimulation of competing clones of cells which produce "blocking" anti-

bodies, often of the IgG or IgA immunoglobulin class. This is likely to be only a partial explanation of the phenomenon, which may depend on several different mechanisms.

SERUM SICKNESS REACTION

Serum sickness reactions to drugs are more common than immediate anaphylactic responses. The clinical features of serum sickness include urticarial skin eruptions, arthralgia or arthritis, lymphadenopathy, and fever. The reactions generally last 6–12 days and usually subside once the offending drug is eliminated. IgE antibodies are likely to be involved in serum sickness, but other immunoglobulin classes (IgG and others) appear to play a role also. Corticosteroids are sometimes useful in attenuating severe serum sickness reactions to drugs.

AUTO-IMMUNE REACTIONS TO DRUGS

Certain auto-immune syndromes can be induced by drugs. Examples of this phenomenon include systemic lupus erythematosus following hydralazine or procainamide therapy, "lupoid hepatitis" due to cathartic sensitivity, auto-immune hemolytic anemia resulting from methyldopa administration, and thrombocytopenic purpura due to quinidine. In these drug-induced auto-immune states, antibodies to tissue constituents or to the drug can be demonstrated. Immune mechanisms also appear to be involved in many additional cases of so-called idiopathic thrombocytopenic purpura, but it is more difficult to demonstrate the specific antibodies. The blood platelet is sometimes an innocent bystander to an immunologic reaction to a drug but manages to be damaged or activated by antigen-antibody complexes, leading to the development of idiopathic thrombocytopenic purpura.

Fortunately, auto-immune reactions to drugs usually subside within several months after the offending drug is withdrawn. Immunosuppressive therapy is not warranted in these reactions unless the auto-immune response is unusually severe.

VASCULITIS DUE TO DRUGS

Vasculitis, presumably on an immune basis, can also be induced by drugs. These reactions frequently appear more like abnormalities in delayed hypersensitivity than of serum antibody formation, and specific antibody has generally not been demonstrated in these disorders. The sulfonamides, penicillin, thiouracil, anticonvulsants, and iodides have all been implicated in the initiation of hypersensitivity angiitis. Erythema multiforme is a relatively mild vasculitic skin disorder which may be secondary to drug hypersensitivity. Stevens-Johnson syndrome is probably a more severe form of this hypersensitivity reaction and includes erythema multiforme, arthritis, nephritis, CNS abnormalities, and myocarditis. It has frequently been associated with sulfonamide therapy.

CLINICAL IDENTIFICATION OF IMMUNOLOGIC REACTIONS TO DRUGS

In view of the multiplicity of drugs that hospitalized patients frequently receive, it is not always easy to determine which drug has initiated an allergic or immune syndrome of drug sensitivity. Careful questioning about the history of prior drug sensitivities is an important part of every patient's medical record, and errors of omission can be dangerous. Since certain commonly used drugs such as the penicillins are frequent offenders, direct questions about penicillin sensitivity should always be included in the patient's history. Skin testing can be very useful in identifying drug allergy when the history is equivocal. Skin testing is considerably less hazardous than a therapeutic trial and is usually indicated where there is an equivocal allergic history and a strong clinical indication for treatment with the drug.

Warnings of known sensitivities should be prominently displayed in the patient's record or hospital chart. Once a drug allergy is defined, this information should always be conveyed in clear language to the patient himself to prevent repeated challenges with the same agent in the future, when the reaction may be much more severe. In the case of known severe sensitivity to common drugs, the patient should be advised to carry a clearly written notice of the sensitivity on his person to lessen the chance that he would be given the agent when he is incapacitated, as might occur after an accident.

• ο •

General References

Current Concepts in Immunology

Amos, B. (editor): *Progress in Immunology: First International Congress of Immunology.* Academic Press, 1971.

Immunosuppressive Agents

Ascari, W.Q., & others: Rh_O (D) immune globulin (human): Evaluation in woman at risk of Rh immunization. JAMA 205:71, 1968.

Denman, A.M.: Anti-lymphocytic antibody and autoimmune disease: A review. Clin Exper Immunol 5:217–249, 1969.

Dixon, F.J.: The pathogenesis of glomerulonephritis. Am J Med 44:493, 1968.

Fahey, J.L., & others: Recent progress in human transplantation immunology. Ann Int Med 71:1177–1196, 1969.

Finn, R., & others: Experimental studies on the prevention of Rh haemolytic disease. Brit MJ 1:1486, 1961.

Hitching, G.H., & G.B. Elion: Chemical suppression of the immune response. Pharmacol Rev 15:365, 1963.

James, K.: Anti-lymphocytic antibody: A review. Clin Exper Immunol 2:615, 1967.

Johnson, M.W., Maibach, H.I., & S.E. Salmon: Skin reactivity in patients with cancer: Impaired delayed hypersensitivity or faulty inflammatory response? New England J Med 284:1255–1257, 1971.

Medawar, P.: Antilymphocyte serum: Its properties and potentials. Hosp Practice 4:26, 1969.

Miller, J.F.A.P., & others: Cell to cell interaction in the immune response. J Exper Med 128:801, 1968.

Moller, G., & H. Wigzell: Antibody synthesis at the cellular level: Antibody-induced suppression of 19S and 7S antibody response. J Exper Med 121:969, 1965.

Moller, G., & C.F. Zukoski: Heterologous antilymphocyte serum: Differential effect on antigen-sensitive and antibody producing cells. Surgery 64:39–47, 1968.

Nossal, G.J.V., Abbott, A., & J. Mitchell: Antigens in immunity. XIV. Electron microscopic radioautographic studies of antigen capture in the lymph node medulla. J Exper Med 127:263, 1968.

Russell, P.S., & A.P. Monaco: Heterologous antilymphocyte sera and some of their effects. Transplantation 5:1086, 1967.

Russell, P.S., & H.J. Winn: Transplantation. New England J Med 282:786, 1970.

Salmon, S.E., Krakauer, R.S., & W.F. Whitmore: Lymphocyte stimulation: Selective destruction of cells undergoing the blastogenic response to transplantation antigens. Science 172:490, 1971.

Santos, G.W., & A.W. Owens, Jr.: 19S and 7S antibody production in the cyclophosphamide or methotrexate treated rat. Nature 209: 622, 1966.

Schwartz, R.S.: Immunosuppression: The challenge of selectivity. Hosp Practice 4:42, 1969.

Schwartz, R.S., Eisner, A., & W. Dameshek: The effect of 6-mercaptopurine on primary and secondary immune responses. J Clin Invest 38:1394, 1959.

Schwartz, R., Stock, J., & W. Dameshek: Effects of 6-mercaptopurine on antibody production. Proc Soc Exper Biol Med 99:164–167, 1958.

Starzl, T.E., & others: The use of heterologous antilymphoid agents in canine renal and liver homotransplantation and in human renal transplantation. Surg Gynec Obst 124:301, 1967.

Swanson, M.A., & R.S. Schwartz: Immunosuppressive therapy: The relation between clinical response and immunological competence. New England J Med 277:163, 1967.

Uhr, J.W., & J.B. Bauman: Antibody formation. 1. The suppression of antibody formation by passively administered antibody. J Exper Med 113:935, 1961.

Uhr, J.W., & G. Moller: Regulatory effects of antibody on antibody formation. Advances Immunol 8:81, 1968.

Unanue, E.R., & J.C. Cerottin: Persistence of antigen on the surface of macrophages. Nature 222:1193–1195, 1969.

Immunologic Reactions to Drugs & Allergy

Ishizaka, K.: The identification and significance of gamma E. Hosp Practice 4:70, 1969.

Ishizaka, K., & T. Ishizaka: Human reaginic antibodies and immunoglobulin E. J Allergy 42:330, 1968.

Ishizaka, T., & others: Histamine release from human leukocytes by anti-E antibodies. J Immunol 102:884, 1969.

Ishizaka, T., & others: Release of histamine and slow reacting substance of anaphylaxis by E system from sensitized monkey lung. J Allergy 43:168, 1969.

Lichtenstein, L.M., & P.S. Norman: Human allergic reactions. Am J Med 46:163, 1969.

47 . . .

Mechanisms of Action of Clinically Used Antimicrobial Drugs

The advent of many effective antimicrobial drugs since 1935 has completely altered the practice of medicine. The outstanding characteristic of this revolution is **selective toxicity**, a feature which is common to all effective and useful antimicrobial drugs which distinguishes them from the disinfectants. The term "selective toxicity" applied to systemically effective antimicrobial drugs means that they are far more toxic for the parasite than for the host cell. This selective action must be based on certain unique features in structure or function of the parasite which set it apart from the host cell. Intensive efforts have been made to define these unique features of microorganisms.

Initially it was believed that most types of antibacterial action could be explained by **competitive antagonism.** The meaning of competitive antagonism is as follows: An enzyme (eg, a bacterial enzyme) usually catalyzes a single reaction. The substrate attaches to the enzyme's active center to be activated, metabolized, and released. A chemical compound (the competitor) similar to but not identical with the substrate may be able to combine with the enzyme's active center, but it cannot be metabolized and released. It remains attached to the active center and blocks its combination with the true substrate. A specific example is given in the discussion of the sulfonamides, below.

More recently, however, it has become apparent that competitive antagonism is rare and that most of the effective antibacterial substances interfere with the synthesis, assembly, or function of the macromolecular components of bacterial cells. In the following paragraphs a brief summary is presented of the established or postulated mechanisms of antimicrobial drug action.

ANTIMICROBIAL ACTION THROUGH INHIBITION OF GROWTH BY MEANS OF COMPETITIVE ANTAGONISM
(*Example:* Sulfonamides.)

For many microorganisms, p-aminobenzoic acid (PABA) is an essential metabolite. It is used by them as a precursor in the synthesis of folic acid, which serves as an important step in the synthesis of purines. The specific mode of action of PABA probably involves an adenosine triphosphate (ATP) dependent condensation of a pteridine with PABA to yield dihydropteroic acid, which is subsequently converted to folic acid. Sulfonamides are structural analogues of PABA.

Sulfonamides can enter into the reaction in place of PABA and compete for the active center of the enzyme. As a result, nonfunctional analogues of folic acid are formed, preventing further growth of the bacterial cell. This is the outstanding example of competitive antagonism among antimicrobial drugs. For a given sulfonamide and a given microorganism, the ratio of the inhibitory concentration of a sulfonamide to different concentrations of PABA is almost constant. This S/PABA ratio is an index of sulfonamide activity and varies greatly with different drugs—eg, it might be 2000 for sulfanilamide and 27 for sulfathiazole. Animal cells cannot synthesize folic acid, and must depend upon exogenous sources. Likewise, some bacteria do not synthesize folic acid but require it for growth. These bacteria, like animal cells, are not inhibited by sulfonamides. Many other bacteria, however, synthesize folic acid as mentioned above, and consequently are susceptible to sulfonamide action. The inhibiting action of sulfonamides on bacterial growth can be counteracted by an excess of PABA in the environment.

Tubercle bacilli are not inhibited markedly by sulfonamides, but their growth is inhibited by PAS (p-aminosalicylic acid). Conversely, most sulfonamide-susceptible bacteria are resistant to PAS. This suggests that the receptor site for PABA differs in different types of organisms.

Trimethoprim (3,4,5-trimethoxybenzyl pyrimidine) inhibits the dihydrofolic acid reductase of bacteria 10,000 times more efficiently than the same enzyme of mammalian cells. These enzymes convert dihydro- to tetrahydrofolic acid, a stage in a sequence

p-Aminobenzoic acid
(PABA)

Sulfonamide

leading to the synthesis of purines and ultimately of DNA. Sulfonamides and trimethoprim produce sequential blocking in the sequence, resulting in a marked enhancement (synergism) of activity in urinary tract infections, enteric fevers, or malaria.

Pyrimethamine (Daraprim) also inhibits dihydrofolate reductase, but it is more active against the mammalian cell enzyme and therefore more toxic than trimethoprim. Pyrimethamine plus sulfonamides is the current treatment of choice in toxoplasmosis.

ANTIMICROBIAL ACTION THROUGH INHIBITION OF CELL WALL SYNTHESIS

In contrast to animal cells, bacteria possess a rigid outer layer, the cell wall. It maintains the shape of microorganisms and "corsets" the bacterial cell, which possesses an unusually high internal osmotic pressure. Removal of the cell wall (eg, by lysozyme) or inhibition of its formation may lead to lysis of the cell. In a hypertonic environment (eg, 20% sucrose), damaged cell wall formation leads to formation of spherical bacterial "protoplasts" limited by the fragile cytoplasmic membrane. If such "protoplasts" are placed in an environment of ordinary tonicity, they may explode.

The cell wall contains a chemically distinct complex polymer "mucopeptide," peptidoglycan, consisting of polysaccharides and a highly cross-linked polypeptide. The polysaccharides regularly contain an amino sugar, acetylmuramic acid, which is found only in bacteria.

Penicillins are selective inhibitors of bacterial cell wall synthesis. Under the influence of low concentrations of penicillin, the formation of dividing cross walls is inhibited, and enormous bizarre forms develop from bacteria. With higher concentrations of penicillin, cell wall formation is completely blocked and cells may lyse or, if the medium is hypertonic, change to protoplasts. In penicillin-inhibited cells, nucleotides accumulate which are cell wall precursors. However, the synthesis of proteins and nucleic acids continues unabated.

All penicillins, including semisynthetic ones, and all cephalosporins act through selective inhibition of cell wall synthesis. The difference in susceptibility of gram-positive and gram-negative bacteria to penicillins may depend upon the chemical differences in cell wall composition which determine penetration or binding of the drugs. Penicillin resistance of organisms which do not produce penicillinase also is attributed to a distinct cell wall composition.

The inhibition of synthesis of cell wall mucopeptide may be due to a structural similarity of penicillins to acyl-D-alanyl-D-alanine. Thus in the presence of penicillin, the terminal cross-linking of linear glycopeptides ("transpeptidation") is inhibited, resulting in a block of cell wall formation. This transpeptidation reaction involves the loss of a D-alanine from the pentapeptide. Earlier it had been proposed that penicillin may be a structural analogue of acetylmuramic acid

and may inhibit muramic acid incorporation into mucopeptide.

The remarkable lack of toxicity of penicillins for animal cells must be due to the absence of bacterial-type cell walls in animal cells.

Several other drugs likewise inhibit bacterial cell wall synthesis, but this may not be their sole mode of action. Among them are bacitracin, vancomycin, ristocetin, novobiocin, and cycloserine. D-Cycloserine, a structural analogue of the amino acid D-alanine, blocks cell wall synthesis by interfering with alanine incorporation into the peptide portion of the polymer.

The susceptibility to penicillins is, in part, determined by the organism's production of penicillin destroying enzyme (β-lactamase). Certain penicillins (eg, methicillin, cloxacillin) have a high affinity for the β-lactamase produced by some gram-negative bacteria, eg, pseudomonas. They bind the enzyme, are not hydrolyzed by it, and thus protect simultaneously present hydrolyzable penicillins (eg, ampicillin) from destruction. This is a form of "synergism" of known mechanism (see Chapter 59).

ANTIMICROBIAL ACTION THROUGH INHIBITION OF CELL MEMBRANE FUNCTION

The cytoplasm of all living cells is bounded by the cytoplasmic membrane, which serves as a selective permeability barrier and thus controls the internal composition of the cell. If the functional integrity of the cytoplasmic membrane is disrupted, purine and pyrimidine nucleotides and proteins escape from the cell and cell damage or death ensues. The cytoplasmic membrane of certain bacteria and fungi can be more readily disrupted by certain agents than the membranes of animal cells. Consequently, selective chemotherapeutic activity is possible.

The outstanding examples of this mechanism are the polymyxins acting on gram-negative bacteria and the polyene antibiotics acting on fungi (see Chapter 55). However, polymyxins are inactive against fungi and polyenes are inactive against bacteria. This is because sterols are present in the fungal cell membrane and absent in the bacterial cell membrane. Polyenes must interact with a sterol in the fungal cell membrane prior to exerting their effect. Bacterial cell membranes do not contain that sterol, and (presumably for this reason) are resistant to polyene action—a good example of cell individuality and of selective toxicity.

ANTIMICROBIAL ACTION THROUGH INHIBITION OF PROTEIN SYNTHESIS

It is established that chloramphenicol, tetracyclines, streptomycins, and erythromycins can inhibit protein synthesis in bacteria. Puromycin is an effective inhibitor of protein synthesis in animal and other cells. The antibacterial effect of these drugs depends, at least partly, on their inhibition of protein synthesis. The concepts of protein synthesis are undergoing rapid change, and the precise mechanism of action is not established for any one drug.

Chloramphenicol does not interfere with either cell wall or nucleic acid synthesis. It acts on the 50 S unit of ribosomes and interferes markedly with the binding of amino acids to nascent peptide chains. It may block the action of peptidyl transferase. Chloramphenicol is bacteriostatic for many bacteria, and its action is readily reversible.

Tetracyclines inhibit protein synthesis in bacteria, perhaps by blocking the binding of charged aminoacyl transfer RNA (tRNA) to the 30 S unit of ribosomes. The macrolides (erythromycin group) and lincomycin also inhibit protein synthesis by competing with amino acids for ribosomal binding sites and by blocking aminoacyl translocation reactions.

Streptomycin effectively inhibits protein synthesis of bacteria and causes a progressive breakdown of polysomes. Streptomycin binds to a surface protein of the 30 S subunit of bacterial ribosomes, distorts the "recognition region" of the ribosome, and causes a misreading of the mRNA message. This results in the insertion of improper amino acids and the synthesis of nonfunctional proteins. In streptomycin-dependent cells, misreading of the genetic message is a requirement for growth. In streptomycin-resistant cells, the specific protein which serves as a ribosomal binding site for streptomycin is missing or altered.

Other aminoglycosides, eg, neomycin, kanamycin, or gentamicin, probably act similarly to streptomycin.

ANTIMICROBIAL ACTION THROUGH INHIBITION OF NUCLEIC ACID SYNTHESIS

Drugs such as the actinomycins are effective inhibitors of DNA synthesis. Actually, they form complexes with DNA by binding to the deoxyguanosine residues. The DNA-actinomycin complex inhibits the DNA-dependent RNA polymerase and blocks mRNA formation. Actinomycin also inhibits DNA virus replication.

Mitomycins result in the firm cross-linking of complementary strands of DNA and consequently block DNA synthesis. Both actinomycins and mitomycin inhibit bacterial as well as animal cells and are not sufficiently selective to be employed in antibacterial chemotherapy. Rifampin inhibits bacterial growth by binding strongly to the DNA-dependent RNA polymerase of bacteria. Thus it inhibits bacterial RNA synthesis. The mechanism of rifampin action on viruses is different and not well understood.

The halogenated pyrimidines, eg, IUDR (5-iodo-2-deoxyuridine, idoxuridine, IDU) can block the synthesis of functionally intact DNA and thus interfere with the replication of infective DNA viruses. IUDR can interfere with the incorporation of thymidine into viral DNA, and IUDR itself may be incorporated to form nonfunctional DNA. Although the systemic administration of IUDR is rarely feasible because of severe toxicity, local application of IUDR to DNA virus-producing cells (especially in herpes simplex keratitis) can result in significant suppression of viral replication in vivo.

Nalidixic acid (NegGram), used principally as a urinary antiseptic, is a potent inhibitor of DNA synthesis. However, it is not known whether its antibacterial action depends on this effect.

.   .   .

RESISTANCE TO ANTIMICROBIAL DRUGS

There are many possible interpretations of the mechanism of microbial drug resistance. The following are possible, but only partly supported by evidence:

(1) Increased destruction of the drug—eg, production of penicillin destroying enzymes (β-lactamase [penicillinase], amidase) by many penicillin resistant organisms; production of aminoglycoside destroying (phosphorylating or adenylating) enzymes by resistant gram-negative bacteria.

(2) Decreased permeability of the organism to the drug.

(3) Increased formation of the metabolite with which the drug competes for an enzyme—eg, increased PABA synthesis in some sulfonamide resistant strains of bacteria.

(4) Increased synthesis of an inhibited enzyme.

(5) Development of an altered enzyme which is still able to perform its metabolic function but is no longer affected by the drug.

(6) An altered structure of ribosomal protein—eg, streptomycin resistance may depend on an alteration or loss of a 30 S ribosomal protein which otherwise serves as binding site for streptomycin; erythromycin resistant units have an altered protein of the 50 S ribosome unit.

(7) Development of an altered metabolic pathway, bypassing the inhibited reaction.

In general, the emergence of drug resistance is a genetic event. Spontaneously arising mutants which are drug resistant are selected out and favored in their survival and proliferation in the presence of the drug. Thus, drug resistant mutants arise independently of exposure to the drug, and the antibiotic or antimicrobial drug serves only to select them from the susceptible organisms in the population. This "selection pressure" of the drug may manifest itself in a single host (patient) or in an environment (eg, hospital).

Mutation to drug resistance is commonly a change at a specific locus on the bacterial chromosome. While it usually arises spontaneously, the locus may also be transferred from one bacterium to another by means of bacteriophage mediated transductions. In addition, drug resistance may be transferred genetically by a nonchromosomal method. A "resistance transfer factor (RTF)," apparently an episome, can be transferred from a resistant to a susceptible organism during bacterial conjugation. This "infective drug resistance" may involve single or, more commonly, multiple drugs. RTF can transmit resistance to different bacterial species or genera, especially among the gram-negative enteric bacteria. Another type of extrachromosomal genetic factor, a plasmid, controls β-lactamase formation in staphylococci and is transferred in this genus through transduction by bacteriophage.

Microorganisms resistant to a certain drug and selected out from the population by that drug may also be resistant to another drug to which they have not been exposed. This is known as cross-resistance.

Such relationships exist principally between agents that are closely related chemically, eg, all tetracyclines, macrolides (erythromycins-oleandomycins), aminoglycosides (neomycin-kanamycin), polymyxins (polymyxin B-colistin).

Drug resistance may also be a nongenetic event. Since active multiplication of bacteria is a requirement for most types of antimicrobial drug actions, bacteria which are metabolically inactive may be drug resistant. Such organisms, called "persisters," may be responsible for the survival of infectious organisms in the face of antimicrobial therapy. The offspring of such "persisters" are fully drug susceptible.

Cell wall defective forms of microorganisms (L forms) can persist in the presence of cell wall inhibitory drugs (eg, penicillins).

• • •

General References

Davis, B.D.: Streptomycin resistance and the study of ribosomal structure and function. New England J Med 283:1405–1406, 1970.

Martin, D.C., & J.D. Arnold: Trimethoprim and sulfalene therapy of *Plasmodium vivax.* J Clin Pharmacol 9:155–159, 1969.

Novick, R.P., & S.I. Morse: In vivo transmission of drug resistance factors between strains of *Staphylococcus aureus.* J Exper Med 125:45–59, 1967.

Pestra S.: Inhibitors of ribosome function. Ann Rev Microbiol 25:487–562, 1971.

Sabath, L. D.: Drug resistance of bacteria. New England J Med 280:91–94, 1969.

Strominger, J.L., & D.J. Tipper: Bacterial cell wall synthesis in relation to the mechanism of action of penicillins and other antibacterial agents. Am J Med 39:708–721, 1965.

Watanabe, T : Infectious drug resistance in enteric bacteria. New England J Med 275:888–894, 1966.

48...

General Principles of Anti-infective Therapy*

Antimicrobial drugs represent one of the most important advances in drug therapy, but unfortunately they have been improperly used on a large scale. The principal disadvantages of improper use are as follows: (1) Most antimicrobial drugs cause toxic reactions. (2) Hypersensitivity may be induced, giving rise to reactions upon repeat administration of the same drug or a related drug. (3) The normal flora is often altered, increasing the opportunity for superinfection. (4) Resistant mutants are selected out of microbial populations, a danger both to the individual and to others (eg, staphylococcal infections, or gram-negative rod infections acquired in hospitals).

Adherence to the principles outlined in the following paragraphs will ensure optimal use of the antimicrobial drugs and minimize the dangers resulting from their abuse:

(1) Before prescribing an antimicrobial drug the physician must **formulate a diagnosis** which is strongly suggestive of the presence of a given **microbial infection**. The therapeutic effect of these drugs depends solely on their ability to inhibit or kill microorganisms.

(2) Most antimicrobial drugs have a specific effect on a very limited range of different types of microorganisms. The physician must attempt to formulate a **specific etiologic diagnosis** before prescribing an antimicrobial drug. On clinical grounds he can often make an intelligent guess about what organism is most likely to be the cause of a given infectious process. He can then choose a drug that is likely to be effective against that organism.

(3) The clinician need not be bewildered by the multiplicity of names for antimicrobial drugs and the strident claims made for them in the promotional literature he receives. In reality there are **only a few types** of drugs among the hundreds now being marketed. It is necessary to be acquainted with only 1−2 drugs in each group.

Sulfonamides (including sulfones)
Chloramphenicol
Macrolides (erythromycins)
Penicillins and cephalosporins
Polymyxins
Aminoglycosides (kanamycin, gentamicin, streptomycin)
Tetracyclines
Urinary antiseptics
Specialized drugs (antistaphylococcal, antituberculosis)
Antifungal drugs

(4) On the basis of a tentative diagnosis—his "informed best guess"—the physician can select the drug **most likely to be effective** against the suspected microorganism. (A brief summary of such "drugs of choice, 1971−1972" is offered in Table 48−1.) Before beginning treatment, however, **specimens for laboratory examination** must be obtained and sent to the laboratory for identification of the causative microorganism. Perhaps days later, after the results of the examination are known, a change in therapy may be required on the basis of laboratory tests and patient response.

(5) **Laboratory results** do not always overrule clinical judgment, however. The recovery of a specific microorganism from appropriate specimens is always an important finding that must be considered, and isolation of an organism that reinforces the clinical impression ("best guess") is useful confirmatory evidence. Conversely, laboratory studies may contradict the initial clinical impression and require a second look at the diagnosis and the treatment being given. If the specimen was obtained from a site which is normally devoid of bacterial flora and not exposed to the external environment (eg, blood, CSF, pleural or joint fluid), the recovery of a microorganism is a significant finding even if different from the clinically suspected etiologic agent. Such a laboratory result may force a change in antimicrobial therapy. On the other hand, the isolation of unexpected microorganisms from respiratory tract, gut, or surface lesions must be critically evaluated before drugs judiciously selected on the basis of an initial "best guess" are abandoned.

(6) When a significant microorganism has been isolated from the patient, laboratory tests for **antimicrobial susceptibility** (sensitivity) are often requested. Some microorganisms need not be subjected to sensitivity tests because they are uniformly susceptible to a given antimicrobial drug. (Eg, group A hemolytic streptococci and clostridia respond predictably to penicillin.)

*Certain specialized aspects of the general principles of antimicrobial therapy are considered in Chapter 59, Combinations of Antimicrobial Drugs, and Chapter 60, Chemoprophylaxis.

TABLE 48–1. Drug selections, 1971–1972.

Suspected or Proved Etiologic Agent	Drug(s) of First Choice	Alternative Drug(s)
Gram-negative cocci		
Gonococcus	Penicillin[1], ampicillin	Erythromycin[2], tetracycline[3]
Meningococcus	Penicillin[1]	Tetracycline, chloramphenicol
Gram-positive cocci		
Pneumococcus	Penicillin[1]	Erythromycin, lincomycin
Streptococcus, hemolytic groups A,B,C	Penicillin[1]	Erythromycin, lincomycin
Streptococcus viridans	Penicillin[1]	Cephalosporin[4], vancomycin
Staphylococcus, nonpenicillinase-producing	Penicillin[1]	Cephalosporin, vancomycin, lincomycin
Staphylococcus, penicillinase-producing	Penicillinase-resistant penicillin[5]	Cephalosporin, vancomycin, lincomycin
Streptococcus faecalis (enterococcus)	Ampicillin plus streptomycin or kanamycin	Penicillin plus kanamycin or gentamicin
Gram-negative rods		
Aerobacter (Enterobacter)	Kanamycin or gentamicin	Tetracycline, chloramphenicol, polymyxin
Bacteroides	Tetracycline	Ampicillin, chloramphenicol
Brucella	Tetracycline plus streptomycin	Streptomycin plus sulfonamide[6]
Escherichia		
E coli sepsis	Kanamycin	Cephalothin, ampicillin
E coli urinary tract infection (first attack)	Sulfonamide[7]	Ampicillin, cephalexin
Hemophilus (meningitis, respiratory infections)	Ampicillin	Chloramphenicol
Klebsiella	Cephalosporin or kanamycin	Gentamicin, chloramphenicol
Mima-Herellea	Kanamycin	Tetracycline, gentamicin
Pasteurella (plague, tularemia)	Streptomycin plus tetracycline	Sulfonamide[6]
Proteus		
P mirabilis	Penicillin or ampicillin	Kanamycin, gentamicin
P vulgaris and other species	Kanamycin or carbenicillin	Chloramphenicol, gentamicin
Pseudomonas		
Ps aeruginosa	Polymyxin or gentamicin	Carbenicillin
Ps pseudomallei (melioidosis)	Chloramphenicol	Rifampin, tetracycline
Ps mallei (glanders)	Streptomycin plus tetracycline	
Salmonella	Chloramphenicol	Ampicillin
Serratia	Gentamicin	Kanamycin
Shigella	Ampicillin	Tetracycline, kanamycin
Vibrio (cholera)	Tetracycline	Chloramphenicol
Gram-positive rods		
Actinomyces	Penicillin[1]	Tetracycline, sulfonamide
Bacillus (eg, anthrax)	Penicillin[1]	Erythromycin
Clostridium (eg, gas gangrene, tetanus)	Penicillin[1]	Tetracycline, erythromycin
Corynebacterium	Erythromycin	Penicillin, cephalosporin
Listeria	Ampicillin	Tetracycline
Acid-fast rods		
Mycobacterium tuberculosis	INH plus PAS plus streptomycin	Other antituberculosis drugs
Mycobacterium leprae	Dapsone or solapsone	Other sulfones
Nocardia	Sulfonamide[6]	Tetracycline, cycloserine
Spirochetes		
Borrelia (relapsing fever)	Tetracycline	Penicillin[1]
Leptospira	Penicillin[1]	Tetracycline
Treponema (syphilis, yaws)	Penicillin[1]	Erythromycin, tetracycline
Mycoplasma	Tetracycline	Erythromycin
Psittacosis-lymphogranuloma-trachoma agents (chlamydiae)	Tetracycline, sulfonamide[6]	Erythromycin, chloramphenicol
Rickettsiae	Tetracycline	Chloramphenicol

[1] Penicillin G is preferred for parenteral injection; penicillin G (buffered) or penicillin V for oral administration. Only highly sensitive microorganisms should be treated with oral penicillin.

[2] Erythromycin estolate and triacetyloleandomycin are the best absorbed oral forms.

[3] All tetracyclines have the same activity against microorganisms and all have comparable therapeutic activity and toxicity. Dosage is determined by the rates of absorption and excretion of different preparations.

[4] Cephalothin and cephaloridine are the best accepted cephalosporins at present.

[5] Parenteral methicillin, nafcillin, or oxacillin. Oral dicloxacillin or other isoxazolylpenicillin.

[6] Trisulfapyrimidines have the advantage of greater solubility in urine over sulfadiazine for oral administration; sodium sulfadiazine is suitable for intravenous injection in severely ill persons.

[7] For previously untreated urinary tract infection, a highly soluble sulfonamide such as sulfisoxazole or trisulfapyrimidines is the first choice.

On the other hand, some organisms are sufficiently variable in their response to antimicrobial drugs that laboratory susceptibility testing is warranted (eg, gram-negative bacteria). In such instances the physician must begin therapy on the basis of experience but must be ready to modify the plan of treatment when laboratory results are reported.

(7) The most common laboratory test for antibiotic susceptibility is the so-called **disk test**. This test measures the ability of a drug that can diffuse through agar to inhibit the growth of microorganisms. The size of the zone of inhibition is not a function of the in vivo activity of the drug. To estimate microbial susceptibility, the zone of microbial growth inhibition by a given drug must be compared with a standard for this drug. Zone sizes are not comparable from one drug to another. The disk test measures only growth inhibition and therefore is of no direct value when bactericidal activity is required (eg, bacterial endocarditis, acute osteomyelitis, or infection in a severely debilitated patient).

(8) In general, disk tests give valuable results. At times, however, there is a marked **discrepancy between the results of the test and the clinical response** of the patient. A few possible explanations for such discrepancies are listed below:

(a) Failure to drain a collection of pus or remove a foreign body: Antimicrobial drugs almost never eradicate microorganisms within an abscess or within necrotic tissue such as a bony sequestrum.

(b) The drug may not reach the site of active infection. The pharmacologic properties of antimicrobial drugs determine their absorption and distribution. Poorly diffusing drugs of a large molecular size reach such areas as joint cavities, dural sac, or pleural space only if injected directly into the area. Similarly, some drugs may penetrate into phagocytic cells poorly and thus not reach intracellular organisms.

(c) Superinfection occurs fairly often in the course of prolonged chemotherapy. The physician must bear in mind that microorganisms may have established themselves against which the originally selected drug is ineffective.

(d) If a microbial strain contains a few resistant mutants in a large susceptible population, these organisms cannot be detected on disk testing although they might be detected in tests employing liquid media.

(e) In occasional cases 2 or more microorganisms participate in an infectious process but only one of them may have been isolated from the specimen. The drug being used may be one that is effective only against the less pathogenic organism.

(9) It may be necessary to determine **serum drug levels** in order to decide whether the proper drug or drugs are being used in the proper dosage. If drug therapy is adequate, the patient's serum will be markedly bactericidal in vitro against the organism isolated from that patient prior to therapy. In infections limited to the urinary tract, **drug levels in urine** may determine treatment results.

(10) The **duration** of antimicrobial drug therapy is judged in part by response and in part by past clinical experience. Ultimate recovery must be proved by careful clinical and laboratory follow-up examinations.

(11) In evaluating the patient's clinical response, the possibility of adverse reactions from antimicrobial drugs must be kept in mind. Such reactions may mimic continuing activity of the infectious process by causing fever, skin rashes, CNS disturbances, and changes in blood and urine. With many drugs it is desirable to perform examinations of blood and urine at intervals, and occasionally also to measure renal and liver function. Abnormal findings may force the physician to alter the dose or even discontinue the use of a given drug.

(12) Renal failure, uremia, and oliguria have an important influence on antibiotic dosage because most antimicrobials are excreted—to a greater or lesser extent—by the kidneys. Only a minor adjustment in frequency of administration is necessary with relatively nontoxic drugs, such as the penicillins, or with drugs that are largely detoxified or excreted by the liver, such as chloramphenicol and erythromycin. On the other hand, the aminoglycosides (streptomycin, kanamycin-neomycin), the tetracyclines, and the polymyxins must be drastically reduced in dosage or frequency of administration if serious cumulation and toxicity are to be avoided. As a general rule, these 3 categories of drugs should be administered in full doses only once every 3—4 days to patients with marked retention of nitrogen or with prolonged oliguria.

Excretory mechanisms for many antimicrobials are undeveloped or deficient in the newborn or premature infant. Special dosage schedules must be applied to such infants in order to avoid toxic cumulation of drugs.

ANTIBIOTICS IN RENAL FAILURE

Infection, antimicrobial treatment, and renal failure are interrelated in several ways. Persons in renal failure are particularly prone to acquire many different types of infections and handle them less well than persons with normal renal function. The treatment of renal failure may involve procedures such as hemodialysis, peritoneal dialysis, high doses of corticosteroids, or even cytotoxic immunosuppressants—all of which favor the introduction or spread of microorganisms. Renal function is an important determinant of treatment with antimicrobial drugs because the excretion of most drugs occurs to a greater or lesser extent through the kidneys. Many antimicrobial drugs are in themselves nephrotoxic and thus may produce or aggravate renal failure.

Patients in renal failure are subject to precisely those infections, eg, with gram-negative enteric bacteria, which must be treated by the administration of potentially nephrotoxic drugs. Thus, it is not practicable to completely avoid the use of such drugs in renal failure. Their administration requires some knowledge of the method of excretion of each drug, its

TABLE 48–2. Use of antibiotics in patients with renal failure.

Drug	Principal Mode of Excretion or Detoxification	Approximate Half-Life in Serum		Proposed Dosage Regimen in Renal Failure	
		Normal	Renal Failure*	Initial Dose†	Give Half the Initial Dose at Interval Of
Penicillin G	Tubular secretion	0.5 hours	10 hours	6 gm IV	8–12 hours
Ampicillin	Tubular secretion	1.5 hours	10 hours	6 gm IV	8–12 hours
Methicillin	Tubular secretion	0.5 hours	10 hours	6 gm IV	8–12 hours
Cephalothin	Tubular secretion	0.8 hours	15 hours	8 gm IV	18 hours
Cephalexin	Tubular secretion and glomerular filtration	1 hour	15 hours	2 gm orally	8–12 hours
Streptomycin	Glomerular filtration	2.5 hours	3–4 days	1 gm IM	3–4 days
Kanamycin	Glomerular filtration	3 hours	3–4 days	1 gm IM	3–4 days
Gentamicin	Glomerular filtration	2.5 hours	2–4 days	2 mg/kg IM	2–3 days
Vancomycin	Glomerular filtration	6 hours	8–9 days	0.5 gm IV	8–10 days
Polymyxin B	Glomerular filtration	5 hours	2–3 days	2.5 mg/kg IV	3–4 days
Colistimethate	Glomerular filtration	3 hours	2–3 days	3.5 mg/kg IM	3–4 days
Tetracycline hydrochloride	Glomerular filtration and liver	8 hours	3 days	1 gm orally or 0.5 gm IV	3 days
Chloramphenicol	Liver and glomerular filtration	3 hours	4 hours	1 gm orally or IV	8 hours
Erythromycin	Liver and glomerular filtration	1.5 hours	5 hours	1 gm orally or IV	8 hours
Lincomycin	Glomerular filtration and liver	4.5 hours	10 hours	1 gm orally or IV	12 hours

*Considered here to be marked by creatinine clearance of 10 ml/minute or less.
†For a 60 kg adult with a serious systemic infection. The "initial dose" listed is administered as an intravenous infusion over a period of 1–8 hours, or as 2 intramuscular injections during an 8-hour period, or as 2–3 oral doses during the same period.

rate of clearance by the kidneys, and the possible cumulation in body fluids and tissues which is likely to produce additional renal damage. In addition, it is desirable to be aware of the removal of each drug in the course of peritoneal dialysis or hemodialysis which is employed in the management of uremia.

An attempt is made here to furnish some general guide lines for the administration of antimicrobial drugs in renal failure based on the following information:

(1) The principal mode of detoxification or excretion of the drug.
(2) The half-life of active drug in serum or blood, ie, the time required for the decline in drug level from peak concentration to half of that concentration.
(3) The type of untoward effects to be expected from cumulation of the drug as a result of impaired renal excretion.

Penicillins & Cephalosporins

These drugs are excreted principally by tubular secretion. Even in far-advanced glomerular failure, they are still excreted to some extent, but significant cumulation may occur. Untoward effects are not prominent even with very high drug levels, except irritation of the CNS, or potassium intoxication as a result of exceedingly high concentrations of a potassium salt of peni-

cillin. Cephaloridine is inherently nephrotoxic and thus should be avoided in renal failure. Cephalothin is the preferred cephalosporin drug for the treatment of sepsis in renal failure. During hemodialysis, only a portion of the circulating drug is removed, so that some antimicrobial drug levels of penicillins and cephalosporins persist. In peritoneal dialysis, penicillin G and cephalothin pass freely into the dialysate and are thus lost to the patient unless the dialysis fluid contains comparable adequate levels of the appropriate drug. However, methicillin is not eliminated by peritoneal dialysis or hemodialysis.

Aminoglycosides (Streptomycin, Neomycin, Kanamycin, Gentamicin)

These drugs are excreted by glomerular filtration. In uremia they tend to cumulate significantly and to exhibit marked nephrotoxicity and ototoxicity. To avoid additional renal damage due to unusually high drug levels, the dosage of aminoglycosides must be drastically reduced in patients with renal failure or the interval between doses must be prolonged, as suggested in Table 48–2. Rapid micro-assays of aminoglycoside concentration in serum can effectively guide treatment (J Lab Clin Med 78:457, 1971). Aminoglycosides are removed to a limited extent by hemodialysis but to a significantly greater extent by peritoneal dialysis. To avoid undue loss of drug in peritoneal dialysis, the

TABLE 48–3. Incompatibilities between antimicrobial drugs and other agents.

Antimicrobial Drug	Other Agent	Results
In Vitro Incompatibilities When Mixed for Intravenous Administration*		
Amphotericin B	Benzylpenicillin, tetracyclines, aminoglycosides	Precipitate
Cephalosporins	Calcium gluconate or calcium chloride, polymyxin B, erythromycin, tetracyclines	Precipitate
Chloramphenicol	Polymyxin B, tetracyclines, vancomycin, hydrocortisone, B complex vitamins	Precipitate
Gentamicin	Carbenicillin	Inactivation
Methicillin	Any acidic solution, tetracyclines	Inactivation in 6 hours
Nafcillin	Any acidic solution, B complex vitamins	Inactivation in 12 hours
Novobiocin	Aminoglycosides, erythromycins	Insoluble precipitate
Oxacillin	Any acidic solution, B complex vitamins	Inactivation in 12 hours
Penicillin G	Any acidic solution, B complex vitamins, amphotericin B, chloramphenicol, tetracyclines, vancomycin, metaraminol, phenylephrine, carbohydrate at pH > 80	Inactivation in 12 hours, precipitate
Polymyxin B	Cephalothin	Precipitate
Tetracyclines	Calcium-containing solutions, amphotericin B, cephalosporins, heparin, hydrocortisone, polymyxin B, chloramphenicol, any divalent cations, iron	Chelation, inactivation, precipitate
Vancomycin	Heparin, penicillins, hydrocortisone, chloramphenicol	Precipitate
Physiologic Drug Interactions		
Chloramphenicol	Diphenylhydantoin, tolbutamide, bishydroxycoumarin	Increased blood concentration of these drugs
Griseofulvin	Anticoagulants	Decreased anticoagulant effect
Kanamycin, streptomycin, neomycin, gentamicin, polymyxins	Curare, anticoagulants	Increased curare effect Increased anticoagulant effect
Sulfonamides, chloramphenicol, tetracyclines	Anticoagulants	Increased anticoagulant effect (probably due to inhibition of intestinal flora, which produces vitamin K)
Sulfonamides	Sulfonylurea	Hypoglycemia
Sulfonamides (oral)	Methenamine (oral)	Insoluble HCOH-sulfonamide compound in urine

*Many other incompatibilities may occur.

drugs must be incorporated in the dialysate in effective concentrations (equivalent to those in serum).

Vancomycin

Vancomycin is excreted mainly by glomerular filtration and tends to cumulate rapidly in the presence of renal failure, exhibiting marked nephrotoxicity and some ototoxicity. The half-life of vancomycin is exceedingly prolonged in the uremic patient, and the drug is not removed to a significant extent by hemodialysis or peritoneal dialysis.

Polymyxin B & Colistimethate

These drugs are excreted mainly by glomerular filtration and cumulate rapidly in renal failure, resulting in marked nephrotoxicity and severe neurotoxic manifestations but little ototoxicity. Uremic patients requiring these drugs are given the usual doses spaced several days apart. Neither one of these polymyxins is removed to a significant extent by either hemodialysis or peritoneal dialysis.

Nitrofurantoin

Nitrofurantoin is normally separated from its serum protein carrier in the renal tubules. Antibacterial activity is demonstrable only in the urine, not in serum. In azotemic patients, nitrofurantoin is excreted into the urine only to a negligible extent, and significant levels in urine can virtually never be attained. Consequently, nitrofurantoin cannot be employed effectively as a urinary antiseptic in oliguric or uremic patients, and there is a greatly enhanced risk of untoward side-effects from the cumulated drug.

Chloramphenicol & Erythromycins

Chloramphenicol and the erythromycins are normally excreted by the kidneys only to a very limited extent; the liver plays a much larger role in detoxification and excretion. Consequently, these drugs can be employed for systemic infections in the usual doses in patients with advanced renal failure. Chloramphenicol may not be useful for the treatment of urinary tract infection in uremic patients because not enough drug for effective antibacterial action may reach the urine. Both chloramphenicol and the erythromycins are removed fairly effectively by hemodialysis or peritoneal dialysis. Chloramphenicol can be incorporated into peritoneal dialysis fluid in the treatment of peritonitis because it is absorbed very little from the peritoneal cavity. Lincomycin is not well removed by dialysis.

Tetracyclines

Different tetracyclines have markedly different half-lives. The rapidly excreted tetracyclines (eg, oxytetracycline, tetracycline hydrochloride) have a half-life of 6–9 hours, whereas the slowly excreted tetracyclines (eg, demeclocycline, doxycycline, methacycline) have a half-life of 13–16 hours in the normal person. The latter drugs should probably not be employed in oliguric or uremic individuals because cumulation of drug to toxic levels may occur. The short-acting tetracyclines can be given to persons with a creatinine clearance of 10 ml/minute in a dose of 0.5 gm orally every 2–4 days. Tetracyclines are removed to a moderate extent by either hemodialysis or peritoneal dialysis. They are absorbed fairly effectively from the peritoneal cavity and could be administered by this route for the achievement of systemic levels.

Special Considerations

The values of dose and time interval between doses suggested in Table 48–2 for patients with a creatinine clearance of 10 ml/minute or less provide only crude and initial guide lines. If persons with renal failure require prolonged administration of antimicrobial drugs, levels of drug must be monitored at frequent intervals by serum assay procedures (see p 491). Great caution must be employed in such patients to avoid cumulation of drug to toxic levels which may further depress renal function.

Intravenous Antibiotics (See Table 48–3.)

When an antibiotic must be administered intravenously (eg, for life-threatening infection or for maintenance of very high blood levels), the following cautions should be observed:

(1) Give in neutral solution (pH 7.0–7.2) of isotonic sodium chloride (0.9%) or dextrose (5%) in water.

(2) Give alone without admixture of any other drug in order to avoid chemical and physical incompatibilities (which can occur frequently).

(3) Administer by intermittent (every 2–6 hours) addition to the intravenous infusion to avoid inactivation (by temperature, changing pH, etc) and prolonged vein irritation from high drug concentration, which favors thrombophlebitis.

(4) The infusion site must be changed every 48 hours to reduce the chance of superinfection.

●   ●   ●

General References

Barnett, J.A., & J.P. Sanford: Bacterial shock. JAMA 209:1514–1517, 1969.

Bauer, A.W., & others: Antibiotic susceptibility testing by a standardized single disc method. Am J Clin Path 45:493–496, 1966.

Bennett, W.M.: Practical guide to drug usage in patients with impaired renal function. JAMA 214:1468–1475, 1970.

Ericsson, H.M., & J.C. Sherris: Antibiotic sensitivity testing. Acta path microbiol scandinav, Suppl. No. 217, 1971.

Finegold, S.M., & others: Chemotherapy guide. California Med 111:362–387, 1969.

Jawetz, E.: Principles of antimicrobial therapy. Mod Treat 1:819–828, 1964.

Levin, H.S., & B.M. Kagan: Antimicrobial agents: Pediatric dosages, routes of administration, and preparation procedures for parenteral therapy. P Clin North America 15:275–290, 1968.

Perkins, R.L., Smith, E.J., & S. Saslaw: Cephalothin and cephaloridine: Comparative pharmacodynamics in chronic uremia. Am J Med Sc 257:116–124, 1969.

Weinstein, L.: Common sense (clinical judgment) in the antibiotic therapy of etiologically undefined infections. P Clin North America 15:141–156, 1968.

Weinstein, L., & A.C. Dalton: Host determinants of response to antimicrobial agents. New England J Med 279:467–473, 524, 580–588, 1968.

49 . . .
Penicillins & Cephalosporins

PENICILLINS

The penicillins comprise a large group of substances some of which are natural products of molds and others semisynthetic compounds. They share a common chemical nucleus, 6-aminopenicillanic acid, and a common mode of antibacterial action, the inhibition of cell wall mucopeptide synthesis. They can be grouped according to different criteria—eg, pH stability, susceptibility to enzymatic hydrolysis, protein binding, spectrum of activity, mode of production.

In 1929, Fleming reported his observation that colonies of streptococci lysed on a plate which had become contaminated with a penicillium mold. His efforts to extract the bacteriolytic substance failed, but in 1940 Chain, Florey, and their associates succeeded in producing significant quantities of the first penicillins from cultures of *Penicillium notatum.* Production methods improved rapidly, so that by 1949 virtually unlimited quantities of penicillin were available for clinical use. Several different fermentation products were obtained and called penicillins F, G, K, X, O, etc. Of these, penicillin G proved to be the best, and the manufacture of the others was discontinued.

The 2 principal limitations of penicillin G were its susceptibility to destruction by β-lactamase (penicillinase) and its relative inactivity against most gram-negative bacteria. A research assault on these problems organized by Chain, Rolinson, and Batchelor led, in 1957, to the isolation of 6-aminopenicillanic acid in bulk amounts. Thus began the development of a long series of semisynthetic penicillins. This resulted in the selective design of drugs resistant to β-lactamase, stable to acid pH, and active against both gram-positive and gram-negative bacteria.

Chemistry

All penicillins share the basic structure shown in Table 49–1. There is a thiazolidine ring (a) attached to a β-lactam ring (b) which carries a free amino group (c). Acidic radicals (R) can be attached to the amino group and can be separated from the amino group by bacterial and other amidases. The structural integrity of the 6-aminopenicillanic acid nucleus is essential to the biologic activity of the molecules. If the β-lactam ring is enzymatically cleaved by bacterial β-lactamases (penicillinases), the resulting product, penicilloic acid, is devoid of antibacterial activity. However, it carries

an antigenic determinant of the penicillins, acts as a sensitizing structure when attached to serum proteins, and can be used as skin testing material when attached to peptide chains. Products of alkaline hydrolysis of the penicillins also contribute to sensitization.

The attachment of different radicals (R) to the free amino group of 6-aminopenicillanic acid determines the essential pharmacologic properties of the resulting molecules. Clinically important penicillins available in 1970 fall into 3 main groups: (1) Highest activity against gram-positive bacteria, inactivated by penicillinase (eg, penicillin G, penicillin V, benzathine penicillin). (2) Somewhat lower activity against gram-positive bacteria but resistant to penicillinase (eg, methicillin, nafcillin, oxacillin, dicloxacillin). (3) Broad-spectrum activity against both gram-positive and gram-negative bacteria, inactivated by penicillinase (eg, ampicillin, carbenicillin).

Some representatives of each group are shown in Fig 49–1, with a few distinguishing characteristics.

Most penicillins are dispensed as the sodium or potassium salt of the free acid. Potassium penicillin G contains about 1.7 mEq of K^+ per million units of penicillin (2.8 mEq/gm). Nafcillin contains Na^+, 2.8 mEq/gm. Procaine salts (procaine penicillin) and benzathine salts (benzathine penicillin, Bicillin) are employed to provide repository forms for intramuscular injection.

In dry crystalline form, penicillin salts are stable for long periods (eg, for years at 4° C). Solutions lose their activity rapidly (eg, 24 hours at 20° C) and must be prepared fresh for administration.

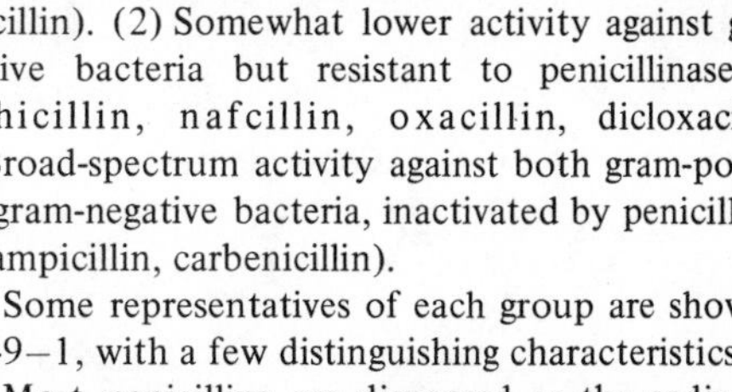

Penicilloic acid

Antimicrobial Activity

All penicillins have the same mechanism of antibacterial action. Penicillins specifically inhibit the synthesis of bacterial cell walls which contain a com-

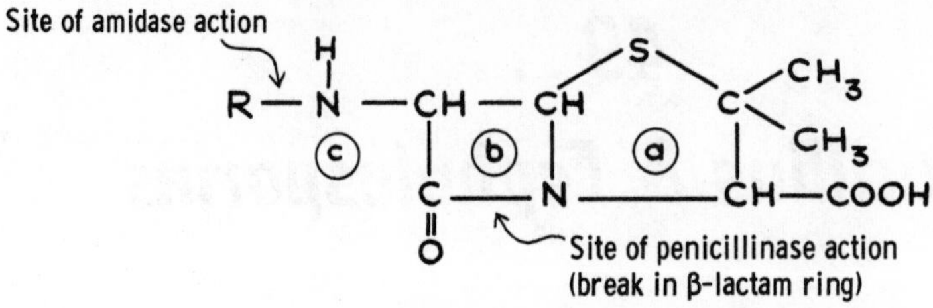

Site of amidase action

6-Aminopenicillanic acid

The following six structures can each be substituted at the R to produce a new penicillin.

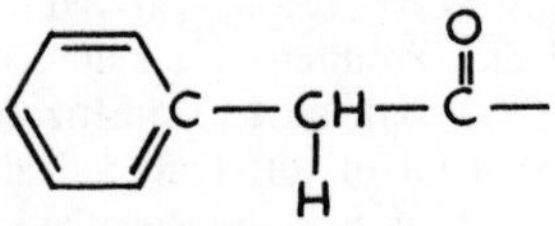

Penicillin G (benzylpenicillin):
High activity against gram-positive bacteria. Low activity against gram-negative bacteria. Acid-labile. Destroyed by β-lactamase.

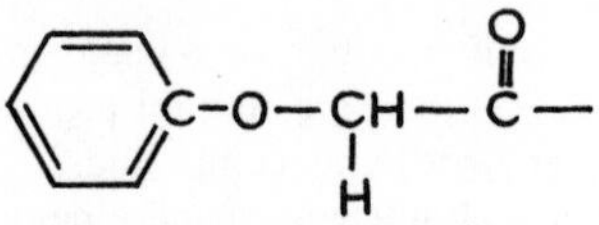

Penicillin V (phenoxymethyl penicillin):
Similar to penicillin G, but relatively acid-resistant.

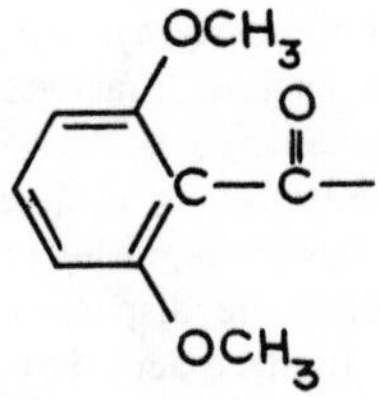

Methicillin (dimethoxyphenylpenicillin):
Lower activity than penicillin G but resistant to penicillinase. Acid-labile. Low protein-binding.

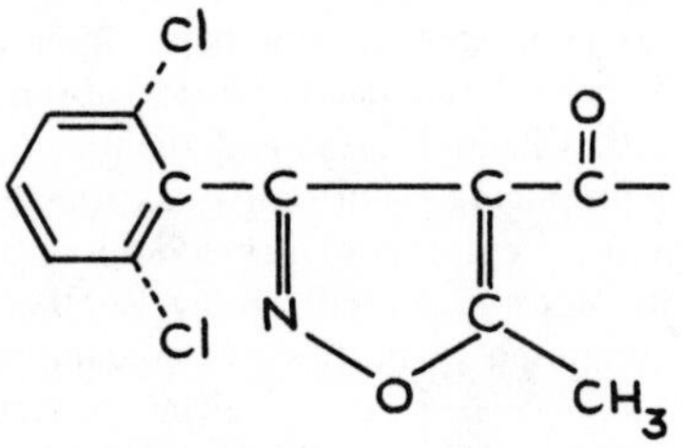

Oxacillin; cloxacillin (one Cl in structure); dicloxacillin (2 Cl's in structure); flucloxacillin (one Cl and one F in structure) (isoxazolyl penicillins); Similar to methicillin in penicillinase resistance, but acid-stable. Highly protein-bound (95–98%).

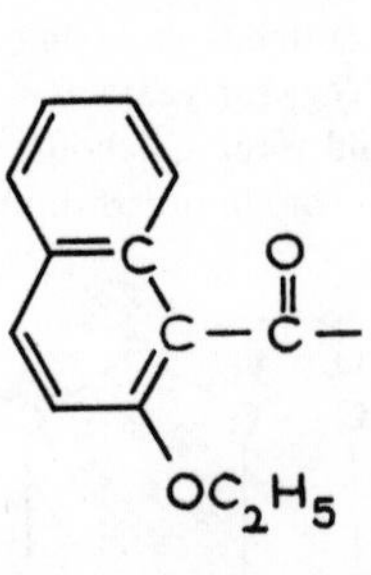

Nafcillin (ethoxynaphthamidopenicillin):
Similar to isoxazolyl penicillins; less strongly protein-bound (90%).

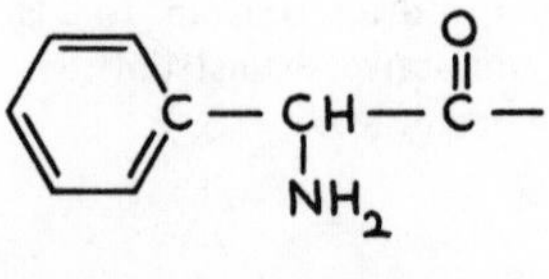

Ampicillin (alpha-aminobenzylpenicillin):
Similar to penicillin G (destroyed by β-lactamase), but acid-stable and more active against gram-negative bacteria. Carbenicillin has —COONa instead of —NH$_2$ group.

FIG 49–1. **Structures of the penicillins.**

plex "mucopeptide" consisting of polysaccharides and a highly cross-linked polypeptide (peptidoglycan).

Penicillin may be a structural analogue of acyl-D-alanyl-D-alanine and may inhibit the terminal cross-linking of linear glucopeptides, thus blocking the complex mucopeptide (peptidoglycan) synthesis.

With low concentrations of penicillin, the formation of dividing bacterial cross walls is inhibited and bizarre and long threads develop from bacteria. With higher concentrations, cell wall formation is completely blocked. Cells either lyse or, if the environment is hypertonic, change into protoplasts or L forms (fragile bacterial forms lacking a cell wall). In an isotonic environment, inhibition of cell wall formation leads to bursting of the cell which results in death. Penicillins are thus mainly bactericidal if active mucopeptide synthesis takes place at the time of exposure to the drug. Metabolically inactive cells are largely unaffected ("persisters"; see p 488).

Most penicillins are much more active against gram-positive than against gram-negative bacteria. Whereas $0.002-1$ $\mu g/ml$ of penicillin G is lethal for a majority of susceptible gram-positive bacteria, concentrations $10-100$ times that are required before gram-negative bacteria are affected. The difference in susceptibility between gram-positive and gram-negative bacteria may depend upon the chemical differences in cell wall composition which determine penetration and binding of drugs, or resistance to rupture. There are exceptions, however. Gram-negative gonococci, for example, are penicillin-susceptible; and ampicillin in vitro is virtually as active against gram-negative as against gram-positive bacteria, although its in vivo activity is more limited.

The activity of penicillin G was originally defined in units. Crystalline sodium penicillin G contains approximately 1600 units/mg (1 unit = 0.6 μg; 1 million units of penicillin = 0.6 gm). Most semisynthetic penicillins are prescribed in gram doses only. Different penicillins have different activities per microgram against susceptible microorganisms. Penicillin G and ampicillin are the most active; methicillin and isoxazolyl penicillins are $5-50$ times less active than penicillin G.

Resistance

Resistance to penicillins falls into several distinct categories.

A. Certain bacteria (eg, many pathogenic staphylococci, *Bacillus subtilis*, coliform organisms) produce an inducible (adaptive) enzyme, β-lactamase (penicillinase). In organisms carrying the genetic trait, all penicillins induce active enzyme formation. This enzyme then destroys penicillin by breaking the β-lactam ring. Apart from producing the enzyme, such organisms may be susceptible to penicillin. Thus they are suppressed by the β-lactamase-resistant penicillins which have a β-lactam ring protected by parts of the R− side chain. The genetic control of β-lactamase formation in staphylococci resides in a plasmid (see Chapter 47).

B. Certain bacteria (eg, coliform organisms) produce an enzyme, amidase, which splits off the R− side chain from the amino group of 6-amino-penicillanic acid. This hydrolysis largely destroys the biologic activity of penicillins.

C. Other bacteria may be resistant to the action of penicillins but do not destroy the drug. The nature of this resistance is not understood, but it must reside in processes related to mucopeptide synthesis. Resistant mutants of this type arise in many penicillin-susceptible bacterial populations in a characteristic stepwise fashion. All mutants in a given step are similarly resistant, and the steps tend to be of very small magnitude. These features explain the exceedingly slow evolution of penicillin resistance in nature among non-β-lactamase-producing organisms.

D. Metabolically inactive organisms (which do not actively synthesize mucopeptide) are phenotypically resistant to penicillins but genotypically fully susceptible. Such organisms can act as "persisters" both in vitro and in vivo and are not killed by penicillins. Protoplasts or L forms can act as "persisters" because they lack cell walls.

E. Organisms resistant to methicillin or an isoxazolyl penicillin tend to be resistant to other penicillins and cephalosporins also. The nature of this cross-resistance is not known; it often involves only a small proportion of a microbial population. Among staphylococci, methicillin resistance occurs in 10% of *S albus* and $1-40\%$ of *S aureus* in different countries.

Absorption, Metabolism, & Excretion

After parenteral administration, absorption of most penicillins is complete and rapid. Because of the irritation and consequent local pain produced by the intramuscular injection of large doses, administration by the intravenous route (continuous infusion, or intermittent addition to a continuous drip) is often preferred. After oral administration only a portion of the dose is absorbed—from 1/3 to 1/20, depending upon acid stability, binding to foods, and the presence of buffers. In order to minimize binding to foods, oral penicillins should not be preceded or followed by food for at least 1 hour.

After absorption, penicillins are widely distributed in body fluids and tissues. This varies to some extent with the degree of protein binding exhibited by different penicillins. Penicillin G, methicillin, and ampicillin are moderately protein bound (depending upon the method of measurement, $40-60\%$), whereas the isoxazolyl penicillins are highly protein bound ($95-98\%$). While the importance of serum binding is far from clear, it is probable that intensive protein binding diminishes the amount of drug available for antibacterial action in vivo and thus delays a therapeutic response. With parenteral doses of $3-6$ gm ($5-10$ million units) of penicillin G, injected by continuous infusion or divided intramuscular injections, average serum levels of the drug reach $1-10$ units ($0.6-6$ μg)/ml. A rough relationship of 6 gm given parenterally per day, yielding serum levels of $1-6$

μg/ml, also applies to other penicillins. Naturally, the highly serum bound isoxazolyl penicillins yield, on the average, lower levels of free drug than less strongly bound penicillins.

Special dosage forms of penicillin have been designed for delayed absorption to yield low blood and tissue levels for long periods. The outstanding example is benzathine penicillin G. After a single intramuscular injection of 1.5 gm (2.4 million units), serum levels in excess of 0.03 unit/ml are maintained for 10 days and levels in excess of 0.005 unit/ml for 3 weeks. The latter is sufficient to protect against beta-hemolytic streptococcal infection; the former to treat an established infection with these organisms. Procaine penicillin also has delayed absorption, yielding levels for 24 hours.

In many tissues penicillin concentrations are equal to those in serum. Much lower levels are found in the joints, eyes, and CNS. However, with active inflammation of the meninges, as in bacterial meningitis, penicillin levels in the CSF exceed 0.2 μg/ml with a daily parenteral dose of 12 gm. Thus, pneumococcal and meningococcal meningitis may be treated with systemic penicillin and there is no need for intrathecal injection.

Most of the absorbed penicillin is rapidly excreted by the kidneys into the urine; small amounts are excreted by other channels. About 10% of renal excretion is by glomerular filtration and 90% by tubular secretion, to a maximum of about 2 gm/hour in an adult. Tubular secretion can be partially blocked by probenecid (Benemid) to achieve higher systemic levels. Renal clearance is less efficient in the newborn, so that proportionately smaller doses result in higher systemic levels and are maintained longer than in the adult. Individuals with impaired renal function likewise tend to maintain higher penicillin levels longer.

Renal excretion of penicillin results in very high levels in the urine. Thus, systemic daily doses of 6 gm of penicillin may yield urine levels of 500–3000 μg/ml—enough to suppress not only gram-positive but also many gram-negative bacteria in the urine (provided they produce no β-lactamase or amidase).

Penicillin is also excreted into sputum and milk to levels of 3–15% of those present in the serum. This is the case in both man and cattle. The presence of penicillin in the milk of cows treated for mastitis presents a problem in allergy.

Clinical Uses

Penicillins are by far the most effective and the most widely used antibiotics. All oral penicillins should be given away from meal times (1 hour before or 1–2 hours after), to reduce binding and acid inactivation. Oxacillin is most strongly food-bound (ie, protein bound), dicloxacillin somewhat less so. Blood levels of all penicillins can be raised by simultaneous administration of probenecid, 0.5 gm every 6 hours orally (10 mg/kg/every 6 hours), which impairs tubular secretion.

A. Penicillin G is the drug of choice for infections caused by gonococci, pneumococci, streptococci, meningococci, non-β-lactamase-producing staphylococci, *Treponema pallidum* and many other spirochetes, *Bacillus anthracis* and other gram-positive rods, clostridia, listeria, bacteroides, and streptobacillus. Most of these infections respond to daily doses of penicillin G, 0.6–5 million units (0.36–3 gm). Intermittent intramuscular injection is the usual method of administration. Much larger amounts (6–120 gm daily) can be given by intravenous infusion in serious or complicated infections due to these organisms. Oral administration of buffered penicillin G or penicillin V is indicated only in minor infections—eg, of the respiratory tract or its associated structures, especially in children (pharyngitis, otitis, sinusitis)—in a daily dose of 1–4 gm. Oral administration is subject to so many variables that it should not be relied upon in seriously ill patients. Many gonococci have developed partial resistance to penicillin, requiring 1–3 units/ml for inhibition. Treatment of gonorrhea now requires procaine penicillin, 2.4–4.8 million units once, or on 2 successive days. In gonococcal prostatitis, arthritis, salpingitis, or other closed lesions, the same dose must be given daily for 7–14 days, combined with drainage when needed.

Penicillin G is inhibitory for enterococci (*Streptococcus faecalis*), but the simultaneous administration of an aminoglycoside is often necessary for bactericidal effects, eg, in enterococcal endocarditis. In actinomycosis, penicillin G is sometimes combined with sulfonamides. In urinary tract infections, large doses of penicillin G (eg, 1–10 million units IM) may provide sufficiently high levels in the urine to inhibit relatively resistant gram-negative coliform bacteria and, in particular, *Proteus mirabilis*. However, this form of treatment is likely to fail in the presence of large numbers of bacteria producing large amounts of β-lactamase.

B. Benzathine penicillin G is a salt of very low water solubility for intramuscular injection which yields low but prolonged drug levels. A single injection of 1.2–2.4 million units IM is satisfactory for treatment of beta-hemolytic streptococcal pharyngitis. A similar injection given intramuscularly once every 3–4 weeks provides satisfactory prophylaxis against reinfection with beta-hemolytic streptococci. Benzathine penicillin G (2.4 million units IM once a week for 3 or 4 weeks) is also useful for the treatment of syphilis. This drug should never be given by mouth.

C. Ampicillin can be given orally in divided doses, 3–6 gm daily, to treat urinary tract infections with gram-negative coliform organisms. An oral dose of 6–12 gm/day of ampicillin may be effective in eliminating salmonellae from certain chronic carriers, although claims are conflicting. Ampicillin is probably only the drug of second choice (after chloramphenicol) in symptomatic salmonellosis. For bacterial meningitis in small children, ampicillin, 150 mg/kg IV, is the present choice, especially for *Hemophilus influenzae*. Ampicillin is also more active against enterococci than penicillin G. In enterococcus endocarditis, ampicillin should be combined with streptomycin, kanamycin, or gentamicin.

Carbenicillin resembles ampicillin but has more marked activity against pseudomonas and proteus, although many klebsiellae are resistant. Resistance emerges rapidly in susceptible populations, and therefore carbenicillin, 12–30 gm/day IV, may be combined with gentamicin in pseudomonas sepsis. Carbenicillin contains Na⁺, 4.7 mEq/gm. Hetacillin is converted in vivo to ampicillin and should not be used.

D. Methicillin, the isoxazolyl penicillins (oxacillin, cloxacillin, dicloxacillin, and flucloxacillin), nafcillin, and several other β-lactamase-resistant penicillins have only a single indication, ie, the treatment of infection with β-lactamase-producing staphylococci. For non-β-lactamase-producing staphylococci, penicillin G remains the drug of choice.

Methicillin is acid-labile and cannot be given by mouth. It may also be inactivated in solution at room temperature. Therefore, methicillin, 8–16 gm daily, is given IV by intermittent addition to a constant infusion of 5% dextrose in water as treatment of choice in serious (β-lactamase-producing) staphylococcal infections. The dose for children is 100 mg/kg/day. Nafcillin, 6–12 gm daily IV, or oxacillin are alternative choices. (For children, 50–100 mg/kg/day.)

For relatively mild infections caused by β-lactamase-producing staphylococci, dicloxacillin or nafcillin capsules can be given by mouth, 2–6 gm daily in divided doses far removed from food intake. These drugs are not the first choice in any other infections. They should not be used in streptococcal pharyngitis when β-lactamase-producing staphylococci may be also present in the throat.

Doses for children are not well established for many newer penicillins, but 25–100 mg/kg/day is the usual pediatric dosage.

Adverse Reactions

The penicillins undoubtedly possess less direct toxicity than any other antibiotics. Most of the serious side-effects are due to hypersensitivity.

A. Allergy: All penicillins are cross-sensitizing and cross-reacting. Any preparation containing penicillin may induce sensitization, including foods or cosmetics. In general, sensitization occurs in direct proportion to the duration and total dose of penicillin received in the past. The responsible antigenic determinants appear to be degradation products of penicillins, particularly penicilloic acid and products of alkaline hydrolysis bound to host protein. Skin tests with penicilloyl-polylysine, with alkaline hydrolysis products, and with undegraded penicillin will identify many hypersensitive individuals. Among positive reactors to skin tests, the incidence of subsequent penicillin reactions is high. Although many persons develop antibodies to antigenic determinants of penicillin, the presence of such antibodies does not appear to be correlated with allergic reactivity (except rare hemolytic anemia), and serologic tests have little predictive value. A history of a penicillin reaction in the past is not always reliable; however, in such cases, penicillin should be administered with caution.

Allergic reactions may occur as typical anaphylactic shock, typical serum sickness type reactions (urticaria, fever, joint swelling, angioneurotic edema, intense pruritus, and respiratory embarrassment occurring 7–12 days after exposure), and a variety of skin rashes (commonest with ampicillin), oral lesions, fever, nephritis, eosinophilia, hemolytic anemia, and other hematologic disturbances, and vasculitis. LE cells are sometimes found. The incidence of hypersensitivity to penicillin is estimated to be 5–10% among adults in the USA, but is negligible in small children.

At times individuals known to be hypersensitive to penicillin can tolerate the drug during corticosteroid administration. "Desensitization" with gradually increasing doses of penicillin is also occasionally attempted but is not without hazard. Anaphylactic reactions are rare but can follow oral as well as parenteral penicillin.

B. Toxicity: Since the action of penicillin is directed against a unique bacterial structure, the cell wall, it is virtually without effect on animal cells. The toxic effects of penicillin G are due to the direct irritation caused by intramuscular or intravenous injection of exceedingly high concentrations (eg, 1 gm/ml). Such concentrations may cause local pain, induration, thrombophlebitis, or degeneration of an accidentally injected nerve. All penicillins are irritating to the CNS and greatly increase the excitability of neurons. For that reason, no more than 20,000 units can be given intrathecally on any one day, but there is little indication for intrathecal administration at present. In rare cases a patient receiving more than 50 gm of penicillin G daily parenterally has exhibited signs of cerebrocortical irritation, presumably as a result of the passage of unusually large amounts of penicillin into the CNS. With doses of this magnitude, direct cation toxicity (Na⁺, K⁺) can also occur (see Chemistry, above), particularly in patients with renal failure.

Large doses of penicillins given orally may lead to gastrointestinal upset, particularly nausea, vomiting, and diarrhea. Oral therapy may also be accompanied by luxuriant overgrowth of staphylococci, pseudomonas, proteus, or yeasts, which may occasionally cause enteritis. Superinfections in other organ systems may occur with penicillins as with any antibiotic therapy. Methicillin and isoxazolyl penicillins have occasionally caused granulocytopenia, especially in children, and nephritis. Carbenicillin can cause transaminase elevation in serum.

Problems Relating to the Use of the Penicillins

The penicillins are by far the most widely used antibiotics. Several hundred tons of these drugs have been administered to humans during the past 20 years. Therefore, penicillins have been responsible for some of the most drastic consequences of antibiotic misuse.

A significant proportion of the population of many countries (perhaps 5–10%) have become hypersensitive to the drug. In many cases there is no doubt that sensitization has occurred when penicillin was administered without proper indication. It would be desirable to have penicillin-hypersensitive individuals definitely identified.

The saturation of certain environments (eg, hospitals) with penicillin has produced a selection pressure against penicillin-sensitive microorganisms and resulted in greater numbers of penicillin-resistant organisms. Hospital environments consequently have become filled with β-lactamase-producing staphylococci. In some instances these organisms were endowed with enhanced ability to disseminate and produce infection. "Hospital staphylococci" have been responsible for outbreaks of lethal disease in newborn nurseries and surgical units.

The suppression of normal flora creates a partial void which is regularly filled with drug-resistant, prevalent organisms. Penicillins are administered to a high proportion of patients in hospitals. These patients are made selectively susceptible to superinfections with microorganisms derived from the hospital environment (proteus, pseudomonas, enterobacter, yeasts, staphylococci, etc). Such organisms become established in organ systems where the normal flora has been suppressed (eg, the respiratory tract, gut, skin) and can cause disease processes there.

The drastic restriction of penicillin abuse in certain hospitals has illustrated man's ability to control the harmful changes in the microflora of the environment. Restricted use of penicillin has led to a return of penicillin-sensitive microorganisms to the environment and reduction of the harmful effects of drug resistant bacteria.

Preparations Available

Ampicillin (Omnipen, Penbritin, Polycillin):
Capsules, 250 and 500 mg
Oral suspension, 60 and 80 ml containing 125 mg/5 ml; 80 ml containing 250 mg/5 ml
Injectable (IM or IV), vials containing 125, 250, 500, and 1000 mg

Benzathine penicillin G (Bicillin):
Tablets, 100,000 and 200,000 units*
Suspension, 150,000 and 300,000 units/5 ml, 60 ml*
Drops, 150,000 units/ml, 10 ml*
Injectable (IM or IV), 300,000 units/ml, 10 ml; 600,000 units/ml, 1, 2, and 4 ml

Cloxacillin sodium (Tegopen, Orbenin):
Capsules, 125 and 250 mg
Granules (suspension), 125 mg/5 ml, 80 and 150 ml

Dicloxacillin monohydrate (Dynapen, Veracillin)
Capsules, 125 and 250 mg

Methicillin (Dimocillin, Staphcillin): 1, 4, and 6 gm vials for IM or IV injection

Nafcillin sodium (Unipen):
Capsules, 250 mg
Oral solution, 125 mg/5 ml, 60 and 80 ml; 250 mg/5 ml, 80 ml
Injectable (IM or IV), vials containing 125, 250, 500, and 1000 mg

Oxacillin sodium (Prostaphlin, Resistopen):
Capsules, 125, 250, and 500 mg
Oral solution, 125 mg/5 ml, 80 and 150 ml
Injectable (IM or IV), vials containing 250, 500, and 1000 mg

Penicillin G potassium: (Various mfrs.)
Tablets, 50,000, 100,000, 200,000, 250,000, 400,000, 500,000, 800,000, and 1 million units
Soluble tablets, 50,000, 100,000, 200,000, 250,000, and 400,000 units
Capsules, 200,000 and 400,000 units
Oral solution, 100,000, 125,000, 200,000, 250,000, 400,000, and 500,000 units/5 ml, 60 ml; 200,000 and 400,000 units/5 ml, 80 and 150 ml
Inhalation, sifter cartridges containing 100,000 units each; packages of 3*
Ointment, 1000, 2000, 5000, and 10,000 units/gm, 1 oz
Ophthalmic ointment, 1000 and 100,000 units/gm, 1/8 oz
Injectable (IM or IV), ampules or vials containing 0.2, 0.5, 1, 5, 10, and 20 million units

Penicillin G procaine:
Ointment, 1000 and 10,000 units/gm, 1 oz
Injectable aqueous suspension (IM or IV):
300,000 units/ml, 5 and 10 ml vials
500,000 units/ml, 10 ml vials
600,000 units/dose (single dose)
1 million units/dose (syringe)
1.2 million units/2 ml ampule

Penicillin G sodium: Vials or ampules for IM or IV injection, 1 and 5 million units

Phenoxymethyl penicillin (penicillin V, Compocillin, Pen-Vee, V-Cillin):
Tablets, 125 and 300 mg; potassium, 125 and 250 mg
Sustained action tablets, 250 mg
Capsules, 125 and 250 mg
Wafers (hydrabamine salt), 125 and 250 mg
Oral solution (potassium), 125 mg/5 ml (flavored or not), 40, 80, and 150 ml; 250 mg/5 ml (flavored), 40 ml

*Dosage forms included for completeness but not recommended for use.

Oral suspension:
> Hydrabamine salt, 180 mg/5 ml, 40, 80, and 150 ml
> Benzathine salt, 180 mg/5 ml, 80 and 150 ml; 90 mg/5 ml, 60 ml

Pediatric suspension:
> Benzathine salt, 250 mg/5 ml
> Fruit flavored, 125 mg/5 ml, 40 and 80 ml; 250 mg/5 ml, 60 ml

Drops:
> Flavored suspension, 125 mg/dropperful, 1.5 gm
> Benzathine salt, 90 mg/ml, 10 ml

7-Aminocephalosporanic acid

CEPHALOSPORINS

In 1945 Brotzu isolated a fungus, *Cephalosporium acremonium,* in Sardinia. This fungus produced several antibiotics, called cephalosporins, which resembled penicillins but resisted the action of penicillinase and were active against both gram-positive and gram-negative bacteria. The chemical structure of cephalosporins was established largely by Abraham and Newton, who showed the similarity of cephalosporin C to penicillins. Methods for the large-scale production of 7-aminocephalosporanic acid were eventually developed, making possible the synthesis of many derivatives by chemical means. Several such semisynthetic derivatives, cephalothin, cephaloridine, cephaloglycin, and cephalexin, are available at present.

Chemistry

The nucleus of the cephalosporins, 7-aminocephalosporanic acid, bears a close resemblance to the nucleus of the penicillins, 6-aminopenicillanic acid (Fig 49–1).

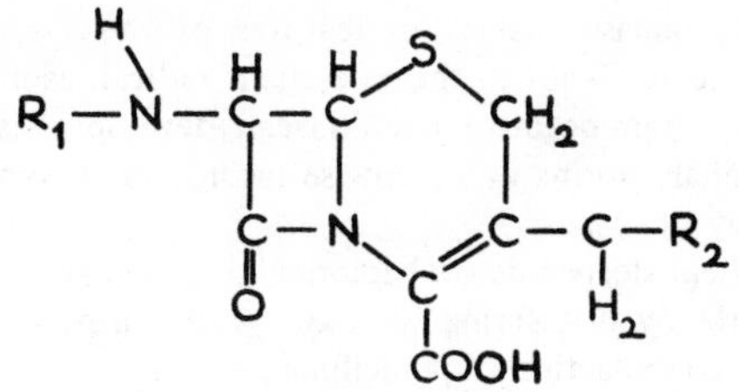

The intrinsic antimicrobial activity of the natural cephalosporins is low. However, the attachment of various R— groups has yielded compounds of high therapeutic activity and low toxicity.

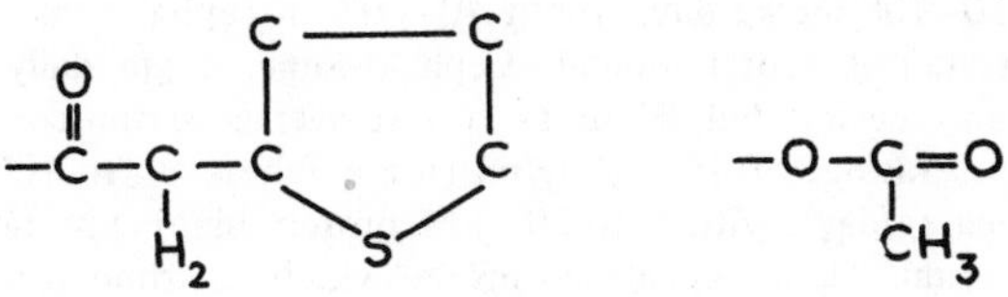

The cephalosporins have molecular weights of 400–450. They are cream-colored crystalline solids, freely soluble in water and relatively stable to temperature, pH, and to degradation by β-lactamase. Cephaloridine is much more readily hydrolyzed by staphylococcal β-lactamase than cephalothin. Solutions can also be degraded by a cephalosporinase produced by certain gram-negative bacteria. The marketed sodium salt contains about 55 mg of sodium per gm of cephalothin. **Fusidic acid** and **helvolic acid** are related to certain cephalosporins and have been used in Great Britain as antistaphylococcal drugs.

Antimicrobial Activity

The cephalosporins are active in vitro in concentrations of 1–10 μg/ml against most gram-positive microorganisms (except *Streptococcus faecalis*), including actinomyces, and in concentrations of 5–30

R_1 R_2

Cephalothin

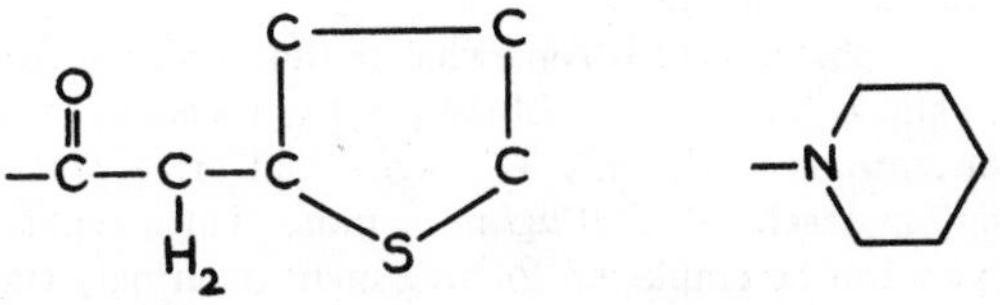

Cephaloridine

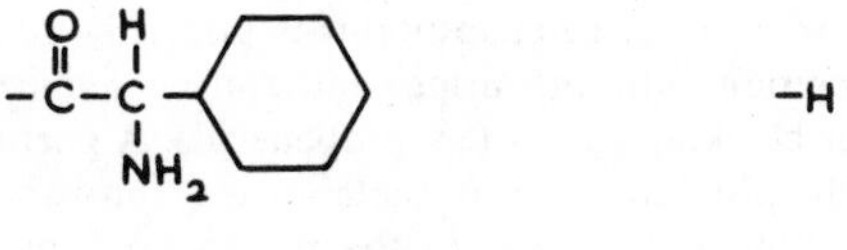

Cephalexin

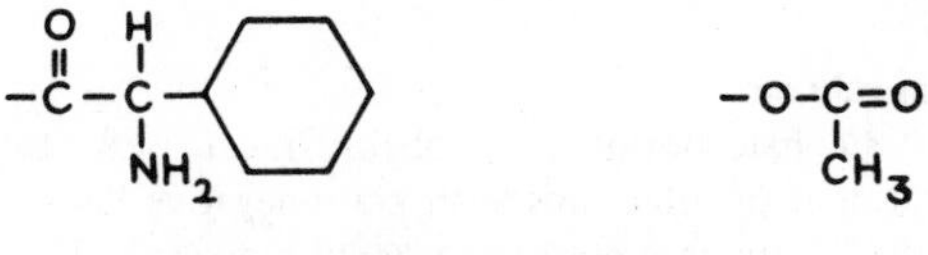

Cephaloglycin

μg/ml against many gram-negative bacteria. All strains of pseudomonas and herellea and many strains of serratia, enterobacter, and proteus are resistant, but the latter may sometimes be susceptible to concentrations of cephalosporins which are reached in the urine (200–1000 μg/ml). There is at least partial cross-resistance between cephalosporins and β-lactamase-resistant penicillins. The resistance of cephalosporins to β-lactamase resides in features of the 7-cephalosporanic acid—not in the side chain radical, as in penicillins. Gram-negative bacteria can develop resistance to cephalosporins in a stepwise fashion, and some can destroy the drugs.

Cephalosporins are bactericidal against susceptible bacteria by interfering with cell wall synthesis (analogous to the action of penicillins).

Absorption, Distribution, & Excretion

Cephalothin and cephaloridine are not absorbed from the gastrointestinal tract sufficiently for systemic therapy. Therefore, they must be injected parenterally. Cephalothin, 8—16 gm daily, is usually injected IV (IM injection is very painful) to give average serum concentrations of 5—20 μg/ml. The dose for children is 50—100 mg/kg/day. About 40—60% of cephalothin in serum is protein-bound. Cephaloridine, 4 gm daily, may be injected IM or IV to give average serum concentrations of 10—25 μg/ml (for children, up to 100 mg/kg/day), with only 20—30% protein binding in the serum. These cephalosporins are widely distributed in tissues and body fluids, including the eye and synovial fluid, but CSF concentrations are negligible following systemic administration. Systemic cephalothin is not a treatment of choice in meningitis. Urine levels may reach 200—1000 μg/ml.

Cephaloglycin is somewhat better absorbed from the gut. After oral doses of 0.5 gm 4 times daily, serum concentrations are only 1—3 μg/ml but urine concentrations reach 50—500 μg/ml or more. Thus, cephaloglycin can be employed for treatment of urinary tract infections.

Cephalexin is well absorbed from the gut; after oral doses of 0.5 gm, the serum level reaches 10 μg/ml; about 15% of cephalexin in serum is protein-bound, and most is excreted into urine.

Excretion of cephalosporins is primarily by tubular secretion into the urine, and can be reduced by tubular blocking agents (eg, probenecid). A portion of the administered dose is metabolized, probably by deacylation in the liver. In the presence of impaired renal excretion very high blood and tissue levels of cephalosporins may accumulate and exert toxic effects.

Clinical Uses

Cephalosporins are probably most useful for the treatment of infections with gram-negative bacteria or with β-lactamase-producing staphylococci. The oral cephalosporins may find a place in the treatment of urinary tract or respiratory tract infections. Cephalosporins are occasionally chosen as penicillin substitutes for known allergic individuals, but some cross-hypersensitivity exists.

Cephalothin, 8—16 gm/day, is commonly given by continuous IV infusion (for children, 50—100 mg/kg/day). Solutions containing 1 mg/ml have occasionally been instilled into joints or surgical wounds. Cephaloridine, 4 gm/day, may be given IM in divided doses (for children, up to 100 mg/kg/day), with monitoring of renal function. Cephaloridine is more susceptible to staphylococcal penicillinase than cephalothin. Cephaloglycin, 0.5 gm orally 4 times daily, may be employed for the treatment of urinary tract infections. Cephalexin, 0.5 gm orally 4—8 times daily (50 mg/kg/day), may be used in urinary or respiratory tract infections caused by susceptible organisms. It could be employed after an initial response to parenteral cephalosporin.

Adverse Reactions

A. Toxicity: Local irritation can produce severe pain after intramuscular injection and thrombophlebitis after repeated intravenous injection. Other toxic reactions include anaphylaxis, urticaria, skin rashes, fever, eosinophilia, granulocytopenia, and hemolytic anemia. Some of these are probably hypersensitivity reactions (see below). Renal toxicity producing tubular necrosis has been demonstrated for cephaloridine but not for cephalothin.

The oral cephalosporins also produce diarrhea, nausea, and vomiting.

B. Allergy: It is established that cephalosporins can be sensitizing and that specific hypersensitivity reactions, including anaphylaxis, can occur. Because of the chemical difference in the drug nucleus structure, the antigenicity of the cephalosporins differs from that of the penicillins. Consequently, some individuals who are hypersensitive to the penicillins can tolerate the cephalosporins. It is estimated that about 10% of penicillin-hypersensitive persons may also be hypersensitive to cephalosporins.

Preparations Available

Sodium cephalothin (Keflin): 10 ml ampules containing 1 gm (dry powder) for IV use

Cephaloridine (Loridine): 5 ml ampules containing 500 mg and 10 ml ampules containing 1 gm for IM or IV use

•　　　•　　　•

General References

Barret, F.F., & others: Methicillin-resistant *Staphylococcus aureus* at Boston City Hospital. New England J Med 279:441–448, 1968.

Bear, D.M., & others: Ampicillin. M Clin North America 54:1145–1159, 1970.

Gilbert, D.N., & J.P. Sanford: Methicillin. M Clin North America 54:1113–1125, 1970.

Kass, E.H.: Carbenicillin: How useful? J Infect Dis 122:S115, 1970.

Rosenblatt, J.E., & others: Mechanisms responsible for the blood level differences of isoxazolyl penicillins. Arch Int Med 121:345–348, 1968.

Saslaw, S.: Cephalosporins. M Clin North America 54:1217–1228, 1970.

Steigbigel, N.H., & others: Clinical evaluation of cephaloridine. Arch Int Med 121:24–38, 1968.

Thoburn, R., & others: The relationship of cephalothin and penicillin allergy. JAMA 198:345–348, 1966.

50 . . .

Chloramphenicol, Erythromycin Group, & Tetracyclines

CHLORAMPHENICOL

Chloramphenicol was first isolated from cultures of *Streptomyces venezuelae* in 1947 and was synthesized in 1949. It is the only available representative of its chemical type and the only completely synthetic antibiotic of importance to be produced commercially.

Chemistry

Crystalline chloramphenicol is a neutral, stable compound with the following structure:

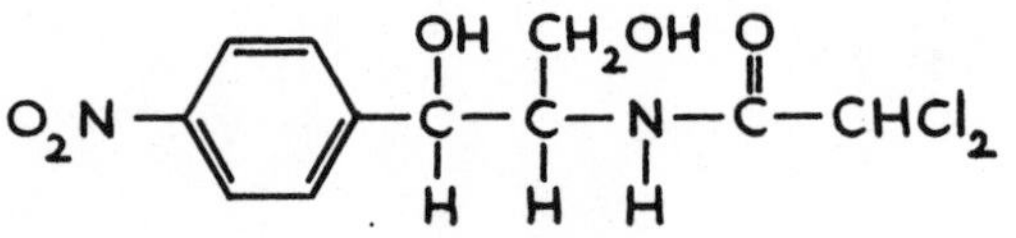

Chloramphenicol

It consists of colorless crystals with an intensely bitter taste. It is highly soluble in alcohol and poorly soluble in water. Saturated aqueous solutions (0.25%) keep their activity for many months at refrigerator or room temperature if protected from light. Chloramphenicol succinate is highly soluble in water and is hydrolyzed in tissues with the liberation of free chloramphenicol; it is used for parenteral injection.

Antimicrobial Activity

Chloramphenicol is a potent inhibitor of protein synthesis and has little effect on other metabolic functions. It acts on the 50 S unit of bacterial ribosomes and interferes markedly with the incorporation of amino acids into newly formed peptides by blocking the action of peptidyl transferase (see Chapter 47). Chloramphenicol also inhibits mitochondrial protein synthesis of mammalian bone marrow cells but does not greatly affect other intact cells.

Chloramphenicol is bacteriostatic for many bacteria and for rickettsiae; its action is reversible by removal of the drug. Most gram-positive bacteria are inhibited by chloramphenicol in concentrations of 1–10 μg/ml, and many gram-negative bacteria by concentrations of 0.2–5 μg/ml. Hemophilus and salmonellae are often highly susceptible.

Resistance

In most bacterial species, large populations of chloramphenicol-susceptible cells contain occasional resistant mutants. These mutants are usually only 2–4 times more resistant than the parent populations; consequently, they emerge slowly in treated individuals. There is no cross-resistance between chloramphenicol and other drugs, but episome-like genetic resistance transfer factors (RTF, "infectious resistance of bacteria") may transmit multiple drug resistance (chloramphenicol, tetracycline, streptomycin, etc) from one bacterium or species to another. Chloramphenicol resistance in some bacterial mutants may be associated with the presence of bacterial enzymes which acetylate chloramphenicol, such as an acetyl transferase.

Absorption, Metabolism, & Excretion

After oral administration, crystalline chloramphenicol is rapidly and completely absorbed. With daily doses of 2 gm orally, blood levels usually reach 20 μg/ml. Chloramphenicol palmitate, administered to children in doses up to 50 mg/kg/day orally, is hydrolyzed in the intestine to yield free chloramphenicol, but the usual blood levels rarely exceed 10 μg/ml. For parenteral injection, chloramphenicol succinate, 25–50 mg/kg/day IM or IV, yields free chloramphenicol by hydrolysis, giving blood levels somewhat lower than those achieved with the orally administered drug.

After absorption, chloramphenicol is widely distributed to virtually all tissues and body fluids, including the CNS and CSF, although about 50% is bound to serum protein. It penetrates cells readily. Most chloramphenicol is inactivated in the body either by conjugation with glucuronic acid (principally in the liver) or by reduction to inactive aryl amines. Excretion of active chloramphenicol (about 10% of the total dose administered) and of inactive degradation products (about 90% of total dose administered) occurs into the urine. It may be that the active drug is cleared mainly by glomerular filtration and the inactive products mainly by tubular secretion. Only small amounts of active drug are excreted into bile or feces.

Clinical Uses

Chloramphenicol is a possible drug of choice in only a few types of infections: (1) symptomatic salmonella infection; (2) *Hemophilus influenzae* meningitis or laryngotracheitis not responding to ampicillin;

(3) occasional bacteremia caused by gram-negative bacteria expected (on the basis of experience) to be resistant to other drugs; (4) severe rickettsial infections.

A. For salmonella infections (eg, typhoid or paratyphoid fever), adults should receive chloramphenicol, 2–3 gm daily orally, and children 30–50 mg/kg/day orally for 14–21 days. Prolonged treatment tends to reduce the frequency of relapses. A similar program may be followed in severe rickettsial infections (eg, scrub typhus or Rocky Mountain spotted fever).

B. For *H influenzae* meningitis or laryngotracheitis (in small children) or pneumonia (in the elderly), chloramphenicol, 50 mg/kg/day orally, has been given for 8–14 days, depending upon clinical response and CSF changes. However, ampicillin is the drug of first choice at present.

C. Other Uses: In severe coliform bacteremias, chloramphenicol, 3 gm/day or 50 mg/kg/day, can be combined with kanamycin, 2 gm/day. Rarely, chloramphenicol is the drug of choice in urinary tract infections caused by organisms resistant to other drugs. The dose is 0.5 gm orally every 6–12 hours. In ophthalmology, topical application of chloramphenicol to the eye has been employed because of the wide antibacterial spectrum of the drug and its penetration of ocular tissues. Sepsis caused by some species of bacteroides and severe melioidosis may respond to chloramphenicol. Chloramphenicol is also effective in meningococcal meningitis in patients hypersensitive to penicillin.

Adverse Reactions

A. Gastrointestinal Disturbances: Adults taking chloramphenicol, 1.5–2.5 gm daily, occasionally develop nausea, vomiting, and diarrhea in 2–5 days. This is rare in children. After 5–10 days, the results of microbial flora alteration may become apparent, with prominent candidiasis of mucous membranes (especially of the mouth and vagina).

B. Bone Marrow Disturbances: Adults taking chloramphenicol in excess of 50 mg/kg/day regularly exhibit disturbances in red cell maturation after 1–2 weeks of blood levels above 25–30 μg/ml. These are characterized by the appearance of markedly vacuolated nucleated red cells in the marrow, anemia, and reticulocytopenia. These anomalies usually disappear when chloramphenicol is discontinued. The disturbance appears to be a maturation arrest associated with a rise in serum iron concentration and a depression of serum phenylalanine levels and is not related to the rare occurrence of aplastic anemia.

Aplastic anemia is a rare consequence of chloramphenicol administration. It probably represents a specific genetically determined idiosyncrasy of the individual. It is not related to dose or time of intake, but is seen more frequently with prolonged use. It tends to be irreversible and fatal. The precise incidence of fatal aplastic anemia as a toxic reaction to chloramphenicol administration is not known, but the disease is estimated to occur 13 times more frequently after the use of the drug than it does spontaneously. Leukemia may follow the development of hypoplastic anemia.

C. Toxicity for Newborn Infants: Newborn infants lack an effective glucuronic acid conjugation mechanism for the degradation and detoxification of chloramphenicol. Consequently, when infants are given doses of 75 mg/kg/day or more, the drug may accumulate, resulting in the "gray syndrome," with vomiting, flaccidity, hypothermia, gray color, shock, and collapse. To avoid this toxic effect, chloramphenicol should be used with caution in infants and the dosage should be limited to 50 mg/kg/day or less in full-term infants and 30 mg/kg/day or less in prematures.

Medical & Social Implications of Overuse

Because of its "broad spectrum" and its apparent lack of toxicity, chloramphenicol was used indiscriminately between 1948 and 1951 without specific indications. It has been estimated that more than 8 million people received the drug for minor complaints, respiratory (usually viral) illnesses, etc. This inappropriate use was followed by a wave of cases of aplastic anemia which, in turn, almost resulted in the complete abandonment of an effective drug.

Preparations Available

Chloramphenicol (Chloromycetin):
    Capsules, 50, 100 and 250 mg
    Injectable: 500 mg/ampule for IV injection, 1 gm/ampule for IM injection
    Cream, 1%, 1 oz
    Ophthalmic powder, 5 ml vial containing 25 mg
    Ophthalmic ointment, 10 mg/gm, 1/8 oz
    Otic, 15 ml containing 0.5% in propylene glycol with 1% benzocaine

Chloramphenicol palmitate:
    Suspension, 60 ml containing 125 mg/4 ml

Chloramphenicol sodium succinate:
    250 mg and 1 gm for IM or IV use

THE ERYTHROMYCIN GROUP
(Macrolides)

This is a group of closely related compounds characterized by a macrocyclic lactone ring to which sugars are attached. The prototype drug, erythromycin, was obtained in 1952 from *Streptomyces erythreus*. Members of the group include carbomycin, oleandomycin, spiramycin, and many others. Troleandomycin (triacetyloleandomycin) was introduced in 1958.

Chemistry

The formula of erythromycin is $C_{37}H_{67}O_{13}N$. Its general structure is shown below with the macrolide ring and the sugars desosamine and cladinose. The molecular weight of erythromycin is 734. It is poorly soluble in water (0.1%) but dissolves readily in organic solvents. Solutions are relatively stable at 4° C but lose activity rapidly at 20° C and at acid pH. Erythromycins are dispensed as various esters and salts.

Antimicrobial Activity

Erythromycins are effective against gram-positive organisms, especially pneumococci, streptococci, staphylococci, and corynebacteria in concentrations of $0.02-2$ $\mu g/ml$. Neisseriae, hemophilus, and mycoplasma are also susceptible.

The antibacterial action of the erythromycins is both inhibitory and bactericidal for susceptible organisms. Activity is enhanced at alkaline pH. Inhibition of protein synthesis occurs by action on the 50 S unit of ribosomes where erythromycin competes with amino acids for ribosomal binding sites, perhaps by blocking the aminoacyl translocation reaction.

Resistance

In most susceptible microbial populations, mutants have arisen which are highly resistant to erythromycin. Resistant mutants are especially frequent among staphylococci, and their emergence in the course of prolonged treatment with erythromycin in highly predictable. Consequently, erythromycin should never be used as the sole drug in treating severe staphylococcal infections. Erythromycin-resistant pneumococci and streptococci are now appearing.

There appears to be virtually complete cross-resistance among all members of the erythromycin group. The basis of erythromycin resistance probably is based on an altered protein on the 50 S unit of the ribosome. Resistance does not involve destruction of drug. There is some cross-resistance to lincomycin.

Absorption, Metabolism, & Excretion

Basic erythromycins are rapidly destroyed by stomach acids. Erythromycin stearate is acid-resistant but not so well absorbed as esters of erythromycin.

Oral doses of 2 gm/day result in serum levels of up to 2 $\mu g/ml$. Large amounts are lost in feces. Absorbed drug is distributed widely in the tissues with the exception of the CNS and CSF.

Erythromycins are excreted largely in the bile, where levels may be 50 times higher than in the blood. A portion of the drug excreted into bile is reabsorbed into the intestines. Only 5% of the administered dose is excreted in the urine.

Clinical Uses

Erythromycins are probably the drugs of choice only in some corynebacterial infections (erythrasma, diphtheria carriers, diphtheroid sepsis) and in disease caused by *Mycoplasma pneumoniae.* Erythromycin is active against many atypical mycobacteria. Otherwise, they are most useful as penicillin substitutes in individuals with streptococcal or pneumococcal infections who are hypersensitive to penicillin. In this group of drugs, erythromycin estolate (the lauryl sulfate of the propionyl ester of erythromycin) and troleandomycin are absorbed with greatest regularity. However, they also produce the most severe adverse reactions. Therefore the less well absorbed base stearate or succinate may be preferred.

A. Oral Dosage: 0.5 gm every 6 hours for adults; 40 mg/kg/day for children.

B. Intravenous Dosage: (Eg, erythromycin gluceptate or lactobionate.) 0.5 gm every 8–12 hours for adults; 40 mg/kg/day for children.

Adverse Reactions

A. Gastrointestinal Effects: Anorexia, nausea, vomiting, and diarrhea occasionally accompany oral administration.

B. Liver Toxicity: Erythromycin estolate and troleandomycin can produce acute cholestatic hepatitis with fever and jaundice or subclinical impaired liver function. It is probable that this is a reaction of

Erythromycin

specific hypersensitivity which can be elicited repeatedly by challenge with the same drugs. Up to 15% of patients receiving these drugs in full doses for more than 2 weeks may have abnormal liver function tests. Some of these abnormal tests (elevated SGOT) may be false positives, but others indicate impairment of liver function. Most patients recover completely, but a few deaths have been reported.

Preparations Available

Erythromycin base (Ilotycin):
Tablets, 100 and 250 mg
Ointment, 1% in petrolatum base, ½ and 1 oz

Erythromycin estolate (Ilosone):
Capsules, 125 and 250 mg
Chewable tablets, 125 mg
Oral suspension, 125 mg/5 ml, 60 and 150 ml
Drops, 100 mg/ml, 10 ml

Erythromycin stearate (Erythrocin):
Tablets, 100 and 250 mg

Erythromycin ethyl succinate (Erythrocin, Pediamycin):
Chewable tablets, 200 mg
Pediatric suspension, 200 mg/5 ml, 60 and 500 ml
Granules, 200 mg/5 ml, 60 ml
Drops, 100 mg/2.5 ml, 30 ml
Injectable (IM), 50 mg/ml, 2 ml ampules and 10 ml vials

Erythromycin gluceptate (Ilotycin IV):
250 mg/20 ml, 500 mg/30 ml, and 1 gm/50 ml for IV injection

Erythromycin lactobionate (Erythrocin IV):
500 mg and 1 gm vials for IV injection

Troleandomycin (triacetyloleandomycin, Cyclamycin, Tao):
Capsules, 125 and 250 mg
Suspension, 125 mg/5 ml, 60 ml
Drops, 100 mg/ml (Tao), 10 ml

TETRACYCLINES

The tetracyclines are a large group of drugs with a common basic structure and activity. Chlortetracycline, isolated from *Streptomyces aureofaciens*, was introduced in 1948. Oxytetracycline, derived from *S rimosus*, was introduced in 1950. Tetracycline (many trade names), obtained either from a streptomycete or by catalytic dehalogenation of chlortetracycline, has

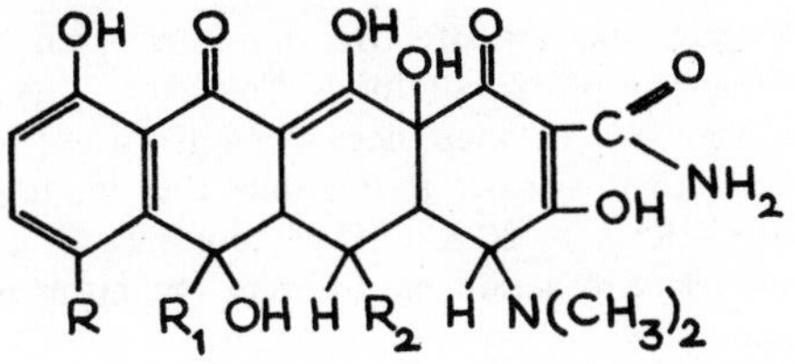

	R	R$_1$	R$_2$	Renal Clearance (ml/min)
Chlortetracycline	−Cl	−CH$_3$	−H	−
Oxytetracycline	−H	−CH$_3$	−OH	90
Tetracycline	−H	−CH$_3$	−H	65
Demeclocycline	−Cl	−H	−H	35
Methacycline	−H	=CH$_2$*	−OH	31
Doxycycline	−H	−CH$_3$*	−OH	16
Minocycline	−N(CH$_3$)$_2$	−H	−H	−

*There is no −OH at position 6 on methacycline and doxycycline.

been available since 1953. Demethylchlortetracycline (demeclocycline) is obtained by demethylation of chlortetracycline.

Chemistry

All of the tetracyclines have the basic structure shown above.

Free tetracyclines are crystalline amphoteric substances of low solubility. They are available as hydrochlorides which are more soluble (about 10% in water). Such solutions are acid and, with the exception of chlortetracycline, fairly stable. Chlortetracycline is very unstable in vitro, losing much of its activity in a few hours; for this reason it is not widely used clinically at present. Tetracyclines combine firmly with divalent metal ions, and this chelation can interfere with absorption and activity of the molecule. Tetracyclines fluoresce bright yellow in ultraviolet light of 3600 A.

Antimicrobial Activity

Tetracyclines are bacteriostatic for many gram-positive and gram-negative bacteria, including anaerobes, and strongly inhibitory for the growth of mycobacteria, rickettsiae, mycoplasmas and L forms, agents of the psittacosis-LGV-trachoma group (chlamydiae), and some protozoa, eg, amebas. Equal amounts of all tetracyclines in serum or tissues have approximately equal antimicrobial activity. Such differences in activity as may be claimed for individual tetracycline drugs are of small magnitude and no practical importance. However, great differences exist in the susceptibility of different strains of a given species of microorganisms to tetracyclines, and laboratory tests are therefore important in determining their usefulness in a given patient.

Tetracyclines are effective inhibitors of phosphorylation and of protein synthesis. The latter is assumed to be the basis of their chemotherapeutic efficacy. Tetracyclines appear to inhibit the binding of aminoacyl-tRNA to 30 S units of ribosomes. The basis of their selective action on different organisms is not understood.

Resistance

Susceptible microbial populations contain small numbers of mutants which are resistant to tetracyclines. The degree of resistance is small, usually only 2–6 times higher than that of the parent population. Among gram-negative bacterial species (especially pseudomonas, proteus, and coliforms), the selection of highly resistant types has already occurred, and tetracyclines have therefore lost some of their usefulness. Tetracycline resistance can be transmitted from one gram-negative species to another by resistance transfer factors (RTF, see Chapter 47). Resistance is increasing even among what were at first highly susceptible bacterial species (eg, pneumococci, hemophilus, streptococci, bacteroides). This is a consequence of the intense selection pressure exerted on microbial populations by the widespread use of the tetracycline drugs.

Absorption, Metabolism, & Excretion

Tetracyclines are absorbed somewhat irregularly from the gastrointestinal tract. Absorption is limited by the low solubility of the drugs, especially at alkaline pH and by chelation with Ca^{++} or Fe^{++}. A large proportion of an orally administered tetracycline remains in the gut lumen, modifies intestinal flora, and is excreted in the feces. Citrates and phosphates are often added to tetracyclines to enhance intestinal absorption. Specially formulated buffered tetracycline solutions can be administered intramuscularly or intravenously.

In the blood stream, 20–50% of absorbed tetracycline is bound to serum protein. With full systemic doses (2 gm/day), the levels of antimicrobially active tetracycline in serum reach 2–10 μg/ml. The drugs are distributed widely in tissues and body fluids, but the levels in the CNS, CSF, and joint fluids are only 3–10% of serum levels.

Tetracyclines are specifically deposited in growing bones and teeth, probably as a result of calcium binding.

Absorbed tetracyclines are excreted mainly in bile and urine. Concentrations in bile are 10 times higher than in serum; some of the drug excreted in bile is probably reabsorbed from the intestine and contributes to maintenance of serum levels. Up to 20% of the oral dose may be excreted in urine, probably by glomerular filtration, resulting in urine levels of 5–50 μg/ml or more. Up to 80% of the oral dose is excreted with feces.

Certain tetracyclines (demeclocycline, methacycline) are more slowly excreted than others and therefore can lead to higher blood levels with comparable doses and even to accumulation to toxic levels. Doxycycline is excreted even more slowly, so that the total daily dose is only 100–200 mg. Minocycline is somewhat better absorbed than other tetracyclines and slowly excreted.

Clinical Uses

Tetracyclines are the most typical "broad spectrum" antibiotics. They are effective against a variety of microorganisms, and for this reason are often used indiscriminately. There is no convincing evidence that any of the many formulations of tetracycline are therapeutically superior to tetracycline hydrochloride, although the slowly excreted members of the group may require less frequent administration and thus be more convenient. Indications and dosages will be given here for tetracycline hydrochloride only. For other tetracyclines, manufacturers' directions should be followed. (See list at end of chapter.)

Tetracyclines may be the drugs of choice in cholera or in infections with *Mycoplasma pneumoniae* or members of the psittacosis-LGV-trachoma group. They are useful in mixed bacterial infections related to the respiratory tract, especially sinusitis and bronchitis. They may be employed in many gram-positive and gram-negative bacterial infections (provided the organism is susceptible); in most rickettsial infections; and in amebiasis. They have been used in pneumonias and in urinary tract and skin infections, particularly acne.

A. Oral Dosage: The minimal effective oral dose for rapidly excreted tetracyclines, equivalent to tetracycline hydrochloride, is 0.25 gm 4 times daily for adults and 20 mg/kg/day for children. For severe systemic infections, a dose 2–3 times larger for at least 3–5 days is indicated. In acne, a dose of 0.25–0.5 gm daily for many months is popular.

The slowly excreted tetracyclines are less reliably absorbed, produce lower levels, and should probably not be employed in severe infections. The minimal effective daily dose is 600 mg for demeclocycline or methacycline, 100 mg for doxycycline, and 200 mg for minocycline. Tetracyclines chelate with divalent ions, eg, Ca^{++}, Mg^{++}, Al^{++}, and should therefore not be given with antacids containing them or with ferrous sulfate.

B. Parenteral Dosage: Several tetracyclines are available for intramuscular or intravenous injection in doses of 0.1–0.5 gm every 6–12 hours; 10–15 mg/kg/day can be used in children.

Adverse Reactions

Hypersensitivity reactions (drug fever, skin rashes) to tetracyclines appear to be uncommon. Most side-effects are due to direct toxicity of the drug or to alteration of microbial flora.

A. Gastrointestinal Side-Effects: Nausea, vomiting, and diarrhea are the commonest reasons for discontinuing tetracycline medication. During the first few days of administration they appear to be attributable to direct local irritation of the intestinal tract.

After a few days of oral use, tetracyclines tend to modify the normal flora. Although some coliform organisms are suppressed, pseudomonas, proteus, staphylococci, resistant coliform mutants, and candida become prominent. This can result in intestinal functional disturbances, in anal pruritus, vaginal or oral candidiasis, or even staphylococcal enterocolitis with shock and death.

Nausea, anorexia, and diarrhea can usually be controlled by administering the drug with food or carboxymethylcellulose, reducing drug dosage, or discontinuing the drug.

B. Bony Structures and Teeth: Tetracyclines are readily bound to calcium deposited in newly formed bone or teeth. When the drug is given during pregnancy it can be deposited in the fetal teeth, leading to fluorescence, discoloration, enamel dysplasia, deformity, or growth inhibition. If the drug is given to small children for long periods, similar changes can result.

C. Liver Toxicity: Tetracyclines can probably impair hepatic function, especially during pregnancy, in patients with preexisting hepatic insufficiency, and when high doses are given intravenously. Hepatic necrosis has been reported with daily doses of 4 gm IV or more.

D. Kidney Toxicity: Renal tubular acidosis and other forms of renal injury resulting in nitrogen retention have been attributed to the administration of outdated tetracycline preparations. This has not been documented for fresh preparations.

E. Local Tissue Toxicity: Intravenous injection can lead to venous thrombosis. Intramuscular injection produces painful local irritation which can lead to infiltration.

F. Photosensitization: Systemic tetracycline administration, especially of demeclocycline, can induce sensitivity to sunlight or ultraviolet light, particularly in blonds.

Medical & Social Implications of Overuse

The widespread use of tetracyclines for minor illnesses has led to the emergence of resistance even among highly susceptible species, eg, pneumococci and group A streptococci. The large-scale use of these drugs in hospitals has resulted in the selection of tetracycline-resistant organisms, particularly staphylococci and pseudomonas, as common superinfecting agents. In some measure tetracyclines (among other antibiotic drugs) must be credited with the rising incidence of mycotic infection in hospitalized, severely ill patients.

On the other hand, tetracyclines have been of great benefit not only for the control of existing infection but also for chemoprophylaxis in chronic bronchitis and bronchiectasis, keeping many persons well and at work.

Preparations Available

Tetracycline hydrochloride: (Various mfrs.)
Capsules, 50, 100, and 250 mg
Tablets, 250 mg
Syrup, 125 mg/5 ml, 60 and 480 ml
Drops, 100 mg/ml, 10 ml
Oral suspension, 250 mg/ml, 30 ml
Injectable (IM), 200 and 250 mg vials
Injectable (IV), 100, 250, and 500 mg ampules

Otic, 10 ml containing 50 mg/ml in propylene glycol with 5% benzocaine
Ointment, 30 mg/gm (3%), ½ and 1 oz
Ophthalmic powder, 25 mg/vial, 5 ml
Ophthalmic ointment (for otic use also), 10 mg/gm, 1/8 oz
Ophthalmic suspension, 1% in oil, 4 ml
Surgical powder, 200 mg/5 gm

Tetracycline buffered:
Phosphate complex:
Capsules, 100, 125, and 250 mg
Syrup, 125 mg/5 ml, 60 and 480 ml
Drops, 100 mg/ml, 10 ml
Glucosamine:
Capsules, 125 and 250 mg
Syrup, 125 mg/ml, 60 and 480 ml
Drops, 100 mg/ml, 10 ml
Citric acid and sodium citrate:
Syrup, 125 mg/5 ml, 60 and 480 ml
Drops, 100 mg/ml (cherry flavored), 10 ml
Potassium metaphosphate:
Syrup, 100 and 125 mg/5 ml, 60 ml and 16 oz

Tetracycline with lidocaine:
Hydrochloride, 100 mg for intramuscular injection
Phosphate complex, 100 and 250 mg for intramuscular injection

Chlortetracycline (Aureomycin):
Capsules, 50, 100, and 250 mg
Soluble tablets, 50 mg
Syrup, 125 mg/4 ml, 4 and 16 oz
Spersoids, 25 dose quantity containing 50 mg/3 gm dispersible powder
Injectable (IV), 500 mg ampules
Otic, 10 ml containing 50 mg in propylene glycol with 5% benzocaine
Ointment, 30 mg/gm (3%), ½ and 1 oz
Ophthalmic powder, 25 mg, 5 ml
Ophthalmic ointment, 10 mg/gm, 1/8 oz
Surgical powder, 200 mg/5 gm

Oxytetracycline (Terramycin):
Capsules, 125 and 250 mg
Tablets, 250 mg
Soluble tablets, 50 mg
Syrup, 125 mg/5 ml, 60 and 480 ml
Drops, 100 mg/ml (20 drops), 10 ml
Injectable (IM), 2 ml ampules and 2 ml Isoject ampules containing 50 and 125 mg/ml with 2% lidocaine; 50 mg/ml also available in 10 ml vials.
Injectable (IV), 250 and 500 mg
Aerosol, 500 mg in 75% propylene glycol, 10 ml
Nasal, 5 mg/5 ml with 0.25% deoxyephedrine hydrochloride

Ointment, 30 mg/gm with polymyxin B sulfate, 10,000 units/gm, ½ and 1 oz

Ophthalmic solution, 5 mg/ml, 5 ml

Ophthalmic ointment (for otic use also), 5 mg/gm plus polymyxin B sulfate, 10,000 units/gm, 1/8 oz

Otic, 5 ml containing 25 mg in propylene glycol plus polymyxin B sulfate, 50,000 units, and benzocaine, 250 mg

Topical powder, 1 oz shaker can containing 30 mg/gm plus polymyxin B sulfate, 10,000 units/gm

Vaginal suppositories, 100 mg with polymyxin B sulfate, 100,000 units; packages of 10

Demeclocycline (Declomycin):
Capsules, 150 mg
Tablets, 75, 150, and 300 mg

Suspension, 900 mg (75 mg/5 ml), 2 oz

Syrup, 75 mg/5 ml, 60 and 480 ml

Drops, 60 mg/ml (cherry flavored), 10 ml

Ointment, 5 mg/gm, 20 gm

Methacycline (Rondomycin):
Capsules, 150 and 300 mg
Syrup, 75 mg/5 ml

Doxycycline (Vibramycin):
Capsules, 50 and 100 mg
Dry powder for oral suspension, 25 mg/5 ml, 60 ml

Minocycline (Minocin):
Capsules, 100 mg

•   •   •

General References

Chloramphenicol

Scott, J.L., &. others: A controlled double-blind study of the hematologic toxicity of chloramphenicol. New England J Med 272:1137–1142, 1965.

Snyder, M.J., & T.E. Woodward: The clinical use of chloramphenicol. M Clin North America 54:1187–1197, 1970.

Wallerstein, R.O., & others: Statewide study of chloramphenicol therapy and fatal aplastic anemia. JAMA 208:2045–2050, 1969.

Erythromycin Group

Garrod, L.P.: The erythromycin group of antibiotics. Brit MJ 2:57–63, 1957.

Sabath, L.D., & others: Serum glutamic oxalacetic transaminase: False elevations during administration of erythromycin. New England J Med 279:1137–1139, 1968.

Tetracyclines

Kunin, C.M.: The tetracyclines. P Clin North America 15:43–56, 1968.

Ory, E.M.: The tetracyclines. M Clin North America 54:1173–1186, 1970.

Steigbigel, N.H., & others: Absorption and excretion of 5 tetracycline analogues in normal young men. Am J Med Sc 255:296–312, 1968.

Wallace, C.K., & others: Optimal antibiotic therapy in cholera. Bull World Health Organ 39:239–245, 1968.

51...

Aminoglycosides & Polymyxins

Aminoglycosides are a group of drugs sharing chemical, antimicrobial, pharmacologic, and toxic characteristics. At present, the group includes streptomycins, neomycin, kanamycin, viomycin, gentamicin, and related drugs. All inhibit protein synthesis by attaching to and inhibiting the function of the 30 S unit of bacterial ribosomes. All are much more active at alkaline pH than at acid pH.

STREPTOMYCINS

Streptomycin was isolated from a strain of *Streptomyces griseus* by Waksman and his associates in 1944. Dihydrostreptomycin can be produced by catalytic reduction of streptomycin- trihydrochloride and has also been isolated from strains of *Str humidus*. Both streptomycin compounds have similar chemical and identical antimicrobial properties. However, dihydrostreptomycin is significantly more ototoxic than streptomycin and has been largely abandoned.

Chemistry

Streptomycin is a triacidic base with the empirical formula $C_{21}H_{39}N_7O_{12}$. It consists of streptidine, streptose, and N-methyl-L-glucosamine. The latter 2 components are referred to as streptobiosamine (see formula below).

Several salts have been prepared from streptomycin, the sulfate being most widely used. Streptomycin sulfate is a white powder, quite soluble in water and insoluble in alcohol. Neutral solutions are stable for weeks at temperatures below 25° C. Streptomycin is more active at alkaline pH. It can be inactivated by hydroxylamine or cysteine.

Antimicrobial Activity

A number of mechanisms have been postulated to account for the antibacterial activity of streptomycin. Experimentally, streptomycin can inhibit an oxaloacetate-pyruvate condensation reaction carried out by some organisms; it can cause progressive breakdown of polysomes, inhibition of polypeptide synthesis, and misreading of the genetic message. This latter mechanism is currently believed to form the basis of the antibacterial action of aminoglycosides in vivo. Streptomycin effectively inhibits protein synthesis of bacteria. It binds to a surface protein of the 30 S subunit of bacterial ribosomes, distorts the "recognition region" of the ribosome, and causes a misreading of the mRNA message. This results in the insertion of improper amino acids and the synthesis of nonfunctional proteins. In streptomycin-dependent cells, misreading of the genetic message is a requirement for growth. In streptomycin-resistant cells, the specific protein which otherwise serves as a binding site for streptomycin is missing or altered.

Resistance

Streptomycin resistance occurs when a mutation alters or eliminates the binding site for the drug on the ribosome. Large microbial populations of all susceptible microorganisms contain resistant mutants. These tend to be selected out rapidly in the presence of streptomycin. A mutant may be 2–6 times or even 1000 times more resistant than the parent population. In

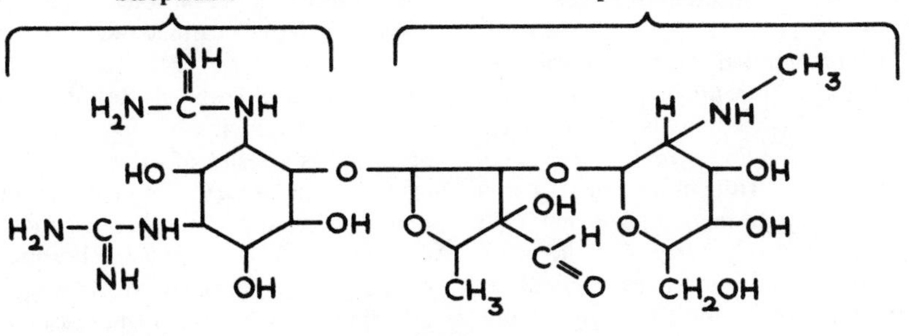

Streptidine   Streptobiosamine

Streptomycin

511

nontuberculous infections, daily treatment with streptomycin for 4—5 days results either in eradication of
the infecting agent or the emergence of resistant,
intractable variants. For this reason, if treatment is to
extend beyond 5 days, streptomycin is usually
employed in combination with another antimicrobial
drug. This is particularly important in mycobacterial
infections, where prolonged treatment is always required. Some streptomycin-resistant organisms can
adenylate or phosphorylate the drug.

Absorption, Metabolism, & Excretion

Streptomycin is not significantly absorbed from
the gastrointestinal tract, but exerts some antibacterial
effect in the bowel lumen until it is excreted in feces.
After intramuscular administration (it is rarely given
intravenously or subcutaneously), streptomycin is
readily absorbed from the injection site. Peak serum
concentrations are achieved in 1—2 hours, and detectable amounts may be present for 6—9 hours in serum
and even longer in tissues. With doses of 2 gm daily,
serum concentrations up to 20 μg/ml are achieved.

Streptomycin is widely distributed in body fluids
and tissues but does not penetrate to a significant
extent into the CNS, the CSF, or joint fluids unless
inflammation is present. Streptomycin penetrates
poorly into living cells and so is only slightly active
against intracellular (phagocytized) bacteria. This may
account in part for its inability to eradicate those
chronic infections in which a majority of organisms are
intracellular.

Streptomycin is excreted principally in the urine,
where the concentration may be 5—50 times higher
than in serum. Excretion is by glomerular filtration
and is unaffected by agents that block tubular secretion. In the presence of renal damage leading to nitrogen retention, the excretion of streptomycin is
impaired and cumulation to toxic levels can occur
rapidly with average doses.

Clinical Uses

**A. Tuberculosis and Other Mycobacterial Infec-
tions:** In pulmonary and other nondisseminated forms
of tuberculosis, streptomycin, 1 gm, is injected IM
twice weekly or daily for months as part of combined
therapy. (When used in the treatment of tuberculosis,
streptomycin is always combined with isoniazid, 5—10
mg/kg/day, or aminosalicylic acid [PAS], 10—14
gm/day [or both], for many months.) In acute tuberculous pneumonia, miliary dissemination, or meningitis
in children, up to 60 mg/kg/day IM should be administered initially in combination with isoniazid and
aminosalicylic acid (PAS). In meningitis, streptomycin,
25 mg dissolved in 10 ml saline, may be injected intrathecally.

B. Nontuberculous Infections: In systemic
infections (eg, plague), streptomycin, 2—4 gm daily
IM, is given in divided doses every 4—8 hours. A
second drug (eg, tetracycline) may also be required.

C. Combined Treatment: In certain infections,
penicillin plus an aminoglycoside may be required for

eradication of organisms even though in vitro the bacteria appear to be resistant to the aminoglycoside
alone. For example, in enterococcal endocarditis,
streptomycin, 1—2 gm IM daily, may be given in addition to penicillin, 24—120 gm IV daily (or ampicillin,
4—12 gm IV daily), to achieve bactericidal levels in
serum and clinical cure.

In certain *Streptococcus viridans* and other infections, the addition of streptomycin may also enhance
the bactericidal action of a penicillin. In tularemia and
plague, streptomycin may be combined with tetracyclines or chloramphenicol.

Adverse Reactions

A. Allergy: Fever, skin rashes, and other allergic
manifestations may result from hypersensitivity to
streptomycin. This occurs most frequently upon prolonged contact with the drug, either in patients who
receive a prolonged course of treatment (eg, for tuberculosis) or in medical personnel who handle the drug.
(Nurses preparing solutions should wear gloves.) Desensitization is occasionally successful.

B. Toxicity: Pain at the injection site is common
but usually not severe; it can be relieved by injecting
the drug with a local anesthetic (eg, procaine hydrochloride). The most serious toxic effect is disturbance
of vestibular function—vertigo and loss of balance. The
frequency and severity of this disturbance are proportionate to the age of the patient, the blood levels of
the drug, and the duration of administration. Vestibular dysfunction may follow a few weeks of unusually
high blood levels (eg, in individuals with impaired renal
function) or months of relatively low blood levels.
After the drug is discontinued, partial recovery frequently occurs. Because streptomycin can impair semicircular canal function, it has been used to treat
Ménière's disease (2—3 gm/day for 1—4 weeks).

With streptomycin, hearing loss is less frequent
than vestibular impairment. With dihydrostreptomycin, auditory impairment is frequent, severe, and
irreversible; for this reason, dihydrostreptomycin has
now been virtually abandoned. The concurrent or
sequential use of other aminoglycosides with streptomycin should be avoided to reduce the likelihood of
ototoxicity.

Streptomycin in high doses can also exert a
nephrotoxic effect. This is most often noted in individuals with preexisting kidney damage in whom streptomycin therapy with elevated blood levels tends to increase nitrogen retention. Experimentally, streptomycin can depress cardiac function.

General Medical Problems Resulting From Overuse

Streptomycin-resistant bacteria have become
prevalent as a result of the widespread use of the drug,
often in unnecessary combination with penicillin. Multiple drug resistance is frequent among bacteria in urinary tract infections, and the hospital transmission of
such organisms aggravates treatment problems. Primary
infection with streptomycin-resistant tubercle bacilli
occurs in up to 5% of cases of pulmonary tuberculosis
studied in the USA.

Preparations Available

Injectable (IM): Multiple dose vials containing 1 gm and 5 gm powder for reconstitution; solution containing 1 gm/2.5 ml and 5 gm/12.5 ml; disposable syringe containing 1 gm 2 ml

Syrup, 4 oz containing 50 mg/ml (Strycin)

THE KANAMYCIN-NEOMYCIN GROUP

These drugs constitute a chemically and biologically closely related group which combine a broad spectrum of antibacterial activity with significant nephrotoxicity and ototoxicity. **Neomycin** was isolated by Waksman in 1949 from *Streptomyces fradiae;* **kanamycin** was isolated by Umezawa in 1957 from *Streptomyces kanamyceticus.* Other members of the group are **framycetin** and **paromomycin.** All have very similar properties.

Chemistry

Each member of this group consists of several components in which amino sugars are coupled by means of glycoside linkages. Kanamycin, the most widely used representative of the group, has the formula $C_{18}H_{36}N_4O_{11}$ and consists of 3-D-glucosamine and 6-D-glucosamine linked to deoxystreptamine. Kanamycin sulfate is a white powder which is readily soluble in water and quite stable at 20° C.

Commercial neomycin is a mixture of 2 related compounds, neomycin B and C. (Neomycin A is not used.) Each contains diaminohexose linked to deoxystreptamine and D-ribose. Neomycin sulfate is a crystalline white substance readily soluble in water and insoluble in alcohol. Solutions are very stable at 20° C. Paromomycin consists of glucosamine and a disaccharide linked to an inositol derivative. All drugs of the group are more active at alkaline pH.

Antimicrobial Activity

Drugs of the neomycin group are bactericidal in concentrations of 1–10 µg/ml for many gram-positive and gram-negative bacteria and mycobacteria. Proteus organisms are often susceptible, but pseudomonas and streptococci are generally resistant. The mechanism of antibacterial action of the neomycin group appears to be similar to that of streptomycin, and they can substitute for streptomycin in streptomycin-dependent organisms.

Kanamycin A

Resistance

In susceptible bacterial populations, rare resistant mutants occur. Most of these are only 2–4 times more resistant than the parent population, but in the presence of the drug gradual selection leads to the emergence of highly resistant mutants. This has occurred particularly among staphylococci in the course of neomycin "prophylaxis" for intestinal surgery. These neomycin-resistant staphylococci have produced outbreaks of enterocolitis. Complete cross-resistance exists among members of the neomycin group, but there is little cross-resistance with gentamicin.

Absorption, Metabolism, & Excretion

Drugs of the neomycin group are not significantly absorbed from the gastrointestinal tract. After oral administration, the intestinal flora is suppressed or modified and the drug is excreted in the feces.

After parenteral injection (0.5 gm IM every 6–12 hours), serum levels may reach 5–10 µg/ml. The drugs are fairly widely distributed, but do not reach significant levels in the CSF or joint or pleural fluid unless injected locally. Excretion is mainly through glomerular filtration into the urine, where levels of 10–50 µg/ml may be reached. Some excretion also occurs in the bile. In the presence of renal insufficiency, drugs of the neomycin group may accumulate and rapidly reach toxic levels. To avoid this the dose or the frequency of injection must be greatly reduced.

Clinical Uses

At present kanamycin is the preferred drug of this group for parenteral administration because it is slightly less toxic than neomycin. The other members of the group are used only topically or orally.

A. Topical: Solutions containing 1–5 mg/ml are used on infected surfaces or injected into joints, the pleural cavity, tissue spaces, or abscess cavities where infection is present. The total amount of drug given in this fashion must be restricted because much of it can be absorbed, giving rise to systemic toxicity. Ointments containing 1–5 mg/gm are applied to infected skin lesions or in the nares for suppression of staphylococci. Some ointments contain polymyxin and bacitracin in addition to neomycin. Aerosols of kanamycin, 1 mg/ml, have been used in lower respiratory tract infections.

B. Oral: For preoperative reduction of gut flora, 1 gm every 4–6 hours is given for 2–3 days before surgery. In hepatic coma the coliform flora can be suppressed for prolonged periods by giving 1 gm every 6–8 hours, together with reduced protein intake, thus reducing ammonia intoxication. Paromomycin (Humatin), 1 gm every 6 hours orally for 2 weeks, has been effective in intestinal amebiasis. All drugs of the neomycin group can suppress intestinal infection with enteropathogenic *Escherichia coli* and other bacteria, but they are not effective in the treatment of shigella or salmonella infections.

C. Parenteral: Kanamycin, 0.5 gm every 6–12 hours IM (15 mg/kg/day), is effective in the treatment of bacteremia caused by gram-negative enteric organisms. It is sometimes combined with a cephalosporin drug or tetracycline. Particularly serious infections of the urinary tract with proteus, enterobacter, or other "difficult" organisms may at times be treated similarly.

Adverse Reactions

All members of the neomycin group are nephro- and ototoxic. Kanamycin is preferred at present because it is somewhat better tolerated.

A. Nephrotoxicity: Proteinuria and renal function impairment with nitrogen retention occur commonly, particularly in patients with preexisting kidney damage. This must be monitored (eg, by means of creatinine clearance determinations) and the dose or frequency of injection adjusted as required (see Chapter 48). In general, these toxic effects are reversible when treatment is discontinued.

B. Ototoxicity: The auditory portion of the eighth nerve can be selectively and irreversibly damaged by members of the neomycin group and also by gentamicin. The development of deafness is proportionate to the dosage and the duration of administration, but it can occur unpredictably even after short-term administration. Loss of perception of high frequencies as shown on audiograms may be a warning sign. Ototoxicity is a particular risk in patients with impaired kidney function and consequent accumulation of the drug.

C. CNS Toxicity: The sudden absorption of large amounts of neomycin drugs can lead to respiratory arrest. This has occurred particularly following the instillation of 3–5 gm of neomycin or kanamycin into the peritoneal cavity after bowel surgery. Neostigmine is a specific antidote.

D. Hypersensitivity: The topical application of neomycins to the skin or eyes can result in allergic reactions.

Preparations Available

Neomycin sulfate: (Various mfrs.)
Tablets, 500 mg (equivalent to 350 mg base)
Solution, 125 mg/5 ml
Injectable (IM): Powder, 0.5 gm
Topical solution: Powder, 5 and 10 gm
Ointment, ½, 1, 4, 8, and 16 oz containing 5 mg/gm
Ophthalmic ointment, 1/8 oz containing 5 mg/gm (equivalent to 3.5 mg base)

Kanamycin sulfate (Kantrex):
Capsules, 500 mg
Injectable (IM): 500 mg in 2 ml; 1 gm in 3 ml

Paromomycin (Humatin):
Capsules, 250 mg (sulfate)
Syrup (pediatric), 60 ml containing 125 mg/5 ml (root beer flavored)

Framycetin: Not commercially available.

GENTAMICIN

Gentamicin is an aminoglycoside antibiotic complex isolated from *Micromonospora purpurea.* It is effective against both gram-positive and gram-negative organisms, and many of its properties resemble those of kanamycin and neomycin.

Chemistry

The 3 active antibiotic components of gentamicin C have molecular weights between 450 and 475 and differ principally in methyl group content. The proposed structural formula is shown below. The sulfate is used for intramuscular injection. It is soluble in water, and such solutions are stable for weeks. The antibacterial activity of the drug is much greater at alkaline than at acid pH.

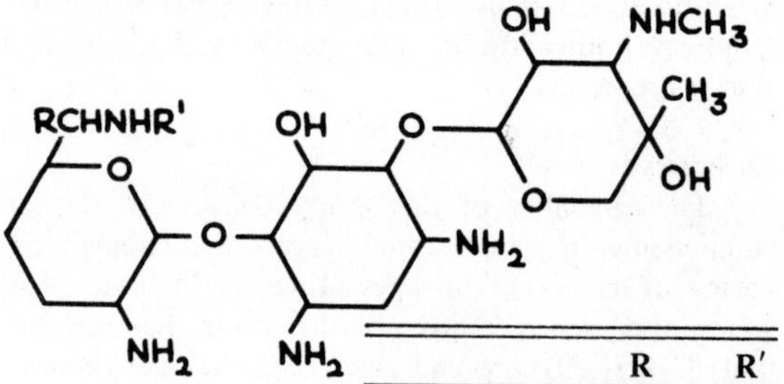

	R	R'
Gentamicin C_1	CH_3	CH_3
Gentamicin C_2	CH_3	H
Gentamicin C_{1a}	H	H

Antimicrobial Activity

In concentrations of 0.5–5 μg/ml, gentamicin is rapidly bactericidal for many gram-positive and gram-negative bacteria. Activity is enhanced at alkaline pH. Gentamicin sulfate, 10 μg/ml, inhibits in vitro most strains of staphylococci, coliform organisms (*E coli,* klebsiella, enterobacter), and *Pseudomonas aeruginosa,* and many strains of proteus and serratia. Bactericidal action is probably due to inhibition of protein synthesis, perhaps by causing a misreading of the mRNA message at the 30 S unit of the ribosome such as is postulated for other aminoglycosides.

The simultaneous use of carbenicillin and gentamicin may result in synergistic enhancement and activity against some strains of *Ps aeruginosa,* and may permit use of smaller doses of gentamicin. However, a penicillin and gentamicin cannot be used in vitro.

Resistance

Enterococci are resistant to gentamicin. Occasional resistant strains have been found among susceptible species, but exposure of bacterial populations in vitro does not generally result in the rapid emergence of resistance except in hospital environments. Gentamicin-resistant bacteria appear to have altered ribosomal proteins. Microorganisms made resistant to gentamicin are usually cross-resistant to kanamycin-neomycin, but the reverse is not the case. Some bacteria inactivate gentamicin by phosphorylation, and this property can be transmitted by resistance transfer factors (RTF) from one bacterial species to another.

Absorption, Metabolism, & Excretion

The drug is not significantly absorbed after oral administration. After intramuscular injection, gentamicin is rapidly absorbed and widely distributed in tissues. About 25–30% of the drug in plasma is protein-bound. With the usual doses, serum levels reach 3–5 µg/ml in persons with normal renal function, but there can be marked cumulation of drug in the presence of azotemia. The drug is excreted largely by glomerular filtration through the kidneys into the urine. Concentrations in urine may be 10–100 times higher than in serum. Gentamicin does not penetrate well into the CNS or the CSF and intrathecal injection is necessary to achieve high CSF concentration. Gentamicin may have to be instilled into joints or abscess cavities, because diffusion into these spaces from the serum is inadequate.

Clinical Uses

A. Intramuscular: Gentamicin is employed in severe infections caused by gram-negative bacteria which are likely, or proved, to be resistant to other less toxic drugs. Included are sepsis, infected burns, pneumonia, and other serious infections due to coliform organisms, klebsiella-enterobacter, proteus, pseudomonas, and serratia. In these disorders, gentamicin is employed in full systemic doses, 2–3 mg/kg/day IM in 3 equal doses for 7–10 days. In some life-threatening infections, 5–8 mg/kg/day has been given for 1–3 days. Renal, auditory, and vestibular functions should be monitored, particularly in patients with preexisting nitrogen retention, which predisposes to drug cumulation and toxic effects. In renal failure, the interval between doses must be lengthened, eg, 1 mg/kg gentamicin can be injected 2–3 times weekly (see Chapter 48).

In urinary tract infections caused by these organisms, 0.8–1.2 mg/kg/day is injected IM in 2 or 3 equal divided doses for 10 days or more.

B. Topical: Creams, ointments, or solutions containing 0.1–0.3% gentamicin sulfate have been used for the treatment of infected burns, wounds, or skin lesions. Ten mg can be injected subconjunctivally.

C. Intrathecal: Meningitis caused by gram-negative bacteria has been treated by the intrathecal injection of 0.1–1 mg gentamicin sulfate per day, with equivocal results. Epidural abscess has been instilled with gentamicin 20 mg/day for 10 days.

Adverse Reactions

Like all aminoglycosides, gentamicin is nephrotoxic and ototoxic, particularly under conditions which lead to excessive blood or tissue levels for prolonged periods. It can produce neuromuscular blockade.

A. Nephrotoxicity: With recommended doses and in the absence of preexisting renal failure, nephrotox-

icity is said to be rare. It should be monitored by means of repeated creatinine clearance determinations. If there is evidence of reduced creatinine clearance or increased nitrogen retention, the dose should be reduced and the interval between injections lengthened. It is believed that nephrotoxic effects of gentamicin are reversible if the drug is discontinued early.

B. Ototoxicity: With recommended doses and in the absence of drug cumulation, it is estimated that 2–3% of patients develop signs of ototoxicity due to gentamicin. This manifests itself mainly as vestibular dysfunction, perhaps attributable to destruction of hair cells. However, loss of hearing also occurs and has occasionally been complete and irreversible.

C. Hypersensitivity: Experience has been insufficient to indicate the incidence of hypersensitivity to be expected with gentamicin.

Preparations Available

Gentamicin sulfate injection (Garamycin), 40 mg/ml

Gentamicin sulfate cream, 0.1%, and ointment, 0.1%

SPECTINOMYCIN

Spectinomycin is an aminocyclitol antibiotic (related to aminoglycosides) dispensed as the dihydrochloride pentahydrate for intramuscular injection. While active in vitro against many gram-positive and gram-negative organisms, spectinomycin is proposed only as an alternative treatment for gonorrhea in patients who might be hypersensitive to penicillin or whose gonococci are resistant to penicillin. About 10% of gonococci may be resistant to spectinomycin, but there is no cross-resistance with other drugs.

Spectinomycin is rapidly absorbed after intramuscular injection. A dose of 2 gm injected into each buttock just once (total, 4 gm) results in serum levels of 100 µg/ml or more and is said to result in 85–90% cure of gonorrhea. There is pain at the injection site and occasionally fever and nausea. Nephrotoxicity and anemia have been observed rarely.

THE POLYMYXIN GROUP

The polymyxins are a group of basic polypeptides selectively active against gram-negative bacilli. Polymyxins A, B, C, D, and E were derived from a spore-forming gram-positive bacillus (*Bacillus polymyxa, B aerosporus*) in 1947. All but polymyxins B and E have been discarded because of excessive nephrotoxicity. Colistin, introduced in 1950, is identical with polymyxin E.

Chemistry

All polymyxins are cationic, basic polypeptides with molecular weights of about 1400. All contain the fatty acid D-6-methyloctan-1-oic acid and the amino acids L-threonine and L-diaminobutyric acid. In addition, polymyxins B and E contain L-leucine; B contains D-phenylalanine; and E contains D-leucine. The sulfates of polymyxins are freely soluble in water and very stable. Methanesulfonate (sulfo-methyl) complexes can be prepared which slowly release the active peptide. One μg of pure polymyxin B sulfate equals 10 units. The relationship between mg and units appears to be variable in the case of methanesulfonate complexes.

Antimicrobial Activity

The activity of polymyxin B sulfate is identical with that of polymyxin E (colistin) sulfate. Similarly, the methanesulfonate complexes of polymyxins B and E have the same activity. However, it is grossly misleading to compare quantitatively the activity of the sulfate of one polymyxin with the methanesulfonate of another. Sulfates are used in disk tests and do not reflect methanesulfonate activity.

Polymyxins are active mainly against gramnegative bacilli, particularly pseudomonas and coliform organisms. They are strongly bactericidal in concentrations of $1-5$ $\mu g/ml$. They act by attaching to the cell membranes of bacteria (perhaps forming a monomolecular layer) and disrupting the osmotic properties of the membrane. This results in leakage of macromolecules and death of the cell. This action is inhibited by cations. Polymyxins may also disturb the exterior layer of the bacterial cell wall.

Resistance

Proteus species, gram-positive organisms, and neisseriae are highly resistant. This is probably due to the impermeability of the outer cell wall structures to polymyxins. In susceptible bacterial populations, resistant mutants are rare. There is complete crossresistance between polymyxin B and polymyxin E (colistin).

Absorption, Metabolism, & Excretion

Polymyxins are not absorbed from the gastrointestinal tract. After oral administration the drug exerts antibacterial effects in the gut lumen and is then excreted in the feces.

Parenterally injected polymyxins are strongly protein-bound. With doses of 2.5 mg/kg/day, blood levels rarely exceed $1-2$ $\mu g/ml$. Tissue concentrations are even lower. Polymyxins pass the placenta but do not reach the CNS or CSF unless injected intrathecally. They do not reach joint fluids or ocular tissues unless injected locally. Polymyxins are also strongly bound by cell debris, acid phospholipids, and purulent exudates. They do not penetrate into cells, and phagocytized or intracellular bacteria are therefore unaffected.

Excretion is mainly in the urine, where concentrations of $25-300$ $\mu g/ml$ may be reached during prolonged administration. Excretion is impaired in renal insufficiency, and toxic levels may be reached quickly unless the dose is restricted. The methanesulfonate complexes are excreted more rapidly than the sulfates; colistimethate gives higher urine levels than other polymyxins.

Clinical Uses

Polymyxins are drugs of choice for the treatment of infections caused by pseudomonas or coliform bacteria resistant to other antimicrobial drugs. Polymyxin treatment is limited by the restricted distribution and penetration of the drug, by its toxicity, and by its binding to many tissue components.

A. Topical: Solutions containing 1 mg/ml of polymyxin B or E sulfate can be applied to wounds, burns, sinuses, and other surfaces infected with *Pseudomonas aeruginosa* or other resistant microorganisms. Similar solutions (up to a total dose of 2.5 mg/kg/day) can be injected intrapleurally or intraperitoneally. Solutions of $1-10$ mg/ml are inhaled as aerosols in pseudomonas infections of the bronchi and lungs. Up to 20 mg of polymyxin B sulfate may be injected subconjunctivally in pseudomonas infections of the eye. Ointments containing 0.5 mg/gm of polymyxin B sulfate in mixture with bacitracin or neomycin (or both) are commonly applied to infected skin lesions. Solutions containing polymyxin B, 20 mg/liter, and neomycin, 40 mg/liter, can be employed as antiseptic for continuous irrigation of the urinary bladder through a 3-way catheter in a closed sterile system. This can delay bacterial contamination of the drainage system.

B. Intrathecal: In pseudomonas meningitis the intrathecal injection of polymyxin B or E sulfate, $2-10$ mg in saline daily for $2-3$ days, and then every other day for $2-3$ weeks, is essential for cure because penetration into the CNS of systemically administered polymyxin is negligible. Polymyxin methanesulfonates should never be given intrathecally.

C. Intramuscular: The intramuscular injection of polymyxin B sulfate or polymyxin E sulfate (colistin sulfate) is painful and requires the simultaneous administration of a local anesthetic. For this reason, the methanesulfonate complex, which sometimes includes a local anesthetic and slowly releases active drug after intramuscular injection, is preferred. The total systemic dose can be $2.5-5$ mg/kg/day. It is most commonly indicated in urinary tract infections with pseudomonas or with enterobacter or other coliforms resistant to less toxic drugs. Salmonella infections do not respond to polymyxins in spite of in vitro susceptibility.

D. Intravenous: The slow absorption of the methanesulfonate complexes diminishes their usefulness in serious, rapidly progressive infection, and the intravenous injection of polymyxin B sulfate is preferable. The intravenous injection by slow drip of 2.5 mg/kg/day of polymyxin B sulfate in 5% dextrose in water is indicated in pseudomonas bacteremia or peritonitis (eg, after peritoneal dialysis). When renal function is impaired, the drug may be administered in full doses once every $3-5$ days. Hemodialysis does not remove polymyxins rapidly.

E. Oral: Polymyxins are not absorbed from the gut. Oral doses of 20 mg/kg/day have been used to suppress shigella in bacillary dysentery, and other gram-negative members of the intestinal flora.

Adverse Reactions

The general toxicity of polymyxin B and polymyxin E limit both the dose and the duration of therapy. The 2 compounds have similar toxicities, and the observed differences are attributable largely to differences between the sulfate and methanesulfonate compounds. However, colistimethate appears to be the least nephrotoxic of all currently available polymyxins. The sulfates produce intense local pain on intramuscular injection and are rapidly absorbed, whereas the methanesulfonates produce (with little pain) a local depot from which absorption proceeds more slowly. The principal side-effects are neurotoxicity and nephrotoxicity. Hypersensitivity appears to be very rare. Very high blood levels ($> 30 \mu g/ml$) of any polymyxin can cause respiratory arrest. Respiratory paralysis caused by polymyxins can be reversed by $CaCl_2$.

A. Neurotoxic Effects: Adequate systemic concentrations of any polymyxin can cause paresthesias (circumoral and stocking or glove distribution), dizziness, flushing, and incoordination. All of these disappear promptly when the drug has been discontinued and excreted. With very high levels, paralysis may occur.

B. Nephrotoxic Effects: Some degree of proteinuria, hematuria, or cylindruria commonly accompanies the administration of polymyxin B or E and is evidence of tubular injury. These urinary signs usually disappear soon after the drug is discontinued. Nitrogen retention may occur, particularly with doses in excess of 2 mg/kg/day. In individuals with preexisting renal disease, nitrogen retention must be monitored (most accurately by endogenous creatinine clearance determinations) and the dose of polymyxin or colistimethate adjusted. Accidental overdosage may result in renal failure, neuromuscular paralysis, and even death.

Laboratory

The large molecules of the polymyxins diffuse poorly through agar. Consequently, disk tests reveal very narrow zones of inhibition even with fully susceptible microorganisms. Colistin disks contain sulfate, not methanesulfonate.

Medical Aspects of Overuse

Polymyxins are becoming more important because of the increasing numbers of patients infected with pseudomonas and enterobacter. These are often hospitalized patients with other diseases and impaired renal function who therefore require careful, individualized adjustments of a polymyxin regimen.

Preparations Available
Polymyxin B sulfate (Aerosporin):
Tablets, 50 mg
Soluble tablets, 25 mg (to make solution)
Injectable (IM), 20 ml vials containing 50 mg (500 thousand units)
Colistimethate (Coly-Mycin):
Injectable (IM), 2 ml vials containing 150 mg colistin and 2 mg dibucaine. Also available without dibucaine.
Pediatric, bottle of 300 mg colistin sulfate (25 mg/5 ml)

• • •

General References

Cox, C.E.: Gentamicin. M Clin North America 54:1305–1315, 1970.

Finland, M. (editor): International symposium on gentamicin: October 30–31, 1968. J Infect Dis 119:335–540, 1969.

Hoeprich, P.H.: The polymyxins. M Clin North America 54:1257–1265, 1970.

Holt, R.J., & R.L. Newman: Gentamicin in urinary infections of children. Arch Dis Childhood 43:329–333, 1968.

Jawetz, E.: Polymyxins, colistin, bacitracin, ristocetin, and vancomycin. P Clin North America 15:85–94, 1968.

Mann, C.H. (editor): Kanamycin: Appraisal after 8 years of clinical application. Ann New York Acad Sc 132:771–1090, 1966.

Ryan, K.J., & others: Colistimethate toxicity: Report of a fatal case. JAMA 207:1099–2101, 1969.

Vinnicombe, J., & T.A. Stamey: The relative nephrotoxicity of polymyxin B sulfate, sodium sulfomethylcolistin and neomycin sulfate. Invest Urol 6:505–519, 1969.

Weinstein, L.: Streptomycin. Pages 1242–1252 in: *The Pharmacological Basis of Therapeutics*, 4th ed. Goodman, L.S., & A. Gilman (editors). Macmillan, 1970.

52...

Antituberculosis Drugs

Streptomycin was the first antimicrobial drug to exhibit striking action against tubercle bacilli. It remains an important agent in the management of severe tuberculosis and has also found a place in other forms of antibiotic therapy (see Table 48–1 and discussion in Chapter 51). The other important antituberculosis drugs in use at the present time—isoniazid, aminosalicylic acid, and ethambutol—are of importance only in tuberculosis. Several agents which are drugs of second choice in the treatment of tuberculosis are mentioned here only briefly.

Singular problems exist in the treatment of tuberculosis and related mycobacterial infections. The infections tend to be exceedingly chronic, but may also give rise to hyperacute, lethal complications. The organisms are frequently intracellular, exhibit long periods of metabolic inactivity, and tend to develop resistance to any drug. All these points contribute to the complexity of antituberculosis therapy.

In extensive pulmonary or other organ tuberculosis, miliary tuberculosis, and tuberculous meningitis, treatment is usually started with 3 drugs (isoniazid + streptomycin + either aminosalicylic acid or ethambutol). With improvement parenteral streptomycin can be omitted and treatment continued with the oral drugs for a total of 24 months or longer.

STREPTOMYCIN

The pharmacologic features of streptomycin have been discussed on p 509. It is assumed that the mechanism of action of streptomycin against mycobacteria is the same as that against other microorganisms. Most tubercle bacilli are inhibited, and may be killed, by streptomycin, 1–10 μg/ml, in vitro. Most "atypical" mycobacteria are resistant to streptomycin in pharmacologic concentrations. All large populations of tubercle bacilli contain some streptomycin-resistant mutants. On the average, 1 in 10^8 to 1 in 10^{10} tubercle bacilli can be expected to be resistant to streptomycin at serum levels of 10–100 μg/ml. Certain of these mutants tend to survive the in vivo exposure to therapeutic concentrations of streptomycin. This results in "treatment resistance" of clinical tuberculosis, and may induce primary streptomycin-resistant

new infections in contacts. Such a sequence may occur within 2–4 months of treatment with streptomycin alone. This is a prime reason for employing streptomycin in combination with another drug effective against tubercle bacilli. Combined treatment can markedly delay the emergence of streptomycin-resistant mutants.

Streptomycin exerts its action mainly on extracellular tubercle bacilli. Only about 10% of the drug penetrates into cells which harbor intracellular organisms. Thus, even if the entire microbial population were streptomycin-susceptible, at any one moment a large proportion of the tubercle bacilli would be unaffected by streptomycin. Treatment for many months is therefore required.

Streptomycin remains one of the "big 3" drugs used in tuberculosis treatment. It is employed principally in individuals with severe, possibly life-threatening forms of tuberculosis, particularly tuberculous meningitis, miliary dissemination, and extensive, active pulmonary or renal involvement. The usual dosage is 1 gm IM daily for adults (30 mg/kg/day for children) for weeks or months, followed by 1 gm IM 2–3 times weekly for several months. Other drugs are always given simultaneously.

Intrathecal injection of streptomycin in tuberculous meningitis has been largely abandoned.

The toxicity for the eighth nerve of streptomycin injected intramuscularly for many weeks manifests itself principally as dysfunction of the labyrinth, resulting in inability to maintain equilibrium and in deafness. The latter is often permanent, but some compensation for the former often occurs. Dihydrostreptomycin has the same antituberculosis action as streptomycin, but it produces irreversible deafness more frequently. Therefore, its use has been abandoned.

Dosage forms of streptomycin are listed in Chapter 51.

AMINOSALICYLIC ACID (PAS)

Among several derivatives of salicylic and benzoic acids, p-aminosalicylic acid has the most marked effect on tubercle bacilli.

Chemistry

The structural formula of PAS reveals its close similarity to *p*-aminobenzoic acid (PABA) and to the sulfonamides (see Chapter 53).

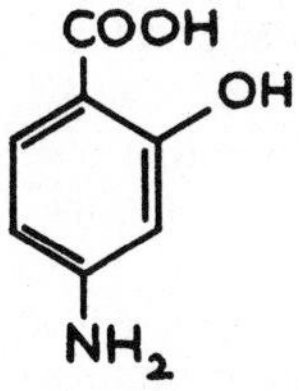

Aminosalicylic acid (PAS)

PAS is a white crystalline powder only slightly soluble in water and rapidly destroyed by heat. The sodium salt is freely soluble in water and relatively stable at room temperature.

Antimycobacterial Activity

Most bacteria are not affected by PAS. Tubercle bacilli are usually inhibited in vitro by PAS, 1–5 μg/ml, but "atypical" mycobacteria are resistant. In susceptible mycobacterial populations, resistant mutants occur and tend to emerge in vitro and in vivo during exposure to PAS. The simultaneous use of a second drug with antimycobacterial activity tends to delay this emergence of resistance.

It is probable that the mode of action of PAS against tubercle bacilli is analogous to the mode of action of sulfonamides against other bacteria. Probably there is competition between PAS and PABA for the active center of an enzyme involved in converting PABA to dihydropteroic acid. The receptors for PABA attachment must be quite specific, because PAS is ineffective against most bacteria whereas sulfonamides are ineffective against tubercle bacilli.

Absorption, Metabolism, & Excretion

PAS is readily absorbed from the gastrointestinal tract. Average daily doses (8–12 gm) tend to give blood levels of 10 μg/ml or more. The drug is widely distributed in body fluids and tissues except the CSF. PAS is rapidly excreted in the urine, in part as active PAS and in part as the acetylated compound and other metabolic products. Very high concentrations of PAS are reached in the urine. To avoid crystalluria, the urine must be kept alkaline.

Clinical Uses

Aminosalicylic acid is employed together with isoniazid or streptomycin, or both, in the long-term treatment of pulmonary tuberculosis with cavitation, or other serious forms of tuberculosis. The dosage for adults is 8–12 gm daily orally in divided doses with meals. The drug is rarely used in children. The dosage in children is 300 mg/kg/day.

Adverse Reactions

A. Direct Toxicity: Gastrointestinal symptoms often accompany full doses of PAS. Anorexia, nausea, diarrhea, and epigastric pain and burning may all be diminished by giving PAS with meals and with antacids. Peptic ulceration and hemorrhage may occur. Kidney or liver damage, thyroid gland injury (goiter with or without myxedema), and metabolic acidosis are rare.

B. Allergic Reactions: Drug fever, joint pains, skin rashes, granulocytopenia, and a variety of neurologic symptoms—all probably attributable to hypersensitivity—often occur from the third to eighth weeks of PAS therapy, making it necessary to stop PAS administration temporarily or permanently.

Preparations Available

Enteric-coated tablets, 500 mg
Powder, 100 gm, ¼ lb, and 1 lb

ISONIAZID (INH)

Isoniazid, introduced in 1952, is the most active tuberculostatic drug.

Chemistry

Isoniazid is the hydrazide of isonicotinic acid, often called INH. It is a white crystalline powder, freely soluble in water. The structural similarity to pyridoxine is shown below.

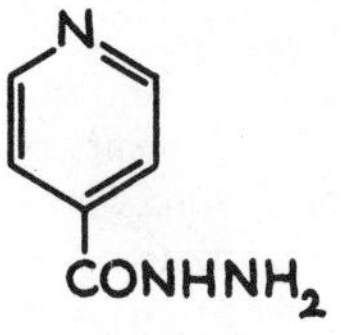

Isoniazid

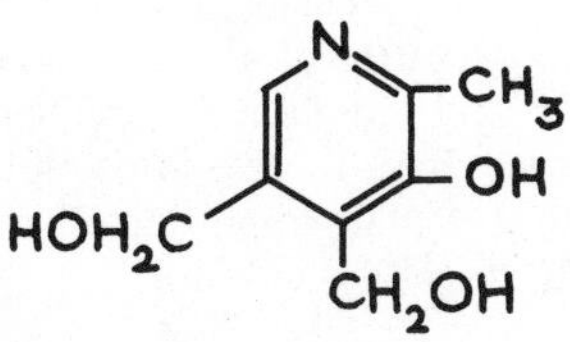

Pyridoxine

Antimycobacterial Activity

In vitro, INH inhibits most tubercle bacilli in a concentration of 0.2 μg/ml or less and is bactericidal for actively growing tubercle bacilli. However, INH has no significant effect on atypical mycobacteria. INH reaches similar concentrations both inside and outside animal cells and thus is able to act on intracellular mycobacteria as well as extracellular ones. Resistant mutants occur in susceptible bacterial populations, and tend to be selected out both in vitro and in vivo in the presence of INH. There is no cross-resistance between INH, streptomycin, PAS, and ethambutol. The simultaneous use of any 2 of these drugs markedly delays the emergence of resistance to one of them. Some isoniazid-resistant tubercle bacilli possess greatly reduced virulence for guinea pigs, but it is probable that they remain virulent for humans.

The mechanism of action of INH is not known. INH apparently combines with an enzyme that is peculiar to INH-susceptible strains of *Mycobacterium tuberculosis,* displacing a pigment precursor molecule and leading to a variety of disorders in cellular metabolism. INH exerts competitive antagonism in pyridoxine-catalyzed reactions in *Escherichia coli.* INH and pyridoxine are structural analogues. However, this mechanism is not involved in the antituberculosis action. The administration of large doses of pyridoxine to patients receiving INH does not interfere with the tuberculostatic action of INH.

Absorption, Metabolism, & Excretion

INH is readily absorbed from the gastrointestinal tract. The administration of 8 mg/kg/day to children results in blood levels of about 2 μg/ml or more. INH diffuses readily into all body fluids and tissues, including the CNS and CSF. Its intracellular and extracellular levels are the same.

The metabolism—particularly the acetylation—of INH is under genetic control. Two groups of people can be recognized: the "slow" and the "rapid" inactivators of the drug, through acetylation. The "slow" inactivator appears to have an autosomal homozygous recessive hereditary trait, whereas the allele controlling the dominant character (rapid inactivation) shows intermediate dominance. Six hours after ingestion of 4 mg/kg of INH, plasma concentrations of more than 0.8 μg/ml are found in persons who acetylate INH slowly, whereas plasma concentrations are 0.2 μg/ml or less in persons who acetylate INH rapidly. "Slow" inactivators tend to develop polyneuritis more often than "rapid" inactivators (see Toxicity, below).

INH is excreted mainly in the urine—partly as unchanged drug, partly as the acetylated form, and partly as other conjugates. The proportion of unchanged, free INH in the urine is higher in the "slow" inactivators; the proportion of acetylated form is higher in the "rapid" inactivators.

Clinical Uses

Isoniazid is probably the most widely useful drug in tuberculosis. In active, clinically manifest disease, it is given in conjunction with streptomycin, aminosalicylic acid, or both. A dose of 8–10 mg/kg/day orally or more (20 mg/kg/day in small children) is employed in tuberculous meningitis, miliary dissemination, or widespread active pulmonary tuberculosis. Following initial improvement, the dosage is usually reduced to 5–7 mg/kg/day orally (10 mg/kg/day in small children).

Children converting from tuberculin negative to positive skin tests may be given INH, 10 mg/kg/day (maximum 300 mg/day), for 1 year as prophylaxis against the 5–15% risk of meningitis or miliary dissemination. For tuberculin converting adults, similar prophylaxis with INH, 4–8 mg/kg/day, is recommended by some. For prophylaxis, INH is given as the sole drug.

INH is usually given by mouth, but can be injected parenterally in the same dosage.

Adverse Reactions

The incidence and severity of untoward reactions to INH are related to dosage and duration of administration.

A. Allergic Reactions: Fever, skin rashes, and hepatitis are occasionally seen.

B. Direct Toxicity: The most common and important toxic effects are on the peripheral and central nervous systems. These have been attributed to a relative pyridoxine deficiency, perhaps resulting from competition of INH with pyridoxal phosphate for an enzyme (apotryptophanase). These toxic reactions include peripheral neuritis, insomnia, restlessness, muscle twitching, urinary retention, and even convulsions and psychotic episodes. Most of these complications can be prevented by the administration of pyridoxine, 100 mg daily.

Preparations Available

Tablets, 50 and 100 mg
Syrup, 50 mg/5 ml
Injectable (IM), 100 mg/ml, 10 ml vials

ETHAMBUTOL

This is a synthetic, water-soluble, heat-stable compound, the D isomer of the structure shown below, dispensed as the hydrochloride.

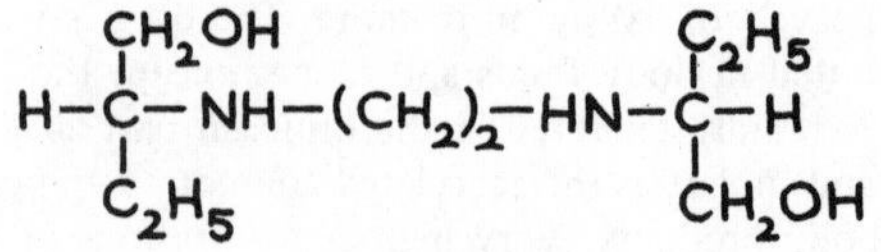

$$H-\underset{\underset{C_2H_5}{|}}{\overset{\overset{CH_2OH}{|}}{C}}-NH-(CH_2)_2-HN-\underset{\underset{CH_2OH}{|}}{\overset{\overset{C_2H_5}{|}}{C}}-H$$

Ethambutol

Many strains of *Mycobacterium tuberculosis* are inhibited in vitro by ethambutol, 1–5 μg/ml. The mechanism of action is not known.

Ethambutol is well absorbed from the gut. Following ingestion of 25 mg/kg, a blood level peak of 2–5 μg/ml is reached in 2–4 hours. About 20% of drug is excreted in feces and 50% in urine, in unchanged form. Excretion is delayed in renal failure.

About 15% of absorbed drug is metabolized by oxidation and conversion to a dicarboxylic acid. In meningitis, ethambutol appears in the CSF.

Resistance to ethambutol emerges fairly rapidly among mycobacteria when the drug is used alone. Therefore, ethambutol is best given in combination with other antituberculosis drugs, most commonly INH. In combined therapy, ethambutol effectively replaces PAS and is better tolerated than PAS by most patients.

Ethambutol, 15 mg/kg, is usually given as a single daily dose in combination with INH. At times, the dose is 25 mg/kg/day.

Hypersensitivity to ethambutol occurs infrequently. The commonest side-effects are visual disturbances: reduction in visual acuity, optic neuritis, and perhaps retinal damage occurs in some patients on full doses given for several months. Most of these changes apparently regress when ethambutol is discontinued. However, period visual acuity testing is mandatory during treatment.

Ethambutol (Myambutol) is available as tablets of 100 mg and 400 mg.

ALTERNATIVE DRUGS IN TUBERCULOSIS TREATMENT

The drugs of first choice in tuberculosis in 1970 are undoubtedly isoniazid, streptomycin, and aminosalicylic acid, both because of their antimicrobial efficacy and their relative clinical safety. The alternative drugs listed below are usually considered only (1) in the case of drug resistance to the drugs of first choice, which occurs with increasing frequency; (2) in case of failure of clinical response to conventional therapy; and (3) when expert guidance is available to deal with the toxic side-effects. In most of the second choice drugs listed (alphabetically) below, the dosage, emergence of resistance, and long-term toxicity have not been fully established.

Capreomycin

Capreomycin (not commercially available) is a peptide antibiotic obtained from *Streptomyces capreolus*. Daily injection of 1 gm IM results in blood levels of 10 μg/ml or more. Such concentrations in vitro are inhibitory for several mycobacteria. Capreomycin (0.5–1.5 gm/day) can perhaps take the place of streptomycin in combined antituberculosis therapy. The most serious toxicity is for the kidney, resulting in nitrogen retention, and for the eighth nerve, resulting in deafness and vestibular disturbances.

Cycloserine

Cycloserine is an antibiotic analogue of D-alanine. Oral doses of 250 mg 3 times daily result in blood levels of 15–25 μg/ml. This is sufficient to inhibit many strains of tubercle bacilli. The most serious toxic

reactions are various CNS dysfunctions and psychotic reactions.

Cycloserine (Seromycin) is available as 250 mg capsules, alone or in combination with isoniazid, 150 mg. The dose is 0.5–1 gm/day in tuberculosis. Cycloserine has been used in urinary tract infections in doses of 15–20 mg/kg/day.

Cycloserine is discussed further in Chapter 56.

Ethionamide

This yellow crystalline substance is stable and almost insoluble in water. It is a close chemical relative of isoniazid.

In spite of this similarity, there is no cross-resistance between isoniazid and ethionamide. Most tubercle bacilli are inhibited in vitro by ethionamide, 2.5 μg/ml, or less. Many photochromogenic mycobacteria are also inhibited by ethionamide, 10 μg/ml.

Ethionamide

Such concentrations in plasma and tissues are achieved by daily oral doses of 1 gm. This dosage is effective in the clinical treatment of tuberculosis, but is poorly tolerated because of the intense gastric irritation and neurologic symptoms it causes. A dose of 0.5 gm orally per day is better tolerated but not very effective. Resistance to ethionamide develops rapidly in vitro and in vivo. Consequently, this drug can be used only in combination with other antituberculosis drugs.

Ethionamide (Trecator) is available in 250 mg tablets.

Pyrazinamide (PZA)

This relative of nicotinamide is stable and sparingly soluble in water.

Pyrazinamide (PZA)

At neutral pH it is inactive in vitro, but at pH 5.0 it strongly inhibits the growth of tubercle bacilli within cells in concentrations of 15 μg/ml. Such concentrations are achieved by daily oral doses of 20–30 mg/kg, usually given as 0.5 gm 4–6 times daily. Pyrazinamide is well absorbed from the gastrointestinal tract and widely distributed in body tissues. Tubercle bacilli develop resistance to pyrazinamide fairly readily, but there is no cross-resistance with isoniazid. Satisfactory clinical effects can be achieved with this drug, but toxicity is marked. The most serious toxic effect is the hepatic injury that frequently results. Pyrazinamide should be considered only as part of a combined drug regimen in patients harboring tubercle bacilli resistant to first choice drugs.

Pyrazinamide (Aldinamide) is available (in hospitals only) as 0.5 gm tablets.

Rifampin

Rifampin is a semisynthetic derivative of rifamycin, an antibiotic produced by *Streptomyces mediterranei*. It is active in vitro against some gram-positive and gram-negative cocci, some enteric bacteria, mycobacteria, chlamydiae, and poxviruses. While many meningococci and mycobacteria are inhibited by less than 1 μg/ml, highly resistant mutants occur in all microbial populations in a frequency of 1 in 10^7 or greater. The prolonged administration of rifampin as a single drug permits the emergence of these highly resistant organisms. There is no cross-resistance to other antimicrobial drugs.

Rifampin binds strongly to DNA-dependent RNA polymerase and thus inhibits RNA synthesis in bacteria and chlamydiae. It blocks a late stage in the assembly of poxviruses, perhaps interfering with envelope formation.

Rifampin is well absorbed after oral administration, widely distributed in tissues, excreted mainly through the liver and to a lesser extent into the urine. With oral doses of 600 mg, serum levels exceed 5 μg/ml for 4–6 hours and urine levels may be 10–100 times higher.

Rifampin (Rifadin, Rimactane) is available in 300 mg capsules. In tuberculosis, a single oral dose of 450–900 mg (usually 600 mg) daily is administered together with ethambutol or another antituberculosis drug in order to delay the emergence of rifampin-resistant mycobacteria. A similar regimen may apply to atypical mycobacteria.

An oral dose of 600 mg once or twice daily can eliminate a majority of meningococci from carriers. Unfortunately, some highly resistant meningococcal strains are selected out by this procedure. In urinary tract infections and in chronic bronchitis, the applicability of rifampin is more doubtful.

Rifampin imparts an orange color to urine and sweat, which is harmless. Occasional adverse effects include rashes, thrombocytopenia, and transient elevations of SGOT, alkaline phosphatase, and serum bilirubin.

Caution: The indiscriminate use of rifampin for minor infections may favor the widespread selection of rifampin-resistant mycobacteria and thus deprive the drug of most of its usefulness.

Viomycin

This antibiotic is produced by certain streptomyces organisms. It is an aminoglycoside and a strong base, dispensed as neutral sulfate which is very soluble in water. Most strains of tubercle bacilli are inhibited in vitro by viomycin, 1–10 μg/ml. Such concentrations can be achieved by the injection of 1 gm IM every 12 hours every third day. Tubercle bacilli resistant to viomycin emerge fairly rapidly. There is also some cross-resistance with streptomycin, kanamycin, and capreomycin. Therefore, viomycin—if used at all—must be used in combination with other drugs to delay the emergence of resistance. The most serious toxic side-effects are damage to the kidney and to the eighth nerve, resulting in loss of equilibrium and deafness. Toxic effects are more serious than with streptomycin.

Viomycin (Vinactane, Viocin) is available in vials containing 1 gm and 5 gm of the sulfate.

Other Antimycobacterial Drugs

Kanamycin and tetracyclines have been employed in combined therapy of tuberculosis. These drugs can inhibit tubercle bacilli in comcentrations which may be achieved in vivo. However, they are much less effective than the drugs of first choice.

• • •

General References

Curry, F.J.: Prophylactic effect of isoniazid in young tuberculin reactors. New England J Med 277:562–567, 1967.

Daniels, T.M.: Rifampin: A major new chemotherapeutic agent for the treatment of tuberculosis. Editorial. New England J Med 280:615–616, 1969.

Dans, P.E., & others: Rifampin: Absorption and excretion in normal young men. Am J Med Sc 259:120–132, 1970.

Deal, W.B., & E. Sanders: Rifampin in treatment of meningococcal carriers. New England J Med 281:641–645, 1969.

Eickhoff, T.C.: Studies of resistance to rifampin in meningococci. J Infect Dis 123:414–420, 1971.

Mitchell, R.S.: Control of tuberculosis. New England J Med 276:842–848, 905–911, 1967.

Place, V.A., & others: Ethambutol in tuberculous meningitis. Am Rev Resp Dis 99:783–785, 1969.

Pyle, M.M.: Ethambutol and viomycin. M Clin North America 54:1317–1327, 1970.

Vall-Spinosa, A., & others: Rifampin in the treatment of drug-resistant *M tuberculosis* infections. New England J Med 283:616–621, 1970.

53...

Sulfonamides & Sulfones

SULFONAMIDES

A red dye, prontosil, synthesized in Germany by Klarer and Mietzsch in 1932, was ineffective against bacteria in vitro; but Domagk reported in 1935 that it was strikingly active in vivo against hemolytic streptococcal and other infections. This was due to the conversion in the body of prontosil to sulfanilamide, the active drug. The sulfonamide molecule was chemically altered by the attachment of many different radicals, and there has been a proliferation of active compounds. Perhaps 150 different sulfonamides have been marketed at one time or another, the modifications being designed principally to achieve greater antibacterial activity, a wider antibacterial spectrum, greater solubility, or more prolonged action. In spite of the advent of the antibiotic drugs, the sulfonamides are among the most widely used antimicrobial agents in the world today, chiefly because of the low cost and their relative efficacy in some common bacterial diseases.

Chemistry

The sulfonamides are a group of compounds whose basic formula and relationship to PABA are shown below.

All have the same nucleus to which various R— radicals in the amido group (SO_2NH_2) have been attached or in which various substitutions of the amino group (NH_2) are made. These changes produce compounds with varying physical, chemical, pharmacologic, and antibacterial properties. In general, the sulfonamides are white, odorless, bitter tasting crystalline powders which are much more soluble at alkaline than at acid pH. In a mixture of sulfonamide drugs, each component drug exhibits its own solubility. Therefore, a mixture may be much more soluble, in terms of total sulfonamide present, than one drug used alone. This is the reason for the use of trisulfapyrimidines, a preparation that permits 3 times higher dosage than a single drug for comparable solubility in urine.

Most sulfonamides can be prepared as sodium salts which are moderately soluble, and these are used for intravenous administration. Such solutions are highly alkaline and not very stable, and may precipitate out of solution with polyionic electrolytes (eg, lactate-chloride-carbonate). Certain sulfonamide molecules are designed for low solubility (eg, succinylsulfathiazole, phthalylsulfathiazole) so that they will stay in the lumen of the bowel for long periods.

Antimicrobial Activity

Different sulfonamides may show quantitative but not necessarily qualitative differences in activity. All can inhibit both gram-positive and gram-negative bacteria, actinomyces, nocardia, the chlamydiae of trachoma and LGV, and certain protozoa. In practice, sulfonamides tend to inhibit gram-negative coliform bacteria with the exception of pseudomonas and proteus; they may inhibit some shigellae, gram-positive cocci, and neisseriae. They are especially useful in the treatment of urinary tract infections (first attack), nocardiosis, toxoplasmosis, and trachoma.

The action of sulfonamides is bacteriostatic and is reversible by removal of the drug or in the presence of an excess of para-aminobenzoic acid (PABA). The mode of action of the sulfonamides is a good example of **competitive inhibition**, which was discussed in Chapter 47. In brief, susceptible microorganisms require extracellular PABA in order to form folic acid, an essential step in the production of purines. Sulfon-

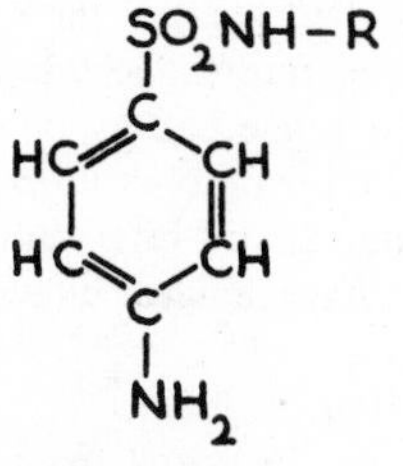

$$SO_2NH-R$$

Sulfonamide
prototype

[R = H in the case of sulfanilamide.]

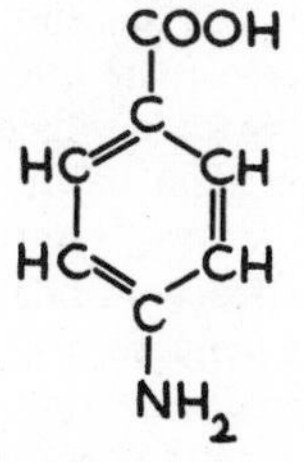

$$COOH$$

Para-aminobenzoic acid
(PABA)

amides can enter into the reaction in place of PABA, compete for the enzyme involved, and form nonfunctional analogues of folic acid. As a result, further growth of the microorganisms is prevented. For a given microorganism and a given sulfonamide, the ratio of the inhibitory concentration of drug(s) to varying amounts of PABA is virtually constant. This S/PABA ratio is an index of drug activity and varies from about 30/1 to 2000/1.

Trimethoprim, a trimethoxybenzylpyrimidine, inhibits the dihydrofolic acid reductase of bacteria and some protozoa far more efficiently than the same enzyme of mammalian cells. Pyrimethamine, another benzylpyrimidine, inhibits the dihydrofolic acid reductase of protozoa more than that of mammalian cells. Dihydrofolic acid reductases are enzymes which convert dihydrofolic acid to tetrahydrofolic acid, a stage leading to the synthesis of purines and ultimately to DNA. Trimethoprim or pyrimethamine, given together with sulfonamides, produce sequential blocking in this metabolic sequence, resulting in a marked enhancement (synergism) of the activity of sulfonamides (see Chapter 47).

Pyrimethamine

Trimethoprim

Resistance

Animal cells (and some bacteria) are unable to synthesize folic acid but depend upon exogenous sources and for this reason are not susceptible to sulfonamide action. Other cells which produce a large excess of PABA are resistant to sulfonamides, and still others may actually destroy sulfonamides. Sulfonamide resistant mutants occur in most susceptible bacterial populations and tend to emerge under suitable selection pressure. Thus, the widespread therapeutic use of sulfonamides against gonorrhea has resulted in the establishment of sulfonamide resistant strains

throughout the world. The widespread use of sulfonamides against beta-hemolytic streptococci similarly aided the emergence of resistant strains. Most recently, sulfonamide resistant meningococci have appeared in military—and have spread to civilian—populations. Other types of microorganisms—eg, many coliform organisms—are also commonly resistant. It should be specifically mentioned that rickettsiae not only are not inhibited by sulfonamides but are actually stimulated in their growth.

Absorption, Metabolism, & Excretion

Sulfonamides are usually given orally. They are rapidly absorbed from the stomach and small intestine and distributed widely to tissues and body fluids (including CNS and CSF), placenta, and fetus. Absorbed sulfonamides become bound to serum proteins to an extent varying from 20% to over 90%. A varying proportion also becomes acetylated or inactivated by other metabolic pathways. Chemical determinations performed on serum may measure free (active) sulfonamide, the acetylated (inactive) sulfonamide, or the total of both. In order to be therapeutically effective after systemic administration, a sulfonamide must generally achieve a concentration of 8–12 mg/100 ml of blood. Peak blood levels generally occur 2–3 hours after oral intake.

Soluble sulfonamides are excreted mainly by glomerular filtration into the urine. Different compounds exhibit different degrees of reabsorption in the tubules. A portion of the drug in the urine is acetylated, but enough active drug remains for effective treatment of infections of the urinary tract (usually 10–20 times the concentration present in the blood).

Sodium salts of sulfonamides are employed for parenteral administration because of their greater solubility. Their distribution and excretion are similar to those of the orally administered drugs.

The "insoluble" sulfonamides (eg, succinylsulfathiazole, phthalylsulfathiazole) are given orally, absorbed only slightly in the intestinal tract, and are excreted largely in the feces. Their action is exerted mainly on the intestinal flora.

"Long-acting" sulfonamides, eg, sulfamethoxypyridazine (Kynex, Midicel), sulfanilamidomethoxypyrimidine (sulfameter) and sulfadimethoxine (Madribon), are rapidly absorbed after oral intake and are distributed widely, but urinary excretion—especially of the free form—is very slow. This results in prolonged drug levels in serum. The slow renal excretion is due in part to the high protein binding (more than 85%) and in part to the extensive tubular reabsorption of the free (unacetylated) drug. These drugs are often inadvisable because instances of severe toxicity have resulted from their use.

Sulfonamides of "intermediate action," eg, sulfamethoxazole, have no clear indication or advantage.

Laboratory Studies

In order to grow bacteria from specimens obtained from patients receiving sulfonamides, culture media must contain an excess of PABA (5 mg/100 ml) to overcome the inhibitory effect of the sulfonamide carried in the specimen. This is particularly important in blood cultures.

Bacterial susceptibility testing with sulfonamide containing disks is generally unreliable and unsatisfactory because traces of PABA may be present in the medium or because uneven distribution of the bacterial inoculum gravely prejudices the results. Reliable susceptibility testing must be performed in well defined liquid media which are completely free of PABA, contain all nutrients required for fastidious microorganisms (eg, meningococci), and permit the use of a moderately small bacterial inoculum.

Clinical Uses

A. Topical: In general, the application of sulfonamides to the skin, in wounds, or on mucous membranes is undesirable because of their low activity and high risk of allergic sensitization. (An exception to the rule against topical application of sulfonamides may be the use of sodium sulfacetamide solution [30%] or ointment [10%] to the conjunctivas.) Oral administration of the "insoluble" sulfonamides, 8–15 gm daily, results in a topical effect—temporary inhibition of the intestinal microbial flora—which is of value in preparing the bowel for surgery; it must be timed so that the lowest microbial levels coincide with the time of the operation (usually on the fifth to seventh day after administration). Mafenide acetate (Sulfamylon) cream is a sulfonamide topically applied to burned skin surfaces. It has been effective in reducing burn sepsis but has led to an increase of burn infections by fungi and resistant bacteria.

Salicylazosulfapyridine has been suggested as a treatment for ulcerative colitis or enteritis, but there is no objective support for this claim.

B. Oral: The highly soluble and rapidly excreted sulfonamides (eg, sulfadiazine, sulfamerazine, sulfisoxazole) are given in initial doses of 2–4 gm (40 mg/kg) followed by a maintenance dose of 0.5–1 gm (15 mg/kg) every 4–6 hours. This regimen is indicated in systemic infections and can also be applied to urinary tract infections. In the latter, sulfisoxazole is often preferred because of its high solubility in urine. The urine should be kept alkaline. Alternatively, a mixture of several sulfonamides (in the total doses given above) can be used (eg, trisulfapyrimidines). After an initial attack of urinary tract infection has been treated with sulfonamides, resistant organisms often prevail. Therefore, in relapses, other drugs must be used. The slowly excreted sulfonamides (sulfamethoxypyridazine, sulfadimethoxine, etc) can be given in daily doses of 0.5–1 gm (10 mg/kg) for the treatment of minor infections (eg, sinusitis, otitis) or for prolonged maintenance therapy.

In protozoal infections, soluble sulfonamides are administered in combination with other agents. Thus, in toxoplasmosis or leishmaniasis, sulfonamides in full systemic doses are combined with pyrimethamine, 50 mg/day. In malaria, sulfonamides and trimethoprim are given together. In nocardiosis, sulfonamides may be given with cycloserine.

C. Intravenous: Sodium salts of many sulfonamides are available for parenteral injection, but because of their marked alkalinity are best injected intravenously (not intramuscularly) in 5% dextrose in water. Intravenous sulfonamides are generally reserved for comatose patients (most commonly patients with meningitis) or patients who are otherwise unable to take medication by mouth.

D. Pyrimethamine and Trimethoprim: Pyrimethamine is the more toxic drug, and is employed in combination with sulfonamides as a treatment of choice for toxoplasmosis. Trimethoprim plus sulfonamides have been used in bacterial urinary tract infections, brucellosis, cholera, and other bacterial infections, and in malaria. Resistance to this combined therapy (inducing a sequential block) emerges very slowly among bacteria or protozoa. Supplemental folates may have to be administered with such combined therapy of falciparum malaria in order to combat folic acid deficiency.

The daily oral dose often includes 300–400 mg of trimethoprim plus 5 times that amount of a sulfonamide. The daily oral dose of pyrimethamine is often 25–50 mg in combination with full doses of a sulfonamide.

Adverse Reactions

The sulfonamides can produce a wide variety of side-effects which are due partly to allergy and partly to direct toxicity, and which must be considered whenever unexplained symptoms or signs occur in a patient who may have received these drugs. Up to 5% of patients may exhibit such reactions. The overall incidence of side-effects is higher with the slowly excreted "long-acting" sulfonamides than with the rapidly excreted ones.

The commonest side-effects are fever, skin rashes, photosensitivity, urticaria; nausea, vomiting, or diarrhea; and difficulties referable to the urinary tract (see below). Others include stomatitis, conjunctivitis, arthritis, hematopoietic disturbances (see below), hepatitis, exfoliative dermatitis, polyarteritis nodosa, Stevens-Johnson syndrome, psychosis, and many more.

A. Urinary Tract Disturbances: Sulfonamides may precipitate in urine, especially at neutral or acid pH, producing crystalluria, hematuria, or even obstruction. This is best prevented by using the most soluble sulfonamides (sulfisoxazole, trisulfapyrimidines), keeping the urine pH alkaline (5–15 gm sodium bicarbonate daily), forcing fluids, and performing urinalysis every 3–5 days.

Sulfonamides have also been implicated in various types of nephrosis and in allergic nephritis.

B. Hematopoietic Disturbances: Sulfonamides can produce anemia (hemolytic or aplastic), granulocytopenia, thrombocytopenia, or leukemoid reactions. In order to prevent these reactions or to be able to withdraw the drug before the reaction has advanced to a severe or life-threatening stage, it is important to check the white blood count and hemoglobin level every 3–5 days. Sulfonamides cause hemolytic reactions especially in patients whose erythrocytes are deficient in glucose-6-phosphate dehydrogenase.

Medical & Social Aspects

Sulfonamides can be made and distributed cheaply and are thus among the principal antimicrobial agents available in many developing areas of the world. They continue to be useful for the treatment of such widespread disorders as urinary tract infections and trachoma, but the emergence of drug resistance has impaired their usefulness in streptococcal, gonococcal, meningococcal, shigella, and other infections. Topical use (skin) on a vast scale has contributed heavily to the sensitization of a significant part of the population.

Preparations Available

"Insoluble" sulfonamides:
  Succinylsulfathiazole (Sulfasuxidine):
    Tablets, 0.5 gm
    Suspension, 0.5 gm/5 ml
  Phthalylsulfathiazole (Sulfathalidine):
    Tablets, 0.5 gm
    Suspension, 1 gm/5 ml

"Highly soluble" sulfonamides:
  Sulfadiazine:
    Tablets, 250, 300, and 500 mg
    Suspension, 0.5 gm/5 ml
    Cream, 5%, 1 oz
    Ointment, 5%, 1 oz
    Ophthalmic ointment, 5%, 1/8 oz
    Lozenges, 200 and 300 mg
    Injectable (IV only), 10 ml ampules
      containing 5 and 25% of sodium
      salt
    Suppositories, 0.6 gm
  Sulfamerazine:
    Tablets, 0.5 gm
  Sulfisoxazole (Gantrisin; various mfrs.)
    Tablets, 0.5 gm
    Syrup, 0.5 gm/5 ml (chocolate flavored)
    Pediatric suspension, 0.5 gm/5 ml
    Injectable (IV), 0.4 gm/ml, 10 ml
    Vaginal cream, 10%
  Trisulfapyrimidines: (Various mfrs.)
    Sulfadiazine, sulfamerazine, and sulfamethazine, 0.167 gm each
  Sodium sulfacetamide (Sodium Sulamyd):
    Ophthalmic ointment, 10%, 1/8 oz
    Ophthalmic solution, 5 and 15 ml of
      30%; 5 and 15 ml of 10% (with
      methylcellulose)

Long-acting sulfonamides:
  Sulfadimethoxine (Madribon):
    Tablets, 500 mg
    Chewable tablets, 250 mg
    Suspension, 250 mg/5 ml, 4 and 16 oz

    Pediatric drops, 250 mg/ml, in 10 ml
      dropper bottle
  Sulfamethoxypyridazine (Kynex, Midicel):
    Tablets, 500 mg
    Suspension (Kynex Acetyl), 250 mg/5
      ml, 4 and 16 oz
  Sulfamethoxazole (Gantanol):
    Tablets, 500 mg
    Suspension, 10%, 500 mg/5 ml, 16 oz
  Trimethoprim (Syraprim): Not available in
    USA.
  Pyrimethamine (Daraprim):
    Tablets, 25 mg

SULFONES USED IN THE TREATMENT OF LEPROSY

A number of drugs closely related to the sulfonamides have been used effectively in the long-term treatment of leprosy. Some are also employed in malaria. The clinical manifestations of both lepromatous and tuberculoid leprosy can often be suppressed by treatment extending over several years.

Absorption, Metabolism, & Excretion

All of the sulfones are well absorbed from the intestinal tract, are distributed widely in all tissues, and tend to be retained in skin, muscle, liver, and kidney. Skin involved by leprosy contains 10 times more drug than normal skin. Sulfones are excreted into the bile and reabsorbed by the intestine. Consequently, blood levels are prolonged. Excretion into the urine is variable and occurs mostly as a glucuronic acid conjugate. Some persons acetylate sulfones slowly, others rapidly. This may require dosage adjustments.

Adverse Reactions

The sulfones may cause any of the side-effects listed above for sulfonamides. Anorexia, nausea, and vomiting are common. Hemolysis, methemoglobinemia, or agranulocytosis may occur.

Clinical Uses

Diaminodiphenylsulfone is the most widely used and least expensive drug. It is given orally, beginning with a dosage of 25 mg twice weekly and gradually increasing to 100 mg 3–4 times weekly and eventually to 300 mg twice weekly.

Sulfoxone sodium is given orally in corresponding dosage.

Solapsone, a complex substituted derivative of DDS, is given initially in a dosage of 0.5 gm 3 times daily orally. The dose is then gradually increased until a total daily dose of 6–10 gm is reached.

Other classes of drugs are used uncommonly. An ethyl mercaptan (Ditophal) may be applied to the skin. Thiosemicarbazones (eg, amithiozone, Tibione) permit the rapid emergence of resistance if used alone. Therefore, if administered, they are given with a sulfone.

Preparations Available

Diaminodiphenylsulfone (DDS, dapsone, Avlosulfon):
  Tablets, 100 mg
Sulfoxone sodium (Diasone):
  Enteric-coated tablets containing 165 mg of a DDS derivative (equivalent to 50 mg of DDS)

Solapsone (Sulphetrone):
  Tablets, 500 mg
  Granules for preparation of injection
  Injectable (deeply subcut or IM), 500 mg/ml, 5 ml ampules

•   •   •

General References

Feldman, H.A.: Toxoplasmosis. New England J Med 279:1370, 1431–1437, 1968.

Modell, W.: Malaria. Science 162:1346–1352, 1968.

Weinstein, L., Madoff, M.A., & C.M. Samet: The sulfonamides. New England J Med 263:900–907, 952–956, 1960.

54...

Specialized Drugs Against
Gram-Positive Bacteria

BACITRACIN

Bacitracin is a complex material obtained from a special strain of *Bacillus subtilis* in 1943. It is active against gram-positive microorganisms. Because of its marked toxicity when used systemically, it is now generally limited to topical use.

Chemistry

Bacitracin consists of a group of polypeptides which are highly water soluble. The material is stable in the dry form or when incorporated into a petrolatum. The unit of activity is defined as the equivalent of 26 μg of a Food and Drug Administration (USA) standard.

Antibacterial Activity

Bacitracin is most active against gram-positive bacteria, including β-lactamase producing staphylococci, in concentrations of 0.1–20 unit/ml. Resistant organisms are rare in susceptible populations, and clinical resistance, if it occurs, emerges slowly. There is no cross-resistance between bacitracin and other antimicrobial drugs.

Bacitracin inhibits cell wall formation but its mode of action is not identical with that of the penicillins. Bacitracin probably interferes with the final dephosphorylation in cycling the phospholipid carrier which transfers mucopeptide to the growing cell wall. Bacitracin binds to the cell membrane and changes its permeability.

Absorption, Metabolism, & Excretion

Like other peptide antibiotics of high molecular weight, bacitracin is not well absorbed from the gut, from skin, wounds, or mucous membrane surfaces, from pleura, or from synovia. Topical application thus results in local effects without significant systemic toxicity. After intramuscular injection bacitracin is fairly well absorbed, widely distributed in the body, and excreted by glomerular filtration into the urine.

Clinical Uses

Because of its systemic toxicity, bacitracin is now used mainly for topical treatment. Bacitracin, 500 units/gm in an ointment base (often combined with polymyxin or neomycin), is useful for the suppression of mixed bacterial flora in surface lesions of the skin, in wounds, or on mucous membranes. Solutions of bacitracin containing 100–200 units/ml in saline can be employed for instillation into joints, wounds, or the pleural cavity—often in conjunction with other drugs given systemically. Rarely, bacitracin, 1000 units/kg/day, is injected IM into small children with bacterial pneumonia.

Adverse Reactions

Bacitracin is markedly nephrotoxic, producing proteinuria, hematuria, and nitrogen retention. Therefore, systemic use has been virtually abandoned. Topical application only rarely causes hypersensitivity reactions (eg, skin rashes) or produces significant systemic toxicity.

Preparations Available

Ointment, 500 units/gm, 15, 30, 120 gm
Sterile powder, 10,000 units/vial and 50,000 units/vial
Ophthalmic ointment, 500 units/gm, 1/8 oz

VANCOMYCIN

Vancomycin is an antibiotic produced by *Streptomyces orientalis,* purified in 1958. It is active against gram-positive bacteria, particularly staphylococci.

Chemistry

Vancomycin hydrochloride is a crystalline material of high molecular weight (3300). It is soluble in water and very stable. The structural formula has not been established.

Antibacterial Activity

Vancomycin is bactericidal for gram-positive bacteria in concentrations of 0.5–3 μg/ml. Most pathogenic staphylococci are killed by 10 μg/ml or less. Resistant mutants are rare in susceptible populations, and clinical resistance emerges very slowly. There is no cross-resistance with other known antibiotics.

The mechanism of action involves inhibition of cell wall mucopeptide synthesis but is different from that of the penicillins. Vancomycin inhibits the utilization of disaccharide(-pentapeptide)-P-phospholipid. Cell membrane function is also damaged.

Absorption, Metabolism, & Excretion

Vancomycin is not absorbed from the intestinal tract and can be given orally only for the treatment of staphylococcal enterocolitis. Systemic doses must be administered intravenously because intramuscular injection is very painful. After IV injection of 0.5 gm, blood levels of 10 μg/ml are reached in 5 minutes and maintained for 1–2 hours. The drug is widely distributed in the body. Excretion is mainly through the kidneys into the urine. In the presence of renal insufficiency, striking accumulation may occur and may have serious toxic consequences.

Clinical Uses

The only indication for the use of vancomycin is serious staphylococcal infection or enterococcal endocarditis not responding to other treatment. For staphylococcal enterocolitis, 3–4 gm are given daily by mouth. For staphylococcal septicemia 0.5 gm is injected IV in 20–30 minutes every 6–8 hours (20–40 mg/kg/day for children).

Adverse Reactions

A. **Allergic Reactions:** Skin rashes and anaphylaxis have been observed infrequently.

B. **Direct Toxicity:** Vancomycin is highly irritating to tissue. Intramuscular injection is very painful. Thrombophlebitis and chills and fever are common following intravenous injection. Nephrotoxicity and ototoxicity are such that vancomycin is used only in those serious staphylococcal sepsis patients who fail to respond to, or cannot be given, the penicillins.

Preparations Available (Vancocin)

Injectable (IV), 10 ml ampules containing 500 mg

LINCOMYCIN & CLINDAMYCIN

Lincomycin is an antibiotic elaborated by *Streptomyces lincolnensis*. Clindamycin is a chlorine-substituted derivative of lincomycin. Both drugs have antimicrobial activity similar to that of erythromycin, but they are chemically quite distinct from erythromycin.

Antibacterial Activity

Many gram-positive cocci are inhibited by lincomycins, 0.5–5 μg/ml. Enterococci, hemophilus, neisseriae, and mycoplasma are usually resistant (in contrast to erythromycin). While lincomycins have little or no action on most gram-negative bacteria, bacteroides are often susceptible. Lincomycins inhibit protein synthesis, perhaps by blocking aminoacyl translocation on the bacterial ribosome. Resistance to lincomycin has been encountered among streptococci, pneumo-

cocci, and staphylococci. There is some cross-resistance between lincomycins and erythromycins.

Absorption, Metabolism, & Excretion

Oral doses of lincomycin, 0.5 gm every 6 hours, are readily absorbed from the gut if taken away from meals, and yield serum concentrations of 2–5 μg/ml. Similar concentrations are obtained with clindamycin, 0.15 gm every 6 hours orally. Lincomycin (but not clindamycin) can be given intramuscularly or intravenously to achieve somewhat higher levels. Lincomycins are widely distributed in the body but do not appear in the CNS in significant concentrations. Excretion is mainly through the liver, bile, and urine.

Clinical Uses

Lincomycin, 0.5 gm every 6 hours, or clindamycin, 0.15–0.3 gm every 6 hours, can be given by mouth to treat streptococcal or staphylococcal infections. These drugs appear to be substitutes for erythromycin, which in turn is principally a substitute for penicillin. Successful use of lincomycin has been reported in bone infections and in actinomycosis. To achieve higher levels, lincomycin can be given intravenously, 0.6 gm every 8 hours, and this route has occasionally been employed in bacterial endocarditis in combination with other drugs. There is, however, no unequivocal clinical indication for the use of lincomycins.

Adverse Reactions

With oral lincomycin, diarrhea is a very frequent disturbance. This is said to be less common with clindamycin. Impaired liver function (with or without jaundice) and neutropenia have occurred infrequently. Large intravenous doses of lincomycin injected rapidly can cause cardiopulmonary arrest.

Preparations Available
Lincomycin (Lincocin)
 Capsules, 250 and 500 mg
 Injectable, 300 mg/ml in 2 and 10 ml vials or
  2 ml disposable syringe
Clindamycin (Cleocin)
 Capsules, 75 and 150 mg

NOVOBIOCIN

Novobiocin (also called streptonivicin, cardelmycin) is an acidic antibiotic produced by *Streptomyces niveus* and purified in 1956. It is active mainly against gram-positive bacteria.

The acidic material is insoluble, but the sodium or calcium salts are readily soluble in water and fairly stable.

Antibacterial Activity

Many gram-positive cocci are inhibited by novobiocin, $1-5$ μg/ml, as are some strains of proteus also. Resistant mutants occur in all susceptible bacterial populations with such frequency (and are of such magnitude) that clinical resistance tends to emerge very rapidly. Therefore, novobiocin can usually not be employed as the sole antimicrobial drug for more than a few days and, if employed at all, it must be given in combination with a second drug. There is no known cross-resistance with other antimicrobials.

The mechanism of action of novobiocin is not fully understood. The drug inhibits the synthesis of cell wall mucopeptide, of protein, and of nucleic acids in a nonselective manner. The primary site of action (metabolic lesion) is not known.

Absorption, Metabolism, & Excretion

Novobiocin is readily absorbed from the gastrointestinal tract. A major portion of the absorbed drug is bound to serum protein. After ingestion of 0.5 gm every 6 hours, the average serum concentration of free (unbound) novobiocin is $2-5$ μg/ml. Novobiocin is fairly widely distributed in body fluids and tissues except the CNS. Excretion is into the urine and bile. A large proportion of the ingested drug is excreted in the feces.

Clinical Uses

Since the newer penicillins became available there is no longer an unequivocal indication for the use of novobiocin. Previously its principal indication was serious staphylococcal infection. At present, novobiocin might occasionally be useful in the treatment of indole-positive proteus infections or of staphylococcal infections in penicillin hypersensitive persons. The oral dose is 0.5 gm every 6 hours (30 mg/kg/day for children). For the prolonged treatment of chronic infection, novobiocin would have to be combined with a second drug selected to delay the emergence of novobiocin resistance.

Preparations of novobiocin for intramuscular or intravenous administration (in the same dosage) are available.

Adverse Reactions

The incidence of side-effects is high (10−20%).

A. Direct Toxicity: Nausea, vomiting, and diarrhea occur following oral intake; pain at the site of injection, liver damage with jaundice, and hemolytic anemia occur following parenteral use.

B. Allergic Reactions: Skin rashes, fever, eosinophilia, granulocytopenia, and thrombocytopenia can occur frequently.

Preparations Available (Cathomycin, Albamycin)

Capsules, 250 mg
Syrup, 125 mg/5 ml, 60 and 480 ml
Injectable (IM or IV), 500 mg vials (sodium salt)

•   •   •

General References

Friedberg, C.K., & others: Vancomycin therapy for enterococcal and *Streptococcus viridans* endocarditis. Arch Int Med 21:134−140, 1968.

Garrod, L.P., & F. O'Grady: *Antibiotic and Chemotherapy*, 3rd ed. Livingstone, 1971.

Jawetz, E.: Polymyxins, colistin, bacitracin, ristocetin, and vancomycin. P Clin North America 15:85−94, 1968.

Riley, H.D.: Vancomycin and novobiocin. M Clin North America 54:1277−1289, 1970.

Sanders, E.: Lincomycin: Fact, fancy and future. M Clin North America 54:1295−1303, 1970.

Wallace, J.F., Smith, R.H., & R.G. Petersdorf: Oral administration of vancomycin in the treatment of staphylococcal enterocolitis. New England J Med 272:1014−1015, 1965.

55...
Antifungal Agents

Most fungi are completely resistant to the action of antibacterial drugs. Only a few substances have been discovered which exert an inhibitory effect on the fungi pathogenic for man, and most of these are relatively toxic. There is a great need for better antifungal drugs.

Amphotericin B is the only antifungal drug which has been used with any success in the treatment of deep mycoses. Other polyene antibiotics are under study. Fluorocytosine has some effect in meningitis or sepsis due to yeasts. Griseofulvin is effective in dermatophytosis. Nystatin, candicidin, and tolnaftate can only be applied topically. Penicillin and sulfonamides are used in the treatment of actinomycosis and nocardiosis.

AMPHOTERICIN B

Amphotericin B is one of 2 antibiotics produced by *Streptomyces nodosus,* purified in 1956. Amphotericin A is not used in therapy.

Chemistry
Amphotericin B is an amphoteric polyene with the empirical formula $C_{46}H_{73}O_{20}N$. The basic moiety is an aminomethylpentose. Amphotericin B is insoluble in water. It is unstable at $37°$ C, but stable for weeks at $4°$ C. Microcrystalline preparations can be applied topically but are not absorbed to a significant extent. For systemic use by intravenous injection, a colloidal preparation is employed. This is a yellow powder containing 0.8 mg of sodium deoxycholate for each mg of amphotericin, with a phosphate buffer, to be dissolved in dextrose solution.

Antifungal Activity
Amphotericin B, 0.1–0.8 μg/ml, inhibits in vitro *Histoplasma capsulatum, Cryptococcus neoformans, Coccidioides immitis, Candida albicans, Blastomyces dermatitidis, Sporotrichum schenckii,* and other organisms producing systemic mycotic disease in man. It has no effect on bacteria. The emergence of resistance to amphotericin B has been observed in vitro with candida.

The mode of action of the polyene antibiotics is fairly well understood. The drug apparently is bound firmly to the cell membrane in the presence of certain sterols and disturbs the permeability characteristics of the membrane. This results in loss of intracellular components (particularly cations) from the cell and produces irreversible damage. It is believed that bacteria are insusceptible to polyenes because they lack the sterol which is essential for attachment to the cell membrane.

Absorption, Metabolism, & Excretion
Amphotericin is poorly absorbed from the gastrointestinal tract. Orally administered amphotericin therefore is effective only on fungi within the lumen of the tract and cannot be used for the treatment of systemic disease. The intravenous injection of 100 mg of amphotericin B per day (0.65 mg/kg/day) results in average blood levels of 1–2 μg/ml. The drug is widely distributed in tissues, but only 2–3% of the blood level is reached in CSF. Consequently, intrathecal administration may be necessary in fungal meningitis. Most of the injected amphotericin is excreted in the urine.

Clinical Uses
For the treatment of systemic fungal infections, amphotericin B is available as a colloidal dry powder to be dissolved with sodium deoxycholate in 5% dextrose in water to a concentration of 0.1 mg/ml; the solution is then given by slow intravenous infusion over a period of 4–6 hours. The initial dose is 1–5 mg/day, increasing daily by 5 mg increments until a final dosage of 1–1.5 mg/kg/day is reached. This is usually continued for 6–12 weeks or longer.

In fungal meningitis, intrathecal injection of 0.5 mg amphotericin B may be given 3 times weekly for up to 10 weeks or longer. Sometimes continuous infusion with an Ommaya reservoir is used. Fungal meningitis relapses commonly.

Adverse Reactions
The intravenous injection of amphotericin usually produces chills, fever, vomiting, and headache. This may be minimized by reducing the dosage temporarily, administering corticosteroids, or stopping injections for several days.

Therapeutically active amounts of amphotericin B commonly impair renal (eg, fall in creatinine clearance) and hepatocellular function and produce anemia. Shock-like fall in blood pressure, electrolyte disturbances, and a variety of neurologic symptoms also occur commonly.

Preparations Available (Fungizone)
    Cream or ointment, 3%, 20 gm
    Lotion, 3%, 30 ml
    Injectable (IV), 50 mg vials

GRISEOFULVIN

Griseofulvin is a substance isolated from *Penicillium griseofulvum* in 1939 and from *P janczewski* in 1946. While ineffective against bacteria, it produced shrinking and stunting of fungal hyphae. It was introduced for the treatment of dermatophytoses in 1957.

Chemistry

The structural formula of griseofulvin is shown below.

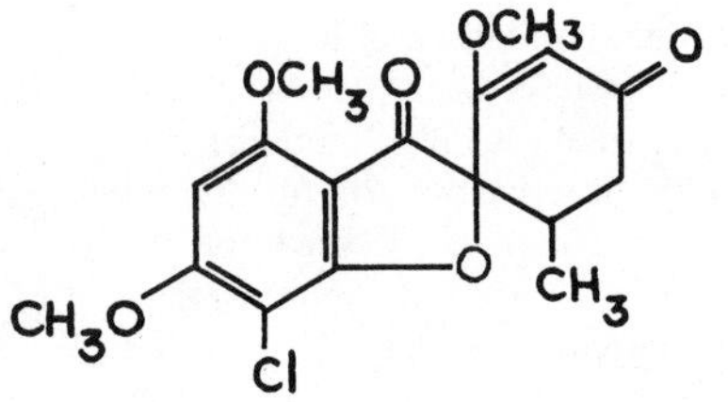

Griseofulvin

The drug is very insoluble in water but quite stable at high temperature, including autoclaving.

Antifungal Activity

Griseofulvin inhibits the growth of dermatophytes, including epidermophyton, microsporum, and trichophyton in concentrations of $0.5-3$ $\mu g/ml$. It has no effect on bacteria, the fungi producing deep mycoses of man, or on certain fungi producing superficial lesions. Resistance can emerge among susceptible dermatophytes.

The mechanism of action has not been established, but it is probable that griseofulvin interferes with nucleic acid synthesis and polymerization. The inhibitory effect may be partially reversed by purines.

Absorption, Metabolism, & Excretion

Absorption of griseofulvin depends greatly on the physical state of the drug and is aided by high-fat foods. Preparations containing microsize particles of the drug are absorbed twice as well as those with larger particles. Microsized griseofulvin, 1 gm daily, gives, in adults, blood levels of $0.5-1.5$ $\mu g/ml$. The absorbed drug has an affinity for diseased skin and is deposited there, bound to keratin. Thus it makes keratin resistant to fungal growth, and the new growth of hair or nails is first freed of infection. As the keratinized structures are shed they tend to be replaced by normal, uninfected ones. Little griseofulvin is present in body fluids or other tissues. The bulk of ingested griseofulvin is excreted in feces and only a small part in urine.

Clinical Uses

Topical use of griseofulvin has little effect.

The microsized preparations of griseofulvin are given orally, $0.5-1$ gm daily, in divided doses ($0.25-0.5$ gm for children weighing over 50 lb, or 15 mg/kg/day). Treatment must be continued for $3-6$ weeks if only the skin is involved and for $3-6$ months if hair and nails are involved. Griseofulvin is indicated for severe dermatophytosis involving skin, hair, or nails, particularly if caused by Trichophyton or Microsporum species, which respond poorly to other measures. Other topical antifungal drugs may have to be used in conjunction with griseofulvin.

Griseofulvin may increase the metabolism of coumarin, so that higher doses of the anticoagulant are required. Phenobarbital reduces absorption of griseofulvin from the gut.

Adverse Reactions

The overall frequency of side-effects is low.

A. Allergic Reactions: Fever, skin rashes, leukopenia, and serum sickness type reactions occur.

B. Direct Toxicity: Headache, nausea, vomiting, diarrhea, hepatotoxicity, photosensitivity, and mental and neurologic difficulties have been reported.

Preparations Available (Fulvicin, Grifulvin, Grisactin)
    Tablets, 250 and 500 mg
    Suspension, 250 mg/5 ml, 4 oz
    Microsize capsules, 125 mg
    Microsize tablets, 125, 250, and 500 mg

NYSTATIN

Nystatin is an intracellular product of *Streptomyces noursei,* described in 1951.

Chemistry

Nystatin is a polyene antibiotic, a very large ring system linked to mycosamine, an amino sugar. The empirical formula is $C_{46}H_{77}NO_{19}$. Nystatin is very slightly soluble in water, but quickly decomposes in the presence of water or plasma. It is stable in dry form.

Antifungal Activity

Nystatin has no effect on bacteria or protozoa, but in vitro it inhibits many fungi, including Candida species, dermatophytes, and organisms producing deep mycoses in man. In vivo its action is limited to surfaces where the nonabsorbed drug can be in direct contact with the yeast or mold. Resistance to nystatin does not develop in vivo, but drug resistant strains of Candida species occur.

The mode of action involves binding of nystatin to the cell membrane in the presence of a specific sterol. This results in drastic changes in the permeability of the cell membrane and loss of cations from the cell.

Absorption, Metabolism, & Excretion

Nystatin is not significantly absorbed from skin, mucous membranes, or the gastrointestinal tract. Virtually all nystatin taken orally is excreted in the feces. There are no significant blood or tissue levels after oral intake.

Clinical Uses

Nystatin can be applied topically to the skin or mucous membranes (buccal, vaginal) in the form of creams, ointments, suppositories, suspensions, or powders for the suppression of local candida infections. Nystatin may be given orally for the suppression of candida in the lumen of the bowel, especially during tetracycline administration. However, there is no disease state associated with prevalence of candida in the bowel in most individuals, and consequently there is no good indication for the use of nystatin for this purpose. An exception may be very small infants or persons with impaired host defenses (diabetes mellitus, leukemia, high doses of steroids), in whom the possibility of disseminated candidiasis exists. In such individuals the "prophylactic" administration of nystatin during tetracycline therapy may be permissible.

Nystatin preparations often contain antibacterial drugs.

Preparations Available (Mycostatin)

Tablets, 500,000 units
Suspension, 100,000 units/ml
Cream, 100,000 units/gm, 15 gm
Ointment, 100,000 units/gm, 15 and 30 gm
Dusting powder, 100,000 units/gm in talc base, ½ oz
Vaginal tablets, 100,000 units

MISCELLANEOUS ANTIFUNGAL DRUGS

1. TOLNAFTATE

Tolnaftate−2-naphthyl-N-methyl-N-(3-tolyl)thionocarbamate−is a topical antifungal drug for use in dermatophytosis. While candida is resistant, many dermatophytes are suppressed, and clinical efficacy is claimed for treatment courses of 1−10 weeks. With topical application, there appears to be no significant systemic absorption. Toxic and allergic reactions appear to be minimal.

Tolnaftate (Tinactin) is available as 1% cream, 1% powder, and 1% solution in polyethylene glycol 400 containing 10 mg/ml.

2. CANDICIDIN

Candicidin is a polyene antibiotic proposed solely as a topical drug for the treatment of candidal vaginitis. It is not absorbed systemically and produces few toxic effects. Its efficacy is currently being tested.

Candicidin (Candeptin) is available as vaginal tablets, 3 mg, or ointment, 75 gm containing 3 mg/5 gm.

3. HYDROXYSTILBAMIDINE

Hydroxystilbamidine isethionate is an aromatic diamidine active against *Blastomyces dermatitidis* and occasionally against *Nocardia asteroides* in vitro and in vivo. It is administered intravenously in a dosage of 225 mg dissolved in 200 ml of 5% dextrose in water, infused over a 2-hour period once daily. It may be severely toxic for liver and kidneys, and has been largely replaced by amphotericin B.

Hydroxystilbamidine is available in 20 ml ampules containing 225 mg.

4. FLUOROCYTOSINE

5-Fluorocytosine is active in vitro against some isolates of candida and cryptococcus. Daily amounts of 3−8 gm (100−200 mg/kg/day) orally have produced clinical remissions in patients unsuccessfully treated with amphotericin. Resistant yeasts sometimes appear during therapy. Toxic effects include loss of hair and bone marrow depression. This drug is in an experimental stage.

5. CYCLOHEXIMIDE

Cycloheximide has been abandoned as an antifungal drug because of its severe systemic toxicity.

6. FATTY ACIDS

Fatty acids, particularly undecylenic acid and its salts, are effective topical antifungal drugs. (See Chapter 58.)

• • •

General References

Bindschadler, D.D., & J.E. Bennett: A pharmacologic guide to the clinical use of amphotericin. J Infect Dis 120:427–436, 1969.

Butler, W.T.: Pharmacology, toxicity and therapeutic usefulness of amphotericin B. JAMA 195:371–375, 1966.

Goldman, L.: Griseofulvin. M Clin North America 54:1339–1345, 1970.

Parker, J.D., & others: Experience with blastomycosis and its treatment with amphotericin B. Am Rev Resp Dis 99:895–902, 1969.

Tassel, D., & M.A. Madoff: Treatment of candida sepsis and cryptococcus meningitis with 5-fluorocytosine. JAMA 206:830–832, 1968.

56...

Urinary Antiseptics*

Urinary antiseptics are drugs that exert anti-bacterial activity in the urine but have little or no systemic antibacterial effect. Their usefulness is limited to urinary tract infections. They have no marked anti-microbial activity in the renal parenchyma, but they may have therapeutic usefulness in pyelonephritis—perhaps by preventing ascending reinfection. Prolonged suppression of bacteriuria by means of urinary anti-septics may be desirable in chronic urinary tract infection where eradication of infection by short-term systemic therapy has not been possible.

With indwelling bladder catheters, microorganisms tend to reach the bladder in 2—3 days unless an aseptic closed system is employed. Such a system may also contain acetic acid, 0.25%, or be irrigated with a solution containing polymyxin B, 20 mg/liter, and neomycin, 40 mg/liter, to prevent ascending infection.

NITROFURANTOIN

Chemistry

Many derivatives of furan possess antibacterial properties. Most of these substances are topical disinfectants (see Chapter 58). Nitrofurantoin is the main urinary antiseptic among nitrofurans.

Nitrofurantoin

Antibacterial Activity

Nitrofurans are bacteriostatic and bactericidal for both gram-positive and gram-negative bacteria in concentrations of 10—500 μg/ml. Although certain strains of microorganisms are resistant (eg, many strains of *Proteus vulgaris* and all strains of *Pseudomonas*

*The sulfonamides are discussed in Chapter 53.

aeruginosa), resistant mutants are rare in nitrofuran-toin susceptible populations. In other words, clinical drug resistance emerges slowly. There is no cross-resistance between nitrofurans and other antimicrobial agents.

The mechanism of action of the nitrofurans is not known. The activity of nitrofurans depends to some extent upon the size of the microbial population. With very high concentrations of bacteria in the urine or in broth, the activity of nitrofurantoin is diminished. The activity of nitrofurantoin is greatly enhanced at pH 5.5 or below.

Absorption, Metabolism, & Excretion

Nitrofurantoin is rapidly and completely absorbed from the gastrointestinal tract, but the absorbed drug is bound so completely to serum protein that no antibacterial effect can be detected in the blood. Nitrofurantoin therefore has no systemic anti-bacterial activity. In the kidneys, the drug is separated from the carrier protein and excreted in the urine both by glomerular filtration and tubular secretion. Tubular reabsorption occurs, and concentration in hilar lymph is high. Significant nitrofurantoin levels may also be found in interstitial tissue. With average daily doses, concentrations of 200 μg/ml are reached in urine; maximum urine levels may be 300—400 μg/ml. In renal failure urine levels are insufficient for antibacterial action, but high blood levels may cause toxicity.

Clinical Uses

The average daily dose for urinary tract infection in adults is 400 mg orally in divided doses (5—8 mg/kg/day for children) taken with meals or after eating. Some persons can tolerate up to 600 mg/day, but this higher dose often results in nausea or vomiting. Gastrointestinal disturbance due to nitrofurantoin can be reduced if the drug is taken with food or milk. Nitrofurantoin must never be given to patients with renal insufficiency. Oral nitrofurantoin can be given for weeks, months, or even years for the suppression of chronic urinary tract infection. An acidifying agent is desirable to keep urinary pH below 5.5 (see Acidifying Agents, below).

It is possible to administer the soluble sodium salt of nitrofurantoin intravenously. From 360—540 mg are injected daily by continuous infusion for a few days. Even the intravenously injected drug has no systemic antimicrobial activity, but this route reduces severe gastrointestinal disturbances.

Another nitrofuran, furazolidone, 400 mg (5–8 mg/kg in children) daily orally, can effectively reduce diarrhea in cholera and perhaps shorten vibrio excretion.

Adverse Reactions

A. Direct Toxicity: Anorexia, nausea, and vomiting are the principal (and frequent) side-effects of orally administered nitrofurantoin. They occur rarely with intravenous administration. Neuropathies and hemolytic anemias (in G6PD deficiency) are rare.

B. Allergic Reactions: Various skin rashes, pulmonary infiltration, and other hypersensitivity reactions have been reported.

Preparations Available (Furadantin)

Tablets, 50 and 100 mg
Suspension, 25 mg/5 ml
Injectable (IV), vials containing 180 mg/20 ml (sodium salt)

NALIDIXIC ACID

Nalidixic acid is a urinary antiseptic for urinary tract infections with gram-negative bacteria which is effective when taken orally. It has no significant systemic activity.

Chemistry

This is a synthetic chemical with the formula shown below. It is stable in the dry form and poorly soluble in water.

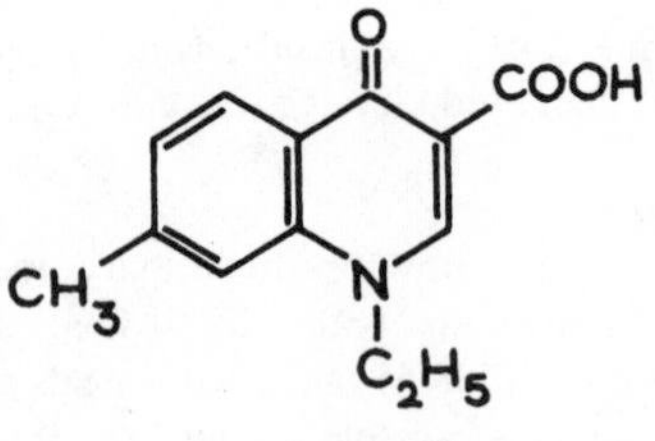

Nalidixic acid

Antibacterial Activity

Nalidixic acid inhibits many gram-negative bacteria in vitro in concentrations of 1–50 μg/ml. Much higher concentrations are necessary to inhibit gram-positive organisms. Most strains of *Escherichia coli* are inhibited, and some strains of aerobacter, klebsiella, and proteus. Pseudomonas species are usually resistant.

The mechanism of the chemotherapeutic effect is not entirely clear. Nalidixic acid may lower the pH of the urine sufficiently to result in inhibition of bacteria.

Nalidixic acid is also a specific and powerful inhibitor of the DNA synthesis of *E coli* but has little effect on the synthesis of protein or RNA. This inhibition of DNA replication may be the basis of the chemotherapeutic action of this compound.

Resistant microorganisms emerge rapidly during nalidixic acid therapy, both by selection of drug-resistant members of the population and by superinfection with drug-resistant microorganisms of another strain or species. There is no cross-resistance with other antimicrobial drugs.

Absorption, Metabolism, & Excretion

After oral administration the drug is readily absorbed from the gut. In the blood, virtually all nalidixic acid is firmly bound to protein. Thus there is no significant systemic antibacterial action. About 20% of the absorbed drug is excreted in the urine in the active form and 80% in an inactive form as a glucuronide conjugate. Levels of active drug in the urine reach 10–150 μg/ml.

Clinical Uses

The only indication for this agent is urinary tract infection with coliform organisms. The dose for adults is 1 gm orally 4 times daily for 1 week or more. The dose for children is 55 mg/kg/day orally in 2–4 divided doses. For prolonged use, the dosage may be reduced.

Adverse Reactions

Nalidixic acid excreted in the urine may give rise to false-positive tests for glucose, but true hyperglycemia and glycosuria may also be produced. There are occasional gastrointestinal disturbances, skin rashes, sensitization to sunlight, visual disturbances in focusing or color perception, and double vision. Convulsions have been reported following overdosage.

Preparations Available

Nalidixic acid (NegGram) is available in 250 and 500 mg tablets.

METHENAMINE MANDELATE & METHENAMINE HIPPURATE

Methenamine mandelate is the salt of mandelic acid and methenamine, and possesses to some extent the properties of both of these urinary antiseptics. Mandelic acid ($C_6H_5CHOHCOOH$) or hippuric acid taken orally is excreted unchanged in the urine, where these drugs are bactericidal for some gram-negative bacteria if the pH can be kept below 5.5. Methenamine is absorbed readily after oral intake and excreted in the urine. If the urine is strongly acid (pH below 5.5), methenamine releases formaldehyde, which is antibacterial.

Methenamine mandelate, 3–6 gm daily orally, or methenamine hippurate, 2–4 gm daily orally, are used only as urinary antiseptics. If necessary, acidifying agents (eg, ascorbic acid, 4–12 gm daily) may be given to lower urinary pH below 5.5. Sulfonamides cannot be given at the same time because they may form an insoluble compound with the formaldehyde released by methenamine. Persons taking methenamine may exhibit falsely elevated tests for catecholamines.

The action of methenamine mandelate or hippurate is nonspecific against many different microorganisms, and consists of the simultaneous effect of formaldehyde and acidity. Microorganisms such as proteus which make a strongly alkaline urine through the release of ammonia from urea usually are insusceptible.

Methenamine mandelate is available in tablets of 0.25, 0.5, and 1 gm; or in suspension, 0.25 gm/5 ml or 0.5 gm/5 ml (forte).

ACIDIFYING AGENTS

In chronic urinary tract infections, eradication of the organisms often fails. It is then important to suppress bacteria for 6–18 months.

Any substance which will produce a urine pH below 5.5 usually inhibits bacterial growth in urine. Ketogenic diets, ammonium chloride, ascorbic acid, mandelic acid, methionine, and hippuric acid (eg, from ingestion of cranberry juice) all can be employed to that end. It is important to check urinary pH frequently and to ascertain by direct microscopic examination that the bacteriuria is actually suppressed. Prolonged suppression (6–18 months) occasionally permits healing of the infection, probably because it blocks the frequent ascending reinfection of the kidneys from the lower tract.

Ammonium chloride is available as 300 mg tablets; as enteric coated tablets containing 0.3, 0.5, and 1 gm; or in 100 ml vials containing 0.6% solution. Methionine is available as 500 mg tablets, and the daily dose for adults is 9–12 gm. Mandelic acid is available in powder form. The daily dose of ascorbic acid is 4–12 gm.

SYSTEMICALLY ACTIVE DRUGS IN URINARY TRACT INFECTION

Many antimicrobial drugs are excreted in the urine in active form. The concentration in urine is often many times higher than the concentration in body fluids or tissues. Effective antibacterial concentrations can therefore be attained in urine with doses too low to be effective in systemic infections. This permits the use of drugs which are relatively toxic. Drugs such as kanamycin-neomycin or the polymyxins can be administered in doses sufficient to achieve high urine levels without risking significant adverse effects. Even more toxic drugs such as cycloserine (see below) can be administered in a dose of 10–15 mg/kg/day. This produces urine levels sufficient to suppress highly resistant organisms, eg, proteus, with only a moderate risk of serious toxicity. Penicillins in systemic doses are excreted in the urine to yield concentrations of 100–5000 units/ml. This may be sufficient to suppress not only gram-positive but also many gram-negative bacteria. Ampicillin and carbenicillin are particularly effective against many gram-negative bacteria in the urinary tract unless they are inactivated by high concentrations of β-lactamase in bladder urine.

Cycloserine

Cycloserine (D-4-amino-3-isoxazolidone) is an antibiotic produced by *Streptomyces orchidaceus* in 1955 and later synthesized.

Cycloserine

The substance is water-soluble and very unstable at acid pH. Cycloserine inhibits many microorganisms, including coliforms, proteus, and mycobacteria. The mode of action involves the inhibition of incorporation of D-alanine into mucopeptide of the bacterial cell wall. After ingestion of 0.25 gm every 6 hours, blood levels reach 20–30 μg/ml—sufficient to inhibit many strains of mycobacteria and gram-negative bacteria. The drug is widely distributed in tissues. Most of the drug is excreted in active form into the urine, where concentrations are sufficiently high to inhibit many organisms causing urinary tract infections.

Cycloserine may produce serious CNS toxicity manifested by headaches, tremor, vertigo, acute psychosis, and convulsions. With careful management of oral dosage (below 0.75 gm/day), these symptoms can usually be avoided. Cycloserine is occasionally employed for the treatment of tuberculosis or urinary tract infections. The dosage is usually 0.25 gm 2–3 times daily by mouth (for children, 20 mg/kg/day). In nocardiosis, cycloserine, 0.25 gm 4 times daily with full systemic doses of a sulfonamide, has been curative.

Cycloserine (Seromycin) is available in 250 mg capsules.

TOPICAL USE OF ANTIMICROBIAL DRUGS IN THE URINARY TRACT

Indwelling catheterization of the urinary bladder has a high risk of producing urinary tract infection. This risk can be markedly reduced if a closed, sterile collection system is employed with strictest asepsis. This is often combined with the use of an irrigating solution which contains bactericidal concentrations of polymyxins and neomycins, administered by 3-way catheter. Such systems may delay infection with indwelling catheterization for several weeks. They have no place in the treatment of urinary tract infections.

•   •   •

General References

Kleeman, C.R., Hewitt, W.L., & L.B. Guze: Pyelonephritis. Medicine 39:3–116, 1960.

Stamey, T.A., Govan, D.E., & J.M. Palmer: The localization and treatment of urinary tract infections: The role of bactericidal urine levels as opposed to serum levels. Medicine 44:1–36, 1965.

Turck, M., Anderson, K.N., & R.G. Petersdorf: Relapse and reinfection in chronic bacteriuria. New England J Med 275:70–73, 1966.

57...

Antiviral Chemotherapy & Prophylaxis

In many viral infections, replication of the virus reaches a maximum before any clinical symptoms appear. In order to be clinically effective, chemicals which block viral replication must be administered prior to the appearance of disease, ie, as chemoprophylaxis. Some outstanding practical examples (amantadine in influenza A, methisazone in smallpox) are discussed in Chapter 60, Chemoprophylaxis, and also below. In some other viral diseases (eg, herpes simplex keratitis), replication of the agent continues for prolonged periods and partial inhibition of virus replication may enhance healing. This is the case with iododeoxyuridine (IDU, IUDR) in herpetic keratitis.

Only a few clinically applicable agents are available for antiviral therapy, but active research in this area is likely to make significant progress. At present, most chemicals which inhibit virus replication also disturb host cell function significantly and therefore are too toxic to be used in chemotherapy.

Inhibitors of viral replication are presented here according to the steps in the replicative process which they inhibit. These steps are (1) adsorption, (2) penetration into susceptible cells, (3) synthesis of early (nonstructural) proteins (eg, nucleic acid polymerases), (4) synthesis of nucleic acids (RNA or DNA), (5) synthesis of late (structural) proteins, (6) maturation (assembly) of viral particles, and (7) release from the cell. No chemicals are available which inhibit steps (1) or (7).

INHIBITORS OF PENETRATION INTO SUSCEPTIBLE CELLS

Gamma Globulin

If gamma globulin contains specific antibodies directed against superficial antigens of a given virus, it can interfere with entry of that virus particle into a cell, probably by blocking penetration rather than adsorption. The intramuscular injection of pooled gamma globulin, 0.02–0.1 ml/lb body weight, during the early incubation period can modify infection with the viruses of measles, hepatitis, rabies, poliomyelitis, and possibly other diseases. The protective effect of a gamma globulin injection lasts 2–3 weeks. For infections which have prolonged incubation periods, injections may have to be given every 2–3 weeks.

It often happens that viral replication is only partially inhibited, so that the development of active immunity may accompany the temporary passive protection conferred by gamma globulin.

Gamma globulin is available in vials containing 2 ml and 10 ml.

Amantadine (Adamantanamine)

Amantadine, a tricyclic symmetric amine, inhibits the penetration into susceptible cells of certain myxoviruses, eg, influenza A (but not influenza B), rubella, and some tumor viruses. It therefore inhibits the replication of these viruses in vitro and in experimental animals. In man a daily oral dose of 200 mg of amantadine hydrochloride for 2–3 days before and 6–7 days after influenza A infection reduces the incidence and severity of symptoms and the magnitude of serologic response. There may also be a slight therapeutic effect if amantadine is started within 18 hours of the onset of symptoms of influenza.

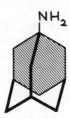

Amantadine

The most marked untoward effects are insomnia, slurred speech, dizziness, ataxia, and other CNS signs.

Amantadine (Symmetrel) is available as 100 mg capsules and as syrup containing 50 mg/5 ml.

INHIBITION OF INTRACELLULAR SYNTHESIS

Inhibition of Synthesis of "Early" Proteins

Guanidine and hydroxybenzylbenzimidazole are both capable of inhibiting the replication of certain RNA enteroviruses, but not of others. Both substances inhibit the formation of RNA polymerases at concentrations which appear to be harmless to host cells in vitro. Mutants resistant to the action of these compounds are frequent and are rapidly selected out in the presence of the drugs. Therefore, as expected, these compounds do not have significant therapeutic activity in vivo. Trials of biguanidines in RNA virus infections in man were not encouraging.

Guanidine hydrochloride

Hydroxybenzylbenzimidazole

Inhibition of Synthesis of Nucleic Acids

Dactinomycin (actinomycin D, Cosmegen) inhibits DNA dependent RNA synthesis (ie, synthesis of messenger RNA) and thus inhibits the multiplication of DNA viruses. However, the effect is not sufficiently specific to permit its application in vivo, as the drug is severely cytotoxic.

Several **halogenated pyrimidines** can inhibit the replication of DNA viruses because they are analogues of the bases which are DNA building blocks. The incorporation of some pyrimidine analogues results in the formation of nonfunctional DNA and noninfectious virus. Other pyrimidine analogues inhibit specific enzymes. All halogenated pyrimidines with antiviral activity possess marked toxic properties for animal cells and therefore cannot be given systemically without serious adverse effects. However, topical administration is possible and can be used as chemotherapy in special circumstances.

5-Fluorouracil and **5-bromouracil** effectively block the replication of DNA viruses in cell culture systems, but they are relatively ineffective in vivo. **Idoxuridine** (5-iodo-2-deoxyuridine, IDU, IUDR) can inhibit the replication of most DNA viruses in vitro, in cell culture. In vivo it inhibits the replication of herpes simplex virus in the cornea and thus aids in the healing of herpetic keratitis in man. This is a special circumstance since herpesvirus proliferates in the avascular corneal epithelium and the topically applied drug remains local and is not rapidly removed by the blood stream. In the vascular conjunctiva the drug has little therapeutic effect; although adenoviruses are readily inhibited by idoxuridine in vitro, adenovirus conjunctivitis cannot be controlled by idoxuridine in vivo.

For the treatment of herpetic keratitis, idoxuridine is applied to the cornea (every 2 hours around the clock) by instilling 1 drop of a 0.1% aqueous solution into the conjunctival sac. This tends to accelerate spontaneous healing. However, DNA synthesis of host cells is also affected, and some toxic effects on corneal cells are occasionaly observed, especially if treatment is continued for more than 10 days. Ointments containing 0.5% idoxuridine have been prepared in order to provide higher drug concentrations.

Most isolates of herpesvirus from untreated cases of herpetic keratitis are strongly inhibited in vitro by idoxuridine, 2 μg/ml. Upon prolonged exposure to idoxuridine in vitro, occasional drug resistant mutants are selected out which are not inhibited by idoxuridine, 20 μg/ml or more. "Drug resistant" cases of herpetic keratitis occur relatively frequently. Such patients fail to improve with prolonged idoxuridine treatment. However, many of the virus isolates from such cases appear to be intrinsically susceptible to idoxuridine inhibition in vitro. It is probable that many such strains escape the inhibitory effect of idoxuridine in vivo because they rapidly penetrate into the depth of the corneal stroma and thus become inaccessible to idoxuridine applied to the corneal surface.

Vaccinial keratitis responds irregularly to idoxuridine.

Idoxuridine (Dendrid, Herplex, Stoxil) is available as solution, 15 ml containing 0.1%, or ointment (Stoxil), 4 gm containing 0.5%.

In early cases of herpetic encephalitis, the intravenous administration of idoxuridine, 0.3%, has been claimed to have curative effects. The recommended dose is 100–430 mg/kg/day for 5 days, not to exceed a total of 30 gm. Topically applied idoxuridine has no effect on skin lesions of herpes simplex or zoster, but therapeutic claims are made for idoxuridine in dimethyl sulfoxide or injected by jet gun.

Another pyrimidine analogue, **cytosine arabinoside** (arabinofuranosylcytosine hydrochloride, cytarabine), also inhibits DNA synthesis and interferes with the replication of DNA viruses. By weight it is about 10 times more effective than idoxuridine, but it is also 10 times more toxic for host cells. Idoxuridine resistant herpesviruses can be inhibited by cytosine arabinoside. Because of its higher toxicity for the cornea, cytosine arabinoside has been employed topically only for patients with herpetic keratitis who have failed to respond to idoxuridine. Cytosine arabinoside, 0.3–2 mg/kg IV as a single daily dose for 5 days, has been used in severe disseminated herpes simplex and in disseminated varicella.

A third pyrimidine analogue, arabinofuranosyladenine (adenine arabinoside), has marked suppressive and curative effects in experimental DNA virus infections. It appears to have low toxicity and is undergoing clinical trial.

Interferon

Interferons are proteins, stable at pH 2.0, with molecular weights of 25–90 thousand, which are induced in cells by various stimuli and interfere with the synthesis of viruses, probably at the level of ribosomes, where interferon may lead to the production of an antiviral protein. Interferons are host species specific but not virus specific—eg, interferon made in chick cells inhibits the synthesis of different viruses in chick but not in mouse or human cells. Inducers of interferon may be viruses, nucleic acids, endotoxins, large polysaccharides, bacteria, synthetic polyanions, and other substances.

In view of the broad range of viruses which are susceptible to interferon inhibition, interferon can be considered a potentially valuable chemotherapeutic agent. However, production of **exogenous** interferon presents great difficulties, and its clinical usefulness is limited at present. The yield from cells grown in vitro is small, and the duration of action of interferon is short. Although the specific activity of purified interferon is high, the problem of how to produce large quantities for repeated administration has not yet been solved. The activity of **endogenously** stimulated interferon is therefore of interest. Thus, parenterally administered double-stranded RNA, synthetic polymers, and other large molecules can induce (or release) into the blood stream significant amounts of circulating interferon which exhibits antiviral effects for several days. Harmless and potent inducers of interferon are currently being sought.

Inhibition of Synthesis of "Late" Proteins

A number of different amino acid analogues (eg, **fluorophenylalanine**) inhibit the synthesis of structural proteins for the coats of virus particles. The antibiotic **puromycin** does likewise. However, these inhibitors of protein synthesis show no specificity for the synthesis of virus protein and impair protein synthesis of the host cell to such degree that they are intensely toxic. Consequently, none of these substances are useful in chemotherapy at present.

In many poxviruses various thiosemicarbazones inhibit virus replication by interfering with the synthesis of a "late" structural protein. As a result, the assembly of normal particles is impaired or blocked. Methisazone can block replication of smallpox (variola) virus in man if administered to contacts within 1–2 days after exposure. Methisazone, 2–4 gm orally daily (100 mg/kg/day for children) for 3–4 days, gives striking protection against clinical smallpox, as shown

Methisazone
(N-methyl-isatin-β-thiosemicarbazone)

in controlled trials. Limited replication of smallpox virus still occurs in treated individuals, as shown by a marked rise in specific antibody to smallpox virus and the development of active immunity.

The above application to smallpox is chemoprophylaxis rather than therapy. In addition, the replication of vaccinia virus can be inhibited by methisazone after symptoms have started, eg, in generalized vaccinia or in progressive vaccinia in immunologically deficient individuals. This is a valid form of antiviral chemotherapy restricted to poxviruses only.

Methisazone is not commercially available in the USA. It is available in Europe as 1.5 gm chewable capsules (Marboran) which can be chewed or swallowed whole. It often induces vomiting.

INHIBITION OF MATURATION

The assembly of intact particles can be inhibited by many agents (eg, **5-fluoro-2-deoxyuridine** or **puromycin**) which induce the synthesis of defective viral constituents—whether nucleic acids or structural proteins.

Rifampin (see Chapter 52) inhibits DNA-dependent RNA polymerase in bacteria and mammalian cells. It also inhibits poxviruses, but by a different mechanism. Rifampin prevents the assembly of enveloped mature particles. The block apparently occurs during the stage of envelope formation and is reversible upon removal of the drug.

Rifampin has not been used in treatment of human poxvirus infections, but topical application can inhibit human vaccinia lesions.

•   •   •

General References

Bauer, D.J.: Clinical experience with the antiviral drug Marboran. Ann New York Acad Sc 130:110–117, 1965.

Eggers, H.J., & I. Tamm: Antiviral chemotherapy. Ann Rev Pharmacol 6:231–250, 1966.

Nolan, D.C., & others: *Herpesvirus hominis* encephalitis: 13 cases, 6 treated with idoxuridine. New England J Med 282:10–13, 1970.

58

Disinfectants & Antiseptics

The antiseptics and disinfectants differ fundamentally from systemically active chemotherapeutic agents in that they possess little or no selective toxicity. Most of these substances are toxic not only for microbial parasites but for host cells as well. Therefore, they may be used to reduce the microbial population in the inanimate environment, but they can usually be applied only topically, not systemically, to man.

The terms disinfectants, antiseptics, or germicides have been used interchangeably by some, and the definitions overlap greatly in the literature. The term **disinfectant** often denotes a substance which kills microorganisms in the inanimate environment. The term **antiseptic** often is applied to substances which inhibit bacterial growth both **in vitro** and **in vivo** when applied to the surface of living tissue under suitable conditions of contact.

The antibacterial action of antiseptics and disinfectants is largely dependent on concentration, temperature, and time. Very low concentrations may stimulate bacterial growth, higher concentration may be inhibitory and still higher concentrations may be bactericidal for certain organisms.

Evaluation of the antiseptics and disinfectants is difficult because methods of testing are controversial and results are subject to different interpretations. Ideally, such substances should be lethal for microorganisms in high dilution, noninjurious to tissues or inanimate substances, inexpensive, stable, nonstaining, odorless, and rapid-acting even in the presence of foreign proteins, exudates, or fibers. No preparation now available combines these characteristics to a high degree.

Many antiseptics and disinfectants were at one time used in medical and surgical practice. Most have now been displaced by chemotherapeutic substances. The 2 remaining areas of use are urinary antiseptics (see Chapter 56) and topical antiseptics. Most topical antiseptics do not aid wound healing but, on the contrary, often impair healing. In general, cleansing of abrasions and superficial wounds by washing with soap and water is far more effective and less damaging than the application of topical antiseptics.

A few chemical classes of disinfectants and antiseptics are briefly characterized in the following paragraphs.

Alcohols

Aliphatic alcohols are antimicrobial in varying degree. Ethyl alcohol in 70% concentration is bactericidal in 1–2 minutes at 30° C but less effective at lower and higher concentrations. Ethyl alcohol, 70%, and isopropyl alcohol, 70–90%, are at present the most satisfactory disinfectants for skin surfaces. They may be useful for sterilizing instruments but have no effect on spores, and better agents are available for this purpose. Aerosols of 70% alcohol with 1 μm size droplets may be the best disinfection for mechanical respirators.

Propylene glycol and other glycols have been used as vapors to disinfect air. Precise control of humidity is necessary for good antimicrobial action. Glycol vapors are rarely employed at present.

Aldehydes

Formaldehyde in a concentration of 1–10% effectively kills microorganisms and their spores in 1–6 hours. It acts by combining with and precipitating protein. It is too irritating for use on tissues, but is widely employed as a disinfectant for instruments. Formaldehyde solution USP contains 37% formaldehyde by weight, with methyl alcohol added to prevent polymerization.

Methenamine taken orally can release formaldehyde into acid urine. It is employed as a urinary disinfectant (see Chapter 56).

Acids

Several inorganic acids have been used for cauterization of tissue. Although they are effective antimicrobial agents, the tissue destruction they cause precludes their use. Benzoic acid, 0.1%, is employed as a food preservative. Esters of benzoic acid are used as antimicrobial preservatives of certain other drugs. Acetic acid, 1%, can be used in surgical dressings as a topical antimicrobial agent; it is particularly active against *Pseudomonas aeruginosa*. Boric acid, 5% in water, or as powder can be applied to a variety of skin lesions as an antimicrobial agent. However, the toxicity of absorbed boric acid is high, particularly for small children, and its use is not advisable. Salicylic acid can serve as a fungicide.

Mandelic acid is excreted unchanged in the urine after oral intake; 12 gm daily taken orally can lower the pH of urine to 5.0, sufficient to be antibacterial. Mandelic acid, methenamine mandelate, and nalidixic acid are used as urinary antiseptics. They are discussed in Chapter 56.

Halogens & Halogen-Containing Compounds

A. Iodine: Elemental iodine is one of the most effective germicides. Its mode of action is unknown. A 1:20,000 solution of iodine kills bacteria in 1 minute and spores in 15 minutes, and its tissue toxicity is relatively low. Iodine tincture USP contains 2% iodine and 2.4% sodium iodide in alcohol. It is the most effective disinfectant available for intact skin and should always be used to disinfect skin when obtaining blood cultures by venipuncture. The principal disadvantage of tincture of iodine is the occasional dermatitis which can occur in hypersensitive individuals. This can be avoided by promptly removing the tincture of iodine with 70% ethyl or 90% isopropyl alcohol. When using iodine for skin preparation, the absorption of iodine from the skin usually does not interfere with PBI determinations in the investigation of thyroid dysfunction.

Iodine can be complexed with polyvinylpyrrolidone to yield povidone-iodine NF. This is a water-soluble complex which liberates free iodine in solution. It is widely employed as a skin disinfectant, particularly for preoperative skin preparation. It is an effective local antibacterial substance, and hypersensitivity reactions are infrequent. Povidone-iodine (Betadine) is available in many forms: solution, ointment, aerosol, surgical scrub, shampoo, skin cleanser, vaginal gel, vaginal douche, and individual cotton swabs.

B. Chlorine: Chlorine exerts its antimicrobial action in the form of undissociated hypochlorous acid (HOCl), which is formed when chlorine is dissolved in water at neutral or acid pH. Chlorine concentrations of 0.25 ppm are effectively bactericidal for many microorganisms. Mycobacteria are 500 times more resistant to chlorine at these concentrations. Organic matter greatly reduces the antimicrobial activity of chlorine. The amount of chlorine bound by organic matter in an environment (eg, water) and thus not available for antimicrobial activity is called the "chlorine demand." The chlorine demand of relatively pure water is low, so that the addition of 0.5 ppm chlorine is sufficient for disinfection. The chlorine demand of grossly polluted water may be very high, so that 20 ppm or more of chlorine may have to be added for effective bactericidal action.

Chlorine gas causes severe poisoning in concentrations of 1:100,000 or less. It was one of the earliest agents employed in chemical warfare, and acts as an intense lung irritant.

Chlorine is used mainly for the disinfection of inanimate objects and particularly for the purification of water. Chlorinated lime forms hypochlorite solution when dissolved. It is a cheap (but unstable) form of chlorine. Halazone USP is a chloramine employed in tablet form for the sterilization of drinking water. The addition of 4–8 mg halazone per liter will sterilize water in 15–60 minutes unless a large quantity of organic material is present.

Sodium hypochlorite solution, 0.5% NaOCl (diluted sodium hypochlorite [modified Dakin's] solution NF), contains about 0.1 gm of available chlorine per 100 ml and can be used as an irrigating fluid for the cleansing and disinfecting of contaminated wounds. Household bleaches containing chlorine can serve as disinfectants for inanimate objects.

Halazone is available in 4 mg tablets.

Oxidizing Agents

Some antiseptics exert an antimicrobial action because they are oxidizing agents. Most are of no practical importance, and only hydrogen peroxide, sodium perborate, and potassium permanganate are occasionally used.

Hydrogen peroxide solution USP contains 3% H_2O_2 in water. Contact with tissues releases molecular oxygen and there is a brief period of antimicrobial action. There is no penetration of tissues, and the main applications of hydrogen peroxide are as a mouthwash and for the cleansing of wounds.

Potassium permanganate USP consists of purple crystals which dissolve in water to give deep purple solutions that stain tissues and clothing brown. A 1:10,000 dilution of potassium permanganate kills many microorganisms in one hour. Higher concentrations are irritating to tissues. The principal use of potassium permanganate solutions is in the treatment of weeping skin lesions.

Heavy Metals

A. Mercury: Mercuric ion precipitates protein and inhibits sulfhydryl enzymes. Microorganisms inactivated by mercury can be reactivated by thiols (sulfhydryl compounds). Mercurial antiseptics inhibit the sulfhydryl enzymes of tissue cells as well as those of bacteria. Therefore, most mercury preparations are highly toxic if ingested. Mercury bichloride NF can be employed in 1:1000 dilution as a disinfectant for instruments or unabraded skin.

Yellow mercuric oxide ointment NF contains 1% of insoluble HgO and can be applied to superficial infected skin lesions. Ammoniated mercury ointment USP contains 5% of the active insoluble compound ($HgNH_2Cl$) and serves as a skin disinfectant in impetigo.

Some organic mercury compounds are less toxic than the inorganic salts and somewhat more antibacterial. Nitromersol NF, thimerosal NF, and phenylmercuric nitrate NF are used as antiseptics for cutaneous and mucosal surfaces in concentrations of 1:1000–1:100,000 and have primarily bacteriostatic activity. They are also used as "preservatives" in various biologic products to reduce the chance of accidental contamination. Merbromin NF (Mercurochrome) is used as a 2% solution which is a feeble antiseptic but stains tissue a brilliant red color. The psychologic effect of this stain has lent support to the (otherwise almost negligible) antiseptic properties of this material.

B. Silver: Silver ion precipitates protein and also interferes with essential metabolic activities of microbial cells. Inorganic silver salts are strongly bactericidal. Silver nitrate, 1:1000, destroys most microorganisms rapidly upon contact. Silver nitrate ophthalmic solution USP contains 1% of the salt, to be instilled into the eyes of newborns to prevent gonococcal ophthalmia. It is effective for this purpose but may cause chemical conjunctivitis by being quite acid; therefore, penicillin ointment has been used instead at times. Other inorganic silver salts are rarely used for their antimicrobial properties because they are strongly irritating to tissues. The use of silver nitrate solution for the treatment of burns has recently been revived. Compresses of 0.5% silver nitrate are effective in reducing infection of the burn wound, in aiding rapid eschar formation, and in reducing mortality. Complexes of silver salts with mafenide may be even more effective (see below).

Colloidal preparations of silver are less injurious to superficial tissues and have significant bacteriostatic properties. Mild silver protein NF contains about 20% silver and can be applied as an antiseptic to mucous membranes. Prolonged use of any silver preparation may result in argyria. If silver nitrate is reduced to nitrite by bacteria in the burn, methemoglobinemia may result.

Other Metals

Other metal salts (eg, zinc sulfate, copper sulfate) have significant antimicrobial properties but are rarely employed in medicine at present.

Phenols & Related Compounds

Phenol denatures protein. It was the first antiseptic employed, as a spray, during surgical procedures by Lister in 1867. Concentrations of at least 1−2% are required for antimicrobial activity, whereas a 5% concentration is strongly irritating to tissues. Therefore, phenol is used mainly for the disinfection of inanimate objects and excreta. Various substituted phenols are more effective, if somewhat more expensive, as environmental disinfectants. Among them are many proprietary preparations containing cresol and other alkyl-substituted phenols.

Other phenol derivatives such as resorcinol, thymol, and hexylresorcinol have enjoyed some popularity in the past as antiseptics. Several chlorinated phenols are much more active antimicrobial agents.

Hexachlorophene USP is a white crystalline powder which is insoluble in water but soluble in organic solvents, dilute alkalies, and soaps and is an effective bacteriostatic agent. Hexachlorophene liquid soap USP and many proprietary preparations are used widely in surgical scrub routines and as deodorant soaps. Single applications of such preparations are no more effective than plain soaps, but daily use results in a deposit of hexachlorophene on the skin which exerts a prolonged bacteriostatic action. Thus the number of resident skin bacteria is lower on the surgeon's hands if he uses hexachlorophene soap daily and does not employ other soaps, which promptly remove the residual hexachlorophene film. Regular use of hexachlorophene

soaps may reduce body odor by the prevention of bacterial decomposition of organic material in apocrine sweat.

Other antiseptic soaps contain carbanilides or salicylanilides and have similar effects. All such preparations may produce allergic reactions or photosensitization. Bathing newborns in 3% hexachlorophene permits absorption and possible toxic effects.

Surface-Active Agents

Surface-active compounds are widely used as wetting agents and detergents in industry and in the home. They act by altering the energy relationship at interfaces. Cationic surface-active agents are bactericidal, probably by altering the permeability characteristics of the cell membrane. Cationic agents are antagonized by anionic surface-active agents and thus are incompatible with soaps. Cationic agents are also strongly adsorbed onto porous or fibrous materials, eg, rubber or cotton, and are effectively removed by them from solutions.

A variety of cationic surface-active agents are employed as antiseptics for the disinfection of instruments, mucous membranes, and skin. Benzalkonium chloride USP (Zephiran, Roccal) and cetylpyridinium chloride NF are among the large number of substances in this group. Aqueous solutions of 1:1000−1:10,000 exhibit good antimicrobial activity but have some disadvantages. These quaternary ammonium disinfectants are antagonized by soaps, and soaps should not be used on surfaces where the antibacterial activity of quaternary ammonium disinfectants is desired. They are adsorbed onto cotton and thereby removed from solution. When applied to skin they form a film under which microorganisms can survive. Because of these properties, these substances have given rise to outbreaks of serious infections due to pseudomonas and other gram-negative bacteria. They cannot be employed safely as skin disinfectants and only rarely as disinfectants of instruments.

Nitrofurans

Many derivatives of furan have antimicrobial properties, especially if a nitro group is in the 5 position of the furan ring. Such compounds are markedly bactericidal for many bacteria in concentrations of 1:20,000 or less. The mechanism of action is not known. Strains of pseudomonas and proteus are often resistant.

Nitrofurantoin USP (Furadantin) is used exclusively as a urinary antiseptic for oral administration. Nitrofurazone NF (Furacin) is used as a topical antimicrobial agent on superficial wounds or skin lesions and as a surgical dressing. The preparations contain about 0.2% of the active drug, and do not interfere with wound healing. However, about 5% of patients may become sensitized and may develop reactions. Furazolidone NF (Furoxone) has only local effects. After ingestion it acts on shigella and vibrios in the gut, and is not absorbed significantly. After insertion into the vagina it acts on trichomonas. Nifuroxime NF inserted into the vagina acts locally on candida.

Miscellaneous Antiseptics

Many synthetic organic dyes have antimicrobial properties. Gentian violet is bacteriostatic but aesthetically unappealing. Acridine dyes have been used as topical antiseptics in 1:2000 concentration. Methylene blue was formerly used as a urinary antiseptic. Pyridium, an azo dye, was used as a urinary antiseptic although it acts primarily as an analgesic in the bladder. Local anesthetics (eg, procaine, lidocaine) have some inhibitory effect on the growth of bacteria and fungi. Thus, they may interfere with growth of an etiologic agent in specimens from tissues or surfaces exposed to these agents.

Sulfur, in various preparations, is employed as a fungicide and parasiticide for topical use. Many fatty acids, especially propionic and undecylenic acids, are important topical antifungal drugs. Undecylenic acid NF, 5%, and zinc undecylenate NF, 20%, are among the least irritating and most fungistatic drugs available for treatment of dermatophytosis.

Mafenide (Sulfamylon) is a topical sulfonamidelike drug applied as a 10% emulsion to burned surfaces. It can inhibit bacterial growth and shorten the delay until skin grafting.

STERILIZATION PROCEDURES

The function of sterilization procedures is to make materials free from viable microorganisms, spores, or viruses. In the past, this was accomplished most commonly by the application of heat under controlled conditions.

Incineration, using controlled burning, is used to dispose of infectious materials. Dry heat (160–170° C for more than 1 hour) is employed to sterilize dry glassware, ceramics, and other materials. Moist heat or autoclaving (121° C for 15 minutes or more at 15 lb/sq inch) is used for many instruments, dressings, linens, and bacteriologic media. All of these procedures must be carefully controlled with respect to time, temperature, size of materials, air circulation, displacement of cold air by steam, permeability of packaging materials, and other features which determine the efficacy of the application of heat.

Many materials which must be sterilized do not tolerate high heat, eg, plastics, optical devices, pump oxygenators, and extracorporeal circulation devices. These materials are "gas sterilized" by exposure to **ethylene oxide**, because irradiation is not readily controllable. Ethylene oxide can destroy the viability of microorganisms, probably by the alkylation of sulfhydryl groups of proteins. Ethylene oxide rapidly penetrates most materials exposed in a vacuum to its action and sterilizes them in 4–12 hours; it then must be removed because it leaves toxic residues, eg, ethylene glycol and ethylene chlorohydrin. For proper ethylene oxide sterilization, materials must be wrapped in cloth, paper, or polyethylene, exposed to the gas for a proper period under controlled temperature, and then evacuated to remove gas and toxic residues and aerated for a prescribed time (often 8–16 hours) before being used.

In most sterilization procedures, indicators of adequate time and temperature exposure and of sterility ("spore strips") must be employed. Careful records are essential and must be kept for years.

•　•　•

General References

Cason, J.S., & E.J.L. Lowbury: Mortality and infection in extensively burned patients treated with silver-nitrate compresses. Lancet 1:651–654, 1968.

Lawrence, C.A., & S.S. Block: *Disinfection, Sterilization, and Preservation.* Lea & Febiger, 1968.

Perkins, J.J.: *Principles and Methods of Sterilization in Health Sciences,* 2nd ed. Thomas, 1969.

Reddish, G.F. (editor): *Antiseptics, Disinfectants, Fungicides, and Chemical and Physical Sterilization.* Lea & Febiger, 1957.

59 ...

Combinations of Antimicrobial Drugs

For 2 decades physicians have been so justifiably impressed with the efficacy and the relative harmlessness of the antimicrobial drugs that many were tempted to reason that, "If one drug is good, 2 should be better, and 3 should cure almost anybody of almost anything." As a result, multiple antibiotic administration flourished. About one-fifth of all patients admitted to hospitals in the USA receive an antibiotic, and about half of these are given 2 or more antimicrobial drugs simultaneously. The use of fixed drug combinations has been promoted by the pharmaceutical industry vigorously and at times unscrupulously.

The indiscriminate use of antimicrobial drugs has several important disadvantages (see Chapter 48). The use of combinations has obvious additional drawbacks. Among them are the increase in adverse reactions and in sensitization to several drugs simultaneously, and the temptations they offer to relax efforts to arrive at an accurate diagnosis promptly. The problems of antibiotic abuse are discussed in Chapter 48. It is the purpose of this chapter to review some basic features of combined antimicrobial drugs.

POSSIBLE INDICATIONS FOR COMBINED ANTIMICROBIAL DRUGS

The possible reasons for employing 2 or more drugs simultaneously instead of a single drug are as follows:

(1) In certain desperately ill patients with suspected infections of unknown etiology it might be desirable to administer more than one antimicrobial drug immediately in an effort to "cover" the most likely pathogenic organisms. Before such treatment is begun it is essential to take appropriate samples so that laboratory tests can be performed to establish an etiologic diagnosis. The drugs are aimed at the organisms most likely to cause the clinical picture observed, and are administered only until the establishment of an etiologic diagnosis permits specific therapy.

(2) In mixed infections it is possible that 2 or more drugs, each acting on a separate portion of a complex microbial flora, may be more effective than one. This applies occasionally to infections of skin, wounds, and body cavities, particularly when poorly absorbed antibacterial drugs with narrow spectra are used topically (eg, polymyxin, neomycin, bacitracin). It may at times apply also to mixed systemic infections, particularly of the cardiovascular system, the respiratory tract, or the urinary tract.

(3) In some clinical situations the rapid emergence of bacteria resistant to one drug may impair the chances for cure. The addition of a second drug sometimes delays the emergence of that resistance. This effect has been demonstrated unequivocally in tuberculosis and is the basis for the frequent use of combinations of streptomycin, isoniazid, aminosalicylic acid, ethambutol, rifampin, or other drugs. It may apply to other chronic infections, and is the basis for the belief that erythromycin, carbenicillin, streptomycin, or similar agents should not be given singly for protracted periods because resistance to each drug is likely to develop. This is the basis for sometimes giving carbenicillin together with gentamicin in pseudomonas sepsis.

(4) Drug combinations may at times reduce the incidence or intensity of adverse reactions. A given microorganism may be susceptible to each of 2 drugs, but only in dosages which are likely to cause severe adverse reactions. If the drugs are used simultaneously, each can be used in half the dosage—below the threshold of adverse reaction. For example, a pseudomonas strain might be inhibited by polymyxin, 5 μg/ml, or chloramphenicol, 30 μg/ml, used singly, or by a combination of polymyxin, 2 μg/ml, and chloramphenicol, 15 μg/ml. The latter levels can be achieved by reasonably well tolerated doses of each drug, whereas a dose of polymyxin sufficient to yield blood levels of 5 μg/ml will give rise to severe adverse effects.

(5) The simultaneous use of 2 drugs may at times achieve an effect not obtainable by either drug alone. One drug enhances the antibacterial activity of the second drug against a specific microorganism. Such an effect could be considered "synergism," a term which has been much abused. Unfortunately, such "synergism" is unpredictable: A given combination of drugs must be specifically tailored, by laboratory test, to fit a certain isolate of a given microorganism. A synopsis of the dynamics of combined antibiotic action is given below. One of the best established examples of "synergism" is the cure of bacterial endocarditis caused by enterococci (*Streptococcus faecalis*) by a combination of a penicillin with an aminoglycoside (eg, streptomycin) as compared to the usual treatment failure with a penicillin alone.

PROBLEMS IN DEFINING & MEASURING COMBINED ANTIMICROBIAL DRUG EFFECTS

Even when technically feasible, chemical estimates of antimicrobial drug concentration usually do not mirror the antibacterial activity. Direct evaluation of bacteriostatic or bactericidal activity is the only meaningful way of measuring the effects of these drugs. Several methods can be employed, and all may be applicable to the measurement of combined drug action.

(1) **Bacteriostatic effect:** Endpoints are expressed as the minimum amount of drug necessary to suppress visible growth for a given time.

(2) **Bactericidal effect as shown by the rate of killing:** Results are expressed as the bactericidal rate, ie, the slope of the plot of viable survivors at various time intervals.

(3) **Bactericidal effect as shown by the completeness of killing:** The results are expressed as the smallest concentration of drug resulting in a given number of viable survivors in a given time.

(4) **Curative effect as shown in therapeutic trials in vivo.**

The results of any one type of examination need not coincide with those of any other type because the different methods may measure different events in the test system. For example, drug A may be markedly inhibitory but only slightly bactericidal in a certain concentration against a given organism. Drug B may have a slow early bactericidal rate but may kill completely at the end of 24 or 48 hours. One result is not necessarily "better" than another. The test may have to be fitted, by experience, to the clinical problem. Even within a given test system the results may depend on concentration of drugs, duration of action, etc, and on the importance attached to a given event. An example, applied to the measurement of combined antibiotic action, is shown in Fig 59–1.

It is evident that at time I fewer bacteria have survived exposure to drug A than to the combination of A + B. Thus, the early bactericidal effect of A + B is less than that of A alone, an example of antibiotic antagonism. At time II, however, there are fewer survivors of A + B than of A alone—perhaps an additive effect. The interpretation of such test results obviously depends on the importance attached to early bactericidal action and to completeness of killing, respectively.

A fallacy in the comparison of single drugs with combinations, on the basis of weight, must also be considered. It is possible to determine experimentally one minimal effective dose (MED) (eg, bacteriostatic, bactericidal, or curative) and express it in weight of drug. The temptation is then great to claim synergism for a combination that contains less than ½ MED of each of 2 drugs and which possesses greater activity than would be expected on the basis of algebraic summation. The fallacy lies in the assumption of a linear relationship between drug weight and effectiveness. The relationship between weight and effect of a single drug can be estimated experimentally only above 1 MED. However, below 1 MED the relationship might lie on X or Y (Fig 59–2). Thus, the effect of ½ MED of drug A + ½ MED of drug B might be greater than, equal to, or less than the effect of 1 MED by weight of either drug alone. Regrettably, this point is frequently not recognized in evaluating synergism and is used as the basis for claiming it.

DYNAMICS OF COMBINED ANTIBIOTIC ACTION

Let us consider that 2 antimicrobial drugs act simultaneously on a homogeneous microbial population. One of 3 effects—indifference, synergism, or antagonism—may be observed as diagrammed in Fig 59–3.

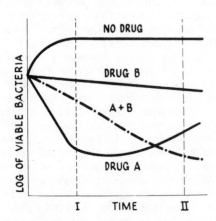

FIG 59–1. Number of viable bacteria after various times of exposure to a single drug or a combination of drugs.

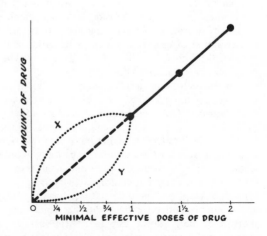

FIG 59–2. Relationship between amount (weight) and antimicrobial effect of a drug.

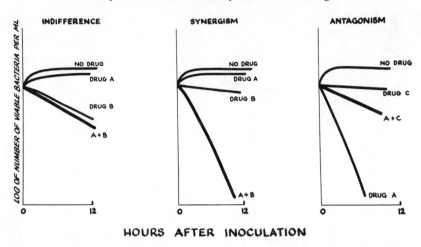

HOURS AFTER INOCULATION

FIG 59–3. Types of combined action of antimicrobial drugs.

Indifference

The most common result is indifference. The combined effect of drugs A and B is equal to that of the single more active component of the mixture A + B, or is equal to the arithmetic sum of the effects of the individual drugs in their chosen doses. The same total effect could be obtained by the use of a single drug in a dose equivalent to that of the mixture. Undoubtedly, the use of drug mixtures by physicians most often belongs in this category. (It must also be recognized, however, that the simultaneous use of 2 drugs in the "indifferent" category may be justified for one of the reasons given above.)

Synergism

At times the simultaneous action of 2 drugs results in an effect (A + B) which is far greater than that of either A alone or B alone in much larger dosages and also greater than could be expected from simple addition of individual drug effects. The measurement of such an event presents problems that are discussed above.

One type of "synergism" is manifested by a striking increase in rate of bactericidal action of the drug combination beyond that accomplished with twice the concentration of each single drug participating in the mixture. The characteristics of this type of "synergism" may be summarized briefly here:

When such "synergism" is found for a given pair of drugs acting on a given microorganism, it usually extends over a fairly wide range of concentrations of each member of the drug pair and is not greatly influenced by the proportion in the mixture. Conditions must be suitable for the organism to multiply in order to demonstrate "synergism." Only one member of the drug pair need exhibit inhibitory activity in the concentration employed in the mixture; the other may appear to be ineffective by itself. The simultaneous presence of the 2 drugs is essential: If the first drug is removed before the second drug is added, no "synergism" occurs.

The mechanism of action of "synergism" is largely speculative at present. It may be that one drug is more active against one portion of the microbial population and the other more active against the remainder of the population. Or the action of one drug may block microbial replication only incompletely, and the action of the second drug may be necessary for bacteriostatic or bactericidal effect. It has been postulated that the combined effect of penicillin with an aminoglycoside on enterococci results in the killing of replicating bacteria by penicillin and killing of L forms by the aminoglycoside. Alternatively, it has been postulated that penicillin damages the cell wall and thus greatly enhances the penetration of the aminoglycoside into enterococcal cells. Two examples of known mechanism for synergistic drug action are given in Chapter 47, ie, sulfonamide-trimethoprim combinations acting on protozoa or bacteria, and methicillin-ampicillin combinations acting on gram-negative bacteria.

Clinical evidence for "synergism": No fixed drug combination regularly results in desirable "synergism." To obtain a "synergistic" combination for use in treating a given patient with an infection, the drugs have to be fitted specifically to the organism isolated from the infection. The best clinical evidence for antibiotic synergism comes from the treatment of bacterial endocarditis, a disease that can be cured only if the infecting organisms are eradicated by bactericidal drugs. The bactericidal action of penicillin on many viridans streptococci is enhanced and accelerated in vitro by the simultaneous presence of streptomycin. Combined treatment with penicillin for 3 weeks and streptomycin for half that period may be optimal for *Streptococcus viridans* endocarditis. Endocarditis caused by enterococci (*S faecalis*) can usually not be cured by penicillin alone, since penicillin is inhibitory but not bactericidal for enterococci. The addition of an aminoglycoside is strikingly bactericidal for many strains of enterococci, and the cure of many such patients with a combination of penicillin or ampicillin with kanamycin or streptomycin is an accepted example of clinical "synergism."

However, not all strains of enterococci behave in this fashion. A few are killed by penicillin alone; others require other drug combinations for cure. Before the availability of methicillin, many patients with endocarditis or sepsis caused by β-lactamase producing staphylococci were cured by drug combinations specifically selected in vitro for their "synergistic" activity, although the individual drugs were often ineffective. In urinary tract infections or sepsis caused by gram-negative bacteria, drug pairs specifically selected in the laboratory provided "synergistic" effects in the patient.

Antagonism

At times the addition of a second drug (C) actually diminishes the antibacterial effectiveness of the first drug (A) (Fig 59–3). This "antagonism" can be manifested by a decrease in the inhibitory activity or in the early bactericidal rate of a drug mixture below that of one or both of its components. Such "antagonism" exhibits the following characteristics.

Antagonism can be demonstrated only when the drugs act on organisms capable of multiplication. Antagonism is most marked when a barely active amount of a bacteriostatic drug is added to a minimal bactericidal amount of a second drug. It is obscured by a large excess of either one of the participating agents. Antagonism is limited not only by dose but also by time relationships. The interfering agent must act either before or simultaneously with the bactericidal drug–not after. The mechanism of antibiotic antagonism must be the result of sequential action whereby the interfering agent reduces the importance or activity of that metabolic pathway which would have been inhibited by the bactericidal drug. Interfering agents (eg, chloramphenicol, tetracyclines, erythromycins) act primarily as inhibitors of protein synthesis. They antagonize actively bactericidal agents such as penicillin which act as inhibitors of cell wall mucopeptide synthesis. It is possible that protein synthesis must proceed actively to permit active mucopeptide synthesis; if so, inhibitors of protein synthesis will antagonize inhibitors of mucopeptide synthesis.

Clinical evidence for antimicrobial drug "antagonism": Antagonism is sharply limited by time-dose relationships in vitro and in vivo. It is readily demonstrated with single dose treatment of animal infections but only with difficulty in multiple dose treatment, where the ever-changing blood and tissue levels make it unlikely that the stringent requirements for antagonism will be met. In clinical practice it is usual to give a large excess of antimicrobial drug in multiple doses. Consequently, antagonism cannot be expected to be a frequent outcome of clinical antimicrobial therapy.

There are few documented examples of clinical antagonism. The combination of penicillin and chlortetracycline cured fewer patients with pneumococcal meningitis than did the same dose of penicillin alone. Similarly, the addition of chloramphenicol to ampicillin resulted in more treatment failures in bacterial meningitis than ampicillin alone. Antagonism was also shown for a tetracycline-penicillin combination and for an erythromycin-penicillin combination in group A hemolytic streptococcal pharyngitis. In urinary tract infections caused by gram-negative rods, antagonistic drug combinations failed to eradicate the causative organisms, whereas synergistic drug combinations succeeded. In all of these instances the observed antagonism fitted into the concepts outlined above. The strict time-dose requirements for the demonstration of antagonism make its observation difficult and suggest that it plays only a minor role in determining the end result of treatment in most infections.

THE SELECTION OF DRUG COMBINATIONS IN CLINICAL PRACTICE

As described above, combined drug action is a specific effect of a given drug combination for a given microorganism. It is completely misleading to describe a given drug pair as "synergistic" without specifying a given microorganism. Thus, desirable drug combinations have to be selected for each strain by appropriate laboratory methods. However, a few general rules for combined antibiotic action can be formulated for the guidance of the clinician.

In the original attempts to provide an experimental basis for combined antibiotic therapy a tentative scheme was suggested which was amplified later. Antimicrobial drugs were placed into 2 groups: (I) Penicillins, streptomycin, bacitracin, neomycins, polymyxins. (II) Tetracyclines, chloramphenicol, erythromycins, novobiocin, sulfonamides.

"Synergism" manifested by in vitro enhancement of bactericidal activity occurred relatively frequently among members of group I, virtually never among members of group II. The effect of a mixture of I and II depended on the behavior of the organism toward the group I drug. If the organism was very rapidly killed by the group I drug, addition of a group II drug might slow the bactericidal rate and result in antagonism. If the organism was relatively resistant to the group I drug, addition of a group II drug might give synergism under some circumstances.

This empirical scheme was intended to serve only as a framework for laboratory studies, and its essential validity has been confirmed in several laboratories. It was never suggested that it should be used as a clinical guide or that the behavior of a microorganism could be predicted a priori. It must therefore be stressed once more that, in the absence of clinical experience and of specific laboratory information, the scheme cannot serve as a guide for combined therapy.

Today the need for combinations of antimicrobial drugs arises infrequently. Apart from enterococcal endocarditis, infections with gram-negative rods and tuberculosis are the most likely candidates for combined antimicrobial therapy. In contrast, most staphylococcal infections can be handled well with the β-lactamase resistant penicillins, and brucella, klebsiella, and pasteurella infections often respond as well to single drugs as to combinations. Above all, the indiscriminate use of drug combinations must never take the place of proper diagnosis or specifically directed antimicrobial therapy.

• • •

General References

Dowling, H.F.: Present status of therapy with çombinations of antibiotics. Am J Med 39:796—803, 1965.

Jawetz, E.: The use of combinations of antimicrobial drugs. Ann Rev Pharmacol 8:151—170, 1968.

60...

Chemoprophylaxis*

Anti-infective chemoprophylaxis is the administration of drugs to prevent the acquisition and establishment of pathogenic microorganisms. In a broader sense it also includes the use of drugs soon after the acquisition of pathogenic microorganisms but before the development of symptoms and disease.

The administration of one or several antimicrobial agents cannot remove all microorganisms or keep away the entire "microbial world." The useful effect of chemoprophylaxis is limited to the action of a specific drug against a specific microorganism. Thus, only sharply "aimed" chemoprophylaxis can be effective. An effort to prevent all types of microorganisms in the environment from establishing themselves invariably fails and only selects the most drug-resistant organism as the cause of the resulting infection. In all forms of proposed prophylaxis, the risk of the patient's acquiring an infection must be weighed against the toxicity, cost, and inconvenience of the proposed prophylactic drug.

ANTIBACTERIAL & ANTIRICKETTSIAL CHEMOPROPHYLAXIS

SPECIFIC PROPHYLAXIS IN PERSONS OF NORMAL SUSCEPTIBILITY EXPOSED TO A SPECIFIC PATHOGEN

The outstanding examples of this type of chemoprophylaxis are the prevention of streptococcal, meningococcal, and gonococcal infections in both military and civilian populations. Syphilis, plague, and the rickettsioses will also be considered here.

Streptococci

Group A streptococcus infections may produce acute illness, suppurative complications, and late nonsuppurative complications such as rheumatic fever or glomerulonephritis. Prevention of primary infection

can prevent illness or complications. Treatment of established infection with group A beta-hemolytic streptococci can prevent nonsuppurative complications if the responsible streptococcal antigens are eliminated quickly and completely. Prevention of reinfection with any type of group A streptococci in persons with a past history of rheumatic fever may prevent exacerbations of the latter and development of rheumatic heart disease. Because of the small number of nephritogenic types and the existence of type-specific postinfectious immunity, prevention of reinfection with streptococci is not indicated in nephritis.

Sulfonamides were first employed on a large scale in military populations to prevent streptococcal infections. This was effective for only a short time because of the rapid emergence and selection of sulfonamide resistant streptococci. Subsequently, penicillin was introduced for mass prophylaxis in military populations, and it has maintained its efficacy: No penicillin-resistant strains of group A beta-hemolytic streptococci have emerged to date. At present the preferred method is the intramuscular injection of benzathine penicillin G, 1.2 million units, once each month.

Reinfection with streptococci in rheumatic patients can be prevented with benzathine penicillin G, 1.2–2.4 million units IM every 3–4 weeks; with oral penicillin, 250,000 units twice daily; or (less certainly) with sulfonamides, eg, sulfadiazine, 1 gm orally daily on arising. The optimal duration of such prophylaxis in rheumatic subjects has not been established. Some authorities believe that in rheumatic children it should be continued for at least 5 years after a rheumatic attack, and perhaps indefinitely. With advancing age, the chance of a damaging reactivation of rheumatic activity diminishes; therefore, the duration of prophylaxis may be shortened. There must be continuous reassessment of this question. Children on continuous penicillin prophylaxis for rheumatic fever regularly carry penicillin-resistant normal flora in their respiratory tract.

Nonsuppurative poststreptococcal complications can be prevented by the prompt eradication of the infecting streptococci from the respiratory tract. Drugs that suppress streptococcal growth but do not kill them (eg, sulfonamides or tetracyclines) should **never** be used in spite of the apparent clinical improvement they produce in streptococcal sore throat. The treat-

*Antiviral prophylaxis is discussed in Chapter 57; antiparasitic prophylaxis in Chapters 62 and 63.

ment of choice is benzathine penicillin G, 1.2 or 2.4 million units (600,000 units for children under 10 years) given IM once. If procaine penicillin G or other salts are used, repeated intramuscular or oral doses must be given to maintain adequate penicillin levels for 10 days. If such eradication of streptococci begins within 5–8 days after the onset of infection, post-streptococcal complications can be prevented. If eradication of streptococci is started later, it is a significantly less effective form of prophylaxis. Penicillin administration in established acute rheumatic fever does not prevent valvular heart disease.

As an alternative to penicillin, erythromycin may be used.

Many streptococcal infections are asymptomatic. The continuous prophylaxis used in rheumatic subjects is directed largely (and effectively) at subclinical infections. Among nonrheumatics, this is not feasible. However, the attack rate of rheumatic fever is about 3% following symptomatic clinical streptococcal infections and only about 0.3% following asymptomatic or very mild streptococcal infections. The attack rate is somewhat proportionate to the severity of the attack preceding the poststreptococcal complication. Thus, early treatment of symptomatic infections will have a major prophylactic effect. The attack rate of acute glomerulonephritis among children with mild or asymptomatic streptococcal infection is near 0.17%.

Meningococci

Meningococcal infections are a particularly severe problem in closed population groups such as military units. In such groups there is a high exchange of respiratory microbial flora and establishment of a high carrier rate of pathogenic meningococci. This in turn is followed by a rise in the incidence of meningococcemia and meningitis.

After World War II the administration of sulfadiazine, 3 gm orally daily for 3 days, effectively reduced the carrier rate in military units and eliminated meningitis because virtually all meningococci were sulfonamide sensitive. Since 1963, sulfonamide resistant meningococci of groups A, B, and C have produced repeated outbreaks in military groups and in civilian populations. Consequently, sulfonamide prophylaxis lost much of its previous effectiveness. All known meningococci remain susceptible to penicillin G to date. Penicillin administration only suppresses the meningococcal carrier state but does not terminate it.

If started very promptly, penicillin in high dosage (eg, 20 million units [12 gm] daily) can cure infection with sulfonamide resistant meningococci. The question of prophylaxis for contacts (family, etc) of such patients is not settled. Since most contacts who acquire the organisms will remain healthy, it might be best to keep contacts under observation and reserve possible massive penicillin treatment for those with persistently positive nasopharyngeal cultures or those who develop symptoms. Rifampin, 600–900 mg daily for 4 days, can eliminate meningococci from 90% of carriers, but in the remaining ones the meningococci

are rifampin resistant. Minocycline, 200 mg daily for 5 days, can reduce carriers by 65%.

Gonococci

Gonococcal infection occurs principally after one of 2 types of contact: the passage of the fetus through the mother's infected cervix, and sexual intercourse. Infection resulting from either type of exposure can be prevented with drugs because of the superficial location of the infecting organisms and their susceptibility to drugs.

The prevention of ophthalmia neonatorum is accomplished by instilling a bactericidal substance into the conjunctival sac of the newborn immediately after delivery. In many countries, 1% silver nitrate is prescribed by law for this purpose. This chemoprophylaxis is effective.

The implantation of gonococci in the mucous membranes of adult genitalia can be prevented by the presence of sufficient tissue levels of penicillin. Two tablets of 800,000 units penicillin G taken 1–2 hours before or after sexual intercourse can provide tissue levels sufficient to kill the limited number of gonococci acquired during contact. Whereas most gonococci were killed by less than 0.02 unit/ml penicillin G in 1945, some strains now require 2 units/ml for the same effect. Larger doses of penicillin or erythromycin may be necessary for prophylaxis in the near future.

Penicillin prophylaxis of gonorrhea may have an effect on the acquisition of syphilis. Multiplication of *Treponema pallidum* may often be inhibited by antigonorrheal prophylaxis, so that the development of clinical syphilis is masked. Prolonged follow-up (serology) is therefore necessary to rule out subclinical syphilitic infection.

Syphilis

Syphilis can be prevented by chemoprophylaxis. The administration of therapeutic doses of benzathine penicillin G (2.4 million units IM) within 24 hours of exposure has a good chance of preventing or aborting infection. Because of the risk of subclinical infection in spite of chemoprophylaxis, prolonged follow-up is mandatory, with serologic tests on blood and spinal fluid.

Plague

Plague is an extremely serious epidemic threat when primary cases of human pneumonic plague have occurred. Under such circumstances the administration of sulfonamides to the entire exposed population (sulfadiazine, 3 gm daily orally for 3 days) has successfully controlled outbreaks.

Rickettsioses

Certain rickettsial infections (eg, scrub typhus) are not always amenable to vector control (eg, elimination of mites). Since rickettsial multiplication can be inhibited by several antibacterial drugs, chemoprophylaxis is feasible. Chloramphenicol or tetracycline, 1 gm orally daily, can provide drug levels that will inhibit rickettsial multiplication in man after infection has occurred. This chemoprophylaxis serves to avoid serious clinical illness in persons who are forced to spend a short time in a hyperendemic area. It does not prevent infection, but prevents the unrestricted multiplication of the rickettsiae which may result in symptoms. Thus, disease is avoided during drug prophylaxis but the individual remains infected. After drugs are discontinued, multiplication of rickettsiae can begin and may result in disease unless a second and more aggressive therapeutic course of the drugs is begun soon after the symptoms have started.

SPECIFIC PROPHYLAXIS IN PERSONS OF INCREASED SUSCEPTIBILITY

Certain individuals with anatomic or functional abnormalities are predisposed toward infections of a serious or even life-threatening nature. It may be feasible to prevent or abort such infections by means of chemoprophylactic drugs given at specific times for short periods.

Prevention of Bacterial Endocarditis

Persons with congenital or acquired (eg, rheumatic) abnormalities of heart valves are unusually susceptible to the implantation of viridans streptococci and other organisms circulating in the blood stream. If recognized promptly, the resulting endocarditis can usually be cured with proper treatment. Nevertheless, endocarditis remains an exceedingly serious disease and efforts to prevent it are worthwhile. Viridans streptococci enter the blood stream from the respiratory tract. Large numbers of these organisms are pushed into the circulation during chewing and especially during dental procedures and operations on the throat (eg, tonsillectomy). At such times the increased risk warrants the use of a chemoprophylactic drug. The present choice is the administration of procaine penicillin G, 600,000 units IM 1–2 hours before the procedure and once daily for 2 days thereafter. An additional dose of 600,000 units aqueous penicillin G IM is given just prior to the procedure. In lieu of injection, oral buffered penicillin G, 400,000–600,000 units, may be given every 6 hours for 6–8 doses. Erythromycin is substituted in persons hypersensitive to penicillin and in those receiving oral penicillin for long-term rheumatic fever prophylaxis. They carry penicillin resistant viridans streptococci in the throat.

Enterococci (*Streptococcus faecalis*) cause about 10% of cases of bacterial endocarditis. These organisms reach the blood stream from the urinary or gastrointestinal tract or from the female genital tract. During surgical procedures in these areas, persons with heart valve lesions can be given chemoprophylactic drugs directed against enterococci. This involves the administration of penicillin G, 5 million units, and streptomycin, 1.5 gm, IM daily beginning on the day of surgery and continuing for 3 days.

During and after cardiac catheterization, blood cultures are positive in 10% to 20% of patients and many of these subsequently have fever. Prophylactically administered antibiotics do not influence this sequence.

Persons With Functional & Anatomic Abnormalities of the Respiratory Tract

Persons with emphysema, bronchiectasis, and other pulmonary disturbances are subject to attacks of "chronic bronchitis," a recurrent bacterial infection which precipitates respiratory decompensation. The commonest organisms involved in "chronic bronchitis" are pneumococci and *Hemophilus influenzae*. Chemoprophylaxis aimed at these and similar organisms consists of the administration of tetracycline or ampicillin, 1 gm daily, or cephaloridine, 2 gm daily, during the season of highest bronchitis incidence. This is successful only if patients are not in a hospital environment, where superinfection with pseudomonas, proteus, or yeasts is very common.

Mucoviscidosis (cystic fibrosis) in children predisposes to frequent and severe bronchopulmonary infections. Before antibiotics became available, such infections were a principal cause of early death. The continuous or intermittent administration of tetracyclines has been remarkably effective in prolonging life and reducing the frequency and severity of respiratory tract infections. Children with mucoviscidosis still get infections even with tetracycline prophylaxis, but their life span is markedly extended. The mechanism of this effect is not fully established. The complicating infections now are mainly caused by pseudomonas and staphylococci.

Chronic Corticosteroid Administration

Patients who are chronically ill with diseases such as systemic lupus erythematosus or pemphigus which are being controlled only by continuous high doses of corticosteroids may be given antibacterial chemoprophylaxis as long as they are outside the hospital environment; in these circumstances the risk of bacterial infection can perhaps be diminished by continuous or intermittent administration of antimicrobial drugs. There is no uniform or accepted method for such "prophylaxis," however, and its efficacy is not established. Such an approach always fails in hospitalized patients because superinfection with drug resistant bacteria occurs promptly.

Postcoital Cystitis

Some women suffer from acute exacerbations of symptoms of urinary tract infection 24–48 hours after sexual intercourse. Although this fact is widely accepted, its mechanism is not established. Marked relief of symptoms is reported if these women take "prophylactic" antimicrobial drugs, eg, 2–3 million units of penicillin G or ampicillin, 2 gm, by mouth within 24 hours, beginning immediately after intercourse. The effect probably is to suppress incipient bacterial multiplication in the bladder. This form of "prophylaxis" is not generally accepted.

ANTIMICROBIAL DRUG PROPHYLAXIS
IN SURGERY

Several well controlled studies have established that the overall incidence of postoperative infections is not diminished by the administration of antimicrobial drugs before, during, or after surgery in either "clean" or potentially contaminated types of operations. Such drug administration may delay the onset of the symptoms and signs of infection, and often tends to select out the more drug resistant types of microorganisms. Thus, it is well accepted that general "antibiotic prophylaxis" to protect against all types of postoperative infection does not exist. However, some specialized, limited forms of "prophylaxis" listed below enjoy favor with some surgeons.

Lower Gastrointestinal Tract Surgery

Before elective operations on the lower gastrointestinal tract, it has been the custom to reduce the bowel flora by the preoperative oral administration of either insoluble sulfonamides (succinylsulfathiazole, phthalylsulfathiazole) or neomycin. It is assumed that the reduction in numbers of intestinal bacteria will reduce the hazard of peritoneal infection after accidental contamination with bowel contents at the site of surgery. It is probable that the skill of the surgeon and strict aseptic technic are far more important in preventing such infections than the action of these drugs. Two particular problems must be considered:

(1) Oral administration of prophylactic drugs suppresses the bowel flora only transiently and partially. The lowest numbers of bacteria are present within 48 hours after starting neomycin and within 5–6 days after starting sulfonamides. Soon thereafter, the numbers return to normal levels even when drugs are continued, but the composition of the flora is changed.

(2) Preoperative administration of neomycin may lead to implantation of neomycin resistant staphylococci in the bowel and increase the chances of the development of staphylococcal enterocolitis, with high morbidity and mortality.

Heart Surgery

In cardiac surgery the endothelium is usually damaged and a high incidence of viridans streptococcus endocarditis might be expected postoperatively. When penicillin is administered for 4 days postoperatively, this complication is virtually unknown. It is assumed that this "prophylactic penicillin" has specifically prevented implantation of viridans streptococci. However, staphylococcal endocarditis and pericarditis can take a considerable toll. The administration of methicillin for 5 days postoperatively is believed to prevent that complication. More recently, pseudomonas and other drug resistant gram-negative rod infections have appeared in cardiac surgery. Some cardiac surgeons now administer cephalosporins, polymyxins, or aminoglycosides as a "prophylactic" drug against those organisms. Each of the drugs can prevent the development

of infection by a particular bacterium but favors the selection of more resistant microorganisms (eg, fungi).

Topical Drug "Prophylaxis"

The local application of drugs directed against the commonest infective organisms has been proposed for certain surgical sites, eg, the eyes, joints, and bones. It is reasoned that these are highly susceptible tissues with poor host defenses and that the locally applied drugs may inactivate the few organisms that inevitably contaminate the operative field during long procedures. There is no conclusive evidence to support this belief.

TREATMENT OF SPECIFIC
ASYMPTOMATIC INFECTION AS
"PROPHYLAXIS" AGAINST DISEASE

This category of "prophylaxis" is more properly considered early treatment since the drugs are administered after infection has been established and the aim is to prevent disease, not infection. One example will suffice. An asymptomatic person converts from a negative to a positive tuberculin skin test. Physical and x-ray examinations are entirely negative. To prevent later clinical tuberculosis such a person is given isoniazid, 6–10 mg/kg/day, for 6–12 months on the assumption that such drug treatment will suppress or even eradicate the small population of tubercle bacilli. (See Chapter 52.)

ANTIVIRAL
CHEMOPROPHYLAXIS

A rapidly increasing number of chemicals are becoming available which interfere with the multiplication of certain specific viruses in man. While these are sometimes referred to as antiviral chemotherapy, they are really active prophylactically because they succeed only if administration of the drug precedes entry and replication of the virus.

Amantadine hydrochloride (adamantanamine, Symmetrel; see Chapter 57) in a daily dose of 200 mg taken 2–3 days before and 6–7 days after infection with influenza A viruses may reduce the incidence and severity of symptoms and the magnitude of the serologic response. This drug is ineffective against influenza B viruses and most other respiratory agents and thus is of little practical concern at present.

Methisazone (N-methyl-isatin-β-thiosemicarbazone, Marboran; see Chapter 57) in a daily dose of 2–4 gm (100 mg/kg/day for children) administered for 3 days to smallpox contacts beginning 1–2 days after exposure has effectively reduced subsequent morbidity and mortality due to smallpox. The drug inhibits viral replication to a limited extent and permits the development of active immunity. It is strikingly effective in areas where smallpox is endemic.

•   •   •

General References

Clark, H.: Antibiotic prophylaxis in cardiac catheterization. Am Heart J 77:767–771, 1969.

Karl, R.C., & others: Prophylactic antimicrobial drugs in surgery. New England J Med 275:305–308, 1966.

Petersdorf, R.G., & others: Symposium on the chemoprophylaxis of infection. J Pediat 58:149–194, 1961.

61...

Biologic Products for Prophylaxis & Therapy

Some biologic products are used for the purpose of inducing active immunity to an infectious disease and are administered before symptoms or signs of that disease appear or even before the individual has been exposed to the infectious agent. Other products are administered for the purpose of providing passive immunity to a toxic or infectious agent; these usually consist of preformed antibodies which have short-lived biologic activity.

Whenever biologic products are administered, the physician must be prepared to recognize and manage their untoward effects. Biologic products are usually labile, with a limited shelf life and a definite expiration date, and require specialized storage. The manufacturer's directions must be followed because changes in dosage schedules occur frequently.

THE INDUCTION
OF PASSIVE IMMUNITY
WITH PREFORMED ANTIBODIES

These products are more or less purified and concentrated antibody solutions derived either from man or animals actively immunized against a given antigen. If the source of antibody is human serum, no precautions against hypersensitivity reactions are usually necessary. However, if the antibodies were derived from animal sera, hypersensitivity reactions are common and must be guarded against. These reactions are of the immediate type, ranging from anaphylaxis to serum sickness. In order to avoid anaphylactic reactions, careful tests for hypersensitivity to the animal serum must be performed. If the tests give evidence of hypersensitivity, it is best to avoid that specific type of foreign protein (eg, horse serum) and obtain antibodies made in another animal (eg, goat, rabbit). If an alternative preparation is not available and administration of the specific antibody is deemed essential and potentially lifesaving, desensitization can be carried out. A summary of tests for hypersensitivity and desensitization with antibody-containing proteins is given on p 565.

Antibodies derived from human serum not only avoid the risk of hypersensitivity reactions but also have a much longer half-life in man (about 23 days for IgG antibodies) than those from animal sources. Consequently, much smaller doses of human than of animal antibody can be administered to provide therapeutic concentrations for several weeks. These advantages point to the desirability of using human antibodies for passive protection whenever possible.

HUMAN GAMMA GLOBULIN
(Immune Serum Globulin USP)

Immune serum globulin USP is a commercial preparation of gamma globulin derived from large pools of human plasma by low temperature ethanol fractionation. The preparation contains about 165 mg of gamma globulin per ml of solution (representing a 25-fold concentration of antibody-containing immunoglobulins of plasma), glycine as stabilizer, and thimerosal as preservative. Such immune serum globulin can be injected intramuscularly or subcutaneously but not intravenously. It has been employed clinically in the following circumstances:

(1) **Hypogammaglobulinemia**: Deficient antibody production occurs in various degrees and in various clinical forms on the basis of defects in antibody-producing cells. There may also be enhanced catabolism of immunoglobulins. Most of these disorders have a genetic basis and manifest themselves in childhood, leading to recurrent bacterial infections, predominantly of the respiratory tract. Such complications can usually be prevented by the injection of 0.3–0.45 ml/lb immune serum globulin (ie, 150 mg gamma globulin per kg) once each month. Antimicrobial drugs are used to control individual episodes of bacterial infection.

(2) **Viral hepatitis**: The manifestations of infectious hepatitis (IH) can be minimized or prevented with immune serum globulin, and the infection can often be kept subclinical. Persons intending to travel to areas where IH is endemic can be given immune serum globulin, 0.01 ml/lb (0.02 ml/kg) every 4–6 weeks, to provide partial passive protection. For nonimmune persons residing in areas where IH is highly endemic, the injection of 0.05 ml/lb (0.1 ml/kg) once every 4–6 months has been recommended.

After suspected or known exposure to IH, immune serum globulin, 0.01 ml/lb (0.02 ml/kg), is injected as promptly as possible, and the injection is repeated 3 weeks later to prevent or modify the disease.

The administration of immune serum globulin does not stop viral multiplication but restricts it somewhat. This favors the development of mild or subclinical disease, which tends to induce active immunity. There is no evidence that passive immunization against viral hepatitis prevents infection; it only modifies the disease.

It has been suggested that immune serum globulin, 0.06 ml/lb (0.12 ml/kg), given to patients who must receive multiple blood transfusions, may reduce the risk of serious serum hepatitis. However, the evidence is not convincing that pooled human gamma globulin can affect serum hepatitis.

(3) Measles: This disease should be prevented by universal vaccination in early childhood. When vaccinating with the "attenuated" (Edmonston) live strain of measles virus, untoward reactions (ie, manifestations of infection such as fever and rash) can be minimized by the simultaneous injection of immune serum globulin, 0.01 ml/lb (0.02 ml/kg), into a separate site. With more highly attenuated measles vaccine strains (eg, Schwarz), globulin is unnecessary.

In nonvaccinated susceptibles, measles can be either prevented or attenuated with immune serum globulin. To *prevent* clinical measles in susceptible persons, 0.01 ml/lb (0.02 ml/kg) of immune serum globulin is injected once during the first 6 days after exposure. This may be indicated in very young or debilitated unvaccinated children, and it interferes with the development of active immunity.

To *attenuate* clinical measles, 0.02 ml/lb (0.04 ml/kg) of immune serum globulin is injected between the sixth and eighth days after exposure. This results in a modified, mild disease, and permits the development of active immunity which is usually lifelong. Administration of immune serum globulin between the eighth and the tenth days after exposure may produce some attenuation of disease, but after the onset of rash there is no effect.

(4) Rubella: The injection of 0.2–0.5 ml/kg serum immune globulin into pregnant women soon after exposure to rubella may modify or prevent the disease. However, it is unlikely that such treatment is able to prevent infection of the fetus with rubella virus.

SPECIFIC HYPERIMMUNE HUMAN GAMMA GLOBULINS

Tetanus

A specific hyperimmune gamma globulin has been prepared from persons repeatedly immunized with tetanus toxoid. This human gamma globulin eliminates the problems of hypersensitivity to animal proteins in persons who must receive passive immunization against tetanus. For prophylaxis after injury in nonimmunized persons, 250–500 units of human hyperimmune tetanus globulin injected IM yield levels of 0.03 unit or more of antitoxin per ml of serum for several weeks.

Ideally, every individual should have active immunization against tetanus, with boosters at suitable intervals (see immunization schedule, p 566). Human antitoxin, 3000–6000 units, has been administered for the treatment of clinical tetanus, but proof of its efficacy is lacking. In tetanus of the newborn, 500 units of human hyperimmune tetanus globulin has some therapeutic benefit.

Vaccinia

Hyperimmune gamma globulin prepared from the plasma of persons recently and successfully revaccinated with vaccinia virus is available from the American Red Cross. Injection of 0.6–1 ml/kg IM can arrest the dissemination of vaccinia lesions in patients with eczema and can stop progressive vaccinia in certain persons.

Chickenpox (Varicella)

Specific immune globulin (ZIG) is prepared from the serum of persons recently recovered from herpes zoster and exhibiting high antibody titer. A dose of 0.12 ml/kg injected into susceptible children within 72 hours of exposure can prevent both infection and disease.

Rabies

A concentrated serum derived from hyperimmunized horses is available (see p 559). Specific immune globulin has been prepared from the serum of persons repeatedly vaccinated against rabies. It contains 165 IU/ml and is being used experimentally for the treatment of severe bites by rabid animals. In the future it should supplant the antirabies horse serum employed at present.

Rh Sensitization; Erythroblastosis Fetalis

When an Rh-negative mother has an Rh-positive child by an Rh-positive father, she may become sensitized by Rh-positive fetal cells—usually at the time of delivery—and develop antibodies to them. A subsequent Rh-positive fetus may suffer hemolytic disease when these anti-Rh antibodies lyse its red cells. Rh sensitization can usually be prevented when an unsensitized Rh-negative mother is injected with specific immune human $Rh_0(D)$ globulin within 72 hours of delivery. The usual dose is 1 vial containing 1–1.5 ml of high titer IgG globulin injected IM. This antibody inhibits active antibody formation to the red blood cell antigens which entered the mother's circulation at delivery.

Pertussis

Specific hyperimmune globulins containing antibodies to *Hemophilus pertussis* and to various other bacteria have been prepared in the past. The clinical

TABLE 61–1. Agents for induction of passive immunity: Preparations available.

Product	Manufacturer	Preparations Available
Immune serum globulin USP (gamma globulin)		
Immune serum globulin, human	Hyland	Vials, 2 and 10 ml
Gamulin	Pitman-Moore	Vials, 2 and 10 ml
Gammagee	Merck Sharp & Dohme	Vials, 2 and 10 ml
Immuglobin	Savage	Vials, 10 ml
Gamastan	Cutter	Vials, 2 and 10 ml
Immune serum globulin	Philips Roxane	Vials, 10 ml
Immu-G	Parke-Davis	Vials, 2 and 10 ml
Poliomyelitis immune globulin	Breon	Vials, 2 and 10 ml
Specific hyperimmune human gamma globulin		
Tetanus		
Gamulin-T	Pitman-Moore	Vials, 250 units
Homo-Tet Injection	Savage	Vials, 250 units, and syringes, 250 units
Hu-Tet	Hyland	Vials, 250 units
Hyper-Tet	Cutter	Vials and disposable syringes, 250 units
Immu-Tetanus	Parke-Davis	Sterilized vials, 250 units
Pro-Tet Injection	Lederle	Vials and disposable syringes, 250 units
T-I-Gammagee	Merck Sharp & Dohme	Disposable syringes, 250 units
Vaccinia hyperimmune gamma globulin	Available from American Red Cross	
Rh sensitization		
Immune globulin, Rh_O (D) (human) (RhoGAM)	Ortho Diagnostics	Single dose vial and 1:1000 dilution for cross-match
Pertussis		
Pertussis immune globulin	Breon, Hyland	Vials, 1.5 ml
Hypertussis (concentrate)	Cutter	Vials, 1.25 ml
Antitoxins and antisera for passive protection of man prepared in animals		
Antirabies serum, equine origin	Lederle	Vials, 1000 units
Botulism antitoxin, bivalent (AB), equine origin	Lederle	Vials containing 10,000 units each of types A and B
Botulism antitoxin, trivalent (ABE)	Connaught	Available from Center for Disease Control, Atlanta
Botulism antitoxin type ABEF	Statens Serum Institute, Copenhagen	
Tetanus antitoxin	National	Vials, 1500, 3000, 5000, 10,000, and 20,000 units
Antivenins		
Antivenin (crotalidae), polyvalent (North and South American antisnakebite serum)	Wyeth	Vials to yield 10 ml serum
Antivenin (*Micrurus fulvius*) (North American coral snake)	Wyeth	Lyophilized vials to yield 10 ml
Antivenin, black widow spider (*Latrodectus mactans*)	Merck Sharp & Dohme	Lyovac vial to yield 2.5 ml, not less than 6000 units/vial
Gas gangrene		
Gas gangrene antitoxin, polyvalent	National	Therapeutic dose vials containing 10,000
Gas gangrene antitoxin, trivalent	Parke-Davis	units each of perfringens and septicum and 1500 units of oedematiens per vial
Gas gangrene antitoxin, polyvalent	Lederle	Therapeutic dose vials containing 10,000 units of perfringens and septicum, 3000 units of histolyticum, and 1500 units of oedematiens and bifermentans per vial

TABLE 61-2. Skin test antigens.

Antigen	Manufacturer	How Supplied
Blastomycin	Parke-Davis	Vials, 0.01 ml, with buffered diluent, 1 ml
Brucellosis	Merck Sharp & Dohme, Parke-Davis	Vials, 1 ml (10 test)
Candida albicans	Hollister-Stier	Vials, 2 ml, 5 ml, 10 ml, undiluted, diluted
Coccidioidin	Bioproducts, Cutter	Vials, 1 ml, 1:10 and 1:100 dilution
Diphtheria toxin (Schick test)	Many manufacturers	Vials (diluted)
Histoplasmin	Lederle, Michigan Dept of Health, Parke-Davis	Vials, 0.01 ml, with buffered diluent, 1 ml
Lymphogranuloma venereum	Squibb	Vial, 1 test with control
Mumps	Lilly	Vials, 1 ml, 10 test
Trichinella extract	Lederle	Vials, 1 ml, with saline control, 1 ml
Tuberculin PPD	Many manufacturers	First strength, 10 test and 50 test Intermediate strength, 10 test and 50 test Second strength, 10 test and 50 test
Tularemia	Center for Disease Control	

efficacy of these preparations is doubtful, and they are rarely used.

ANTITOXINS & ANTISERA FOR PASSIVE PROTECTION OF MAN PREPARED IN ANIMALS

These are concentrated antibody preparations derived from specifically immunized animals, usually horses, sheep, rabbits, or goats, standardized as units. For the production of antitoxins, animals are injected repeatedly with toxoids, ie, toxins detoxified by formaldehyde. The resulting antitoxins can neutralize toxins prior to their attachment to a receptor site. Thus, antitoxins must be administered as promptly as possible to neutralize toxins **before** they are irreversibly bound. The following antitoxins are available:

Diphtheria Antitoxin

A concentrated globulin fraction of pooled sera of animals immunized with diphtheria toxoid. When the presumptive clinical diagnosis of diphtheria is made, antitoxin, 10,000–100,000 units, is injected IM or IV after suitable tests for hypersensitivity. Except for the mildest cases, the antitoxin is given without waiting for laboratory confirmation of diphtheria infection.

Botulism Antitoxin

Concentrated globulin fraction of sera of animals immunized with the toxin of *Clostridium botulinum*, type A, B, or E. Antitoxin is usually available as pooled polyvalent antitoxin. It must be injected as promptly as possible after the diagnosis of botulism is strongly suspected. After testing for hypersensitivity, give in the dosage and by the route directed by the manufacturer.

Tetanus Antitoxin

Concentrated globulin fractions of sera of horses or cattle immunized with the toxoid of *Clostridium tetani*. This preparation should be employed only if human hyperimmune antitetanus globulin is not available. Furthermore, under ideal circumstances, all persons should receive active immunization with tetanus toxoid in childhood and suitable booster injections thereafter.

Antivenins

Concentrated globulin fraction of sera of animals immunized with the venoms of poisonous snakes (rattlesnakes, vipers, cobras, and others), spiders, and scorpions. Follow the manufacturer's directions for dosage and route of administration and test for hypersensitivity.

Gas Gangrene Antitoxin

Concentrated globulin fraction of sera of animals immunized with the toxins of various clostridia, including *Cl welchii (perfringens), Cl septicum,* and *Cl oedematiens.* These trivalent or polyvalent preparations have been injected into patients who are suspected of developing gas gangrene as a result of sustaining contaminated wounds. However, their efficacy is very doubtful. It is probably preferable to rely on thorough surgical debridement and treatment with penicillin or other antimicrobial drugs. Hyperbaric oxygen therapy is a possibly useful adjunct.

Rabies Antiserum

Rabies antiserum is a concentrated globulin fraction of serum of horses immunized with rabies virus. It must be injected soon after the bite of a rabid animal, both systemically and into the area of the wound. Directions on dosage are given by The World Health Organization.

THE INDUCTION
OF ACTIVE IMMUNITY

INACTIVATED (KILLED) VACCINES

1. BACTERIAL INACTIVATED VACCINES

A variety of products are used in the induction of active immunity to infectious agents or their toxic products. The method of preparation of these biologic products, their nature, and their effects change frequently. Consequently, the manufacturer's directions must be consulted regarding dosage regimen and anticipated untoward effects. The following pages offer only a general description of these biologic products and a summary of recommendations for 1970 regarding immunization of children and travelers.

Products for the induction of active immunity fall into 3 general categories: (1) toxoids, (2) inactivated (killed) vaccines, and (3) live attenuated vaccines. Each of these categories is briefly summarized below.

TOXOIDS

Toxoids are prepared from the exotoxins of bacteria by treatment with formaldehyde and purification. This treatment results in a material which has lost its toxic properties but maintains the antigenic specificity of the active toxin. Antitoxins formed against toxoids will neutralize the active toxins. Toxoids can be dispensed as fluid toxoids, as toxoids adsorbed onto aluminum hydroxide or similar colloid for slower absorption from tissues, or as toxoids alum-precipitated from the original solution and resuspended in saline.

The most universally employed toxoids are those of diphtheria and tetanus. They are often used together (DT), and sometimes combined with pertussis vaccine (DPT). In the immunization of children, alum-precipitated or adsorbed toxoids are injected intramuscularly 3 times at intervals of 4–6 weeks during the first year of life, with subsequent boosters. Children tolerate such slowly absorbed preparations well, but many adults develop fairly severe local and systemic reactions. These reactions can be anticipated by prior testing by means of intradermal injection of 0.1 ml of a 1:20 dilution of diphtheria toxoid (Moloney test). Because of the relative frequency of such reactions, adults should be given (with caution) only specially purified toxoids (Td adult) designated "for adult immunization." Following the primary course of immunization with toxoids, antitoxin levels rise and then fall, but booster injections induce a rapid secondary rise of antibody levels to clinically protective levels (for tetanus, more than 0.02 unit/ml of serum) which persist for long periods. Consequently, years after initial immunization, persons at risk from tetanus or diphtheria are protected by an additional booster injection given immediately after injury or exposure.

Pertussis (Whooping Cough)

Suspensions of inactivated phase I *Bordetella pertussis*, adsorbed onto aluminum hydroxide or precipitated with alum, are injected intramuscularly into children during the first year of life. This effectively prevents or modifies disease due to this organism. Pertussis vaccine is usually combined with diphtheria and tetanus toxoids. The vaccine may produce febrile reactions but is usually well tolerated.

Plague

Suspensions of inactivated *Pasteurella pestis* are injected intramuscularly repeatedly in order to stimulate partial resistance to plague infection in areas where epidemiologic control of plague is not feasible. The vaccine often induces marked local pain, swelling, and heat, and a febrile response. Its efficacy is probably not great.

Cholera

Suspensions of inactivated cholera and El Tor vibrios can be injected repeatedly intramuscularly to stimulate partial resistance to cholera infection in countries where the disease is likely to occur. The vaccine often induces marked local pain, swelling, and heat, and a febrile response. Protection depends largely on frequent booster injections (the WHO certificate is valid for only 6 months) and is, at best, of intermediate degree.

Typhoid

Suspensions of acetone-killed *Salmonella typhi* are injected repeatedly subcutaneously to stimulate partial resistance to typhoid infection in countries where the disease is likely to occur. The vaccine often induces marked local pain, swelling, and heat, and a febrile response. The degree of protection against *S typhi* infection is fairly good; paratyphoid vaccines are almost worthless.

2. RICKETTSIAL INACTIVATED VACCINES

Epidemic Typhus

Suspensions of inactivated *Rickettsia prowazeki* grown in the yolk sacs of embryonated eggs and purified to reduce the content of egg antigens are injected repeatedly intramuscularly. This vaccine can induce a moderate degree of protection against louse-borne typhus. The efficacy of this vaccine is relatively good provided frequent booster injections are given. The vaccine is indicated only for persons likely to have contact with louse-borne typhus.

Rocky Mountain Spotted Fever

Suspensions of inactivated purified *Rickettsia rickettsi* grown in embryonated eggs can be injected repeatedly intramuscularly into persons likely to be exposed to tick bites in endemic areas. This vaccine and others against spotted fevers in other parts of the world are moderately effective in protecting against severe disease.

Other Vaccines

Other vaccines against rickettsial infections (eg, Q fever, scrub typhus) have been prepared. These inactivated preparations probably have moderate protective value in very specialized situations. They are not commercially available.

3. VIRAL INACTIVATED VACCINES

A variety of inactivated viral vaccines have been prepared and proposed for general use. Most have little merit when compared to effective live vaccines.

Adenovirus

Suspensions of inactivated cell culture grown adenovirus types 3, 4, and 7 were proposed for the prevention of respiratory disease in military recruits and children. They are not available in the USA at present because of fears of tumorigenicity, SV40 contamination, etc.

Arbovirus

Suspensions of inactivated Japanese B, western equine, and eastern equine encephalomyelitis viruses have been prepared. They are used principally in occupationally exposed persons and are probably not highly protective. They are not commercially available.

Influenza

Suspensions of inactivated egg-grown influenza viruses of the prevailing types and subtypes can be injected intramuscularly to provide a marginal degree of protection against natural infection. Such vaccines induce little nasal IgA antibody response in spite of good circulating antibody response. They are recommended only for high-risk patients, eg, elderly persons with chronic respiratory disease, patients with serious mitral valve disease, and children with cystic fibrosis. Such individuals should be injected every year with polyvalent vaccine.

Measles

Inactivated measles virus vaccine should not be used because it induces significant hypersensitivity without causing effective immunity. Use live virus vaccine.

Mumps

Suspensions of inactivated mumps virus repeatedly injected intramuscularly may induce partial resis-tance to natural infection. However, the inactivated vaccine is not very effective, and live virus vaccine should be used. Inactivated mumps vaccine has been used as a skin test: A positive delayed reaction (maximum at 18–30 hours) suggests that the person has experienced mumps before and, therefore, may be immune if exposed to the natural disease. Inactivated vaccine has also been used in adults to demonstrate that the individual is capable of giving a positive delayed skin reaction.

Poliomyelitis

Suspensions of cell culture grown, formalin-inactivated poliovirus of types I, II, and III (Salk vaccine) can be injected repeatedly intramuscularly. This can induce effective circulating antibodies and gives protection against the CNS manifestations of poliomyelitis if boosters are given regularly. However, this vaccine does not alter the susceptibility to intestinal infection with poliovirus and does not tend to eradicate poliovirus from the community. Oral, live virus vaccines are preferable because they can accomplish these ends.

Rabies

Suspensions of tissues from rabies infected animals, inactivated with phenol, are used for repeated injection into persons bitten by animals suspected of having rabies. Occasionally they are given prior to exposure. The efficacy of inactivated rabies vaccine is not established, and all preparations may induce an allergic encephalomyelitis because of their content of CNS tissue. At present, rabies virus vaccine is prepared in embryonated duck eggs. Effective live rabies vaccine is used in animals.

LIVE ATTENUATED VACCINES

These consist of suspensions of infectious bacteria or viruses which are attenuated and proved to produce infection but only in a mild, self-limited form or one with no clinical manifestations of illness at all. The aim of such vaccines is to stimulate all aspects of cellular and humoral immunity which occur as part of the response to the natural infection but to avoid the risk of serious disease from fully virulent microorganisms. Thus, a planned mild infection is substituted for an unpredictable, possibly severe one. The most effective vaccines for the induction of active immunity are in this category.

Possible disadvantages of such live vaccines are the difficulty of maintaining a stable, attenuated strain of living agent; manufacturing, standardization, and storage problems; control over contaminating living agents; the threat of mutation toward virulence; and the production of disease in debilitated recipients. In spite of these difficulties, more and more viral vaccines employ live attenuated infectious agents.

TABLE 61−3. Agents for induction of active immunity: Preparations available.

Product	Manufacturer	Preparations Available
Toxoids		
Diphtheria toxoid, adsorbed		
Diphtheria toxoid, alum-precipitated	National	Vials, 5 ml
Diphtheria toxoid, aluminum phosphate adsorbed	Parke-Davis	Vials, 5 ml
Diphtheria toxoid, aluminum phosphate adsorbed, ultrarefined	Wyeth	Vials, 5 ml
Tetanus toxoid, adsorbed		
Tetanus toxoid	Various mfrs	Disposable syringes, 0.5 ml, or vials, 0.5, 1.5, 7.5, and 15 ml
Tetanus toxoid, alum-precipitated	Merck Sharp & Dohme, Lilly, National	Disposable syringes, 0.5 ml, or vials, 0.5, 1, and 5 ml
Tetanus toxoid, aluminum phosphate adsorbed	Lederle, Parke-Davis, Wyeth	Disposable syringes, 0.5 ml, or vials, 1 and 5 ml
Tetanus toxoid, aluminum hydroxide adsorbed (Alhydrox)	Cutter	Vials, 5 ml
Diphtheria and tetanus toxoids, combined (for pediatric use)		
Plain	Lilly, Parke-Davis	Vials, 7.5 ml
Diphtheria and tetanus toxoids, adsorbed (for pediatric use)		
Alum-precipitated	Lilly, National, Pitman-Moore	Vials, 5 ml
Diphtheria and tetanus toxoids, aluminum phosphate adsorbed	Lederle, Wyeth Parke-Davis	Disposable syringes, 0.5 ml, and vials, 5 ml
Diphtheria and tetanus toxoids, adsorbed (for adult use)		
Alum-precipitated	Lilly, National	Vials, 5 ml
Aluminum phosphate adsorbed	Lederle, Wyeth	Disposable syringes, 0.5 ml, and vials, 5 ml
Diphtheria and tetanus toxoids and pertussis vaccine, plain	National, Parke-Davis	Vials, 7.5 ml
Diphtheria and tetanus toxoids and pertussis vaccine combined, adsorbed		
Alum-precipitated	National	Vials, 1.5 and 7.5 ml
Tri-Solgen (alum-precipitated, purified)	Lilly	Disposable syringes, 0.5 ml, and vials, 7.5 ml
Aluminum phosphate adsorbed		
Infagen	Pitman-Moore	Vials, 7.5 ml
Tri-Immunol	Lederle	Vials, 7.5 ml
Triogen	Parke-Davis	Disposable syringes, 0.5 ml, and vials, 1.5 and 7.5 ml
Triple Antigen	Wyeth	
Quadrigen (0.33 ml fluid poliomyelitis vaccine and 0.5 ml Triogen)		
Inactivated (killed) bacterial vaccines		
Pertussis vaccine	Lederle, Lilly, Parke-Davis	Vials, 7.5 ml
Pertussis vaccine, aluminum phosphate adsorbed	Parke-Davis	Vials, 7.5 ml
Plague vaccine (2 billion killed *Pasteurella pestis* per ml)	Cutter	Vials, 2 and 20 ml
Cholera vaccine (8 billion killed cholera vibrios of Asiatic strain per ml)	Lederle, Lilly National, Wyeth	Vials, 1.5 ml Vials, 20 ml
Typhoid vaccine (1 billion killed typhoid bacilli per ml)	Lilly	Vials, 1.5 and 15 ml
Inactivated (killed) rickettsial vaccines		
Typhus vaccine, epidemic	Lederle Lilly	Vials, 1 and 10 ml Vials, 2 and 20 ml
Rocky Mountain spotted fever vaccine	Lederle	Vials, 3 and 15 ml
Inactivated (killed) viral vaccines		
Adenovirus vaccine, types 3, 4, and 7 (temporarily unavailable in USA)	Parke-Davis	Vials, 5 ml

TABLE 61–3 (cont'd). Agents for induction of active immunity: Preparations available.

Product	Manufacturer	Preparations Available
Influenza vaccines		
Influenza vaccine virus, bivalent (each ml containing 700 CCA units: 400 CCA units of A_2/Aichi/2/68 Hong Kong variant, and 300 CCA units B/Mass./3/68)	Lederle, National Wyeth Merck Sharp & Dohme (Fluax)	Vials, 10 ml Vials, 10 ml, and Tubex, 1 ml
Each 0.5 ml of above, specially purified		
Fluogen	Parke-Davis	Disposable syringes, 0.5 ml, and vials, 5 ml
Zonomune Bivalent	Lilly	Vials, 2.5 ml
Mumps virus vaccine, inactivated	Lederle, Lilly	Disposable syringes, 1 ml, and vials, 2 and 10 ml
Poliomyelitis virus vaccine, parenteral (containing equal parts types I [Mahoney], II [MEF-1], and III [Saukett])		
Poliomyelitis vaccine, purified	Parke-Davis	Vials, 10 ml
Rabies virus vaccine	National Lilly	Vials (1 dose), 0.5 ml Vials (1 dose)
Bacterial live attenuated vaccines		
Tuberculosis vaccine, bacterial (BCG vaccine) (Living culture of bacillus Calmette-Guérin strain of *Mycobacterium tuberculosis* var *bovis*, freeze-dried.)	Lilly	1 ml
Viral live attenuated vaccines		
Smallpox vaccine (from lymph of calves)	National, Lilly, Wyeth	In capillary tubes for 1, 5, or 10 vaccinations
Smallpox vaccine, avianized (propagated in chick embryos)	Lederle	In capillary tubes for 1, 5, or 10 vaccinations
Poliomyelitis virus vaccine, oral (Sabin strains types 1, 2, and 3)		
Poliovirus vaccine, live, oral, monovalent	Pfizer, Wyeth	Types 1, 2, or 3 in 1, 10, or 100 dose dropper containers
Orimune	Lederle	Types 1, 2, or 3 in 100 dose size
Poliovirus vaccine, live, oral, trivalent	Pfizer, Wyeth	Types 1, 2, and 3 combined in various dose containers
Orimune	Lederle	
Measles (rubeola) virus vaccine, live attenuated		
Edmonston strain (grown in chick embryo)	Lilly	1 dose package
M-Vac	Lederle	1 dose package
Max Measles-L	Pfizer	1 dose package
Rubeovax Lyovac	Merck Sharp & Dohme	1 dose package
Edmonston strain (in canine renal tissue)	Parke-Davis Philips Roxane	1 dose vial
Schwarz strain Lirugen	Pitman-Moore	1 dose vial
German measles (rubella) virus vaccine, live		
Meruvax Lyovac	Merck Sharp & Dohme	Single dose vials of lyophilized vaccine containing 1000 TCID rubella virus
Mumps virus vaccine, attenuated Mumpsvac Lyovac	Merck Sharp & Dohme	Single dose vials
Yellow fever vaccine (available only through USPHS facilities, military hospitals and clinics, and other government authorized agencies)		Vials, 5 and 20 dose
Adenovirus vaccine (available only through USPHS and military hospital facilities)		

1. BACTERIAL LIVE VACCINES

Live attenuated bacteria are used to immunize animals against anthrax and brucella infections. These vaccines are not used for humans.

Plague

While the most widely accepted plague vaccines are killed bacterial suspensions, live attenuated plague bacillus vaccines have been used for immunization campaigns in hyperendemic areas, particularly in the face of threatened epidemics. They appear to be fairly effective live vaccines but are not widely available.

Tuberculosis

Live, avirulent tubercle bacilli, strain BCG (bacille Calmette-Guérin), have been injected into many millions of persons in an attempt to induce partial resistance to infection with virulent tubercle bacilli. Such vaccination usually results in conversion of the tuberculin skin test from negative to positive, and BCG organisms may survive for 3–7 years in the subject. Thus, vaccination results in the loss of the tuberculin test as a sensitive indicator of primary virulent infection and its possible prompt treatment. In many developed countries, BCG vaccination is now recommended only for tuberculin-negative persons who are heavily exposed to infectious cases of tuberculosis (eg, children in a family with active disease) who can be observed medically at frequent intervals. The use of BCG in leprosy has been suggested on the basis of experimental evidence.

2. VIRAL LIVE VACCINES

Most effective viral vaccines are in this category at present.

Smallpox

Active vaccinia virus in the form of glycerolated calf lymph or grown in chick embryos is dispensed in capillary tubes. The virus loses viability unless stored below 0° C. After cleansing, the dry skin is inoculated by the multiple pressure method or by scarification. For proper immunization, the virus must multiply locally, producing vesicles or pustules. Properly performed vaccination results in resistance to smallpox for up to 3 years (WHO certificate). It is recommended that routine smallpox vaccination in the USA be limited to health personnel and travelers. In other persons, it is to be an elective immunization.

More stable lyophilized vaccines and vaccines grown in cell culture are not generally available. A contraindication to vaccination is the presence of eczema or other widespread skin disease in the patient or family contacts, because this may predispose to generalized vaccinia, a serious disease. Vaccination should also be avoided in persons with known immunologic defects–agammaglobulinemia, Hodgkin's disease, etc.

Poliomyelitis

Attenuated strains of poliomyelitis virus types 1, 2, and 3, grown in cell culture, are administered orally either as single type or (repeatedly) as a trivalent mixture to small children. A trivalent booster dose is given orally 1–2 years later and another 3–5 years later. The ingested live virus replicates in the intestine, and some is excreted in feces and spread to contacts. Intestinal virus multiplication is accompanied by both systemic and intestinal antibody formation and induces solid immunity to subsequent virulent poliovirus exposure.

Measles (Rubeola)

Attenuated strains of measles virus, grown in cell culture, are injected intramuscularly once. This produces a mild systemic infection which results in long-term resistance to the natural infection. With the "Edmonston" strain, fever and rash often occur as untoward effects. This can be minimized by the simultaneous injection of human immune serum globulin. Immune serum globulin is not required with the further attenuated strains (eg, Schwarz) of measles virus, which usually result in asymptomatic infection. Live measles vaccines are highly effective. Inactivated measles vaccines induce hypersensitivity without permanent immunity and are undesirable.

German Measles (Rubella)

Attenuated strains of rubella virus, grown in cell culture, are injected subcutaneously. This produces a systemic infection perhaps followed by long-term immunity to the natural infection. Children tolerate the vaccine well, but fever and arthralgia are common in adults. Rubella vaccine must not be given to pregnant women because the vaccine strain may infect the fetus.

Some physicians prefer to administer rubella vaccine only to prepubertal girls. If given to seronegative adolescent girls and women it must be ascertained that pregnancy will not occur for 3 months after immunization.

Mumps

Attenuated strains of mumps virus, grown in cell culture and dispensed in lyophilized form, are injected subcutaneously or intramuscularly. This produces an asymptomatic infection which probably induces long-term systemic immunity to natural infection. The vaccine appears to be well tolerated by children.

Yellow Fever

An attenuated strain (17D) of yellow fever virus grown in embryonated eggs is dispensed in lyophilized form and injected subcutaneously. It produces an asymptomatic infection and solid immunity to natural infection and disease for 10 years or more. It has been used in many millions of persons and is an excellent vaccine.

Rabies

An attenuated strain of rabies virus grown in embryonated eggs (high egg passage Flury strain) has been widely used for immunization of animals. After injection, this virus produces an asymptomatic systemic infection and good immunity to natural infection and disease for at least 1—2 years. While this live vaccine is not now accepted for human use, its efficacy is so much greater than that of the traditional inactivated rabies vaccine that it might be very valuable for persons at high risk of exposure to virulent rabies, an almost invariably fatal infection.

Adenovirus

Strains of adenovirus type 4 and type 7 grown in cell culture and ingested in an enteric-coated capsule produce asymptomatic intestinal infection. This infection induces systemic immunity to the potentially debilitating respiratory infection and pneumonitis caused by the same type of adenovirus. This vaccine is being used only in military personnel, where adenovirus respiratory disease is a serious problem.

HYPERSENSITIVITY TO ANIMAL PROTEINS & DESENSITIZATION

Many persons are hypersensitive to animal proteins or drugs. If they are given such material by injection, there is a chance that anaphylaxis may develop. Therefore, tests for hypersensitivity are indicated prior to any such injection. Serum sickness can develop in anyone, independently of prior sensitization. The following steps are desirable as a safeguard against anaphylactic reactions, and must be observed with biologic products administered for prophylaxis or therapy, particularly with animal sera.

(1) **Past history**: Has the patient received a similar material before? Does he have known allergy, eg, to egg protein?

(2) **Materials available must include**: Epinephrine, 1:1000 solution, in sterile syringe; airway, soluble corticosteroid, tourniquet, antihistamine drug (eg, diphenhydramine) for injection, oxygen.

(3) **Intradermal test**: Diluted test material (eg, 1:10 diluted animal serum) is injected intradermally so that 0.1 ml raises a bleb, and the site is observed for 15 minutes. The appearance of erythema and edema with wheal formation suggests specific hypersensitivity.

(4) **Conjunctival test**: May be done as an alternative to the intradermal test. Instillation of 1 drop of 1:10 dilution of test material into a normal conjunctiva results in itching, lacrimation, and redness within 5 minutes if the person is hypersensitive. One drop of physiologic saline is instilled into the other eye as a control.

When the skin test or conjunctival test indicates hypersensitivity, it is preferable to avoid injection of the material in question and substitute another product. Thus, in place of diphtheria antitoxin in horse serum, diphtheria antitoxin in goat serum might be administered. If an alternative product is not available, desensitization may be attempted as follows:

Inject gradually increasing doses of the product every 30—60 minutes, observing for possible significant reactions. Begin with 0.1 ml of product diluted 1:100. If there is no reaction, give 0.1 ml diluted 1:10. If there is still no reaction, inject 0.1 ml undiluted. If a significant local reaction occurs, inject the same dose, or a smaller dose together with epinephrine, 1:1000, 0.5 ml. Increase the doses of the product gradually but steadily until 2 or 3 ml of undiluted product have been administered without significant reaction. Repeat this dose every 30—60 minutes until the full prophylactic or therapeutic dose has been given.

Desensitization often permits the administration of an animal protein to which the person exhibits moderate hypersensitivity. However, if major reactions occur during the procedure, desensitization attempts should be abandoned.

ACTIVE IMMUNIZATION AGAINST INFECTIOUS DISEASES

Biologic products used for active immunization are frequently modified. The schedule of administration, dose, and recommended route vary with the product and change often. Always consult the manufacturer's package insert and follow its recommendations. A schedule for active immunization of children is shown in Table 61—4.

RECOMMENDED IMMUNIZATION OF ADULTS FOR TRAVEL

Every adult, whether traveling or not, must be immunized with tetanus toxoid. Purified toxoid "for adult use" must be used to avoid reactions. Every adult should also have primary vaccination for poliomyelitis (oral live trivalent vaccine), for diphtheria (use purified toxoid "for adult use"), and perhaps for smallpox. Every traveler must fulfill the immunization requirements of the health authorities of the countries he visits. These are listed in *Immunization Information for International Travel*, US Public Health Service, Division of Foreign Quarantine, 7915 Eastern Avenue, Silver Spring, Maryland 20910.

The following are suggestions for travel in different parts of the world.

TABLE 61–4. Recommended schedule for active immunization and skin testing of children.

Age	Product Administered	Test Recommended
2–3 months	DPT[1] Oral poliovaccine[2], trivalent or type 2	
4–5 months	DPT Oral poliovaccine, trivalent or type 1	
6–7 months	DPT Oral poliovaccine, trivalent or type 3	
12 months	Measles vaccine[3]	
15–19 months	DPT Oral poliovaccine, trivalent Smallpox vaccine[4] (elective)	Read primary take of smallpox after 1 week
2 years	Mumps vaccine[5]	Tuberculin test[6]
4–6 years	DPT Smallpox vaccine (elective) Oral poliovaccine, trivalent	Tuberculin test[6]
8–10 years	Rubella vaccine[7]	Tuberculin test[6]
12–14 years	Td[8] Smallpox vaccine (elective)	Tuberculin test[6]

[1] **DPT**: Toxoids of diphtheria and tetanus, alum-precipitated or aluminum hydroxide adsorbed, combined with pertussis bacterial antigen. Suitable for young children. Three doses of 0.5 ml IM at intervals of 4–8 weeks. Fourth injection of 0.5 ml IM given about 1 year later.

[2] **Oral live poliomyelitis virus vaccine:** Either trivalent (types 1, 2, and 3 combined) or single type. Trivalent given 3 times at intervals of 6–8 weeks and then as a booster 1 year later. Monovalent type 2, then type 1, then type 3 given at 6-week intervals, and then a booster of trivalent vaccine 1 year later. Inactive (Salk type) trivalent vaccine is available but not recommended. *Note:* The sequence of monovalent vaccines given here (type 2, then 1, then 3) is in accord with the recommendations of the US Public Health Service Advisory Committee on Immunization Practices. The American Academy of Pediatrics recommends the sequence 1, 3, 2.

[3] **Live measles virus vaccine,** 0.5 ml IM. When using attenuated (Edmonston) strain, give human gamma globulin, 0.01 ml/lb, injected into the opposite arm at the same time, to lessen the reaction to the vaccine. This is not advised with "further attenuated" (Schwarz) strain vaccine. Inactivated measles vaccine should not be used.

[4] **Live smallpox vaccine (vaccinia virus),** usually supplied as calf lymph, must be used fresh, before the expiration date, and must be stored at low temperature. It is administered by multiple pressure technic. Site must be inspected at 7 days for evidence of "primary take" or at 3–4 days for evidence of "accelerated reaction." Some vesicles must be found to indicate immunizing proliferation of virus. Papules without vesication are not acceptable as evidence of "take." Do not vaccinate in the presence of eczema in the child or his siblings, during pregnancy, or when there is known immunologic deficiency. The US Public Health Service recommends that routine smallpox vaccination be abandoned in the USA because the risk of contracting the disease is less than the risk of complications from vaccination. Smallpox vaccination should be limited to those who may travel to places where smallpox has not been eradicated and to health personnel.

[5] **Live mumps virus vaccine (attenuated),** 0.5 ml IM.

[6] The frequency with which **tuberculin tests** are administered depends on the risk of exposure, ie, the prevalence of tuberculosis in the population group.

[7] **Rubella live virus vaccine (attenuated)** can be given between age 1 year and puberty. Some physicians recommend rubella vaccine only for prepubertal girls. The entire contents of a single dose vaccine vial, reconstituted from the lyophilized state, are injected subcutaneously. The vaccine must **not** be given to women who are pregnant or are likely to become pregnant within 3 months of vaccination. Adult women must also be warned that there is a 40% likelihood of developing arthralgias and arthritis (presumably self-limited) within 4 weeks of vaccination.

[8] **Tetanus toxoid and diphtheria toxoid,** purified, suitable for adults.

Tetanus

Booster injection of 0.5 ml tetanus toxoid, for adult use, every 5–7 years, assuming completion of primary immunization. (All countries.)

Smallpox

Revaccination with live smallpox vaccine (vaccinia virus) by multiple pressure method every 3 years. WHO certificate requires registration of batch number of vaccine. The physician should ascertain a "take" by observing vesicle formation, after administration of either liquid or freeze-dried effective vaccine. (Many countries.)

Typhoid

Suspension of killed *Salmonella typhi*. For primary immunization, inject 0.5 ml subcut twice at intervals of 4–6 weeks (0.25 ml for children under 10 years). For booster, inject 0.5 ml subcut (or 0.1 ml intradermally) every 3 years. (All countries.) Paratyphoid vaccines are probably ineffective and not recommended at present.

Yellow Fever

Live attenuated yellow fever virus, 0.5 ml, injected subcut. WHO certificate requires registration of batch number of vaccine. Vaccination available in USA only at approved centers. Vaccination must be repeated at intervals of 10 years or less. (Africa, South America.)

Cholera

Suspension of killed vibrios, including prevalent antigenic types. Two injections of 0.5 and 1 ml are given IM 4–6 weeks apart. This must be followed by 0.5 ml booster injections every 6 months of possible exposure. Protection depends largely on booster doses. WHO certificate is valid for 6 months only. (Middle Eastern countries, Asia, occasionally others.)

Plague

Suspension of killed plague bacilli given IM, 2 injections of 0.5 ml each, 4–6 weeks apart, and a third injection 6 months later. (Middle Eastern countries, Asia, occasionally South America and others.)

Typhus

Suspensions of inactivated typhus rickettsiae given IM, 2 injections of 0.5 ml each, 4–6 weeks apart. Booster doses of 0.5 ml every 6 months may be necessary. (Southeastern Europe, Africa, Asia.)

Hepatitis

No active immunization available. Temporary passive immunity may be induced by the IM injection of human gamma globulin, 0.01 ml/lb every 2–3 months. It is better to give 0.05 ml/lb every 4–6 months.

•   •   •

General References

Ascari, W.Q., & others: Rh$_O$(D) immune globulin (human). Evaluation in women at risk of Rh immunization. JAMA 205:1–5, 1968.

Brunnel, P.A., & others: Prevention of varicella by zoster immune globulin. New England J ·Med 280:1191–1194, 1969.

Committee on Control of Infectious Diseases: *Report,* 16th ed. American Academy of Pediatrics, 1970.

Grady, G.F., & A.J. Bennett: Prevention of post-transfusion hepatitis by γ-globulin. JAMA 214:139–142, 1970.

Janeway, C.A., & F.S. Rosen: The gamma globulins. New England J Med 275:826–831, 1966.

Lane, J.A., & others: Complications of smallpox vaccination, 1968. New England J Med 281:1201–1208, 1969.

Woodson, R.D., & J.J. Clinton: Hepatitis prophylaxis abroad. JAMA 209:1053–1056, 1969.

62 . . .

Antiprotozoal Drugs

J.F. Catchpool, MB, BS (Lond), LRCP, MRCS

THE CHEMOTHERAPY & CHEMOSUPPRESSION OF MALARIA

The choice of a drug or combinations of drugs for the chemotherapy or chemosuppression* of malaria depends on the following factors:

The Prevalence of Drug-Resistant Strains of Plasmodia

Strains of malaria resistant to chloroquine and other antimalarials are now rapidly spreading throughout Southeast Asia and Latin America, where a combination of heavy drug pressure, the introduction of large numbers of nonimmune persons, and the partial eradication of the disease have destabilized the ecology of malaria. However, in Africa, where much of the population is still exposed to malaria from birth and has acquired a considerable degree of immunity, the use of antimalarial drugs has not yet been sufficiently widespread to bring about the preferential emergence of chloroquine-resistant strains.

The choice of chemosuppressive antimalarial drugs must therefore take into consideration the geographic area that the nonimmune subject is going to visit, and the chemotherapy of acute malaria must be based on a knowledge of the prevalence of drug-resistant strains in the area where the infection was acquired.

The Species of the Infecting Parasite

Human malaria can be caused by 4 species of protozoal parasites. Three of the 4, *Plasmodium vivax*, *P malariae*, and *P ovale*, are classified as "relapsing

Dr. Catchpool is Assistant Research Epidemiologist, G.W. Hooper Foundation, University of California, San Francisco.
Section on amebiasis by Robert S. Goldsmith, MD, DTM&H, Associate Professor of Tropical Medicine and Epidemiology, University of California, San Francisco.
*The term chemosuppression is preferable to chemoprophylaxis because, in the strict sense, no drugs are yet available that can prevent all stages of parasitization by killing all the sporozoites. Several drugs, however, prevent expression of the disease by attacking the parasites at various stages of the plasmodial life cycle. The chemotherapy and chemoprophylaxis of the rapidly emerging drug-resistant strains of malaria consist of administering a combination of drugs, which is discussed under a separate heading below.

malarias" because they have a secondary or persisting stage of their life cycle. This secondary exo-erythrocytic stage of development provides a reservoir of parasites for the reinfection of the erythrocytes that can give rise to a recrudescence of symptoms months or even years after a clinical cure has been obtained by the destruction of the asexual forms in the blood.

P falciparum, the most lethal form of malaria, has no exo-erythrocytic stages. If the strain is not resistant, it readily responds to treatment, and a radical cure can be achieved. Malaria caused by this parasite is sometimes called "malignant tertian malaria" because it produces a fulminating infection in nonimmune victims with spikes of fever every third day corresponding to the bursting of the erythrocytes and the release of the merozoites. Untreated falciparum malaria in nonimmune individuals may rapidly progress to a fatal conclusion. In Vietnam, 84% of cases of malaria in Americans are due to *P falciparum*.

Malaria caused by *P vivax* is sometimes called "benign tertian malaria" because there are spikes of fever every third day and it runs a more benign and chronic course than *P falciparum* infections. Of the 3000 cases of malaria with onset within the USA reported during 1971, 85% were due to *P vivax* infections.

The disease caused by *P malariae* is sometimes called "quartan malaria" because the spikes of fever come every fourth day. In West Africa, quartan malaria is associated with a high incidence of nephrotic syndrome.

A rare form of relapsing malaria is caused by *P ovale*. Its periodicity is similar to that of *P vivax*, but it runs a milder course and is more easily treated.

Therapy for the relapsing malarias must be continued for several weeks after the last exposure to infection.

The Stage of Parasitization

Different antimalarial drugs exert their effects at different stages of the parasite's life cycle. Therapy or suppression may be aimed at (1) the pre-erythrocytic stages (sometimes called "primary exo-erythrocytic" or "tissue" stages), which take place in the liver; (2) the erythrocytic stages, in which the parasites multiply rapidly in erythrocytes; or (3) the exo-erythrocytic or secondary tissue stages of the relapsing malarias *(P vivax, P malariae,* and *P ovale)*, which also take place in the liver. In addition, some drugs may have a selectively toxic effect on the gametocytes that form in the erythrocytes and are responsible for transferring the infection to the mosquito. Other drugs, when ingested in the blood by the mosquito, may prevent the transmission of malaria to another victim by preventing multiplication (sporogony) in the mosquito gut and salivary glands.

Antimalarial drugs are sometimes classified as follows:

(1) Primary tissue schizonticides: Drugs that destroy the primary (pre-erythrocytic) tissue schizonts in the liver soon after infection (eg, primaquine).

(2) Blood schizonticides: ("Clinically curative" drugs.) Drugs that suppress the symptoms of malaria by destroying the schizonts and merozoites in the erythrocytes (eg, quinine, quinacrine, chloroquine, and amodiaquine).

(3) Gametocides: Drugs that prevent infection of mosquitoes and therefore the spread of infection by mosquitoes by destroying gametocytes in the blood (eg, primaquine).

(4) Sporonticides: Drugs that could help to eradicate the disease by preventing sporogony and multiplication of the parasites in the mosquito when ingested with the blood of the human host (eg, chloroguanide and pyrimethamine).

(5) Secondary tissue schizonticides: ("Radically curative" drugs.) Drugs used to cure the chronic relapsing fevers due to infection by *P vivax, P malariae,* and *P ovale* by destroying the secondary (exo-erythrocytic) tissue schizonts developing in the liver (eg, primaquine).

The Frequency of Administration

The antimalarial drugs presently available offer a range in speed and duration of drug action. Rapid-acting drugs are needed for therapy of acute attacks. For suppressive therapy, drugs taken once a week or once a month are convenient, but drugs taken daily may have advantages. It is usually easier to form a daily habit than to remember something once a month. In households with young children the dangers of double dosage or of dose omission are fewer if tablets are taken once daily; antimalarials are often kept, as vitamins often are, on the family breakfast table. The frequency of dosage for troops operating in the tropics is different from that for a family with small children living in the tropics. Tests of the urine of troops stationed in Vietnam have shown that many neglect to take their prophylactic antimalarials.

The Race of the Recipient

US blacks not previously exposed to malaria are notably less susceptible to *P vivax* malaria than US whites. Fifteen percent of US blacks are liable to suffer an acute self-limiting hemolysis when treated with primaquine. Certain unfavorable genetic polymorphisms have been maintained in populations living in malarial areas by conferring a greater tolerance to *P falciparum* malaria. For example, heterozygosity for the sickle cell gene provides a measure of protection against *P falciparum* infection, and it is likely that glucose-6-phosphate dehydrogenase (G6PD) deficiency, hemoglobin C disease, hemoglobin E disease, and β-thalassemia do so also.

The Degree of Host Immunity

In many parts of the world, the malaria death rate of children under the age of 4 is frequently as high as 15%. Chronic malarial infection may significantly impair the growth and development of the survivors. However, neonates born to immune mothers are partially immune by virtue of transplacentally acquired antibodies. This protection decreases in the first few months of life, and a partial immunity is acquired by repeated mild attacks of malaria. By age 5, this ability to acquire immunity largely disappears. Chemosuppression of malaria during these first few years may deprive a child of the ability to form active immunity.

Continuous protection of nonimmune persons with antimalarial drugs is mandatory. Continuous regular chemosuppression in children born in malarious areas will not only reduce the high morbidity and mortality due to malaria but will also enhance their physical development.

Epidemiologic Factors

Mass chemosuppression of malaria must also take into account the danger of resistant strain emergence. Intermittent and inadequate chemosuppression of nonimmune and partially immune populations who are constantly being reinfected from indigenous reservoirs of parasites greatly favors the emergence and spread of drug-resistant strains of malaria.

Immune populations should not be given chemosuppressive drugs unless the dosage regimens are adequate and strictly adhered to. Areas now cleared of malaria but having suitable anopheline mosquitoes may become reinfected by individuals carrying inadequately treated resistant strains of relapsing malaria. Therefore, personnel returning from Southeast Asia should be adequately treated with a tissue schizonticide (such as primaquine) for 4 weeks to obtain a radical cure of the relapsing malarias.

Malaria Following Blood Transfusion

An increasing number of cases of malaria (some fatal) have resulted from transfusions of infected blood. In most cases, a donor is incriminated by the presence in his serum of fluorescent antibodies to malaria, but often no parasites can be found in his blood. Subsequent inquiry always reveals that the infected donor once lived in a malarious area. Most of these infections are due to *P vivax* malaria, but infections with *P malariae* and *P ovale,* and even *P falciparum,* have been reported. Vietnam veterans should be rejected as blood donors for at least 2 years after leaving the tropics. Recent outbreaks of malaria in the USA have occurred in groups sharing equipment to "mainline" narcotic drugs.

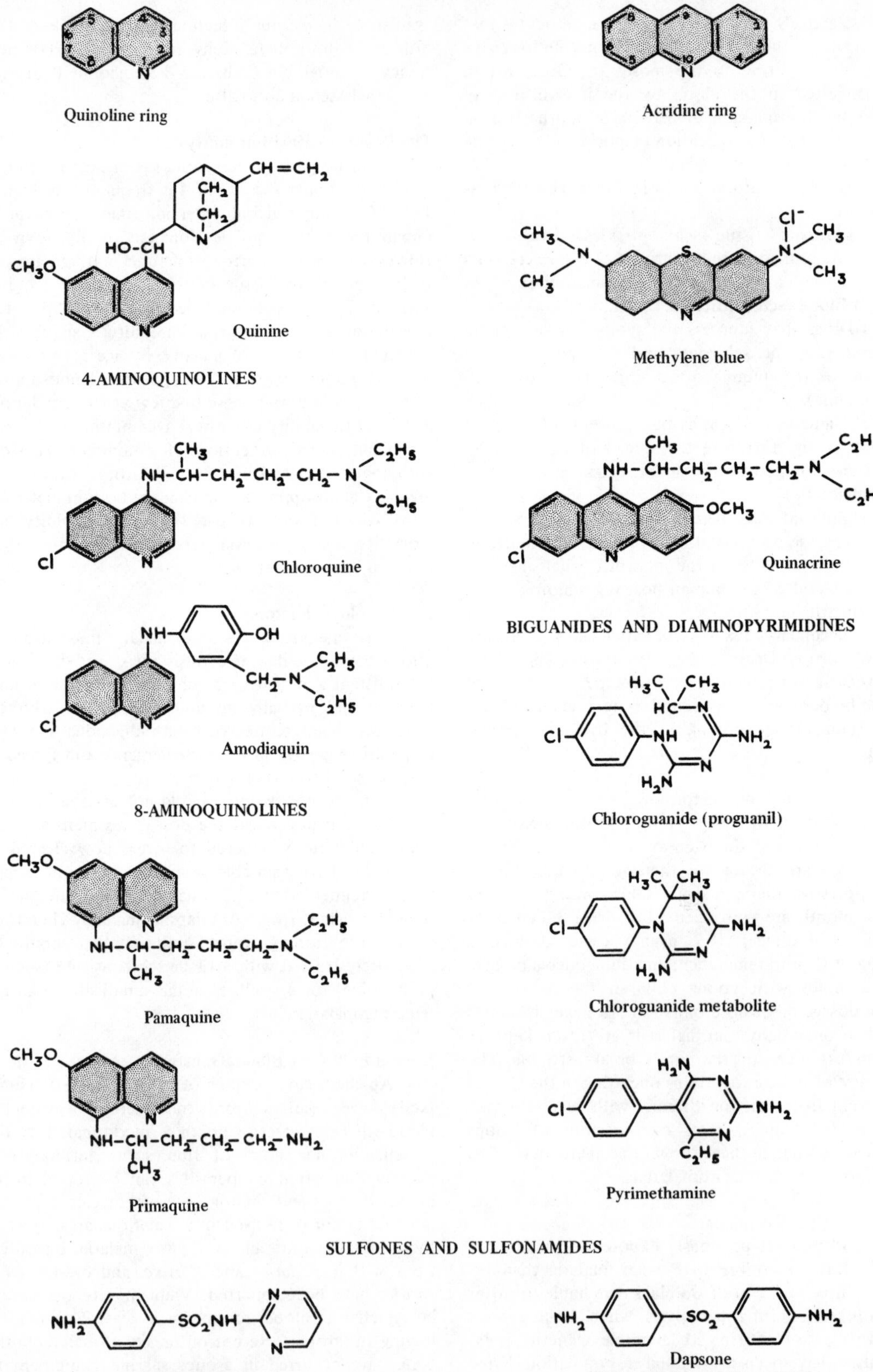

Quinoline ring

Acridine ring

Quinine

4-AMINOQUINOLINES

Methylene blue

Chloroquine

Quinacrine

Amodiaquin

BIGUANIDES AND DIAMINOPYRIMIDINES

Chloroguanide (proguanil)

8-AMINOQUINOLINES

Pamaquine

Chloroguanide metabolite

Primaquine

Pyrimethamine

SULFONES AND SULFONAMIDES

Sulfadiazine

Dapsone
(diaminodiphenylsulfone, DDS)

FIG 62–1. Structural formulas of antimalarial drugs. Arranged to show structural relationships and historical development of the compounds.

QUININE

History

Quinine is the principal alkaloid found in the bark of the South American cinchona tree. The use of cinchona bark for the treatment of malarial fevers dates back to the 17th century. Its discovery and introduction into Europe is usually credited to the Jesuits. Without quinine, the European colonization of tropical Africa would have been impossible. For 300 years until the Japanese occupation of the Javanese cinchona plantations early in World War II intensified the search for synthetic antimalarial drugs, the powdered bark was the only drug that could effectively suppress the symptoms of malaria. Although quinine can now be synthesized, it and the other cinchona alkaloids are still extracted from cinchona bark.

Chemistry

The 4 principal cinchona alkaloids (quinine, quinidine, cinchonidine, and cinchonine) all contain a quinoline ring linked by a secondary alcohol at its fourth position to a quinuclidine ring. Quinidine is the dextrorotatory optical isomer of quinine; cinchonidine is quinine minus a methoxy group; and cinchonine is the D isomer of cinchonidine. All 4 cinchona alkaloids have schizonticidal activity, but quinine is the only one used in the treatment of malaria because its absorption is much better.

Absorption, Metabolism, & Excretion

Quinine is rapidly absorbed from the small intestine, and peak plasma concentrations are obtained 1–3 hours after ingestion. Quinine can be detected in the urine as early as 15 minutes after ingestion. Excretion reaches a maximum after 4 hours, tapers off after another 4 hours, and is almost complete in 24 hours. Only 10% of the oral dose is excreted in the urine; the rest is metabolized. Given by subcutaneous or intramuscular injection, quinine is poorly absorbed because it is often precipitated. Inflammation and sloughing may occur at the site of injection.

Pharmacologic Effects

A. Mechanism of Action: The exact mechanism of quinine's antimalarial action is uncertain. Quinine can form a hydrogen-bonded complex with double-stranded DNA which inhibits protein synthesis by preventing strand separation and therefore DNA replication and transcription to RNA. Quinine has been observed to depress so many enzyme systems that it has in the past been described as a "general protoplasmic poison."

B. Effects on Malaria: Quinine, along with quinacrine, chloroquine, and amodiaquine, is classed as a "blood schizonticide." It has no effect on the primary or secondary exo-erythrocytic "tissue" forms of the parasites and cannot therefore bring about a radical cure of malaria caused by *P vivax, P malariae,* or *P ovale;* neither is it effectively gametocidal or sporonti-cidal to *P falciparum.* Although quinine cannot prevent infection, it can suppress the symptoms of malaria and also bring about rapid control of an acute attack. Quinine by intravenous drip is now once again the treatment of choice for nonimmunes suffering an acute attack of falciparum malaria in areas where chloroquine-resistant strains of *P falciparum* are known to exist.

C. Other Effects: The actions of quinine on the cardiovascular system are similar to those of quinidine (see Adverse Reactions, below). Quinine has little effect on smooth muscle other than a slight oxytocic action on the gravid uterus, especially during the third trimester of pregnancy. Clinically, it has no effect until labor has started, although dangerously toxic amounts may cause abortion.

In skeletal muscle, quinine has a curare-like effect on the motor endplate and causes a lengthening of the refractory period. Tetanic contractions associated with various conditions may be diminished by quinine, and the drug has been used to lessen the contractions of myotonia congenita and to provide a diagnostic test for myasthenia gravis by aggravating the symptoms. Quinine was used for centuries to abate fevers due to any cause; its antipyretic action was due mostly to peripheral vasodilation.

Clinical Uses

A. Use in Acute Malaria: For 300 years, quinine was the drug of choice for the treatment and chemosuppression of malaria. By 1959, quinine as an antimalarial had been totally superseded by synthetic antimalarials. However, 3 years later, chloroquine-resistant strains of *P falciparum* were being reported from Colombia and Brazil, and later from Southeast Asia. By 1965, 80% of the chloroquine-treated Americans in Vietnam were relapsing with malaria resistant to chloroquine; quinine appeared to be the only drug that could control this chloroquine-resistant malaria, but radical cures could be achieved in only 10–30% of cases treated with quinine alone. By 1969, US Army hospitals in Vietnam were reporting that prompt treatment with quinine combined with pyrimethamine had reduced the relapse rate to less than 1%. Unfortunately, a strain of *P falciparum* (Smith strain) appeared in 1968 that does not respond to quinine-pyrimethamine treatment. Infections with the Smith strain induced in volunteers in US prisons either relapsed after or were completely refractory to treatment with combinations of quinine, chloroquine, pyrimethamine, proguanil, and trimethoprim but were sensitive to a combination of quinine and sulphametopyrazine (Sulfalene). For cerebral malaria, which occurs in 2% of attacks of *P falciparum* malaria occurring in nonimmunes, intravenous quinine should be preceded by corticosteroids such as dexamethasone, 4–6 mg every 4–6 hours.

B. Other Uses: Quinine has been used for the symptomatic relief of headache, myalgia, arthralgia, and neuralgia, but as an analgesic it is more toxic and no more effective than aspirin. Muscle spasm (eg, leg cramps) and tetanic contractions associated with myotonia congenita may be relieved by quinine. It has also been used in diagnostic tests to aggravate the symptoms of myasthenia gravis which can then be relieved with neostigmine. In trace amounts, its intensely bitter taste is made use of in tonic waters and stomachics. In an emergency, quinine can be used as a substitute for quinidine, and vice versa.

Adverse Reactions

A. Side-Effects:

1. **Cinchonism**—This term denotes the mild toxic state that usually develops when the plasma level of quinine exceeds 10–12 mg/liter. Symptoms include flushed and sweaty skin, tinnitus, blurred vision, impaired hearing, dizziness, nausea, vomiting, and diarrhea. With severe cinchonism, there may be papular or urticarial skin rashes, deafness, somnolence, diminished visual acuity or blindness (toxic amblyopia) due to ischemia of the retinal vessels, abdominal pain, and disturbances in cardiac rhythm or conduction. Widening of the QRS complex of the ECG and hypotension are among the earliest signs of quinine toxicity.

2. **Local irritant effect**—Quinine is an irritant to the gastric mucosa, causing nausea and pain. Painful sterile abscesses frequently result from intramuscular injections. Intravenous injections may cause thrombophlebitis.

3. **Hematologic effects**—Hemolysis directly attributable to quinine occurs in 0.05% of people treated for acute malaria. A brown pigment consisting of an albumin-hematin complex consistently appears in the serum of patients receiving quinine and pamaquine concurrently. Quinine inhibits phagocytosis and may rarely cause leukopenia, agranulocytosis, thrombocytopenic purpura, and Schönlein-Henoch purpura.

4. **Blackwater fever**—Blackwater fever is a dread syndrome of excessive intravascular hemolysis, hemoglobinuria, azotemia, intravascular sludging and coagulation, renal failure, uremia, and death in 25–50% of cases. It is seldom seen in immune populations unless they have been treated with quinine. A recent study of renal involvement in malaria reported that all of the cases of hemoglobinuria occurred in patients who were receiving quinine and who were also G6PD-deficient. However, irregular or heavy therapy with any antimalarial, repeated infections, sensitization to the parasite, fatigue, chilling, and possibly idiosyncrasy to quinine may all be predisposing factors. The indications for quinine should be reviewed at the first sign of hemolysis. It is at times necessary to continue quinine therapy in spite of the hemolytic reaction if the infection is due to a resistant strain that cannot be treated with another drug. Every effort must be made to maintain fluid and electrolyte balance. Corticosteroids, heparinized low molecular weight dextran, and extracorporeal hemodialysis (when available) may help. Transfusion of whole blood should be avoided because the transfused cells are rapidly hemolyzed. The concomitant use of quinacrine or any 8-aminoquinoline drug is contraindicated in blackwater fever.

B. Overdosage Toxicity: Quinine is a neurotoxic agent which has specific effects on the ganglion cells. The lethal dose of quinine for adults is about 8 gm, but survival has been reported after much larger doses. After overdosage, prompt gastric lavage with an alkaline solution is imperative because the drug is rapidly absorbed and death may ensue within a few hours. There is usually a profound fall of blood pressure due to the peripheral vasodilation and myocardial depression. Respiration soon becomes slow and shallow, and cyanosis develops. The quinidine-like action produces ventricular tachycardia and, sometimes, transient bouts of ventricular fibrillation. Caffeine, ephedrine, and corticosteroids should be used to support the blood pressure, and oxygen and artificial respiration to relieve the cyanosis. After an overdose, the chances of survival improve with time because quinine is rapidly degraded in the body. Doses greater than 4 gm in 24 hours usually lead to visual impairment, usually transient. Vasodilating drugs such as intravenous sodium nitrite, inhalations of amyl nitrite or oxygen with 5% CO_2, and even stellate ganglion block help to produce dilatation of the retinal vessels.

Massive intravascular hemolysis followed by ischemic tubular necrosis and acute renal failure have occurred when large doses of quinine were given in an attempt to terminate pregnancy.

Preparations & Dosages

A. Oral: Quinine sulfate is available in 0.3 gm tablets. For the treatment of acute attacks, give 0.6 gm 3 times a day for 14 days. Doses should be taken after meals in order to minimize the gastric irritation.

B. Intravenous: Quinine hydrochloride in 2 ml ampules (300 mg/ml) is diluted with 300 ml of glucose in saline and administered slowly by intravenous drip in 30–60 minutes. Blood pressure and ECG should be monitored to detect hypotension or cardiac arrhythmias. Oral therapy should be substituted as soon as possible.

For recrudescences of the acute attack, the above dosage may be repeated.

The dose (to be given 3 times a day) for children under 1 year is 30 mg; 1–2 years, 60 mg; 2–3 years, 120 mg; 3–5 years, 200 mg; 5–7 years, 250 mg; 7–9 years, 300 mg.

THE 4-AMINOQUINOLINE DERIVATIVES

1. CHLOROQUINE

History

Originally synthesized in 1934 in Germany (Resochine), chloroquine was tested for antimalarial activity, but in 1935 it was reported to be too toxic for human use. In April 1942, following the fall of the

Javanese cinchona plantations to the Japanese, the US War Production Board instigated a crash program of research for synthetic antimalarial drugs. By late 1944, US workers had synthesized 25 different 4-amino-quinoline derivatives, finally selecting a compound designated SN 7618 (later named chloroquine) as the most promising—only to discover a few months later that it was identical with the compound patented in Germany and the USA under the name of Resochine.

By 1946, chloroquine had become the drug of choice for the treatment of malaria the world over.

Chemistry & Nomenclature

Chloroquine (Aralen) is 7-chloro-4-(4'-diethyl-amino-1'-methylbutylamino)quinoline.

Trade names and code designations for chloroquine diphosphate are: Aralen, Avloclor, Bemaphate, Chinamine, Gontochin, Imagon, Iroquine, Klorokin, Luprochin, Resochin, Resoquine, Sanoquin, Tanakan, Tresochin, Trochin, SN 7618, and Win 244.

Chloroquine sulfate: Nivaquine, Nivaquine B, 3377 RP.

Chloroquine methylene-bis-β-hydroxynaphthoate: Chloroquine "embonate," Resochin "tasteless."

Hydroxychloroquine sulfate: Plaquenil, Plaquinol, Win 1258, SN 16,168.

Oxychloroquine diphosphate: SN 8137.

Sontoquine disulfate: SN 6911, Santoquine, Santochin, Sontochin, Nivaquine C (3038 RP) (dihydrochloride), Nivaquine M (3032 RP) (methylene bis-hydroxynaphthoate), Nivaquine R (Resorcine Carbonate).

Chloroquine diphosphate is a bitter, colorless, dimorphic crystalline powder soluble in water at pH 4.5 but with diminishing solubility at more neutral or alkaline pH. The D and L isomers are equally potent, but the D isomer is slightly less toxic. Chloroquine has a quinoline ring like that of quinine with a side chain identical to that of quinacrine. The Cl atom in the seventh position appears to be crucial to the antimalarial activity of the 4-aminoquinolines and quinacrine.

Absorption, Metabolism, & Excretion

Absorption of chloroquine from the gastrointestinal tract is rapid and complete; maximum plasma concentrations are reached in 1–2 hours. The half-life of chloroquine in the body is about 5 days. Chloroquine is rapidly removed from the plasma and concentrated in those tissues where active protein synthesis and cell multiplication are greatest. The liver, spleen, kidneys, lungs, and leukocytes often contain 200–700 times the plasma concentration (whereas the brain and spinal cord contain only 10–30 times the plasma concentration). For this reason, whenever an effectively schizonticidal plasma level is urgently needed, a loading dose should be given. The concentration of chloroquine in the erythrocytes is about 10–20 times greater than that of the plasma and in parasitized erythrocytes about 25 times greater than in normal erythrocytes. Only 10–25% of the oral dose is excreted in the urine. The rate of excretion may be increased by acidification

of the urine or decreased by alkalinization of the urine. Concomitant administration of other 4-amino-quinolines or 8-aminoquinolines prolongs and potentiates plasma levels of chloroquine.

Pharmacologic Effects

A. Mechanism of Action: Chloroquine and its congeners block the enzymatic synthesis of DNA and RNA. These drugs form a complex with DNA which prevents it from acting as a template for its own replication or transcription to RNA. It has been postulated that the quinoline ring of chloroquine is inserted between the base pairs of the DNA double helix so that the chlorine atom in position 7 of the quinoline ring lies in close proximity to the 2-amino group of guanine in a guanine-cytosine base pair. The diamino-aliphatic side chain of chloroquine lying across the minor groove of the DNA helix ties the 2 strands together by interacting ionically with the phosphoric acid groups of both strands. The electronegativity of the substituent at position 7 of the quinoline ring appears to be critical to the stability of the complex. The length of the side chain bridging the minor groove of the DNA helix is also critical; antimalarial activity is maximal when there are 4 carbon atoms between the 2 N atoms in the side chain, whereas a side chain with 3 or 5 carbon atoms instead of 4 has only two-thirds of the antimalarial activity of chloroquine, and a chain with 2 or 6 carbon atoms instead of 4 exhibits only a third the activity. The selective toxicity for the malarial parasites must therefore depend on a chloroquine-concentrating mechanism.

B. Effects:

1. In malaria—Chloroquine is an excellent blood schizonticidal drug for all 4 types of malaria. The fever and parasitemia produced by nondrug-resistant strains of plasmodia are usually controlled within 24–48 hours, and in *P falciparum* infections a complete cure can be obtained. However, the drug has no effect on secondary tissue schizonts of relapsing malarias and thus cannot effect a "radical" cure of malaria caused by *P vivax, P malariae,* or *P ovale.*

Chloroquine, like quinine, is not lethal to the gametocytes or sporozoites of *P falciparum,* so that the blood of falciparum-infected chloroquine-treated humans can remain infective to mosquitoes for months. This may favor the emergence of drug-resistant strains of *P falciparum* in endemic areas.

Mechanism of chloroquine resistance. Parasites grown for many months in the presence of steadily increasing but sublethal doses of chloroquine will eventually become partially or totally resistant to the drug, and no concentration of chloroquine in the parasitized red cells can be demonstrated.

Plasmodial resistance to chloroquine is probably due to an impaired mechanism of drug transport across the parasite cell wall so that the concentration of chloroquine in resistant schizonts never reaches a level sufficient to arrest nucleic acid synthesis.

2. On cardiovascular system—Chloroquine has a slight quinidine-like effect on the cardiovascular system, and changes in the T wave of the ECG may be noticeable during therapy. Chloroquine depresses myocardial excitability to approximately the same extent as quinidine, but it has hardly any effect on the conduction velocity. It has on occasion been used in place of quinidine. Toxic doses depress vasomotor function and induce circulatory collapse, shock, respiratory paralysis, and death.

3. Anti-inflammatory effects—Chloroquine has anti-inflammatory effects which have been useful in the treatment of rheumatoid arthritis and discoid lupus erythematosus. The mechanism of this effect is not understood.

The mechanism of chloroquine's therapeutic effect on extra-intestinal amebiasis (see below) is presumably the same as the mechanism of its effect on the erythrocytic schizonts.

Clinical Uses

A. Malaria, Acute Attacks: Chloroquine usually terminates the fever and parasitemia of acute attacks of nonresistant strains of falciparum malaria within 24–48 hours, and complete cures are usually obtained because *P falciparum* has no secondary tissue stage. If an acute attack does not respond to chloroquine within 24 hours, a resistant strain may be involved and other antimalarial drugs must be tried. For acute attacks of *P vivax* malaria, chloroquine is the drug of choice; however, because it has no effect on the exo-erythrocytic stages, a radical cure is not possible and the symptoms are likely to recur after chloroquine therapy is stopped.

B. Suppression of Malaria: Chloroquine effectively suppresses all types of malaria; however, if the drug is discontinued too soon after *P vivax* infections, parasitemia may recur after several days. Chloroquine is more potent, less toxic, better tolerated, and more easily administered than quinine or quinacrine. Complete suppression may be obtained with a plasma level of 5–8 μg/liter. The prophylactic use of chloroquine or other 4-aminoquinolines involves the risk of the development of resistant strains. Perhaps chloroquine should be used only for the treatment of acute disease and chloroguanide or pyrimethamine for routine prophylaxis except in areas where resistance to these drugs has been reported.

C. Amebiasis: Chloroquine can bring about rapid and complete clinical cures of extra-intestinal amebiasis, although it is slightly less effective than emetine, which is directly toxic to the myocardium. The conventional course for hepatic amebiasis is 250 mg 4 times daily for 2 days followed by 250 mg twice daily for 2–3 weeks. Chloroquine does not reach amebas in the lumen of the colon because the drug is rapidly absorbed from the upper part of the small intestine, and amebas in the intestinal wall are not affected because chloroquine is not concentrated in intestinal epithelium. Iodochlorhydroxyquin or some other luminal amebicide must therefore be given with chloroquine to prevent reinfection of the liver by amebas remaining in the gut. The risk of incurring severe retinal lesions with prolonged high dosage has made chloroquine less than ideal for the treatment of extra-intestinal amebiasis.

D. Fluke Infections: See Chapter 63.

E. Other Uses: Chloroquine has been used in lupus erythematosus and arthritis, but the danger of prolonged high dosages outweighs the therapeutic advantages. Chloroquine may suppress skin cancers induced by ultraviolet light. It has occasionally been used for the treatment of cardiac arrhythmias, but tolerance quickly develops and quinidine is much more effective.

Adverse Reactions

A. Side-Effects: When used for the chemosuppression of malaria, chloroquine has essentially no toxic effects. During chloroquine therapy, there is occasionally vertigo, malaise, anorexia, diarrhea, headache, blurring of vision, pruritus, and urticaria. The mechanism of this toxicity is unknown, and it resembles mild cinchonism. Oral ammonium chloride may be given to acidify the urine and thereby increase renal excretion of chloroquine.

After high dosage there may be macropapular eruptions, desquamation, or exfoliative lesions of the skin, and alopecia or graying of the hair. Lupus erythematosus, lichenoid skin eruptions, and leukopenia induced by chloroquine have been reported.

Toxic psychoses with hallucinations and agitation and peripheral neuropathies with loss of reflexes and muscle power in the lower limbs can occur. ECG changes, particularly flattening or inversion of the T waves, are frequent with high doses.

Congenital deafness and mental retardation have been reported in children born to mothers who were taking large doses of chloroquine during pregnancy. Permanent nerve deafness in adults has followed high-dose chloroquine therapy.

B. Ocular Toxicity: Severe and often permanent eye damage may be caused by the prolonged administration of chloroquine in high dosage.

1. Corneal changes—Chloroquine, secreted in tears, is absorbed by the corneal epithelium. The cornea at first becomes insensitive, and diffuse white granules appear in the epithelium. These granules later aggregate into curved lines just below the center of the cornea. Between 10 and 33% of patients taking large doses of chloroquine develop these symptomless corneal deposits, which always regress when the drug is discontinued.

2. Retinal changes—These are nearly always permanent and often progress after withdrawal of the drug. Early visual symptoms include halos around lights and ill-defined blurring of vision. Ophthalmoscopic examination at this time may reveal a slight edema with fine degrees of pigment clumping, and frequently small pericentral scotomas causing reading discomfort. These scotomas later coalesce into ring scotomas causing large visual field defects. A characteristic ophthalmoscopic picture consists of a granular or stippled hyperpigmentation of the macula, surrounded by a clear zone of depigmentation encircled by another ring of pigment so that the whole pattern has been likened to a bull's eye. Most recorded cases have occurred after more than 300 mg have been given daily for more than a year. Retinal thresholds were abnormal in all patients who had received a total of more than 100 gm of chloroquine. More than 13% of patients with rheumatoid arthritis treated with chloroquine have retinal changes.

All patients on a prolonged course of chloroquine in high dosage must have vision tested and retinas examined at least every 3 months. Electroretinograms may provide an early index of retinal change.

C. Overdosage Toxicity: Each year the number of sudden deaths after accidental or intentional overdosage with chloroquine increases. At least 40 recorded suicides have been attributed to chloroquine. After a toxic dose there are visual disturbances, hyperexcitability, convulsions, atrial arrest, nodal rhythm, and death within 2 hours. At autopsy, no abnormalities can be demonstrated except (sometimes) the presence of undissolved tablets in the stomach and tissue levels of chloroquine that are 20 times as high as the prophylactic tissue levels.

There is no antidote. Because chloroquine is rapidly absorbed, gastric lavage must be done before symptoms occur if it is to be of any value.

Contraindications & Cautions

Chloroquine crosses the placenta and may damage the fetus when large doses have been taken during pregnancy. Patients with porphyria and psoriasis should not use chloroquine because it may precipitate an acute attack, and chloroquine should not be combined with other drugs known to cause dermatitis.

Chloroquine should be used with caution in patients with a history of liver damage, or neurologic or hematologic disorders.

Many malariologists condemn the use of chloroquine for mass chemotherapy because of the danger of resistant strain selection. Resistance to chloroquine always extends to the other 4-aminoquinolines and quinacrine, and often to chloroguanide and pyrimethamine as well.

Therapy of acute attacks should never be attempted with combined chloroquine-primaquine tablets, because an adequate therapeutic dose of chloroquine cannot be achieved without also giving toxic amounts of primaquine.

Dosages

A. Malaria Chemosuppression: Chloroquine and the other 4-aminoquinolines are usually given in doses of 500 mg (300 mg base)/week, which provide a plasma level ranging from 20–40 mg/liter to 150–250 mg/liter. A blood level of at least 10 μg/liter must be maintained for effective suppression.

Unless chloroquine is continued for a full 10 weeks after the last exposure to *P vivax*, or unless it is combined with primaquine, evident *P vivax* parasitemias may develop at any time from 5–10 weeks after the last dose of chloroquine.

B. Acute Attacks of Malaria: Because chloroquine is rapidly concentrated in the tissues, a 1 gm (600 mg base) priming dose of chloroquine is necessary to achieve effective plasma levels. The priming dose should be followed by 500 mg (300 mg base) 6 hours later and 500 mg on 2 successive days to a total of 2.5 gm (1.5 gm base) in 3 days. For critically ill patients with delirium or coma, one 250 mg ampule of chloroquine hydrochloride (150 mg base in 5 ml distilled water) may be given IM (2.5 ml in each buttock). In dire emergencies, such as blackwater fever, the drug may be given intravenously (very slowly) diluted with 40 ml saline. For pediatric emergencies, 5 mg chloroquine per kg may be given IM followed 6 hours later by an equal oral dose. The total daily dose should not exceed 10 mg/kg.

Pediatric dosages. The WHO recommended dose of chloroquine for infants and children is a loading dose of 10 mg/kg body weight followed by 5 mg/kg/day.

All cases of malaria showing no reduction of parasitemia after 12 hours of chloroquine therapy must be assumed to be due to a resistant strain, and quinine therapy should be started. Advice can be obtained from the Center for Disease Control in Atlanta, Georgia.

C. Other Uses: For extra-intestinal amebiasis, 500 mg of chloroquine are given twice daily for 2 days followed by 250 mg twice daily for 2–3 weeks.

Preparations Available

Chloroquine (Aralen) is available as the phosphate salt for oral administration in tablets containing 125 mg (75 mg base) and 250 mg (150 mg base); and as the hydrochloride for intramuscular administration, 50 mg (40 mg base)/ml in 5 ml ampules.

Chloroquine silicate has an antimalarial activity similar to that of chloroquine phosphate. It is almost without a bitter taste and therefore less likely to induce vomiting, and is more acceptable to small children.

2. THE CHLOROQUINE CONGENERS

None of the 200 known derivatives of 4-aminoquinoline with proved schizonticidal activity have been conclusively shown to be superior to chloroquine; therefore, chloroquine, whose potency and side-effects have been abundantly documented, is the preferred preparation.

Amodiaquine

Amodiaquine dihydrochloride (CAM-AQ1, Camoquinal, Camoquine, Flavoquine, Fluroquine, Miaquin, SN 10,751) is 7-chloro-4-(3'-diethylaminomethyl-4'-hydroxyanilino)quinoline. Chloroquine and amodiaquine are similar, and their pharmacologic properties are identical. Amodiaquine is also effective only

against the erythrocytic stages of malaria and cannot
cure the relapsing fevers of *P vivax, P malariae,* and *P
ovale.* Plasmodia resistant to chloroquine are always
resistant to amodiaquine.

The toxic effects of amodiaquine are similar to
those of chloroquine, but yellow pigmentation of the
skin has been reported as well as a blue-gray pigmentation of the face, nails, hands, and palate simulating
cyanosis; 11 cases of agranulocytosis have occurred.

For the therapy of acute malaria, the dosage of
amodiaquine hydrochloride is 200 mg every 6 hours
for 3 doses followed by 200 mg twice daily for 2 days.
For chemosuppression, the dosage is 300 mg of base
weekly.

Cycloquine

Cycloquine (Ciklochin, Halochin), 7-chloro-4-
(3′,5′,-bis[diethylamino-methyl]-4′-hydroxyanilino)
quinoline, is one of the three 4-aminoquinolines listed
in the WHO report on chemotherapy of malaria as in
common use.

Amopyroquin (Propoquin)

Amopyroquin, 7-chloro-4-(3′-pyrrolidyl-4′-hy-
droxyanilino)quinoline, is said to be an effective
schizonticide and less toxic than chloroquine. It has
been successfully used for single-dose treatment of
acute malaria.

THE 8-AMINOQUINOLINES

History & Chemical Characteristics

Guttmann and Ehrlich observed in 1891 that
methylene blue had a weak activity against vivax
malaria. German workers in 1926 replaced the acridine
ring of methylene blue with a quinoline ring similar to
that of quinine to create an 8-aminoquinoline (pamaquine) which was 60 times more potent than quinine
but too toxic for prophylactic use. Later, Atabrine
(designated quinacrine in the USP and mepacrine in
the BP) was synthesized by combining the side chain
of pamaquine with the acridine ring of methylene blue.
During World War II, Atabrine became the first
synthetic to be used for the mass chemosuppression of
malaria.

In the search for an effective cure of the relapsing
malarias, the 8-aminoquinolines were restudied, but
only pentaquine, isopentaquine, and finally primaquine were found sufficiently nontoxic to be of use.
Primaquine has the highest therapeutic index of all the
8-aminoquinolines synthesized and tested. It is the
only one now used.

1. PRIMAQUINE

Chemistry

Primaquine diphosphate (SN 13,272, Neo-
Quipenyl), the primary amine form of pamaquine, is a
6-methoxy-8-(4′-amino-1′-methylbutylamino)quino-
line. It is an orange-red crystalline powder with a solubility of 6 gm/100 ml of water.

Absorption, Metabolism, & Excretion

Absorption from the intestine is essentially complete, and peak plasma levels are reached in 6 hours.
Only trace amounts can be detected in the plasma 24
hours later, and only about 1% is excreted in the urine
unchanged.

Effective clearance of the tissue schizonts does
not begin until primaquine has undergone biodegrada-
tion by demethylation and oxidation to quinoline-
quinone derivatives, which are the active antimalarial
and hemolytic agents. The highest tissue concentrations of primaquine are found in the liver and lungs,
but primaquine is also concentrated in brain, heart,
and skeletal muscles.

Pharmacologic Action

A. Mechanism of Action: Unlike the 4-amino-
quinolines, the 8-aminoquinolines do not inhibit DNA
replication and transcription.

Primaquine undergoes biotransformation to quin-
oline-quinone intermediates that are electron-carrying
redox compounds capable of acting as oxidants. The
intermediate metabolites probably account for the
hemolysis and methemoglobinemia as well as the
schizonticidal action of the drug.

B. Effects: Although the 8-aminoquinolines structurally resemble the 4-aminoquinolines, their actions
on malaria parasites are quite different. The 8-amino-
quinolines act on the exo-erythrocytic stages and have
practically no effect on the erythrocytic stages. Their
mode of action is probably related to the mechanism
by which they produce an acute self-limiting intravascular hemolysis in individuals with an inherited
glucose-6-phosphate dehydrogenase (G6PD) deficiency.

It is postulated that, in contrast to the erythrocytic schizonts, both the tissue schizonts and the
G6PD-deficient erythrocytes have a deficiency of an
enzyme or cofactor involved in the pentose phosphate
pathway, making them especially susceptible to oxidative damage.

Primaquine also has an effect on the gametocytes;
some are destroyed in the blood, and others cannot
later mature in the mosquito gut. Primaquine is therefore a "tissue schizonticide" and the only antimalarial
able to bring about "radical cures" of the relapsing
malarias. Its gametocidal activity also makes it the best
available drug to interrupt the transmission of malaria.

Primaquine given orally in therapeutic doses has
no pharmacologic effects other than its antimalarial
action and its toxic effect on erythrocyte metabolism.

It is never given parenterally because it can produce ECG changes and a profound fall of blood pressure.

Clinical Uses

Primaquine is highly active against the primary exo-erythrocytic stages of falciparum and vivax malaria and the secondary exo-erythrocytic forms of the relapsing malarias (*P vivax, P malariae,* and *P ovale*). It is also highly active against the gametocytes of all 4 species of human malaria and is therefore used to limit the transmission of malaria. It has only a slight effect on the blood schizonts and cannot be used to relieve the fever and parasitemia of acute attacks. Primaquine is at the moment the only drug able to attack the late tissue stages of *P vivax, P malariae,* or *P ovale* and therefore able to effect a radical cure. Unfortunately, strains of *P vivax* have now appeared in Southeast Asia that are partially resistant to primaquine.

Several programs of mass chemoprophylaxis with primaquine have been carried out in areas of heavy malaria endemicity by WHO and other public health authorities.

Adverse Reactions

A. Primaquine Sensitivity: G6PD deficiency, sometimes called primaquine sensitivity, is an inherited error of metabolism, transmitted by a gene of partial dominance located on the X chromosome. It is estimated that over 100 million people are affected. Red cells deficient in G6PD are sensitive in various degrees to the 8-aminoquinolines and many other drugs, eg, sulfonamides, PAS, aspirin, certain vitamin K derivatives, nitrofurans, and fava beans.

Normal red cells require glucose for survival. Of the glucose metabolized by red cells, 90% is broken down via the Embden-Meyerhof pathway and the other 10% is metabolized by the pentose phosphate pathway. The enzyme G6PD is necessary for the regeneration of NADPH, which in turn is required for the reduction of oxidized glutathione. One of the functions of reduced glutathione is to protect sulfhydryl-dependent enzymes and other cellular proteins against oxidation. The level of reduced glutathione in the red cells of G6PD-deficient individuals fluctuates and is usually lower than normal. Cells with a low level of reduced glutathione and an impaired mechanism for the regeneration of NADPH are particularly vulnerable to the oxidizing effects of substances such as the quinolinequinones derived from primaquine. When primaquine brings about a further reduction of the level of reduced glutathione in cells that already have an impaired mechanism for the regeneration of NADPH, glucose metabolism may be so deranged that the red cells undergo hemolysis.

The amount of hemolysis occurring with primaquine therapy is therefore dependent on 3 factors:

1. The degree of G6PD deficiency—Because the disease is carried on the X chromosome, affected males and the rare females who are homozygous for the trait have the full expression of the disease. Female carriers of the disease are heterozygous for the trait and have a variable expression of the disease. For some reason not yet fully understood, affected whites (especially those whose ancestors inhabited the Mediterranean littoral) have a much more severe expression of primaquine sensitivity than G6PD-deficient blacks.

2. Age of the erythrocyte population—The older erythrocytes have a lower level of G6PD than younger cells, and will be the first to hemolyze. Therefore, if aging susceptible cells have already been removed by hemolysis, the remaining younger population of red cells, which are relatively more resistant, will suffer less hemolysis. For this reason, the hemolysis produced by small doses, eg, 15 mg of primaquine per day, is usually self-limiting. Hemolysis occurring at the inception of primaquine therapy can cause a flu-like febrile episode consisting of malaise, weakness, and chills lasting 2–3 days.

3. Dose size—The amount of primaquine-induced hemolysis is dose-dependent and self-limiting. Daily doses of 15 mg of primaquine are well tolerated by young G6PD-deficient blacks, and only minor hemolytic disturbances are encountered; with a daily dose of 30 mg, the incidence and severity of the reactions increase sharply.

In some populations, over 20% of those who live in (or whose ancestors came from) areas of endemic falciparum malaria carry the G6PD deficiency trait. The distribution of this potentially lethal gene can be explained by the fact that it confers a small degree of protection against falciparum malaria.

Other less common types of inherited enzyme deficiencies involving erythrocyte metabolism (eg, glutathione reductase deficiency) may also be expressed as primaquine sensitivity.

B. Side-Effects: Toxic reactions, often seen when large doses (60–240 mg) are given, include nausea, headache, disturbances of visual accommodation, pruritus, and abdominal cramps (which may be relieved with antacids). Severe reactions associated with high-dose therapy include leukopenia and methemoglobinemia usually presenting as cyanosis. All patients receiving primaquine should be told to report any signs of hemolysis, such as reddening or darkening of the urine.

Contraindications & Cautions

Blacks, Greeks, Sephardic Jews, Sardinians, and Iranians who are known to have a high incidence of G6PD deficiency should be watched for signs of hemolysis during primaquine therapy. Patients with active rheumatoid arthritis, lupus erythematosus, or any grave systemic disease should not receive primaquine therapy. Nor should primaquine be given at the same time as quinacrine or other drugs known to have depressant effects on the bone marrow.

When primaquine was used for mass chemosuppression, drug resistance of *P falciparum* was induced. In the laboratory, strains of *P berghei* made resistant to primaquine show significant cross-resistance to cycloguanil, pyrimethamine, and dapsone.

Preparations & Dosages

The usual tablet of primaquine contains 26.3 mg primaquine phosphate, which is equivalent to 15 mg primaquine base. For suppressive therapy in endemic areas, the US Army uses a combined chloroquine/primaquine (CP) tablet (300 mg chloroquine base and 45 mg primaquine base) to be taken once weekly and continued for 8 weeks after leaving endemic areas. These combined tablets cannot be used for therapy of acute attacks of malaria. To obtain a radical cure after an acute attack of relapsing malaria, give primaquine, 15 mg base, once daily orally for 14 days.

In Southeast Asia, where chloroquine-resistant strains are frequently encountered, dapsone (diaminodiphenylsulfone, DDS, Avlosulfon) in a daily dose of 25 mg orally is given in addition to the regular weekly CP tablet.

There are no indications or preparations for intravenous or intramuscular primaquine therapy.

2. QUINOCIDE

The only other 8-aminoquinoline now used is quinocide dihydrochloride (Chinocide, CN 1115, Win 10,448), a 6-methoxy-8-(4'-amino-4'-methylbutylamino)quinoline. Three hundred and thirty thousand US troops returning from Korea by ship were given a single 15 mg daily dose of quinocide for the duration of the 14-day Pacific crossing. Although the regimen was well tolerated and successfully prevented the introduction of malaria into the USA, quinocide has no clear-cut superiority over primaquine.

To obtain a radical cure of *P vivax,* give 15 mg base once daily for 14 days combined with 2 weekly 300 mg doses of chloroquine base.

QUINACRINE

Quinacrine, also known as Atabrine and mepacrine, was the first effective synthetic antimalarial of low toxicity. Until the introduction of chloroquine, it was the principal drug used for antimalarial prophylaxis by both the Allied and the Axis armies in World War II.

The standard (100 mg) malaria suppressive oral dose of quinacrine is readily absorbed from the intestinal tract, and peak plasma levels are reached 8 hours later. Four to 6 weeks after discontinuing therapy, quinacrine can still be detected in the plasma. The drug is concentrated in the pancreas, lungs, bone marrow, liver, and erythrocytes. Quinacrine crosses the placenta, and fetal tissue levels are nearly the same as the maternal levels.

Quinacrine, like quinine and the 4-aminoquinolines, is a blood schizonticide. Continuous therapy can effectively suppress all 4 types of human malaria and can effect a radical cure of nonresistant strains of *P falciparum.* Malaria due to *P vivax, P malariae,* and *P ovale* will relapse a few weeks or months after discontinuing the drug because quinacrine has no effect on the exo-erythrocytic schizonts. There is cross-resistance between chloroquine and quinacrine.

Quinacrine can be a cerebrocortical stimulant, producing heightened awareness, increased physical activity, restlessness, and insomnia.

Clinical Uses

A. Treatment and Chemosuppression of Malaria: Quinacrine as an antimalarial agent was superseded in 1945 by the far more potent and less toxic 4-aminoquinolines.

B. Taeniasis: Quinacrine is one of the drugs of choice for the treatment of beef tapeworm *(Taenia saginata),* pork tapeworm *(T solium),* fish tapeworm *(Diphyllobothrium latum),* and dwarf tapeworms *(Hymenolepis nana* and *H diminuta)* infections. (See Chapter 63.) Quinacrine (100 mg daily for 3 days) can also be used to eliminate most of the organisms and symptoms of giardiasis.

C. Other Uses: See Chapters 29, 45, and 63.

Adverse Reactions

When used in low dosages as an antimalarial, quinacrine produces yellow staining of the skin and infrequent incidence of minor psychotic reactions. A grayish-blue discoloration of the ears, nasal cartilages, and fingernail beds that can be mistaken for cyanosis is sometimes seen.

For the adverse reactions that can occur when quinacrine is used in high dosages as a taeniacide, see Chapter 63.

Dosages

A. For Malaria Chemosuppression: The dose for adults and for children over 8 years is 100 mg daily. Chemosuppression with quinacrine should be started 2 weeks before arriving in areas of endemic malaria and continued for at least 1 month after leaving the area.

B. For Helminthic Infestations: See Chapter 63.

THE ANTIFOLICS: CHLOROGUANIDE (PROGUANIL), PYRIMETHAMINE, & TRIMETHOPRIM

History

British wartime research for a completely nontoxic antimalarial for mass chemoprophylaxis resulted, in 1946, in chloroguanide (proguanil); however, its effectiveness was soon compromised by the emergence of resistant strains. In 1948, a number of 2,4-diaminopyrimidines had been shown, like guanidine, to antagonize folic acid metabolism. Pyrimethamine, because of its resemblance to the active metabolite of guanidine (see structural formulas, p 570), was tested and found to be a highly effective antimalarial. Trimethoprim, an antifolic originally developed as an antibacterial agent, was not tested for antimalarial activity until the desperate search in 1968 and 1969 for drugs effective against the Southeast Asian strains of *P falciparum* resistant to chloroguanide, chloroquine, and pyrimethamine. The recent discovery of the synergistic potentiation of the antimalarial activity of the antifolics when combined with sulfonamides such as sulfamethoxypyridazine and sulfamethoxazole and with sulfones such as dapsone (DDS) has opened a whole new field of antimalarial therapy which is now being evaluated. However, because of the rapid development of resistance, with cross-resistance to other combinations of antifolics and sulfonamides, it is now recommended that these combinations be used only for the treatment of chloroquine-resistant strains.

Chemistry & Nomenclature

A. Chloroguanide (Proguanil) Hydrochloride: Chloroguanide is N^1-(*p*-chlorophenyl)-N-isopropyl-biguanide hydrochloride (Balusil, bigumal, biguanide, chlorguanide, Chloroguanil, Diguanyl, Drinupal, Guanatol, Lepadina, Paludrine, Palusil, Plasin, Proguanide, and Tirian).

B. Pyrimethamine: Pyrimethamine is a 2,4-diamino-5-*p*-chlorophenyl-6-ethylpyrimidine. It is also known by the proprietary names Chloridin, Darapram, Daraprim, Erbaprelina, and Malocide.

C. Trimethoprim: Trimethoprim (Syraprim) is a 2,4,-diamino-5-(3,4,5,-trimethoxybenzyl)pyrimidine. It is not yet available in the USA but is available elsewhere as a combination of trimethoprim and sulfamethoxazole in the ratio of 1:5, known as Bactrim and Septrim.

Absorption, Metabolism, & Excretion

Chloroguanide, pyrimethamine, and trimethoprim are slowly but adequately absorbed from the gastrointestinal tract. Peak plasma levels are reached in 3–7 hours after an oral dose, and loading doses are not necessary. Chloroguanide is so rapidly eliminated from the body that it must be administered daily; pyrimethamine is excreted more slowly. Trimethoprim is excreted more slowly than sulfamethoxazole, with which it is combined.

Unlike the quinoline drugs, chloroguanide, pyrimethamine, and trimethoprim do not accumulate in the tissues. Only very low levels of chloroguanide can be detected in the plasma 24 hours after an oral dose, but significant quantities of pyrimethamine and its metabolites—and of trimethoprim—can be found in the tissues 9 days after an oral dose. Between 40–60% of the oral dose of chloroguanide is excreted in the urine and 10% in the feces; 60% is excreted unchanged and 30% as the triazine metabolite. Sufficient pyrimethamine is excreted in maternal milk so that chemosuppressive levels of the drug may be reached in wholly breast-fed infants.

Pharmacologic Effects

When the antifolics are given in therapeutic doses, no effects are seen other than the intended antiprotozoal or antibacterial effects. In excessive doses, abdominal pain, diarrhea, hematuria, and a macrocytic anemia like that of folic acid deficiency may occur.

Antimalarial Effects

All 3 of these drugs are strongly sporonticidal. Pyrimethamine, the most potent of the three, has been calculated to be 2000 times as toxic to the malarial parasite as to the host. These drugs can also prevent sporogony in the mosquito gut, and a single dose of pyrimethamine given to a nonimmune person can interrupt transmission for several weeks. All 3 can provide effective and nontoxic antimalarial chemoprophylaxis provided they are continued for at least 10 weeks after the last infected mosquito bite and that there are no resistant strains in the area. They should not be used for the treatment of acute attacks because their blood schizonticide action is too slow.

Mode of Action of the Antifolics

Chloroguanide itself is not active, only its triazine metabolite which is rapidly excreted. The selective toxicity of all 3 antifolics depends on the fact that plasmodia, unlike man and many other animals, have not lost the enzymes needed for the synthesis of folic acid from para-aminobenzoic acid (PABA), glutamic acid, and pteridine but yet cannot make use of preformed folic acid. The plasmodicidal effects of these 3 antimalarials are due to a deficiency of tetrahydrofolate that results in the inhibition of cell division and schizogony. This interference with folic acid metabolism therefore explains the marked synergistic enhancement of potency that occurs when any of these drugs are combined with sulfonamides or sulfones, causing a sequential blockade of folic acid synthesis at 2 different stages along the metabolic pathway (see Chapter 53).

Clinical Uses

A. Malaria Chemosuppression: Chloroguanide is the least toxic of all the antimalarials, but it must be taken in daily 100 mg doses because of its rapid excretion. Pyrimethamine is the most potent chemoprophylactic available (requiring only 25 mg weekly), but, like chloroguanide, it must be taken for 10 weeks after leaving the endemic area. Cures of acute attacks of malaria in nonimmunes should not be attempted with these drugs because their ability to reduce fever and parasitemia is much too slow.

B. Combination Therapy of Chloroquine-Resistant Falciparum Malaria: In 1969, 12 cases of agranulocytosis occurred among 200,000 soldiers in Vietnam who were taking the standard CP (chloroquine, 300 mg base; primaquine, 45 mg base) tablet once a week plus 25 mg of dapsone weekly. Various other combinations such as pyrimethamine plus quinine and pyrimethamine plus sulfadoxine are advocated and have been found to be effective, but malaria resistance to these new combinations soon develops. For this reason, combinations of antifolics and sulfonamides should only be used for chloroquine-resistant malaria.

C. Endemic Malaria: Pyrimethamine has been used to interrupt the transmission of malaria in communities of partial immunes. Such eradication programs should always follow a course of a quick-acting blood schizonticide to minimize the risk of resistant strain emergence. Endemic malaria control has been attempted by the addition of pyrimethamine to cooking salt supplies. However, when this is done the dosage levels in children under 6 are extremely variable and the emergence of resistant strains is practically assured.

D. Toxoplasmosis: Pyrimethamine, 25 mg, combined with trisulfapyrimidines, 1 gm, given orally 4 times a day for 6 weeks, can be used for the treatment of toxoplasmosis. However, if toxoplasmic chorioretinitis is present or if there is a danger of congenital toxoplasmosis, corticosteroids should also be given.

Adverse Reactions

Chloroguanide occasionally induces anorexia but is the least toxic of all the antimalarials.

Pyrimethamine is also well tolerated. Large doses of pyrimethamine given for long periods sometimes lead to folic acid deficiency. Supplementary folic acid can correct the hematologic defect without impairing the drug's therapeutic effect.

Contraindications & Cautions

Cross-resistance to chloroguanide and pyrimethamine may develop when these drugs are given singly in low doses and for long periods of chemosuppression.

Preparations & Dosages

Chloroguanide hydrochloride (proguanil, Paludrine) is available as tablets of 25, 50, 100, and 300 mg containing 87% of the base. For the chemosuppression of malaria, 100–200 mg daily are usually sufficient.

Pyrimethamine is available as 25 mg tablets. For the chemosuppression of malaria, the dosage is 1 or 2 tablets per week. For children under 14, give pyrimethamine elixir (6.25 mg/ml), 2 ml weekly. The first dose should be taken before entering endemic areas, and suppressive therapy must be continued for 10 weeks after leaving the area.

For the treatment of drug-resistant falciparum malaria, 25 mg of pyrimethamine can be given every 8 hours for the first 3 days of a 14-day course of quinine (650 mg every 8 hours). One gram of sulphormethoxine, a long-acting sulfonamide, has been combined with 50 mg of pyrimethamine to produce a single-dose cure of chloroquine-resistant malaria. Because of the true synergism between these 2 drugs, 1/10 of the curative dose of pyrimethamine plus 1/4 of the curative dose of sulfadiazine add up to one curative dose for the treatment of *P falciparum* malaria.

THE TREATMENT OF AMEBIASIS

Amebiasis may present as a severe intestinal infection (dysentery or severe diarrhea), a mild symptomatic intestinal infection, an asymptomatic intestinal infection, or as an ameboma or liver abscess, or in the form of other extra-intestinal infections.

Drugs available for therapy can be classified according to their site of antiamebic action. Luminal amebicides such as diiodohydroxyquin and diloxanide furoate are active against luminal organisms but are ineffective against parasites in the bowel wall or tissues. The parenterally administered tissue amebicides, dehydroemetine and emetine, are effective against parasites in the bowel wall and tissues but not against luminal organisms. Chloroquine, administered orally or parenterally, acts only against organisms in the liver. Antibiotics taken orally are indirect-acting luminal amebicides that exert their effects against bacterial associates of *E histolytica* in the bowel lumen and in the bowel wall but not in other tissues. Given parenterally, antibiotics have little antiamebic activity at any site. Metronidazole is uniquely effective against organisms at 3 sites: the bowel lumen, bowel wall, and tissues.

The following is a partial list of useful antiamebic drugs:

(1) Tissue amebicides (drugs that act primarily in the bowel wall, liver, and other extra-intestinal tissues):

(a) Dehydroemetine, emetine.

(b) Chloroquine (active principally in the liver).

(2) Luminal amebicides (drugs that act primarily in the bowel lumen):

(a) Halogenated hydroxyquinolines: Diiodohydroxyquin (Diodoquin), iodochlorhydroxyquin (Vioform), chiniofon.

(b) Pentavalent arsenicals: Glycobiarsol (Milibis), carbarsone.

(c) Alkaloids: Emetine-bismuth-iodide (EBI).

(d) Amides: Clefamide (Mebinol), diloxanide furoate (Furamide).

(e) Antibiotics (act also in bowel wall): Tetracyclines, paromomycin (Humatin).

(3) Tissue and luminal amebicides: Metronidazole (Flagyl).

Treatment may require the concomitant or sequential use of several drugs. Table 62–1 outlines 2 methods of treatment for each clinical type of amebiasis. No drugs are recommended as safe or effective for chemoprophylaxis.

Asymptomatic Intestinal Infection

When infection is confined to the bowel lumen, cure may be obtained by use of luminal amebicides alone. Of the many drugs available, none is completely reliable in eradicating the infection, but diiodohydroxyquin is probably the most effective and least toxic.

TABLE 62–1. Treatment of amebiasis.

	Drug(s) of Choice	Alternative Drug(s)
Asymptomatic intestinal infection	Diiodohydroxyquin, 650 mg 3 times daily for 21 days	Diloxanide furoate,* 500 mg 3 times daily for 10 days
Mild intestinal infection	(1) Diiodohydroxyquin, 650 mg 3 times daily for 21 days, **plus** (2) Oxytetracycline, 250 mg 4 times daily for 10 days, **plus** (3) Chloroquine, 500 mg (salt) twice daily for 2 days and then 250 mg twice daily for 19 days	(1) Diloxanide furoate,* 500 mg 3 times daily for 10 days, **plus** (2) Oxytetracycline, 250 mg 4 times daily for 10 days, **plus** (3) Chloroquine, 500 mg (salt) twice daily for 2 days and then 250 mg twice daily for 19 days
Severe intestinal infection	(1) Metronidazole,† 750 mg 3 times daily for 5 days, **followed by** (2) Diiodohydroxyquin, 650 mg 4 times daily for 21 days	(1) Dehydroemetine,‡ 1–1.5 mg/kg IM or subcut daily for the least number of days necessary to control symptoms (usually 4–6 days; maximum 10 days) (maximum total dose, 1 gm) **or** Emetine (see text for dosage) **plus** (2) Oxytetracycline, 250 mg 4 times daily for 10 days, **plus** (3) Diiodohydroxyquin, 650 mg 4 times daily for 21 days, **followed by** (4) Chloroquine, 500 mg (salt) twice daily for 2 days and then 250 mg twice daily for 19 days
Hepatic abscess	(1) Metronidazole,† 750 mg 3 times daily for 5 days, **followed by** (2) Diiodohydroxyquin, 650 mg 3 times daily for 21 days	(1) Dehydroemetine,‡ 1–1.5 mg/kg daily IM or subcut for 10 days (maximum total dose, 1 gm), **or** Emetine (see text for dosage) **plus** (2) Chloroquine, 500 mg (salt) twice daily for 2 days and then 250 mg twice daily for 26 days **plus** (3) Diiodohydroxyquin, 650 mg 3 times daily for 21 days
Ameboma or extra-intestinal infection	As for hepatic abscess	As for hepatic abscess, but not including chloroquine

*Not approved by the FDA for use in the USA.

†At present approved by the FDA for use in the USA for trichomoniasis but not for amebiasis.

‡Available in the USA for investigational use only from the Parasitic Disease Drug Service, Center for Disease Control, Atlanta, Georgia 30333.

Mild Intestinal Infection

In addition to clearing amebas from the bowel lumen, treatment of mild intestinal disease should eradicate trophozoites from the bowel wall and liver. Metronidazole is effective against both luminal and tissue parasites and may become the simplest form of therapy. However, until additional reports assess the effectiveness of metronidazole in mild intestinal disease, diiodohydroxyquin remains the drug of choice for initiating treatment. Concomitant use of oxytetracycline enhances cure rates. Chloroquine is given concurrently with the intestinal amebicides to eradicate trophozoites carried to the liver.

Severe Intestinal Infection

Metronidazole alone will cure approximately 90% of patients with one course of treatment. To further increase the cure rate, it is at present suggested that a course of diiodohydroxyquin follow metronidazole.

For patients too ill to take oral medications, the drug of choice is emetine (or dehydroemetine) given intramuscularly or subcutaneously.

Emetine should be used for the minimum number of days (usually 4–6) needed to control severe symptoms. Significant toxicity usually does not occur in this period. Concurrently, the patient is given a full course of oxytetracycline and diiodohydroxyquin. Chloroquine must also be administered to ensure the destruction of trophozoites carried to the liver that are not killed by the short course of emetine.

Opiates to control bowel motility and bed rest are necessary adjuncts in severe amebic dysentery.

Hepatic Abscess

The simplest and safest treatment is metronidazole, 750 mg orally 3 times daily for 5 days. Alternatively, emetine plus chloroquine is effective but potentially more toxic. Small liver abscesses do not require drainage, but large abscesses should be aspirated with a wide-bore needle under strict aseptic conditions.

Diiodohydroxyquin should be given even when parasites have not been identified in the stool.

Ameboma or Extra-intestinal Disease

Metronidazole is the drug of choice, but emetine may be used. Chloroquine does not reach sufficiently high tissue concentrations (except in the liver) to be effective. A simultaneous course of intestinal amebicides should also be given.

DEHYDROEMETINE

Racemic 2-dehydroemetine dihydrochloride is a synthetic substance which can substitute for emetine as an equally effective and probably less toxic drug. It has the same limitations of activity against amebas as emetine. At present, it is not approved for general use in the USA, but it is available from the Parasitic Disease Drug Service, Center for Disease Control, Atlanta, Georgia.

In laboratory animals, dehydroemetine is less toxic on an equal weight basis than emetine, although qualitatively their toxicities are alike. In man, the therapeutic action of dehydroemetine is equal to that of emetine, but greater clinical experience is needed to establish that dehydroemetine is indeed less toxic in man.

In experimental animals, dehydroemetine disappears more rapidly from the heart (but not from the liver) than emetine, and is excreted more rapidly. If this also occurs in man, it could account for the fewer ECG changes that dehydroemetine causes when identical doses of the 2 drugs are given.

The clinical uses of dehydroemetine are similar to those of emetine: treatment of severe intestinal amebi-

asis that cannot be treated by orally administered metronidazole and treatment of amebic liver abscess in conjunction with chloroquine if metronidazole cannot be used.

The adverse reactions, cautions, and contraindications are currently the same as those for emetine.

Dehydroemetine is available for injection in 1 and 2 ml ampules containing 30 mg/ml. The dosage for severe intestinal disease is 1–1.5 mg/kg IM or subcut daily for the least number of days necessary to control symptoms (usually 4–6 days; maximum, 10 days). The maximum total dose is 1 gm.

Oxytetracycline and diiodohydroxyquin should be given in conjunction with dehydroemetine, and chloroquine should follow if dehydroemetine has been used for less than 10 days.

For liver abscess, dehydroemetine is given in conjunction with chloroquine and diiodohydroxyquin. The dosage of dehydroemetine is 1–1.5 mg/kg daily IM or subcut for 10 days. The maximum total dose is 1 gm.

EMETINE HYDROCHLORIDE

Emetine hydrochloride, used for more than 50 years for the treatment of *Entamoeba histolytica* infection, remains one of the principal drugs for the treatment of extra-intestinal amebiasis (including liver abscess) and severe intestinal amebiasis.

Chemistry

Emetine is the methyl ester of cephaeline. It can be synthesized or derived from ipecac, which in turn is prepared from dried rhizomes and roots of *Cephaelis ipecacuanha*. Since emetine has 4 asymmetric centers, several stereoisomers are possible, but the structure below is generally accepted as the configuration of the natural (−) alkaloid.

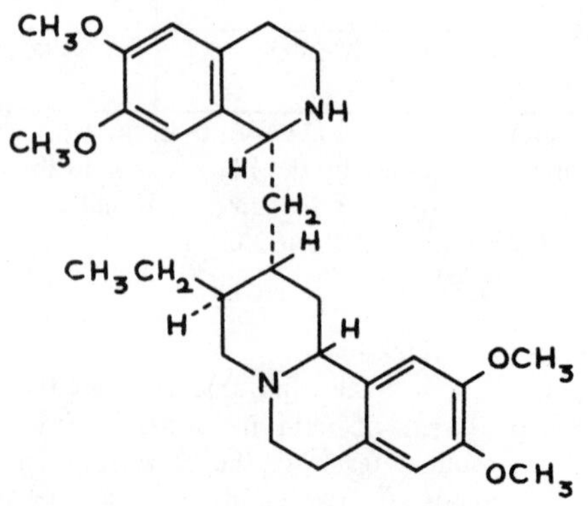

Emetine

Emetine is usually employed as the hydrochloride, a stable white or yellowish crystalline powder that is freely soluble in water.

Absorption, Metabolism, & Excretion

Emetine is not administered orally because it is absorbed erratically from the gastrointestinal tract and may induce emesis as a result of its local irritant effect on the intestinal mucosa even when given in enteric-coated tablets.

When given parenterally, emetine is stored primarily in the liver, lungs, spleen, and kidneys; only a small amount is found in other tissues, including cardiac, striated, and intestinal muscle. Because emetine is eliminated only slowly via the kidney, toxicity can be cumulative; trace amounts of the drug are detectable in the urine 1–2 months after stopping therapy.

Pharmacologic Effects

Emetine is a general protoplasmic poison. In experimental animals, emetine given parenterally in toxic doses causes hyperemia, cloudy swelling, and cellular damage in the liver and kidneys and in skeletal and cardiac muscle. In the myocardium, there is cloudy swelling and necrosis of myocardial fibers with focal areas of cellular infiltration and interstitial proliferation resembling Aschoff bodies. Small parenteral doses increase intestinal peristalsis; large doses produce edema, congestion, and hemorrhages of the intestinal mucosa and, occasionally, ulcerations.

Toxic doses of the drug weaken cardiac contraction and depress conduction, and this may result in a variety of atrial and ventricular arrhythmias, cardiac dilatation, and death. In vitro emetine has an adrenergic neuron blocking action. A similar action of the drug in vivo may be responsible for the hypotension and diarrhea that frequently accompany its use. A form of myositis probably occurs in man that is similar to that reported in animals. Nausea and vomiting commonly develop even after small doses of emetine and are considered central in origin. Emetine may cause a disturbance in potassium metabolism, reducing serum potassium levels in some patients.

Antiamebic Effects

Emetine in therapeutic dosages acts only against trophozoites. At high doses (beyond those tolerated by man), the drug may be active against cysts.

Clinical Uses

A. Amebic Dysentery or Severe Diarrhea: Parenterally administered emetine rapidly alleviates severe intestinal symptoms but is rarely curative even if a full course is given. For this reason and because of its toxicity, emetine should be given for the minimum period needed to relieve severe symptoms (usually 4–6 days; maximum, 10 days). Marked toxicity is unlikely when treatment is less than 7 days.

In addition to emetine, the full therapeutic regimen for severe intestinal amebiasis includes the concurrent administration of a full course of oxytetracycline, followed by a course of diiodohydroxyquin plus chloroquine. Chloroquine need not be used if emetine has been given for 10 days.

Severe intestinal disease in children should be treated first with oxytetracycline; emetine should not be used unless symptoms fail to improve rapidly.

Emetine should not be used to treat mild or asymptomatic amebiasis.

B. Amebic Liver Abscess: Emetine followed by chloroquine (or taken concurrently) is a treatment of choice for amebic liver abscess. A course of diiodohydroxyquin should also be given.

C. Amebomas and Extra-intestinal Amebiasis: Emetine is effective in treating amebomas and extra-intestinal amebiasis; chloroquine is not effective.

D. Other Parasites: Emetine has occasionally been useful in the treatment of infections with *Balantidium coli, Fasciola hepatica,* and *Paragonimus westermani.*

Adverse Reactions

Emetine is cumulative in its toxic action. Side-effects develop in most patients but are usually not severe if the dosage does not exceed 65 mg daily for 10 days. Few and (usually) mild side-effects appear if the drug is given for 3–4 days; additional mild to severe side-effects appear if the drug is given for up to 10 days; serious toxicity is common if it is given for more than 10 days.

A. Acute Toxicity: Acute toxicity induces nausea, vomiting, diarrhea, prostration, hypotension, arrhythmias, and death from heart failure. The lethal dose of emetine in man is 10–20 mg/kg.

B. Local Reactions: Pain, tenderness, and muscle weakness in the area of the injection are frequent, often starting 24–48 hours after the injection, and may persist for 1–2 weeks. Occasionally, sterile abscesses develop after subcutaneous or intramuscular injection.

C. Gastrointestinal Effects: Diarrhea is induced or exacerbated in many patients, generally beginning several days after the onset of therapy. In the treatment of severe symptoms, there may be a short period of emetine-induced improvement followed by a relapse. The diarrhea may then be accompanied by abdominal cramps and by blood and mucus in the stools. Transient nausea occurs in over 30% of patients, but vomiting is rare. A course of treatment can usually be completed in spite of gastrointestinal symptoms. If they are too severe, therapy must be discontinued.

D. Cardiovascular Effects: Emetine may cause tachycardia, hypotension, precordial pain, dyspnea, ECG abnormalities, gallop rhythm, cardiac dilatation, congestive heart failure, and death. Most deaths from emetine have been in patients given total doses over 1200 mg; some deaths have been reported in patients given the standard total dose of 650 mg or less. ECG changes induced in more than 50% of patients include flattening and inversion of P and T waves, lengthening of the P–R and Q–T intervals, ST elevation, premature beats, nodal rhythm, and transient atrial fibrillation. These changes usually appear about 7 days after the onset of treatment but occasionally not until 2–3 weeks after the last injection. They are generally reversible, requiring about 6 weeks to return to normal. In rare instances, emetine-induced abnormalities have persisted for several years.

Opinion differs about the occurrence of permanent myocardial damage following therapeutic doses. ECG patterns resembling those of myocardial infarction have been reported, but only degenerative changes in the myocardium have been found in cases of fatal emetine intoxication.

E. Neuromuscular Effects: Generalized muscular weakness—sometimes associated with tenderness, stiffness, aching, or tremors—is reported by many patients. At therapeutic doses, the weakness is usually mild and reversible, but it may persist for several weeks after treatment is stopped. At high doses, marked weakness and even paralysis may occur. These symptoms are attributed to a direct action of emetine on the muscles and not to neuritis. Although mild paresthesias are reported by patients, a true polyneuritis with objective signs of nerve damage occurs rarely, if ever.

F. Other Side-Effects: Many other mild and often transient side-effects may occur, including fatigue, headache, dizziness, and urticarial, eczematous, or purpuric skin lesions. Proteinuria may also be present.

Contraindications & Cautions

Since emetine is a potentially dangerous drug, careful hospital supervision is essential. Considerable caution should be observed to avoid inadvertent intravenous administration.

Patients should be kept at bed rest with bathroom privileges during treatment and for several days afterward. They should be examined daily for cardiovascular, neuromuscular, and gastrointestinal signs or symptoms. Pulse and blood pressure should be recorded 3 times a day and ECGs taken prior to the first injection, on the fifth and tenth days of therapy, and weekly for 2 weeks after the last injection.

The drug should be discontinued if the resting pulse (or, particularly, the sleeping pulse) exceeds 110/minute or if marked hypotension, precordial pain, or generalized weakness or other neuromuscular symptoms develop. Generalized weakness and muscular aching (to be distinguished from local reactions due to injections) tend to develop before more serious toxic symptoms and thus can be used as a guide for avoiding overdosage.

ECG criteria for discontinuing therapy have not been established. Some clinicians believe that prolongation of the P–R or Q–T interval is an indication for stopping treatment; conduction defects or ectopic rhythms, although extremely rare, clearly require cessation of therapy.

Patients should remain sedentary for about 4 weeks after completion of therapy, and surgery is inadvisable for at least 6 weeks after emetine therapy.

Great care should be exercised in administering the drug to aged or debilitated people; dosage is usually reduced by half for such patients.

Emetine should not be used in pregnancy or in patients with cardiac or renal disease or a recent history of polyneuritis.

Preparations & Dosages

Aqueous solutions of emetine hydrochloride are supplied in ampules containing 32 or 65 mg.

The daily dose of emetine for adults and children is 1 mg/kg subcut or IM. The maximum daily dose for adults is 65 mg; for children under 8 years, 10 mg.

For the treatment of severe dysentery or diarrhea, injections are generally given for 4–6 days (not more than 10 days). They are given for the minimum number of days needed to control severe symptoms. For severe intestinal disease in children, oxytetracycline should be used first and emetine employed subsequently only if symptoms are not responsive to oxytetracycline.

For the treatment of ameboma and extra-intestinal disease, including hepatic abscess, the same doses of emetine are used but for a total of 10 days. Patients should not be treated beyond 10 days.

If a second course of therapy is needed, an intervening period of 6 weeks is required.

THE HALOGENATED HYDROXYQUINOLINES
(Chiniofon, Iodochlorhydroxyquin, Diiodohydroxyquin)

The halogenated hydroxyquinolines were among the first synthetic drugs active in amebiasis. Chiniofon (introduced in 1921), iodochlorhydroxyquin (in 1931), and diiodohydroxyquin (in 1936) are effective against organisms in the bowel lumen but not against trophozoites in the intestinal wall or extra-intestinal tissues.

Chemistry

Three synthetic halogen-substituted 8-hydroxyquinolines have had extensive clinical use—chiniofon (8-hydroxy-7-iodoquinoline-5-sulfonic acid), iodochlorhydroxyquin (5-chloro-8-hydroxy-7-iodoquinoline), and diiodohydroxyquin (8-hydroxy-5,7-diiodoquinoline).

Chiniofon is a yellow powder with a bitter taste, containing about 28% iodine. It is prepared as a mixture containing 20% sodium bicarbonate and is soluble 1:25 in water. The solid is stable if protected from light, but solutions are not stable and should be freshly prepared before use.

Iodochlorhydroxyquin, containing approximately 40% iodine and 12% chlorine, and diiodohydroxyquin, containing approximately 64% iodine, are yellow-brown, tasteless powders that are almost insoluble in water.

Absorption, Metabolism, & Excretion

Iodochlorhydroxyquin is the most readily absorbed, diiodohydroxyquin is next, and chiniofon is

Chiniofon

Iodochlorhydroxyquin
(Vioform)

Diiodohydroxyquin
(Diodoquin)

the least well absorbed (about 13%). After administration of daily therapeutic doses, the highest blood iodine levels occur on the seventh day, averaging 87 μg/100 ml for chiniofon, 444 μg/100 ml for iodochlorhydroxyquin, and 692 μg/100 ml for diiodohydroxyquin.

The peak blood level for chiniofon occurs about 2 hours after oral administration of the drug in man. The bulk of the absorbed drug is excreted in the urine in the first 12 hours. Chinofon is partly broken down after absorption, iodine being split off. A portion of the free iodine fraction is then detectable in the thyroid gland. The unabsorbed portion of chiniofon is eliminated in the feces. Little is known about the metabolic fate of iodochlorhydroxyquin and diiodohydroxyquin in man.

Antiamebic Effects

The mechanism of action of diiodohydroxyquin, iodochlorhydroxyquin, and chiniofon against amebas is not known. The drugs apparently act only against trophozoites; cysts are eliminated by passage in the feces.

Clinical Uses

A. Amebiasis: Diiodohydroxyquin and iodochlorhydroxyquin are the drugs of choice for the treatment of mild or asymptomatic intestinal amebiasis but are not indicated for chemoprophylaxis. They are not effective in the initial treatment of severe intestinal disease, but are used in the subsequent eradication of the infection. The drugs are not effective against amebomas or extra-intestinal forms of the disease, including hepatic amebiasis, but are used in the eradication of concurrent intestinal infection. Reported cure rates for each of the 2 compounds are as high as 80%. Diiodohydroxyquin may cause less diarrhea and gastric irritation than iodochlorhydroxyquin and has been preferred in the USA.

Chiniofon, given rectally by high retention enema, has been used (along with oral therapy) for severe or refractory intestinal amebiasis. The discomfort of enemas restricts their use.

B. *Trichomonas Vaginalis* Vaginitis: Iodochlorhydroxyquin, given in vaginal inserts or insufflation powders, has been used for the topical treatment of this infection.

C. Other Intestinal Parasites: Diiodohydroxyquin has been reported to be effective in the treatment of some cases of *Giardia lamblia* and *Balantidium coli* infection.

Adverse Reactions

Diarrhea occurs infrequently but usually stops after several days. Other side-effects include nausea, vomiting, gastritis, abdominal discomfort, constipation, pruritus ani, headache, malaise, slight enlargement of the thyroid gland, and iodine sensitivity.

Iodochlorhydroxyquin has recently been implicated as a cause of subacute myelo-optic neuropathy (SMON) when used to prevent "travelers' diarrhea." Although evidence is not yet available to confirm this association, there is no acceptable evidence that iodochlorhydroxyquin or the other halogenated hydroxyquinolines are effective for this purpose, and they should not be so used.

Contraindications & Cautions

These drugs should be discontinued in patients in whom they produce a persistent diarrhea or signs of iodine sensitivity. They are contraindicated in patients with known intolerance to iodine, in renal disease, and probably in severe liver disease not due to amebiasis.

Preparations & Dosages

The drugs are taken orally after meals. A course should not be repeated without an intervening period of 2–3 weeks.

A. Diiodohydroxyquin (Diodoquin, Embequin, Lanodoxin, Savorquin, Sebaquin, Yodoxin): Diiodohydroxyquin is available as uncoated tablets containing 650 mg. The adult dosage is 650 mg orally 3 times a day (mild disease) or 4 times a day (severe disease) for 21 days. The pediatric dosage is 10 mg/kg 4 times a day for 21 days. The medication is well accepted by young children when it is crushed and mixed with applesauce or chocolate syrup.

B. Iodochlorhydroxyquin (Entero-Vioform, Nioform, Vioform): Iodochlorhydroxyquin is available as enteric-coated tablets or vaginal inserts containing 250 mg and as a powder for vaginal insufflation. The oral dosage is 250 mg 3 times a day (mild disease) or 4 times a day (severe disease) for 10 days. Enemas are prepared by suspending 2 gm in 200 ml of water and instilling on alternate nights for a total of 5 times.

C. Chiniofon (Anayodin, Avlochin, Quinoxyl, Yatren): Chiniofon is prepared as enteric-coated tablets containing 250 mg or as a powder. The dosage is 0.5 gm orally 3 times a day for 3 days and then 1 gm 3 times a day for 7 days. Chiniofon high retention enemas, prepared fresh by dissolving 6 gm of the drug in 200 ml of warm water, may be given each night for

7–10 days. Oral doses should be reduced to half the usual dose when enemas are given.

THE ARSENICALS
(Carbarsone, Glycobiarsol)

The arsenical drugs have been used for many years for the treatment of intestinal amebiasis. Trivalent arsenicals are more effective, but they are also more toxic; therefore, only the pentavalent arsenicals are used.

Chemistry

Carbarsone (*p*-ureidobenzenearsonic acid), a pentavalent arsenical, contains 29% arsenic. It is a white powder, nearly insoluble in water, with a slightly acid taste.

Carbarsone

Glycobiarsol
(Milibis)

Glycobiarsol (bismuth *p*-glycolylarsanilate), a pentavalent arsenical, contains 15% arsenic and 42% bismuth. It is a yellowish-white compound, slightly soluble in water.

Absorption, Metabolism, & Excretion

Carbarsone is absorbed from the gastrointestinal tract whether taken orally or by retention enema, and is slowly excreted in the urine.

Glycobiarsol is poorly absorbed. In man, only 2–4% of the orally administered drug is excreted in the urine. Significant amounts of arsenic have not been detected in the tissues of experimental animals.

Antiamebic Effects

Both carbarsone and glycobiarsol are thought to exert their antiamebic action against trophozoites but not against cysts. The exact mode of action is not known. Because carbarsone is absorbed, it may exert some of its action systemically.

Clinical Uses

A. **Amebiasis**: Glycobiarsol and carbarsone are used for the treatment of mild intestinal amebiasis and asymptomatic infections. Neither drug, alone, can be relied upon to give a high cure rate. The drugs are not effective for the immediate management of severe amebic dysentery but are employed for the eradication of the infection after severe symptoms have been stopped by other drugs. The drugs are also ineffective in the treatment of ameboma or extra-intestinal infections, but they may be used to eradicate concurrent intestinal infections.

Controversy exists about whether the moderate effectiveness of these drugs warrants the risk of their toxicity.

Carbarsone enemas may be prepared by dissolving 2 gm in 200 ml of a 2% sodium bicarbonate solution. This is instilled after a cleansing enema and retained for several hours and may be repeated for 5–6 nights. Carbarsone enemas are probably less effective than chiniofon enemas.

B. *Trichomonas Vaginalis:* Both carbarsone and glycobiarsol vaginal inserts, creams, or powders have been used for the treatment of trichomoniasis.

Adverse Reactions

The side-effects of glycobiarsol and carbarsone are due to arsenical reactions. Although infrequent, the most common signs and symptoms are nausea, vomiting, diarrhea, epigastric distress, and skin rashes, which start after several days of therapy. Glycobiarsol turns the stools black.

More severe toxicity includes weight loss and polyuria. Exfoliative dermatitis, agranulocytosis, encephalitis, and hepatitis are very rare; a few fatalities have been reported.

At the first indication of toxic symptoms, the drug should be discontinued. If symptoms are severe, treatment with dimercaprol (BAL) should be started as for arsenic poisoning.

Contraindications & Cautions

The drugs are contraindicated in the presence of hepatic disease (whether or not due to amebiasis), renal disease, and abnormalities of visual fields, and in patients with a history of arsenic sensitivity.

If treatment is to be repeated with an arsenical drug, at least 7–14 days should elapse between courses.

Preparations & Dosages

Both carbarsone and glycobiarsol are administered orally after meals, usually to outpatients.

Glycobiarsol (Amoebicon, Milibis, Wia, Wintodon) is supplied in tablets containing 250 and 500 mg. The adult dosage is 500 mg orally 3 times daily for 7 days. Glycobiarsol is also supplied as a vaginal cream (Broxolin) which contains 250 mg/5 ml and as 250 mg vaginal inserts. Glycobiarsol is no longer marketed in the USA.

Carbarsone (Amabevan, Aminarsone, Leucarsone) is supplied in tablets and capsules containing 250 mg. The dosage for adults and children is 4 mg/kg (maximum 250 mg) orally twice a day for 10 days. Carbarsone vaginal inserts—each containing 130 mg of the drug—are supplied for the treatment of *Trichomonas vaginalis* infection.

METRONIDAZOLE
(Flagyl)

Metronidazole was introduced in 1959 for the treatment of trichomoniasis, but it is also very effective for the oral treatment of amebiasis and giardiasis. It is free of serious toxicity and has the unique property of being highly effective against organisms in the intestinal tract, intestinal wall, and extra-intestinal tissues. It has become the drug of choice for treatment of severe intestinal disease, liver abscess, ameboma, and other forms of extra-intestinal disease. It probably will become the drug of choice for the treatment of mild and asymptomatic intestinal infections and possibly for chemoprophylaxis and mass chemotherapy, but few published reports establishing its efficacy, dosage, and safety for these purposes are available. Although the drug is administered at 3 times the dosage used for trichomoniasis, it appears to be free of serious toxic effects. Little information is available on its use in children under 2 years; therefore, it should be used with caution in this age group.

In the USA, metronidazole is approved by the FDA for the treatment of trichomoniasis but not yet for amebiasis.

Pharmacologic actions, adverse reactions, contraindications, and cautions are described on pp 591–592.

Clinical Uses; Preparations & Dosages

Metronidazole (Flagyl) is marketed as 250 mg tablets for oral use.

A. Severe Intestinal Disease: Metronidazole is the drug of choice for the oral treatment of severe intestinal amebiasis. It is given in a dosage of 750 mg orally 3 times daily for 5 days. Powell reported cure rates of 93% when patients were treated with 800 mg of metronidazole 3 times daily for 5 days.

B. Liver Abscess, Ameboma, and Other Forms of Extra-intestinal Infection: Metronidazole replaces other drugs as the simplest and safest preparation for the oral treatment of these infections. The dosage is 750 mg orally 3 times daily for 5 days. Powell reported that 100% of patients with liver abscess were cured. However, single doses as small as 2.4 gm can be curative.

THE TREATMENT OF LEISHMANIASIS

THE PENTAVALENT ANTIMONIAL DRUGS

Antimony compounds have been used since antiquity. Trivalent antimonials were introduced in 1908 for the treatment of trypanosomiasis and are still drugs of choice in schistosomiasis. Pentavalent antimony compounds can be administered more easily and are the choice in the treatment of leishmania infections.

Chemistry

In sodium antimony gluconate or sodium stibogluconate (Pentostam, Bayer 561, Solustibosan, Glucatamime, Pentahexonate, Solyusurmin, Stibinol, Stibanose, Stibatin, and antimony V hexonate (Myostibin), as with many of the organic compounds of antimony, the point of attachment of the antimony is uncertain. Sodium antimony gluconate is a colorless amorphous powder of which about a third is antimony. It is soluble in water, chemically stable in the dark, and deteriorates in sunlight.

Ethylstibamine (Neostibosan, Von Heyden 693, Stibosamine, Astaril, and Bayer 693B) is a complex of para-aminophenylstibonic acid, para-acetylaminophenylstibonic acid, antimonic acid, and diethylamine in the molar ratio of 1:2:1:3. Ethylstibamine is a pale, brownish-yellow powder containing 41–44% antimony. It forms a colloidal solution in water which precipitates on standing or heating.

Urea stibamine (Stiburea, Carbostibamide, Ureastibol, Aminostibune, Stiburamine) contains symdiphenylcarbamido-4,4-distibonic acid and other unidentified substances. It is a pale brown, amorphous powder, soluble in water and unstable in air, containing 39–42% antimony.

Meglumine antimoniate (Glucantime, Protostib, 2168RP), an N-methylglucamine antimoniate, is closely related to sodium stibogluconate, but the location of the antimony atom in the molecule is not yet known. It is the leishmanicide most commonly used in those parts of Africa and Asia where French influence is dominant. It is a white powder, of which a third is antimony, and is soluble in water.

Sodium stibogluconate (Solustibosan, Pentostam)

$$CH_2OH$$
$$(CHOH)_4$$
$$CH_2NHCH_3 \, , \quad Sb = O$$

with an OH group and an O double bond

Meglumine antimoniate
(Glucantime, Protostib)

The in vivo activity of the antimonials correlates well with the concentration of antimony in the spleen. It is probable that the pentavalent antimonial compounds undergo metabolic reduction to the trivalent form before they become active leishmanicidal agents. In vitro, the pentavalent antimonials have little effect on the leptomonads of leishmanias, which can grow on culture media containing 1:200 ethylstibamine.

Absorption, Metabolism, & Excretion

Both the trivalent and pentavalent antimonials are much too irritating to the intestinal mucosa to be given orally. (Tartar emetic is so called because it was once used as an emetic.) After intravenous injection, the trivalent antimonials leave the circulation rapidly and are concentrated in the liver and thyroid. The pentavalent antimonials become concentrated mostly in the spleen. The trivalent compounds are excreted into the intestine; up to 50% of the first dose is excreted within a few hours, although some antimony can be detected in the urine up to 100 days after the last dose. The pentavalent antimonials reach much higher blood concentrations than the trivalents and are excreted in the urine in a pentavalent state at a rate proportionate to the amount injected. Fecal excretion of the pentavalent antimonials is negligible. A portion of injected pentavalent antimonials can be detected in the tissues in a reduced trivalent state.

Pharmacologic Effects

The activity and toxicity of the various pentavalent antimonials are difficult to standardize because the composition and potency vary with the age and pH of the preparation. The sensitivity of the parasites and the resistance of the host to the toxic effects of the drugs is also variable.

Sodium stibogluconate, ethylstibamine, and urea stibamine have approximately equal leishmanicidal potencies, but only half that of the trivalent stibamine glucosamide. Most trypanosomes are said to have high carbohydrate requirements, and the antimonials have been shown to interfere with the utilization of glucose by trypanosomes. Antimonials inhibit hexokinase, ATPase, glyceraldehyde-3-phosphate dehydrogenase, and other enzymes essential to the anaerobic metabolism of glucose. This inhibition can be partially reversed by cysteine. The antimonials reduce the production of lactic acid by inhibiting the formation of fructose diphosphate from fructose-6-phosphate. The selective toxicity of the antimonials for schistosomes,

trypanosomes, and leptomonads may be due to the fact that the fructose enzyme system of these parasites is more susceptible than the mammalian fructose enzyme system to inhibition by antimony compounds.

Other Pharmacologic & Toxicologic Actions

Applied locally, antimony compounds are more caustic than arsenic. They cause papular eruptions that frequently become vesicular and pustular, especially at the orifices of cutaneous glands. Intravenous injections of antimony compounds cause many transitory cardiovascular changes. The force and amplitude of ventricular contractions are diminished, and cardiac output and blood pressure fall. The venous and pulmonary arterial pressures rise, and the heart dilates. These effects are manifest on the ECG, and are experienced as a feeling of faintness and constriction of the chest. The vessels of the intestines, spleen, and liver are dilated, and the engorgement of these organs may be felt as abdominal fullness by the patient.

Clinical Uses

The principal use of the trivalent antimonials is for the treatment of schistosomiasis (see Chapter 63).

Of the pentavalent antimonials, sodium stibogluconate is usually cited as the drug of first choice for the treatment of infections with *L donovani* (visceral leishmaniasis, kala-azar) and *L tropica* (cutaneous leishmaniasis, Oriental sore). Mucocutaneous leishmaniasis (espundia), caused by *L braziliensis,* is best treated with ethylstibamine, which can also be used as an alternate drug for the treatment of visceral leishmaniasis.

It is hoped that less toxic drugs will replace pentavalent antimonials for the treatment of leishmaniasis.

Adverse Reactions

Marked side-effects are common during antimony therapy. The toxicity of the various preparations may vary with each batch of a drug and is not related to the antimony content. The trivalent antimonials are more toxic than the pentavalent compounds. Immediately after an intravenous injection of antimony, there may be coughing or vomiting, headache, dyspnea, facial edema, abdominal pain, urticarial rashes, and vascular collapse. Anaphylactic reactions are particularly likely to occur several days after treatment is started.

During antimony therapy, the patient may lapse into a shock-like state with a precipitous drop in blood pressure due to dilatation of splanchnic vessels and depression of the myocardium. The ECG shows a slow beat, increased amplitude of the P wave, fusion of the S–T segment, lengthening of the Q–T interval, and flattening of the T waves. The ECG pattern usually returns to normal after 30–60 days.

Liver function may be depressed, sometimes for months after termination of therapy. If hepatitis develops, immediate cessation of therapy is indicated.

If severe toxic reactions develop during therapy with any antimonial, heavy metal detoxification with chelating agents such as dimercaprol (BAL) should be considered (see Chapter 64).

Contraindications & Cautions

Antimonials should be avoided in persons with diseases of the heart, liver, or kidneys. Trivalent antimonials are extremely irritating and should only be given by intravenous injection so that they will be rapidly diluted. The pentavalent compounds may be given by intramuscular injection.

Preparations & Dosages

For *L donovani* infections (kala-azar, visceral leishmaniasis) and *L tropica* infections (cutaneous leishmaniasis), give sodium stibogluconate, 600 mg IV or IM for 10 days. It is sometimes infiltrated into the tissues surrounding the lesions. An alternative is to give ethylstibamine, 200 mg IV followed (if tolerated) with 300 mg IV daily or every other day for 16 doses.

For *L braziliensis* infections (mucocutaneous leishmaniasis, espundia), give ethylstibamine, 200 mg IV followed (if tolerated) with 300 mg IV daily or every other day for 16 doses.

Sodium stibogluconate is available from the Center for Disease Control, Atlanta.

Meglumine antimoniate (Glucantime) is given in courses of 12–15 daily doses of 60–100 mg/kg IM.

Apparent failures with antimonial therapy may reflect the wide variation of drug sensitivity of the Leishmania species in different parts of the world.

OTHER DRUGS USED FOR THE TREATMENT OF LEISHMANIASIS

Amphotericin B (Fungizone), 25–50 mg in 500 ml 5% glucose-saline solution, given by slow intravenous drip on alternate days for periods of weeks and even months, has led to complete healing of the lesions of mucocutaneous leishmaniasis which were resistant to antimony therapy.

The suggested daily dose of amphotericin B is 0.25–1 mg/kg. (For toxicity, see Chapter 55.) In cultures of *L braziliensis,* amphotericin B, 0.1 mg/ml, completely immobilizes the leptomonads within 10 minutes. Amphotericin B may be more potent as a leishmanicide than the antimonials.

Cures of *L braziliensis* and *L tropica* infections have also been obtained with intramuscular injections of the antimalarial repository drug **cycloguanil embonate** (cycloguanil pamoate), an insoluble salt of the dihydrotriazine metabolite of chloroguanide (pro-

guanil). One or 2 IM injections of 350 mg (2.5 ml) of the base have given cure rates of up to 85%.

Oral dehydroemetine resinate (Mebadin) in doses of 1.5 mg/kg orally after meals (to a total dose of 0.85–7 gm) gave a 70% cure rate of *L tropica* infections in a study carried out in Iraq.

Metronidazole (Flagyl), 250 mg twice daily orally for 15 days, produced an excellent cure rate of Mexican cutaneous leishmaniasis.

THE TREATMENT OF TRYPANOSOMIASIS

THE AROMATIC DIAMIDINES: PENTAMIDINE, STILBAMIDINE, & PROPAMIDINE

History

Pentamidine, stilbamidine, and propamidine are the only aromatic diamidine derivatives that are sufficiently potent as trypanosomicides and have toxicities low enough to be used for the treatment of trypanosomiasis (sleeping sickness). Pentamidine is now the drug of choice for the treatment and prevention of *Trypanosoma rhodesiense* and *T gambiense* infection and is an alternative to sodium stibogluconate for the treatment of leishmaniasis. Propamidine and the dihydroxyl derivative of stilbamidine are occasionally used.

Chemistry

Pentamidine isethionate (Lomidine) is a 4,4'-diamidinophenoxypentane. It is a white, hygroscopic, crystalline powder soluble 1:10 in water.

The in vitro trypanosomicidal activity of the guanidine derivatives is associated with the terminal amidine and guanidine groups, and the activity is maximal when the amidine groups are connected by an undecane methylene chain.

Absorption, Metabolism, & Excretion

Diamidine compounds are not well absorbed from the gastrointestinal tract, but absorption after parenteral administration is satisfactory. Following intravenous injection, the drug rapidly leaves the circulation and only small amounts appear in the urine. The liver, spleen, kidneys, and adrenals maintain high levels of

Pentamidine

the diamidines for months after treatment. Single injections of pentamidine can prevent infection by *T gambiense* for up to 6 months. A portion of the drug is metabolized in the body, and part is excreted in the urine. Intermediary metabolic products are not known.

Diamidine compounds cross the placenta but are not excreted in milk. Only trace amounts appear in the CNS, so that other trypanosomicides such as tryparsamide or one of the melanyl arsenicals must be used for the treatment of late stages of African trypanosomiasis with CNS involvement.

Pharmacologic Effects

The aromatic diamidines are highly toxic to certain species of protozoa and only slightly toxic to others. *T rhodesiense* and *T gambiense* infections in man and *T donovani* infections in hamsters can be cured with pentamidine, but the drug has no effect on *T cruzi* infection in mice. The diamidines have some plasmocidal, bactericidal, and fungicidal activity and have been used for the treatment of systemic blastomycosis (see p 533).

Intravenous injections of the diamidines produce a sharp fall of blood pressure which can be only partially blocked by atropine. The peripheral vasodilatation is probably due to a release of tissue-bound histamine and peripheral adrenergic blockade.

After injection of a diamidine drug, the trypanosomes quickly take up the drug to a concentration about 1400 times that of the surrounding tissues. Trypanosomicidal effects appear only after a long latent period. The trypanosomicidal action of the diamidines is antagonized by glucose, and the addition of insulin to cultures slows trypanosome multiplication. Diamidines may interfere with glycolysis in a susceptible protozoon.

Clinical Uses

Pentamidine is the drug of choice for the prevention and treatment of both *T gambiense* and *T rhodesiense* infection. In the early stages pentamidine can clear the organisms from the blood and lymph nodes. Diamidines cannot be given intrathecally, and do not reach the CNS in sufficient quantities to have any therapeutic effect. Thus, other drugs such as melarsoprol or suramin must be used. In early trypanosomiasis, propamidine and stilbamidine can also be employed.

The diamidines are also used for visceral leishmaniasis (kala-azar) in patients who do not respond to or cannot tolerate antimonials.

Adverse Reactions

The diamidines may result in initial respiratory stimulation followed by respiratory depression. Intravenous injections usually produce a fall of blood pressure, dizziness, and headache together with breathlessness, tachycardia, and vomiting. Respiratory failure and death occur rarely.

The diamidines are nephrotoxic and occasionally neurotoxic, causing nystagmus, ataxia, convulsions, and death.

Delayed toxicity of stilbamidine (but not pentamidine) consists of paralysis of the trigeminal nerve and other peripheral neuropathies.

Preparations & Dosages

Pentamidine isethionate (Lomidine) is marketed as a dry powder in ampules containing 200 mg.

For the early stages of *T rhodesiense* and *T gambiense* infections, pentamidine, 4 mg/kg IM, is given every 1–2 days for 10 doses. For chemoprophylaxis, give 3 mg/kg IM every 3–6 months.

For *L donovani* infections (kala-azar, visceral leishmaniasis), give pentamidine, 2–4 mg/kg IV or IM daily for up to 15 days.

For the late CNS stages of *T rhodesiense* and *T gambiense* infections, melarsoprol must be given.

There are no effective drugs for the treatment of *T cruzi* infection (Chagas' disease). However, some encouraging results have been reported with metronidazole (Flagyl).

MELARSOPROL

Melarsoprol (Mel B), an organic arsenical, is a 2-*p*-(4,6-diamino-1,3,5-triazin-2-ylamino)phenyl-4-hydroxymethyl-1,3,2-dithioarsolan.

Pharmacologic Effects

Melarsoprol is formed by condensing a toxic trivalent arsenical trypanosomicide (melarsen oxide) with an arsenic antagonist (BAL). In the product, the trypanosomicidal activity is retained while the toxicity of arsenic is mitigated. Its mode of action is probably related to an interaction with the sulfhydryl groups of enzymes essential to trypanosome metabolism.

Absorption, Metabolism, & Excretion

Melarsoprol is well absorbed from the gastrointestinal tract, but it is given only intravenously. The drug is quickly excreted.

Clinical Uses

Unlike pentamidine, melarsoprol appears in the CSF in sufficient amounts to exert a trypanosomicidal effect on the late meningoencephalitic stages of human trypanosomiasis. It is also effective in the earlier stages of the disease, but it is used only for the rare pentamidine-refractory cases.

Adverse Effects

The most serious side-effect of melarsoprol therapy, usually occurring at the end of the first week of therapy, is a reactive encephalopathy which may be fatal. Patients in the most advanced stages of the disease are most severely affected.

If the intravenous injections are given too fast, vomiting and colicky abdominal pains occur.

Hypersensitivity reactions can be relieved with corticosteroids.

Preparations & Dosages

Melarsoprol (Mel B) is available for intravenous injection as a solution containing 3.6% (w/v) in propylene glycol. For the therapy of the late stages of *T rhodesiense* and *T gambiense* infections, three 3-day courses are given with an interval of 7 days between courses. Daily injections of 90 mg are given very slowly for the first 3 days; 90–180 mg for the second 3-day course; and 180 mg for the last 3-day course.

Leakage at injection sites causes intense pain and sometimes sloughing.

In the USA, melarsoprol is available only from the Center for Disease Control, Atlanta.

THE TREATMENT OF TRICHOMONIASIS

METRONIDAZOLE
(Flagyl)

Chemistry

Metronidazole, 1-(2-hydroxyethyl)-2-methyl-5-nitroimidazole, is a crystalline nonhygroscopic powder, slightly soluble in water and alcohol. In 1959, the trichomonacidal properties of metronidazole were demonstrated, and human trials showed that the drug is excreted in the semen and urine, making possible high cure rates of chronically infected but asymptomatic males.

Metronidazole (Flagyl)

Pharmacologic Actions

Apart from the trichomonacidal effect achieved by the recommended doses on human infections of *Trichomonas vaginalis,* the drug has so few actions that it appears to be pharmacologically inert. It may produce disulfiram-like aversion to alcohol and thus may also inhibit several enzymes concerned with the metabolism of alcohol. In vitro studies have demonstrated that alcohol dehydrogenase (an NAD-linked enzyme), xanthine oxidase (an FAD-linked enzyme), and uricase (the enzyme converting uric acid to allantoin in subprimate mammals) are all reversibly inhibited by metronidazole. Because metronidazole can inhibit 3 different classes of oxidases but not monoamine oxidase and diamine oxidase, it has been postulated that the drug acts as a nonspecific electron trap.

In humans, metronidazole (10 mg/kg orally) is a highly effective systemic trichomonacide that does not disturb the normal vaginal flora. In vitro, metronidazole in concentrations of 2.5 μg/liter destroys 99% of the parasites in cultures of *T vaginalis* within 24 hours, but concentrations as high as 250 μg/liter do not affect the growth of Döderlein's bacillus *(Lactobacillus acidophilus)* or *Candida albicans.*

In dogs, large doses (125–150 mg/kg) have produced tremor, ataxia, muscle spasticity, convulsions, and death within 7–28 days. In humans, metronidazole is pharmacologically inert, and doses of up to 800 mg 3 times a day for 10 days for the treatment of intestinal and extra-intestinal amebiasis are commonly used without any major side-effects. It is possible that metronidazole is acting on a metabolic pathway in nonprimate mammals that has no counterpart in humans (eg, the uricase enzyme system).

Absorption, Metabolism, & Excretion

Metronidazole is rapidly and almost completely absorbed from the gastrointestinal tract. Although only trace amounts of the ingested dose can be recovered in the feces, metronidazole is a potent amebicide for the luminal and hepatic forms of *Entamoeba histolytica.* Metronidazole's ability to heal colonic ulcer and cure chronic cyst passers may be due to a metabolite which is formed in the liver and then excreted into the bowel.

After ingestion, the plasma level rises rapidly; effective serum levels are reached in 2–3 hours and maintained for 12 hours after a single oral dose. Approximately 69% of the drug is excreted in the urine unchanged, 26% as a carboxylic metabolite, and 5% as a glucuronic acid-ether conjugate of metronidazole. The urine is often colored a deep red brown. There is no evidence of the metabolic reduction of the nitroimidazole group. Metronidazole crosses the placenta and is excreted in the saliva, milk, semen, and vaginal secretions.

Clinical Uses

A. Extra-intestinal and Luminal Amebiasis: Metronidazole is now the drug of choice. See p 581.

B. Urogenital Trichomoniasis: Systemic therapy makes possible the delivery of effective trichomonacidal concentrations of the drug to foci of infections in the genitourinary tract that cannot be reached by local applications. Approximately 90% of *T vaginalis* infections can now be cured with a single course of metronidazole. Although partial resistance has recently been reported, about 90% of the treatment failures will respond to retreatment. Most recrudescences are due to a failure to eradicate the organism from the paraurethral glands of sexual partners; therefore, the treatment of asymptomatic sexual consorts is advised.

C. Mexican Cutaneous Leishmaniasis: If the reported 75% cure rates of *Leishmania mexicana* infections are substantiated, metronidazole may soon become the treatment of choice for this disfiguring disease.

D. Chagas' Disease: Considerable amelioration of this virtually untreatable South American form of trypanosomiasis has followed 3-month courses of metronidazole, 250 mg orally 3 times daily.

E. Giardiasis: In the treatment of *Giardia lamblia* and *T hominis* infections, 2 courses of metronidazole (500 mg daily for 5 days repeated after a 15-day interval) appear to be as effective as and less toxic than quinacrine therapy. Cure rates of up to 94% have been obtained.

F. Other Uses: In studies purporting to show that metronidazole has a disulfiram-like effect, control of the withdrawal symptoms of chronic alcoholism is claimed.

Acute ulcerative gingivitis of Vincent's stomatitis has been cured with 200 mg orally 3 times daily for 7 days.

Metronidazole is able to bring about a significant decrease in endocrine exophthalmos without producing any significant changes in thyroid function.

Adverse Reactions

Metronidazole has been extensively used for about 10 years, and few significant side-effects have yet been reported. The most commonly noted side-effects are a disagreeable metallic taste, furred tongue, mild nausea, and darkening of the urine. Very rarely, anorexia, diarrhea, weakness, fatigue, abdominal discomfort, headache, dizziness, vertigo, glossitis, or stomatitis may necessitate discontinuing the drug. Hematologic studies have failed to reveal any evidence of blood dyscrasias despite the fact that the nitro group of the imidazole ring has, in other compounds, been associated with serious blood dyscrasias. No cardiotoxicity has been found, and cases of Chagas' disease with severe myocardial involvement have been improved with metronidazole. The drug is well tolerated during pregnancy, and no instances of fetal damage have been recorded. Most apparent treatment failures and relapses of *T vaginalis* infections are due to reinfection. Trichomonads taken from seemingly resistant cases have all thus far proved to have the usual in vitro sensitivity to metronidazole; however, certain organisms, including *Proteus vulgaris, P mirabilis, Streptococcus faecalis, E coli, Pseudomonas aeruginosa,* and mimeae, can inactivate metronidazole. Several instances of attempted suicide with doses of 4—10 gm attest to the low toxicity of this drug.

Contraindications & Cautions

Although dogs develop severe neurologic disorders with large doses of metronidazole and rats develop testicular damage, there are no reports of serious toxicity to humans. Moderate leukopenias returning to normal after completion of treatment have been reported. Other careful studies have failed to confirm this finding.

Alcohol should be avoided during treatment. Coexistent candidiasis may be aggravated during therapy, especially when vaginal inserts are used.

Preparations & Dosages

Metronidazole is available in uncoated cream-colored 250 mg tablets for oral administration and 500 mg vaginal inserts. For *T vaginalis* infections, metronidazole, 250 mg 3 times a day for 10 days for females or 250 mg twice a day for 10 days for males, will effect a radical cure in 90% of cases. Should retreatment be necessary, intervals of 4—6 weeks should be allowed between courses. There is no evidence that the concurrent use of vaginal inserts with oral therapy brings about any improvement in the cure rate.

For amebiasis dosages, see p 581.

●   ●   ●

General References

Malaria

General

Bartelloni, P.J., Sheehy, T.W., & W.D. Tigertt: Combined therapy for chloroquine-resistant *Plasmodium falciparum* infection. JAMA 199:173—177, 1967.

Clyde, D.F., & others: Treatment of falciparum malaria caused by strain resistant to quinine. JAMA 213:2041—2045, 1970.

Dover, A.S.: Malaria in a heroin user. JAMA 215:1987, 1971.

Fisher, G.U., & others: Malaria in soldiers returning from Vietnam: Epidemiologic, therapeutic, and clinical studies. Am J Trop Med 19:27—39, 1970.

Hinman, E.H.: Malaria: The changing outlook. M Clin North America 51:729—734, 1967.

Jelliffe, D.B.: The therapy of cerebral malaria in children. Trop Pediat 69:483—484, 1966.

Neva, F.A.: Malaria: Recent progress and problems. New England J Med 277:1241—1252, 1967.

Powell, R.D.: The chemotherapy of malaria. Clin Pharmacol Therap 7:48—76, 1966.

Sitprija, V.: Renal involvement in malaria. Tr Roy Soc Trop Med Hyg 64:695—699, 1970.

Treatment of acute malaria. Med Lett Drugs Ther 8:22—23, 1966.

US Departments of the Army, the Navy, and the Air Force: *Malaria (Clinical Features, Treatment, Control and Prevention).* Pages 1—27. Washington, DC, July 14, 1967.

World Health Organization: *Chemotherapy of Malaria.* Report of a WHO Scientific Group. Technical Report Series No. 375, 1967.

Quinine

Lang, P.A., & C.C. Jones: Acute renal failure precipitated by quinine sulfate in early pregnancy. JAMA 188:464—466, 1964.

Sheehy, T.W., & R.C. Reba: Complications of falciparum malaria and their treatment. Ann Int Med 66:807—809, 1967.

Smitskamp, H., & F.H. Walthus: New concepts in treatment of malignant tertian malaria with cerebral involvement. Brit MJ 1:714—716, 1971.

Chloroquine

Blount, R.D.: Chloroquine-resistant falciparum malaria. JAMA 200:886, 1967.

Burns, R.P.: Delayed onset of chloroquine retinopathy. New England J Med 275:693–696, 1966.

Carson, J.W., Barringer, M.L., & R.E. Jones, Jr.: Fatal chloroquine ingestion: An increasing hazard. Pediatrics 40:449–450, 1967.

Ciak, J., & F.E. Hahn: Chloroquine: Mode of action. Science 151:347–349, 1966.

Congeners of Chloroquine

Booth, K., Larkin, K., & I. Maddocks: Agranulocytosis coincident with amodiaquine therapy. Brit MJ 3:32–33, 1967.

Lucasse, C.: Single-dose treatment of acute malaria. J Trop Med 66:280–282, 1963.

8-Aminoquinolines

Cahn, M.M., & E.J. Levy: The tolerance to large weekly doses of primaquine and amodiaquine in primaquine-sensitive and non-sensitive subjects. Am J Trop Med 11:605–606, 1962.

Peters, W.: The possible role of primaquine in inducing multiple drug resistance in *Plasmodium falciparum.* Tr Roy Soc Trop Med Hyg 60:140–141, 1966.

Quinacrine

Sapp, O.L., III: Toxic psychosis due to quinacrine and chloroquine. JAMA 187:373–375, 1964.

Proguanil, Pyrimethamine, & Trimethoprim

Bushby, S.R.M., & G.H. Hitchings: Trimethoprim, a sulphonamide potentiator. Brit J Pharmacol 33:72–90, 1968.

Greenberg, J., & H.W. Bond: Further studies on cross-resistance between pyrimethamine and related compounds. Am J Trop Med 5:14–18, 1956.

Laing, A.B.G.: Treatment of acute falciparum malaria with sulphorthodimethoxine (Fanasil). Brit MJ 1:905–907, 1965.

McGregor, I.A., Williams, K., & L.G. Goodwin: Pyrimethamine and sulphadiazine in treatment of malaria. Brit MJ 2:728–729, 1963.

Amebiasis

General

Powell, S.J.: Drug therapy of amoebiasis. Bull WHO 40:953–956, 1969.

Powell, S.J.: The cardiotoxicity of systemic amebicides: A comparative electrocardiographic study. Am J Trop Med 16:447–450, 1967.

Wilmot, A.J.: *Clinical Amoebiasis.* Blackwell, 1962.

Woodruff, A.W., & S. Bell: The evaluation of amoebicides. Tr Roy Soc Trop Med Hyg 61:435–439, 1967.

Woolfe, G.: The chemotherapy of amoebiasis. Progr Drug Res 8:13–52, 1965.

World Health Organization Expert Committee: Amoebiasis. Technical Report Series No. 421, 1969.

Emetine & Dehydroemetine

Klatskin, G., & H. Friedman: Emetine toxicity in man: Studies on the nature of early toxic manifestations, their relation to the dose level, and their significance in determining safe dosage. Ann Int Med 28:892–915, 1948.

Pain, A., & A. Wingfield: Electrocardiographic changes due to emetine therapy. Tr Roy Soc Trop Med Hyg 62:221–226, 1968.

Powell, S.J., & others: A comparative trial of dehydroemetine and emetine hydrochloride in identical dosage in amoebic liver abscess. Ann Trop Med 61:26–28, 1967.

Scragg, J.N., & S.J. Powell: Emetine hydrochloride and chloroquine in the treatment of children with amoebic liver abscess. Arch Dis Childhood 41:549–550, 1966.

Arsenicals & Halogenated Hydroxyquinolines

Knight, A.A., & J. Miller: Comparative studies on the iodine absorption of Anayodin, Chiniofon, Diodoquin and Vioform in man. Ann Int Med 30:1180–1187, 1949.

Radke, R.A., & W.G. Baroody: Carbarsone toxicity: A review of the literature and report of 45 cases. Ann Int Med 47:418–427, 1957.

Metronidazole

Powell, S.J., & others: Metronidazole in amoebic dysentery and amoebic liver abscess. Lancet 1:1329–1331, 1966.

Powell, S.J., Wilmot, A.J., & R. Elsdon-Dew: Further trials of metronidazole in amoebic dysentery and amoebic liver abscess. Ann Trop Med 61:511–514, 1967.

Leishmaniasis

Beltran, H.F., Gutierrez, F.M., & F.F. Biagi: [Treatment of Mexican cutaneous leishmaniasis with metronidazole.] Bull Soc path exot 60:61–64, 1967.

Chavarria, A.P., & E. Kotcher: Preliminary evaluation of cycloguanil pamoate in dermal leishmaniasis. JAMA 194:1142–1144, 1965.

Hassan Abd-Rabbo: Dehydroemetine in leishmaniasis (Oriental sore). J Trop Med 69:171–174, 1966.

Prata, A.: Treatment of kala-azar with amphotericin B. Tr Roy Soc Trop Med Hyg 57:266–268, 1963.

Reinhard, M., & H. Wacker: [Treatment of cutaneous leishmaniasis with cycloguanil pamoate.] Deutsch Med Wschr 95:2380–2382, 1970.

Salem, H.H., & others: The treatment of cutaneous leishmaniasis with oral dehydroemetine. Tr Roy Soc Trop Med Hyg 61:776–780, 1967.

Trypanosomiasis

Gutteridge, W.E.: Chemotherapy and drug sensitivity: Further investigations on the mode of action of pentamidine. Tr Roy Soc Trop Med Hyg 60:120, 1966.

Trichomoniasis

Metronidazole

Baker, R.M., & A.L. Kennan: Therapy of trichomoniasis. Wisconsin MJ 66:370–371, 1967.

Diddle, A.W.: *Trichomonas vaginalis:* Resistance to metronidazole. Am J Obst Gynec 98:583–585, 1967.

McLoughlin, D.K.: Drug tolerance by *Trichomonas foetus.* J Parasitol 53:646–648, 1967.

63 . . .

Anthelmintic Drugs

Robert S. Goldsmith, MD, DTM&H

CHEMOTHERAPY OF HELMINTHIC INFECTIONS

Anthelmintic drugs are a group of compounds used to eradicate or reduce in numbers helminthic parasites in the gastrointestinal tract or tissues of man. Table 63–1 lists the major helminthic infections and provides a guide to the drug of choice and alternate drugs for each infection. In the text that follows, these drugs are arranged alphabetically.

Most anthelmintics in use today are active against specific parasites, and some are toxic. Therefore, parasites must be accurately identified before treatment is started, usually by finding the parasite, ova, or larvae in the feces, urine, blood, sputum, or tissues of the host.

Administration of Anthelmintic Drugs

Unless otherwise indicated, oral drugs should be taken with water during or after meals. If pre- or post-treatment purges are necessary in conjunction with a specific drug, magnesium or sodium sulfate may be used. The usual dose, 15–30 gm for an adult and 1–2 gm/10 lb body weight for children, is dissolved in a glass of water. The intensely bitter taste may be partially masked by giving the salts in lemon juice. Magnesium sulfate must not be given to individuals with impaired renal function, and sodium sulfate may be contraindicated in patients with congestive heart failure. Other contraindications to severe purgation are signs of intestinal obstruction, debilitation, and pregnancy.

Dosages for Children

Dosages for infants and children are on a less secure basis than for adults; when not shown in milligrams per kilogram of body weight (or otherwise specified), the dosage should be calculated as a fraction of the adult dose, as follows:

Under 15 lb: 1/8 of adult dose
15–30 lb: 1/4 of adult dose
30–60 lb: 1/2 of adult dose
Over 60 lb: Approximately adult dose

Dr. Goldsmith is Assistant Professor of Tropical Medicine and Epidemiology, University of California, San Francisco.

Contraindications

Pregnancy and ulcers of the gastrointestinal tract are contraindications for most of the drugs listed. Specific contraindications are given in the discussions that follow.

New Drugs

During the past 2 decades, many older anthelmintic drugs have been replaced by far safer and more effective compounds. This constitutes a remarkable revolution in the treatment of a group of infections that remain among the most common diseases of man. Excellent drugs are now available for the treatment of most gastrointestinal parasites. For many of the parasites found in the tissues, however, we are still without highly effective nontoxic drugs. New remedies are particularly needed for schistosomiasis, onchocerciasis, clonorchiasis, trichuriasis, and hydatid disease. Greater knowledge of the physiology and biochemistry of parasitic worms, as well as of the structure-activity relationships of compounds to be tested, is needed to make rational choices in the development of effective anthelmintics.

Efforts continue toward the development of a broad-spectrum anthelmintic that would permit simultaneous treatment of many gastrointestinal parasites, particularly on a mass basis. No drug is as yet available that meets all the criteria: safety with minimal side-effects, a high degree of effectiveness for many parasites, low cost, and palatability.

Included in the text are several new drugs not yet fully accepted and still undergoing clinical trials. Not included are other new drugs in early stages of clinical investigation that may eventually become valuable anthelmintics—eg, trichlorophone (Dipterex) and tris (p-aminophenyl)carbonium pamoate for schistosomiasis, Mel W for onchocerciasis, and pyrantel pamoate, a broad-spectrum anthelmintic.

Older Drugs Not Included

Many older drugs are not included because of their toxicity or low therapeutic effects. Carbon tetrachloride, oil of chenopodium, and thymol, formerly used for hookworm infections; gentian violet for strongyloidiasis and pinworm; santonin for ascariasis; and pelletierine for tapeworm have been replaced by more satisfactory drugs.

Dithiazanine iodide and hexachloroparaxyol have recently been withdrawn because of their toxicity.

ANTIMONY COMPOUNDS

The trivalent antimony compounds have long been the principal and most widely used drugs for individual and mass treatment of schistosomiasis (bilharziasis). Antimony potassium tartrate (tartar emetic) was introduced in 1918, antimony pyrocatechol sodium disulfonate (stibophen) in 1929, and antimony sodium dimercaptosuccinate (stibocaptate) in 1954. Less frequently used antimony preparations include antimony sodium thioglycollate, antimony lithium thiomalate (anthiomaline), antimony thioglycollamide, and antimony sodium gluconate (Triostam).

Antimony drugs are not completely satisfactory since each possesses one or more major defects, including severe toxicity, difficulty of administration, length of treatment, or low effectiveness. Tartar emetic is superior to the other antimonials in the treatment of *Schistosoma japonicum* infection, but it is the most toxic drug of the group. Also, it is unstable in solution and requires intravenous administration. Stibophen and stibocaptate are the preferred antimonials for the treatment of *S mansoni* and *S haematobium* infections because they are stable, moderately effective, can be given intramuscularly, and are less toxic than comparable doses of tartar emetic. A course of stibocaptate can generally be completed in a shorter period than stibophen.

Reports from different parts of the world on the effectiveness of various antimony preparations are far from uniform even when workers have used the same drug and followed the same treatment schedule. These variations reflect, in part, different criteria of cure and perhaps also varying susceptibility of different strains of parasite; host factors such as nutritional status, age, sex, race, and immunity; and the intensity and duration of infection. Many observers have failed to take into account pre- and post-treatment egg output; cure rates tend to be higher in patients with lower intensities of infection.

Pharmacologic Effects

A. Actions on Man: Little information is available concerning the physiologic and biochemical effects of the trivalent antimonials or the mechanisms of their toxicity, except that antimonials may cause respiratory and cardiac depression as well as irritation of the CNS, liver, and kidneys.

B. Anthelmintic Actions: In animals and probably in man, trivalent antimony compounds damage intrauterine eggs and inhibit phosphofructokinase, an enzyme necessary for glycolysis, a major source of energy for the parasites. In addition, the drugs paralyze schistosome adults, which then shift from the mesenteric veins to the liver. When antimony concentrations fall below a threshold level, the worms return to the mesenteric veins and the inhibition of the enzyme is reversed. Death of the worms is ultimately achieved by continued paralysis through repeated administration of the drug.

Absorption, Distribution, & Excretion

Trivalent antimonials, when given orally, irritate the gastrointestinal tract and are slowly absorbed. Therefore, they are administered parenterally, achieving high but transient blood levels. Most circulating antimony shifts rapidly to the tissues; the remainder is largely fixed to the erythrocytes. Little is known about the distribution of antimony in the tissues of man, but high concentrations are found in the liver, thyroid, heart, and kidneys of experimental animals.

In man, antimony is excreted mainly via the kidneys; a small amount appears in the feces. Excretion varies according to the drug, dosages, and the individual responsiveness of the patient. Schulert & others reported that after a single parenteral dose of tartar emetic (2.5 mg/kg), 49% of the antimony was excreted in the urine in 24 hours and 56% in 1 week. After a single injection of stibocaptate (3.1 mg/kg), 14% of the antimony was excreted in 24 hours and 27% in 1 week.

1. STIBOCAPTATE
(Astiban, Antimony Sodium Dimercaptosuccinate)

Chemistry

Stibocaptate is antimony sodium dimercaptosuccinate (antimony III sodium meso 2,3-dimercaptosuccinate; TWSb/6; Astiban). It is a trivalent antimonial which differs from antimony tartrate in that the oxygen atoms of the hydroxyl groups are replaced by sulfur.

Stibocaptate is a stable, white crystalline substance containing 25−26% antimony. It is readily soluble but unstable in water and should be used shortly after being placed in solution.

Clinical Uses

Stibocaptate is a drug of choice for *Schistosoma haematobium* and *S mansoni* infections and an alternative drug for *S japonicum* infection.

A wide range of effectiveness has been reported for stibocaptate in different clinical trials. Reported cure rates for *S mansoni* infection are 29−91%; for *S haematobium* infection, 12−100%. There are relatively few studies on the use of stibocaptate for *S japonicum* infections; a cure rate of 58% was reported for 111 patients who received a total dose of 40−60 mg/kg, divided into equal amounts and injected over 12 days.

Adverse Reactions

These are common in adults, but the drug is better tolerated by children. Pain at the injection site

TABLE 63–1. **Drugs for the treatment of helminthic infections.**

Infecting Organism	Drug of Choice	Alternative Drugs
Roundworms (Nematodes)		
Ascaris lumbricoides (roundworm)	Piperazine citrate	Hexylresorcinol
Trichuris trichiura (whipworm)	Hexylresorcinol by retention enema	None
Necator americanus (hookworm)	Tetrachloroethylene	Bephenium
Ancylostoma duodenale (hookworm)	Bephenium	Tetrachloroethylene
Strongyloides stercoralis (threadworm)	Thiabendazole	Pyrvinium pamoate* or niridazole*†
Enterobius (Oxyuris) vermicularis (pinworm)	Piperazine citrate or pyrvinium pamoate	None
Trichinella spiralis (trichinosis)	ACTH, corticosteroids, or thiabendazole*	None
Cutaneous larva migrans (creeping eruption)	Thiabendazole	Diethylcarbamazine*
Visceral larva migrans	Thiabendazole*	None
Angiostrongylus cantonensis	None	None
Wuchereria bancrofti (filariasis) *W (Brugia) malayi* Tropical eosinophilia *Gnathostoma spinigerum*	Diethylcarbamazine	None
Onchocerca volvulus (onchocerciasis) *O caecutiens*	Suramin† plus diethylcarbamazine	None
Dracunculus medinensis (guinea worm)	Niridazole†	Thiabendazole
Intestinal capillariasis	Thiabendazole	None
Flukes (Trematodes)		
Schistosoma haematobium (bilharziasis)	Niridazole† or stibocaptate† (see antimony compounds)	Stibophen or lucanthone‡ (only for children 16 and under)
S mansoni	Stibophen or stibocaptate† (see antimony compounds)	Niridazole† or lucanthone‡ (only for children 16 and under)
S japonicum	Tartar emetic (see antimony compounds)	Stibophen or stibocaptate† (see antimony compounds)
Clonorchis sinensis (liver fluke) Opisthorchis species	Chloroquine phosphate*	Bithionol*†
Paragonimus westermani (lung fluke)	Bithionol†	Chloroquine phosphate*
Fasciola hepatica (sheep liver fluke)	Bithionol†	Emetine or dehydroemetine†
Fasciolopsis buski (large intestinal fluke)	Hexylresorcinol	Tetrachloroethylene
Heterophyes heterophyes *Metagonimus yokogawai*	Tetrachloroethylene	Hexylresorcinol or bephenium
Tapeworms (Cestodes)		
Taenia saginata (beef tapeworm) *Diphyllobothrium latum* (fish tapeworm)	Niclosamide† or dichlorophen‡	Quinacrine or paromomycin
Taenia solium (pork tapeworm)	Niclosamide† or dichlorophen‡	Quinacrine or paromomycin
Cysticercosis (pork tapeworm larval stage)	None	None
Hymenolepis nana (dwarf tapeworm) *H diminuta* (rat tapeworm) *Dipylidium caninum*	Niclosamide† or paromomycin	Quinacrine or hexylresorcinol or chloroquine
Echinococcus granulosus (hydatid disease) *E multilocularis*	None	None

*Effectiveness not established or of a low order.

†Available in the USA, for clinical investigational use only, from the Parasitic Disease Drug Service, Parasitic Diseases Branch, Center for Disease Control, Atlanta, Georgia 30333.

‡Not available in the USA.

can be reduced by prior administration of 1% lidocaine (Xylocaine) through the same needle used for the drug. Vomiting tends to start late in the course of treatment, usually 2–4 hours after injection. Its severity can sometimes be reduced by belladonna, antacids, or antiemetics. Other frequent side-effects are headache, dizziness, fatigue, prostration, nausea, abdominal pain, myalgia, arthralgia, fever, and skin rashes. Less common are a metallic taste, pruritus, herpetic lesions, facial edema, tachycardia, and hypotension. Most side-effects are not severe and disappear within 1–2 days after the last injection. The drug should be discontinued, however, in the event of severe vomiting, progressive proteinuria, substernal pain, or purpura. Reversible ECG changes similar to those produced by other antimonial drugs occur in most patients, and it may take several months for the ECG to return to normal. These changes are not an indication to discontinue therapy. Acute liver injury is rare. Several deaths have occurred unexpectedly during or shortly after treatment.

Contraindications & Cautions

Some workers advise clearing intestinal helminth infections, particularly ascarids, before treatment with stibocaptate. Although most patients can be treated on an ambulatory basis, their cardiac and renal status should be carefully followed. Stibocaptate is contraindicated in the presence of tuberculosis, acute febrile conditions, herpes simplex and zoster, severe anemia, cardiac, renal, and hepatic insufficiency, terminal forms of schistosomiasis, and for patients treated with antimonials within the previous 2 months. It should be used with caution in debilitated patients.

Preparations & Dosages

Stibocaptate (Astiban) is supplied in vials containing 0.5 gm of the lyophilized drug, to be dissolved in 5 ml of sterile water or normal saline. The resultant 10% solution should be refrigerated and used within 24 hours. The intramuscular route is preferred, but slow intravenous injections can be used. The drug is not licensed for use in the USA but can be obtained from the Parasitic Disease Drug Service, Center for Disease Control, Atlanta, for investigational use.

The total dose for treatment of *S haematobium* or *S mansoni* infections is 40 mg/kg body weight and for *S japonicum* infection 50 mg/kg (maximum total 2.5 gm). The total dose is divided into 5 equal injec-

tions given once a week for 5 weeks. If given at shorter intervals, side-effects are more severe. After each injection, the patient should rest for half an hour.

2. STIBOPHEN
(Antimony Pyrocatechol Sodium Disulfonate)

Chemistry

Stibophen (sodium antimony III bis-pyrocatechol-2,4-disulfonate) is a crystalline, white powder containing 13.6% of trivalent antimony. It is freely soluble and stable in water; may dissociate and become toxic after prolonged storage; and oxidizes when exposed to the air.

Clinical Uses

A. *Schistosoma Mansoni* **and** *S Haematobium:* Shookhoff reported 74 cures among 81 adult Puerto Rican patients treated for *S mansoni* infection who were given 70–100 ml of stibophen. Most & others observed no relapses in 28 Puerto Rican patients infected with *S mansoni* who were treated with 70 ml of stibophen.

B. *Schistosoma Japonicum:* Stibophen can be used if tartar emetic (the drug of choice) is not well tolerated, but an intensive course of treatment involving administration of a highly toxic amount of stibophen is required. Most & others reported that when 100 ml of stibophen were given during a 14-day period, the drug failed to cure 13 of 64 patients.

Adverse Reactions

Intramuscular injections may cause pain at the site of injection, but necrosis does not occur. Shortly after injection, the pulse rate is generally slowed about 10 beats per minute.

During treatment, anorexia, nausea, vomiting, arthralgia, myalgia, and trace amounts of protein in the urine are common side-effects. Headache, bradycardia, weakness, cough, abdominal pain, skin rashes, and conjunctivitis are less frequent. Some patients develop hepatomegaly and laboratory evidence of liver dysfunction early in treatment. Rare side-effects include peripheral neuritis, herpes zoster, retrobulbar neuritis with central scotomas, hematuria, thrombocytopenia, hemolytic anemia (of the autoimmune type), and

Stibophen

hypotension. ECG changes similar to those caused by tartar emetic are frequent but are generally less pronounced. Sudden deaths, presumably due to ventricular fibrillation, have been reported, particularly from Egypt during mass campaigns. Fatalities have also been reported associated with thrombocytopenia and hemolytic anemia.

Mild nausea may be reduced by 6–10 ml of aluminum hydroxide gel given before the injection, or by 15–20 minims of tincture of belladonna, given 3 times a day before meals. Hypotension responds to subcutaneous injections of epinephrine.

Contraindications & Cautions

Muscle or joint pains, nausea, or ECG changes are not indications to stop or modify treatment. If pains or nausea are severe or vomiting develops, however, the interval between injections should be increased or the dosage reduced. Discontinue therapy if vomiting persists or if an intercurrent febrile reaction or precordial pain occurs. Urine and blood should be examined weekly and the drug discontinued in the event of hematuria, progressive proteinuria, thrombocytopenia, or signs of hemolytic anemia.

Inadvertent intravenous administration may intensify side-reactions. The dosage should be reduced in poorly nourished patients.

During repeat courses of treatment, patients should be closely watched for the development of hemolytic anemias, which may be preceded by a marked febrile reaction.

Stibophen is contraindicated in the presence of renal and cardiac disease and hepatic disease not due to schistosomiasis.

Preparations & Dosages

Stibophen (Fuadin, Fouadin, Neoantimosan, Repodral) is available in ampules, each containing 5 ml of a 6.3% aqueous solution with not more than 0.1% sodium bisulfite as preservative. Each milliliter contains the equivalent of 8.5 mg of trivalent antimony. Once an ampule has been opened, the solution should be used promptly as it oxidizes when exposed to the air for any length of time; unused portions should be discarded.

Treatment is generally on an outpatient basis. A test dose of 1.5 ml IM should be given on the first day to detect the occasional patient who may have an idiosyncratic reaction. Give 3.5 ml the second day, 5 ml the third day, and then 5 ml every second or third day into alternate buttocks until 40 ml have been given. After a rest period of 1–2 weeks the course should be repeated.

If stibophen is used for the treatment of *S japonicum* infection, an intensive (and very toxic) course is required. Inject the drug daily into alternate buttocks as follows: 2, 4, and 6 ml on days 1–3 inclusive, followed by 8 ml daily for 11 doses, the entire course taking 14 days.

A course of treatment may be repeated after 2 months if live schistosome eggs are detected on reexamination of the stool or urine or mucosal biopsy.

3. TARTAR EMETIC
(Antimony Potassium Tartrate)

Chemistry

Antimony potassium tartrate (tartar emetic) takes the form of colorless transparent crystals or a white powder that contains 36.5% of trivalent antimony. It is soluble 1:12 in water. The sodium salt may be more stable and less toxic than the potassium preparation.

Antimony potassium tartrate
(tartar emetic)

Clinical Uses

A. *Schistosoma Japonicum:* Tartar emetic is the drug of choice for treatment of *S japonicum* infection. Most & others reported 13 failures among 79 patients treated with a total of 1.8 gm and 2 failures among 50 patients treated with 2.08 gm during a course of 25–33 days. Ata & Mousa reported the use of a longer course of 12–16 injections given at weekly intervals; the drug was well tolerated and the therapeutic results were similar to those of the standard course.

B. *Schistosoma Mansoni* **and** *S Haematobium:* Although tartar emetic is effective for the treatment of *S mansoni* and *S haematobium* infections, other less toxic drugs are preferred. Most reported that a total of 1.8 gm of tartar emetic would cure more than 90% of infections with *S mansoni* and that 1.5–1.7 gm would cure more than 90% of *S haematobium* infections.

Adverse Reactions

Each injection must be given intravenously with scrupulous care since leakage of even small amounts into the perivascular tissues causes severe necrosis. Phlebitis is a frequent sequel of intravenous administration. The speed of injection should be very slow to reduce the incidence of immediate side-effects: cough, dyspnea, a sense of chest constriction, tachycardia, dizziness, vomiting, and hypotension. Paroxysms of coughing occur in most patients but usually subside within a few minutes after the injection. Hypotension responds promptly to stopping the injection and giving epinephrine subcutaneously.

Other side-effects can be anticipated in most patients during the course of treatment. Nausea, vomiting, and arthralgia are most common. Less frequent are a metallic taste, toothache, conjunctivitis, papular rash, herpes simplex or zoster, facial edema, colic, diarrhea, myalgia, weakness, dizziness, fever, and depression. ECG changes develop in most patients and may last up to 2 months after completion of the course but are not associated with evidence of permanent cardiac injury. These changes include increased amplitude of P waves, prolonged Q–T intervals, depressed S–T segments, inverted T waves, and fusion of the ST segment with the T wave. Amphojel is sometimes useful to reduce nausea.

Sudden deaths have occurred, particularly in malnourished individuals but also in some healthy patients, due to ventricular arrhythmias and circulatory collapse. Some patients develop abnormal liver function during treatment that persists for several months afterward. Jaundice, pneumonia, and peripheral neuritis are rare.

Contraindications & Cautions

The drug must be given very slowly by the intravenous route, taking great care to avoid leakage into the perivascular tissues. Patients should be under continuous observation during administration, and a syringe containing epinephrine (1:1000) should be immediately available during each injection. Muscle and joint pains and ECG changes usually occur during treatment but require no alteration of dosage. If other toxic symptoms develop, the drug may be temporarily stopped or the interval between injections lengthened. The drug should be permanently discontinued in the presence of jaundice or syncopal attacks or when diarrhea or vomiting is severe and persistent.

Tartar emetic is contraindicated in the presence of renal and cardiac disease and in hepatic disease not due to schistosomiasis.

Preparations & Dosages

Antimony potassium tartrate (tartar emetic) is available as a granular powder. A 0.5% solution that contains 1.8 mg of metallic antimony or 5 mg of tartar emetic per milliliter should be freshly prepared in 5% glucose, physiologic saline solution, or distilled water, and sterilized by filtration or by gentle boiling for 5 minutes. Boiling for more than 5 minutes and autoclaving should be avoided. The resultant solution should be crystal clear, free of sediment, and used within 2 hours.

Patients should be hospitalized and should refrain from vigorous exercise during the course of treatment. The drug is best given 2–3 hours after a light meal, and the patient should remain recumbent for several hours afterward.

The drug is administered intravenously very slowly through a fine needle over a 10-minute period. The initial dose is 8 ml of the 0.5% solution. Subsequent doses of 12, 16, 20, 24, and 28 ml are given on alternate days. Thereafter, continue 28 ml on alternate days until a total of 360 ml (1.8 gm) has been given. If a second course is required, a few months should elapse before resuming treatment.

ASPIDIUM OLEORESIN
(Extract of Male Fern)

One dose of aspidium oleoresin, formerly the major drug for the treatment of tapeworm infections, will eradicate *Taenia saginata, T solium,* and *Diphyllobothrium latum* in more than 80% of patients. However, because of its unpredictable toxicity in some patients, the drug has been superseded first by quinacrine and, more recently, by niclosamide and dichlorophen. Aspidium should not be used if these safer drugs are available; the drug is rarely available in the USA.

Aspidium oleoresin (male fern) is a dark-green liquid with an unpleasant smell and taste that is extracted from the rhizomes of *Dryopteris filix-mas.* It should be used fresh and should contain 25% (w/w) of the active ingredient filicin.

Aspidium is absorbed from the gastrointestinal tract of man and partially excreted unchanged in the urine. Mild side-effects include nausea, vomiting, diarrhea, abdominal colic, and headache. Unpredictable variations in absorption and susceptibility may occasionally produce severe toxic effects, including bloody diarrhea, jaundice, bilirubinemia, proteinuria, vertigo, tremors, severe muscle cramps, tonic convulsions, bradycardia, and death due to respiratory or cardiac failure. Optic neuritis also occurs and may be followed by yellow vision and temporary or permanent blindness.

Aspidium is contraindicated in the presence of ulcers of the gastrointestinal tract, marked anemia, and renal, hepatic, or cardiac disease. It should also be avoided in pregnancy, in elderly or debilitated patients, and for infants; it must be used with caution in older children.

Patients should be hospitalized for 2 days before treatment and should receive only bland fluids, without milk or fats. Absorption of the drug is increased by lipids. Each morning, a small saline purge is given. On the third morning, aspidium is administered to the fasting patient, the total adult dose of 4–8 gm (average 5 gm) being divided into 3 parts and given at 15-minute intervals. A satisfactory draught may be prepared by combining 8 ml of aspidium, 8 gm of acacia, 14 ml of glycerin, and 35 ml of cinnamon water. (When given to children, the dosage is 0.3 gm/year of age, not to exceed 3 gm.) A large saline purge (30 gm $MgSO_4$) should be given 30 minutes after the last dose of aspidium to remove both the paralyzed tapeworm and the unabsorbed drug. The patient should remain at bed rest for 2 hours thereafter.

An alternative procedure is to deliver the drug in divided doses via a duodenal tube. Thirty minutes later, the purge is given also via the tube, and the tube is removed. Use of the tube reduces vomiting; therefore, in treating *T solium* infection, only the duodenal tube procedure should be used since drug-induced vomiting may give rise to cysticercosis.

BEPHENIUM HYDROXYNAPHTHOATE
(Alcopara)

Bephenium hydroxynaphthoate, synthesized in 1958, is now the drug of choice for hookworm infections due to *Ancylostoma duodenale* and an alternative drug for the treatment of hookworm due to *Necator americanus.* The drug is moderately effective in ascariasis, has a low order of activity in trichuriasis, and is ineffective in strongyloidiasis.

Chemistry

The bephenium salts are quaternary ammonium compounds. Bephenium hydroxynaphthoate (benzyl-dimethyl-2-phenoxyethyl-ammonium hydroxynaphthoate) is a pale yellow crystalline substance with an aqueous solubility of 0.02–0.03%.

Bephenium base

Absorption, Metabolism, & Excretion

Bephenium hydroxynaphthoate is poorly absorbed after oral administration. In man, less than 0.5% of an oral dose of 1 gm (of base) was recovered in the urine within 24 hours.

Pharmacologic Effects

Embryopathy was observed when 250–500 mg/kg was given to pregnant rabbits. The water-soluble chloride salt, when inoculated parenterally into dogs and cats, had ganglion blocking properties and caused a brief fall in blood pressure.

Anthelmintic Actions

The mode of action of bephenium hydroxynaphthoate against susceptible parasites is not yet established, but its effects on ascarid musculature have been shown to be those of excitation followed by paralysis, associated with a loss of muscular reactivity to acetylcholine. These effects are not reversible.

Clinical Uses

Bephenium hydroxynaphthoate is a safe, well tolerated drug. It may be used in the very young and also in the presence of diarrhea or marked anemia, either of which may accompany severe hookworm disease. The drug's deficiencies are its bitter taste and a high incidence of vomiting after its use.

A. *Ancylostoma Duodenale:* Bephenium hydroxynaphthoate is the drug of choice for the treatment of hookworm infections due to *A duodenale.* Many studies indicate that a single course of treatment results in a cure rate of 76–98% and that the worm burden in the remaining patients is sharply reduced.

B. *Necator Americanus:* Hookworm infections due to *N americanus* (the species prevalent in the USA) are more resistant than those due to *A duodenale,* and therefore require treatment on 3 successive days.

C. *Ascaris Lumbricoides:* Bephenium hydroxynaphthoate is moderately effective against roundworms. The reported cure rate after one dose varies from 30–82%, which is less satisfactory than the results obtained with piperazine.

D. Mixed Ascaris and Hookworm Infections: Bephenium hydroxynaphthoate paralyzes roundworms. Therefore, it can be used to treat mixed infestations of hookworms and roundworms without the risk of stimulating ascaris migration as reported for tetrachloroethylene.

E. *Trichostrongylus Orientalis:* Single treatments have resulted in the eradication of the infection from 75–82% of patients.

Adverse Reactions

Bephenium hydroxynaphthoate has a very low toxicity at therapeutic doses. Nausea and vomiting, the only common side-effects, occur more frequently in young children. Other symptoms—dizziness, headache, cramping abdominal pain, and diarrhea—are infrequent, mild, and short-lasting.

Contraindications & Cautions

Patients with marked anemia, diarrhea, or dehydration should have the condition partially corrected before the drug is given. In the presence of severe diarrhea due to hookworm disease, it may be necessary to continue daily treatments for 4–7 days.

The drug probably should not be used in pregnancy. In hypertensive patients it should be used with caution because, if appreciably absorbed, it might produce a brief but marked fall in blood pressure.

Dosages

The drug should be given orally on an empty stomach and food then withheld for 2 hours. Since it is bitter when mixed with water, it can be made more palatable (and less vomiting occurs) when mixed in chocolate milk, orange juice, flavored syrups, or milk. No purgatives should be used.

The dosage for adults and older children is 5 gm of the granules, mixed with water or other liquid, taken twice a day; children weighing less than 22 kg take 1/2 of the adult dosage. One day of treatment results in a high cure rate for *Ancylostoma duodenale* and *Trichostrongylus orientalis* infections. The same daily dosage should be repeated for 3 days if the drug is used for *Necator americanus* infections. If the species of hookworm is not known, this 3-day course of treatment is given rather than making the cumbersome laboratory diagnosis of the species. Two weeks after the course of treatment, the stools should be reexamined; if still infected, the patient can be treated again. It is not always possible or essential to completely eradicate hookworm infection. If iron deficiency anemia accompanies severe hookworm disease, it should be treated with iron medication and a high-protein diet.

Preparations Available

Bephenium hydroxynaphthoate (Alcopara) is prepared as granules in 5 gm packets (5 gm of the granules contain 4.3 gm of bephenium hydroxynaphthoate equivalent to 2.5 gm of bephenium base).

BISCOMATE
(Jonit)

Biscomate (phenylene-diisothiocyanate [1,4]) is currently undergoing clinical investigation for the treatment of both hookworm species. It is a colorless, tasteless compound that is used without dietary preparation or purges. In 7 clinical trials of 263 persons treated with a standard dosage (100 mg given orally 3 times at 12 hour intervals), 212 persons (80%) were cured of hookworm infections due to *Ancylostoma duodenale* or *Necator americanus*. The drug also produced substantial reductions in egg counts in most of the remaining patients. Side-effects, although short-lasting and usually mild, are often reported by more than 50% of patients who take the drug. They are mainly gastrointestinal symptoms, dizziness, and headache.

BITHIONOL
(Actamer, Lorothidol, Bithin)

Bithionol is the drug of choice for treatment of *Paragonimus westermani* (lung fluke) infections and has been reported to be effective for *Fasciola hepatica* (liver fluke) and several tapeworm species. The drug is not licensed for use in the USA, but it can be obtained from the Parasitic Disease Drug Service, Center for Disease Control, Atlanta, for investigational use.

Bithionol (2,2'-thiobis[4,6-dichlorophenol]) is a tasteless white crystalline powder, poorly soluble in water. The drug reaches peak blood levels in man in 4–8 hours. At a daily dosage of 50 mg/kg in 3 divided doses for 5 days, a serum level of 50–200 µg/ml is maintained. Excretion appears to be mainly via the kidney. The mode of action of bithionol against *Paragonimus westermani* has not been established, but the drug does inhibit oxidative phosphorylation.

The recommended dosage for pulmonary and cerebral paragonimiasis and for subcutaneous paragonimiasis (*P skrjabini*) is 30–50 mg/kg by mouth on alternate days for 10–15 doses. The daily dose should be divided into a morning and evening dose. From 1961–1967, clinical reports indicated that 97% of 420 patients were cured of pulmonary paragonimiasis using a dosage schedule ranging from 10–50 mg/kg, on alternate days, for a total of 5–15 doses. The drug may be of value in acute cerebral paragonimiasis, sometimes requiring more than one course of treatment, but is less effective in chronic cerebral infections.

Side-effects are frequent but are generally mild and transient. They include nausea, vomiting, diarrhea, colic, headache, dizziness, and urticaria and other skin rashes. Diarrhea occurs in more than 65% of patients, particularly during the first few days of treatment, but may then stop with continued drug administration.

Bithionol sulfoxide (Bithin-S) is a new compound that appears to be as effective as bithionol for paragonimiasis. It can be used in smaller doses because of its greater intestinal absorption and may cause fewer and less severe side-effects.

CHLOROQUINE PHOSPHATE
(Aralen)

For general pharmacologic discussion, see Chapter 62.

Clinical Uses

A. *Clonorchis Sinensis*, Opisthorchis Species: No satisfactory treatment is available for clonorchiasis or opisthorchiasis, and the use of chloroquine for these parasites is controversial. Many other drugs have been used, including gentian violet and antimony preparations. Dithiazanine and hexachloroparaxyol have been withdrawn because of toxic effects.

The recommended course of treatment with chloroquine is 250 mg 3 times a day for 6–8 weeks. Although cure rates are low, particularly in heavy or chronic infections, treatment may provide symptomatic relief. Egg production usually decreases or stops after treatment, but patients should not be regarded as cured until at least a 6-month follow-up has been completed.

Adverse reactions at the recommended dosage are frequent, particularly in the first few weeks, and may necessitate temporary reduction in dosage or discontinuation of therapy. Side-effects include nausea, headache, pruritus, dizziness, and diarrhea. The ocular damage that may develop during long-term administration of the drug for other conditions has not been reported when chloroquine is used for 6–8 weeks.

B. *Paragonimus Westermani*: Chloroquine is an unsatisfactory alternative drug for the treatment of paragonimiasis. Bithionol is the drug of choice wherever it is available.

The dosage of chloroquine is 250 mg twice a day for 6 weeks. Pulmonary paragonimiasis is sometimes cured, but the drug has no effect on cerebral infections.

C. *Hymenolepis Nana, H Diminuta*: Chloroquine may be used as an alternative to quinacrine for the treatment of infections with these small tapeworms of man. The dosage schedule is 250 mg twice a day for 20 days.

DICHLOROPHEN
(Anthiphen)

Dichlorophen (2,2'-dihydroxy-5,5'-dichloro-diphenylmethane) is effective and safe for the treatment of several tapeworms. Reported cure rates for *Taenia saginata* infection range from 70–90% for doses greater than 5 gm. Cure rates for *T solium* infection are probably similar, but few reports are available. Biagi treated 64 patients infected with *Hymenolepis nana* with 62 mg/kg, resulting in a 70% reduction in egg counts in 80% of his patients. Waris reported 64% of 73 patients cured of *Diphyllobothrium latum* infection using 6 gm daily for 2 days.

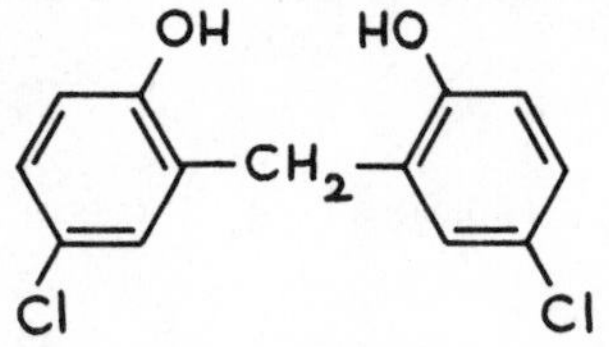

Dichlorophen

Dichlorophen has a consistent laxative effect; mild nausea, vomiting, and colic may also occur. Lassitude is rare, and jaundice has been reported.

The same cautions should be observed for the treatment of *Taenia solium* infection with dichlorophen as are described for niclosamide with respect to the theoretical risk of cysticercosis after release of ova from disintegrating tapeworm segments. Dichlorophen is contraindicated in the presence of liver disease.

Dichlorophen (Anthiphen) is prepared as 0.5 gm tablets. The dosage is 70 mg/kg taken on an empty stomach in the morning without prior dietary restrictions or purgatives. Breakfast may follow in 2 hours. Some physicians repeat the dose the following morning. No post-treatment purge is necessary even if a search for the scolex is intended, because the drug itself has a laxative action. Since the disintegrated scolex can rarely be identified, the results of treatment are not known with certainty until stools are reexamined 3–4 months later when worms, if not expelled, will have regenerated and begun to shed new segments.

Dichlorophen is not approved for use in the USA.

DICHLORVOS
(Dichlorman)

Dichlorvos (2,2'-dichlorovinyldimethyl phosphate), previously used in veterinary medicine, is in the experimental stage for use in man as a single-dose oral broad-spectrum anthelmintic.

It is an organophosphate compound supplied in a granular-resin formulation for slow release in the intestine. It regularly reduces plasma cholinesterase and in a few patients causes brief, mild headache, but no serious side-effects have been seen in as yet limited clinical trials.

Additional experience is needed to establish the safety of dichlorvos, which could become an important broad-spectrum anthelmintic and the drug of choice for trichuriasis. No other drug equals its reported cure rates for trichuriasis of 88–95% of patients treated with a single 12 mg/kg dose. At the same dose, 86–91% of hookworm infections and 78% of ascaris infections were cured.

DIETHYLCARBAMAZINE CITRATE
(Banocide, Hetrazan, Notezine)

Diethylcarbamazine was discovered in 1948 as a result of a search for new antifilarial drugs after World War II.

Chemistry

Diethylcarbamazine citrate (N,N-diethyl-4-methyl-1-piperazinecarboxamide dihydrogen citrate), a piperazine derivative, is a white crystalline powder, readily soluble in water, and has an unpleasant sweetish taste.

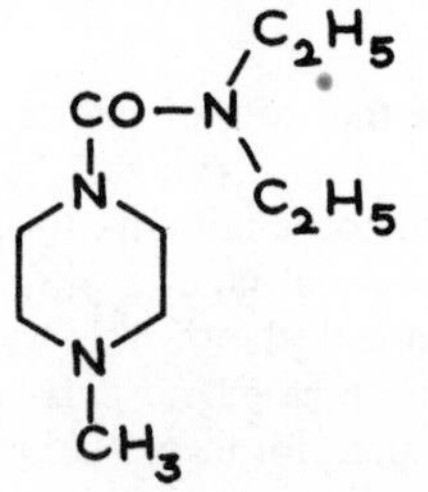

Diethylcarbamazine base

Absorption, Metabolism, & Excretion

When given orally, diethylcarbamazine is rapidly absorbed from the gastrointestinal tract. A single oral dose of 10 mg/kg of base produces a peak blood level of 4–5 μg/ml in 3 hours; the blood level then falls to zero within 48 hours. The minimum effective blood concentration appears to be 0.8–10 μg/ml.

Distribution studies indicate that the drug rapidly equilibrates with all tissues (including blood cells) except fat, but that neither microfilariae nor adult worms concentrate the drug. More than 95% of a ^{14}C-labeled preparation was excreted within 30 hours in the urine, either as unchanged drug or as a variety of degradation products. There is little tendency to accumulation when repeated doses are given.

Pharmacologic Effects

A. Actions on Laboratory Animals: Diethylcarbamazine is mildly diuretic and analgesic. When injected intravenously into dogs, it stimulates respiration and a brief rise in blood pressure occurs followed by a brief fall.

Toxicity in experimental animals is low. The acute LD_{50} after oral administration in mice was 560 mg/kg; in rats, 395 mg/kg. Chronic toxicity did not occur in cotton rats when 170 mg/kg were given intraperitoneally twice daily for more than 12 doses.

B. Anthelmintic Actions: Diethylcarbamazine is not active against microfilariae or adult filarial worms in vitro. However, when the drug is administered to patients infected with *Wuchereria bancrofti, Brugia malayi,* or *Loa loa,* microfilariae disappear rapidly from the blood. Microfilariae also disappear from the skin of patients infected with *Onchocerca volvulus* and *Dipetalonema streptocerca,* but the drug is less effective against microfilariae of *Dipetalonema perstans.* Microfilariae in hydroceles caused by *W bancrofti* infections or in nodules due to *O volvulus* are not killed by diethylcarbamazine since they are outside the general circulation.

Experiments in cotton rats infected with Litomosoides show that 80% of the microfilariae disappear from the blood in 1 minute after intravenous injection and are trapped primarily in the sinusoids of the liver, where they are destroyed by phagocytes. Hawking suggests that the surfaces of the microfilariae may be sensitized in some way so that they become susceptible to phagocytosis by the fixed macrophages of the reticuloendothelial system.

The extent to which adult worms of *W bancrofti* and *B malayi* are killed by diethylcarbamazine in man is not known. However, if therapy is adequate, microfilariae do not reappear in the majority of patients, which suggests that the adult worms are killed or at least permanently sterilized. The death of adult worms has been confirmed by experimental studies on *B malayi* infection in cats, direct observations of *Loa loa* infection in man, and biopsies of *W bancrofti* infections in man. No conclusion can be drawn, however, about the mode of action of diethylcarbamazine against adult worms.

Diethylcarbamazine is ineffective against adult *O volvulus;* microfilariae reappear after therapy is terminated.

Clinical Uses

A. *Wuchereria Bancrofti, Brugia Malayi, Loa Loa*: Diethylcarbamazine is the drug of choice for treatment of these parasites. In view of its oral effectiveness, high order of therapeutic efficacy, and relative lack of serious toxicity, diethylcarbamazine is preferable to older antifilarial drugs containing antimony or arsenic.

Microfilariae are rapidly killed by diethylcarbamazine. Adults are killed more slowly, often requiring several courses of treatment.

B. *Onchocerca Volvulus*: The use of diethylcarbamazine for onchocerciasis is controversial. Although the drug kills microfilariae in the skin, it causes severe, sometimes violent reactions. Furthermore, the reduction in microfilariae is only temporary since the drug does not kill adult worms.

The preferred treatment of onchocerciasis consists of surgical removal of accessible nodules (particularly those on the head) and the use of suramin to kill adult worms. A course of diethylcarbamazine can be given before and after suramin to destroy the microfilariae, or the latter can be left to die naturally, a process that is probably complete in several months. Diethylcarbamazine should be given, however, if microfilariae are producing symptoms in the skin or in the area around the eyes.

C. Other Parasites: Diethylcarbamazine is effective against tropical eosinophilia when given orally in a variety of dosage schedules including 4 mg/kg 3 times a day for 4 days. The drug is not effective against *Dipetalonema perstans* or *Mansonella ozzardi* infections. It has been used for ascaris infections, and cutaneous larva migrans, but other drugs are superior.

D. Mass Therapy: One important application of diethylcarbamazine therapy has been its use on a mass basis for *W bancrofti* infections to treat patients, reduce transmission, and, it is hoped, to achieve eradication in some areas. Various regimens have been used, a common one being 5–6 mg/kg orally 1 day each week or month for 6–12 doses. Often, because of side-effects, cooperation is not obtained for repeated doses.

E. Prevention of *Loa Loa*: For the prevention of *Loa loa* infections, a regimen of 200 mg twice daily for 3 consecutive days once a month may be tried.

Adverse Reactions

Diethylcarbamazine is a safe drug at therapeutic levels. Only a few mild side-effects can be attributed directly to the drug: headache, lassitude, malaise, anorexia, and nausea and vomiting. Mild to severe "allergic" reactions are frequent, however, as a result of the release of foreign protein from dying microfilariae or adult worms. These reactions are usually mild for *W bancrofti* infection, more intense for *B malayi* infection, occasionally severe for *Loa loa* infection, and often very severe for *O volvulus* infection. Reactions are also more likely in patients with high pretreatment microfilaria counts. Side-effects may start within hours after the initial dose of diethylcarbamazine, and include hyperpyrexia (up to 39° C), headache, tachycardia, nausea and vomiting, malaise, joint pains, papular rash, intense pruritus, urticaria, and inflammatory reactions of lymph nodes, scrotal contents, and lymphatics, particularly in the groin or thigh. An allergic encephalitis has occurred rarely in patients treated for loiasis. Leukocytosis and an intensification of eosinophilia are usually present.

These symptoms persist for 3–7 days. If allergic reactions are severe, the dosage should be reduced or treatment interrupted. Thereafter, treatment may be continued without new reactions occurring, except for an occasional local reaction at the site of a dying adult worm.

Diethylcarbamazine has been administered to several million persons, and no fatalities due to drug idiosyncrasy have been reported. Recently, however, Oomen reported 7 deaths from one hospital in Ethiopia among 49 very debilitated patients treated for onchocerciasis. After taking a small amount of the drug, and without allergic symptoms, the patients lapsed into coma followed by death.

Contraindications & Cautions

In patients infected with onchocerciasis, severe reactions may be provoked early in therapy and damage to the eye may result as microfilariae are killed. Particular caution should be employed if microfilariae are producing symptoms in the skin or if microfilariae or nodules are close to the eyes.

Patients with attacks of lymphangitis due to *W bancrofti* or *B malayi* infection should be treated in a quiescent period between attacks.

Patients suspected of having malaria should be treated with chloroquine before they are given diethylcarbamazine, since the latter drug may provoke a relapse in nonsymptomatic malaria infections.

There are no contraindications to the use of diethylcarbamazine.

Preparations & Dosages

Diethylcarbamazine citrate (Banocide, Hetrazan, Notezine) is available as 50 mg tablets or as a syrup containing 24 mg/ml. The citrate salt contains 51% of the active base.

A. Wuchereria Bancrofti, Brugia Malayi, Loa Loa: These infections are treated orally with 2 mg of the citrate salt per kg body weight given orally 3 times a day after meals for 21–28 days. To reduce the incidence of allergic reactions from dying microfilariae, a single dose (2 mg/kg) is administered on the first day, 2 doses on the second day, and 3 doses on the third day and thereafter. It is common practice to give antihistamines daily for the first 4–5 days of diethylcarbamazine therapy to reduce "allergic" reactions. Corticosteroids may be started and doses of diethylcarbamazine lowered temporarily if severe reactions occur.

Blood should be checked for microfilariae several days after treatment is completed; if any are still present, a course may be repeated at intervals of 3–4 weeks. However, since the initial treatment does not kill all adult worms, microfilariae may reappear in 3–12 months. Cure may require subsequent shorter courses of treatment over 1–2 years.

B. Onchocerca Volvulus: If diethylcarbamazine is used to kill microfilariae, severe reactions should be anticipated. Treatment should be started with 25 mg of diethylcarbamazine and the dosage only slowly increased until the reaction subsides. In lightly infected cases, or where suramin is contraindicated, a 3-week course of diethylcarbamazine may be given at a dosage of 2 mg/kg 3 times daily. If both drugs are used, a 1-week course of diethylcarbamazine may precede and a 2-week course follow treatment with suramin. Premedication with antihistamines may reduce symptoms.

Severe ocular allergic reactions should be treated with 0.5% hydrocortisone eye drops and corticosteroids. If ocular lesions are pronounced before therapy, it is often advantageous to give cortisone acetate, 25 mg 4 times a day, for 2 days in advance of treatment and for 4 days thereafter. Serotonin antagonists such as cyproheptadine are being tested to reduce allergic reactions.

DITHIAZANINE IODIDE
(Delvex, Telmid)

The production of dithiazanine iodide has been discontinued because of its unpredictable toxicity. It is a cyanine dye which, if absorbed, results in bluish discoloration of the scleras and skin; 8 deaths have been associated with its use.

EMETINE HYDROCHLORIDE

Emetine is an alternative drug for the treatment of *Fasciola hepatica* infection. It is administered by deep subcutaneous injection in doses of 1 mg/kg (maximum 65 mg daily) for 10 days. This treatment program is fairly effective in removing the parasite and in this dosage schedule is relatively safe. General pharmacologic information and the precautions necessary in treatment with emetine are presented in Chapter 62.

HEXYLRESORCINOL
(Crystoids)

Hexylresorcinol, introduced in 1931 for use against roundworms, later came to be used for other gastrointestinal parasites, including hookworms, pinworms, whipworms, and tapeworms.

Chemistry

Hexylresorcinol (1,3-dihydroxy-4-hexylbenzene) is a phenol derivative. It is a pale yellow crystalline substance with a pungent odor and a sharp astringent taste. It is only slightly soluble in water but freely soluble in alcohol.

Absorption, Metabolism, & Excretion

After ingestion, approximately 1/3 of hexylresorcinol is absorbed from the gastrointestinal tract and then eliminated rapidly in the urine.

Since the drug is soluble in fat and combines with protein, food should not be present in the upper gastrointestinal tract.

Clinical Uses

Although hexylresorcinol taken orally is less effective against specific parasites than several newer anthelmintics, its broad spectrum of antiparasitic activity associated with low toxicity on occasion makes it a useful alternative preparation. It can be used to treat young children and debilitated patients and can be administered on an outpatient basis.

A. *Trichuris Trichiura:* Hexylresorcinol by retention enema is the drug of choice in the treatment of trichuriasis. However, it is recommended only for patients with significant gastrointestinal symptoms (diarrhea, abdominal pain, rectal prolapse), anemia, or weight loss. No satisfactory treatment is available for asymptomatic patients, but these patients do not need to be treated.

B. *Ascaris Lumbricoides:* Two oral treatments with hexylresorcinol are effective in removing about 95% of the ascarids (roundworms). In the presence of infections with roundworms and hookworms, hexylresorcinol can be used to treat the 2 parasites simultaneously.

C. Hookworms: Hexylresorcinol removes 50–75% of hookworms (*N americanus* or *A duodenale*). The variability of its effectiveness may be due in part to the rapidity with which the pill passes through the upper gastrointestinal tract. As a result, it may fail to release the drug in those areas in which most hookworms are attached.

D. *Hymenolepis Nana:* Hexylresorcinol is an alternative drug in the treatment of dwarf tapeworm infections.

E. Others: Hexylresorcinol's vermicidal action against other parasites has been reported to be 47% for *Taenia saginata* infection and 50% for *Fasciolopsis buski* infection.

Adverse Reactions

Hexylresorcinol is nearly devoid of systemic toxicity at therapeutic levels, but topically it is corrosive to the oral mucosa and perianal skin. When given orally, mucosal ulceration may occur in the mouth unless the crystals are incorporated into hard gelatin-coated pills. Although the mucosa of the intestinal tract is protected by its mucous secretions, the drug may cause epigastric discomfort, vomiting, or diarrhea in a few individuals. Perianal skin irritation that develops when hexylresorcinol is used as a retention enema may be prevented by the application of a film of petrolatum.

Contraindications & Cautions

To protect the oral mucosa, considerable care must be taken to ensure that pills are swallowed immediately and not chewed. Children should be supervised to be certain that the pills are not retained between the teeth and cheeks or under the tongue. For uncooperative children, hexylresorcinol crystals dissolved in 20 ml of water may be delivered through a duodenal tube.

Hexylresorcinol is contraindicated in the presence of peptic ulcers, ulcerative colitis, and intestinal obstruction.

Preparations & Dosages

Hexylresorcinol is available as pills (Crystoids) for oral use or in bulk form for preparation of enemas. The pills are gelatin-coated and contain 0.2 gm of the drug.

A. Treatment of Trichuriasis (Whipworm, Trichocephaliasis): Heavy infestations with *Trichuris trichiura* may be treated with hexylresorcinol enemas. In addition, some physicians give hexylresorcinol orally.

In the evening, a warm soapsuds enema is followed by a 0.2% hexylresorcinol enema (volume, 20–30 ml/kg of body weight up to 1200 ml). The enema should be retained for 30 minutes; retention is facilitated by taping the buttocks together. If necessary, a small saline enema may be used to initiate expulsion. Two or more treatments at weekly intervals may be necessary to reduce worm loads and stop symptoms, but removal of all the parasites is not necessary and should not be attempted. *Caution:* The anal region and adjacent skin should be well coated with petrolatum to prevent irritation.

B. Treatment of Roundworms, Hookworms, and Dwarf Tapeworms: Alcohol should be avoided for 24 hours before and after treatment. Pretreatment purges are generally omitted. The day before treatment, the total diet should be reduced and the evening meal limited to soft, fat-free foods. Breakfast should be omitted on the morning of treatment and the drug administered with water. No food should be taken for 5 hours, but water is permissible. A saline purge (for adults use 30 gm magnesium sulfate) should be given 2 hours after the treatment to remove the dead worms. Repeat the treatment in 3 days and reexamine stool specimens in 1 week. If ova are still present, an additional course of treatment can be given.

Adults and children over 12 years receive 1 gm; children 8–12 years, 0.8 gm; children 6–8 years, 0.6 gm; and infants and children up to 6 years, 0.1 gm/year of age. A minimum dose of 0.4 gm is usually necessary for small children, who tolerate it well. Smaller doses are markedly less effective.

C. Treatment of Fasciolopsiasis and Taeniasis: These conditions have been treated with moderate success by delivering 1 gm of hexylresorcinol in 20 ml of water through a duodenal tube. Two hours later, the patient is given a saline purge. Pretreatment purgation is needed to facilitate elimination of *Fasciolopsis buski.*

HYCANTHONE
(Etrenol)

Hycanthone methanesulfonate (Etrenol), a recently introduced thioxanthone compound for the treatment of schistosomiasis, is the hydroxymethyl analogue and natural metabolite of lucanthone. Hycanthone given by injection·or orally is more active than its parent compound and is free of the latter's neuropsychiatric side-effects. Hycanthone's important contribution is its high degree of effectiveness in a single, intramuscular injection. If oral therapy is used, it must be continued for 3–5 days and produces more side-effects. Reported parasitologic cure rates range from 28% to more than 90% for *Schistosoma mansoni* infections, and more than 90% for *S haematobium* infections. Activity against *S japonicum* has not been demonstrated.

Early confidence in the safety of hycanthone has been shaken recently by reports of fatalities associated with its use. Most deaths were apparently characterized by hepatic failure. Minor side-effects from the drug include local induration at the injection site, nausea, vomiting (frequent), abdominal cramps, headache, myalgia, dizziness, skin rashes, and pruritus. Transient changes in liver function and ECG have been reported. Contraindications to the use of hycanthone are not well established, but the drug should not be given to children under 2 years old, patients with severe malnutrition, or when other drugs, particularly phenothiazines, are being taken. Relative contraindications are the presence of acute or chronic infectious diseases and advanced renal, cardiac, and hepatic disease.

The recommended dose is 3 mg of base per kg (±0.5 mg/kg) up to a maximum adult dose of 200 mg of base. It is given as a single injection deep into the gluteus minimus, high under the iliac crest. Peak concentration in the blood is reached in 30 minutes, and in tissues in 60 minutes. More than 60% of the drug is excreted through bile and feces, in the form of conjugated metabolites, and a small amount in the urine.

LUCANTHONE HYDROCHLORIDE
(Miracil D, Nilodin)

Lucanthone hydrochloride is a thioxanthone derivative used orally for the treatment of schistosomiasis. It is no longer marketed in the USA.

Chemistry, Absorption, Metabolism, & Excretion

Lucanthone is the hydrochloride of 1-methyl-4-β-diethylaminoethylaminothioxanthone. Absorption from the gastrointestinal tract is rapid and almost complete; little appears in the feces. Most of the ingested dose is also rapidly degraded in the tissues, with the result that less than 7% is excreted in the urine. After a single dose, maximum blood concentrations are reached within 3 hours and the drug nearly disappears from the blood in 24 hours. With repeated doses, blood concentrations tend to be highest on the second day. The drug ceases to appear in the urine approximately 3 days after the last dose.

Clinical Uses

Reported cure rates from various parts of the world range from 27–90% for *S mansoni* infection and 33–95% for *S haematobium* infection. Lucanthone is not effective against *S japonicum* infection.

Adverse Reactions

In general, side-effects from lucanthone are less frequent and milder in children than in adults, and also less frequent in Negroes than in Caucasians. Symptoms commonly begin after 2–3 days of treatment and include anorexia, vomiting, epigastric or abdominal pain, dizziness, and yellow discoloration of the skin, scleras, and urine. Less frequent are diarrhea, constipation, headache, fever, vertigo, tinnitus, tremors, prostration, insomnia, urticaria, and nonspecific T wave changes on the ECG. Convulsions, depression, confusion, and psychosis are rare. No fatalities have been reported. Symptoms are often so severe in adults that they are unwilling or unable to continue therapy. Most symptoms disappear rapidly after treatment is completed, but skin discoloration takes about 4 weeks to clear.

Side-effects may be reduced by various methods. Some reports indicate the successful use of antihistamines (cyclizine and meclizine) or belladonna alkaloids. Enteric-coated tablets and lucanthone resinates have been tested, but they reduce the effectiveness of the drug.

Contraindications & Cautions

Most authorities restrict the use of lucanthone to children under 16, since side-effects in adults are more frequent and more severe (although not dangerous). The drug should be administered cautiously to patients with impaired renal or hepatic function. It is contraindicated in severe renal or hepatic disease except for hepatic disease due to schistosomiasis.

Preparations & Dosages

Lucanthone hydrochloride (Miracil D, Nilodin) is marketed outside the USA as tablets containing 250 mg of the hydrochloride. The dosage is 5 mg/kg body weight 3 times a day after meals for 6–8 days, although a 3-day course may be sufficient for *S haematobium* infections. For critically ill patients, low doses of the drug spaced every second or third day—for 2–4 weeks for children, or 500 mg weekly for 10 weeks for adults—may be curative in some cases and reduce ova counts in others.

NICLOSAMIDE
(Yomesan)

Niclosamide, introduced in 1960, is the drug of choice for the treatment of infection with several tapeworm species. It is not yet licensed for use in the USA, but it can be obtained from the Parasitic Disease Drug Service, Center for Disease Control, Atlanta, for use on an investigational basis.

Chemistry

Niclosamide (N-[2'-chloro-4'-nitrophenyl]-5-chlorosalicylamide) is a yellowish-white tasteless powder that is virtually insoluble in water.

Niclosamide

Absorption & Metabolism

Niclosamide is apparently not absorbed from the gastrointestinal tract. The unaltered drug has not been recovered from the blood or urine, but the possibility of its conversion to degradation products remains unsettled.

Pharmacologic Effects

A. Actions on Laboratory Animals and Man: Oral administration of niclosamide is well tolerated. Single oral doses (5 gm/kg) and multiple smaller doses (0.1–2.5 gm/kg) have been given to animals for periods ranging from 11 days to a year without serious injury.

The drug is toxic by parenteral administration, however. The LD_{50} in rats by intraperitoneal injection was 0.75 gm/kg; and in mice, by intravenous injection, 0.0075 gm/kg.

B. Anthelmintic Actions: Both in vitro and in vivo, the scoleces and proximal segments of cestodes are rapidly killed on contact with niclosamide. This may be due to the drug's inhibition of oxidative phosphorylation in the mitochondria of the parasites. Associated with the death of the parasite is release of the scolex from the intestinal wall. Even if a purge is used to expel the tapeworm, the scolex may be disintegrated and difficult to identify due to the action of intestinal proteolytic enzymes.

Clinical Uses

Niclosamide has far fewer and less severe side-effects than quinacrine or aspidium oleoresin and is equally or more effective. Dichlorophen, another new taeniacide, is also highly effective but has given variable results. Its side-effects are also mild but may be more frequent than those of niclosamide.

A. *Taenia Saginata* (Beef Tapeworm): The cure rate for 781 documented cases reported in the literature is 89%. Cure rates in individual case studies range

from 58–100%. Adults received 2 gm and children smaller doses.

B. *Taenia Solium* (Pork Tapeworm): Niclosamide is probably equally effective for *T solium* infection, but few cases have been reported.

C. *Diphyllobothrium Latum* (Fish Tapeworm): Kahra & others treated 297 patients; adults received 2 gm in a single dose. When tablets were swallowed whole, cure rates were 73%; when chewed, 87%.

D. *Hymenolepis Nana* (Dwarf Tapeworm): Approximately 350 cases have been reported in the literature, with an overall cure rate of 75%. Ahkami & Hajian have recently reported 100% cure rates using only one dose which was approximately double the usual daily dose. They used 100–130 mg/kg once only for children and 70–80 mg/kg once only for adults.

E. Other Tapeworms: Results have been promising on the few patients treated for *Hymenolepis diminuta* and *Dipylidium caninum* infections. Niclosamide is not effective against tapeworm species in man that are parasites of extra-intestinal tissues (cysticercosis or hydatid disease).

Adverse Reactions

The drug rarely produces side-effects. Nausea, vomiting, and intestinal colic have been reported infrequently.

Contraindications & Cautions

Niclosamide does not kill ova that may be released from disintegrating tapeworm segments. Therefore, cysticercosis is theoretically possible after treatment of *Taenia solium* infections, for larvae may be released from the ova, penetrate the intestinal wall, and reach the tissues. Some investigators feel that niclosamide should not be used in this infection, but the hazard may be overemphasized since no cases of cysticercosis have been reported after its use. If the drug is used for *T solium* infection, an effective purge should be given within 1–2 hours after treatment in an attempt to eliminate all mature segments before ova can be released. Niclosamide should be used cautiously in children under 2 years since experience with the drug in this age group is very limited.

There are no contraindications to the use of niclosamide.

Preparations and Dosages

Niclosamide (Yomesan) is prepared as chewable tablets, each containing 0.5 gm of the drug. Tablets are flavored with saccharin and vanillin.

Treatment is on an outpatient basis. Breakfast should be omitted, but the patient may eat 2 hours after taking the medication.

A. *T Saginata* and *D Latum*: The adult dosage is 4 tablets (2 gm). Children weighing more than 75 lb are given 3 tablets; children 25–75 lb, 2 tablets. The tablets **must** be chewed thoroughly and swallowed with water. For small children, the tablets should be pulverized and then mixed with water. Pre- and post-treatment purges are not necessary; the worm is passed by normal peristalsis. Unless the intact worm is eliminated shortly after treatment, segments or ova may continue to be passed for about a week; if present thereafter, treatment has failed and should be repeated.

A purge may be given 2 hours after treatment in an attempt to recover and identify the scolex before it disintegrates, thus indicating that the entire worm has passed and will not regenerate. If the scolex is not found, cure can be presumed only if regenerated segments have not reappeared 3–4 months after treatment.

B. *H Nana:* Hymenolepiasis requires extended treatment because infection is multiple, some parasites are in the larval stage in the intestinal wall, and children may auto-infect themselves. For adults, give 2 gm daily for 7 days. Children weighing more than 75 lb are given 3 tablets the first day and 2 tablets for the next 6 days; children 25–75 lb are given 2 tablets the first day and 1 tablet for the next 6 days. Purgatives should not be given. Stools should be rechecked for ova in 2 weeks since surviving scolices regenerate rapidly.

NIRIDAZOLE
(Ambilhar)

Niridazole, introduced in 1964, is a useful oral drug for the treatment of schistosomiasis and dracontiasis. It is not licensed for use in the USA but may be obtained from the Parasitic Disease Drug Service, Center for Disease Control, Atlanta, for use on an investigational basis.

Chemistry
Niridazole is 1-(5-nitro-2-thiazolyl)-2-imidazolidinone, a nitrothiazole derivative. It is a yellow, tasteless, crystalline powder, stable to heat and light and nearly insoluble in water.

Niridazole

Absorption, Metabolism, & Excretion
The drug is absorbed over several hours following oral administration. The concentration of the unmetabolized compound (the active agent) is 5 times higher in the portal blood than in the peripheral circulation, since most of the drug is rapidly metabolized in the liver. Metabolites are then largely eliminated in the urine and feces. In patients with hepatic dysfunction,

limited evidence indicates that metabolic degradation of niridazole is impaired. In the presence of portalsystemic shunts, higher concentrations of the unmetabolized drug are found in the peripheral circulation. Threshold doses of the unmetabolized drug are probably responsible for many side-effects.

Pharmacologic Effects
A. Actions in Experimental Animals and Man: The drug produces temporary inhibition of spermatogenesis in experimental animals, but inhibition is reversible with no subsequent interference in fertility and no post-treatment teratogenic effect. In animals, signs of damage to the hematopoietic system have been noted following niridazole therapy for several weeks, but similar effects have not been described in man. Niridazole has been shown to have a glycogen-lowering effect in monkey muscle; such glycogen depletion may be responsible for some of the side-effects in man.

B. Anthelmintic Actions: In experimental animals infected with *S mansoni*, adequate oral doses of niridazole cause a "liver shift" of adult worms that is followed by their death. Niridazole is rapidly concentrated in adult worms resulting in the inhibition of phosphorylase inactivation, and followed by glycogen depletion of the parasite.

Clinical Uses
A. *Schistosoma Haematobium*, *S Mansoni*, and *S Japonicum:* In the treatment of *S haematobium* infections, cure rates of 90–100% in both adults and children have been reported by various investigators in more than 3500 patient trials. Those not cured showed a marked reduction in egg output (about 90%). The drug was generally well tolerated, particularly by children.

Parasitologic cure rates for *S mansoni* are not consistently high. Among 2100 patients studied, cure rates ranged from 70–100% for adults but only 30–70% for children. Ova reduction in patients not cured exceeded 80%. Opinions vary on whether increased dosages in young children result in higher cure rates. Although niridazole was well tolerated by children with *S mansoni* infections, adults—particularly those with liver dysfunction—often had significant symptoms.

S japonicum infections appear to be least responsive to niridazole; of the few studies reported, cure rates ranged from 0–70%, but with high reduction in egg output in those not cured.

B. *Dracunculus Medinensis:* Niridazole provides effective treatment for dracontiasis (guinea worm). Reduction of swelling and rapid relief of pain follow treatment, and the worms can then be pulled out relatively easily.

C. *Entamoeba Histolytica:* Niridazole and metronidazole (Flagyl) given orally are the first drugs that are effective against both intestinal and extraintestinal amebiasis. Metronidazole is the superior drug because of its freedom from significant side-effects. If niridazole is used for amebiasis, the recommended dosage is 25 mg/kg (maximum 1.5 gm) for 7–10 days in divided daily doses.

Adverse Reactions

Minor side-effects occur in more than 70% of patients but may diminish in intensity as therapy is continued. These include asthenia, anorexia, nausea, vomiting, diarrhea, abdominal discomfort or cramps, headache, dizziness, myalgia, arthralgia, sweating, and palpitations. Although these symptoms are not dangerous and are not an indication for stopping the drug, they often cause patients to discontinue the full course. Analgesics and antispasmodics may alleviate some symptoms. Antihistamines may be useful in controlling infrequent allergic manifestations (skin rashes, pruritus) caused by release of foreign proteins from disintegrating worms. In general, children tolerate niridazole better than adults. The urine may become yellow-brown with an unpleasant musty odor. Epistaxis and gastrointestinal hemorrhage have been reported during niridazole therapy, but the drug has not been incriminated as a cause of bleeding tendencies. However, niridazole can provoke hemolysis in persons with red cells deficient in glucose-6-phosphate dehydrogenase.

The following toxic manifestations are mild, reversible, and not a cause for stopping therapy. Tachycardia and minor ECG changes (flattening or inversion of T waves and ST depression) may occur in more than 50% of patients. Niridazole inhibits spermatogenesis in some males but has no effect on potency. Concern has been expressed about possible teratogenic effects, but none have been reported.

Neuropsychiatric symptoms have been reported in 1–2% of patients infected with *S haematobium* and in up to 5% of patients infected with *S mansoni* who are free of hepatic dysfunction, but in up to 21% of patients with either advanced liver disease (including that due to schistosomiasis) or vascular shunts that bypass the liver. Mild symptoms include paresthesias, insomnia, and anxiety.

If the following occur, the drug should be discontinued: marked mood changes (excitability, anxiety, depression), slurred speech, psychosis, and convulsions. The administration of phenobarbital or diazepam throughout niridazole therapy appears to improve tolerance of the drug and in particular to diminish the CNS reactions.

Contraindications & Cautions

Normally, niridazole may be used on an outpatient basis. There are no absolute contraindications to its use. However, it should be used with considerable caution and under closely supervised hospital conditions for the elderly and very young and for patients who have advanced liver disease from any cause, portacaval shunts, coronary artery disease, or a history of psychiatric disorders, epilepsy, or gastrointestinal hemorrhage or ulcer. If such patients are given smaller doses for a longer period (12 mg/kg daily in divided doses for 15 days), side-effects may be less severe but therapeutic results are equal to those for the standard dose. Patients with marked anemia, malnutrition, or concomitant infections or parasitoses should

have these conditions corrected before niridazole therapy is begun.

Preparations & Dosages

Niridazole (Ambilhar) is prepared in 100 and 500 mg tablets. The dosage for schistosomiasis and dracontiasis is 25 mg/kg (maximum, 1.5 gm) daily for 7 days divided into 2–3 fractions and given with meals. Adult patients should receive phenobarbital, 100–150 mg daily in divided doses, to reduce the incidence of CNS side-effects. For *S japonicum* infections it is currently recommended that the course of treatment be stopped after 5 days.

PIPERAZINE

Piperazine salts were introduced as anthelmintics in 1949 by Fayard. Piperazine citrate and other piperazine salts have since been used extensively and are drugs of choice in the treatment of roundworms and pinworms. Piperazine is not useful for the treatment of hookworm infection, trichuriasis, or strongyloidiasis.

Chemistry

Piperazine (diethylenediamine) is available as a hexahydrate (which contains about 44% of the base) and as a variety of neutral salts: citrate, phosphate, adipate, tartrate, and others. The salts are stable white crystals, freely soluble in water.

Piperazine citrate

Absorption, Metabolism, & Excretion

A portion of the absorbed salt is metabolized in the body. The remainder is excreted in the urine, but the rate of excretion varies widely for different persons.

Anthelmintic Actions

In vivo studies indicate that piperazine causes a paralysis of *Ascaris lumbricoides* muscle and a decrease in the production of succinic acid by the worms. The paralytic action occurs because the drug blocks the stimulating effects of acetylcholine at the myoneural junction of ascaris. Piperazine has a similar myoneural blocking action on mammalian skeletal muscle, but of a low order. When the drug is used in man, the paralyzed roundworms are unable to maintain their position in the host and are expelled by normal peristalsis. Since the worms are alive when passed, disintegration products do not accumulate in the intestines.

Piperazine's mode of action against *Enterobius vermicularis* infection has not been established.

Clinical Uses

Several properties of the piperazine salts combine to make these drugs nearly ideal for the treatment of *Ascaris lumbricoides* and *Enterobius vermicularis* infections: palatability, a high order of effectiveness, low cost, an almost complete lack of toxicity at therapeutic levels, and the lack of need for pre- or post-treatment purges.

A. *Ascaris Lumbricoides:* Piperazine is the drug of choice for roundworm infections. When patients are treated once daily for 2 days, cure rates are over 90%. Longer courses are needed for equivalent cure rates in patients with heavy infections. Piperazine syrup, administered via an intestinal drainage tube, has also been successfully used for the nonsurgical management of intestinal obstruction due to heavy ascaris infection.

B. Enterobius (Oxyuris) Vermicularis: Piperazine is a drug of choice for pinworm infections; cure rates of 95% or higher usually require daily treatment for 7 days.

Adverse Reactions

There is a wide range between therapeutic and toxic doses of piperazine. Mild drug reactions occur occasionally, including nausea, vomiting, mild diarrhea, abdominal pain, and headache. Rarely reported are transitory vertigo, incoordination, difficulty in focusing, muscular weakness, erythema multiforme, urticaria, and lethargy. Patients with a predisposition to grand mal or petit mal may have an exacerbation of seizures.

Contraindications & Cautions

Piperazine compounds should be administered with caution in the presence of renal disease, since the drugs may be cumulative when impaired renal excretion is present. There are no contraindications to the use of piperazine, but alternative drugs are best used for patients with a history of epilepsy. Piperazine may be used during the last trimester of pregnancy.

Preparations & Dosages

The therapeutic effectiveness of the various piperazine salts is about the same; in solution, all form piperazine hexahydrate. Among the many preparations available as tablets, wafers, or syrups are piperazine citrate (Antepar, Anthecole, Multifuge, Vermago, Vermidol, Pipizan), piperazine phosphate (Antepar wafers, Pripsen), piperazine calcium edetate (Perin), piperazine tartrate (Piperat, Veroxil), piperazine adipate (Entacyl, Oxurasin, Oxyzin), and piperazine hexahydrate (Arpezine, Dispermin).

Piperazine citrate (Antepar) is prepared as a syrup which contains 110 mg/ml (the equivalent of 100 mg of piperazine hexahydrate), or as tablets which contain 550 mg (the equivalent of 500 mg of piperazine hexahydrate).

A. Treatment of Ascariasis: Many dosages and treatment schedules for piperazine have been tested and found effective. An accepted dosage for piperazine (as the hexahydrate) is 75 mg/kg body weight up to a maximum dose of 3.5 gm. The usual procedure is to repeat this dosage for 2 days in succession, giving the drug orally before or after breakfast. For heavy infestations, treatment should be continued for 4 days in succession. No pre- or post-treatment cathartics are used. In most cases, cure is obtained, but stools should be reexamined at 2-week intervals and treatment repeated until ova are no longer found.

In circumstances where mass treatment of ascaris is desirable and repeated therapy is impracticable, one dose of 150 mg/kg, up to a maximum dose of 6 gm, has been used.

B. Treatment of Enterobiasis: The daily oral dose of piperazine (as the hexahydrate) is 65 mg/kg up to a maximum dose of 2 gm. This dosage should be repeated for 7 days, given before or after breakfast. Cathartics are not used. Although eradication is usually possible with one course of treatment, a second course may be instituted after 1 week if reexamination shows continued egg production. To prevent reinfection of the patient, all members of the household may need treatment concurrently, since for each overt case there are usually several inapparent cases. Nevertheless, recurrences are frequent in children, because of continued exposure outside the home.

PYRVINIUM PAMOATE
(Povan)

Several pyrvinium compounds are effective for the treatment of pinworm. Pyrvinium chloride (Vanquin) was used initially but has since been replaced by pyrvinium pamoate (Povan), which causes fewer side-effects.

Chemistry

Pyrvinium pamoate (pyrvinium embonate), a cyanine dye, is the bis-6-dimethylamino-2(2-[2,5-dimethyl-1-phenyl-3-pyrrolyl] vinyl)-1-methylquinolinium salt of pamoic acid (4,4'-methylene-bis-[3-hydroxy-2-naphthoic acid]). It is a crystalline powder ranging in color from bright orange to almost black. It is stable to heat, light, and air, almost insoluble in water, and tasteless.

Absorption, Metabolism, & Excretion

Pyrvinium pamoate is not appreciably absorbed from the gastrointestinal tract when taken orally.

Anthelmintic Actions

As a group, the cyanine dyes contain the amidinium ion system which may be responsible for their anthelmintic activity. Pyrvinium pamoate is highly effective against *Enterobius vermicularis* infection; it appears to exert its effect by preventing the parasite from using exogenous carbohydrates. The parasite dies when its endogenous reserves are depleted. Although the drug may be useful for the treatment of *Strongyloides stercoralis* infection, it has only a low order of anthelmintic action against *Trichuris trichiura* and hookworm infections, and is not effective against *Ascaris lumbricoides* infection.

There are no contraindications to the use of pyrvinium pamoate. However, it is preferable not to use the drug in the presence of inflammatory conditions of the gastrointestinal tract which theoretically might facilitate absorption, resulting in untoward reactions. Povan tablets should not be used (the syrup may be used) for individuals sensitive to aspirin because of the cross-sensitivity between tartrazine contained in the tablet coating and aspirin.

Dosage

For the treatment of pinworms, a single dose is administered orally before or after meals. The dosage is 5 mg of pyrvinium base per kg body weight up to a

Pyrvinium base

Clinical Uses

A. *Enterobius Vermicularis* (Pinworm): Pyrvinium pamoate is a drug of choice for pinworm infections. It is effective after a single treatment as compared to the 7-day course required for piperazine, although side-effects occur more frequently from pyrvinium. Reported cure rates after a single dose of 5 mg/kg of pyrvinium range from 90–100%. Smaller doses (2 mg/kg) have been reported to be equally effective and may result in fewer side-effects.

B. *Strongyloides Stercoralis* (Dwarf Threadworm): There are few reports on the use of pyrvinium pamoate in the treatment of strongyloidiasis. Wang & Galli reported clearing larvae from the stools of 11 of 12 patients using 2–6.4 mg/kg of pyrvinium pamoate suspension for 7 days. The safety and effectiveness of this extended treatment has yet to be confirmed.

Adverse Reactions

Pyrvinium pamoate is well tolerated, but it may cause nausea, vomiting, diarrhea, or dizziness in some persons, particularly young children. Emesis occurs more often with the suspension than the tablet formulation. One case of an allergic reaction and one of possible photosensitization have been reported. Parents and patients should be told that post-treatment stools are often stained red for several days.

Contraindications & Cautions

Tablets should be swallowed intact to avoid staining the teeth. The drug should be used cautiously in children weighing less than 22 lb, for experience is limited on its use in young children.

maximum of 250 mg. No pre- or post-treatment purges are used. To increase the cure rate, treatment may be repeated once in 2 weeks. When one member of a household is treated for pinworms, it may be necessary for all other members to be treated concurrently to eradicate infections in asymptomatic carriers, who may otherwise perpetuate the infection in the family. In spite of these measures, however, reinfection from the outside occurs frequently.

Preparations Available

Pyrvinium pamoate (Povan) is available in tablets containing 50 mg of pyrvinium base and as a pediatric suspension (Povan Suspension) containing 10 mg of base per ml.

QUINACRINE HYDROCHLORIDE
(Mepacrine, Atabrine)

Quinacrine is one of the drugs of choice for the treatment of tapeworm infections. During World War II it was extensively used for the chemosuppression and treatment of malaria, for which it has since been replaced by less toxic antimalarial drugs.

The use of quinacrine in the treatment of metastatic cancer is discussed in Chapter 45. The chemistry, absorption, metabolism, excretion, and pharmacologic effects are discussed in Chapter 62.

Anthelmintic Actions

The mode of action of quinacrine against tapeworms is unknown. It does not kill the worm, but instead causes the scolex to temporarily detach from the intestinal wall; the worm is then expelled by means of a purge.

Clinical Uses

A. *Taenia Saginata, T Solium, Diphyllobothrium Latum:* When quinacrine is used for *Taenia saginata* (beef tapeworm) infections, reported cure rates after a single treatment range from 40–96%. Niclosamide is a superior drug for *T saginata* and *D latum* infections because of its freedom from side-effects, but at present quinacrine is still recommended for *T solium* infection (see Niclosamide).

B. *Hymenolepis Nana, H Diminuta, Dipylidium Caninum:* Quinacrine is an alternative drug for the treatment of these tapeworms.

Adverse Reactions

Quinacrine commonly causes nausea and vomiting in the high dosage used for tapeworm therapy (8 times the daily dose used for malaria suppression). An antiemetic taken before treatment and sodium bicarbonate taken concurrently reduce this tendency. However, in the occasional patient unable to retain the drug orally, it should be administered by duodenal tube. Additional side-effects include dizziness, mild diarrhea, colic, headache, urticaria, and CNS stimulation. The latter may be manifested by restlessness, confusion, anxiety, euphoria, aggressive behavior, or psychotic reactions. Chronic toxicity may rarely cause aplastic anemia, hepatitis, contact dermatitis, convulsions, and psychotic reactions. The incidence of psychotic reactions among patients receiving quinacrine daily for malaria prophylaxis was 1.4 cases/1000 patients treated.

Contraindications & Cautions

When quinacrine is used to treat *Taenia solium* infections, it should be administered by duodenal tube to prevent vomiting. The vomiting that frequently follows oral administration of the drug is potentially dangerous in the presence of *T solium* since it may result in segments being regurgitated into the stomach, followed by release of ova from the segments. Larvae may then be freed from the ova and penetrate the gut wall, resulting in cysticercosis.

Quinacrine should also be used with caution in the elderly, in young children, and in patients with a history of psychosis.

Psoriasis, exfoliative dermatitis, and concurrent treatment with primaquine are contraindications to the use of quinacrine.

Preparations & Dosages

Quinacrine (mepacrine, Atabrine) is supplied as tablets containing 100 mg of the dihydrochloride.

A. *Taenia Saginata, T Solium, Diphyllobothrium Latum:* Patients may be treated at home, but pretreatment preparation of the bowel, observation of the patient for untoward drug reactions, and collection of stool specimens is facilitated by hospitalization. Preparation of the bowel is important and involves freeing the intestines of food, which would keep the drug from coming in contact with the head of the worm (scolex), the small but vital portion of the tapeworm. Patients should receive a nonresidue fluid diet for at least 24 hours before treatment; some authorities urge 48 hours. A saline purge such as magnesium sulfate (15–30 gm) is given each morning for 1–2 days preceding treatment.

On the morning of treatment, the patient remains fasting except for water. An enema is administered, and the patient then takes 10 mg of prochlorperazine to reduce vomiting (substitute a barbiturate for children). When the latter has taken effect, 4 doses of quinacrine, 200 mg each, are given 10 minutes apart for a total of 0.8 gm (adult dose). Each dose should be swallowed with about 75 ml of water containing 600 mg of sodium bicarbonate. Two hours after the last dose of quinacrine, the patient should receive sufficient magnesium sulfate (30 gm) to produce a copious evacuation to remove the worm and the unabsorbed drug. If there are no results in 3–4 hours, the enema should be repeated. Additional laxative may also be required. Food may be given after the purge has become effective.

Use of a duodenal tube, although uncomfortable for the patient, precludes vomiting and may provide a higher cure rate than oral treatment for the large tapeworms. A duodenal tube is required for the treatment of *T solium* infection and should be used for other tapeworms if the patient is unable to retain the drug orally. Duodenal intubation is accomplished by having the patient lie on his right side after swallowing 65 cm of a Rehfuss tube. Two to 3 hours later, when aspirated material is alkaline, the correct positioning of the tube in the duodenum should be ascertained by fluoroscopy. The full dose of quinacrine (0.8 gm) is then dissolved in 100 ml of warm water, delivered all at once via the tube, and then washed through with additional water. The purgative is given 30 minutes later via the tube and the tube is removed. Usually in taenia infections, only one worm is present, and it is passed within 4–10 hours, alive and stained yellow, in one piece or fragmented. The entire stool specimen should be collected for 48 hours and passed through a sieve or cheese cloth to find the scolex. Search is facilitated by ultraviolet light, since quinacrine absorbed by the worm causes it to fluoresce under ultraviolet radiation. Toilet paper should not be placed in the bedpan, as it makes the search more difficult.

If the scolex is found, and only one worm is present, the patient is cured. If long segments are passed but the scolex is not found, a cure can be presumed only if segments do not reappear in the stool 3 or 4 months later. Treatment may be repeated in 2–3 weeks.

B. *Hymenolepis Nana, H Diminuta, Dipylidium Caninum:* The initial dose on the first day is given as for taeniasis, including pre- and post-treatment purges. Thereafter, 100 mg (adult dose) are given 3 times daily on days 2, 3, and 4 without purges. A repeat course of treatment is often necessary in 2 weeks.

C. Pediatric Dosage: Children should be given reduced doses of quinacrine and sodium bicarbonate calculated according to weight.

SURAMIN
(Belganyl, Germanin, Naphuride)

Suramin is the drug of choice for treatment of the adult parasites of *Onchocerca volvulus* and *O caecutiens* infections and is one of the drugs used to treat African trypanosomiasis. It is not licensed for use in the USA, but can be obtained from the Parasitic Disease Service, Center for Disease Control, Atlanta, for use on an investigational basis.

Anthelmintic Actions

Suramin acts principally on adult female worms, causing them to die and degenerate by the fifth week of treatment; male worms live much longer. Some microfilariae (but not all) are also killed. The mode of action of the drug against the parasites is not known.

Chemistry, Absorption, Metabolism, & Excretion

Suramin, a complex derivative of urea, is a white, finely crystalline powder freely soluble in water.

Because it is poorly absorbed from the gastrointestinal tract and causes local irritation when given subcutaneously or intramuscularly, it should be given intravenously. Suramin persists in the plasma firmly bound to plasma protein and apparently enters cells and CSF only in small amounts. The plasma concentration, which falls during the first few hours to become constant for a period of days, is followed by a period of low concentrations for up to 3 months. Repeated doses are cumulative since metabolic changes are minimal and excretion is slow and only via the kidneys.

Clinical Uses

Suramin and Mel W (melarsonyl potassium) are the only effective drugs against adult onchocerca worms. Because of the unpredictable occurrence of fatal arsenical encephalopathy in a few patients receiving Mel W, suramin remains the preferred drug. An effective therapeutic program for individual patients consists of nodulectomy for accessible onchocerca nodules (particularly those on the head) plus drug therapy in the form of suramin against adult worms and diethylcarbamazine to kill the microfilariae. A 1-week course of diethylcarbamazine may precede and a 2-week course follow the suramin treatment. Some physicians prefer to treat with suramin alone in heavy infections to avoid severe reactions that may follow the deaths of microfilariae during treatment with diethylcarbamazine. In lightly infected cases, or where suramin is contraindicated, a 3-week course of diethylcarbamazine may be given.

Adverse Reactions

Side-effects of suramin are attributable both to the drug and to the death of adult worms or microfilariae. Immediate reactions may include nausea, vomiting, and, rarely, circulatory collapse and loss of consciousness. A few hours after the injection, a new set of reactions may occur: low-grade fever, headache, joint pains, abdominal cramps, myalgia, ocular symptoms (photophobia, lacrimation, burning, itching, iritis), edema of the face or limbs, papular eruptions, and cutaneous hyperesthesia of the soles and palms that may be accompanied by fissuring and peeling. Still later, protein, casts, and occult blood may appear in the urine. Late in the course of treatment, pruritus and other symptoms similar to those described for diethylcarbamazine therapy may occur as parasites die or degenerate and foreign proteins are released. Rare and sometimes fatal reactions have been recorded in patients who develop prolonged high fever, severe prostration, arthritis, exfoliative dermatitis, ulceration of the buccal mucosa, or severe diarrhea. When very large doses of suramin have been used for the treatment of pemphigus, fatalities associated with degeneration of the adrenal cortex have been reported, but similar pathologic findings have not been described in patients treated for onchocerciasis.

Reported differences in the frequency and severity of reactions may represent differences in brands of suramin, effects of drug storage, nutritional status of the host, or other factors. Most reactions are not severe but are so annoying that many patients refuse to complete a course of treatment. Antihistamines may partially relieve allergic reactions due to dying parasites.

Contraindications & Cautions

Patients receiving suramin must be closely watched, preferably in the hospital. The drug is contraindicated in the presence of renal insufficiency. Therapy should be discontinued in patients showing marked intolerance to the initial test dose.

Urine should be examined for protein, red cells, and casts twice a week during the course of treatment. Slight proteinuria is not an indication to stop therapy, as it clears several weeks after excretion of the drug and there is no residual damage to the kidneys. However, the presence of considerable protein or formed elements in the urine calls for skipping a dose or ceasing therapy. Other indications for discontinuation of treatment are prolonged high fever, severe prostration, arthritis, exfoliative dermatitis, ulceration of the buccal mucosa, and severe diarrhea.

Preparations & Dosages

Suramin (Antrypol, Belganyl, Germanin, Naphuride) is marketed in ampules containing 0.5 gm dry powder that must be kept dry, cool, and sealed in dark bottles during storage. A 10% solution should be prepared for injection in cold, pyrogen-free distilled water or saline and must be used within 30 minutes.

Injections must be given slowly intravenously. An initial dose of 0.1 gm is given intravenously to test for idiosyncrasy. The subsequent course is 1 gm to be given intravenously each week for 5–6 weeks.

TETRACHLOROETHYLENE

Tetrachloroethylene, introduced in 1925, replaced the more toxic carbon tetrachloride for the treatment of hookworm infections due to *Necator americanus* or *Ancylostoma duodenale*. Tetrachloroethylene is the most effective drug available for the treatment of *N americanus* infection, but bephenium hydroxynaphthoate is the drug of choice for the treatment of infection with *A duodenale*.

Chemistry

Tetrachloroethylene (perchloroethylene; $Cl_2C=CCl_2$) is an unsaturated halogenated hydrocarbon. It is a clear, colorless, volatile liquid with a characteristic ethereal odor, and is slowly decomposed by light and by various metals in the presence of moisture. To guarantee its therapeutic potency, it should be stored in a cool dark place; broken capsules should not be used.

Although the drug is nearly insoluble in water, its solubility is increased by the presence of alcohol or lipids in the gastrointestinal tract.

Tetrachloroethylene

Absorption, Metabolism, & Excretion

Absorption of tetrachloroethylene is minimal in a normal gastrointestinal tract if the drug is taken in the absence of lipids or alcohol. The small amount absorbed is excreted in the expired air.

Anthelmintic Actions

Tetrachloroethylene is more effective against *Necator americanus* than against *Ancylostoma duodenale*. Its mode of action has not been clearly established; it may depress muscle cells or neighboring nerve structures. Paralysis results, causing the hookworms to release their attachment to the intestinal mucosa.

Tetrachloroethylene does not paralyze or kill *Ascaris lumbricoides*. Instead it is thought that the drug stimulates these worms, causing their migration and rarely leading to fatal obstruction or perforation of the gut.

Clinical Uses

A. *Necator Americanus:* Up to 80% of patients infected with this hookworm species will be cured after one treatment with tetrachloroethylene; the worm load in the remaining patients is generally reduced. Tetrachloroethylene is particularly useful in the mass treatment of *N americanus* infection since it is effective, relatively nontoxic, and inexpensive.

B. *Ancylostoma Duodenale:* The drug of choice for the treatment of hookworm infection due to *A duodenale* is bephenium hydroxynaphthoate. The reported cure rates after a single treatment with bephenium are 76–98%, compared to a 25–65% cure rate after one treatment with tetrachloroethylene. Several additional treatments with tetrachloroethylene are usually required if it is used to eradicate this parasite.

C. Intestinal Flukes: Tetrachloroethylene is often effective in the eradication of the small intestinal flukes, *Heterophyes heterophyes* and *Metagonimus yokogawai,* the large intestinal fluke, *Fasciolopsis buski,* Echinostoma species, and *Gastrodiscoides hominis.* The drug is used in the same dosages and in the same manner as for hookworm infections.

Adverse Reactions

Tetrachloroethylene has had extensive use without serious side-effects. Not infrequent, however, are mild gastrointestinal symptoms: nausea, vomiting, epigastric burning, and abdominal cramps; and CNS symptoms: dizziness, vertigo, headache, and drowsiness. Transient loss of consciousness has been reported, and hypotensive episodes have occurred in severely anemic patients. Therefore, when feasible, the patient should be kept at bed rest and under observation for 4 hours after administration of the drug.

Contraindications & Cautions

Tetrachloroethylene may be contraindicated in the presence of ascaris infections. Therefore, in mixed infections with both roundworms and hookworms, the roundworms should be eliminated first by the use of piperazine or by the use of hexylresorcinol or bephenium hydroxynaphthoate. The latter drugs affect both parasites. When roundworm eggs are no longer found in the stool, tetrachloroethylene can be used to eradicate the remaining hookworms.

The drug is contraindicated in the treatment of small, severely ill children. It should be avoided in pregnancy, hepatic diseases, gastroenteritis, alcoholism, severe constipation, and patients undergoing heavy metal therapy.

Patients with severe anemia should have this condition partially corrected before administration of the drug.

Preparations & Dosages

Tetrachloroethylene USP, while approved for human use, is available in the USA only as a veterinary preparation; however, this preparation is safe and effective for use in man. It is available in a liquid form or in soft gelatin capsules containing 0.2, 1, and 5 ml.

The gelatin capsules prevent irritation of the oral mucous membranes.

The patient should be told to avoid alcohol and fatty foods for 24 hours before and 3 days after medication. Food, but not water, is withheld the morning the drug is administered. The dosage is 0.12 ml/kg up to a maximum of 5 ml, and is taken orally in capsule form. The patient should be kept at bed rest for 4 hours following treatment, and then food may be started. Purgation following treatment is no longer advised for it may increase side-effects and decrease the effectiveness of the drug. An alternative time to give the drug is at bedtime, but 6 hours after the last meal. Stool specimens should be examined at the end of 1 week. Two or more treatments at intervals of 4–7 days may be required to clear the infection or reduce the worm burden to levels at which the remaining parasites cause no significant blood loss. If iron deficiency anemia is present, it should be treated with ferrous sulfate and a high-protein diet.

Occasionally the gelatin capsules containing tetrachloroethylene may not rupture in the upper intestines, the area in which most of the worms are attached. If suspected, the liquid form of the drug may be used by emulsifying an appropriate dosage in mucilage, flavoring it with peppermint, and bringing the final volume to 2 oz with water.

TETRAMISOLE

Tetramisole, introduced in 1966 in veterinary medicine, is undergoing clinical trials in man. The drug eradicates ascarids from most patients with a single treatment and therefore may be particularly useful for mass treatment programs. However, before tetramisole can challenge piperazine as the drug of choice for ascariasis, additional comparative studies are needed to assess further the safety of tetramisole and to compare the effectiveness and freedom from side-effects of the 2 drugs. Some investigators report fewer side-effects from tetramisole. The drug is only moderately effective in hookworm infections and has a low order of activity in trichuriasis and pinworm infections.

Tetramisole (Decaris), the racemic mixture, is 2,3,5,6-tetra-hydro-6-phenylimidazo-(2,1-b) thiazole hydrochloride, a synthetic, white, water-soluble compound. Since its anthelmintic activity is apparently limited to the levorotatory isomer levamisole (Ketrax), use of levamisole rather than tetramisole permits a reduction in dosage and hence in side-effects.

Most studies reported cure rates of 90–100% plus a substantial reduction in ova passed by patients not cured when one dose of levamisole (2.5–5 mg/kg) was used to treat ascariasis. Some studies reported lower cure rates, however, particularly in the presence of heavy infections.

The action of the drug on *Ascaris lumbricoides* is first to paralyze and then to kill the worm, possibly by inhibiting the enzyme succinic dehydrogenase.

In man, mild and infrequent side-effects reported for tetramisole and levamisole include nausea, abdominal pain, dizziness, headache, and malaise.

THIABENDAZOLE
(Mintezol)

Thiabendazole has a broad spectrum of anthelmintic action. It is the drug of choice for the treatment of strongyloidiasis and cutaneous larva migrans and may also be useful in trichinosis and visceral larva migrans infections.

Thiabendazole

Chemistry

Thiabendazole (2-[4'-thiazolyl]-benzimidazole) is a white, crystalline, tasteless, colorless compound that has no staining qualities. It is stable as a solid or in solution and is nearly insoluble in water at neutral pH. Although thiabendazole is a chelating agent that forms stable complexes with a number of metals, including iron, it does not bind calcium.

Absorption, Metabolism, & Excretion

Studies in man have shown that thiabendazole is rapidly absorbed after an oral dose. Drug concentrations in plasma peak within 1 hour and are barely detectable after 8 hours. Excretion is mainly via the urine, 90% appearing in 1 hour. The drug is almost completely metabolized to the 5-hydroxy form which appears in the urine largely as the glucuronide or sulfate conjugate. Thiabendazole is also absorbed from the skin.

Pharmacologic Effects & Toxicity Studies

Thiabendazole given to cats and dogs in large doses orally (4 gm/kg) and intravenously (40 mg/kg) did not produce significant effects on the cardiovascular or respiratory systems.

Acute toxicity studies in various animal species have shown that this drug is relatively well tolerated at dosages far above those used therapeutically in man. Repeated daily oral doses at high levels for 2 years have resulted in a mild normochromic anemia in dogs and hemosiderosis in rats and dogs.

Clinical Uses

Thiabendazole may be used for the following parasites when found singly or in combination:

A. *Strongyloides Stercoralis* (**Threadworm**): Thiabendazole is the drug of choice for the treatment of strongyloidiasis. Most & others, using 25 mg/kg for 2 days, eradicated the infection in all of 17 children treated. Of 134 patients treated in 9 studies, 125 (93%) were cured with a dosage of 25 mg/kg twice daily for 2–3 days.

B. *Enterobius Vermicularis* (**Pinworms**): Thiabendazole eradicates pinworms in over 95% of patients treated. However, because of its potential toxicity the equally effective drugs, piperazine or pyrvinium pamoate, should be used instead.

C. **Cutaneous Larva Migrans (Creeping Eruption)**: Thiabendazole is the first effective systemic drug for the treatment of cutaneous larva migrans, an infection caused by *Ancylostoma braziliense* or *A caninum.* Most larvae are killed by the first treatment; some, however, are only temporarily inactivated, requiring retreatment in 1–2 weeks. Recently, excellent results were reported following application of a cream containing 15% thiabendazole in a hygroscopic base.

D. *Trichuris Trichiura* (**Whipworm**): Reported cure rates for whipworm infections range from 5–35% when thiabendazole is used for 2 days. Cure rates increase when the drug is continued for 3–5 days, but side-effects also increase. However, only symptomatic infections with trichuris require treatment.

E. **Trichinosis**: Thiabendazole has been used successfully to prevent *Trichinella spiralis* infections in experimentally inoculated swine and mice. Sensitivity to the drug declines once infection has begun, but both enteric adult worms and parenteral larvae can be killed by large doses.

Information is limited on the effect of thiabendazole on the intestinal phase of trichinosis in man. During the invasive stage, however, biopsy evidence is increasing that the drug destroys larvae in muscle, especially during the first 2 months of the disease. In this acute phase amelioration or remission of signs and symptoms is usual without equivalent improvement in abnormal laboratory findings. Hennekeuser & others treated 23 patients with thiabendazole, giving 50 mg/kg daily for 10 days (maximum 3 gm/day). Before treatment 15 of 20 patients showed living larvae; afterward, only one patient had live larvae and 8 showed dead, degenerated larvae.

ACTH or corticosteroids are also effective in controlling the clinical manifestations of trichinosis and may be lifesaving in severe infections.

F. *Ascaris Lumbricoides:* When a dosage of 25 mg/kg is used twice daily for 2–3 days, the mean cure rate as reported by various investigators is 75%. Piperazine will clear over 90% of ascaris infections when used for 2 days and has fewer side-effects.

G. **Other Intestinal Infections**: For the treatment of hookworm infections, more information is needed to clarify the comparative effectiveness of thiabendazole, tetrachloroethylene, and bephenium hydroxynaphthoate. When 25 mg/kg of thiabendazole was used twice daily for 2–3 days, the mean cure rate among 488 patients in 14 trials was 77% (range, 30–100%). The available data do not permit definite conclusions about the relative susceptibility of the 2 genera of hookworm to thiabendazole.

Intestinal capillariasis has been successfully treated with thiabendazole at a dosage of 12 mg/kg given twice daily for 30 days.

In doses of 50–100 mg/kg daily for 2–3 days in divided doses, excellent responses have been obtained for the treatment of dracunculiasis. Local inflammation subsides rapidly, followed by death of the worms in 3–4 days. The worms can often be withdrawn or are eliminated by superficial abscess formation followed by incision or rupture.

The effectiveness of thiabendazole in visceral larva migrans has not been determined, but an extended course of treatment may alter the normal course of the disease.

Adverse Reactions

Side-effects from thiabendazole are common but generally mild and transient. They tend to occur 3–4 hours after ingestion of the drug and last 2–8 hours. Reports on their incidence vary from 7% to more than 30% of patients treated with 25 mg/kg twice daily for 2 days. Higher doses or extension of treatment beyond 2 days increases symptoms.

The most common side-effects are dizziness, anorexia, nausea, and vomiting. Less frequent are abdominal cramping pain, diarrhea, headache, drowsiness, lethargy, and pruritus. Perianal rashes, tinnitus, paresthesias, bradycardia, hypotension, and visual disturbances are rare.

Other side-effects have been reported, but some may represent manifestations of the disease or reactions to dying parasites rather than drug reaction. They include fever, chills, conjunctival injection, angioneurotic edema, lymphadenopathy, and skin rashes. Several cases of erythema multiforme, including Stevens-Johnson syndrome (with 2 fatal cases), have been associated with thiabendazole therapy in children.

No significant biochemical abnormalities have been found in toxicity studies in animals. In therapeutic studies in man, several transient abnormalities have only rarely been noted; eg, hyperglycemia, cholestasis, and SGOT and cephalin flocculation elevations.

Some patients may excrete a metabolite that imparts an odor to the urine during therapy and for 24 hours thereafter.

Occasionally reported during thiabendazole treatment have been leukopenia, crystalluria, and hematuria, all of which subsided when therapy was discontinued.

Contraindications & Cautions

Experience with thiabendazole is limited in children weighing less than 15 kg. It may be best to use alternative drugs in patients with hepatic dysfunction. The drug should be used with caution where drug-induced vomiting may be dangerous and there are a few reports of ascarids becoming hypermotile after treatment and appearing at the nose or mouth.

Since the drug makes some patients dizzy or drowsy, it should not be used during the day for patients whose work or activity requires complete mental alertness.

Preparations & Dosages

Thiabendazole (Mintezol) is available as a white suspension containing 100 mg of the drug per ml. It should be given after meals. Pre- and post-treatment purges and dietary restrictions are not necessary.

For the treatment of strongyloidiasis, cutaneous larva migrans, ascariasis, hookworm, trichuriasis, or mixed infections with these parasites, the recommended dosage is 25 mg/kg twice daily for 2 days. The maximum single dose should not exceed 1.5 gm, and the total daily dose should not exceed 3 gm. A second course of treatment may be given 1 week later if indicated.

Thiabendazole is no longer recommended for the treatment of pinworms. Formerly, the dosage used was 25 mg/kg twice daily for 1 day only, to be repeated in 1 week, the total daily dose not to exceed 3 gm.

The current recommendation for the treatment of trichinosis is 25 mg/kg twice daily for 2–4 days. However, as experience is gained, longer courses of therapy may be shown to be necessary. The total daily dose should not exceed 3 gm.

• • •

General References

Antimony Compounds

Ata, A-H., & A.H. Mousa: Treatment of bilharziasis by the slow method. J Egyptian MA 43:746–761, 1960.

Díaz-Rivera, R.S., & others: The treatment of schistosomiasis. Arch Int Med 101:1151–1158, 1958.

Farid, Z., & others: Urinary schistosomiasis treated with sodium antimony tartrate–a quantitative evaluation. Brit MJ 3:713–714, 1968.

Forsyth, D.M., & C. Rashid: Treatment of urinary schistosomiasis. Lancet 1:130–133, 1967.

Jordon, P.: Chemotherapy of schistosomiasis. Bull New York Acad Med 44:245–258, 1968.

Lämmler, G.: Chemotherapy of trematode infections. Pages 153–251 in: *Advances in Chemotherapy*. Vol D. Goldina, A., Hawking, F., & R.J. Schnitzer (editors). Academic Press, 1968.

Lu, Sung-Ts'e & H. Liu: A survey of short-course antimony tartrate therapy for schistosomiasis japonicum in China. Chinese MJ 82:46–54, 1963.

Most, H.: Treatment of schistosomiasis. Am J Trop Med 4:455–459, 1955.

Most, H., & others: Schistosomiasis japonica in American military personnel: clinical studies of 600 cases during the first year after infection. Am J Trop Med 30:239–299, 1950.

Nagaty, H.F., & M.A. Rifaat: Treatment of schistosomiasis, past and present. J Egyptian MA 43:659–707, 1960.

Schulert, A.R., & others: Biological disposition of antibilharzial antimony drugs. II. Antimony fate and uptake by *Schistosoma haematobium* eggs in man. Exper Parisitol 18:397–402, 1966.

Shookhoff, H.B.: Treatment of schistosomiasis. Am J Gastroenterol 44:254–259, 1965.

Standen, O.D.: Chemotherapy of helminthic infections. Chap 20, pp 701–892, in: *Experimental Chemotherapy*. Vol 1. Schnitzer, R.J., & F. Hawking (editors). Academic Press, 1963.

Wolfe, M.S.: Treatment of urinary schistosomiasis in Ghanaians with TWSb (Astiban). Am J Trop Med 13:811–815, 1964.

WHO: Chemotherapy of bilharziasis. WHO Tech Rep Ser No. 317, 1966.

Zaki, M.H., & others: Astiban in schistosomiasis mansoni: A controlled therapeutic trial in a nonendemic area. Am J Trop Med 13:803–810, 1964.

Aspidium Oleoresin

Jopling, W.H., & A.W. Woodruff: Treatment of tapeworm infections in man. Brit MJ 2:542–544, 1959.

Bephenium

Jayewardene, G., Ismail, M.M., & Y. Wijayaratnam: Bephenium hydroxynaphthoate in treatment of ascariasis. Brit MJ 2:268–271, 1960.

Krotov, A.I., & S.N. Fedorova: Effect of bephenium hydroxynaphthoate on ascarids. Fed Proc (Trans Suppl) 23:55–58, 1964.

Salem, H.H., Morcos, W.M., & H.M. el-Ninny: Clinical trials with bephenium hydroxynaphthoate against *Ancylostoma duodenale* and other intestinal helminths. J Trop Med 68:21–24, 1965.

Standen, O.D.: Chemotherapy of helminthic infections. Chap 20, pp 701–892, in: *Experimental Chemotherapy*. Vol 1. Schnitzer, R.J., & F. Hawking (editors). Academic Press, 1963.

Biscomate

Botero, R.D., & A. Perez: Clinical evaluation of a new drug for the treatment of ancylostomiasis. Am J Trop Med 19:471–475, 1970.

Bithionol

D'Sa, C.J.: Human fascioliasis. Proc Roy Soc Med 63:285–286, 1970.

Kim, J.S.: Treatment of *Paragonimus westermani* infections with bithionol. Am J Trop Med 19:940–942, 1970.

Oh, S.J.: Bithionol treatment in cerebral paragonimiasis. Am J Trop Med 16:585–590, 1967.

Yang, S-P., & C-C. Lin: Treatment of paragonimiasis with bithionol and bithionol sulfoxide. Dis Chest 52:220–232, 1967.

Yokogawa, M.: Paragonimus and paragonimiasis. Pages 99–158 in: *Advances in Parasitology*. Vol 3. Dawes, B. (editor). Academic Press, 1965.

Yoshida, Y., & others: Two cases of human infection with Fasciola sp and the treatment with bithionol. Jap J Parasitol 11:75–84, 1962.

Chloroquine Phosphate

El-Din, G.N.: Recent advances in the treatment of intestinal parasites. J Egyptian MA 34:449–461, 1951.

Komiya, Y.: Clonorchis and clonorchiasis. Pages 53–106 in: *Advances in Parasitology*. Vol 4. Dawes, B. (editor). Academic Press, 1966.

Yokogawa, M.: Paragonimus and paragonimiasis. Pages 99–158 in: *Advances in Parasitology*. Vol 3. Dawes, B. (editor). Academic Press, 1965.

Dichlorophen

Biagi, F., Gómez Orozco, L., & E. Robledo: [Efficacy of dichlorophen against *Hymenolepis nana*.] Bol Méd Hosp Infantil Mexico 16:113–116, 1959.

Seaton, D.R.: On the use of dichlorophen as a taenifuge for *Taenia saginata*. Ann Trop Med 54:338–340, 1960.

Standen, O.D.: Chemotherapy of helminthic infections. Chap 20, pp 701–892, in: *Experimental Chemotherapy*. Vol 1. Schnitzer, R.J., & F. Hawking (editors). Academic Press, 1963.

Turner, P.P.: The treatment of tapeworm infestation with "Anthiphen." J Trop Med 66:259–260, 1963.

Dichlorvos

Cervoni, W.A., & others: Dichlorvos as a single-dose intestinal anthelmintic therapy for man. Am J Trop Med 18:912–919, 1969.

Diethylcarbamazine Citrate

Hawking, F.: Chemotherapy of filariasis. Pages 191–222 in: *Progress in Drug Research*. Vol 9. Jucker, E. (editor). Birkhäuser (Basel), 1966.

Hewitt, R., & others: Follow-up observations on the treatment of Bancroftian filariasis with Hetrazan in British Guiana. Am J Trop Med 30:217–237, 1950.

Murgatroyd, F., & A.W. Woodruff: Loiasis treated with Hetrazan (Banocide). Lancet 2:147–149, 1949.

Narang, R.K., & S.C. Jain: Oral diethylcarbamazine in tropical pulmonary eosinophilia. Brit J Dis Chest 60:93–100, 1966.

Oomen, A.P.: Fatalities after treatment of onchocerciasis with diethylcarbamazine. Tr Roy Soc Trop Med Hyg 63:548, 1969.

Santiago-Stevenson, D., Oliver-González, J., & R.I. Hewitt: Treatment of filariasis bancrofti with 1-diethylcarbamyl-4-methylpiperazine hydrochloride ("Hetrazan"). JAMA 135:708–712, 1947.

Emetine

Hadden, J.W., & E.F. Pascarelli: Diagnosis and treatment of human fascioliasis. JAMA 202:149–151, 1967.

Hexylresorcinol

Brown, H.W.: The treatment of ascariasis and trichuriasis with hexylresorcinol pills. Am J Hyg 16:602–608, 1932.

Jung, R.C.: Use of a hexylresorcinol tablet in the enema treatment of whipworm infection. Am J Trop Med 3:918–921, 1954.

Lamson, P.D., Brown, H.W., & C.B. Ward: Anthelmintic studies on alkylhydroxybenzenes. J Pharmacol Exper Therap 53:198–217, 1935.

Hycanthone

Cook, J.A., & P. Jordan: Clinical trial of hycanthone in schistosomiasis mansoni in St. Lucia. Am J Trop Med 20:84–88, 1971.

Katz, N., & others: Further clinical trials with hycanthone, a new antischistosomal agent. Am J Trop Med 18:924–929, 1969.

Lucanthone Hydrochloride

Blair, D.M.: Lucanthone hydrochloride: A review. Bull WHO 18:989–1010, 1958.

Einhorn, A., & others: *Schistosoma mansoni* infection in children. Am J Dis Child 104:62–67, 1962.

Janssens, P.G., De Muynck, A., & J. Sieniawski: Treatment of intestinal schistosomiasis with lucanthone. Trop Geogr Med 17:112–120, 1965.

McMahon, J.E.: Non-intensive chemotherapy in bilharziasis with lucanthone hydrochloride. Preliminary report. Tr Roy Soc Trop Med Hyg 64:433–438, 1970.

Niclosamide

Ahkami, S., & A. Hajian: Radical treatment of *Hymenolepis nana* with niclosamide. J Trop Med 73:258–259, 1970.

Perera, D.R., Western, K.A., & M.G. Schultz: Niclosamide treatment of cestodiasis. Clinical trials in the United States. Am J Trop Med 19:610–612, 1970.

Shah, P.M., & V.G. Joshi: N(2′-chlor 4′-nitrophenyl)-5-chlorsalicylamide in *Taenia saginata* infestations in children. Indian Pediat 1:400–404, 1964.

Niridazole

Faigle, J.W., & others: The metabolism of niridazole (Ambilhar) in man. Ann Trop Med 64:383–393, 1970.

Fontanilles, F.: Risks versus benefits in antischistosomal therapy. Ann New York Acad Sc 160:811–820, 1969.

Kanani, S.R., Knight, R., & A.W. Woodruff: The treatment of schistosomiasis with niridazole in Britain. J Trop Med 73:162–169, 1970.

Kothari, M.L., & others: Niridazole in dracontiasis: A controlled study. Tr Roy Soc Trop Med Hyg 63:608–612, 1969.

The pharmacological and chemotherapeutic properties of niridazole and other antischistosomal compounds. Conference. Ann New York Acad Sc 160:426–946, 1969.

Paromomycin

Wittner, M., & H. Tanowitz: Paromomycin therapy of human cestodiasis with special reference to hymenolepiasis. Am J Trop Med 20:433–435, 1971.

Piperazine

Biagi, F., & O. Rodriguez: A study of ascariasis eradication by repeated mass treatment. Am J Trop Med 9:274–276, 1960.

Brown, H.W., Chan, K.F., & K.L. Hussey: Treatment of enterobiasis and ascariasis with piperazine. JAMA 161:515–520, 1956.

Bumbalo, T.S., & L.J. Plummer: Piperazine (Antepar) in the treatment of pinworm and roundworm infections. M Clin North America 41:575–585, 1957.

Farid, Z., & others: Single-dose treatment for Ascaris infection with piperazine citrate: With a study of the egg-parasite ratio. Am J Trop Med 15:516–518, 1966.

Nickey, L.N.: Possible precipitation of petit mal seizures with piperazine citrate. JAMA 195:1069–1070, 1966.

Pyrvinium Pamoate

Beck, J.W., & others: The treatment of pinworm infections in humans (enterobiasis) with pyrvinium chloride and pyrvinium pamoate. Am J Trop Med 8:349–352, 1959.

Beck, J.W.: Treatment of pinworm infections with reduced single dose of pyrvinium pamoate. JAMA 189:511, 1964.

Desser, K.B., & M. Baden: Allergic reaction to pyrvinium pamoate. Am J Dis Child 117:589, 1969.

Turner, J.A., & P.E. Johnson, Jr.: Pyrvinium pamoate in the treatment of pinworm infection (enterobiasis) in the home. J Pediat 60:243–251, 1962.

Wang, C.C., & G.A. Galli: Strongyloidiasis treated with pyrvinium pamoate. JAMA 193:847–848, 1965.

Quinacrine

Engel, G.L.: Quinacrine effects on the central nervous system. JAMA 197:515, 1966.

Jopling, H.W., & A.W. Woodruff: Treatment of tapeworm infections in man. Brit MJ 2:542–544, 1959.

Schapiro, M.: Observations on the treatment of human teniasis with quinacrine hydrochloride (Atabrine). Am J Trop Med 31:833–835, 1951.

Standen, O.D.: Chemotherapy of helminthic infections. Chap 20, pp 701–892, in: *Experimental Chemotherapy.* Vol 1. Schnitzer, R.J., & F. Hawking (editors). Academic Press, 1963.

Suramin

Burch, T.A., & L.L. Ashburn: Experimental therapy of onchocerciasis with suramin and Hetrazan: Results of a three-year study. Am J Trop Med 31:617–623, 1951.

Duke, B.O.L.: The effects of drugs on *Onchocerca volvulus:* Trials of suramin at different dosages and a comparison of the brands Antrypol, Moranyl, and Naganol. Bull WHO 39:157–167, 1968.

Hawking, F.: Chemotherapy of trypanosomiasis. Chap 5, pp 129–256 in: *Experimental Chemotherapy.* Vol 1. Schnitzer, R.J., & F. Hawking (editors). Academic Press, 1963.

WHO Expert Committee on Onchocerciasis, 2nd report. WHO Tech Rep Ser No. 335, pp 32–39, 1966.

Tetrachloroethylene

Bueding, E., & C. Swartzwelder: Anthelmintics. Pharmacol Rev 9:329–365, 1957.

Carr, H.P., Sardá, M.E.P., & N.A. Nuñez: Anthelmintic treatment of uncinariasis. Am J Trop Med 3:495–503, 1954.

Council on Pharmacy & Chemistry: Report on the present status of tetrachloroethylene. JAMA 107:1132–1133, 1936.

Tetramisole

Lionel, N.D.W., & others: Levamisole in the treatment of ascariasis in children. Brit MJ 4:340–341, 1969.

Thienpont, D., & others: Tetramisole in the treatment of nematode infections in man. Am J Trop Med 18:520–525, 1969.

Vakil, B.J., & others: Clinical trials with a new anthelminthic, tetramisole. Tr Roy Soc Trop Med 64:717–722, 1970.

Thiabendazole

Aur, R.J.A., Pratt, C.B., & W.W. Johnson: Thiabendazole in visceral larva migrans. Am J Dis Child 121:226–229, 1971.

Botero, R.D. Treatment of human intestinal helminthiases with thiabendazole. Am J Trop Med 14:618–621, 1965.

Campbell, W.C., & A.C. Cuckler: Thiabendazole in the treatment and control of parasitic infections in man. Texas Rep Biol Med 27 (Suppl 2):665–692, 1969.

Hennekeuser H.H., & others: Thiabendazole for the treatment of trichinosis in humans. Texas Rep Biol Med 27 (Suppl 2):581–596, 1969.

Mathies, A.W., Jr.: Thiabendazole in the treatment of *Enterobius vermicularis.* Texas Rep Biol Med 27 (Suppl 2):611–614, 1969.

Most, H., & others: The treatment of *Strongyloides* and *Enterobius* infections with thiabendazole. Am J Trop Med 14:379–382, 1965.

Robinson, H.J., Silber, R.H., & O.E. Graessle: Thiabendazole: Toxicological, pharmacological, and antifungal properties. Texas Rep Biol Med 27 (Suppl 2):537–560, 1969.

Stone, O.J.: Systemic and topical thiabendazole for creeping eruption. Texas Rep Biol Med 27 (Suppl 2):659–663, 1969.

Part VIII. Toxicology

64 . . .

Management of Acute Intoxications

The acute and chronic toxicity of the various classes of drugs have been discussed in earlier chapters, and these data about therapeutic agents provide a significant fraction of the information needed by the physician in handling cases of poisoning. However, a large number of poisons that are not used in therapy are encountered in the environment because they are used in household, factory, or farm or are present in food, air, or water. Data on such environmental toxins will be presented in Chapters 65 and 66, and a distinction between acute and chronic effects will often be made.

The management of acute poisoning and a procedure applicable to the management of most poisonings, medicinal or environmental, is presented below. The treatment of definite or possible acute intoxication is a frequent demand on all physicians and must often be carried out with limited or only presumptive information about the nature of the poison and the severity of exposure.

SOURCE & INCIDENCE OF ACUTE POISONINGS

Considering not only accidental but also suicidal, criminal, and industrial exposures, there are about 1½ million cases—8000 of which are fatal—each year in the USA in which a physician will have to initiate treatment for poisoning or decide that emergency treatment is or is not necessary. Of these, about half will be accidental and account for at least 1500 deaths in children, of which 80% will be children 1–4 years of age. Children under age 5 account for 2/3 of the reported accidental poisonings. The agents involved are those that are accessible to the normally curious child. In half of the cases, medicines are involved—most often those commonly around the home, eg, aspirin, iron pills, tranquilizers, sedatives, oral contraceptives, and thyroid. Bleaches and other cleaning products, pesticides, and petroleum products are also common toxic agents despite their unpleasant flavors and aromas.

PREVENTION OF ACCIDENTAL POISONING

A large percentage of acute poisonings, including even suicides, are preventable. Most accidental poisonings conform to familiar patterns, and the home can be made much safer if the physician provides (and the parents accept) some common sense safety instructions. The instructions are designed to prevent selection of the wrong container by an adult and to keep potential poisons out of the reach of children. Keeping aspirin on a high shelf and taking bleaches out of the cabinet under the sink would by themselves reduce the incidence of poisonings significantly. Parents should be asked to search the home for dangerous chemicals before a child begins to creep.

Rules for Prevention of Poisoning

(1) Medicines should be stored in a high or locked cabinet. Medications used regularly—eg, aspirin, sedatives, iron, and contraceptive pills—should not be kept in an easily accessible handbag or on a table or low shelf if young children are in the home.

(2) Patients should be told not to save unused prescription medications. Because very few will act on this advice, prescribed medications should be labeled with the name of the drug, prescribed in the smallest practical amount, and stored with care.

(3) Children should not be cajoled into taking medicine by comparing it with candy. "Candy" medicine tablets and flavored syrups are dangerous for children.

(4) Do not store poisons (cleaners, etc) in the same cabinet as foodstuffs.

(5) Do not store poisons (paint thinner, insecticides, etc) in cups, soft drink bottles, or other food containers. Do not bring insecticides or other chemicals home from work in such containers.

(6) Label all stored materials carefully.

(7) Use the following check list to locate dangers and warn children and parents. These items should be kept locked up or stored out of reach.

    a. In the kitchen or laundry—

      All medicines

      Ammonia

      Bleach

      Caustics (lye, Drano, Liquid-Plumr, washing soda, etc)

      Disinfectants

TABLE 64–1. Management of acute intoxications (summary).

When Not in Attendance (Phone Call)	When in Attendance (Hospital or Emergency Room)

1. Brief history.
2. Disposition:
  a. Treatment or close observation not necessary.
  b. Immediate home treatment followed by hospitalization.
  c. Meet patient at hospital or emergency room.
  d. Call to emergency service (fire department or ambulance service).
3. Immediate home treatment:
  a. Remove from exposure–
    (1) Skin–Remove contaminated clothing, wash skin. Flood acid or alkali burns with water for 5 minutes.
    (2) Eyes–Flood with water 5 minutes (20 minutes if alkali) with lids held apart.
    (3) Inhalation–Remove from contaminated area.
  b. Give artificial respiration if necessary.
  c. Dilute and adsorb poison with 1–2 glasses of milk, beaten eggs, flour or starch suspension, or water.
  d. Attempt to induce emesis unless the patient is comatose, convulsing, or has ingested a corrosive substance (acid or alkali) or petroleum distillate.
	1. Remove any source of continuing exposure–eg, remove contaminated clothing, wash skin, wash eyes.
	2. Maintain patent airway and support respiration and circulation.
	3. Brief history and necessary physical examination.
	4. Consider gastric lavage or induced emesis for orally ingested toxins if there are no contraindications.
	5. Specific therapy if available.
	6. Increase rate of excretion of poisons–eg, fluids, osmotic diuretics, alkalies.
	7. Symptomatic treatment of shock, convulsions, etc.
	8. Definitive history and physical examination. Identify agent if possible.
	9. Collect laboratory samples for identification and determination of levels of poison, both for control of treatment and for legal purposes.
	10. Preach prevention.

Furniture polish and wax
Moth balls
Oven cleaner
Spot remover, rug cleaner
  b. In the garage–
Fire starter
Gasoline, kerosene, etc
Insecticide
Paint remover
Paint, shellac, etc
Paint thinner
Rodenticide
Snail and slug bait
Turpentine
Weed killer
Wood bleach (oxalic acid)
  c. In the bathroom and bedroom–
All medicines
Cold wave preparations
Hair dyes and bleaches
Lighter fluid
Nail polish remover
  (8) All gas heaters and stoves should be vented.

  (9) Write down emergency phone numbers before the need arises.

  (10) If occupational exposure is a hazard, follow the manufacturer's cautions about the storage and handling of toxic materials and the use of protective equipment.

TREATMENT OF ACUTE POISONING

Treatment may begin when the patient is brought to the physician or when a parent phones for advice. The points discussed below are summarized in Table 64–1.

WHEN NOT IN ATTENDANCE

Disposition

The history provided by the parent or other person phoning the physician will usually establish what poison has been taken. The container will usually be at hand, and, if the product is unfamiliar to the physician, the label will usually identify toxic ingredients. The parent will less often be able to provide dependable information on the amount taken but can often describe how quickly the symptoms (if any) appeared.

The most common decision at this point is to suggest that no treatment or a period of close observation is necessary. Not every child who has alarmed his mother by chewing on his crayons need be hospitalized.

At the other extreme is the situation that is so grave (because of respiratory depression or convulsions) that the immediate response is to phone the emergency service in order to provide equipment to support respiration.

Unless some unusual difficulty with transport or distance exists or unless there is an indication for the immediate home treatment outlined below, the patient should be brought to the hospital or emergency room for definitive treatment.

Immediate Home Treatment

A. Remove From Continued Exposure: Treatment should not be delayed but should be started at home if the skin or eyes have been in contact with a corrosive substance or if contamination of the clothing or skin is resulting in continued contact with the poison. Contaminated clothing should be removed and the skin washed. Acid or alkali burns should be flooded with water for 5 minutes. If the eyes have been exposed to a caustic substance, they should be washed while the lids are held apart for 5 minutes (acid) or 20 minutes (alkali) before the patient is moved to the hospital.

In cases of inhalation poisoning (most commonly carbon monoxide), removal to open air is obviously of first importance.

B. Give artificial respiration if necessary.

C. Dilute and Adsorb Poison: The administration of oral fluids, except in the case of ingested caustic or irritant poisons, should be avoided because the additional fluid promotes gastric emptying. When emptying has occurred the poison cannot be removed by lavage or emesis, and greater quantities may be absorbed.

Activated charcoal is an effective adsorbent for some poisons and can be given **after** emesis is induced, but it is seldom available when needed. "Universal antidote"—2 parts powdered charcoal, 1 part tannic acid, 1 part magnesium oxide—is now seldom used because the ingredients are mutually inactivating.

D. Induce Emesis: Most authorities agree that efforts to induce emesis at home merely delay treatment and that the patient should instead be brought promptly to the hospital. Stimulating the back of the throat with a finger or the handle of a spoon or giving salt or mustard are not dependable ways of causing vomiting. If syrup of ipecac is immediately available, it should be given at once.

WHEN IN ATTENDANCE

The order in which the following procedures are carried out will vary with the nature of the poison and with the urgency of the situation.

Terminate Exposure

If the skin or eyes are contaminated, there is more urgency in carrying out this step. If the poison has been taken orally and is not a caustic, termination of continuing exposure is accomplished by inducing emesis or by gastric lavage as described below.

A. Skin Contamination: Water, from whatever source available (shower, faucet, hose, or bucket), should be used to remove poisons from the skin and to dilute and neutralize corrosive substances. Clothing should be removed with concern for the operator—ie, with the protection of gloves or running water. Acids and alkalies should be removed by using large amounts of water but not by chemical neutralization since the exothermic reaction may add damage by heat to the chemical injury.

B. Eyes: Chemical neutralization of acids or alkalies should not be attempted. Any delay in removing caustic substances from the eye is extremely dangerous. Treatment should be started immediately and close to the place of exposure by washing the corneal surface for 5 minutes with flowing water with the lids held apart. As soon as the patient is brought to the emergency service, irrigation should be resumed with sterile saline solution or water for 5 minutes if the substance is acid and 20 minutes if an alkali.

Artificial Respiration

Maintain a patent airway and support respiration in depressed or comatose patients.

Brief History & Cursory Physical Examination

Eliciting the history and performing a physical examination should not unduly delay gastric emptying or other treatment but must provide enough information to allow a decision about whether or not lavage should be performed.

Gastric Lavage or Emesis

The conditions under which the stomach should be emptied are not clearly defined, and opinion also differs about whether gastric lavage or induced emesis is preferable.

A. Gastric Lavage: Lavage is performed by passing a soft rubber tube into the stomach and repeatedly adding and withdrawing 4 oz portions of tap water. Once the toxic material has left the stomach, of course, lavage is of no value. It is generally held that lavage should not be done if more than 2–4 hours have elapsed since exposure, but many poisons cause pylorospasm and slow gastric emptying and lavage may be profitable up to 12 hours after ingestion of the poison.

There appears to be a growing preference for emptying the stomach by inducing vomiting with syrup of ipecac, a procedure that is less difficult for physician and patient.

The value of gastric lavage is not supported by some experimental studies, which suggest that gastric emptying into the intestine is hastened by lavage. However, in these studies a small (nasogastric) tube was used rather than a tube of adequate size (30 gauge) passed through the mouth. Critics of the use of ipecac point out that the mere occurrence of vomiting tells nothing about the completeness of gastric emptying.

The decision to perform lavage or induce vomiting is often based on a desire to protect the physician from recrimination and possible legal action rather than on any belief in its value. When the time from ingestion to treatment is brief enough to justify emptying the stomach, the use of an emetic is convenient and requires no equipment. In the emergency room, conservative practice probably still favors a properly performed gastric lavage.

Clear **contraindications** to the performance of gastric lavage are the following:

1. If more than 30 minutes have elapsed since ingestion of acid or alkali. Necrosis of the esophagus results in an increased hazard of perforation.

2. Ingestion of petroleum distillate (kerosene, paint thinner, spot remover, etc). Regurgitated amounts of these hydrocarbons are aspirated into the lungs and cause chemical pneumonia.

3. Coma, stupor, and delirium are contraindications because of the hazard of aspiration. If, however, a cuffed endotracheal tube is put in place, lavage may be performed on comatose patients.

4. Convulsions, unless or until they are controlled by other medication. The stimulation associated with intubation may precipitate convulsions.

B. Induced Emesis: The indications for and contraindications to inducing emesis are the same as listed above for gastric lavage. The question of which of the 2 technics is preferable is not completely resolved.

1. Ipecac syrup—Syrup of ipecac, 15–20 ml, is given by mouth, followed by as much milk, water, or fruit juice as the patient will drink. The dose may be repeated in 15–20 minutes if the first dose is without effect. Vomiting usually occurs within 10 minutes even if the poison is a drug generally credited with antiemetic properties, eg, antipsychotic tranquilizers.

Syrup of ipecac may be sold without a prescription in 1 oz bottles with directions for use in causing vomiting. It should be kept in every home. Only the specially labeled syrup of ipecac should be used in order to avoid any possible confusion with fluidextract of ipecac. Inadvertent use of the fluidextract has been responsible for at least 7 deaths.

2. Apomorphine—Ipecac syrup has been characterized as a slow emetic, and it has been suggested that apomorphine is preferable because of its more rapid action after injection. The dosage of apomorphine in adults is 6 mg IM; in children, 0.05 mg/kg IM. The action of apomorphine can be terminated with levallorphan (Lorfan), 0.02 mg/kg IM, or nalorphine (Nalline), 0.1 mg/kg IM.

Specific Therapy If Available

The specific antidote should be employed in those few cases in which one is available. These include the following:

Antisera
Ethyl alcohol for methanol
Amyl nitrite for cyanide
Atropine and PAM for phosphate insecticides
Calcium salts for fluoride

Epinephrine for anaphylactic reactions
Methylene blue for methemoglobinemia
Nalorphine for narcotic analgesics
Chelating agents for metals including iron

Symptomatic & Supportive Treatment

If no specific therapy is available, treatment is designed to support the patient during the period of detoxification and to shorten this period by increasing the rate of excretion of the poison. Ill-advised or unduly vigorous symptomatic treatment can be quite damaging to the patient and should be based on experience in treating the specific poison. Pain, vomiting, diarrhea, fluid and electrolyte derangements, and other symptoms are controlled in the usual ways. There are, in addition, a few special problems in treating acute intoxication.

A. Shock: Since the phenothiazine tranquilizers and the related antidepressant drugs are common causes of intoxication, it must be emphasized that hypotension is not necessarily the same as shock. Patients with a predominantly postural hypotension associated with a dilated, warm periphery usually require no treatment other than the recumbent position. Shock or impending shock frequently occurs in intoxication with barbiturates and other depressant drugs and should be treated by reexpansion of the plasma volume rather than with vasopressors such as norepinephrine. Experience with vasodilators such as isoproterenol or phenoxybenzamine is still limited and investigational, but preliminary reports are promising.

B. Coma: The treatment of intoxication with barbiturates or other hypnotics has been discussed in Chapter 23, where the rationale for the conservative or physiologic method of treatment is presented in detail. Analeptic or stimulant drugs are not used because their use is both hazardous and ineffective.

C. Convulsions: Convulsions must be distinguished from the violent dystonias seen in children after intoxication with one of the antipsychotic tranquilizers. Convulsions must then be classified into one or the other of 2 large classes: those that originate in the spinal cord, as after strychnine poisoning or during tetanus; and the more common type that is suprasegmental in origin.

Local anesthetic toxicity is perhaps the most familiar example of convulsions that originate in a suprasegmental site. The treatment of such convulsions is discussed in Chapter 22, where it is emphasized that convulsions are usually well tolerated, especially if oxygen is available between paroxysms, and that treatment with CNS depressants to control the convulsions may add dangerously to the postconvulsant depression. If an anesthetist and the requisite equipment are available, succinylcholine may be used to control convulsions through its peripheral action. An inhalation anesthetic or intravenous thiopental may be used if convulsions persist. If the convulsant poison has a very prolonged duration of action, diphenylhydantoin may be given as an anticonvulsant.

D. Toxic Psychosis: The most common cause of toxic psychosis or paranoid or hallucinatory states

TABLE 64–2. Partial list of drugs and poisons removed by peritoneal dialysis or hemodialysis.

Sedative-hypnotics
    Barbiturates
    Piperidinedione derivatives:
        Methyprylon (Noludar) (but not glutethi-
            mide [Doriden])
    Carbamates:
        Meprobamate (Equanil, Miltown)
        Ethinamate (Valmid)
    Alcohols:
        Chloral hydrate
        Ethanol
        Ethchlorvynol (Placidyl)
        Ethylene glycol
        Methanol
    Others:
        Paraldehyde

Nonnarcotic analgesics
    Aspirin
    Methyl salicylate
    Phenacetin

Narcotic analgesics (*Note:* Specific antagonist availa-
    ble.)
    Dextropropoxyphene (Darvon)
    Heroin

CNS stimulants and antidepressants
    Dextroamphetamine (Dexedrine)
    Tranylcypromine (Parnate)
    Imipramine (Tofranil)
    Amitriptyline (Elavil)
    Phenelzine (Nardil)
    Pargyline (Eutonyl)

Metals and metal ions

Arsenic	Mercury
Calcium	Potassium
Iron	Sodium
Lead	Strontium
Magnesium	

Halides
    Bromide
    Iodide

Miscellaneous
    Boric acid
    Chlorates
    Carbon tetrachloride
    Ergotamine
    Nonhalogenated aromatic hydrocarbons

today is the deliberate use of LSD or methamphetamine (see Chapter 7). A toxic psychosis can be caused
by other CNS stimulants; by parasympatholytics such
as are in stramonium leaves; by bromides; by abrupt
withdrawal of alcohol or other sedatives; by some
industrial poisons; and by infection and fever. Experience with people who take drugs in search of hallucinatory experiences has shown that reassurance and
explanation can greatly reduce the intensity of the
reaction. Chlorpromazine can be used to reduce hallucinatory, paranoid, or excited behavior if necessary
and if the state is due to a stimulant drug. Chlorpromazine will intensify the effects of the atropine-like
drugs, and the sedatives are preferable to the antipsychotic tranquilizers in such situations. The sedatives
are also preferable if anxiety rather than distortion of
perception is the predominant symptom and in the
withdrawal states.

Definitive History & Physical Examination;
    Identification of Agent

The history and physical examination are developed to the extent that the need for emergency treatment permits and the need for information requires.
After essential therapy has been given, a detailed
history should be taken and a careful examination
performed.

Determination of the extent and mechanism of
exposure may require a long period of investigation.
Toxic ingredients in commercial products are usually
printed on the label. Trade names, ingredients, and
much additional useful information are included in the
references listed at the end of this chapter. If the
physician has no references available, the nearest
Poison Control Center can usually provide the information.

Suspected criminal poisoning must always be
reported, and occupational exposures must be reported
in most states.

Increase Rate of Excretion of Poison

The use of osmotic diuretics and alkalies to
shorten the period of detoxification has been discussed
in the sections on the barbiturates and the salicylates.

Peritoneal dialysis or hemodialysis (artificial kidney) may be used in special situations to remove a drug
or poison (Table 64–2). The procedures are themselves
slightly hazardous and are used only in very severe
intoxications and in centers where equipment and
experienced personnel are available.

Collect Samples for Laboratory

The poison can usually be identified on clinical
grounds and the conclusion supported by simple urine
tests for the most common agents done in the emergency room. In chronic intoxications definitive laboratory work may be of great importance, but in acute
poisonings most decisions are made before laboratory
data become available. Nevertheless, vomitus or lavage
fluid and urine should be collected in clean containers
and carefully labeled, sealed, and refrigerated in the

event that they are needed for legal purposes or to identify the agent. Blood and urine samples should be collected in known or suspected poisoning with agents for which analytical methods are useful—especially alcohol, barbiturates, and salicylates. Data on blood gases and electrolytes are of value in managing intoxications.

●   ●   ●

General References

Texts & Manuals for Identification of Agents

Dreisbach, R.H.: *Handbook of Poisoning: Diagnosis & Treatment,* 7th ed. Lange, 1971.

Fairhall, L.T.: *Industrial Toxicology,* 2nd ed. Williams & Wilkins, 1957.

Gleason, M.N., & others: *Clinical Toxicology of Commercial Products,* 3rd ed. Williams & Wilkins, 1969. (Composition of 17,000 products.)

Johnstone, R.T., & S.E. Miller: *Occupational Diseases and Industrial Medicine.* Saunders, 1960.

Kingsbury, J.M.: *Poisonous Plants of the United States and Canada.* Prentice-Hall, 1964.

Moeschlin, S.: *Poisoning.* Grune & Stratton, 1965.

Patty, F.A. (editor): *Industrial Hygiene and Toxicology.* 2 vol. Interscience, 1948, 1949.

Plunkett, E.R.: *Handbook of Industrial Toxicology.* Chemical Publishing Co., 1966.

Treatment

Gosselin, R.E., & R.P. Smith: Trends in the therapy of acute poisonings. Clin Pharmacol Therap 7:279–299, 1966.

Matthew, H., & others: Gastric aspiration and lavage in acute poisoning. Brit MJ 2:1333–1336, 1966.

Matthew, H.: Acute poisoning: Some myths and misconceptions. Brit MJ 1:519–522, 1971.

Matthew, H., & A.A.H. Lawson: *Treatment of Common Acute Poisonings,* 2nd ed. Livingstone, 1970.

Thoman, M.E., & H.L. Verhulst: Ipecac syrup in antiemetic ingestion. JAMA 196:433–434, 1966.

65...

Heavy Metals & Chelating Agents

The metallic poisons or heavy metals are discussed separately from other environmental poisons to simplify the presentation of the many toxic agents that must be identified and to emphasize chelation as a mechanism of drug action. Chelating or sequestering agents remove metallic ions from solution, and the resulting nonionic organometallic complex is often less toxic and more rapidly excreted than the metallic ions.

CHELATION

In the formation of the covalent or ionic bond, each atom contributes one electron to the shared pair in the common molecular orbital. A coordinate-covalent bond is formed when both shared electrons are contributed by one atom. Chelate formation involves formation of coordinate-covalent bonds between an electrophilic, electropositive atom of a metal and nucleophilic atoms or ligands (usually N, O, or S) of an organic molecule so as to form a ring containing the metal atom and 2, 3, or 4 atoms from the organic molecule.

Fig 65–1, for example, represents a common chelating or sequestering agent. The polycarboxylic acid can form salts utilizing covalent or ionic bonds as in the disodium salt (1a). However, when the disodium-calcium salt is formed (1b), additional bonding is possible. Calcium has unfilled **d** orbitals that can accept electron pairs from the nitrogen. The calcium is then held firmly in the heterocyclic organometallic rings that result and can no longer provide calcium ions. In fact, if the tetrasodium salt is added to blood or other material, calcium ions are sequestered by the "claw-like" hold of the chelate. The lead-EDTA chelate is even more stable and is formed preferentially even in the presence of calcium ions. In the compound shown in 1c, all 6 of the ligands of EDTA have contributed to the formation of partially fused, 5-membered rings.

The stability of metal chelates depends upon properties of the metal and of the chelating agent, and compounds can therefore be selected to bind certain metals with a degree of specificity sufficient to make them therapeutically useful in the treatment of intoxications. The stability of the chelate is greatest—ie, the dissociation into metal ion and ligand is least—when the ligand molecule contains more than one electron-donating atom, in which case it is said to be polydentate. Stability is also increased if the metal becomes part of several fused rings when the chelate is formed, and complex, naturally occurring chelates such as hemoglobin are very stable. The chelate is most stable if the ring formed contains 5 atoms and is saturated or consists of 6 atoms with 2 double bonds and the size of the metal atom is such that the rings are strainless.

The chelate formed has chemical and biologic properties different from either of the precursors. The metal is no longer present in an ionized form and is not biologically available. The chelates formed in the course of therapy must be nontoxic and very water-soluble, so that they may be more rapidly excreted than the offending metal. All chelating agents remove or inactivate some of the trace metals present in the organism, and it has been suggested (but not yet established) that some drugs may exert their pharmacologic action through this mechanism.

CHELATING AGENTS
(See Table 65–1.)

A variety of chelating agents are available. In some cases—eg, deferoxamine and iron—a single chelating agent is related to a single metal. As a rule, however, several possible pairs are involved. The pharmacology of the individual chelating agents will, therefore, be discussed separately before the discussion of heavy metal toxicity.

1. DIMERCAPROL (BAL)

Chemistry

Arsenical vesicants were developed late in World War I to supplement sulfur mustard gases. Early in World War II, before it became apparent that the nitrogen mustards would replace the arsenical vesicants should chemical warfare be attempted, the British developed an antagonist to the toxic effects of arsenic.

(a)

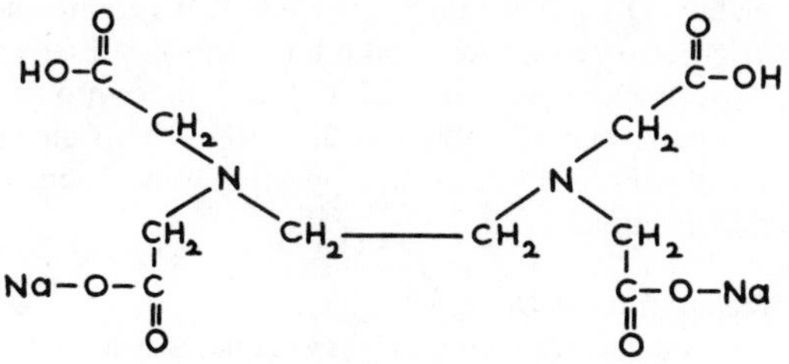

(b)

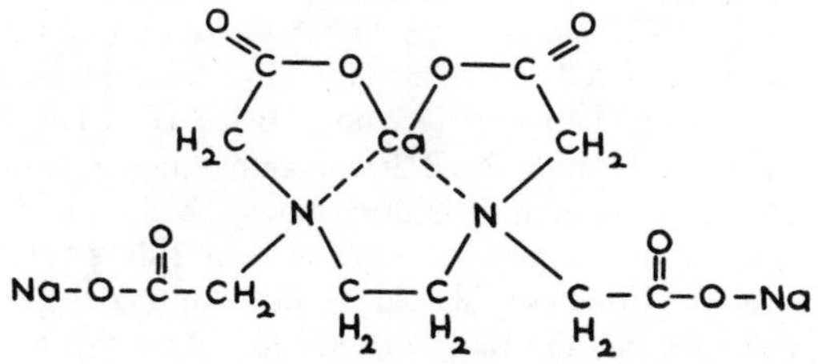

(c)

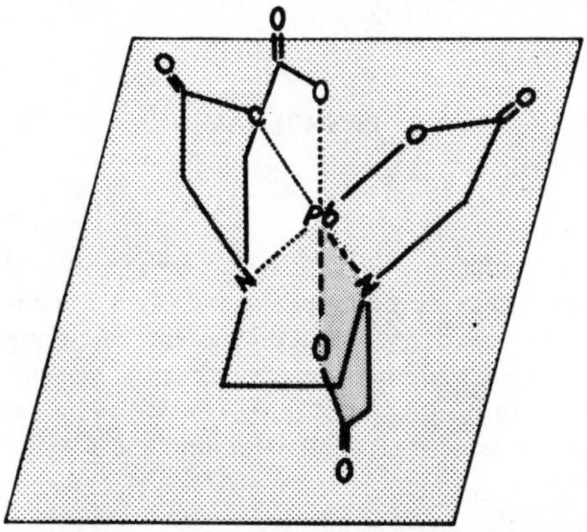

FIG 65—1. **Salt and chelate formation with ethylenediaminetetraacetic acid (EDTA).** Broken lines represent coordinate-covalent bonds. *(a)* In a solution of the disodium salt of EDTA, the sodium and hydrogen ions are chemically and biologically available. *(b)* In solutions of calcium disodium edetate, calcium is bound by coordinate-covalent bonds with nitrogen as well as by the usual ionic bonds. Calcium ions are effectively removed from solution. *(c)* In the lead-edetate chelate, lead is incorporated into 5 heterocyclic rings.

Since the prototype of the arsenic mustard gas was lewisite, the new compound was called British antilewisite, or BAL.

The reaction of arsenic with sulfhydryl groups was well known, Ehrlich having suggested that the thiol group was the "arsenic receptor." In studying the combination of arsenic with the protein keratin, the British workers observed that, generally, one equivalent of arsenic reacted with 2 equivalents of sulfhydryl group. They introduced dimercaprol, a simple dithiol (Fig 65—2), to similarly react with arsenic, neutralizing its toxic effects and hastening its excretion. It is still the primary agent used in the treatment of arsenic and mercury poisoning.

Dimercaprol has an offensive odor similar to that of other mercaptans or thiols. It is not soluble in water, and is dispensed as a solution in peanut oil.

Adverse Reactions

Dimercaprol may reactivate sulfhydryl-containing enzymes that have been inactivated by a heavy metal, but it may inactivate other enzymes, presumably by chelating trace metals. Perhaps for this reason it causes a great variety of side-effects when given in more than the minimal dose described below. However, its acute effects are not dangerous, and chronic toxic effects have not been reported. Side-effects include local pain at the injection site, fever, nausea, salivation, and paresthesias in the mouth and throat.

Preparations & Dosages

Dimercaprol is available as a 10% solution in oil for deep IM administration. Each ampule contains 3 ml, or 300 mg. The dose usually recommended is 2.5 mg/kg (or 0.25 ml/10 kg) every 4 hours for the first 2 days and then every 12 hours for a total of 10 days or until recovery. Treatment can be less intensive if the situation permits—eg, 100 mg 4 times on the first day; 2 times on days 2, 3, and 4; and once on days 5 and 6.

2. CALCIUM DISODIUM EDETATE

Chemistry

Ethylenediaminetetraacetic acid itself—ie, the acid rather than any salt—is the form of this agent most potent in removing calcium from solutions. It may be added to shed blood to prevent clotting, but when so used it is a chemical reagent rather than a drug. Salts of the acid when used as drugs are known under their generic names as edetates. Disodium edetate and trisodium edetate also bind calcium and for this reason have only investigative uses. Given acutely and in large amounts, they are toxic because they lower serum calcium. During chronic administration, the calcium chelate formed may be damaging to the kidneys. During administration of a dose of intermediate size, the plasma calcium level may be maintained by mobilization of calcium from the skeleton and other stores.

Calcium disodium edetate will, on the other hand, exchange calcium for lead and a few other heavy metals. Calcium disodium edetate has been given by mouth in the past; however, it is poorly absorbed, and penicillamine (Cuprimine) is preferable for oral administration in the treatment of lead poisoning. Edetate is still used parenterally during the treatment of lead encephalopathy.

Adverse Reactions

CaNa$_2$ EDTA should be given in dilute solutions to prevent thrombophlebitis and should be given in interrupted dosage to prevent depletion of essential

TABLE 65–1. Summary of metallic poisons, and chelating agents effective against each.

	Chelating Agent of Choice	Alternative Chelating Agent or Other Antidotal Therapy
Antimony	Dimercaprol	
Arsenic	Dimercaprol	
Barium		Precipitate with sulfate
Beryllium	. . .	. . .
Bismuth	Dimercaprol	
Cadmium	Dimercaprol	Edetate
Calcium	Edetate	
Chromium	Dimercaprol	
Cobalt	. . .	. . .
Copper	Penicillamine	
Gold	Dimercaprol	
Iron	Deferoxamine	Edetate
Lead	Penicillamine	Edetate
Manganese		Edetate (?)
Mercury	Dimercaprol	N-Acetylpenicillamine*
Nickel	Dithizon,* dithiocarb*	
Silver		Precipitate with chlorides
Thallium	Dithizon (?)*	
Uranium	Edetate (?)	Bicarbonate prevents renal damage
Vanadium	Edetate (?)	Ascorbic acid
Zinc	Edetate	Dimercaprol

*Investigational drug.

metals. Dosage should not exceed that recommended in order to avoid the renal tubular damage observed in experimental situations. If these precautions· are observed, the side-effects will be limited to an occasional febrile flu-like state appearing some hours after the injection.

Preparations & Dosages

Edetate (Versenate) is available as 5 ml ampules of a 20% solution (1 gm). For intravenous administration, 15–25 mg/kg (0.08–0.125 ml/kg of a 20% solution) are added to 250 or 500 ml of 5% dextrose and given over a period of 1–2 hours twice daily. The daily dose should not exceed 50 mg/kg/day in adults or 30 mg/kg in children. The drug should be given in 5-day courses with a rest period of at least 2 days between courses. Urinalyses should be done during the treatment period, and the dosage reduced if changes appear in the urinary sediment.

3. PENICILLAMINE

Chemistry

Penicillamine (Fig 65–2) is an amino acid that occurs only as a product of the hydrolysis of penicillin. It can be considered a dimethylcysteine or a thiovaline. The D-isomer is much less toxic than the racemate and is the form used as a drug. Penicillamine is well absorbed after oral administration, and very little is

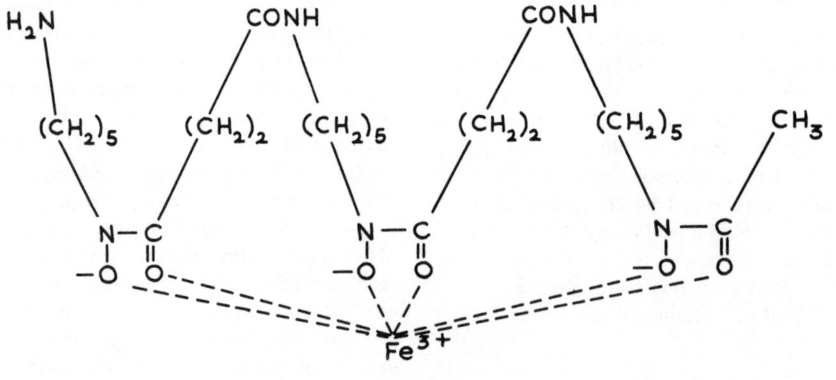

Ferroxamine

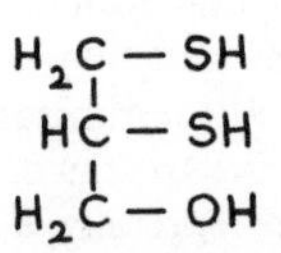

Dimercaprol
(2,3-dimercaptopropanol)

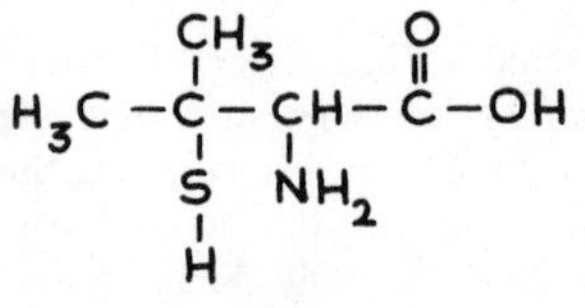

Penicillamine

FIG 65–2. Chemical structures of several chelating agents. Ferroxamine without the chelated iron is deferoxamine (Desferal). Dotted lines represent coordinate-covalent bonds.

metabolized in the body. Its prime advantage is its suitability for chronic oral administration. It is useful as a chelator of copper, lead, and probably mercury. In addition, it combines chemically with cysteine to form a cysteine-penicillamine disulfide that is much more soluble than cystine (cysteine-cysteine disulfide). It is used as an investigative drug in the treatment of cystinuria.

N-Acetylpenicillamine is even more stable than the parent compound and offers advantages over penicillamine, especially as a chelator of mercury. It is still an investigational drug.

Adverse Reactions

A. Side-Effects: These are limited to occasional signs of gastrointestinal irritation.

B. Chronic Toxicity: During the long-term administration of penicillamine to prevent the accumulation of copper in the tissues of patients with hepatolenticular degeneration (Wilson's disease), optic neuritis and nephrotic syndrome have occurred. Both of these processes are reversible, and their causes are not established. The neuritis cannot be explained on the basis of pyridoxine depletion if the D-isomer of penicillamine is used.

C. Allergic Reactions: There is a high incidence (1/3 of cases) of acute allergic reactions shortly after therapy is started, with fever, rash, adenopathy, and leukopenia.

Preparations & Dosages

D-Penicillamine (Cuprimine) is supplied as 250 mg capsules. Except in children, the initial dose is 250 mg 4 times a day, but the optimal dose must be determined with the aid of urinary copper determinations. In the treatment of Wilson's disease, potassium sulfide is given with each meal to reduce absorption of copper by the formation of the sulfide. The use of penicillamine as a deleading agent is under investigation.

4. OTHER CHELATING AGENTS

Deferoxamine (Desferal) is used in the treatment of intoxication with iron (see Chapter 42). Sodium dithiocarb (sodium diethyldithiocarbamate) and diphenylthiocarbazone (dithizon) are investigational drugs used in the treatment of nickel and thallium poisoning.

METALLIC POISONS

LEAD

Inhalation of lead is a hazard in industry when metals or painted metals are cut or burned. Lead pigments are no longer present in the usual house paints, but many old buildings in slum and rural areas have peeling layers of old paint and putty which may be eaten by children. Lead from pipes or ceramic glaze has contaminated water and food.

The discussion below pertains to inorganic lead. Organic lead in the form of tetraethyl lead added to gasoline is a powerful and prolonged CNS stimulant and convulsant. Tetraethyl lead is also a source of inorganic lead that can accumulate in air and even in the surface waters of areas of the ocean close to concentrations of automobiles. The problem at this time is potential rather than immediate.

Clinical Findings

A. Acute Intoxication: When a soluble, rapidly absorbed compound of lead is ingested or when contact with an organic lead compound occurs, the symptoms—eg, lead encephalopathy or abdominal pain—may be rapid in onset. However, the manifestations are the same as those described for chronic intoxication. The onset of symptomatic chronic lead poisoning may be acute, and a chronic course may be interrupted by acute episodes. Therefore, the usual distinction between acute and chronic intoxication is not easily made.

B. Chronic Intoxication:

1. Red blood cells—Anemia is usually present due in part to an inhibition by lead of at least 2 steps in the synthesis of heme: (1) Delta-aminolevulinic acid (ALA) is not converted to porphobilinogen and appears in the urine in abnormal and diagnostically useful amounts. (2) Protoporphyrin is not converted to heme and hemoglobin, and its immediate precursor appears in the urine in increased amounts. In addition, the period of survival of red cells is reduced.

2. Smooth muscle—Intestinal smooth muscle is stimulated. Spasm and hypermotility cause intense cramping pain or "lead colic." Blood vessel constriction causes pallor and an acute, reversible hypertension.

3. Encephalopathy—In adults, symptoms may be limited to irritability. In children and following exposure to organic lead compounds, cerebral edema with delirium and convulsions may be prominent.

4. Lead palsy or myopathy—It is still not established whether changes in muscle function are neural or muscular in origin. Fatigability and weakness are common. Wrist drop and involvement of the extraocular muscles occur. Sensory changes do not occur.

5. Lead line—A finely stippled deposit may occur in the margins of the gingival tissues. The procedure for identification consists of expressing blood from the area and observing with a hand lens.

6. X-ray findings—Radiopaque material may be demonstrable upon x-ray examination of the abdomen.

7. Laboratory findings—The following technics are available:

a. Lead in urine or blood.

b. Response of urinary lead to test dose of penicillamine or edetate.

c. Increased amount of erythrocyte stippling.

d. Increase in urinary coproporphyrin excretion.

e. Increase in amounts of aminolevulinic acid excretion in urine.

Treatment

A. Chelation: If the intoxication is acute, treatment should be initiated with injections of both dimercaprol and edetate in order to avoid the increased toxic effects sometimes precipitated by edetate. Thereafter, treatment can be continued with edetate or the combination of both drugs.

In less acute situations, deleading can be accomplished with repeated courses of a chelating agent—eg, edetate—given as described above, but oral penicillamine (Cuprimine) is far more convenient.

B. Calcium Gluconate: In the past, calcium was given to hasten the deposition of lead with the extra calcium in bone. There is no question but that lead is retained in bone, but the relief of colic afforded by injected calcium salts is apparently due to its action on smooth muscle.

C. Encephalopathy: Chelating agents are of doubtful immediate value. Urea or a similar osmotic diuretic may be used to reduce cerebral edema (see Chapter 17).

ARSENIC

Arsenic is a transition element or metalloid. Its oxides are hydrated to acids, but it also reacts with nonmetals.

Inorganic arsenicals were for several hundred years the favorite agents of poisoners. Paris green (copper acetoarsenite) was the first pesticide, and organic arsenicals were the primary agents in the therapy of syphilis until penicillin became available. The toxicology of arsenic has lost much of its practical importance, but of the metals only lead causes more deaths. Industrial exposure still occurs during the refining and smelting of other metals, and some pesticides (snail and rat bait, herbicides) contain arsenic.

Clinical Findings & Treatment

A. Acute Intoxication: Because arsenic damages all capillaries, many organ systems are affected, but gastrointestinal symptoms are most prominent. After overwhelming doses the symptoms reflect a violent gastroenteritis: pain and difficulty in swallowing, epigastric and abdominal pain, vomiting, and watery or bloody diarrhea. Blood pressure falls, and death is due to shock. Jaundice or oliguria may appear in 1–3 days. Smaller single doses cause some of the same symptoms together with muscle cramps, irritability, dizziness, and weakness that last for about 2 weeks.

Specific treatment is with dimercaprol.

B. Chronic Intoxication: The onset may be insidious and may simulate many diseases. Appetite is well maintained; thus, when arsenic was used criminally, ingestion continued to the end. The manifestations include peripheral or optic neuritis, pigmentation of the skin, localized edema, conjunctivitis, diarrhea, nausea and vomiting, nephritis, jaundice, cirrhosis, anemia, and dependent edema.

Specific treatment is with dimercaprol.

C. Carcinogenicity: Arsenic has long been said to cause palmar and plantar keratoses and subsequent carcinomas. Most observations are in conflict with the traditional belief. Carcinomas do not follow industrial exposures, and many of the cases reported earlier were probably due to coal tar. Since 1952, when arsenicals were withdrawn from use as insecticides in tobacco fields, the level of arsenic in the soil has fallen to negligible levels. There has been no change in the rising incidence of carcinoma of the lung.

D. Arsine: Arsine is a gas that results from the action of acid on arsenic metal or arsenic compounds in the presence of a reducing agent—eg, another active metal. It can cause severe hemolysis.

MERCURY

Opportunities for contact with salts of mercury are fortunately becoming rare. Mercuric (bi)chloride is now rarely used as a disinfectant or homicidal agent. Metallic mercury has become comparatively more important as a toxic agent. Orally ingested, it is poorly absorbed and virtually nontoxic in adults. However, it volatilizes at room temperature and is a hazard in laboratories. Metallic mercury from the clinical laboratory has also been accidentally and suicidally injected.

Mercury is excreted by the kidneys, colon, salivary glands, and liver. Many of the toxic effects appear at these sites of greatest concentration.

Clinical Findings & Treatment

A. Acute Intoxication: The immediate danger (first day) is shock due to fluid loss from local damage to the gastrointestinal tract. Colitis with bloody diarrhea follows when mercuric ions are excreted by the large bowel. Necrosis of the proximal renal tubule may follow. Recovery begins in about 1 week.

Specific treatment is with dimercaprol as described above.

B. Chronic Intoxication: Signs are related to the kidney (eg, proteinuria), the mouth (eg, stomatitis, excessive salivation, and blue gum line), and the CNS (eg, anxiety, depression, headache, weakness, insomnia, and irritability). Treatment consists of dimercaprol, 2.5 mg/kg IM twice daily for a prolonged period as determined by the course of the patient.

C. Acrodynia: Small amounts of mercury in infants and young children—eg, from teething powders, diaper rinses, ammoniated mercury ointment, or paint—may cause a hypersensitivity reaction with generalized erythema. It is responsive to treatment with dimercaprol.

D. Alkyl Mercury Poisoning: The toxicity of alkyl mercury compounds is different from that of inorganic mercury and cannot be treated with chelating agents or any other specific therapy. The manifestations may include ataxia and slurred speech, impaired vision and hearing, paralysis, disturbed or retarded behavior, and coma. These may be irreversible or lethal due to degenerative changes in the brain.

Fungicides have been responsible for a few poisonings. In the early 1950s, methyl mercury was discharged into Minamata Bay and taken up by fish and shellfish. Among the families who depended upon the seafood there were 111 cases of illness with 41 deaths. The current concern is based on the demonstration that inorganic mercury in industrial waste can be converted to methyl and dimethyl mercury by bacteria and enter the food chain. The alkyl mercury is converted to the mercurous ion, which, if not innocuous, is much less toxic.

ANTIMONY

Antimony occurs in type metal and other alloys, batteries, ceramics, and drugs such as tartar emetic. Its properties are similar to those of arsenic. Like arsenic, upon reaction with acid it evolves a gas, stibine (SbH_3), that causes hemolysis. The MLD of antimony is 100 mg.

Clinical Findings & Treatment

A. Acute Intoxication: Antimony is more irritating locally than arsenic but is more rapidly excreted. Manifestations include nausea, vomiting, diarrhea, nephritis, and hepatitis. In addition to general measures, treat with dimercaprol; its effectiveness is established for inorganic antimonial and trivalent organic compounds.

B. Chronic Intoxication: Manifestations include itching skin pustules, bleeding gums, conjunctivitis, laryngitis, headache, weight loss, and anemia.

BERYLLIUM

Beryllium salts were used until 1949 in the phosphors of fluorescent lamps. Contact also occurs during its smelting. Beryllium and its alloys are being used more and more in airframes, but no problems of toxicity have yet been reported.

The hazards of even minimal contact with beryllium salts were acknowledged only reluctantly and after needless delay had prolonged an epidemic of intoxications.

Clinical Findings & Treatment

Beryllium acts locally to produce a granulomatous response. Three clinical patterns are seen:

A. Indolent Ulcers: Contact with beryllium salts causes an eczematoid dermatitis. With heavier exposure or (especially) if some of the material is deposited in the tissue, as in a cut from a broken fluorescent lamp, an indolent ulcer occurs that does not heal until the irritant material is excised.

B. Respiratory Tract Irritation: Signs of upper respiratory tract irritation and acute pulmonary edema occur.

C. Chronic Pulmonary Granulomatoses: Over 200 fatal cases of chronic obliterative pulmonary disease have been identified. The extent of the underlying exposure may be very slight; some cases resulted from handling the clothes of workers, and a latent period of up to 5 years may be present. Treatment with corticosteroids may have a temporary effect but does not alter the variable and unpredictable course.

The properties of beryllium should be related to those of silica and other particulate matters that cause pulmonary fibrosis.

BISMUTH

Soluble bismuth compounds are a very rare cause of chronic intoxication. Manifestations include skin eruptions, weakness, joint pains, diarrhea, metal line on the gums, and stomatitis.

Treatment is with dimercaprol.

CADMIUM

Poisoning by ingestion of cadmium is rare now that cadmium-plated cooking utensils are no longer used. Cadmium poisoning still occurs following the inhalation of cadmium oxide dusts or fumes during the smelting of zinc ores or welding or cutting cadmium-plated metal.

Clinical Findings & Treatment

A. Acute Inhalation: Initial symptoms are as for other metal fume fevers followed in a few hours by dyspnea, chest pain, and pulmonary edema. Permanent pulmonary fibrotic changes may follow.

B. Chronic Intoxication: The onset is insidious and is delayed at least 2 years after first exposure. Symptoms may first become apparent when exposure is no longer present. Progressive obstructive respiratory disease develops. Renal tubular damage with proteinuria is less threatening.

Chelating agents do not influence the chronic state. During acute intoxication, cadmium excretion is increased by administration of dimercaprol or EDTA. The complex may, however, cause additional renal damage.

CHROMIUM & CHROMATES

Chromium, chromium salts, and chromates are used in alloying, in tanning, in the manufacture of rust- and corrosion-resistant paints, and in many other industrial processes.

No treatment of established value is available for the acute or the topical reaction.

Clinical Findings

A. Topical Effects: Skin contact, especially with the strongly oxidizing chromates, leads to incapacitating eczematous dermatitis and ulceration. Ulceration and perforation of the nasal septum also occur.

B. Carcinogenicity: The incidence of lung cancer is increased up to 15 times normal in workers exposed to chromite, chromic oxide, and chromium ores.

C. Acute Intoxication: Gastroenteritis, nephritis, hepatitis.

GOLD

Various gold salts are still occasionally used in the treatment of rheumatoid arthritis. Toxic reactions are common. Skin rashes may progress to a potentially fatal exfoliative dermatitis. Hepatitis, agranulocytosis, and aplastic anemia also occur.

The serious reactions respond to treatment with dimercaprol.

MANGANESE

Manganese toxicity occurs as a consequence of exposure to dusts in mining or alloying.

Clinical Findings

A. Acute Intoxication: Metal fume fever.

B. Chronic Pulmonary Effects: Recurrent chemical pneumonitis.

C. Chronic Neurologic Effects: Damage to basal ganglia with permanent changes similar to those of parkinsonism. After the worker leaves the source of the exposure, the manganese excess is excreted but the neurologic defect persists. Chelating agents are of no value, but levodopa is effective as in other parkinsonian states.

NICKEL & NICKEL CARBONYL

Metallic nickel can cause a contact (allergic) dermatitis.

Nickel carbonyl—$Ni(CO)_4$—is a volatile pulmonary irritant and carcinogenic substance generated during the purification of nickel.

Immediate symptoms are cough, dizziness, and weakness; these are followed by dyspnea and pulmonary edema.

Treat dyspnea with 100% oxygen by mask. Treat pulmonary edema. Sodium diethyldithiocarbamate, 50—100 mg/kg orally or IM, is an investigative drug.

THALLIUM

The oral administration of thallium salts as depilatories in the treatment of ringworm led to many cases of toxicity prior to 1940. Sporadic cases of intoxication still occur from the mistaken ingestion of rodent or ant bait that contains thallium sulfate or acetate.

With large doses, signs of intense gastrointestinal irritation, headache, and tachycardia appear in 12 hours. Delirium, convulsions, coma, and respiratory paralysis can occur in 2—7 days.

With smaller doses, the onset of signs of intoxication may be delayed. They include ataxia, paresthesias and neuropathy, lethargy, confusion, and depilation.

Thallium can be detected in the urine for as long as 2 months after exposure.

No specific treatment is available. Claims are made that large doses of dimercaprol are effective. Diphenylthiocarbazone (dithizon) is used in veterinary practice but is an investigational drug (although easily available as a chemical reagent) in the treatment of human intoxication.

•   •   •

General References
(See also texts and manuals listed in Chapter 64.)

Chelating Agents

Chenoweth, M.B.: Clinical uses of metal-binding drugs. Clin Pharmacol Therap 9:365–387, 1968.

Sternlieb, I.: Penicillamine and the nephrotic syndrome. JAMA 198:1311–1312, 1966.

Stokes, G.S., & others: New agent in the treatment of cystinuria: N-acetyl-D-penicillamine. Brit MJ 1:284–288, 1968.

Lead

Coffin, R., & others: Treatment of lead encephalopathy in children. J Pediat 69:198–206, 1966.

Greengard, J.: Lead poisoning in childhood: Signs, symptoms, current therapy, clinical expressions. Clin Pediat 5:269–276, 1966.

Hardy, H.L., & others: Lead as an environmental poison. Clin Pharmacol Therap 12:982–1002, 1971.

Jacobziner, H.: Lead poisoning in childhood: Epidemiology, manifestations, and prevention. Clin Pediat 5:277–286, 1966.

Selander, S.: Treatment of lead poisoning: Effects of sodium calcium edetate and penicillamine administered orally and intravenously. Brit J Indust Med 24:272–282, 1967.

Mercury

Buxton, J.T., Jr., & others: Metallic mercury embolism: Report of cases. JAMA 193:573–575, 1965.

Goldwater, L.J., Nicolau, A., & S.J. Da Madeira: Absorption and excretion of mercury in man. Arch Envir Health 12:196–198, 1966.

Hill, D.M.: Self-administration of mercury by subcutaneous injection. Brit MJ 1:342–343, 1967.

Hirschman, S.Z., Feingold, M., & G. Boylen: Mercury in house paint as a cause of acrodynia. Effect of therapy with N-acetyl-D,L-penicillamine. New England J Med 269:889–892, 1963.

Noe, F.E.: Mercury as a potential hazard in medical laboratories. New England J Med 261:1002–1006, 1959.

Other Metals (See Chapter 42 for iron and deferoxamine.)

Cadmium poisoning. Leading article. Brit MJ 2:392, 1967.

Cotzias, G.C.: Chronic manganese poisoning: Clearance of tissue manganese concentrations with persistence of neurological picture. Neurology 18:376–382, 1968.

Frost, D.V.: Arsenicals in biology: Retrospect and prospect. Fed Proc 26:194–208, 1967.

Hardy, H.L.: Beryllium poisoning: Lessons in control of man-made disease. New England J Med 273:1188–1198, 1965.

Jenkins, R.B.: Inorganic arsenic and the nervous system. Brain 89:479–498, 1966.

McCarty, D.J., & others: Aplastic anemia secondary to gold-salt therapy. Report of fatal case and a review of literature. JAMA 179:655–657, 1962.

Mena, I., & others: Chronic manganese poisoning: Clinical picture and manganese turnover. Neurology 17:128–136, 1967.

Sternlieb, I., & I.H. Scheinberg: Prevention of Wilson's disease in asymptomatic patients. New England J Med 278:352–359, 1968.

66...

Common Environmental Toxic Agents

Much of the material in prior chapters is relevant to a discussion of toxicology. For convenience in organizing our approach to the practical problems that arise, the toxicity of agents used in therapy was discussed in Chapter 6 independently of other environmental hazards. Therapeutic agents are, of course, involved in many accidental poisonings as well as in therapeutic misadventures. Furthermore, a study of the effects of therapeutic agents is an essential preliminary to the study of environmental poisons that may act through the same mechanism—eg, cholinesterase inhibition and CNS stimulation or depression.

At this point, the problem is to somehow organize the many poisons not anticipated by the discussions of therapeutic agents. It will become obvious that an organized discussion cannot include the name, composition, and special properties of the thousands of industrial and household products involved; for such data the practitioner, no matter what his specialty, will have to keep at hand one of the books listed at the end of the chapter and use other resources such as the nearest Poison Control Center. The properties of the most common industrial and household poisons are presented in an outline that can be expanded by experience and need.

A number of aspects of toxicology are not discussed below, and mention of them would serve to emphasize the many disciplines participating in this field. Analytical chemists, industrial hygienists, agricultural engineers, and criminologists supplement the work of physicians in this field, and other public health workers and regulatory agencies deal with populations as well as with individual patients. The establishment of permissible levels of toxic contaminants in the environment, the use of protective equipment, and the surveillance of exposed workers are problems too varied to include here.

INSECTICIDES

ORGANIC PHOSPHATE INSECTICIDES

The organic phosphate and carbamate types of insecticide—parathion, malathion, demeton, and many others—are irreversible inhibitors of cholinesterase (see Chapter 8). The acute toxicity of the cholinesterase inhibitors is great, but they are not stable in the presence of water and are, therefore, not persistent. Exceptions to that generalization are parathion, which is not water-soluble and may be present for 1–3 weeks after application; and demeton, which may persist for a month and be present as a residue on harvested foods.

CHLORINATED HYDROCARBON INSECTICIDES

The chlorinated hydrocarbon insecticides (introduced in 1939) act slowly to kill insects and are persistent; residues from a single application to an open surface remain active for 2–12 months. They have been valuable in the control of disease vectors—eg, body lice and mosquitoes—and huge amounts have been applied to food plants.

Chemistry & Identification

The compounds are cyclic hydrocarbons that contain a large amount of chlorine. They are very soluble in fat but water insoluble and comparatively stable.

They can be placed in several chemical classes and their names listed (Fig 66–1).

A. Chlorobenzene Derivatives: Chlorophenothane (DDT), DDD, TDE, DFDT (parafluoro analogue of DDT), Neotran, Dimite (DMC), Dilan.

B. Benzene Hexachloride: There are 4 isomers of this compound. The pure gamma isomer is called lindane. Benzene hexachloride and DDT are used topically as parasiticides (see Chapter 5).

C. Chlorinated Camphenes: Toxaphene and a closely related mixture, Strobane.

D. Chlorinated Polycyclic Hydrocarbons: Chlordane (a mixture), heptachlor (a component of chlordane), aldrin, mirex, dieldrin, endrin, isodrin, and methoxychlor.

Properties as Insecticides

The chlorinated hydrocarbons are prepared for use as sprays, aerosols, solutions, emulsions, wettable powders, and dusts. Different insects and different stages of their life cycles have different susceptibilities, and a particular insecticide is selected for a specific

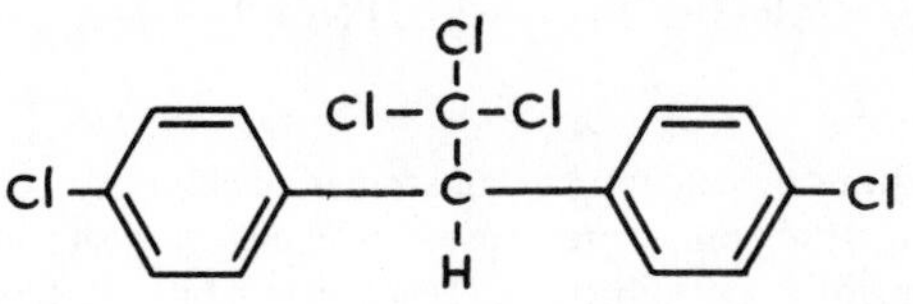

DDT

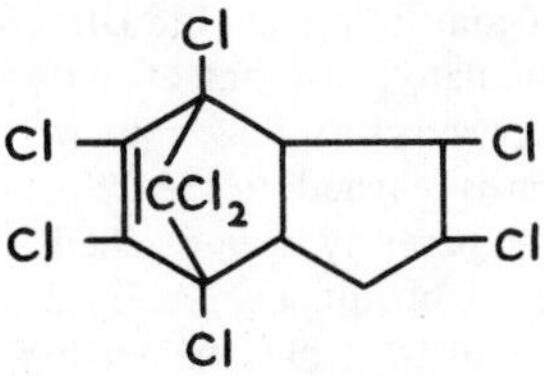

Chlordane

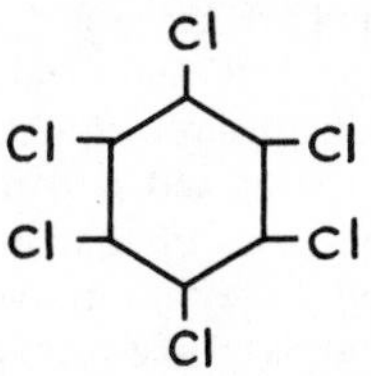

Benzene hexachloride

FIG 66–1. Chemical structure of representative chlorinated hydrocarbon insecticides.

purpose. They act on the insect nervous system to produce convulsions following absorption across the chitinous exoskeleton.

One of the great advantages—and also the basis for the ecologic damage—is the chemical stability and biologic persistence of these fat-soluble substances. Applied to a wall or other surface, they may persist in concentrations lethal to insects for 2–12 months; they may also remain as residues on food plants and in the meat and dairy products of animals that ingest the plants. They are destroyed by microorganisms in the soil only over a period of years; leaching by water, of course, simply contaminates another phase of the environment—eg, the soil from one estuary studied contained 32 lb/acre of DDT and its metabolite DDE.

The persistent insecticides are concentrated as they pass through the food cycle, and fish, reptiles, and birds—and perhaps other forms of life—can accumulate lethal amounts.

Acute Human Intoxication

The chlorinated hydrocarbon insecticides cause a generalized stimulation of the CNS. The sequence of effects may include vomiting, paresthesias, irritability,

undue reactions to auditory and other stimuli, tremors, convulsions, and death from respiratory paralysis.

Treatment is general rather than specific—ie, gastric lavage and control of convulsions.

The above description applies to DDT and related chlorobenzenes. Reactions to toxaphene proceed to convulsions without intervening signs. The estimated oral lethal dose of DDT is probably around 0.3 gm/kg; for toxaphene, pure lindane, or chlordane, about 50 mg/kg.

Recovery from an acute episode may take 2 or more months.

The clinical picture during a possible acute toxic reaction is often complicated by the effects of the solvents—usually petroleum distillate—simultaneously ingested or inhaled.

Possible Chronic Human Intoxication

No pattern of chronic human intoxication has been established—ie, the above state of acute intoxication may be reached slowly, but no separate chronic effects are authenticated.

Understandably, there has been great concern about the chronic effects of insecticides. Residues on

TABLE 66–1. Occupational diseases (excluding eye irritation and chemical burns) and deaths (both accidental and occupational) attributed to agricultural chemicals in the state of California, 1953–63. (Modified and reproduced from: *Occupational Health in California*, California Department of Public Health, 1965.)

Year	All Conditions Attributed to Agricultural Chemicals	Systemic Poisoning				Deaths
		Total	Organic Phosphate Pesticides	DDT, Lindane, Chlordane, Endrin, Dieldrin	Other Agricultural Chemicals	
Total	8566	3066	2277	117	672	109
1963	1013	345	267	14	64	5
1962	827	219	140	21	58	5
1961	911	268	194	14	60	6
1960	975	368	283	7	78	4
1959	1093	499	407	10	82	18
1958	910	328	227	14	87	13
1957	749	252	189	12	51	12
1956	789	281	197	11	73	18
1955	531	183	126	4	53	6
1954	391	122	101	1	20	12
1953	377	201	146	9	46	10

food are controlled, but DDT and its metabolite DDE (and BHC and dieldrin) accumulate in the fat of individuals until equilibrium between the slow rate of ingestion and slow metabolism is reached. In the USA, this point of equilibrium has apparently been reached, and the concentration in the fat of humans remained at about 9–12 parts per million of DDT plus its metabolite until the restrictions on its use were recently imposed.

Volunteers have been given DDT in dosages about 200 times the usual dietary intake for as long as 18 months without detectable toxicity.

The controls on the use of DDT now being put into effect can be justified on the basis of environmental damage other than human toxicity. Federal regulations are still being formulated. In California, where half of the insecticides used in the USA are applied, DDT is no longer used. In that state, each operator using any but the safest agricultural chemicals must be licensed and each application approved. Table 66–1 reflects experience prior to the initiation of the controls.

OTHER INSECTICIDES

A number of older insecticides are still in use. DDT and similar compounds act slowly on the insect, and most household preparations contain, in addition, a rapidly acting insecticide, usually a pyrethrin.

Pyrethrin, an extremely fine powder from pyrethrum flowers, and rotenone have very low toxicity. Thiocyanate insecticides—eg, Lethane and Thanite— also have almost negligible toxicity, although convulsions have been precipitated.

Nicotine, discussed in Chapter 8, is very dangerous. Fortunately, the availability of newer insecticides has reduced its use.

FOOD ADDITIVES & RESIDUES

Food additives may defer the time at which a foodstuff becomes stale or spoiled and thus prevent wastage and add enjoyment. They may also be used to mislead the consumer—eg, the use of nitrites to maintain the red color of meat—or to compensate for poor processing methods. There is, therefore, a Food Additive Amendment to the Food and Drug Act, and pretesting of new additives for safety is required and product surveillance constantly carried out. The regulatory agency determines, for example, that food colorings are not carcinogenic, establishes the limits for residues of insecticides, and prescribes the time before slaughter when a medicated feed must be discontinued.

ARTIFICIAL SWEETENERS

Sodium or calcium cyclamate has advantages over saccharin, the only previously available noncaloric sweetener or sugar substitute. It leaves no bitter aftertaste, and, since it is stable to acid and heat, it can be added to processed foods. Its use had consequently grown until 3.5% of the sugar intake in the USA had been replaced by this synthetic substance. Use of the cyclamates was not limited to individuals with a clear need to restrict total calories or those from carbohydrate but use was extended to foods for general use, including even meats such as bacon and ham.

The only clearly established adverse effect of cyclamate or the cyclamate-saccharin mixtures during the period of common use was the appearance of soft stools or even diarrhea. This effect was apparently caused by less than the 5 gm/day usually said to be necessary. (A single can of a carbonated drink contained as much as 0.5 gm of cyclamate.)

No chronic toxic effects have been demonstrated in humans. Deleterious effects on growth in animals require doses in excess of those used in humans. A rare case of photosensitization has been reported.

However, feeding experiments established that cyclamate is carcinogenic in animals. The demonstration that it is in part metabolized to cyclohexylamine, a known inducer of bladder cancer, intensified the concern. Consequently, its use was suspended.

INDUSTRIAL & HOUSEHOLD SOLVENTS

HYDROCARBONS

The hydrocarbons are all general anesthetics but may in addition have toxic effects on the lungs, liver, heart, and bone marrow. Because of these secondary effects, they are classified here into 3 groups.

1. PETROLEUM DISTILLATES

Petroleum distillates with various boiling points are used in a variety of industrial and household solvents. The many cleaning and polishing preparations are second only to therapeutic agents as causes of accidental intoxication.

Source of Exposure

Petroleum ether (naphtha, benzine, mineral spirits), kerosene, and gasoline are the aliphatic hydrocarbons included in this class. They are used as such and in paint thinner, dry cleaners or spot removers, furniture polish, and countless other products. They may be combined with other toxic solvents—eg, methanol in gun cleaner—or contain toxic solutes such as insecticides.

Mechanism of Action

These hydrocarbons are general anesthetics. In addition, they are pulmonary irritants. They have low surface tensions, and even a small amount will spread over a wide area, causing a chemical interstitial pneumonitis or acute pulmonary edema. The hydrocarbon can reach the lung by aspiration during ingestion of the irritant substance or during vomiting, whether caused by the gastric irritation of the toxin, by efforts to pass a stomach tube, or induced to empty the stomach. The danger of aspiration is greatest with the low boiling point petroleum ether and less with kerosene.

Acute Intoxication

A. Manifestations: Nausea, vomiting, cough, pulmonary edema, pneumonitis, and, with large doses, CNS depression.

B. Treatment: Lavage adds to the risk of aspiration. It may be used if the less volatile substances have been ingested or if a cuffed endotracheal tube can be placed.

The CNS depression may require that respiration be assisted. Pneumonitis should be treated with oxygen and antibiotics.

Corticosteroids are often given to reduce pulmonary fibrosis. There is no evidence for or against their effectiveness. If the patient survives, resolution of the pulmonary infiltrate is usually complete regardless of the treatment.

Chronic Intoxication

A state of chronic intoxication occurs in workers exposed for long periods to low concentrations and possibly in individuals who inhale hydrocarbons habitually. The resulting state is variable, but general slowing (depression), loss of memory, ataxia, and disturbances of speech are reported. Treatment consists entirely of removal from exposure.

2. AROMATIC HYDROCARBONS

Other hydrocarbons are generally anesthetics but lack the specific pulmonary toxicity.

Benzol

Benzol (benzene) and possibly toluene, an ingredient of the cement used in glue sniffing, can cause aplastic anemia. The bone marrow aplasia is not allergic in origin (see Chapter 6) but graded and dose-related. Long exposure is required, and a long latent period may be present.

Naphthalene

Naphthalene is a solid, and significant exposure requires ingestion. In individuals with a deficiency of glucose-6-phosphate dehydrogenase, it can cause hemolysis with anemia and renal tubular damage. Naphthalene can also cause dermatitis after industrial exposure. Toxicity is now uncommon since dichlorobenzene balls or insecticide sprays have replaced naphthalene as moth repellents.

3. HALOGENATED (CHLORINATED) HYDROCARBONS

These solvents are general anesthetics and are also hepatotoxic. Moreover, as was discussed in relation to halogenated hydrocarbons used as general anesthetics, they may be cardiotoxic. High concentrations in inspired air at the beginning of exposure may cause bradycardia or cardiac arrest. They also may sensitize the myocardium to the effects of epinephrine and norepinephrine in causing ventricular arrhythmias. However, the danger of arrhythmias after the use of sympathomimetic amines should be assumed to be present after the ingestion or inhalation of any of the hydrocarbons, whether halogenated or not.

Carbon Tetrachloride

Carbon tetrachloride is a nonflammable solvent, cleaner, and degreaser that is dangerous when inhaled, ingested, or absorbed through the skin. Its use in products sold for household use is now prohibited.

A. Acute Toxicity: The immediate effects are nausea, vomiting, signs of CNS depression ranging from confusion to coma, and respiratory depression. After 2 days to 2 weeks, signs of liver and kidney damage may appear. Fat accumulation in liver cells and centrilobular necrosis is manifest as jaundice and an enlarged, tender liver. Necrosis may be massive enough to be fatal. Oliguria or anuria results from renal tubular damage.

B. Chronic Toxicity: The above changes may occur following repeated smaller exposures.

C. Treatment: No specific treatment is available. As little as one swallow—perhaps as little as 4 ml by mouth—of carbon tetrachloride may be fatal. The toxicity is greatly increased by prior or concurrent ingestion of alcohol.

Other Halogenated Hydrocarbons

Trichloroethylene, which is used to some extent as a general anesthetic (or at least analgesic), is a substitute for carbon tetrachloride in household cleaners and in industry. It has caused hepatic damage but only after heavy exposure in industrial situations.

Tetrachloroethylene is a more potent CNS depressant than carbon tetrachloride and is also hepatotoxic.

Ethylene dichloride is a laboratory and industrial solvent which is as toxic as carbon tetrachloride. It is also a pulmonary irritant and can cause pulmonary edema.

Methyl bromide is a fumigant for grain that is also a pulmonary irritant.

The Freons used as propellants in spray cans are similar in effect to halothane (see Chapter 20). They are occasionally inhaled from a plastic bag for the pleasurable disinhibition provided. In at least 40 cases, death has resulted, presumably because the high initial concentration led to cardiac arrest.

ESTERS, KETONES, ETHERS

These compounds all produce some degree of CNS depression. Most cause irritation of the skin and mucous membranes. The number of compounds that may be encountered is very large, and one of the references listed at the end of Chapter 64 should be consulted for the toxicity of a specific poison. Innocuousness should not be assumed, although serious intoxication is unusual.

CAUSTICS & CORROSIVES

Many substances are local irritants but also exert important systemic effects. Identification of an environmental poison as having only local effects greatly simplifies treatment, but unfortunately some substances cause prolonged morbidity or death by a purely local action.

Substances that act as pulmonary or upper respiratory tract irritants are discussed in the next section. The remaining agents act on the cornea, the skin, or the gastrointestinal tract depending upon the nature of the exposure.

STRONG ACIDS & BASES

Ingestion of strong acids invariably causes death or prolonged morbidity; the estimated lethal dose is about 1 ml. Drain cleaners (Drano) contain sodium hydroxide; washing powders and dishwashing machine powders contain strongly alkaline phosphates; and ammonia is found in most households.

Ingestion

The results of ingestion of any caustic substance include burning pain in the mouth, pharynx, and abdomen, vomiting of material that contains blood, stains or burns around the mouth, shock, and (later) signs of perforation and peritoneal irritation.

Treatment must be immediate. Dilute the acid or alkali by forcing the patient to swallow large amounts of whatever is available—eg, water or milk. Fluids should be given repeatedly even if the patient is vomiting until the poison is diluted several hundred times. Gastric lavage can be performed only within the first hour; thereafter, the risk of perforation is too great. If a gastric tube is passed, it should be left in place until the possibility of perforation has been assessed. After extensive lavage or oral fluids, the poison can be neutralized with milk of magnesia (acid) or with fruit juice (alkali). Chemical neutralization applied prematurely will generate heat and increase damage.

Treat pain and shock as required. A demulcent such as milk or beaten eggs can be given hourly.

The danger of esophageal or gastric perforation is present for several weeks until the tissue destroyed by the caustic is replaced. Corticosteroids should be given (parenterally if necessary) to reduce fibrosis and the chance of an esophageal stricture.

Eye & Skin Contact

Follow the general directions provided in Chapter 64—eg, flood the eyes with water for 15 minutes while holding the lids apart.

OTHER LOCAL IRRITANTS

Bleaches

Common bleaching solutions are 3–6% sodium hypochlorite in water and are less dangerous than the strong bases just discussed. Esophageal damage is rare, and stricture has not been reported. The lethal dose for children is estimated as 15–30 ml. Bleaching solutions are discussed separately from the other alkalies to emphasize that a specific treatment is available. Sodium thiosulfate, 5–10 gm in 200 ml of water, decomposes hypochlorite in the stomach and obviates the need for lavage. Bleach is an alkali, but no attempt should be made to neutralize it since, in the presence of acid, the even more irritant hypochlorous acid is formed.

Soaps & Detergents

Because they are easily accessible in every household, soaps and detergents are often accidentally ingested. Serious reactions are very rare.

A. Anionic and Nonionic Detergents: Anionic detergents are the ordinary soaps—ie, sodium or potassium salts of fatty acids—or the sulfonated hydrocarbon type of detergent found in many familiar household brands. In these compounds the anion rather than the sodium or other cation is responsible for the lowering of surface tension. By themselves they have not been dangerous. Nonionic detergents or surfactants are even less toxic.

However, these detergents are sold as mixtures with other ingredients, and in any individual case it must be determined whether the product contains dangerous amounts of alkali. Liquid detergents (for dishwashing) and granules (for laundry and general purposes) contain phosphate, silicates, and carbonates and are alkaline enough to cause gastroenteritis. It is difficult to imagine the ingestion of a dose large enough to justify lavage, but the material should be diluted with water or milk. Persistent vomiting or diarrhea may require care.

Powders for electric dishwashers contain more alkali, and immediate dilution with large volumes of fluid is required. Ingestion of large amounts of polyphosphate may bind calcium and cause tetany.

B. Cationic Detergents: These substances are used as disinfectants rather than cleaners. They are quaternary ammonium derivatives—ie, the surface active cation contains a charged nitrogen. Examples are methylbenzethonium (Diaparene) and benzalkonium (Zephiran). They are absorbed after ingestion and can cause systemic toxicity due to CNS stimulation (restlessness, confusion, convulsions, and coma) and muscle weakness progressing to respiratory paralysis. The effects are to some degree suggestive of the action of nicotine.

The cation of this type of detergent can be neutralized or antidoted by the anion of soaps just as the germicidal action of one is destroyed by the other. A mild soap solution should be given by mouth. Other treatment is symptomatic.

AGENTS ACTING ON THE RESPIRATORY TRACT

GASES

An inhaled gas may simply be absorbed across the alveolar membrane and exert a systemic effect. However, there are gases that can act on the respiratory tract to cause serious or even lethal local effects without the appearance of systemic toxicity. It is these irritant gases that are emphasized in this section.

Gases may be classified according to their toxic effects as follows:

(1) Gases that are absorbed and exert anesthetic or other systemic effects.

(2) Asphyxiant gases: Simple asphyxiants exclude oxygen from the atmosphere and the lungs. Chemical asphyxiants—eg, cyanide or carbon monoxide—interfere with the transport or utilization of oxygen.

(3) Pulmonary irritants—eg, phosgene or nitric oxide—are agents that act on the lungs after a latent period to produce acute pulmonary edema with minimal or no irritation to the upper respiratory tract or other structures.

(4) Upper respiratory tract irritants—eg, ammonia, formaldehyde, sulfur dioxide—are irritant at once to the upper airway, the eyes, and even the skin.

(5) Upper respiratory tract and pulmonary irritant gases—eg, chlorine—can act in both ways.

1. PULMONARY IRRITANT GASES

Nitric oxide (brown N_2O_4 at room temperature; colorless NO_2 at elevated temperatures) is present in the smoke or fumes from some fires. It is evolved from fresh silage from heavily fertilized fields, and exposure in the confines of a silo can cause "silo-filler's disease." It is formed at the high temperatures that are reached in the cylinders of gasoline engines. The oxides of nitrogen emitted by automobile exhaust probably do not act as pulmonary irritants. They do, however, react with hydrocarbon fragments in the presence of ozone and sunlight to form the eye irritants of smog. **Chlorine** is not only used in industry but is occasionally generated in potentially dangerous amounts in the home by mixing bleach (hypochlorite) and vinegar or acid type toilet bowl cleaners. In a partially closed space—eg, a shower stall—dangerous concentrations can be reached. **Methyl bromide,** a fumigant, **ozone,** and **phosgene** are also pulmonary irritants.

Following exposure there is a latent period of 3 or more hours during which areas of hyperemic consolidation develop in the lungs that are apparent on x-ray as diffuse, granular changes. If the exposure was minimal, the patient may experience some dyspnea and feelings of tightness or oppression in the chest but will recover quickly. After greater exposures, the dyspnea may become intense and be accompanied by cyanosis and the production of frothy, bloody fluid as transudation fills the alveoli.

No specific treatment is agreed upon for this state. Oxygen and bronchial dilators may be used.

Recovery, if it occurs, involves a period of severe bronchial pneumonia. In a few patients who receive an exposure that is barely sublethal, a chronic obliterative pulmonary fibrosis may occur.

2. UPPER RESPIRATORY TRACT IRRITANTS

Chlorine, ammonia, and sulfur dioxide cause conjunctivitis, pharyngitis, laryngitis, and tracheitis. With some concentrations, the irritation may be so intense that laryngospasm may occur. The mucosa may be edematous and hyperemic or, in the most severe cases, may slough.

3. CYANIDE

The cyanide ion stops cellular respiration and causes death so quickly that, practically speaking, treatment is possible only if the exposure is expected and treatment is at hand.

Hydrogen cyanide is used as a fumigant. Its salts are used in industry in synthetic, photographic, plating, and other processes. Exposure may be by ingestion or by inhaling hydrogen cyanide gas generated by the action of acids on sodium or potassium cyanide.

Cyanide can be released from glycosides that occur in plants. Other industrial or laboratory compounds may release cyanide—eg, cyanogen. Cyanide is not liberated by cyanamide, ferricyanide, or ferrocyanide.

The cyanide ion complexes with many metals. It combines with the ferric iron of cytochrome oxidase, which can then no longer act in electron transport. In the absence of cytochrome oxidase activity, oxygen is not utilized and organ function persists only as long as anaerobic metabolism can sustain it. Other metalloenzymes are less sensitive, but inhibition does occur.

Treatment
A. Inhalation: The crucial treatment for inhalation of hydrocyanic acid vapors is removal from the contaminated atmosphere. If the victim has a perceptible pulse or both a pulse and spontaneous respiration, he will probably recover if oxygen and assisted respiration are provided. If he is apneic and pulseless, resuscitation is attempted before the specific treatment (nitrites, sodium thiosulfate) described below is initiated.

B. Ingestion: After a brief period of respiratory stimulation due to an action on carotid chemoreceptors, dizziness, headache, fall in blood pressure, unconsciousness, convulsions, and respiratory arrest follow. Depending upon the dose, 1–15 minutes may be available for treatment.

Cyanide ingestion is one of the few situations in which specific treatment precedes general measures. Treatment includes the following:

1. Oxygen—Oxygen (100%) by mask should be provided. If the period of hyperpnea has passed, the victim should be artificially respired. There is no theoretical reason why oxygen should be of value in this situation, but both laboratory and clinical experience support its use.

2. Inhalation of amyl nitrite—Amyl nitrite is given by inhalation from a crushed ampule. The nitrite is rapidly absorbed in the lungs and converts some hemoglobin to methemoglobin, an oxidized form with iron in the ferric form. Cyanide complexes with such ferric iron and is not transferred to intracellular cytochrome oxidase.

3. Sodium nitrite—Amyl nitrite acts rapidly but forms methemoglobin less actively than sodium nitrite. As soon as possible, give sodium nitrite, 10 ml of 3% solution IV over a period of 2 minutes.

4. Sodium thiosulfate—Cyanide is converted in the liver to thiocyanate, which is virtually nontoxic. The reaction is governed by a transsulfurase, and the rate depends upon the amount of sulfur available. Thiosulfate permits the rapid transformation of cyanide (CN^-) to thiocyanate (SCN^-). Give 50 ml of 25% sodium thiosulfate IV over a period of 10 minutes.

4. CARBON MONOXIDE

Carbon monoxide is still among the most common causes of death by poisoning. Furthermore, it may be or may become an environmental hazard affecting whole populations.

The automobile engine and unvented gas heaters are the important nonindustrial sources of carbon monoxide. Smoking cigarettes or cigars adds to the exposure of the individual. Following explosions or fires, accumulation of carbon monoxide is more often a danger than is exhaustion of oxygen.

Carbon monoxide combines reversibly with hemoglobin at the same site (the ferrous iron) needed for the transport of oxygen. The affinity of carbon monoxide for this site is 200 times greater than that of oxygen. Carbon monoxide can therefore accumulate in the blood even when ambient concentrations are low.

The carboxyhemoglobin formed cannot carry oxygen and, in addition, further reduces the supply of oxygen to the tissues by shifting the dissociation curve of the remaining oxyhemoglobin to reduce transfer of oxygen to tissues. As a result, the dysfunction caused by changing 50% of the hemoglobin to carboxyhemoglobin is much greater than the effect of reducing the hemoglobin concentration 50% in an ordinary anemia.

The principal signs of carbon monoxide intoxication are those of hypoxia. The bright pink color imparted to the skin and mucous membranes by high concentrations of carboxyhemoglobin is seen only at autopsy. With prolonged severe exposure, bullous skin lesions may appear.

The symptoms of acute intoxication depend upon the fraction of hemoglobin converted to carboxyhemoglobin. The progression can be approximated as follows: (1) Decreased psychomotor ability. (2) Headache and a feeling of tightness in the temporal area. (3) Headache progresses and becomes throbbing, with confusion and loss of visual acuity. (Approximately 20–30% carboxyhemoglobin or exposure to 500 ppm.) (4) Tachycardia, tachypnea, syncope, coma. (5) Deep coma, convulsions, shock, respiratory failure. (Approximately 60–90% carboxyhemoglobin or exposure to 1000 ppm.)

Treatment
Treatment consists of removing the patient from the exposure. The patient should be put at rest to reduce oxygen need. Oxygen should be given under positive pressure. Hyperbaric oxygen is probably the best treatment but is not generally available.

Recovery occurs in a few hours but is not necessarily complete. A few patients have persistent neurologic defects as a result of prolonged hypoxia.

DUSTS

Dusts may settle on the surface of the body and cause irritation or allergic reactions, or may be inhaled and absorbed from the mucous membranes of the upper tract and cause systemic toxicity. There are, however, important problems in environmental medicine that are due to suspended particles small enough to be carried to the alveoli with inhaled air. In this context dusts can be defined as solid particles 0.5–10 μm in size dispersed in air.

Dusts may then be classified according to their toxic effects:

(1) Dusts causing systemic poisoning: If the solid is soluble or the particle small enough, it may be absorbed and cause systemic toxicity—eg, the dusts of the heavy metals and insecticides already discussed.

(2) Dusts causing a febrile reaction—eg, the several metal fume fevers already discussed or the reaction to cotton dust.

(3) Dusts causing extensive pulmonary fibrosis—eg, silica and asbestos.

(4) Dusts causing minimal or no pulmonary fibrosis.

The states due to the inhalation of dusts that remain in the lungs are called pneumoconioses. A given pneumoconiosis may be malignant—eg, silicosis—or may not be symptomatic. The malignant pneumoconiosis or pulmonary fibrosis of berylliosis was discussed with the metallic poisons. Silicosis and asbestosis are the other dangerous forms of dust disease.

Silicosis

Dusts of silica (silicon dioxide, SiO_2, quartz) are thrown into the air during rock cutting or grinding, abrasive manufacture, sandblasting, hard rock mining or tunneling, and pottery making. With the exception of the silicates in asbestos, mica, and talc, only silica causes progressive pulmonary fibrosis.

To be damaging, particles must be small enough to be carried to the alveolus—ie, less than 5–10 μm in size and most dangerous in the 1–3 μm range. If the particles are less than 0.5 μm in size, they are dissolved rapidly and a pulmonary reaction does not occur. Depending upon the concentration and characteristics of the dust, exposures of 6 months to 25 years may lead to symptomatic silicosis, sometimes 5 years after the end of exposure.

Silica particles are removed by phagocytic cells. Not all of the silica reaches the lymph nodes, but some particles accumulate in the peribronchial and perivascular spaces. A fibrotic reaction is stimulated as the silica dissolves over a period of many years. The process, as seen on x-ray, is first diffusely granular, then more linear, and finally nodular.

The clinical picture is that of progressive obliterative pulmonary disease—ie, cough and exertional dyspnea. Tuberculosis superimposed on silicosis is more likely to be progressive.

There is no specific treatment. Positive pressure breathing with bronchial dilators may be helpful. Exposure to silica should be reduced to permissible levels.

Silicosis is only very slowly progressive.

Silicate Dusts

Asbestos (chrysotile, hydrated magnesium silicate) causes a pneumoconiosis in which the fibrosis is dense but linear rather than nodular. Asbestos bodies are found in the lungs and sputum. Asbestos is widely used as a fireproofing and insulating material, and recent studies of groups of construction workers establish that asbestosis is not only far more common than was previously realized but that the presently established limit or maximal allowable concentration of fibers in the air is dangerously high. Asbestos or ferruginous bodies are seen in the lungs of urban residents who have had no known exposure.

Workers exposed to asbestos in the mines or working with asbestos insulation have an unexpectedly high incidence of mesothelioma of the pleura or peri-

TABLE 66–2. Effects of inhalation of miscellaneous dusts not discussed in the text.

	Clinical Findings	X-Ray Pattern	Prognosis
Barium sulfate (barite) Iron oxide Tin oxide	None	Stippled or nodular pattern due to radiopacity of insoluble metal salt	Nonprogressive
Cotton dust	Emphysema, bronchitis (byssinosis)	Emphysema	Nonprogressive if exposure terminated
Moldy hay or grain*	Dyspnea, fever, bronchial pneumonia (farmer's lung)	Diffuse mottling	Nonprogressive
Sugar cane dust (bagasse*)	Chills and fever, pneumonitis, dyspnea	Diffuse mottling	Nonprogressive after acute episode
Glass fiber, rock wool	Dermatitis, folliculitis	. . .	Tolerance develops

*Reaction, probably allergic, to contaminating actinomycete.

toneum and of bronchogenic carcinoma. If they also smoke cigarettes, the incidence of carcinomas of the lung is about 92 times the expected rate.

Mica dust (aluminum silicates and other metals) and talc (magnesium silicate) can also cause pulmonary fibrosis.

Coal Workers' Pneumoconiosis

The idea that coal dust containing no silica could lead to slowly progressive, fatal pulmonary disease has been difficult to establish. Yet the "black lungs" of coal miners show a high incidence of pulmonary fibrosis and an emphysema localized in areas of the lungs where dust has accumulated. For many years in this country the relation to occupation was generally denied and compensation withheld. In 1969, federal legislation acknowledged the relationship to employment that had been accepted in Britain since 1934 and at the same time required programs of dust suppression in the mines.

Other Dusts

Bauxite (an aluminum ore) is converted in electric furnaces to alundum or corundum (Al_2O_3). Inhalation of fumes from this source has caused a progressive, linear fibrosis complicated by episodes of pneumothorax. Silica is present in the fumes and in the lungs, and the role of the aluminum oxide is not known.

The effects of some additional dusts are summarized in Table 66–2.

• • •

General References
(See also texts and manuals listed in Chapter 64.)

Hydrocarbons

Baldachin, B.J., & R.N. Melmed: Clinical and therapeutic aspects of kerosene poisoning: A series of 200 cases. Brit MJ 2:28–30, 1964.

Jamison, K.E., & E.R. Wallace: Kerosene pneumonitis treated with adrenal steroids. California Med 100:43–47, 1964.

Knox, J.W., & J.R. Nelson: Permanent encephalopathy from toluene inhalation. New England J Med 275:1494–1496, 1966.

Vigliani, E.C., & G. Saita: Benzene and leukemia. New England J Med 271:872–876, 1964.

Dusts & Gases

Bodansky, O.: Methemoglobinemia and methemoglobin-producing compounds. Pharmacol Rev 3:144–196, 1951.

Cope, C.: The importance of oxygen in the treatment of cyanide poisoning. JAMA 175:1061–1064, 1961.

Finck, P.A.: Exposure to carbon monoxide: Review of the literature and 567 autopsies. Mil Med 131:1513–1539, 1966.

Ivanhoe, F., & F.H. Meyers: Phosgene poisoning as an example of neuroparalytic acute pulmonary edema: The sympathetic vasomotor reflex involved. Dis Chest 46:211–218, 1964.

Kleinfeld, M., Messite, J., & J. Shapiro: Clinical, radiological, and physiological findings in asbestosis. Arch Int Med 117:813–819, 1966.

Lave, L.B. & E.P. Seskin: Air pollution and human health. Science 169:723–733, 1970.

McCarroll, J., & W. Bradley: Excess mortality as an indicator of health effects of air pollution. Am J Pub Health 56:1933–1942, 1966.

Murphy, R.L.H., & others: Effects of low concentrations of asbestos. New England J Med 285:1271–1278, 1971.

Ryder, R., & others: Emphysema in coal workers' pneumoconiosis. Brit MJ 2:481–487, 1970.

Selikoff, I.J., Hammond, E.C., & J. Churg: Asbestos exposure, smoking, and neoplasia. JAMA 204:106–112, 1968.

Stern, A.C. (editor): *Air Pollution*, Academic Press, 1968.

Pesticides

Frazer, A.C.: Pesticides. Ann Rev Pharmacol 7:319–342, 1967.

Hayes, W.J., Jr., Durham, W.F., & C. Cueto, Jr.: The effect of known repeated oral doses of chlorphenothane (DDT) in man. JAMA 162:890–897, 1956.

Hoffman, W.S., & others: The relation of pesticide concentrations in fat to pathological changes in tissues. Arch Envir Health 15:758–765, 1967.

Quinby, G.E., & others: DDT storage in the US population. JAMA 191:175–179, 1965.

Upholt, W.M., & P.C. Kearney: Pesticides. New England J Med 275:1419–1426, 1966.

Woodwell, G.M., Wurster, C.F., Jr., & P.A. Isaacson: DDT residues in an east coast estuary: A case of biological concentration of a persistent insecticide. Science 156:821–824, 1967.

Other Agents

Arena, J.M.: Poisonings and other health hazards associated with use of detergents. JAMA 190:56–58, 1964.

Coon, J.M., & E.A. Maynard (editors): Problems in toxicology. Fed Proc 19(3)(Suppl):1–52, 1960.

Gerarde, H.W.: Toxicology: Organic. Ann Rev Pharmacol 4:223–246, 1964.

Roush, G., Jr., & R.A. Kehoe: Toxicology: Inorganic. Ann Rev Pharmacol 4:247–264, 1964.

Appendix

THE EFFECTS OF DRUGS ON COMMON CLINICAL LABORATORY PROCEDURES
(Table 1)

With the increasing number of available drugs and the increasing number and complexity of tests performed by the clinical laboratory, drug-induced interference with test results is occurring with greater frequency. Table 1 has been prepared to assist clinicians and laboratory personnel in identifying such drug effects. In an effort to keep the information clinically relevant, no information from in vitro or animal studies has been included.

Although an effort has been made to cover each area thoroughly, it is inevitable that a listing of this type will be incomplete. The reader may wish to add to the chart on the basis of his own reading and experience. Comments on and additions to the chart sent to the publisher (Postoffice Drawer L, Los Altos, California) will be gratefully received and acknowledged by the author.

Types of Drug Interference

Alterations in clinical laboratory results caused by drugs may be grouped into 2 general categories:

A. Effects Due to Pharmacologic or Toxic Properties of Drugs: Here, a physiologic change is produced in the level of the parameter being measured. In Table 1, changes of this nature are designated as increase (+) or decrease (−). The magnitude of the change depends upon a variety of factors such as dosage of drug, duration of administration, condition of patient, etc.

B. Effects Due to Interference With the Testing Procedure: In this case the drug or its metabolite becomes a contaminant which may alter the value obtained or interfere with the measurement. This type of interference is indicated in Table 1 as increase (●) or decrease (○). It should be noted that drugs may affect one method of performing a given laboratory procedure and have no effect on another. For this reason, the specific testing method affected has been specified whenever possible.

By Philip Hansten, PharmD, Research Associate, Division of Clinical Pharmacology, Stanford University School of Medicine, Palo Alto, California.

Arrangement of Table 1

Table 1 lists the drugs that may affect the results of the laboratory tests indicated at the top. Tests that are less commonly influenced by drug administration are included in the column headed Other Tests.

All drugs are listed alphabetically by generic name with common trade names and other names in parentheses. Some general drug classifications have been used. If a drug falls into one of the categories listed below, it should be sought under that general classification.

Aluminum antacids
Anabolic steroids
Anthraquinone derivatives
Barbiturates
Calcium antacids
Contrast media, iodine-containing
Corticosteroids
Estrogens
Gold salts
Indandiones
Inorganic iodides
Iron, oral
Magnesium antacids
Mercurial diuretics
Monoamine oxidase inhibitors
Oral contraceptives
Phenothiazines
Progestogens
Salicylates
Sulfonamides
Tetracyclines
Thiazide diuretics

DRUGS HAZARDOUS FOR USE DURING PREGNANCY
(Table 2)

The teratogenic and other ill effects on the fetus of drugs taken during pregnancy are of concern to obstetricians and other physicians and to the regulatory agencies that must authorize the manufacture and distribution of drugs that may be used by this group of patients. Evidence of safety during pregnancy may be more difficult to establish than evidence of teratogenicity, and a conservative attitude toward the use of drugs in pregnant women errs, if at all, in the right ·direction.

Drugs that have been shown or are assumed to be dangerous during pregnancy are listed in Table 2.

TABLE 1. Effects of drugs on common laboratory tests.

+ = Increase (pharmacologic or toxic effect)   ● = Increase (test interference)
− = Decrease (pharmacologic or toxic effect)   ○ = Decrease (test interference)
N = See notes (below)   ★ = Present

DRUG	Amylase	BSP Retention	Cholesterol	Creatinine	Glucose	LE Cells	Methemoglobin	PBI	Phosphatase, Alk.	Potassium	Prothrombin Time	RaI Uptake	SGOT and SGPT	Urea Nitrogen	Uric Acid	Color	Glucose (Benedict)	5-HIAA	Porphyrins	Protein	PSP Excretion	Steroids	VMA	OTHER TESTS
																								BLOOD, SERUM, OR PLASMA / URINE
Acetaminophen					N		★						+											Urine ketones (N)
Acetanilid							★									●	●							Serum bilirubin (N)
Acetazolamide (Diamox)										−				+	−									Urine ketones (N)
Acetohexamide (Dymelor)					−				+				+		−									Blood ammonia +
Acriflavine																								
Alcohol, ethyl	+																							Urine catecholamines +
Allopurinol (Zyloprim)									+				+		−									
Aluminum antacids											N													Diagnex Blue (N)
Aminocaproic acid (Amicar)										+					−									
Aminophylline											N				−									Urine catecholamines +
Aminopyrine															N	N		N						Coombs (direct) (N)
Aminosalicylic acid (PAS)	N	−				★	★		+	−	+	+	+		N	N	●	N						Urine urobilinogen (N)
Amitriptyline (Elavil)								−	+		−													Serum bilirubin +
Amphotericin B (Fungizone)										−				+					★					Serum CPK (N)
Ampicillin													+			N								Serum bilirubin +
Anabolic steroids		N										N			N							N		
Anileridine (Apodol, Leritine)																							N	
Antipyrine					N		★									N								Urine ketones (N)
Anthraquinone derivatives																N					●			Urine urobilinogen (N)
Ascorbic acid			●																			N		
Bacitracin			●											+										
Barbiturates	N	+						N										N						Metyrapone response (N)
Barium sulfate								N																Diagnex Blue (N)

NOTES

Acetaminophen:

Large doses may cause hypoglycemia.

Overdose may produce liver damage with hyperbilirubinemia.

May produce interfering color in ferric chloride test for acetoacetic acid.

Acetanilid:

May produce interfering color in ferric chloride test for acetoacetic acid.

Acriflavine:

May color urine yellow-green.

May produce falsely high readings in the assay of porphyrins by spectrophotofluorimetry.

Alcohol, ethyl:

Large amounts may increase serum uric acid.

The diuresis produced results in a lighter urine.

Attacks of acute intermittent porphyria may be precipitated by ethanol ingestion.

Aluminum antacids:

The absorption of coumarins (weak acids) may be inhibited by concomitant antacid administration.

May displace Diagnex Blue from its resin, and thus could produce false-positive results in patients with achlorhydria.

Aminophylline:

Changes in maintenance doses of oral anticoagulants may be required during xanthine administration.

May produce false increases in serum uric acid when done by an adaptation of the method of Bittner (Am J Clin Path 40:423, 1963).

Aminopyrine:

Possibly involved in producing false-positive direct Coombs tests.

Aminosalicylic acid:

Reportedly may produce acute pancreatitis with elevated serum amylase.

May cause discoloration of the urine.

Will produce yellow color with Ehrlich's reagent test for porphobilinogen or urobilinogen.

Amitriptyline:

May turn urine a blue-green color.

Ampicillin:

Intramuscular ampicillin may result in increased serum CPK levels.

Anabolic steroids:

BSP retention is associated mainly with 17-alpha-alkylated agents (eg, norethandrolone, methandrostenolone).

May decrease blood glucose in diabetic patients.

Norethandrolone (Nilevar) may elevate SGOT.

Testosterone treatment increases urinary excretion of 17-ketosteroids, whereas methyltestosterone does not appear in the urine.

Anileridine:

A preliminary report indicates that screening methods for VMA may yield false positives; confirmation is needed.

Antipyrine:

May produce interfering color in ferric chloride test for acetoacetic acid.

May interfere with test for urine urobilinogen.

Anthraquinone derivatives:

May color urine pink to red or red-brown.

Ascorbic acid:

May produce false elevations in uric acid determinations (except enzymatic methods).

Large doses may produce false negatives in glucose oxidase methods (eg, Clinistix, Testape).

May interfere with the determination of urinary 17–hydroxycorticosteroids by a modification of the Reddy, Jenkins, Thorn procedure (Metabolism 1:511, 1952; 3:489, 1954).

Barbiturates:

Serum amylase may be decreased in barbiturate poisoning.

May stimulate the metabolism of coumarin anticoagulants.

Attacks of acute intermittent porphyria may be precipitated by barbiturates.

Barium sulfate:

May contain inorganic iodine contaminants which can elevate the PBI.

May displace Diagnex Blue from its resin, and thus could produce false-positive results in patients with achlorhydria.

TABLE 1 (cont'd). Effects of drugs on common laboratory tests.

+ = Increase (pharmacologic or toxic effect)   ● = Increase (test interference)
− = Decrease (pharmacologic or toxic effect)   ○ = Decrease (test interference)
N = See notes (below)   ★ = Present

DRUG	Amylase	BSP Retention	Cholesterol	Creatinine	Glucose	LE Cells	Methemoglobin	PBI	Phosphatase, Alk.	Potassium	Prothrombin Time	RaI Uptake	SGOT and SGPT	Urea Nitrogen	Uric Acid	Color	Glucose (Benedict)	5-HIAA	Porphyrins	Protein	PSP Excretion	Steroids	VMA	OTHER TESTS
Bromides			N					N																Urine ketones (N)
Bromsulphalein (BSP)				●				●													●			Urine urobilinogen ●
Caffeine					+																		●	Urine catecholamines +
Calcium antacids																								Serum calcium (N); Diagnex Blue (N)
Carbamazepine (Tegretol)	N					★			+				+											Serum bilirubin (N)
Cephaloridine (Loridine)									+				+	N						★				Coombs (direct) positive
Cephalothin (Keflin)								●					+											Coombs (direct) positive
Chiniofon																	N							
Chloral hydrate											N			N			●		N			N		Urine catecholamines (N)
Chloramphenicol (Chloromycetin)																	●							
Chlordiazepoxide (Librium)											−	−							N			N		Urine urobilinogen −
Chlorobutanol (Chloretone)														N										Serum bilirubin +
Chloroquine (Aralen)													+			N			N					
Chlorpropamide (Diabinese)	N		−		−				+										N					Blood ammonia +
Chlorthalidone (Hygroton)					+					−				+	+									
Chlorzoxazone (Paraflex)																N								
Cholestyramine (Cuemid)			−								N				−									
Clofibrate (Atromid-S)		+	−									+	+											Serum CPK +
Clomiphene (Clomid)		+																						
Cloxacillin (Tegopen)												+	N											
Codeine	N																							
Colchicine			−				N																	
Colistin (Coly-Mycin)				+										+						★				

NOTES

Bromide:
May cause false elevations of cholesterol (direct methods).
Small increases in PBI have been reported, perhaps due to iodine contamination.

Bromsulphalein (BSP):
May interfere with alkaline phosphatase determinations.
May produce false-positive tests for acetone by reacting with sodium nitroprusside.

Calcium antacids:
Large doses of calcium carbonate may produce hypercalcemia.
May displace Diagnex Blue from its resin, and thus could result in false-positives in patients with achlorhydria.

Carbamazepine:
BSP retention has occurred.
Jaundice has occurred; incidence must await further trials.

Cephaloridine:
Larger doses (eg, over 4 gm/day) may adversely affect renal function with elevation of the BUN.

Cephalothin:
May form an interfering dark color in Benedict's tests for urinary glucose.

Chloral hydrate:
May stimulate the metabolism of coumarin anticoagulants.
Large doses reportedly may cause false elevation of BUN (nesslerization technic), but more study is needed.
Attacks of acute intermittent porphyria may be precipitated.
May interfere with the determination of urinary 17-hydroxycorticosteroids by a modification of the Reddy, Jenkins, Thorn procedure (Metabolism 1:511, 1952; 3:489, 1954).
May interfere with fluorimetric test for urine catecholamines.

Chlordiazepoxide:
Has produced variable effects on prothrombin time in patients taking oral anticoagulants.
May falsely increase the reading for 17-hydroxycorticosteroids (modified Glenn-Nelson technic).

Chlorobutanol:
Large doses reportedly may cause false elevation of BUN (nesslerization technic), but more study is needed.

Chloroquine:
May color urine rusty yellow or brown.
May be a precipitating factor in porphyria.

Chlorpropamide:
May be a precipitating factor in porphyria.

Chlorthalidone:
Has produced pancreatitis, with resultant increase in serum amylase.

Chlorzoxazone:
May color urine orange or purplish-red.

Clofibrate:
May enhance the effects of coumarin anticoagulants.

Codeine:
May elevate serum amylase, but less potent than other opiates (eg, morphine) in this regard.
May produce elevated transaminase levels in certain patients.

Colchicine:
Reported to have an unpredictable antithyroid effect.

TABLE 1 (cont'd). Effects of drugs on common laboratory tests.

+ = Increase (pharmacologic or toxic effect)   ● = Increase (test interference)
− = Decrease (pharmacologic or toxic effect)   ○ = Decrease (test interference)
N = See notes (below)   ★ = Present

DRUG	Amylase	BSP Retention	Cholesterol	Creatinine	Glucose	LE Cells	Methemoglobin	PBI	Phosphatase, Alk.	Potassium	Prothrombin Time	RaI Uptake	SGOT and SGPT	Urea Nitrogen	Uric Acid	Color	Glucose (Benedict)	5-HIAA	Porphyrins	Protein	PSP Excretion	Steroids	VMA	OTHER TESTS
Contrast media, iodine-containing	N	N						●				−					N			N				
Corticosteroids	+	N	−	N	+	N		−	−	−	N	−			N		+							Diagnex Blue (N)
Cyproheptadine (Periactin)					N																			
Dehydrocholic acid		+																						
Dextrothyroxine (Choloxin)			−		+						N													
Diazepam (Valium)												−												
Diazoxide (Hyperstat)					+								+		+									
Dicumarol											+			+										
Diiodohydroxyquin								●																
Diphenylhydantoin (Dilantin)					N	★		−			N	−				N						N		Metyrapone response −
Dithiazanine iodide (Delvex)								●												★				Serum bilirubin (N)
Epinephrine					+			N						+	+								N	Urine catecholamines (N)
Erythromycin									+				+											Urine catecholamines ● Serum bilirubin (N)
Estrogens		+	−		+			+	+						N							N		
Ethacrynic acid (Edecrin)	N				N					−												N		
Ethchlorvynol (Placidyl)											N													
Ethinamate (Valmid)																						N		
Ethoxazene (Serenium)		●														N			N		●			
Ethyl aminobenzoate (Benzocaine)							★																	
Florantyrone (Zanchol)		+					N																	
Fluoride (large doses)					−																			
Furazolidone (Furoxone)																								
Furosemide (Lasix)	N				+				+	−				+	+									
Gentamicin (Garamycin)													+	+										

NOTES

Contrast media, iodine-containing:

Iopanoic acid (Telepaque) and BSP are thought to compete for excretion by the liver, resulting in BSP retention.

Sodium diatrizoate (Hypaque) may form a black color in Benedict's tests for glucose.

Iodoalphionic acid (Priodax), iopanoic acid (Telepaque), and sodium diatrizoate (Hypaque) may give false-positives with sulfosalicylic acid and nitric acid, but not with heat and acetic acid.

Corticosteroids:

Have produced pancreatitis, with resultant increase in serum amylase.

It is recommended that corticosteroid treatment be stopped before creatinine clearance is measured.

May reverse positive LE cell tests in patients with systemic lupus erythematosus.

May increase the requirement for coumarin anticoagulants.

Corticosteroids are weak uricosurics, but may produce severe hyperuricemia in patients with acute leukemia.

Reported to produce positive Diagnex Blue tests.

Cyproheptadine:

Although depression of fasting blood glucose has been reported, subsequent studies have not confirmed this.

Dextrothyroxine:

Enhances the effect of coumarin anticoagulants.

Diphenylhydantoin:

Large doses may elevate blood glucose. This has occurred in both diabetics and nondiabetics.

May enhance effect of coumarin anticoagulants.

May color urine pink or red to red-brown.

Slightly decreases excretion of 17-ketosteroids and 17-hydroxycorticosteroids.

Jaundice is a rare complication of diphenylhydantoin therapy.

Epinephrine:

May cause slight decrease in PBI.

Epinephrine and related agents used in asthma by inhalation may increase urinary catecholamines and urinary VMA.

Erythromycin:

The estolate salt may produce cholestatic hepatitis with elevated bilirubin levels.

Estrogens:

May increase cortisol-binding proteins, resulting in moderate decrease in urinary 17-ketosteroids and 17-hydroxycorticosteroids.

May produce false elevation in fluorimetric determinations for urinary catecholamines.

Ethacrynic acid:

Has been implicated in the production of pancreatitis, with resultant increase in serum amylase.

Both hypoglycemia (in uremic patients) and hyperglycemia (in diabetics) have been reported.

May cause uricosuria if given intravenously and urate retention if given orally.

May slightly decrease urinary cortisol excretion.

Ethchlorvynol:

May depress the anticoagulant activity of the coumarin anticoagulants.

Ethinamate:

May markedly increase the absorption of 17-ketosteroid determinations (modified Zimmermann reaction).

Ethoxazene:

May color urine orange to orange-red.

May produce falsely high readings in the assay of porphyrins by spectrophotofluorimetry.

Fluoride:

Large doses may decrease PBI.

Furazolidone:

May color urine brown.

Furosemide:

Has precipitated pancreatitis, with resultant increase in serum amylase.

TABLE 1 (cont'd). Effects of drugs on common laboratory tests.

+ = Increase (pharmacologic or toxic effect)
− = Decrease (pharmacologic or toxic effect)
N = See notes (below)
● = Increase (test interference)
○ = Decrease (test interference)
★ = Present

Column groups: columns *Amylase* through *Uric Acid* = **BLOOD, SERUM, OR PLASMA**; columns *Color* through *VMA* = **URINE**.

DRUG	Amylase	BSP Retention	Cholesterol	Creatinine	Glucose	LE Cells	Methemoglobin	PBI	Phosphatase, Alk.	Potassium	Prothrombin Time	RaI Uptake	SGOT and SGPT	Urea Nitrogen	Uric Acid	Color	Glucose (Benedict)	5-HIAA	Porphyrins	Protein	PSP Excretion	Steroids	VMA	OTHER TESTS
Glucose					+												N							Blood ammonia (N)
Glutethimide (Doriden)							★				N												N	Serum calcium (N)
Glyceryl guaiacolate (Robitussin)																		●						
Gold salts				N		★		○			N									★				
Griseofulvin (Fulvicin, Grifulvin)					N														N	★				Urine catecholamines −
Guanethidine (Ismelin)													+										−	
Haloperidol (Haldol)					N						N							N						
Heparin		●	−		N						+													Coombs (direct) positive (N)
Histamine	N																							
Hydralazine (Apresoline)						★																		
Hydroxyzine (Atarax, Vistaril)																						N		
Indandiones															−	N								
Indomethacin (Indocin)	N	N							+		N		+							★		N		Serum calcium −
Insulin					−					−														Serum calcium −
Iodides, inorganic								●			−	−												
Iodochlorhydroxyquin (Vioform)								●				−												
Iodopyrine								●																
Iothiouracil (Itrumil)								●																
Iron, oral																								Benzidine (N)
Iron sorbitex (Jectofer)					+	★	★						+		N	N				★				Diagnex Blue (N)
Isoniazid (INH)															N	N	N							Blood ammonia (N); Coombs (direct) positive
Kanamycin (Kantrex)			N																					
Levodopa (L-dopa)															N	N	N			★			+	Urine ketones (N)
Levothyroxine (Synthroid)								N																

NOTES

Glucose:

Intravenous glucose may produce glycosuria in some patients.

Some studies have shown that a large glucose load may increase blood ammonia in patients with cirrhosis and portasystemic shunts; however, further studies have indicated that this effect is small.

Glucose tolerance tests may produce small changes in serum calcium.

Glutethimide:

May enhance metabolism of coumarin anticoagulants.

Glyceryl guaiacolate:

May cause a color change during screening methods for VMA, but final measurement apparently is not affected.

Griseofulvin:

May depress anticoagulant activity of coumarin anticoagulants.

May precipitate acute attack in patients with porphyria.

Guanethidine:

Has antidiabetic activity and may decrease insulin requirements.

Haloperidol:

May antagonize the anticoagulant effect of phenindione.

Heparin:

Reportedly may increase blood glucose; confirmation is needed.

In acquired hemolytic anemia, heparin may cause the direct Coombs test to become negative.

Reversal of the LE cell test has occurred in patients receiving heparin.

May decrease urinary 5-HIAA excretion in patients with carcinoid syndrome.

Histamine:

May precipitate pancreatitis in patients who have recently had an attack of pancreatitis.

Hydroxyzine:

May falsely increase the reading for 17-hydroxycorticosteroids (modified Glenn-Nelson technic).

Indandiones:

May color the urine orange.

Indomethacin:

Has produced pancreatitis, with resultant increase in serum amylase.

May cause minimal elevations in BSP retention.

May increase the effect of coumarin anticoagulants.

Inorganic iodides:

May interfere with the determination of urinary 17-hydroxycorticosteroids by a modification of the Reddy, Jenkins, Thorn procedure (Metabolism 1:511, 1952; 3:489, 1954).

Iron, oral:

Administration of ferrous sulfate and ferrous fumarate has resulted in false-positive benzidine tests for occult blood in the stools.

May displace Diagnex Blue from its resin, and thus could result in false-positives in patients with achlorhydria.

Iron sorbitex:

Urine may darken on standing.

Isoniazid:

Although isoniazid is reported to increase blood ammonia, some studies have failed to confirm this.

Both true glycosuria and false-positive Benedict tests have been reported.

Levodopa:

May produce false increases for serum uric acid by colorimetric methods but not when uricase is used.

Urine may darken on standing.

Both false-positive Clinitest and false-negative glucose oxidase reactions may occur, especially with large doses.

May interfere with ferric chloride tests for urine ketones, Ketostix, and possibly Acetest.

Levothyroxine:

It is recommended that thyroxine treatment be stopped before creatinine clearance is measured.

PBI levels increased to normal or above normal in adequately treated patients.

TABLE 1 (cont'd). Effects of drugs on common laboratory tests.

+ = Increase (pharmacologic or toxic effect)
− = Decrease (pharmacologic or toxic effect)
N = See notes (below)
● = Increase (test interference)
○ = Decrease (test interference)
★ = Present

DRUG	BLOOD, SERUM, OR PLASMA															URINE								OTHER TESTS
	Amylase	BSP Retention	Cholesterol	Creatinine	Glucose	LE Cells	Methemoglobin	PBI	Phosphatase, Alk.	Potassium	Prothrombin Time	RAI Uptake	SGOT and SGPT	Urea Nitrogen	Uric Acid	Color	Glucose (Benedict)	5-HIAA	Porphyrins	Protein	PSP Excretion	Steroids	VMA	
Lithium carbonate					+			−				+								★			N	
Magnesium antacids																								Diagnex Blue (N)
Mechlorethamine (HN2, nitrogen mustard, Mustargen)								N			N													
Mefenamic acid (Ponstel)		+											N							★				Coombs (direct) positive (N)
Meperidine (Demerol)	+																	●					N	
Mephenesin (Sinan, Tolserol)						★																		
Mephenytoin (Mesantoin)											−											N		Metyrapone response −
Meprobamate (Equanil, Miltown)								N																
Mercurial diuretics															+					N				
Metaxalone (Skelaxin)		+														N	●							
Methadone (Dolophine)		+																						Urine catecholamines ●
Methenamine (Uritone)																		○						Urine urobilinogen (N)
Methenamine mandelate (Mandelamine)																				★				
Methicillin (Dimocillin, Staphcillin)													+	N	N			●					N	
Methocarbamol (Robaxin)		+											+	+		N								Serum bilirubin +
Methotrexate		+												+	N	N							N	Serum bilirubin +
Methyldopa (Aldomet)		+		N		★			+		N			+	N	N	●					N	N	Coombs (direct) positive; Urine catecholamines ●
Methylene blue							−																	
Metrecal																N								
Metronidazole (Flagyl)					−																		−	Blood ammonia (N)
Monoamine oxidase inhibitors (MAOI)		+															●							Metyrapone response (N)
Morphine	+	+											N						N				N	
Nafcillin (Unipen)	+												+											

NOTES

Lithium carbonate:
Preliminary studies indicate that urinary VMA excretion may be somewhat increased.

Magnesium antacids:
The absorption of coumarins (weak acids) may be inhibited by concomitant antacid administration.
May displace Diagnex Blue from its resin, and thus could result in false-positives in patients with achlorhydria.

Mechlorethamine:
Reported to have an unpredictable antithyroid effect.

Mefenamic acid:
Autoimmune hemolytic anemia may occur after prolonged therapy.

Meperidine:
May elevate transaminase levels in certain patients.

Mephenesin:
May cause color changes during screening methods for VMA, but final measurement apparently is not affected.

Meprobamate:
May increase the absorbance in measurements for 17-ketosteroids (Zimmermann reaction).

Mercurial diuretics:
May decrease PBI as measured by the acid distillation and chloric acid methods (alkaline ash method is apparently not affected).
Meralluride (Mercuhydrin) may produce false-negatives for urinary glucose as measured by glucose oxidase methods (eg, Clinistix, Testape).

Metaxalone:
Implicated in the production of proteinuria.

Methenamine:
Produces false elevation in urinary 17-hydroxycorticosteroids by method of Reddy (Metabolism 3:489, 1954).
May interfere with tests for urinary urobilinogen.

Methocarbamol:
Parenteral preparations may contain polyethylene glycol, which may increase urea retention in patients with renal impairment.
Urine may darken on standing.
May produce false increases in urinary VMA by screening method of Gitlow but not in quantitative procedure of Sunderman.

Methotrexate:
May inhibit uric acid synthesis in leukemic patients.

Methyldopa:
May produce false increases in alkaline picrate method of performing creatinine test.
Abnormalities in prothrombin time have been noted.
May produce false increases in uric acid determinations (phospho-tungstate method).
Does not appreciably affect VMA determinations.

Methylene blue:
Colors the urine blue.

Metronidazole:
May cause darkening of urine.

Monoamine oxidase inhibitors:
Although MAO inhibitors have been reported to reduce blood ammonia, some of these agents have produced hepatotoxicity and thus could be dangerous in patients with impaired liver function.
Nialamide may decrease the response to metyrapone.

Morphine:
May elevate transaminase levels in certain patients.
Attacks of acute intermittent porphyria may be precipitated.

TABLE 1 (cont'd). Effects of drugs on common laboratory tests.

+ = Increase (pharmacologic or toxic effect)
− = Decrease (pharmacologic or toxic effect)
N = See notes (below)
● = Increase (test interference)
○ = Decrease (test interference)
★ = Present

DRUG	Amylase	BSP Retention	Cholesterol	Creatinine	Glucose	LE Cells	Methemoglobin	PBI	Phosphatase, Alk.	Potassium	Prothrombin Time	RAI Uptake	SGOT and SGPT	Urea Nitrogen	Uric Acid	Color	Glucose (Benedict)	5-HIAA	Porphyrins	Protein	PSP Excretion	Steroids	VMA	OTHER TESTS
Nalidixic acid (NegGram)		+			N								+	+			●							Blood ammonia −
Neomycin		+	−								+			+						★				Urine urobilinogen −
Nicotinic acid (large doses)		+	−		+								+	+			N							Urine catecholamines ●; Diagnex Blue ●
Nitrofurantoin (Furadantin)													+			N								Serum bilirubin (N)
Nitroglycerin																							+	Urine catecholamines +
Novobiocin (Albamycin)		+																						Serum bilirubin (N)
Oral contraceptives		+				★		+	+		−	+	+						N			N		Metyrapone response −
Oxacillin (Prostaphlin)		+			+						N		+	N					N	N				
Pancreozymin	+																							
Para-aminobenzoic acid (PABA)							−																	
Pargyline (Eutonyl)					−	★																		
Penicillamine (Cuprimine)																				★				
Penicillin	N																●			N	−	N		Coombs (direct) positive
Pentazocine (Talwin)	N				N																			
Phenacetin (acetophenetidin)					N		★						+				●							Urine ketones (N)
Phenaglycodol (Ultran)																						●		
Phenazopyridine (Pyridium)		●														N			N		●			Urine urobilinogen (N)
Phenformin (DBI)		●	−																		●			
Phenolphthalein		●		●																				Urine ketones (N)
Phenolsulfonphthalein (PSP)		N			N	N		N	−				+		N	N						N		Urine catecholamines (N); Urine ketones (N)
Phenothiazines		N			+	N		N	+						N	N	○	N				N	N	Metyrapone response −; Serum bilirubin +; Serum CPK (N)

NOTES

Nalidixic acid:

Large doses or overdoses may produce false elevations in blood glucose (Somogyi-Nelson procedure).

Nicotinic acid:

May impair glucose tolerance, resulting in glycosuria.

Nitrofurantoin:

May color urine yellow or brown.

Cholestatic jaundice occasionally occurs following nitrofurantoin.

Novobiocin:

May produce jaundice with an increase in unconjugated but not conjugated bilirubin in plasma; also, a yellow pigment may occur in the plasma which interferes with icterus index and bilirubin determinations.

Oral contraceptives:

Oral contraceptives have been reported to elevate serum cholesterol.

A decrease in the hypoprothrombinemic effect of bishydroxycoumarin may occur.

May affect the handling of porphyrins by the liver; urinary coproporphyrin excretion may be increased.

The estrogenic component may increase cortisol-binding proteins, resulting in a moderate decrease in urinary 17-ketosteroids and 17-hydroxycorticosteroids.

Oxacillin:

High doses in infants may cause azotemia and proteinuria.

Penicillin:

Massive doses may yield false-positive results for proteinuria when turbidity measures are used (eg, heat and acetic acid, sulfosalicylic acid).

Intravenous doses may produce false elevations of 17-ketogenic steroids and a less marked increase in 17-ketosteroid determinations.

Pentazocine:

Causes sphincter of Oddi spasm, indicating that elevations of serum amylase may occur.

Phenacetin:

Large doses may cause hypoglycemia.

May produce interfering color in ferric chloride test for acetoacetic acid.

Phenazopyridine:

May color urine orange to orange-red.

May produce falsely high readings in the assay of porphyrins by spectrophotofluorimetry.

May yield a pink to red color in Ehrlich's test for urobilinogen.

Phenolsulfonphthalein (PSP):

May color urine pink (in alkaline urine).

May produce false-positive test for acetone.

Phenothiazines:

Phenothiazines have been noted to increase serum cholesterol.

Chlorpromazine reportedly may produce false-positive LE cell tests.

Large doses may cause slight decrease in PBI.

Chlorprothixene may result in significant uricosuria.

May color urine pink to red or red-brown.

May cause false increase in 17-ketosteroids (Zimmermann reaction).

Chlorpromazine may produce moderate decreases in urinary VMA excretion.

Chlorpromazine may result in high apparent values for methoxycatecholamines; an actual increase in urinary catecholamines has also been reported.

May interfere with diacetic acid determinations.

Intramuscular chlorpromazine may result in increased CPK levels.

TABLE 1 (cont'd). Effects of drugs on common laboratory tests.

+ = Increase (pharmacologic or toxic effect)   ● = Increase (test interference)
− = Decrease (pharmacologic or toxic effect)   ○ = Decrease (test interference)
N = See notes (below)   ★ = Present

DRUG	BLOOD, SERUM, OR PLASMA																URINE							OTHER TESTS
	Amylase	BSP Retention	Cholesterol	Creatinine	Glucose	LE Cells	Methemoglobin	PBI	Phosphatase, Alk.	Potassium	Prothrombin Time	RaI Uptake	SGOT and SGPT	Urea Nitrogen	Uric Acid	Color	Glucose (Benedict)	5-HIAA	Porphyrins	Protein	PSP Excretion	Steroids	VMA	
Phensuximide (Milontin)	N															N								
Phenylbutazone (Butazolidin)						★		N			N	−			N									Serum Bilirubin (N)
Polymyxin B (Aerosporin)				+										+						★				
Prilocaine (Citanest)							★																	
Primaquine							★									N								
Primidone (Mysoline)						★																		
Probenecid (Benemid)		+													−		●				−	N		
Procainamide (Pronestyl)						★																		
Procaine																			N					Urine urobilinogen (N)
Progestogens		+						N	+															
Propoxyphene (Darvon)					N								+											
Propranolol (Inderal)					−																			
Propylthiouracil						★		−			+	−				N								
Pyrazinamide (PZA)								+			N		+	+	+							N		Serum bilirubin +
Quinacrine (Atabrine)																								
Quinethazone (Hydromox)														+	+									
Quinidine, quinine											+											N		Coombs (direct) positive; Urine catecholamines ●; Diagnex Blue (N)
Reserpine																N		N				N	N	Urine catecholamines (N)
Riboflavin													+											Urine catecholamines ●; Diagnex Blue ●
Rifampin (Rifadin)		+											+											Serum bilirubin +
Salicylates	N		N		N	★				−	+				N		●			★			●	Urine ketones (N)
Spironolactone (Aldactone)									+	+														
Stibophen (Fuadin)																								Coombs (direct) positive

NOTES

Phensuximide:
May color urine pink to red or red-brown.

Phenylbutazone:
Parotitis with resultant elevation of serum amylase is a rare complication of phenylbutazone therapy.
Decrease or no change in PBI.
Phenylbutazone is a weak uricosuric.
May occasionally produce hepatitis with hyperbilirubinemia.

Primaquine:
May color urine rusty yellow or brown.

Probenecid:
May decrease 17-ketosteroid excretion.

Procaine:
May react with Ehrlich's reagent in test for porphyrins or urobilinogen.

Progestogens:
May cause slight decrease in PBI.

Propoxyphene:
Has produced hypoglycemia in a patient with impaired renal function.

Pyrazinamide:
May decrease plasma prothrombin levels due to its hepatotoxicity.
Urinary 17-ketosteroids may be decreased followed by a return to normal.

Quinacrine:
May color the urine yellow.

Quinidine, quinine:
May interfere with the determination of urinary 17-hydroxycorticosteroids by a modification of the Reddy, Jenkins, Thorn procedure.
May produce false-positive results in Diagnex Blue test.

Reserpine:
May cause slight initial increase in excretion of 5-HIAA.
May cause slight increase in absorbance in 17-hydroxycorticosteroid measurements (modified Glenn-Nelson technic).
Chronic administration decreases urinary catecholamine and VMA excretion; however, increases in both may be seen during the first day or 2 of therapy.

Riboflavin:
Large doses may produce yellow-green fluorescence to urine.

Salicylates:
Salicylism has resulted in pancreatitis with resultant increase in serum amylase.
Large doses may decrease serum cholesterol.
The salicylates have variable effects on blood glucose; a hypoglycemic action may be seen (especially in diabetics) and both hyperglycemia and hypoglycemia have occurred from salicylate intoxication.
Large doses (eg, 3–5 gm/day) can cause uricosuria, smaller doses result in urate retention.
May produce an interfering color in ferric chloride test for acetoacetic acid.

TABLE 1 (cont'd). Effects of drugs on common laboratory tests.

+ = Increase (pharmacologic or toxic effect)   ● = Increase (test interference)
– = Decrease (pharmacologic or toxic effect)   ○ = Decrease (test interference)
N = See notes (below)   ★ = Present

DRUG	BLOOD, SERUM, OR PLASMA															URINE								OTHER TESTS
TEST	Amylase	BSP Retention	Cholesterol	Creatinine	Glucose	LE Cells	Methemoglobin	PBI	Phosphatase, Alk.	Potassium	Prothrombin Time	RaI Uptake	SGOT and SGPT	Urea Nitrogen	Uric Acid	Color	Glucose (Benedict)	5-HIAA	Porphyrins	Protein	PSP Excretion	Steroids	VMA	
Streptomycin	N	N																		★				
Succinylcholine (Anectine)		+								+														
Sulfinpyrazone (Anturane)						N					+		+		–						–			
Sulfonamides	N	N	N		N	★	★	N				–				N	●		N	N	–			Serum bilirubin (N); Urine urobilinogen (N)
Tetracyclines	N				N						N		+	+			N							Urine catecholamines ●; Urine urobilinogen –
Thiabendazole (Mintezol)													+											
Thiazide diuretics	+				+	★				–				+	+		N							Blood ammonia +
Thyroglobulin (Proloid)				N				N				–												
Thyroid, desiccated				N				N				–												
Tolazamide (Tolinase)					–				+															
Tolbutamide (Orinase)					–			–					+			N				N				
Triamterene (Dyrenium)					+					+				+	+							N		
Triiodothyronine (Cytomel)								–				–												
Trimethadione (Tridione)						★							+									N		
Troleandomycin (TAO)													+							★				Serum bilirubin +
Viomycin (Vanactane, Viocin)																				★				Serum calcium –

NOTES

Sulfonamides:

Reports have appeared describing pancreatitis with elevated serum amylase following salicylazosulfapyridine and sulfamethizole.

Sulfadiazine, sulfamethoxypyridazine, and sulfadimethoxine have precipitated lupus-like syndromes.
May cause slight decrease in PBI.
May color urine rusty yellow or brownish.
May react with Ehrlich's reagent in test for porphyrins or urobilinogen.
May also precipitate an attack of acute intermittent porphyria.

Sulfisoxazole may lead to false-positive results for proteinuria by turbidity, and heat and acid methods; also, many sulfonamides may result in crystalluria with true proteinuria.
Jaundice has been produced, due to both acute hemolytic anemia and hepatotoxicity.

Tetracyclines:

Prolonged high doses have resulted in pancreatitis in certain patients.
Chlortetracycline may cause BSP retention.
Oral chlortetracycline may reduce serum cholesterol.
Oxytetracycline has produced hypoglycemic effects in diabetics, but apparently not in normal subjects.
Intravenous tetracycline may decrease plasma prothrombin activity; also, tetracyclines may reduce the vitamin K producing bacteria in the gut.
Parenteral forms which contain ascorbic acid may cause false negatives in urinary glucose by glucose oxidase methods (eg, Clinistix, Testape).

Thiabendazole:

Hyperglycemia may occur (incidence is low).

Thiazide diuretics:

May cause hyperglycemia and glycosuria in patients predisposed to diabetes.
May cause slight decrease in urinary cortisol excretion.

Thyroglobulin; desiccated thyroid:

It is recommended that thyroxine therapy be stopped before creatinine clearance is measured.

Effects on PBI will be consistent with metabolic effects. In the patient requiring thyroid therapy, the PBI increases about $1-2$ µg/100 ml for each grain of thyroid given daily.

Tolbutamide:

A metabolite may cause false-positive tests for proteinuria when turbidity procedures are used (eg, heat and acetic acid, sulfosalicylic acid).

Triamterene:

May produce a pale blue fluorescence in the urine.

Troleandomycin (triacetyloleandomycin):

May cause false elevations of 17-ketosteroids (Drekter) and 17-hydroxycorticosteroids (Porter-Silber).

TABLE 2. Drugs hazardous for use during pregnancy.

During First Trimester

    A. Antineoplastic Agents:

        Aminopterin

        Chlorambucil (Leukeran)

        Melphalan (Alkeran)

        Methotrexate

        Radioiodine

    B. Antinauseants (Antihistamines): OTC preparations containing these drugs must bear a warning against their use by women who are pregnant or who may become pregnant:

        Chlorcyclizine (Perazil)

        Cyclizine (Marezine)

        Meclizine (Bonine)

    C. Incompletely Studied Drugs: Animal studies do not establish risk or freedom from risk of teratogenicity. Adequate epidemiologic studies are available for only a few drugs. The labeling of a large number of drugs, therefore, includes a statement that the safety of use during pregnancy has not been established or that significant information is not available. The physician is cautioned to weigh the need for any drug during pregnancy against the possible hazard. Such a disclaimer is almost invariably present on the labels of recently introduced drugs, eg—

        Carbamazepine (Tegretol)

        Cholestyramine (Questran)

        Furosemide (Lasix)

        Pargyline (Eutonyl)

        Phenylbutazone (Butazolidin)

        Propranolol (Inderal)

Throughout Pregnancy

    A. Antidiabetic Agents (Oral):

        Acetohexamide (Dymelor)

        Chlorpropamide (Diabinese)

        Phenformin (DBI)

        Tolbutamide (Orinase)

    B. Anti-infective Agents:

        Ethionamide (Trecator)

        Streptomycin

        Tetracyclines

    C. Endocrine Agents:

        Androgens

        Anti-inflammatory (adrenocortical) steroids

        Antithyroid drugs

            Methimazole (Tapazole)

            Propylthiouracil

        Diethylstilbestrol

        Progestins

        Protein anabolic steroids

            Oxandrolone (Anavar)

            Oxymetholone (Adroyd, Anadrol)

            Stanozolol (Winstrol)

Late in Pregnancy

        Ergot alkaloids

        Laxatives (except for mild agents)

        Quinine, quinidine

Close to Time of Delivery

Some drugs transferred to the fetal circulation may have adverse effects on the newborn.

    A. CNS Depressants:

        Barbiturates and other sedative-hypnotics if given in larger than sedative doses

        General anesthetics (except nitrous oxide) if given in more than analgesic concentrations

        Narcotic analgesics

    B. Vitamin K

    C. Chemotherapeutic Agents:

        Chloramphenicol (Chloromycetin)

        Long-acting (protein-bound) sulfonamides, eg, sulfamethoxypyridazine (Kynex, Midicel)

        Novobiocin (?)

    D. Rauwolfia alkaloids

    E. Anticoagulants:

        Dicumarol (bishydroxycoumarin)

        Ethyl biscoumacetate (Tromexan)

        Warfarin (Coumadin)

    F. Agents listed above as hazardous throughout pregnancy.

FDA EVALUATION OF EFFECTIVENESS OF DRUGS INTRODUCED BETWEEN 1938 & 1962

The Food, Drug, & Cosmetic Act of 1938 requires that, before marketing a drug, the producer must provide the Food & Drug Administration with adequate evidence of its safety. The Kefauver-Harris Amendment of 1962 added the authority to require substantial evidence—ie, adequate and well controlled clinical investigations—that a new drug is efficacious in regard to all claims made in labeling and advertising.

Drugs first marketed after 1962 have been approved by the FDA under their expanded authority —ie, evidence of efficacy was presumably supplied. Drugs in continuous use since before 1938 are not subject to review, but drugs first marketed between 1938 and 1962 which may or may not be effective are now being reevaluated. Panels of experts from outside the FDA have examined the approximately 16,000 claims made for 4000 drugs and mixtures. Following the advice of the consultants, the FDA is currently reclassifying the drugs in the following categories:

(1) **Effective:** A drug may be judged effective for at least one of its claimed indications for use, and no question of its continued marketing is raised. For other suggested uses, the drug may be placed in one of the categories described below, in which case the manufacturer must either provide additional information or change the labeling at some future time.

(2) **Probably effective:** The presumption is that the drug is effective for the claimed indication but adequate data are lacking. The manufacturer is given 12 months to provide additional data or develop a protocol for collecting the information.

(3) **Possibly effective:** There is little evidence of effectiveness and small expectation that such evidence can be collected. The manufacturer is given 6 months to develop a satisfactory protocol for further study. The drug may remain on the market in the meantime.

(4) **Ineffective or**

(5) **Ineffective in fixed combination:** In these cases, the data are available and establish that the claims are unsubstantiated or that a hazard exists. The product has either been removed from the market or is in the process of being removed.

The following list includes most of the preparations ruled ineffective thus far. The list of possibly effective drugs would be many times longer.

General

Azacyclonol (Frenquel)
Bemegride
Betahistine (Serc)
Bioflavonoids (Rutin, Quercetin, Hesperidin)
Chlorzoxazone (Paraflex)
Chymotrypsin, injection (Chymar)
Emylcamate (Striatran)
Hexamethonium
Lututrin (Lutrexin, Trexinest)

Mephenesin (Tolserol, Dioloxol)
Mephenesin carbamate (Tolseram)
Mephenoxalone (Trepidone, Lenetran)
Oxalic-malonic acid and ethyl esters (Koagamin)
Oxanamide (Quiactin)
Oxyphenisatin
Phenyramidol (Analexin)
Poison oak extract for injection (Anergex)
Protamide
Sodium ethasulfate (Tergemist)
Sodium succinate
Styramate (Sinaxar)
Tolonium chloride (Blutene)
Trypsin injection (Parenzyme)
Urethane
Valethamate (Murel)

Antimicrobials

Sulfaguanidine
Sulfathiazole
Dental cones and pastes containing erythromycin or oxytetracycline
Topical (dermatologic) sulfonamide preparations, including nasal drops, lozenges, gargles, and gum
Cepacol lozenges
Phemerol tincture, solution, topical
Penicillin for inhalation or topical use

Antibiotics in Fixed Combinations

Tetracycline-sulfonamides
Chlortetracycline-sulfonamides
Penicillin-sulfonamide (Gantricillin, Pentid-Sulfas, Neopenzine, Pen-Vee Sulfas, etc)
Novobiocin-sulfamethizole (Albamycin G.U.)
Erythromycin-sulfonamides (Erythrosulfa, Ilosone Sulfa, Ilotycin Sulfa)
Novobiocin-tetracycline (Panalba)
Penicillin-streptomycin
Tetracycline-oleandomycin or troleandomycin (triacetyloleandomycin) (Signemycin)
Cycloserine-isoniazid
Tetracycline-amphotericin B (Mysteclin-F)
Tetracycline-nystatin (Mysteclin-V, Achrostatin V, Comycin)
Oxytetracycline-nystatin (Terrastatin)
Demethylchlortetracycline-nystatin (Declostatin)

Antibiotics in Combination With Antihistamines, Analgesics, Decongestants, or Vitamins

Tain
Novahistine with penicillin
Achrocidin Compound
Achromycin Nasal Suspension
TAO-Ac
Tetracydin
Tetrex-APC
V-Kor
Pen-Vee-Cidin
Syndecon
Tetracycline with vitamins (Achromycin SV)
Oxytetracycline with vitamins (Terramycin SF)

Miscellaneous Proprietary Combinations
Alertonic
Amplus
Amril
Bilcain
Dactil-OB
Delfeta-SED
Geroniazol
Mesulfin
Myospaz
Neuro-Centrine
Nicozol
Piptal pediatric with phenobarb
Retonic
Strexate

Anti-inflammatory Corticosteroids in Combination With Analgesics
Aristogesic
Artamide-HC
Mephosal with hydrocortisone
Neocyclone
Pabalate-HC
Pabicort AC
Pabirin AC
Predniscorb
Salcort-Delta

Sequential Oral Contraceptives
C-Quens
Provest

Thiazide Diuretic-Potassium Chloride Mixtures

Index*

---

*When the British and USA generic names differ only by a consistent and recognizable convention (eg, British phenobarbitone, USA phenobarbital) or spelling (eg, British oestradiol, USA estradiol), the British name has not been indexed. The British generic name has been indexed when it varies markedly from the USA name—eg, Pethidine (Brit): See Meperidine.

Violotin